KAPLAN & SADOCK'S

Concise
Textbook of Clinical Psychiatry

Third **Edition**

Contributing Editors, *Synopsis of Psychiatry, Tenth Edition*

Jack A. Grebb, M.D.
Caroly S. Pataki, M.D.
Norman Sussman, M.D.

KAPLAN & SADOCK'S

Concise

Textbook of Clinical Psychiatry

Third **Edition**

Benjamin James Sadock, M.D.

Menas S. Gregory Professor of Psychiatry and Vice Chairman,
Department of Psychiatry, New York University School of Medicine;
Attending Psychiatrist, Tisch Hospital;
Attending Psychiatrist, Bellevue Hospital Center;
Consulting Psychiatrist, Lenox Hill Hospital,
New York, New York

Virginia Alcott Sadock, M.D.

Professor of Psychiatry, Department of Psychiatry,
New York University School of Medicine;
Attending Psychiatrist, Tisch Hospital;
Attending Psychiatrist, Bellevue Hospital Center,
New York, New York

Wolters Kluwer | Lippincott Williams & Wilkins
Health
Philadelphia · Baltimore · New York · London
Buenos Aires · Hong Kong · Sydney · Tokyo

Acquisitions Editor: Charles W. Mitchell
Managing Editor: Sirkka E. Howes
Marketing Manager: Kimberly Schonberger
Production Editor: Bridgett Dougherty
Manufacturing Manager: Kathleen Brown
Design Coordinator: Steve Druding
Compositor: Aptara, Inc.

Library of Congress Cataloging-in-Publication Data
Sadock, Benjamin J., 1933–
    Kaplan & Sadock's concise textbook of clinical psychiatry / Benjamin James Sadock, Virginia Alcott Sadock—3rd ed.
        p. ; cm.
    Includes index.
    ISBN-13: 978-0-7817-8746-8 (alk. paper)
    ISBN-10: 0-7817-8746-7 (alk. paper)
    1. Mental illness. 2. Psychiatry.   I. Sadock, Virginia A.   II. Kaplan, Harold I., 1927–1998   III. Title.   IV. Title: Kaplan and Sadock's concise textbook of clinical psychiatry.   V. Title: Concise textbook of clinical psychiatry.
    [DNLM: 1. Mental Disorders.   WM 140 S126ka 2008]
    RC454.K349 2008
    616.89—dc22

                                                                      2008002514

Care has been taken to confirm the accuracy of the information presented and to describe generally accepted practices. However, the authors, editors, and publisher are not responsible for errors or omissions or for any consequences from application of the information in this book and make no warranty, expressed or implied, with respect to the currency, completeness, or accuracy of the contents of the publication. Application of this information in a particular situation remains the professional responsibility of the practitioner.

The authors, editors, and publisher have exerted every effort to ensure that drug selection and dosage set forth in this text are in accordance with current recommendations and practice at the time of publication. However, in view of ongoing research, changes in government regulations, and the constant flow of information relating to drug therapy and drug reactions, the reader is urged to check the package insert for each drug for any change in indications and dosage and for added warnings and precautions. This is particularly important when the recommended agent is a new or infrequently employed drug.

Some drugs and medical devices presented in this publication have Food and Drug Administration (FDA) clearance for limited use in restricted research settings. It is the responsibility of the health care provider to ascertain the FDA status of each drug or device planned for use in their clinical practice.

To purchase additional copies of this book, call our customer service department at (800) 638-3030 or fax orders to (301) 223-2320. International customers should call (301) 223-2300.

Visit Lippincott Williams & Wilkins on the Internet: at LWW.com. Lippincott Williams & Wilkins customer service representatives are available from 8:30 am to 6 pm, EST.

10 9 8 7 6

Dedicated to
Jack Grebb, M.D.
1953–2007

Preface

This textbook evolved from our experience editing a larger volume, *Kaplan & Sadock's Synopsis of Psychiatry,* tenth edition, which covers both the basic behavioral sciences and all of the clinical psychiatric disorders in children and adults. This book, *Concise Textbook Psychiatry,* is smaller and covers only the diagnosis and treatment of mental disorders *without* a review of the behavioral sciences. The reader will find detailed information about the diagnosis and treatment of every mental disorder listed in the latest fourth revised edition of the American Psychiatric Association's *Diagnostic and Statistical Manual of Mental Disorders* (DSM-IV-TR). The elimination of the section on the behavioral sciences accounts for this book's smaller and more manageable size. It is designed to meet the needs of the reader who requires a compact coverage of clinical psychiatry.

As with *Synopsis,* the goal of this book is to foster professional competence and ensure the highest quality care to those with mental illness. An eclectic, multidisciplinary approach has been its hallmark; thus, biological, psychological, and sociological factors are equitably presented as they affect the person in health and disease. Each edition is thoroughly updated and the textbook has the reputation of being an independent, consistent, accurate, objective, and reliable compendium of new events in the field of psychiatry.

TEACHING SYSTEM

This textbook forms one part of a comprehensive system we have developed to facilitate the teaching of psychiatry and the behavioral sciences. At the head of the system is the *Comprehensive Textbook of Psychiatry,* which is global in depth and scope. It is designed for and used by psychiatrists, behavioral scientists, and all workers in the mental health field. *Synopsis of Psychiatry* is a relatively compact, highly modified, original, and current text useful for medical students, psychiatric residents, practicing psychiatrists, and mental health professionals. Another part of the system is *Study Guide and Self-Examination Review of Psychiatry,* which consists of multiple-choice questions and answers. It is designed for students of psychiatry who are preparing for a variety of examinations. Other parts of the system are the pocket handbooks: *Pocket Handbook of Clinical Psychiatry, Pocket Handbook of Psychiatric Drug Treatment,* and *Pocket Handbook of Emergency Psychiatric Medicine.* Those books cover the diagnosis and the treatment of psychiatric disorders, psychopharmacology, and psychiatric emergencies, respectively, and are compactly designed and concisely written to be carried in the pocket by clinical clerks and practicing physicians, whatever their specialty, to provide a quick reference. Finally, *Comprehensive Glossary of Psychiatry and Psychology* provides

simply written definitions of all terms used in psychiatry including a complete glossary of signs and symptoms. Taken together, those books create a multipronged approach to the teaching, study, and learning of psychiatry.

NEW AND REVISED AREAS

Every section on clinical psychiatry has been updated to include all the latest information about diagnosing and treating mental illness. New advances since the publication of *Synopsis of Psychiatry* in 2007 have been added, particularly in the ever-changing area of psychopharmacology. The reader will find completely updated material on medication such as dosages, methods of use, and side effects, including information about all drugs approved since the last edition was published. Particular attention should be paid to several sections that have been newly written and updated: *Palliative Care and Pain Management* reflects the important role that psychiatrists play in the clinical specialty of palliative care and pain medicine. *Psychiatry and Reproductive Medicine* discusses the advances in women's health and describes in detail the disorders surrounding the antepartum and postpartum periods. *Euthanasia and Physician Assisted Suicide* is covered in a separate section in view of its important and controversial status in medicine today. The section on psychotherapy has been expanded to cover new forms of treatment, such as dialectical-behavior therapy. Brain stimulation therapies are covered in detail, including updated discussions of vagal nerve and deep brain stimulation.

Childhood Disorders

The section of childhood disorders has been completely updated, and the section on biological therapies has been newly written to cover the rapid changes and cautionary notes in the psychopharmacological treatment of children. Data about posttraumatic stress disorders in children includes the latest information about the psychological effects on children exposed to terrorist activities and natural disasters. The section on anxiety disorders in children and adolescents was completely reorganized.

FORMAT
Case Histories

Case histories are an integral part of this book and are included to make the clinical disorders more interesting and vital for the student. All cases in this edition are new, derived from various sources: *ICD-10 Casebook, DSM-IV-TR Casebook, DSM-IV-TR*

Case Studies, from contributors to the *Comprehensive Textbook of Psychiatry*, and from the authors' clinical experience at New York's Bellevue Hospital Center. We especially wish to thank the American Psychiatric Press and the World Health Organization for permission to use many of their cases. Cases appear in tinted type to help to the reader find them easily.

References

To conserve space, references were not included at the end of each section. The interested reader can find a complete bibliography for each section by referring to either *Synopsis of Psychiatry* or the *Comprehensive Textbook of Psychiatry*. Those texts will also provide an in-depth, thorough, and detailed discussion of all the topics in this book. We are mindful of the fact that modern-day readers consult internet sources, such as PsychInfo and Medline to stay abreast of the most current literature and encourage that trend.

ACKNOWLEDGMENTS

We deeply appreciate the work of our distinguished group of contributing editors, who gave generously of their time and expertise. Caroly Pataki, M.D. was responsible for updating and revising the section on childhood and adolescent disorders. We thank her for her tremendous help in this area. Norman Sussman, M.D. updated the section on psychopharmacology, enabling us to provide the reader with the current material in this ever-changing and rapidly expanding field. We thank the late Jack Grebb, M.D. to whom this book is dedicated, who guided us throughout and who was co-author of the seventh edition of *Synopsis*. He will be greatly missed. We thank Dorice Viera, Associate Curator of the Frederick L. Ehrman Medical Library at the New York University School of Medicine, for her valuable assistance in the preparation of this and previous editions in which she was so very helpful. Samoon Ahmad, M.D. deserves special thanks for his role as Consulting Editor in the field of biological psychiatry.

Nitza Jones played a key and invaluable role as Project Editor, as she has for many of our other books. Her vast knowledge of every aspect of book publishing was indispensable and she contributed heavily to editing the text. She was ably assisted by Regina Furner and Sara Brown. They worked with enthusiasm, alacrity, and intelligence. Among the many others to thank are René Robinson, M.D., Caroline Press, M.D., Michael Stanger, M.D., Rajan Bahl, M.D., Seeba Anam, M.D., and Jay K. Kantor, Ph.D., all of whom contributed to the text.

We also wish to acknowledge the contributions of James Sadock, M.D. and Victoria Gregg, M.D. for their help in their areas of expertise: emergency adult and emergency pediatric medicine, respectively. We also want to thank Alan and Marilyn Zublatt for the generous support and for their friendship.

We want to take this opportunity to acknowledge those who have translated this and other *Kaplan & Sadock* books into foreign languages, including Chinese, Croatian, French, German, Greek, Indonesian, Italian, Japanese, Polish, Portuguese, Romanian, Russian, Spanish, and Turkish, in addition to a special Asian and international student edition.

Additionally, we wish to acknowledge our great and obvious debt to the more than 2,000 psychiatrists and behavioral scientists who contributed to the various editions of the *Comprehensive Textbook of Psychiatry* and allowed us to synopsize their work. At the same time, we must accept responsibility for the modifications and changes in the new work. The staff at Lippincott Williams & Wilkins was most efficient.

Finally, we wish to thank Katey Millet and Sirkka Howes of Lippincott Williams & Wilkins. Chris Miller of Aptara also deserves our thanks. Joyce Murphy, Associate Director of Development, and Charley Mitchell, Publisher, Medical Practice & Education, have been loyal friends over the years and their encouragement and enthusiasm have been most welcome.

B.J.S.
V.A.S.

Contents

KAPLAN & SADOCK TEXTBOOKS
Published by Lippincott Williams & Wilkins

Comprehensive Textbook of Psychiatry
1st Edition, 1967 (with A.M. Freedman)
2nd Edition, 1975 (with A.M. Freedman)
3rd Edition, 1980 (with A.M. Freedman)
4th Edition, 1985
5th Edition, 1989
6th Edition, 1995
7th Edition, 1998 (with V.A. Sadock)
8th Edition, 2005 (with V.A. Sadock)

Synopsis of Psychiatry
1st Edition, 1972 (with A.M. Freedman)
2nd Edition, 1976 (with A.M. Freedman)
3rd Edition, 1981
4th Edition, 1985
5th Edition, 1988
6th Edition, 1991
7th Edition, 1994 (with J. Grebb)
8th Edition, 1998
9th Edition, 2003 (with V.A. Sadock)
10th Edition, 2007 (with V.A. Sadock)

Study Guide and Self-Examination Review of Psychiatry
1st Edition, 1983
2nd Edition, 1985
3rd Edition, 1989
4th Edition, 1991
5th Edition, 1994
6th Edition, 1999 (with V.A. Sadock)
7th Edition, 2003 (with V.A. Sadock and R.M. Jones)
8th Edition, 2007 (with V.A. Sadock and Z. Levin)

Comprehensive Group Psychotherapy
1st Edition, 1971
2nd Edition, 1983
3rd Edition, 1993

The Sexual Experience
1976 (with A.M. Freedman)

Concise Textbook of Clinical Psychiatry
1st Edition, 1996 (with V.A. Sadock)
2nd Edition, 2004 (with V.A. Sadock)

Pocket Handbook of Clinical Psychiatry
1st Edition, 1990
2nd Edition, 1996
3rd Edition, 2001 (with V.A. Sadock)
4th Edition, 2005 (with V.A. Sadock)

Comprehensive Glossary of Psychiatry and Psychology
1991

Pocket Handbook of Psychiatric Drug Treatment
1st Edition, 1993
2nd Edition, 1996
3rd Edition, 2001 (with V.A. Sadock)
4th Edition, 2006 (with V.A. Sadock and N. Sussman)

Pocket Handbook of Emergency Psychiatric Medicine
1993

Pocket Handbook of Primary Care Psychiatry
1996

Various editions of the above books have been translated and published in Bulgarian, Croatian, French, German, Greek, Indonesian, Italian, Japanese, Polish, Portuguese, Russian, Spanish, and Turkish.

In addition, an International Asian edition has been published in English.

BY OTHER PUBLISHERS

Studies in Human Behavior, 1–5
1972 (with A.M. Freedman)
Athenaeum
1. Diagnosing Mental Illness: Evaluation in Psychiatry and Psychology
2. Interpreting Personality: A Survey of Twentieth-Century Views
3. Human Behavior: Biological, Psychological, and Sociological
4. Treating Mental Illness: Aspects of Modern Therapy
5. The Child: His Psychological and Cultural Development

Volume 1: Normal Development and Psychological Assessment
Volume 2: The Major Psychological Disorders and their Treatment

Modern Group Books I–VI
1972
E.P. Dutton
I. Origins of Group Analysis
II. Evolution of Group Therapy
III. Groups and Drugs
IV. Sensitivity through Encounter and Motivation
V. New Models for Group Therapy
VI. Group Treatment of Mental Illness

The Human Animal
1974 (with A.M. Freedman)
K.F.S. Publications
Volume 1: Man and His Mind
Volume 2: The Disordered Personality

ABOUT THE AUTHORS

BENJAMIN JAMES SADOCK, M.D., is the Menas S. Gregory Professor of Psychiatry and Vice Chairman of the Department of Psychiatry at the New York University (NYU) School of Medicine, New York, New York. He is a graduate of Union College, received his M.D. degree from New York Medical College, and completed his internship at Albany Hospital. After finishing his residency at Bellevue Psychiatric Hospital, he entered military service, serving as Acting Chief of Neuropsychiatry at Sheppard Air Force Base, Wichita Falls, Texas. He has held faculty and teaching appointments at Southwestern Medical School and Parkland Hospital in Dallas and at New York Medical College, St. Luke's Hospital, the New York State Psychiatric Institute, and Metropolitan Hospital in New York. Dr. Sadock joined the faculty of the NYU School of Medicine in 1980 and served in various positions: Director of Medical Student Education in Psychiatry, Co-Director of the Residency Training Program in Psychiatry, and Director of Graduate Medical Education. Currently, Dr. Sadock is Co-Director of Student Mental Health Services, Psychiatric Consultant to the Admissions Committee, and Co-Director of Continuing Education in Psychiatry at the NYU School of Medicine. He is on the staff of Bellevue Hospital and Tisch Hospital and is a consulting psychiatrist at Lenox Hill Hospital. Dr. Sadock is a Diplomate of the American Board of Psychiatry and Neurology and served as Associate Examiner for the Board for more than a decade. He is a Distinguished Life Fellow of the American Psychiatric Association, a Fellow of the American College of Physicians, a Fellow of the New York Academy of Medicine, and a member of Alpha Omega Alpha Honor Society. He is active in numerous psychiatric organizations and is founder and president of the NYU-Bellevue Psychiatric Society. Dr. Sadock was a member of the National Committee in Continuing Education in Psychiatry of the American Psychiatric Association; he served on the Ad Hoc Committee on Sex Therapy Clinics of the American Medical Association, was a delegate to the conference on Recertification of the American Board of Medical Specialists, and was a representative of the American Psychiatric Association Task Force on the National Board of Medical Examiners and the American Board of Psychiatry and Neurology. In 1985, he received the Academic Achievement Award from New York Medical College and was appointed Faculty Scholar at NYU School of Medicine in 2000. He is the author or editor of more than 100 publications, a book reviewer for psychiatric journals, and he lectures on a broad range of topics in general psychiatry. Dr. Sadock maintains a private practice for diagnostic consultations and psychiatric treatment. He has been married to Virginia Alcott Sadock, M.D., Professor of Psychiatry at NYU School of Medicine, since completing his residency. Dr. Sadock enjoys opera, golf, skiing, and traveling, and is an enthusiastic fly fisherman.

VIRGINIA ALCOTT SADOCK, M.D., joined the faculty of the New York University (NYU) School of Medicine in 1980, where she is currently Professor of Psychiatry and Attending Psychiatrist at the Tisch Hospital and Bellevue Hospital. She is Director of the Program in Human Sexuality at the NYU Medical Center, one of the largest treatment and training programs of its kind in the United States. Dr. Sadock is the author of more than 50 articles and chapters on sexual behavior and was the developmental editor of *The Sexual Experience*, one of the first major textbooks on human sexuality, published by Williams & Wilkins. She serves as a referee and book reviewer for several medical journals, including the *American Journal of Psychiatry* and the *Journal of the American Medical Association*. She has long been interested in the role of women in medicine and psychiatry and was a founder of the Committee on Women in Psychiatry of the New York County District Branch of the American Psychiatric Association. She is active in academic matters, has served as Assistant and Associate Examiner for the American Board of Psychiatry and Neurology for more than 15 years; she was a member of the Test Committee in Psychiatry for both the American Board of Psychiatry and the Psychiatric Knowledge and Self-Assessment Program (PKSAP) of the American Psychiatric Association. She has chaired the Committee on Public Relations of the New York County District Branch of the American Psychiatric Association and has participated in the National Medical Television Network series *Women in Medicine* and the Emmy Award-winning PBS television documentary *Women and Depression*. She has been Vice-President of the Society of Sex Therapy and Research and a regional council member of the American Association of Sex Education Counselors and Therapists; she is currently President of the Alumni Association of Sex Therapists. She lectures extensively in the United States and abroad on sexual dysfunction, relational problems, and depression and anxiety disorders. She is a Distinguished Fellow of the American Psychiatric Association, a Fellow of the New York Academy of Medicine, and a Diplomate of the American Board of Psychiatry and Neurology. Dr. Sadock is a graduate of Bennington College; she received her M.D. degree from New York Medical College, and trained in psychiatry at Metropolitan Hospital. She maintains an active practice that includes individual psychotherapy, couples and marital therapy, sex therapy, psychiatric consultation, and pharmacotherapy. She lives in Manhattan with her husband Dr. Benjamin Sadock. They have two children, James William Sadock, M.D., and Victoria Anne Gregg, M.D., both emergency physicians, and two grandchildren, Emily Alcott and Celia Anne. In her leisure time, Dr. Sadock enjoys theater, film, golf, reading fiction, and traveling.

1 ▲

Psychiatric History and Mental Status Examination

PSYCHIATRIC HISTORY

The psychiatric history is the record of the patient's life; it allows a psychiatrist to understand who the patient is, where the patient has come from, and where the patient is likely to go in the future. The history is the patient's life story told to the psychiatrist in the patient's words from his or her point of view. Many times, the history also includes information about the patient obtained from other sources, such as a parent or spouse. Obtaining a comprehensive history from a patient and, if necessary, from informed sources is essential to making a correct diagnosis and formulating a specific and effective treatment plan.

The most important technique for obtaining a psychiatric history is to allow patients to tell their stories in their own words in the order that they consider most important. As patients relate their stories, skillful interviewers recognize the points at which they can introduce relevant questions about the areas described in the outline of the history and mental status examination.

The structure of the history and mental status examination presented in this section is not intended to be a rigid plan for interviewing a patient; it is meant to be a guide for organizing the patient's history when it is written up. Each topic is discussed below.

Identifying Data

The identifying data provide a succinct demographic summary of the patient by name, age, marital status, sex, occupation, language (if other than English), ethnic background, and religion, insofar as they are pertinent, and current circumstances of living. The information can also include the place or situation in which the current interview took place, the source(s) of the information, the reliability of the source(s), and whether the current disorder is the first episode for the patient. The psychiatrist should indicate whether the patient came in on his or her own, was referred by someone else, or was brought in by someone else. The identifying data are meant to provide a thumbnail sketch of potentially important patient characteristics that may affect diagnosis, prognosis, treatment, and compliance. An example of the written report of the identifying data follows:

> Mr. John Jones is a 25-year-old single, white, Protestant male who works as a department store clerk. He is a college grad-
> uate living with his parents. He was referred by his internist for psychiatric evaluation.

Chief Complaint

The chief complaint, in the patient's own words, states why he or she has come or been brought in for help. It should be recorded verbatim in the section on the chief complaint. The other individuals present as sources of information can then give their versions of the presenting events in the section on the history of the present illness.

If the patient is comatose or mute, that should be noted in the chief complaint as such. Examples of chief complaints follow:

> "I am having thoughts of wanting to harm myself"
> "People are trying to drive me insane"
> "I feel I am going mad"
> "I am angry all the time"

History of Present Illness

The history of present illness provides a comprehensive and chronological picture of the events leading up to the current moment in the patient's life. This part of the psychiatric history is probably the most helpful in making a diagnosis: When was the onset of the current episode, and what were the immediate precipitating events or triggers? An understanding of the history of the present illness helps to answer the following questions: Why now? Why did the patient come to the doctor at this time? What were the patient's life circumstances at the onset of the symptoms or behavioral changes, and how did they affect the patient so that the presenting disorder became manifest? Knowing the previously well patient's personality also helps to give perspective on the currently ill patient.

The evolution of the patient's symptoms should be determined and summarized in an organized and systematic way. Symptoms not present should also be delineated. The more detailed the history of the present illness, the more likely it is that the clinician can make an accurate diagnosis. What past precipitating events were part of the chain leading up to the immediate events? In what ways has the patient's illness affected his or her life activities (e.g., work, important relationships)? What is the nature of the dysfunction (e.g., details about changes in such factors as personality, memory, speech)? Are there psychophysiological symptoms? If so, they should be described in terms of location, intensity, and fluctuation. Any relation between physical and psychological symptoms should be noted. A description of the patient's current anxieties, whether they are generalized and nonspecific (free floating) or are specifically related to particular situations, is helpful. How does the patient handle these anxieties? Frequently, a relatively open-ended question such as "How did this all begin?" leads to an adequate unfolding of the history of the present illness. A well-organized patient is generally able to present a chronological account of the history, but a disorganized patient is difficult to interview because the chronology of events is confused. In this case, contacting other informants, such as family members and friends, can be a valuable aid in clarifying the patient's story.

Past Illnesses

The past illnesses section of the psychiatric history is a transition between the story of the present illness and the patient's personal history (also called the anamnesis). Past episodes of both psychiatric and medical illnesses are described. Ideally, a detailed account of the patient's preexisting and underlying psychological and biological substrates is given at this point, and important clues to, and evidence of, vulnerable areas in the patient's functioning are provided. The patient's symptoms, extent of incapacity, type of treatment received, names of hospitals, length of each illness, effects of previous treatments, and degree of compliance should all be explored and recorded chronologically. Particular attention should be paid to the first episodes that signaled the onset of illness because first episodes can often provide crucial data about precipitating events, diagnostic possibilities, and coping capabilities.

With regard to medical history, the psychiatrist should obtain a medical review of symptoms and note any major medical or surgical illnesses and major traumas, particularly those requiring hospitalization. Episodes of craniocerebral trauma, neurological illness, tumors, and seizure disorders are especially relevant to psychiatric histories, as is a history of testing positive for the human immunodeficiency virus (HIV) or having acquired immune deficiency syndrome (AIDS). Specific questions need to be asked about the presence of a seizure disorder, episodes of loss of consciousness, changes in usual headache patterns, changes in vision, and episodes of confusion and disorientation. A history of infection with syphilis is critical and relevant.

Causes, complications, and treatment of any illness and the effects of the illness on the patient should be noted. Specific questions about psychosomatic disorders should be asked and the answers noted. Included in this category are hay fever, rheumatoid arthritis, ulcerative colitis, asthma, hyperthyroidism, gastrointestinal upsets, recurrent colds, and skin conditions. All patients must be asked about alcohol and other substances used, including details about the quantity and frequency of use. It is often advisable to frame questions in the form of an assumption of use, such as, "How much alcohol would you say you drink in a day?" rather than "Do you drink?" The latter question may put the patient on the defensive, concerned about what the physician will think if the answer is yes. If the physician assumes that drinking is a fact, the patient is likely to feel comfortable admitting use.

The importance of a thorough, accurate medical history cannot be overstated. Many medical conditions and their treatments cause psychiatric symptoms that without an attentive medical history may be mistaken for a primary psychiatric disorder. Endocrinopathies such as hypothyroidism or Addison's disease may manifest with depression. Treatment with corticosteroids may precipitate manic and psychotic symptoms. In addition, the coexistence of physical disease may result in secondary psychiatric symptoms. A middle-aged man in the aftermath of a heart attack may suffer from anxiety and depression. A patient's medical status will also guide psychiatric treatment decisions. A depressed patient with cardiac conduction abnormalities will not be treated (at least initially) with a tricyclic antidepressant. A bipolar disorder patient with kidney disease will receive an anticonvulsant mood stabilizer rather than lithium. The names and dosing schedules for all currently prescribed nonpsychiatric drugs should be obtained to avoid adverse interactions with prescribed psychiatric medication.

Family History

A brief statement about any psychiatric illness, hospitalization, and treatment of the patient's immediate family members should be placed in the family history part of the report. Is there a family history of alcohol or other substance abuse or of antisocial behavior? In addition, the family history should provide a description of the personalities and intelligence of the various persons living in the patient's home from childhood to the present as well as a description of the various households in which the patient lived. The psychiatrist should also define the role each person played in the patient's upbringing and this person's current relationship with the patient. What were and are the family ethnic, national, and religious traditions? Informants other than the patient may be available to contribute to the family history, and the source should be cited in the written record. Various members of the family often give different descriptions of the same persons and events. The psychiatrist should determine the family's attitude toward, and insight into, the patient's illness. Does the patient feel that the family members are supportive, indifferent, or destructive? What is the role of illness in the family?

Other questions that provide useful information in this section include the following: What is the patient's attitude toward his or her parents and siblings? The psychiatrist should ask the patient to describe each family member. Who is mentioned first? Who is left out? What does each parent do for a living? What do the siblings do? How do the siblings' occupations compare with the patient's work, and how does the patient feel about it? Who does the patient feel most similar to in the family and why?

Personal History (Anamnesis)

In addition to studying the patient's present illness and current life situation, the psychiatrist needs a thorough understanding of the patient's past and its relation to the present emotional problem. The anamnesis, or personal history, is usually divided into perinatal, early childhood, late childhood, and adulthood. The predominant emotions associated with the different life periods (e.g., painful, stressful, conflictual) should be noted. Depending on time and situation, the psychiatrist may go into detail with regard to each of the following.

Perinatal History.

The psychiatrist considers the home situation into which the patient was born and whether the patient was planned and wanted. Were there any problems with the mother's pregnancy and delivery? What was the mother's emotional and physical state at the time of the patient's birth? Were there any maternal health problems during pregnancy? Was the mother abusing alcohol or other substances during her pregnancy?

Early Childhood (Birth through Age 3 Years).

The early childhood period consists of the first 3 years of the patient's life. The quality of the mother–child interaction during feeding and toilet training is important. Frequently one can learn whether the child presented problems in these areas. Early disturbances in sleep patterns, including episodes of head banging and body rocking, provide clues about possible maternal deprivation or developmental disability. In addition, the psychiatrist should obtain a history of human constancy and attachments during the first 3 years. Was there psychiatric or medical illness present in the parents that may have interfered with parent–child interactions? Did persons other than the mother care for the patient? Did the patient exhibit problems at an early period such as severe stranger anxiety or separation anxiety? Explore the patient's siblings and the details of his or her relationship to them. The emerging personality of the child is a topic of crucial importance. Was the child shy, restless, overactive, withdrawn, studious, outgoing, timid, athletic, friendly? Seek data about the child's ability to concentrate, to tolerate frustration, and to postpone gratification. Also note the child's preference for active or passive roles in physical play. What were the child's favorite games or toys? Did the child prefer to play alone, with others, or not at all? What is the patient's earliest memory? Were there any recurrent dreams or fantasies during this period? A summary of the important areas to be covered follows.

FEEDING HABITS.   Breast-fed or bottle-fed, eating problems

EARLY DEVELOPMENT.   Walking, talking, teething, language development, motor development, signs of unmet needs, sleep pattern, object constancy, stranger anxiety, maternal deprivation, separation anxiety, other caretakers in the home

TOILET TRAINING.   Age, attitude of parents, feelings about it

SYMPTOMS OF BEHAVIOR PROBLEMS.   Thumb sucking, temper tantrums, tics, head bumping, rocking, night terrors, fears, bed-wetting or bed soiling, nail biting, masturbation

PERSONALITY AS A CHILD.   Shy, restless, overactive, withdrawn, persistent, outgoing, timid, athletic, friendly, patterns of play

Middle Childhood (Ages 3 to 11 Years).

In addressing middle childhood, the psychiatrist focuses on such important subjects as gender identification, punishments used in the home, and the persons who provided the discipline and influenced early conscience formation. The psychiatrist must inquire about the patient's early school experiences, especially how the patient first tolerated being separated from his or her mother. Data about the patient's earliest friendships and personal relationships are valuable. The psychiatrist should determine the number and the closeness of the patient's friends, describe whether the patient took the role of a leader or a follower, and describe the patient's social popularity and participation in group or gang activities. Was the child able to cooperate with peers, to be fair, to understand and comply with rules, and to develop an early conscience? Early patterns of assertion, impulsiveness, aggression, passivity, anxiety, or antisocial behavior emerge in the context of school relationships. A history of the patient's learning to read and developing other intellectual and motor skills is important. A history of learning disabilities, their management, and their effects on the child is of particular significance. The presence of nightmares, phobias, bed-wetting, fire setting, cruelty to animals, and excessive masturbation should also be explored.

Late Childhood (Puberty through Adolescence).

During late childhood, persons begin to develop independence from their parents through relationships with peers and group activities. The psychiatrist should attempt to ascertain the values of the patient's social groups and to determine who were the patient's idealized figures. This information provides useful clues about the patient's emerging self-image.

It is helpful to explore the patient's school history, relationships with teachers, and favorite studies and interests, both in school and in extracurricular areas. Ask about the patient's participation in sports and hobbies and inquire about any emotional or physical problems that may have first appeared during this phase. Examples of the types of questions that are commonly asked include the following: What was the patient's sense of personal identity? How extensive was the use of alcohol and other substances? Was the patient sexually active, and what was the quality of the sexual relationships? Was the patient interactive and involved with school and peers, or was he or she isolated, withdrawn, and perceived as odd by others? Did the patient have a generally intact self-esteem, or was there evidence of an inferiority complex? What was the patient's body image? Were there suicidal episodes? Were there problems in school, including excessive truancy? How did the patient use private time? What was the relationship with the parents? What were the feelings about the development of secondary sex characteristics? If the patient is female, what was the response to menarche? What were the attitudes about dating, petting, crushes, parties, and sex games? One way to organize the diverse and large amount of information is to break late childhood into subsets of behavior (e.g., social relationships, school history, cognitive and motor development, emotional and physical problems, and sexuality), as described next.

SOCIAL RELATIONSHIPS.   Attitudes toward sibling(s) and playmates, number and closeness of friends, leader or follower, social popularity, participation in group or gang activities, idealized figures, patterns of aggression, passivity, anxiety, antisocial behavior

SCHOOL HISTORY.   How far the patient progressed, adjustment to school, relationships with teachers—teacher's pet versus rebel—favorite studies or interests, particular abilities or assets, extracurricular activities, sports, hobbies, relations of problems or symptoms to any social period

COGNITIVE AND MOTOR DEVELOPMENT.   Learning to read and other intellectual and motor skills, minimal cerebral dysfunction, learning disabilities—their management and effects on the child

EMOTIONAL AND PHYSICAL PROBLEMS.   Nightmares, phobias, bed-wetting, running away, delinquency, smoking, alcohol or other substance use, anorexia, bulimia, weight problems, feelings of inferiority, depression, suicidal ideas and acts

Adulthood

OCCUPATIONAL HISTORY.   The psychiatrist should describe the patient's choice of occupation, the requisite training and preparation, any work-related conflicts, and the long-term ambitions and goals. The interviewer should also explore the patient's feelings about his or her current job and relationships at work (with authorities, peers, and, if applicable, subordinates) and describe the job history (e.g., number and duration of jobs, reasons for job changes, and changes in job status). What would the patient do for work if he or she could choose freely?

A 40-year-old physician in a successful general practice also had many business ventures in which he invested a great deal of the money he had earned from property development. The ventures frequently entangled him in legal disputes. He spent 12 to 14 hours in his medical office each day seeing patients, completed his charting and paperwork on weekends, and snatched odd moments to conduct complicated business transactions with his attorney. He was snappy and irritable with his family; he expected them to be at his beck and call and to notice his "self-sacrificing" on their behalf. Reducing his practice, taking on an associate, and limiting his business activities were all unacceptable to him.

MARITAL AND RELATIONSHIP HISTORY.   The psychiatrist elicits a history of each marriage, legal or common law. Significant relationships with persons with whom the patient has lived for a protracted period are also included. The story of the marriage or long-term relationship should describe the evolution of the relationship, including the age of the patient at the beginning of the relationship. The areas of agreement and disagreement—including the management of money, housing difficulties, the roles of in-laws, and attitudes toward raising children—should be described. Other questions include the following: Is the patient currently in a long-term relationship? How long is the longest relationship that the patient has had? What is the quality of the patient's sexual relationship (e.g., is the patient's sexual life experienced as satisfactory or inadequate)? What does the patient look for in a partner? Can the patient initiate a relationship or approach someone he or she feels attracted to or compatible with? How does the patient describe the current relationship in terms of its positive and negative qualities? How does the patient perceive failures of past relationships in terms of understanding what went wrong and who was or was not to blame?

A 32-year-old woman had a series of relationships in which she was ultimately abused, always emotionally and often physically and sexually. Despite her conscious intent to find a caring man with whom she could have a less abusive relationship, the pattern repeated itself. Her mother had been chronically beaten by her abusive father. She recalled that her mother warned her repeatedly, "A woman's role is to give in to her husband and put up with the crap as best we can."

MILITARY HISTORY.   The psychiatrist should inquire about the patient's general adjustment to the military, whether he or she saw combat or sustained an injury, and the nature of the discharge. Was the patient ever referred for psychiatric consultation, and did he or she incur any disciplinary action during the period of service?

A 22-year-old soldier returning from combat claimed to have no memory of his last month in combat. He had been assigned to a squad conducting a long-range patrol; only three of eight soldiers returned alive. Through repeated amobarbital interviews conducted in a supportive setting, gradually and with much emotion he recalled that his squad had been ambushed, that early in the firefight he had killed two or three 12- or 13-year-old combat boys who were in the attacking group, and that at a certain point he turned and ran away, leaving one or two of his wounded buddies behind, pleading with him to help them.

EDUCATION HISTORY.   The psychiatrist needs to have a clear picture of the patient's educational background. This information can provide clues about the patient's social and cultural background, intelligence, and motivation and any obstacles to achievement. For instance, a patient from an economically deprived background who never had the opportunity to attend the best schools and whose parents never graduated from high school shows strength of character, intelligence, and tremendous motivation by graduating from college. A patient who dropped out of high school because of violence and substance use displays creativity and determination by going to school at night to obtain a high school diploma while working during the day as a drug counselor. How far did the patient go in school? What was the highest grade or graduate level attained? What did the patient like to study, and what was the level of academic performance? How far did the other members of the patient's family go in school, and how do they compare with the patient's progress? What is the patient's attitude toward academic achievement?

RELIGION.   The psychiatrist determines the religious background of both parents and the details of the patient's religious instruction. Was the family's attitude toward religion strict or permissive, and were there any conflicts between the parents over the child's religious education? The psychiatrist should trace the evolution of the patient's adolescent religious practices to present beliefs and activities. Does the patient have a strong religious affiliation, and, if so, how does this affiliation affect the patient's life? What does the patient's religion say about the treatment of psychiatric or medical illness? What is the religious attitude toward suicide?

SOCIAL ACTIVITY.   The psychiatrist elicits information about the patient's social life and the nature of friendships, with an emphasis on the depth, duration, and quality of human relationships. What social, intellectual, and physical interests does the patient share with friends? What relationships does the patient have with persons of the same sex and the opposite sex? Is the patient essentially isolated and asocial? Does the patient prefer isolation, or is the patient isolated because of anxieties and fears about other people? Who visits the patient in the hospital and how frequently?

CURRENT LIVING SITUATION.   Ask the patient to describe where he or she lives in terms of the neighborhood and the residence as well as the number of rooms, the number of family members living in the home, and the sleeping arrangements. Inquire how issues of privacy are handled, with particular emphasis on parental and sibling nudity and bathroom arrangements. Also ask about the sources of family income and any financial hardships. If applicable, inquire about public assistance and the patient's feelings about it. If the patient has been hospitalized, have provisions been made so that he or she will not lose a job or an apartment? Ask who is caring for the children at home, who visits the patient in the hospital, and how frequently.

LEGAL HISTORY.   Has the patient ever been arrested and, if so, for what? How many times? Was the patient ever in jail? For how long? Is the patient on probation, or are charges pending? Is the patient mandated to be in treatment as part of a stipulation of probation? Does the patient have a history of assault or violence? Against whom? Were weapons used? What is the patient's attitude toward the arrests or prison terms? An extensive legal history, as well as the patient's attitude toward it, may indicate antisocial trends or a litigious personality. An extensive history of violence may alert the psychiatrist to the potential for violence in the future.

Sexual History

Much of the history of infantile sexuality is not recoverable, although many patients can recall curiosities and sexual games played from the ages of 3 to 6 years. The psychiatrist should ask how the patient learned about sex and what he or she felt were parents' attitudes about sexual development. Also inquire whether the patient was sexually abused in childhood. Some material discussed in this section may also be covered in the section on adolescent sexuality. It is not important where in the history it is covered, as long as it is included.

The onset of puberty and the patient's feelings about this milestone are important. Adolescent masturbatory history, including the nature of the patient's fantasies and feelings about them, is of significance. Attitudes toward sex should be described in detail. Is the patient shy, timid, aggressive? Does the patient need to impress others and boast of sexual conquests? Did the patient experience anxiety in the sexual setting? Was there promiscuity? What is the patient's sexual orientation?

The sexual history should include any sexual symptoms, such as anorgasmia, vaginismus, erectile disorder (impotence), premature or retarded ejaculation, lack of sexual desire, and paraphilias (e.g., sexual sadism, fetishism, voyeurism). Attitudes toward fellatio, cunnilingus, and coital techniques may be discussed. The topic of sexual adjustment should include a description of how sexual activity is usually initiated, the frequency of sexual relations, and sexual preferences, variations, and techniques. It is usually appropriate to inquire whether the patient has engaged in extramarital relationships and, if so, under what circumstances and whether the spouse knew of the affair. If the spouse did learn of the affair, the psychiatrist should ask the patient to describe what happened. The reasons underlying an extramarital affair are just as important as understanding its effect on the marriage. Attitudes toward contraception and family planning are important. What form of contraception does the patient use? The psychiatrist, however, should not assume that the patient uses birth control. If an interviewer asks a lesbian patient to describe what type of birth control she uses (on the assumption that she is heterosexual), the patient may surmise that the interviewer will not understand or accept her sexual orientation. A more helpful question is "Do you need to use birth control?" or "Is contraception something that is part of your sexuality?"

The psychiatrist should ask whether the patient wants to mention other areas of sexual functioning and sexuality. Is the patient aware of the issues involved in safe sex? Does the patient have a sexually transmitted disease, such as herpes or AIDS? Does the patient worry about being HIV positive?

Fantasies and Dreams

Freud stated that dreams are the royal road to the unconscious. Repetitive dreams have particular value. If the patient has nightmares, what are their repetitive themes? Some of the most common dream themes are food, examinations, sex, helplessness, and feelings of impotence. Can the patient describe a recent dream and discuss its possible meanings? Fantasies and daydreams are another valuable source of unconscious material. As with dreams, the psychiatrist can explore and record details of the fantasy and attendant feelings.

What are the patient's fantasies about the future? If the patient could make any change in his or her life, what would it be? What are the patient's most common or favorite current fantasies? Does the patient experience daydreams? Are the patient's fantasies grounded in reality, or is the patient unable to tell the difference between fantasy and reality?

Values

The psychiatrist may inquire about the patient's system of values—both social and moral—including values about work, money, play, children, parents, friends, sex, community concerns, and cultural issues. For instance, are children a burden or a joy? Is work a necessary evil, an unavoidable chore, or an opportunity? What is the patient's concept of right and wrong?

MENTAL STATUS EXAMINATION

The mental status examination is the part of the clinical assessment that describes the sum total of the examiner's observations and impressions of the psychiatric patient at the time of the interview. Whereas the patient's history remains stable, the patient's mental status can change from day to day or hour to hour. The mental status examination is the description of the patient's appearance, speech, actions, and thoughts during the interview. Even when a patient is mute, is incoherent, or refuses to answer questions, the clinician can obtain a wealth of information through careful observation.

General Description

Appearance.   In this category, the psychiatrist describes the patient's appearance and overall physical impression, as reflected by posture, poise, clothing, and grooming. If the patient appears particularly bizarre, the clinician may ask, "Has anyone ever commented on how you look?" "How would you describe how you look?" "Can you help me understand some of the choices you make in how you look?"

Examples of items in the appearance category include body type, posture, poise, clothes, grooming, hair, and nails. Common terms used to describe appearance are healthy, sickly, ill at ease, poised, old looking, young looking, disheveled, child-like, and bizarre. Signs of anxiety are noted: moist hands, perspiring forehead, tense posture, wide eyes.

Attitude toward Examiner.   The patient's attitude toward the examiner can be described as cooperative, friendly, attentive, interested, frank, seductive, defensive, contemptuous, perplexed, apathetic, hostile, playful, ingratiating, evasive, or guarded; any number of other adjectives can be used. Record the level of rapport established.

Speech Characteristics.   This part of the report describes the physical characteristics of speech. Speech can be described in terms of its quantity, rate of production, and quality. The patient may be described as talkative, garrulous, voluble, taciturn, unspontaneous, or normally responsive to cues from the interviewer. Speech may be rapid or slow, pressured, hesitant, emotional, dramatic, monotonous, loud, whispered, slurred, staccato, or mumbled. Speech impairments, such as stuttering, are included in this section. Any unusual rhythms (termed *dysprosody*) or accent should be noted. The patient's speech may be spontaneous.

Overt Behavior and Psychomotor Activity.   Here are described both the quantitative and qualitative aspects of the patient's motor behavior. Included are mannerisms, tics, gestures, twitches, stereotyped behavior, echopraxia, hyperactivity, agitation, combativeness, flexibility, rigidity, gait, and agility. Describe restlessness, wringing of hands, pacing, and other physical manifestations. Note psychomotor retardation or generalized slowing of body movements. Describe any aimless, purposeless activity.

Mood and Affect

Mood.   *Mood* is defined as a pervasive and sustained emotion that colors the person's perception of the world. The psychiatrist is interested in whether the patient remarks voluntarily about feelings or is it necessary to ask the patient how he or she feels. Statements about the patient's mood should include depth, intensity, duration, and fluctuations. Common adjectives used to describe mood include depressed, despairing, irritable, anxious, angry, expansive, euphoric, empty, guilty, hopeless, futile, self-contemptuous, frightened, and perplexed. Mood may be labile, fluctuating or alternating rapidly between extremes (e.g., laughing loudly and expansively one moment, tearful and despairing the next).

Affect.   *Affect* may be defined as the patient's present emotional responsiveness, inferred from the patient's facial expression, including the amount and the range of expressive behavior. Affect may or may not be congruent with mood. Affect can be described as within normal range, constricted, blunted, or flat. In the normal range of affect, there is variation in facial expression, tone of voice, use of hands, and body movements. When affect is constricted, the range and intensity of expression are reduced. In blunted affect, emotional expression is further reduced. To diagnose flat affect, there should be virtually no signs of affective expression; the patient's voice should be monotonous, and the face should be immobile. Note the patient's difficulty in initiating, sustaining, or terminating an emotional response.

Appropriateness of Affect.   The psychiatrist can consider the appropriateness of the patient's emotional responses in the context of the subject the patient is discussing. Delusional patients who are describing a delusion of persecution should be angry or frightened about the experiences they believe are happening to them. Anger or fear in this context is an appropriate expression. Psychiatrists use the term *inappropriate affect* for a quality of response found in some schizophrenia patients in which the patient's affect is incongruent with what the patient is saying (e.g., flattened affect when speaking about murderous impulses).

Perception

Perceptual disturbances, such as hallucinations and illusions, may be experienced in reference to the self or the environment. The sensory system involved (e.g., auditory, visual, taste, olfactory, or tactile) and the content of the illusion or the hallucinatory experience should be described. The circumstances of the occurrence of any hallucinatory experience are important; hypnagogic hallucinations (occurring as a person falls asleep) and hypnopompic hallucinations (occurring as a person awakens) have much less serious significance than other types of hallucinations. Hallucinations can also occur in particular times of stress for individual patients. Feelings of depersonalization and derealization (extreme feelings of detachment from the self or the environment) are other examples of perceptual disturbance. Formication—the feeling of bugs crawling on or under the skin—is seen in cocainism.

Examples of questions used to elicit the experience of hallucinations include the following: "Have you ever heard voices or other sounds that no one else could hear or when no one else was around?" "Have you experienced any strange sensations in your body that others do not seem to feel?"

> A young man with schizophrenia heard an insistent voice repeatedly telling him to stop his antipsychotic medication. After resisting the command for many weeks, the patient felt that he could no longer fight the voice, and he discontinued treatment. Two months later, he was hospitalized involuntarily and near cardiovascular collapse. He later said that once he stopped the medication, the voice further insisted that he should stop eating and drinking to purify himself.

> A terrified 37-year-old man in acute delirium tremens glanced agitatedly about the room. He pointed out the window and said, "My God, the Spanish armada is on the lawn. They're about to attack." He experienced the hallucination as real, and it persisted intermittently for 3 days before abating. Subsequently, the patient had no memory of the experience.

Thought Content and Mental Trends.   Thought can be divided into process (or form) and content. *Process* refers to the way in which a person puts together ideas and associations, the form in which a person thinks. Process or form of thought may be logical and coherent or completely illogical and even incomprehensible. *Content* refers to what a person is actually thinking about: ideas, beliefs, preoccupations, obsessions.

Thought Process (Form of Thinking).   The patient may have either an overabundance or a poverty of ideas. There may be rapid thinking, which, if carried to the extreme, is called a *flight of ideas*. A patient may exhibit slow or hesitant thinking.

Thought can be vague or empty. Do the patient's replies really answer the questions asked, and does the patient have the capacity for goal-directed thinking? Are the responses relevant or irrelevant? Is there a clear cause-and-effect relation in the patient's explanations? Does the patient have *loose associations* (e.g., do the ideas expressed seem unrelated and idiosyncratically connected)? Disturbances of thought continuity include statements that are tangential, circumstantial, rambling, evasive, or perseverative.

Blocking is interruption of the train of thought before an idea has been completed; the patient may indicate an inability to recall what was being said or intended to be said. *Circumstantiality* indicates the loss of capacity for goal-directed thinking; in the process of explaining an idea, the patient brings in many irrelevant details and parenthetical comments but eventually does get back to the original point. *Tangentiality* is a disturbance in which the patient loses the thread of the conversation, pursues divergent thoughts stimulated by various external or internal irrelevant stimuli, and never returns to the original point. Thought process impairments may be reflected by incoherent or incomprehensible connections of thoughts (*word salad*), *clang associations* (association by rhyming), *punning* (association by double meaning), and *neologisms* (new words created by the patient by combining or condensing other words).

Thought Content.   Disturbances in content of thought include delusions, preoccupations (which may involve the patient's illness), obsessions ("Do you have ideas that are intrusive and repetitive?"), compulsions ("Are there things you do over and over, in a repetitive manner?" "Are there things you must do in a particular way or order?" "If you do not do them that way, must you repeat them?" "Do you know why you do things that way?"), phobias, plans, intentions, recurrent ideas about suicide or homicide, hypochondriacal symptoms, and specific antisocial urges.

> A patient had the compulsion to do everything eight times, which permeated all his behavior whether it was brushing his teeth or locking the door to his house, each of which he had to do eight times. He knew his behavior was irrational but could not stop himself from this activity.

Does the patient have thoughts of doing self-harm? Is there a plan? A major category of disturbances of thought content involves delusions. Delusions—fixed, false beliefs out of keeping with the patient's cultural background—may be mood congruent (thoughts that are in keeping with a depressed or elated mood, e.g., a depressed patient thinks he is dying or an elated patient thinks she is the Virgin Mary) or mood incongruent (e.g., an elated patient thinks he has a brain tumor). The psychiatrist should describe the content of any delusional system and attempt to evaluate its organization and the patient's conviction about its validity. The manner in which it affects the patient's life is appropriately described in the history of the present illness. Delusions can be bizarre and may involve be-

liefs about external control. Delusions can have themes that are persecutory or paranoid, grandiose, jealous, somatic, guilty, nihilistic, or erotic. The clinician should describe ideas of reference and of influence. Examples of *ideas of reference* include a person's belief that the television or radio is speaking to or about him or her. Examples of *ideas of influence* are beliefs about another person or force controlling some aspect of one's behavior.

> A young man with schizophrenia—a college dropout who could work only part-time at low-level jobs and who lived with his high-achieving family—believed he was the Messiah. He was fully convinced that his struggles and lack of occupational success were merely God's tests until the patient's true identity would be revealed. As he improved, he would, if asked, say that he was God's chosen but, when questioned further, would admit the slight possibility that he was wrong. On reaching his best clinical state, he would muse on the possibility that he was the Messiah but state that he was not sure.

Sensorium and Cognition

The sensorium and cognition portion of the mental status examination seeks to assess brain function, including intelligence, capacity for abstract thought, and level of insight and judgment.

Consciousness.   Disturbances of consciousness usually indicate organic brain impairment. Clouding of consciousness is an overall reduced awareness of the environment. A patient may be unable to sustain attention to environmental stimuli or to maintain goal-directed thinking or behavior. Clouding or obtunding of consciousness is frequently not a fixed mental state. A patient typically exhibits fluctuations in the level of awareness of the surrounding environment. The patient who has an altered state of consciousness often shows some impairment of orientation as well, although the reverse is not necessarily true. Some terms used to describe the patient's level of consciousness are *clouding, somnolence, stupor, coma, lethargy,* and *alert*.

Orientation and Memory.   Disorders of orientation are traditionally separated according to time, place, and person. Any impairment usually appears in this order (i.e., sense of time is impaired before sense of place); similarly, as the patient improves, the impairment clears in the reverse order. The psychiatrist must determine whether a patient can give the approximate date and time of day. In addition, if hospitalized, does the patient know how long he or she has been there? Does the patient seem to be oriented to the present? In questions about orientation to place, patients should be able to state the name and the location of the hospital correctly and to behave as though they know where they are. In assessing orientation for person, the psychiatrist asks patients whether they know the names of the people around them and whether they understand their roles in relationship to them. Do they know who the examiner is? Only in the most severe instances do patients not know who they are.

A 42-year-old alcoholic man in delirium tremens examined in a California hospital in 1995 was asked the date and where he was. He replied, "I'm standing on a street corner in Kansas City in 1966 minding my own business. Why don't you mind yours?"

Memory functions have traditionally been divided into four areas: remote memory, recent past memory, recent memory, and immediate retention and recall. Recent memory may be checked by asking patients about their appetite and then about what they had for breakfast or for dinner the previous evening. Patients may be asked at this point if they recall the interviewer's name. Asking patients to repeat six digits forward and then backward is a test of immediate retention. Remote memory can be tested by asking patients for information about their childhood that can be later verified. Asking patients to recall important news events from the prior few months checks recent past memory. Often in cognitive disorders, recent or short-term memory is impaired first, and remote or long-term memory is impaired later. If there is impairment, what efforts are made to cope with it or to conceal it? Is denial, confabulation, or circumstantiality used to conceal a deficit? Reactions to the loss of memory can give important clues to underlying disorders and coping mechanisms. For instance, a patient who appears to have memory impairment but, in fact, is depressed is more likely to be concerned about memory loss than is someone with memory loss secondary to dementia. The clinician must also determine whether a catastrophic reaction is present (anxious crying when unable to remember).

A 40-year-old chronically alcoholic man whose memory on the mental status examination was markedly impaired frantically demanded to be released from the hospital, saying that his wife had just been in an automobile accident and that he had to rush to another hospital to see her. He said it with sincere conviction and appropriate fearful concern; for the patient, at least, the story was real. In fact, his wife had been dead for 15 years. The patient told the same story over and over, always with evident conviction, despite the fact that staff members confronted him with the reality that his wife had been dead for years. The patient was never influenced by their assertions because he could not register new memories. Although his past memory was patchy at best, he could repeatedly recall the story of his wife's emergency.

Confabulation (unconsciously making up false answers when memory is impaired) is most closely associated with cognitive disorders.

Concentration and Attention.   A patient's concentration can be impaired for many reasons. A cognitive disorder, anxiety, depression, and internal stimuli, such as auditory hallucinations, all may contribute to impaired concentration. Subtracting serial 7s from 100 is a simple task that requires intact concentration and cognitive capacities. Could the patient subtract 7 from 100 and keep subtracting 7s? If the patient could not subtract 7s, could 3s be subtracted? Were easier tasks accomplished—4 × 9,

5 × 4? The examiner must always assess whether anxiety, some disturbance of mood or consciousness, or a learning deficit (dyscalculia) is responsible for the difficulty.

Attention is assessed by calculations or by asking the patient to spell the word *world* (or others) backward. The patient can also be asked to name five things that start with a particular letter.

During his most recent manic episode, a 48-year-old man with bipolar disorder had intense, grandiose, psychotic ideas. He was convinced that he could control the traffic in Los Angeles by driving on certain freeways at specified times and willing others to leave the road. After the manic episode ended and during the depressive episode that immediately followed, he could recall virtually no details of his previous thought content while he was manic. Later, when euthymic, he remembered only a few hazy images. A year later, the beginning of a new hypomanic period was heralded by the patient's spontaneously remembering and describing in great detail the psychotic plans of the previous episode.

Reading and Writing.   The psychiatrist should ask the patient to read a sentence (e.g., "Close your eyes") and then to do what the sentence says. The patient should also be asked to write a simple but complete sentence.

Visuospatial Ability.   The patient should be asked to copy a figure, such as a clock face or interlocking pentagons.

Abstract Thought.   Abstract thinking is the ability to deal with concepts. Patients can have disturbances in the manner in which they conceptualize or handle ideas. Can the patient explain similarities, such as those between an apple and a pear or between truth and beauty? Are the meanings of simple proverbs, such as "A rolling stone gathers no moss," understood? Answers may be concrete (giving specific examples to illustrate the meaning) or overly abstract (giving too generalized an explanation). The appropriateness of answers and the manner in which they are given should be noted. In a catastrophic reaction, brain-damaged patients become extremely emotional and cannot think abstractly.

When asked to explain the proverb "People in glass houses should not throw stones," a schizophrenic patient replied, "That's easy, you can break the glass."

Information and Intelligence.   If a possible cognitive impairment is suspected, does the patient have trouble with mental tasks, such as counting the change from $10 after a purchase of $6.37? If this task is too difficult, are easy problems (such as how many nickels are in $1.35) solved? The patient's intelligence is related to vocabulary and general fund of knowledge (e.g., the distance from New York to Paris, presidents of the United States). The patient's educational level (both formal and self-education) and socioeconomic status must be taken into account. Handling difficult or sophisticated concepts can reflect intelligence, even in the absence of formal education or an extensive fund of information. Ultimately, the psychiatrist estimates the patient's intellectual capability and capacity to function at the level of basic endowment.

Impulsivity

Is the patient capable of controlling sexual, aggressive, and other impulses? An assessment of impulse control is critical in ascertaining the patient's awareness of socially appropriate behavior and is a measure of the patient's potential danger to self and others. Patients may be unable to control impulses secondary to cognitive and psychotic disorders or because of chronic characterological defects, as observed in the personality disorders. Impulse control can be estimated from information in the patient's recent history and from behavior observed during the interview.

Judgment and Insight

Judgment.   During the course of history taking, the psychiatrist should be able to assess many aspects of the patient's capability for social judgment. Does the patient understand the likely outcome of his or her behavior, and is he or she influenced by this understanding? Can the patient predict what he or she would do in imaginary situations (e.g., smelling smoke in a crowded movie theater)?

> When asked what she would do if she found a stamped addressed envelope on the street, the patient replied, "Well, I would open it of course and read what it said. Maybe there would be money in it."

Insight.   Insight is a patient's degree of awareness and understanding about being ill. Patients may exhibit complete denial of their illness or may show some awareness that they are ill but place the blame on others, on external factors, or even on organic factors. They may acknowledge that they have an illness but ascribe it to something unknown or mysterious in themselves.

> An 18-year-old man went to an emergency room with the belief that he was controlled by a computer on an *Enterprise-like* starship, an elaboration from the television series *Star Trek*. He was convinced that all his thoughts, actions, and feelings were being programmed onboard the starship, which was located light-years away and, therefore, could never be detected by anyone else.

Intellectual insight is present when patients can admit that they are ill and acknowledge that their failures to adapt are partly because of their irrational feelings. Patients' inability to apply their knowledge to alter future experiences, however, is the major limitation to intellectual insight. True emotional insight is present when patients' awareness of their motives and deep feelings leads to a change in their personality or behavior patterns.

A summary of six levels of insight follows:

1. Complete denial of illness
2. Slight awareness of being sick and needing help but denying it at the same time
3. Awareness of being sick but blaming it on others, on external factors, or on organic factors
4. Awareness that illness is due to something unknown in the patient
5. Intellectual insight: admission that the patient is ill and that symptoms or failures in social adjustment are due to the patient's particular irrational feelings or disturbances without applying this knowledge to future experiences
6. True emotional insight: emotional awareness of the motives and feelings within the patient and the important persons in his or her life, which can lead to basic changes in behavior

Reliability

The mental status part of the report concludes with the psychiatrist's impressions of the patient's reliability and capacity to report his or her situation accurately. It includes an estimate of the psychiatrist's impression of the patient's truthfulness or veracity. For instance, if the patient is open about significant active substance abuse or about circumstances that the patient knows may reflect badly (e.g., trouble with the law), the psychiatrist may estimate the patient's reliability to be good.

PSYCHIATRIC REPORT

The psychiatric report is a written document that details the findings obtained from the psychiatric history and mental status examination. It includes a final summary of both positive and negative findings and an interpretation of the data. It has more than descriptive value; it has meaning that helps to provide an understanding of the case. The examiner addresses critical questions in the report: Are future diagnostic studies needed, and, if so, which ones? Is a consultant needed? Is a comprehensive neurological workup needed, including an electroencephalogram or computerized tomography scan? Are psychological tests indicated? Are psychodynamic factors relevant? The report includes a diagnosis made according to the text revision of the fourth edition of the *Diagnostic Statistical Manual of Mental Disorders* (DSM-IV-TR) which uses a multiaxial classification scheme consisting of five axes, each of which should be covered. A prognosis is also discussed in the report, with both good and bad prognostic factors listed. Finally, a treatment plan discusses, and makes firm recommendations about, management issues.

2

Physical Illness and Psychiatric Disorder

Confronted with a patient who has a mental disorder, the psychiatrist must decide whether a medical, surgical, or neurological condition may be the cause. Once the physician is satisfied that no disease process can be held accountable, then the diagnosis of mental disorder not attributable to a medical illness can be made. Although psychiatrists do not perform routine physical examinations on their patients, a knowledge and understanding of physical signs and symptoms is part of their training, which enables them to recognize signs and symptoms that may indicate possible medical or surgical illness. For example, palpitations may be associated with mitral valve prolapse, which is diagnosed by cardiac auscultation. Psychiatrists are also able to recognize and treat the adverse effects of psychotropic medications, which are used by an increasing number of patients seen by psychiatrists and nonpsychiatric physicians.

Some psychiatrists insist that every patient have a complete medical workup; others do not. Whatever their policy, psychiatrists should consider patients' medical status at the outset of a psychiatric evaluation. Psychiatrists must often decide whether a patient needs a medical examination and, if so, what it should include—most commonly, a thorough medical history, including a review of systems, a physical examination, and relevant diagnostic laboratory studies. A study of 1,000 medical patients found that in 75 percent of cases no cause of symptoms (i.e., subjective complaints) could be found, and a psychological basis was assumed in 10 percent of those cases.

HISTORY OF MEDICAL ILLNESS

In the course of conducting a psychiatric evaluation, information should be gathered about known bodily diseases or dysfunctions, hospitalizations and operative procedures, medications taken recently or at present, personal habits and occupational history, family history of illnesses, and specific physical complaints. Information about medical illnesses should be gathered from the patient, the referring physician, and the family if necessary.

Information about previous episodes of illness may provide valuable clues about the nature of the present disorder. For example, a distinctly delusional disorder in a patient with a history of several similar episodes that responded promptly to diverse forms of treatment strongly suggests the possibility of substance-induced psychotic disorder. To pursue this lead, the psychiatrist should order a drug screen. The history of a surgical procedure may also be useful; for instance, a thyroidectomy suggests hypothyroidism as the cause of depression.

Depression is an adverse effect of several medications prescribed for hypertension. Medication taken in a therapeutic dose occasionally reaches high concentrations in the blood. Digitalis intoxication, for example, may occur under such circumstances and result in impaired mental functioning. Proprietary drugs may cause or contribute to an anticholinergic delirium. Therefore, the psychiatrist must inquire about over-the-counter remedies as well as prescribed medications. A history of herbal intake and alternative therapy is essential in view of their increased use.

An occupational history may also provide essential information. Exposure to mercury may result in complaints suggesting a psychosis, and exposure to lead, as in smelting, may produce a cognitive disorder. The latter clinical picture can also result from imbibing "moonshine" whiskey with a high lead content.

In eliciting information about specific symptoms, the psychiatrist brings medical and psychological knowledge into full play. For example, the psychiatrist should elicit sufficient information from the patient complaining of headache to predict whether the pain results from intracranial disease that requires neurological testing. In addition, the psychiatrist should be able to recognize that the pain in the right shoulder of a hypochondriacal patient with abdominal discomfort may be the classic referred pain of gallbladder disease.

REVIEW OF SYSTEMS

A review of systems is performed by many psychiatrists as part of the initial workup. It often yields information that relates to the patient's psychiatric complaint.

An inventory by systems should follow the open-ended inquiry. The review may be organized according to organ systems (e.g., liver, pancreas), functional systems (e.g., gastrointestinal), or a combination of the two, as in the following outline. In all cases, the review should be comprehensive and thorough. Even if a psychiatric component is suspected, a complete review of systems may still be indicated.

Head

Many patients give a history of headache; its duration, frequency, character, location, and severity should be ascertained. Headaches often result from substance abuse, including alcohol, nicotine, and caffeine. Vascular (migraine) headaches are precipitated by stress. Temporal arteritis causes unilateral throbbing headaches and may lead to blindness. Brain tumors are associated with headaches as a result of increased intracranial pressure, but some may be silent for long periods, the first signs being a change in personality or cognition. A head injury can result in subdural hematoma and in boxers can cause progressive dementia with extrapyramidal symptoms. The headache of subarachnoid hemorrhage is sudden, severe, and associated with changes in the sensorium. Normal pressure hydrocephalus can follow a head injury or encephalitis and be associated with dementia, shuffling gait, and urinary incontinence. Dizziness occurs in up to 30 percent of persons, and determining its cause is challenging and often difficult. A change in the size or shape of the head may be indicative of Paget's disease.

Eye, Ear, Nose, and Throat

Visual acuity, diplopia, hearing problems, tinnitus, glossitis, and bad taste are covered in this area. A patient taking antipsychotics who gives a history of twitching about the mouth or disturbing movements of the tongue may be in the early and potentially reversible stage of tardive dyskinesia. Impaired vision may occur with thioridazine (Mellaril) in high doses (greater than 800 mg a day). A history of glaucoma contraindicates drugs with anticholinergic effects. Aphonia may be hysterical in nature. The late stage of cocaine abuse can result in perforations of the nasal septum and difficulty breathing. A transitory episode of diplopia may herald multiple sclerosis. Delusional disorder is more common in hearing-impaired persons than in those with normal hearing. Complaints of bad odors may be a symptom of temporal lobe epilepsy rather than schizophrenia. Blue-tinged vision may occur transiently when using sildenafil (Viagra) or similar drugs. The teeth of patients with bulimia can be etched as a result of acid vomitus.

Respiratory System

Cough, asthma, pleurisy, hemoptysis, dyspnea, and orthopnea are considered in this section. Hyperventilation is suggested if the patient's symptoms include all or a few of the following: onset at rest, sighing respirations, apprehension, anxiety, depersonalization, palpitations, inability to swallow, numbness of the feet and hands, and carpopedal spasm. Dyspnea and breathlessness may occur in depression. In pulmonary or obstructive airway disease, the onset of symptoms is usually insidious, whereas in depression, it is sudden. In depression, breathlessness is experienced at rest, shows little change with exertion, and may fluctuate within a matter of minutes; the onset of breathlessness coincides with the onset of a mood disorder and is often accompanied by attacks of dizziness, sweating, palpitations, and paresthesias.

In obstructive airway disease, patients with the most-advanced respiratory incapacity experience breathlessness at rest. Most striking and of greatest assistance in making a differential diagnosis is the emphasis placed on the difficulty in inspiration experienced by patients with depression and on the difficulty in expiration experienced by patients with pulmonary disease. Bronchial asthma has sometimes been associated with a childhood history of extreme dependence on the mother. Patients with bronchospasm should not receive propranolol (Inderal) because it may block catecholamine-induced bronchodilation; propranolol is specifically contraindicated for patients with bronchial asthma because epinephrine given to such patients in an emergency will not be effective. Patients taking angiotensin-converting enzyme (ACE) inhibitors may develop a dry cough as an adverse effect of the drug. Thiazide diuretics may cause hypokalemia with attendant muscle spasm and generalized weakness that may mimic depression or anxiety.

Cardiovascular System

Tachycardia, palpitations, and cardiac arrhythmia are among the most common signs of anxiety about which the patient may complain. Pheochromocytoma usually produces symptoms that mimic anxiety disorders, such as rapid heartbeat, tremors, and pallor. Increased urinary catecholamines are diagnostic of pheochromocytoma. Patients taking guanethidine (Ismelin) for hypertension should not receive tricyclic drugs, which reduce or eliminate the antihypertensive effect of guanethidine. A history of hypertension can preclude the use of monoamine oxidase inhibitors (MAOIs) because of the risk of a hypertensive crisis if such hypertensive patients inadvertently ingest foods high in tyramine. Patients with a suspected cardiac disease should have an electrocardiogram before tricyclics or lithium (Eskalith) is prescribed. A history of substernal pain should be evaluated, and the clinician should keep in mind that psychological stress can precipitate angina-type chest pain in the presence of normal coronary arteries. Patients taking opioids should never receive MAOIs; the combination can cause cardiovascular collapse. Mitral valve prolapse has been associated with anxiety attacks.

Gastrointestinal System

This area covers such topics as appetite, distress before or after meals, food preferences, diarrhea, vomiting, constipation, laxative use, and abdominal pain. A history of weight loss is common in depressive disorders, but depression may accompany the weight loss caused by ulcerative colitis, regional enteritis, and cancer. Atypical depression is accompanied by hyperphagia and weight gain. Anorexia nervosa is accompanied by severe weight loss in the presence of normal appetite. Avoidance of certain foods may be a phobic phenomenon or part of an obsessive ritual. Laxative abuse and induced vomiting are common in bulimia nervosa. Constipation can be caused by opioid dependence and by psychotropic drugs with anticholinergic side effects. Cocaine or amphetamine abuse causes a loss of appetite and weight loss. Weight gain can occur under stress or in association with atypical depression. Polyphagia, polyuria, and polydipsia are the triad of diabetes mellitus. Polyuria, polydipsia, and diarrhea are signs of lithium toxicity. Some patients take enemas routinely as part of paraphilic behavior, and anal fissures or recurrent hemorrhoids may indicate anal penetration by foreign objects. Some patients may ingest foreign objects that produce symptoms that can only be diagnosed by X-ray.

Genitourinary System

Urinary frequency, nocturia, pain or burning on urination, and changes in the size and the force of the stream are some of the signs and symptoms in this area. Anticholinergic adverse effects associated with antipsychotics and tricyclic drugs may cause urinary retention in men with prostate hypertrophy.

Erectile difficulty and retarded ejaculation are also common adverse effects of these drugs, and retrograde ejaculation occurs with thioridazine. A baseline level of sexual responsiveness before using pharmacological agents should be obtained. A history of sexually transmitted diseases—for example, gonorrheal discharge, chancre, herpes, and pubic lice—may indicate sexual promiscuity or unsafe sexual practices. In some cases, the first symptom of acquired immune deficiency syndrome (AIDS) is the gradual onset of mental confusion leading to dementia. Incontinence should be evaluated carefully, and if it persists, further investigation for more extensive disease should include a workup for human immunodeficiency virus (HIV) infection. Drugs with anticholinergic adverse effects should be avoided in men with prostatism. Urethral eroticism in which catheters or other objects are inserted into the urethra may cause infection or laceration.

Orgasm causes prostatic contractions, which may artificially raise prostate-specific antigen (PSA) and give a false-positive test for prostatic cancer. Men scheduled to have a PSA test should avoid masturbation or coitus for 7 to 10 days prior to the test.

Menstrual History

A menstrual history should include the age of the onset of menarche and menopause; the interval, regularity, duration, and amount of flow of periods; irregular bleeding; dysmenorrhea; and abortions. Amenorrhea is characteristic of anorexia nervosa and also occurs in women who are psychologically stressed. Women who are afraid of becoming pregnant or who have a wish to be pregnant may have delayed periods. *Pseudocyesis* is false pregnancy with complete cessation of the menses. Perimenstrual mood changes (e.g., irritability, depression, and dysphoria) should be noted. Painful menstruation can result from uterine disease (e.g., myomata), psychological conflicts about the menses, or a combination of the two. Some women report a premenstrual increase in sexual desire. The emotional reaction associated with abortion should be explored because it can be mild or severe.

GENERAL OBSERVATION

An important part of the medical examination is subsumed under the broad heading of general observation—visual, auditory, and olfactory. Such nonverbal clues as posture, facial expression, and mannerisms should also be noted.

Visual Inspection

Scrutiny of the patient begins at the first encounter. When the patient goes from the waiting room to the interview room, the psychiatrist should observe the patient's gait. Is the patient unsteady? Ataxia suggests diffuse brain disease, alcohol or other substance intoxication, chorea, spinocerebellar degeneration, weakness based on a debilitating process, and an underlying disorder, such as myotonic dystrophy. Does the patient walk without the usual associated arm movements and turn in a rigid fashion, like a toy soldier, as is seen in early Parkinson's disease? Does the patient have asymmetry of gait, such as turning one foot outward,

dragging a leg, or not swinging one arm, suggesting a focal brain lesion?

As soon as the patient is seated, the psychiatrist should direct attention to grooming. Is the patient's hair combed, are the nails clean, and are the teeth brushed? Has clothing been chosen with care, and is it appropriate? Although inattention to dress and hygiene is common in mental disorders—in particular, depressive disorders—it is also a hallmark of cognitive disorders. Lapses—such as mismatching socks, stockings, or shoes—may suggest a cognitive disorder.

The patient's posture and automatic movements or the lack of them should be noted. A stooped, flexed posture with a paucity of automatic movements may be due to Parkinson's disease or diffuse cerebral hemispheric disease or be an adverse effect of antipsychotics. An unusual tilt of the head may be adopted to avoid eye contact, but it can also result from diplopia, a visual field defect, or focal cerebellar dysfunction. Frequent quick, purposeless movements are characteristic of anxiety disorders, but they are equally characteristic of chorea and hyperthyroidism. Tremors, although commonly seen in anxiety disorders, may point to Parkinson's disease, essential tremor, or adverse effects of psychotropic medication. Patients with essential tremor sometimes seek psychiatric treatment because they believe the tremor must be due to unrecognized fear or anxiety, as others often suggest. Unilateral paucity or excess of movement suggests focal brain disease.

The patient's appearance is then scrutinized to assess general health. Does the patient appear to be robust, or is there a sense of ill health? Does looseness of clothing indicate recent weight loss? Is the patient short of breath or coughing? Does the patient's general physiognomy suggest a specific disease? Men with Klinefelter's syndrome have a feminine fat distribution and lack the development of secondary male sex characteristics. Acromegaly is usually immediately recognizable by the large head and jaw.

What is the patient's nutritional status? Recent weight loss, although often seen in depressive disorders and schizophrenia, may be due to gastrointestinal disease, diffuse carcinomatosis, Addison's disease, hyperthyroidism, and many other somatic disorders. Obesity may result from either emotional distress or organic disease. Moon facies, truncal obesity, and buffalo hump are striking findings in Cushing's syndrome. The puffy, bloated appearance seen in hypothyroidism and the massive obesity and periodic respiration seen in Pickwickian syndrome are easily recognized in patients referred for psychiatric help. Hyperthyroidism is indicated by exophthalmos.

The skin frequently provides valuable information. The yellow discoloration of hepatic dysfunction and the pallor of anemia are reasonably distinctive. Intense reddening may be due to carbon monoxide poisoning or to photosensitivity resulting from porphyria or phenothiazines. Eruptions may be manifestations of such disorders as systemic lupus erythematosus (e.g., the butterfly rash on the face), tuberous sclerosis with adenoma sebaceum, and sensitivity to drugs. A dusky purplish cast to the face, plus telangiectasia, is almost pathognomonic of alcohol abuse.

Careful observation may reveal clues that lead to the correct diagnosis in patients who create their own skin lesions. For example, the location and shape of the lesions and the time of their appearance may be characteristic of dermatitis factitia.

The patient's face and head should be scanned for evidence of disease. Premature whitening of the hair occurs in pernicious anemia, and thinning and coarseness of the hair occur in myxedema. In alopecia areata, patches of hair are lost, leaving bald spots; trichotillomania presents a similar picture. Pupillary changes are produced by various drugs—constriction by opioids, and dilation by anticholinergic agents and hallucinogens. The combination of dilated and fixed pupils and dry skin and mucous membranes should immediately suggest the likelihood of atropine use or atropine-like toxicity. Diffusion of the conjunctiva suggests alcohol abuse, cannabis abuse, or obstruction of the superior vena cava. Flattening of the nasolabial fold on one side or weakness of one side of the face—as manifested in speaking, smiling, and grimacing—may be the result of focal dysfunction of the contralateral cerebral hemisphere or of Bell's palsy. A drooping eyelid may be an early sign of myasthenia gravis.

The patient's state of alertness and responsiveness should be evaluated carefully. Drowsiness and inattentiveness may be due to a psychological problem, but they are more likely to result from brain dysfunction, whether secondary to an intrinsic brain disease or to an exogenous factor, such as substance intoxication.

Listening

Listening intently is just as important as looking intently for evidence of somatic disorders. Slowed speech is characteristic not only of depression but also of diffuse brain dysfunction and subcortical dysfunction; unusually rapid speech is characteristic not only of manic episodes and anxiety disorders but also of hyperthyroidism. A weak voice with monotonous tone may be a clue to Parkinson's disease in patients who complain mainly of depression. A slow, low-pitched, hoarse voice should suggest the possibility of hypothyroidism; this voice quality has been described as sounding like a drowsy, slightly intoxicated person with a bad cold and a plum in the mouth. A soft or tremulous voice accompanies anxiety.

Difficulty initiating speech may be owing to anxiety or stuttering or may indicate Parkinson's disease or aphasia. Easy fatigability of speech is sometimes a manifestation of an emotional problem, but it is also characteristic of myasthenia gravis. Patients with these complaints are likely to be seen by a psychiatrist before the correct diagnosis is made.

Word production, as well as the quality of speech, is important. Mispronounced or incorrectly used words suggest a possibility of aphasia caused by a lesion of the dominant hemisphere. The same possibility exists when the patient perseverates, has trouble finding a name or a word, or describes an object or an event in an indirect fashion (paraphasia). When not consonant with patients' socioeconomic and educational levels, coarseness, profanity, or inappropriate disclosures may indicate loss of inhibition caused by dementia.

Smell

Smell may also provide useful information. The unpleasant odor of a patient who fails to bathe suggests a cognitive disorder or a depressive disorder. The odor of alcohol or of substances used to hide it is revealing in a patient who attempts to conceal a drinking problem. Occasionally, a uriniferous odor calls attention to bladder dysfunction secondary to a nervous system disease. Characteristic odors are also noted in patients with diabetic acidosis, flatulence, uremia, and hepatic coma. Precocious puberty can be associated with the smell of adult sweat produced by mature apocrine glands.

PHYSICAL EXAMINATION

Patient Selection

The nature of the patient's complaints is critical to determine whether a complete physical examination is required. Complaints fall into the three categories of body, mind, and social interactions. Bodily symptoms (e.g., headaches and palpitations) call for a thorough medical examination to determine what part, if any, somatic processes play in causing the distress. The same can be said for mental symptoms such as depression, anxiety, hallucinations, and persecutory delusions, which can be expressions of somatic processes. If the problem is clearly limited to the social sphere (e.g., long-standing difficulties in interactions with teachers, employers, parents, or a spouse), there may be no special indication for a physical examination. Personality changes, however, may result from a medical disorder (e.g., early Alzheimer's disease) and cause interpersonal conflicts.

Psychological Reaction to the Physical Examination

Even a routine physical examination may evoke adverse reactions; instruments, procedures, and the examining room may be frightening. A simple running account of what is being done can prevent much needless anxiety. Moreover, if the patient is consistently forewarned of what will be done, the dread of being suddenly and painfully surprised recedes. Comments such as "There's nothing to this" and "You don't have to be afraid because this won't hurt" leave the patient in the dark and are much less reassuring than a few words about what actually will be done.

Although the physical examination is likely to engender or intensify a reaction of anxiety, it can also stir up sexual feelings. Some women with fears or fantasies of being seduced may misinterpret an ordinary movement in the physical examination as a sexual advance. Similarly, a delusional man with homosexual fears may perceive a rectal examination as a sexual attack. Lingering over the examination of a particular organ because an unusual but normal variation has aroused the physician's scientific curiosity is likely to raise concern in the patient that a serious pathological process has been discovered. Such a reaction may be profound in an anxious or hypochondriacal patient.

The physical examination occasionally serves a psychotherapeutic function. Anxious or hypochondriacal patients may be relieved to learn that, in spite of troublesome symptoms, there is no evidence of the serious illness that they fear. The young person who complains of chest pain and is certain that the pain heralds a heart attack can usually be reassured by the report of normal findings after a physical examination and electrocardiogram. The reassurance relieves only the worry occasioned by the immediate episode, however. Unless psychiatric treatment succeeds in dealing with the determinants of the reaction, recurrent episodes are likely.

Sending a patient who has a deeply rooted fear of malignancy for still another test that is intended to be reassuring is usually unrewarding. Some patients may have a false fixed belief that a disorder is present.

During the performance of the physical examination, an observant physician may note indications of emotional distress. For instance, during genital examinations, a patient's behavior may reveal information about sexual attitudes and problems, and these reactions may be used later to open this area for exploration. A chaperone may be a useful accommodation during certain parts of the examination.

Timing of the Physical Examination

Circumstances occasionally make it desirable or necessary to defer a complete medical assessment. For example, a delusional or manic patient may be combative or resistive or both. In this instance, a medical history should be elicited from a family member if possible, but unless there is a pressing reason to proceed with the examination, it should be deferred until the patient is tractable.

For psychological reasons, it may be ill advised to recommend a medical assessment at the time of an initial office visit. For example, a young man may complain about his failure to consummate a first coital attempt. After taking a detailed history, the psychiatrist may conclude that the failure was due to situational anxiety. If so, neither a physical examination nor psychotherapy need be recommended; they would have the undesirable effect of reinforcing the notion of pathology. Reassurance and education might be all that is needed. Should the problem be recurrent, further evaluation would be warranted.

Neurological Examination

If the psychiatrist suspects that the patient has an underlying somatic disorder, such as diabetes mellitus or Cushing's syndrome, referral is usually made to a medical physician for diagnosis and treatment. The situation is different when a cognitive disorder is suspected. The psychiatrist often chooses to assume responsibility in these cases. At some point, however, a thorough neurological evaluation may be indicated.

During the history-taking process in such cases, the patient's level of awareness, attentiveness to the details of the examination, understanding, facial expression, speech, posture, and gait are noted. It is also assumed that a thorough mental status examination will be performed. The neurological examination is carried out with two objectives in mind: to elicit (1) signs pointing to focal, circumscribed cerebral dysfunction and (2) signs suggesting diffuse, bilateral cerebral disease. The first objective is met by the routine neurological examination, which is designed primarily to reveal asymmetries in the motor, perceptual, and reflex functions of the two sides of the body caused by focal hemispheric disease. The second objective is met by seeking to elicit signs that have been attributed to diffuse brain dysfunction and to frontal lobe disease. These signs include the sucking, snout, palmomental, and grasp reflexes and the persistence of the glabella tap response. Computed tomography (CT), magnetic resonance imaging (MRI),

and positron emission tomography (PET) have become the gold standard for the evaluation of neurological, including cognitive, disorders.

Other Findings

Psychiatrists should be able to evaluate the significance of findings uncovered by consultants. With a patient who complains of a lump in the throat (globus hystericus) and who is found on examination to have hypertrophied lymphoid tissue, it is tempting to wonder about a causal relation. How can a clinician be sure that the finding is not incidental? Has the patient been known to have hypertrophied lymphoid tissue at a time when no complaint was made? Do many persons with hypertrophied lymphoid tissue never experience the sensation of a lump in the throat?

With a patient with multiple sclerosis who complains of an inability to walk but, on neurological examination, has only mild spasticity and a unilateral Babinski sign, it is tempting to ascribe the symptom to the neurological disorder, but the complaint may be aggravated by emotional distress. The same holds true for a patient with profound dementia in whom a small frontal meningioma is seen on a CT scan. Dementia is not always correlated with the findings. Significant brain atrophy could cause very mild dementia, and minimal brain atrophy could cause significant dementia.

A lesion is often found that can account for a symptom, but the psychiatrist should make every effort to separate an incidental finding from a causative one and to distinguish a lesion merely found in the area of the symptom from a lesion producing the symptom.

PATIENTS UNDERGOING PSYCHIATRIC TREATMENT

While patients are being treated for psychiatric disorders, psychiatrists should be alert to the possibility of intercurrent illnesses that call for diagnostic studies. Patients in psychotherapy, particularly those in psychoanalysis, may be all too willing to ascribe their new symptoms to emotional causes. Attention should be given to the possible use of denial, especially if the symptoms seem to be unrelated to the conflicts currently in focus.

Not only may patients in psychotherapy be prone to attribute new symptoms to emotional causes, but sometimes their therapists do so as well. The danger of providing psychodynamic explanations for physical symptoms is ever present.

Symptoms such as drowsiness and dizziness and signs such as a skin eruption and a gait disturbance, common adverse effects of psychotropic medication, call for a medical reevaluation if the patient fails to respond in a reasonable time to changes in the dose or the kind of medication prescribed. If patients who are receiving tricyclic or antipsychotic drugs complain of blurred vision (usually an anticholinergic adverse effect) and the condition does not recede with a reduction in dose or a change in medication, they should be evaluated to rule out other causes. In one case, the diagnosis proved to be Toxoplasma chorioretinitis. The absence of other anticholinergic adverse effects, such as a dry mouth and constipation, is an additional clue alerting the psychiatrist to the possibility of a concomitant medical illness.

Early in an illness, there may be few if any positive physical or laboratory results. In such instances, especially if the evidence of psychic trauma or emotional conflicts is glaring, all symptoms are likely to be regarded as psychosocial in origin, and new symptoms are also seen in this light. Indications for repeating portions of the medical workup may be missed unless the psychiatrist is alert to clues suggesting that some symptoms do not fit the original diagnosis and point, instead, to a medical illness. Occasionally, a patient with an acute illness, such as encephalitis, is hospitalized with the diagnosis of schizophrenia, or a patient with a subacute illness, such as carcinoma of the pancreas, is treated in a private office or clinic with the diagnosis of a depressive disorder. Although it may not be possible to make the correct diagnosis at the time of the initial psychiatric evaluation, continued surveillance and attention to clinical details usually provide clues leading to the recognition of the cause.

The likelihood of intercurrent illness is greater with some psychiatric disorders than with others. Substance abusers, for example, because of their life patterns, are susceptible to infection and are likely to suffer from the adverse effects of trauma, dietary deficiencies, and poor hygiene. Depression decreases the immune response.

When somatic and psychological dysfunctions are known to coexist, the psychiatrist should be thoroughly conversant with the patient's medical status. In cases of cardiac decompensation, peripheral neuropathy, and other disabling disorders, the nature and degree of impairment that can be attributed to the physical disorder should be assessed. It is important to answer the following question: Does the patient exploit a disability, or is it ignored or denied with resultant overexertion? To answer this question, the psychiatrist must assess the patient's capabilities and limitations rather than make sweeping judgments based on a diagnostic label.

Special vigilance about medical status is required for some patients in treatment for somatoform and eating disorders. Such is the case for patients with ulcerative colitis who are bleeding profusely and for patients with anorexia nervosa who are losing appreciable weight. These disorders can become life threatening.

Importance of Medical Screening

Numerous articles have called attention to the need for thorough medical screening of patients seen in psychiatric inpatient services and clinics. (A similar need has been demonstrated for the psychiatric evaluation of patients seen in medical inpatient services and clinics.) The concept of *medical clearance* remains ambiguous and has meaning in the context of psychiatric admission or clearance for transfers from different settings or institutions. It implies that no medical condition exists to account for the patient's condition.

Among identified psychiatric patients, from 24 to 60 percent have been shown to suffer from associated physical disorders. In a survey of 2,090 psychiatric clinic patients, 43 percent were found to have associated physical disorders; of these, almost half of the physical disorders had not been diagnosed by the referring sources. (In this study, 69 patients were found to have diabetes mellitus, but only 12 of these patients had been diagnosed before referral.)

Expecting all psychiatrists to be experts in internal medicine is unrealistic, but expecting them to recognize or have high suspicion of physical disorders that are present is realistic. Moreover, they should make appropriate referrals and collaborate in treating patients who have both physical and mental disorders.

Psychiatric symptoms are nonspecific; they can herald medical as well as psychiatric illness. They often precede the appearance of definitive medical symptoms. Some psychiatric symptoms (e.g., visual hallucinations, distortions, and illusions) should evoke a high level of suspicion of a medical toxicity.

The medical literature abounds with case reports of patients whose disorders were initially considered emotional but ultimately proved to be secondary to medical conditions. The data in most of the reports revealed features pointing toward organicity. Diagnostic errors arose because such features were accorded too little weight.

3

Laboratory Tests in Psychiatry

Psychiatrists depend more on the clinical examination and the patient's signs and symptoms to make a diagnosis than do other medical specialists. No laboratory tests in psychiatry can confirm or rule out diagnoses such as schizophrenia, bipolar I disorder, and major depressive disorder. With the continuing advances in biological psychiatry and neuropsychiatry, laboratory tests have become increasingly valuable both to the clinical psychiatrist and to the biological researcher.

In clinical psychiatry, laboratory tests can help rule out potential underlying organic causes of psychiatric symptoms—for example, impaired copper metabolism in Wilson's disease and a positive result on an antinuclear antibody (ANA) test in systematic lupus erythematosus (SLE). Laboratory work is then used to monitor treatment, such as measuring the blood levels of antidepressant medications and assessing the effects of lithium on electrolytes, thyroid metabolism, and renal function. Laboratory data, however, can serve only as an underlying support for the essential skill of clinical assessment.

BASIC SCREENING TESTS

Before initiating psychiatric treatment, a clinician should undertake a routine medical evaluation for the purposes of screening for concurrent disease, ruling out organicity, and establishing baseline values of functions to be monitored. Such an evaluation includes a medical history and routine medical laboratory tests, such as a complete blood count (CBC); hematocrit and hemoglobin; renal, liver, and thyroid function; electrolytes; and blood sugar.

Thyroid disease and other endocrinopathies may present as a mood disorder or a psychotic disorder; cancer or infectious disease can present as depression; infection and connective tissue diseases may present as short-term changes in mental status. In addition, a range of medical and neurological conditions may present initially to the psychiatrist. Those conditions include multiple sclerosis, Parkinson's disease, dementia of the Alzheimer's type, Huntington's disease, dementia due to a human immunodeficiency virus (HIV) disease, and temporal lobe epilepsy. Any suspected medical or neurological condition should be thoroughly evaluated with appropriate laboratory tests and consultation.

NEUROENDOCRINE TESTS

Thyroid Function Tests

Several thyroid function tests are available, including tests for thyroxine (T_4) by competitive protein binding (T_4D) and by ra-

dioimmunoassay (T_4RIA) involving a specific antigen–antibody reaction. More than 90 percent of T_4 is bound to serum protein and is responsible for thyroid-stimulating hormone (TSH) secretion and cellular metabolism. Other thyroid measures include the free T_4 index (FT_4I), triiodothyronine uptake, and total serum triiodothyronine measured by radioimmunoassay (T_3RIA). These tests are used to rule out hypothyroidism, which can appear with symptoms of depression. In some studies, up to 10 percent of patients complaining of depression and associated fatigue had incipient hypothyroid disease. Other associated signs and symptoms common to both depression and hypothyroidism include weakness, stiffness, poor appetite, constipation, menstrual irregularities, slowed speech, apathy, impaired memory, and even hallucinations and delusions. Lithium can cause hypothyroidism and, more rarely, hyperthyroidism. Neonatal hypothyroidism results in mental retardation and is preventable if the diagnosis is made at birth.

The thyrotropin-releasing hormone (TRH) stimulation test is indicated for patients whose marginally abnormal thyroid test results suggest subclinical hypothyroidism, which can account for clinical depression. The test is also used for patients with possible lithium-induced hypothyroidism. The procedure entails an intravenous (IV) injection of 500 mg of TRH, which produces a sharp rise in serum TSH when measured at 15, 30, 60, and 90 minutes. An increase in serum TSH from 5 to 25 IU/mL above baseline is normal. An increase of less than 7 IU/mL is considered a blunted response, which may correlate with a diagnosis of a depressive disorder. Eight percent of all patients with depressive disorders have some thyroid illness.

Dexamethasone-Suppression Test

The dexamethasone-suppression test (DST) is used to help confirm a diagnostic impression of major depressive disorder.

The patient is given 1 mg of dexamethasone (a long-acting synthetic glucocorticoid) by mouth at 11 PM, and the plasma cortisol level is measured at 8 AM, 4 PM, and 11 PM. Plasma cortisol concentrations above 5 mg/dL (known as nonsuppression) are considered abnormal (i.e., a positive result). Suppression of cortisol indicates that the hypothalamic-adrenal-pituitary axis is functioning properly. Since the 1930s, dysfunction of this axis has been known to be associated with stress.

The problems associated with the DST include varying reports of sensitivity and specificity. False-positive and false-negative results are common, and many medical conditions and pharmacological agents can interfere with results. Some evidence indicates that patients with a positive DST result (especially 10 mg/dL) will have a good response to somatic treatment, such as electroconvulsive therapy (ECT) or cyclic antidepressant therapy.

Other Endocrine Tests

Many other hormones affect behavior. Exogenous hormonal administration has been shown to affect behavior, and known endocrine diseases have associated mental disorders. In addition to thyroid hormones, these hormones include the anterior pituitary hormone prolactin, growth hormone, somatostatin, gonadotropin-releasing hormone (GnRH), the sex steroids, luteinizing hormone (LH), follicle-stimulating hormone (FSH), testosterone, and estrogen. Melatonin from the pineal gland has been implicated in seasonal affective disorder. Symptoms of anxiety or depression in some patients may be explained on the basis of unspecified changes in endocrine function or homeostasis.

PROLACTIN. Prolactin levels may become elevated in response to the administration of antipsychotic agents. Elevations in serum prolactin result from blockade of dopamine receptors in the pituitary. This blockade produces an increase in prolactin synthesis and release. Elevated prolactin levels are associated with galactorrhea, menstrual abnormalities, and alterations in libido and bone calcium concentrations.

Prolactin may briefly rise after a seizure. For this reason, prompt measurement of a prolactin level after possible seizure activity may assist in differentiating a seizure from a pseudoseizure.

Catecholamines

The level of serotonin metabolite 5-hydroxyindoleacetic acid (5-HIAA) is elevated in the urine of patients with carcinoid tumors. Elevated levels are noted at times in patients who take phenothiazine medication and in those who eat foods high in serotonin (e.g., walnuts, bananas, and avocados). The concentration of 5-HIAA in cerebrospinal fluid is low in some persons who are in a suicidal depression and in postmortem studies of those who have committed suicide in particularly violent ways. Low 5-HIAA levels in cerebrospinal fluid are associated with violence in general. Norepinephrine and its metabolic products—metanephrine, normetanephrine, and vanillylmandelic acid (VMA)—can be measured in urine, blood, and plasma. Plasma catecholamine levels are markedly elevated in pheochromocytoma, which is associated with anxiety, agitation, and hypertension. Some patients with chronic anxiety may exhibit elevated blood norepinephrine and epinephrine levels. Some depressed patients have a low urinary norepinephrine-to-epinephrine ratio (NE : E).

High levels of urinary norepinephrine and epinephrine have been found in some patients with posttraumatic stress disorder. The norepinephrine metabolite 3-methoxy-4-hydroxyphenylglycol (MHPG) concentration is decreased in patients with severe depressive disorders, especially those patients who attempt suicide.

Kidney Function Tests

Creatinine clearance detects early kidney damage and can be serially monitored to follow the course of renal disease. Blood urea nitrogen (BUN) is also elevated in renal disease and is excreted via the kidneys; serum BUN and creatinine levels are monitored in patients taking lithium. If the serum BUN or creatinine level is abnormal, the patient's 2-hour creatinine clearance and ultimately the 24-hour creatinine clearance are tested.

Liver Function Tests

Total bilirubin and direct bilirubin values are elevated in hepatocellular injury and intrahepatic bile stasis, which can occur with phenothiazine or tricyclic medication and with alcohol and other substance abuse. Certain drugs (e.g., phenobarbital [Luminal]) may lower the serum bilirubin concentration. Liver damage or disease, which is reflected by abnormal findings in liver function tests (LFTs), may manifest with signs and symptoms of a cognitive disorder, including disorientation and delirium. Impaired hepatic function can increase the elimination half-lives of certain drugs, including some benzodiazepines, so that the drug may stay in a patient's system longer than it would under normal circumstances. LFTs must be monitored routinely when using certain drugs, such as carbamazepine (Tegretol) and valproate (Depakene).

Lipids Fasting Blood Sugar and Glycosylated Hemoglobin

Some atypical antipsychotic agents have been associated with abnormalities in serum glucose levels, including the development of diabetes mellitus. Patients who take atypical antipsychotic agents should be monitored for the development of hyperglycemia by obtaining fasting blood glucose levels and glycosylated hemoglobin levels on a quarterly or semiannual basis. In addition, extremes in serum glucose concentrations have been associated with delirium. Hypoglycemia has also been associated with agitation and anxiety. Evaluation for diabetes or other abnormalities in glucose metabolism is usually best done by specialists.

BLOOD TEST FOR SEXUALLY TRANSMITTED DISEASES

The Venereal Disease Research Laboratory (VDRL) test is used as a screening test for syphilis. If positive, the result is confirmed by using the specific fluorescent treponemal antibody-absorption test (FTA-ABS test), in which the spirochete *Treponema pallidum* is used as the antigen. A central nervous system (CNS) VDRL test is performed in patients with suspected neurosyphilis. A positive HIV test result indicates that a person has been exposed to infection with the virus that causes acquired immune deficiency syndrome (AIDS).

TESTS RELATED TO PSYCHOTROPIC DRUGS

In caring for patients receiving psychotropic medication, the trend is to measure the concentration of the prescribed drug in plasma regularly. For some drugs, such as lithium, the monitoring is essential; for other drugs, such as antipsychotics, it is mainly of academic or research interest. A clinician need not practice defensive medicine by insisting that all patients receiving psychotropic drugs have blood levels determined for medicolegal purposes. The current status of psychopharmacological treatment is such that a psychiatrist's clinical judgment and experience, except in rare instances, are better indications of a drug's therapeutic efficacy than determination of its level in plasma. The reliance on plasma levels cannot replace clinical skills.

The major classes of drugs and the suggested guidelines are outlined in what follows.

Benzodiazepines

No special tests are needed for patients taking benzodiazepines. Among the benzodiazepines metabolized in the liver by oxidation, impaired hepatic function increases the half-life. Baseline LFTs are indicated for patients with suspected liver damage. Urine is tested routinely for benzodiazepines in patients being treated for substance abuse.

Antipsychotics

No special tests are needed for patients taking antipsychotics, although it is a good idea to obtain baseline values for liver function and a complete blood cell count. Antipsychotics are metabolized primarily in the liver, with metabolites excreted primarily in urine. Many metabolites are active. Peak plasma concentration usually is reached 2 to 3 hours after an oral dose. Elimination half-life is 12 to 30 hours but may be much longer. Steady state requires at least 1 week at a constant dose (months at a constant dose of depot antipsychotics). With the exception of clozapine (Clozaril), all antipsychotics cause a short-term elevation in serum prolactin concentration (secondary to tuberoinfundibular activity). A normal prolactin level often indicates either noncompliance or nonabsorption. Adverse effects include leukocytosis, leukopenia, impaired platelet function, mild anemia (both aplastic and hemolytic), and agranulocytosis. Bone marrow and blood element adverse effects can occur abruptly, even when the dose has remained constant. Low-potency antipsychotics are most likely to cause agranulocytosis, which is the most common bone marrow adverse effect. These agents may cause hepatocellular injury and intrahepatic biliary stasis (indicated by elevated total and direct bilirubin and elevated transaminases). They also can cause electrocardiographic changes (not as frequently as with tricyclic antidepressants), including a prolonged QT interval; flattened, inverted, or bifid T waves; and U waves. The relation of dose to plasma concentration differs widely among patients.

Clozapine.   Clozapine (Clozaril) levels are determined in the morning before administration of the morning dose of medication. Weekly CBCs are required during the first 6 months of treatment with clozapine because of the risk of agranulocytosis. After the first 6 months of treatment, CBCs are checked every 2 weeks. Results must be sent to a pharmacy for the patient to receive his or her medication. Clozapine should be held for a white blood cell count (WBC) of less than 3,000 per mm^3 or a neutrophil count of less than 1,500 per mm^3.

A therapeutic range for clozapine has not been established; however, a level of 100 nanograms per milliliter (ng/mL) is widely considered to be a minimum therapeutic threshold. Although concentrations between 200 and 700 ng/mL correlate

more with response, nonresponse does occur within this range. At least 350 ng/mL of clozapine is considered to be necessary to achieve a therapeutic response in patients with refractory schizophrenia. The likelihood of seizures and other side effects increases with clozapine levels greater than 1,200 ng/mL or doses greater than 600 mg per day, or both.

Physicians and pharmacists who provide clozapine must be registered through the Clozaril National Registry (1-800-448-5938).

Tricyclic and Tetracyclic Drugs

An electrocardiogram (ECG) may be taken before starting a regimen of cyclic drugs to assess for conduction delays, which may lead to heart block at therapeutic levels. Some clinicians believe that all patients receiving prolonged cyclic drug therapy should have an annual ECG. At therapeutic levels, the drugs suppress arrhythmias through a quinidine-like effect.

Blood levels should be determined routinely when using imipramine (Tofranil), desipramine (Norpramin), or nortriptyline (Pamelor) in the treatment of depressive disorders. Blood level determinations may also be useful for patients with a poor response at normal dose ranges and with high-risk patients for whom there is an urgent need to know whether a therapeutic or toxic plasma level of the drug has been reached. Blood level determinations should also include the measurement of active metabolites (e.g., imipramine is converted to desipramine, amitriptyline [Elavil] to nortriptyline). Some characteristics of tricyclic drug plasma levels are described as follows.

Imipramine.   The percentage of favorable responses correlates with plasma levels in a linear manner between 200 and 250 ng/mL, but some patients may respond at a lower level. Levels above 250 ng/mL yield no improved favorable response, and adverse effects increase.

Nortriptyline.   The therapeutic window (the range within which a drug is most effective) is between 50 and 150 ng/mL. The response rate decreases at levels above 150 ng/mL.

Desipramine.   Levels above 125 ng/mL correlate with a higher percentage of favorable responses.

Amitriptyline.   Different studies have produced conflicting results with regard to blood levels, but they range from 75 to 175 ng/mL.

PROCEDURE FOR DETERMINING BLOOD CONCENTRATIONS. The blood specimen should be drawn 10 to 14 hours after the last dose, usually in the morning after a bedtime dose. Patients must have received a stable daily dose for at least 5 days for the test to be valid. Some patients who metabolize cyclic drugs unusually poorly may have levels as high as 2,000 ng/mL while taking normal doses and before showing a favorable clinical response. Such patients must be monitored closely for cardiac adverse effects. Patients with levels above 1,000 ng/mL are generally at risk for cardiotoxicity.

Monoamine Oxidase Inhibitors

Patients taking monoamine oxidase inhibitors (MAOIs) are instructed to avoid tyramine-containing foods because of the danger of a hypertensive crisis. A baseline normal blood pressure

(BP) must be recorded, and the BP must be monitored during treatment. MAOIs may also cause orthostatic hypotension as a direct drug adverse effect unrelated to diet. Other than their potential for elevating BP when taken with certain foods, MAOIs are relatively free of other adverse effects. A test used both in a research setting and in current clinical practice involves correlating the therapeutic response with the degree of platelet MAO inhibition.

Lithium

Patients receiving lithium should have baseline thyroid function tests, electrolyte monitoring, a WBC, renal function tests (specific gravity, BUN, and creatinine), and a baseline ECG. The rationale for these tests is that lithium can cause renal concentrating defects, hypothyroidism, and leukocytosis; sodium depletion can cause toxic lithium levels; and about 95 percent of lithium is excreted in the urine. Lithium has also been shown to cause ECG changes, including various conduction defects.

Lithium is most clearly indicated in the prophylactic treatment of manic episodes (its direct antimanic effect may take up to 2 weeks), and it is commonly coupled with antipsychotics for the treatment of acute manic episodes. Lithium itself may also have antipsychotic activity. The maintenance level is 0.6 to 1.2 mEq/L, although acutely manic patients can tolerate up to 1.5 to 1.8 mEq/L. Some patients may respond at lower levels; others may require higher levels. A response below 0.4 mEq/L is probably a placebo effect. Toxic reactions may occur with levels above 2.0 mEq/L. Regular lithium monitoring is essential; there is a narrow therapeutic range beyond which cardiac problems and CNS effects can occur.

Blood for lithium level determination is drawn 8 to 12 hours after the last dose, usually in the morning after the bedtime dose. The level should be measured at least twice a week while stabilizing the patient and may be determined monthly thereafter.

Carbamazepine

A pretreatment CBC, including a platelet count, should be done. Reticulocyte count and serum iron tests are also desirable. These tests should be repeated weekly during the first 3 months of treatment and monthly thereafter. Carbamazepine can cause aplastic anemia, agranulocytosis, thrombocytopenia, and leukopenia. Because of the minor risk of hepatotoxicity, LFTs should be done every 3 to 6 months. The medication should be discontinued if the patient shows any signs of bone marrow suppression as measured with periodic CBC. The therapeutic level of carbamazepine is 8 to 12 ng/mL, with toxicity most often reached at levels of 15 ng/mL. Most clinicians report that levels as high as 12 ng/mL are hard to achieve.

Valproate

Serum levels of valproic acid and divalproex (Depakote) are therapeutic in the range of 45 to 50 ng/mL. Above 125 ng/mL, adverse effects occur, including thrombocytopenia. Serum levels should be determined periodically, and LFTs should be run every 6 to 12 months.

Tacrine

Tacrine (Cognex) may cause liver damage. A baseline of liver function should be established, and follow-up serum transaminase levels should be determined every other week for about 5 months. Patients who develop jaundice or who have bilirubin levels above 3 mg/dL must be withdrawn from the drug.

PROVOCATION OF PANIC ATTACKS WITH SODIUM LACTATE

Up to 72 percent of patients with panic disorder have a panic attack when administered IV injection of sodium lactate. Therefore, lactate provocation is used to confirm a diagnosis of panic disorder. Lactate provocation has also been used to trigger flashbacks in patients with posttraumatic stress disorder. Hyperventilation, another known trigger of panic attacks in predisposed persons, is not as sensitive as lactate provocation in inducing panic attacks. Carbon dioxide (CO_2) inhalation also precipitates panic attacks in those so predisposed. Panic attacks triggered by sodium lactate are not inhibited by peripherally acting β-adrenergic receptor antagonists (β-blockers) but are inhibited by alprazolam (Xanax) and tricyclic drugs.

DRUG-ASSISTED INTERVIEW

Interviews with amobarbital (Amytal) administration have both diagnostic and therapeutic indications. Diagnostically, the interviews are helpful in differentiating nonorganic and organic conditions, particularly in patients with symptoms of catatonia, stupor, and muteness. Organic conditions tend to worsen with infusions of amobarbital, but nonorganic or psychogenic conditions tend to get better because of disinhibition, decreased anxiety, or increased relaxation. Therapeutically, amobarbital interviews are useful in disorders of repression and dissociation—for example, in the recovery of memory in psychogenic amnestic disorders and fugue, in the recovery of function in conversion disorder, and in facilitation of emotional expression in posttraumatic stress disorder. Benzodiazepines can be substituted for amobarbital in the infusion.

LUMBAR PUNCTURE

Lumbar puncture is useful in patients who have a sudden manifestation of new psychiatric symptoms, especially changes in cognition. The clinician should be especially vigilant if there is

Table 3–1
Substances of Abuse That Can Be Tested in Urine

Substance	Length of Time Detected in Urine
Alcohol	7–12 hrs
Amphetamine	48 hrs
Barbiturate	24 hrs (short-acting)
	3 wks (long-acting)
Benzodiazepine	3 days
Cannabis	3 days to 4 wks (depending on use)
Cocaine	6–8 hrs (metabolites 2–4 days)
Codeine	48 hrs
Heroin	36–72 hrs
Methadone	3 days
Methaqualone	7 days
Morphine	48–72 hrs
Phencyclidine (PCP)	8 days
Propoxyphene	6–48 hrs

fever or neurological symptoms such as seizures. Lumbar puncture is of use in diagnosing CNS infection (e.g., meningitis).

URINE TESTING FOR SUBSTANCE ABUSE

A number of substances may be detected in a patient's urine if the urine is tested within a specific (and variable) period after ingestion of the substance. Knowledge of urine substance testing is becoming crucial for practicing physicians in view of the controversial issue of mandatory or random substance testing. Table 3–1 provides a summary of substances of abuse that can be detected in urine. Laboratory tests are also used in the detection of substances that may be contributing to cognitive disorders.

4 ▲

Signs and Symptoms in Psychiatry

Signs are objective; symptoms are subjective. Signs are the clinician's observations, such as noting a patient's agitation; symptoms are subjective experiences, such as a person's complaint of feeling depressed. In psychiatry, signs and symptoms are not as clearly demarcated as in other fields of medicine; they often overlap. Because of this, disorders in psychiatry are often described as syndromes—a constellation of signs and symptoms that together make up a recognizable condition. Schizophrenia, for example, is more often viewed as a syndrome than as a specific disorder. This concept is expressed in the use of the terms *schizophrenic spectrum* or *the group of schizophrenias*.

GLOSSARY OF SIGNS AND SYMPTOMS

abreaction A process by which repressed material, particularly a painful experience or a conflict, is brought back to consciousness; in this process, the person not only recalls but also relives the repressed material, which is accompanied by the appropriate affective response.

abstract thinking Thinking characterized by the ability to grasp the essentials of a whole, to break a whole into its parts, and to discern common properties. To think symbolically.

abulia Reduced impulse to act and to think, associated with indifference about consequences of action. Occurs as a result of neurological deficit, depression, and schizophrenia.

acalculia Loss of ability to do calculations; not caused by anxiety or impairment in concentration. Occurs with neurological deficit and learning disorder.

acataphasia Disordered speech in which statements are incorrectly formulated. Patients may express themselves with words that sound like the ones intended but are not appropriate to the thoughts, or they may use totally inappropriate expressions.

acathexis Lack of feeling associated with an ordinarily emotionally charged subject; in psychoanalysis, it denotes the patient's detaching or transferring of emotion from thoughts and ideas. Also called *decathexis*. Occurs in anxiety, dissociative, schizophrenic, and bipolar disorders.

acenesthesia Loss of sensation of physical existence.

acrophobia Dread of high places.

acting out Behavioral response to an unconscious drive or impulse that brings about temporary partial relief of inner tension; relief is attained by reacting to a present situation as if it were the situation that originally gave rise to the drive or impulse. Common in borderline states.

aculalia Nonsense speech associated with marked impairment of comprehension. Occurs in mania, schizophrenia, and neurological deficit.

adiadochokinesia Inability to perform rapid alternating movements. Occurs with neurological deficit and cerebellar lesions.

adynamia Weakness and fatigability, characteristic of neurasthenia and depression.

aerophagia Excessive swallowing of air. Seen in anxiety disorder.

affect The subjective and immediate experience of emotion attached to ideas or mental representations of objects. Affect has outward manifestations that may be classified as restricted, blunted, flattened, broad, labile, appropriate, or inappropriate. *See also* **mood**.

ageusia Lack or impairment of the sense of taste. Seen in depression and neurological deficit.

aggression Forceful, goal-directed action that may be verbal or physical; the motor counterpart of the affect of rage, anger, or hostility. Seen in neurological deficit, temporal lobe disorder, impulse-control disorders, mania, and schizophrenia.

agitation Severe anxiety associated with motor restlessness.

agnosia Inability to understand the import or significance of sensory stimuli; cannot be explained by a defect in sensory pathways or cerebral lesion; the term has also been used to refer to the selective loss or disuse of knowledge of specific objects because of emotional circumstances, as seen in certain schizophrenic, anxious, and depressed patients. Occurs with neurological deficit. For types of agnosia, see the specific term.

agoraphobia Morbid fear of open places or leaving the familiar setting of the home. May be present with or without panic attacks.

agraphia Loss or impairment of a previously possessed ability to write.

ailurophobia Dread of cats.

akathisia Subjective feeling of motor restlessness manifested by a compelling need to be in constant movement; may be seen as an extrapyramidal adverse effect of antipsychotic medication. May be mistaken for psychotic agitation.

akinesia Lack of physical movement, as in the extreme immobility of catatonic schizophrenia; may also occur as an extrapyramidal effect of antipsychotic medication.

akinetic mutism Absence of voluntary motor movement or speech in a patient who is apparently alert (as evidenced by eye movements). Seen in psychotic depression and catatonic states.

alexia Loss of a previously possessed reading facility; not explained by defective visual acuity. *Compare with* **dyslexia**.

alexithymia Inability or difficulty in describing or being aware of one's emotions or moods; elaboration of fantasies associated with depression, substance abuse, and posttraumatic stress disorder.

algophobia Dread of pain.

alogia Inability to speak because of a mental deficiency or an episode of dementia.

ambivalence Coexistence of two opposing impulses toward the same thing in the same person at the same time. Seen in schizophrenia, borderline states, and obsessive-compulsive disorders (OCDs).

amimia Lack of the ability to make gestures or to comprehend those made by others.

amnesia Partial or total inability to recall past experiences; may be organic (*amnestic disorder*) or emotional (*dissociative amnesia*) in origin.

amnestic aphasia Disturbed capacity to name objects, even though they are known to the patient. Also called *anomic aphasia*.

anaclitic Depending on others, especially as the infant on the mother; anaclitic depression in children results from an absence of mothering.

analgesia State in which one feels little or no pain. Can occur under hypnosis and in dissociative disorder.

anancasm Repetitious or stereotyped behavior or thought usually used as a tension-relieving device; used as a synonym for obsession and seen in obsessive-compulsive (anankastic) personality.

androgyny Combination of culturally determined female and male characteristics in one person.

anergia Lack of energy.

anhedonia Loss of interest in and withdrawal from all regular and pleasurable activities. Often associated with depression.

anomia Inability to recall the names of objects.

anorexia Loss or decrease in appetite. In *anorexia nervosa*, appetite may be preserved, but the patient refuses to eat.

anosognosia Inability to recognize a physical deficit in oneself (e.g., patient denies paralyzed limb).

anterograde amnesia Loss of memory for events subsequent to the onset of the amnesia; common after trauma. *Compare with* **retrograde amnesia**.

anxiety Feeling of apprehension caused by anticipation of danger, which may be internal or external.

apathy Dulled emotional tone associated with detachment or indifference; observed in certain types of schizophrenia and depression.

aphasia Any disturbance in the comprehension or expression of language caused by a brain lesion. For types of aphasia, see the specific term.

aphonia Loss of voice. Seen in conversion disorder.

apperception Awareness of the meaning and significance of a particular sensory stimulus as modified by one's experiences, knowledge, thoughts, and emotions. *See also* **perception**.

appropriate affect Emotional tone in harmony with the accompanying idea, thought, or speech.

apraxia Inability to perform a voluntary purposeful motor activity; cannot be explained by paralysis or other motor or sensory

impairment. In *constructional apraxia*, a patient cannot draw two- or three-dimensional forms.

astasia abasia Inability to stand or to walk in a normal manner, even though normal leg movements can be performed in a sitting or lying down position. Seen in conversion disorder.

astereognosis Inability to identify familiar objects by touch. Seen with neurological deficit. *See also* **neurological amnesia.**

asthenopia Pain or discomfort of the eyes, for example, pressure, grittiness.

asyndesis Disorder of language in which the patient combines unconnected ideas and images. Commonly seen in schizophrenia.

ataxia Lack of coordination, physical or mental. (1) In neurology, refers to loss of muscular coordination. (2) In psychiatry, the term *intrapsychic ataxia* refers to lack of coordination between feelings and thoughts; seen in schizophrenia and in severe OCD.

atonia Lack of muscle tone. *See* **waxy flexibility.**

attention Concentration; the aspect of consciousness that relates to the amount of effort exerted in focusing on certain aspects of an experience, activity, or task. Usually impaired in anxiety and depressive disorders.

auditory hallucination False perception of sound, usually voices, but also other noises, such as music. Most common hallucination in psychiatric disorders.

aura (1) Warning sensations, such as automatisms, fullness in the stomach, blushing, and changes in respiration; cognitive sensations; and mood states usually experienced before a seizure. (2) A sensory prodrome that precedes a classic migraine headache.

autistic thinking Thinking in which the thoughts are largely narcissistic and egocentric, with emphasis on subjectivity rather than objectivity, and without regard for reality; used interchangeably with autism and dereism. Seen in schizophrenia and autistic disorder.

automatism A state following a seizure in which the person performs movements or actions without being aware of what is happening.

behavior Sum total of the psyche that includes impulses, motivations, wishes, drives, instincts, and cravings, as expressed by a person's behavior or motor activity. Also called *conation*.

bereavement Feeling of grief or desolation, especially at the death or loss of a loved one.

bizarre delusion False belief that is patently absurd or fantastic (e.g., invaders from space have implanted electrodes in a person's brain). Common in schizophrenia. In nonbizarre delusion, content is usually within the range of possibility.

blackout Amnesia experienced by alcoholics about behavior during drinking bouts; usually indicates reversible brain damage.

blocking Abrupt interruption in train of thinking before a thought or idea is finished; after a brief pause, the person indicates no recall of what was being said or was going to be said (also known as *thought deprivation* or *increased thought latency*). Common in schizophrenia and severe anxiety.

blunted affect Disturbance of affect manifested by a severe reduction in the intensity of externalized feeling tone; one of the fundamental symptoms of schizophrenia, as outlined by Eugen Bleuler.

bradykinesia Slowness of motor activity, with a decrease in normal spontaneous movement.

bradylalia Abnormally slow speech. Common in depression.

bradylexia Inability to read at normal speed.

bruxism Grinding or gnashing of the teeth, typically occurring during sleep. Seen in anxiety disorder.

carebaria Sensation of discomfort or pressure in the head.

catalepsy Condition in which persons maintain the body position into which they are placed; observed in severe cases of catatonic schizophrenia. Also called *waxy flexibility* and *cerea flexibilitas*. *See also* **command automatism.**

cataplexy Temporary sudden loss of muscle tone, causing weakness and immobilization; can be precipitated by a variety of emotional states and is often followed by sleep. Commonly seen in narcolepsy.

catatonic excitement Excited, uncontrolled motor activity seen in catatonic schizophrenia. Patients in a catatonic state may suddenly erupt into an excited state and may be violent.

catatonic posturing Voluntary assumption of an inappropriate or bizarre posture, generally maintained for long periods of time. May switch unexpectedly with catatonic excitement.

catatonic rigidity Fixed and sustained motoric position that is resistant to change.

catatonic stupor Stupor in which patients ordinarily are well aware of their surroundings.

cathexis In psychoanalysis, a conscious or unconscious investment of psychic energy in an idea, concept, object, or person. *Compare with* **acathexis.**

causalgia Burning pain that may be organic or psychic in origin.

cenesthesia Change in the normal quality of feeling tone in a part of the body.

cephalagia Headache.

cerea flexibilitas Condition of a person who can be molded into a position that is then maintained; when an examiner moves the person's limb, the limb feels as if it were made of wax. Also called *catalepsy* or *waxy flexibility*. Seen in schizophrenia.

chorea Movement disorder characterized by random and involuntary quick, jerky, purposeless movements. Seen in Huntington's disease.

circumstantiality Disturbance in the associative thought and speech processes in which a patient digresses into unnecessary details and inappropriate thoughts before communicating the central idea. Observed in schizophrenia, obsessional disturbances, and certain cases of dementia. *See also* **tangentiality.**

clang association Association or speech directed by the sound of a word rather than by its meaning; words have no logical connection; punning and rhyming may dominate the verbal behavior. Seen most frequently in schizophrenia or mania.

claustrophobia Abnormal fear of closed or confining spaces.

clonic convulsion An involuntary, violent muscular contraction or spasm in which the muscles alternately contract and relax. Characteristic phase in grand mal epileptic seizure.

clouding of consciousness Any disturbance of consciousness in which the person is not fully awake, alert, and oriented. Occurs in delirium, dementia, and cognitive disorder.

cluttering Disturbance of fluency involving an abnormally rapid rate and erratic rhythm of speech that impedes intelligibility; the affected individual is usually unaware of communicative impairment.

cognition Mental process of knowing and becoming aware; function is closely associated with judgment.

coma State of profound unconsciousness from which a person cannot be roused, with minimal or no detectable responsiveness to stimuli; seen in injury or disease of the brain, in systemic conditions such as diabetic ketoacidosis and uremia, and in intoxications with alcohol and other drugs. Coma may also occur in severe catatonic states and in conversion disorder.

coma vigil Coma in which a patient appears to be asleep but can be aroused (also known as *akinetic mutism*).

command automatism Condition associated with catalepsy in which suggestions are followed automatically.

command hallucination False perception of orders that a person may feel obliged to obey or unable to resist.

complex A feeling-toned idea.

complex partial seizure A seizure characterized by alterations in consciousness that may be accompanied by complex hallucinations (sometimes olfactory) or illusions. During the seizure, a state of impaired consciousness resembling a dreamlike state may occur, and the patient may exhibit repetitive, automatic, or semipurposeful behavior.

compulsion Pathological need to act on an impulse that, if resisted, produces anxiety; repetitive behavior in response to an obsession or performed according to certain rules, with no true end in itself other than to prevent something from occurring in the future.

conation That part of a person's mental life concerned with cravings, strivings, motivations, drives, and wishes as expressed through behavior or motor activity.

concrete thinking Thinking characterized by actual things, events, and immediate experience rather than by abstractions; seen in young children, in those who have lost or never developed the ability to generalize (as in certain cognitive mental disorders), and in schizophrenic persons. *Compare with* **abstract thinking.**

condensation Mental process in which one symbol stands for a number of components.

confabulation Unconscious filling of gaps in memory by imagining experiences or events that have no basis in fact, commonly seen in amnestic syndromes; should be differentiated from lying. *See also* **paramnesia.**

confusion Disturbances of consciousness manifested by a disordered orientation in relation to time, place, or person.

consciousness State of awareness, with response to external stimuli.

constipation Inability to defecate or difficulty in defecating.

constricted affect Reduction in intensity of feeling tone that is less severe than that of blunted affect.

constructional apraxia Inability to copy a drawing, such as a cube, clock, or pentagon, as a result of a brain lesion.

conversion phenomena The development of symbolic physical symptoms and distortions involving the voluntary muscles or special sense organs; not under voluntary control and not explained by any physical disorder. Most common in conversion disorder, but also seen in a variety of mental disorders.

convulsion An involuntary, violent muscular contraction or spasm. *See also* **clonic convulsion** *and* **tonic convulsion.**

coprolalia Involuntary use of vulgar or obscene language. Observed in some cases of schizophrenia and in Tourette's syndrome.

coprophagia Eating of filth or feces.

cryptographia A private written language.

cryptolalia A private spoken language.

cycloplegia Paralysis of the muscles of accommodation in the eye; observed, at times, as an autonomic adverse effect (anticholinergic effect) of antipsychotic or antidepressant medication.

decompensation Deterioration of psychic functioning caused by a breakdown of defense mechanisms. Seen in psychotic states.

déjà entendu Illusion that what one is hearing one has heard previously. *See also* **paramnesia.**

déjà pensé Condition in which a thought never entertained before is incorrectly regarded as a repetition of a previous thought. *See also* **paramnesia.**

déjà vu Illusion of visual recognition in which a new situation is incorrectly regarded as a repetition of a previous experience. *See also* **paramnesia.**

delirium Acute reversible mental disorder characterized by confusion and some impairment of consciousness; generally associated with emotional lability, hallucinations or illusions, and inappropriate, impulsive, irrational, or violent behavior.

delirium tremens Acute and sometimes fatal reaction to withdrawal from alcohol, usually occurring 72 to 96 hours after the cessation of heavy drinking; distinctive characteristics are marked autonomic hyperactivity (tachycardia, fever, hyperhidrosis, and dilated pupils), usually accompanied by tremulousness, hallucinations, illusions, and delusions. Called *alcohol withdrawal delirium* in the text revision of the fourth edition of the *Diagnostic and Statistical Manual of Mental Disorders. See also* **formication.**

delusion False belief, based on incorrect inference about external reality, that is firmly held despite objective and obvious contradictory proof or evidence and despite the fact that other members of the culture do not share the belief.

delusion of control False belief that a person's will, thoughts, or feelings are being controlled by external forces.

delusion of grandeur Exaggerated conception of one's importance, power, or identity.

delusion of infidelity False belief that one's lover is unfaithful. Sometimes called *pathological jealousy.*

delusion of persecution False belief of being harassed or persecuted; often found in litigious patients who have a pathological tendency to take legal action because of imagined mistreatment. Most common delusion.

delusion of poverty False belief that one is bereft or will be deprived of all material possessions.

delusion of reference False belief that the behavior of others refers to oneself or that events, objects, or other people have a particular and unusual significance, usually of a negative nature; derived from idea of reference, in which persons falsely feel that others are talking about them (e.g., belief that people on television or radio are talking to or about the person). *See also* **thought broadcasting.**

delusion of self-accusation False feeling of remorse and guilt. Seen in depression with psychotic features.

dementia Mental disorder characterized by general impairment in intellectual functioning without clouding of consciousness; characterized by failing memory, difficulty with calculations, distractibility, alterations in mood and affect, impaired judgment and abstraction, reduced facility with language, and disturbance of orientation. Although irreversible when it is due to underlying progressive degenerative brain disease, dementia may be reversible if the cause can be treated.

denial Defense mechanism in which the existence of unpleasant realities is disavowed; refers to keeping out of conscious awareness any aspects of external reality that, if acknowledged, would produce anxiety.

depersonalization Sensation of unreality concerning oneself, parts of oneself, or one's environment that occurs under extreme stress or fatigue. Seen in schizophrenia, depersonalization disorder, and schizotypal personality disorder.

depression Mental state characterized by feelings of sadness, loneliness, despair, low self-esteem, and self-reproach; accompanying signs include psychomotor retardation or, at times, agitation, withdrawal from interpersonal contact, and vegetative symptoms, such as insomnia and anorexia. The term refers to a mood that is so characterized or a mood disorder.

derailment Gradual or sudden deviation in train of thought without blocking; sometimes used synonymously with *loosening of association.*

derealization Sensation of changed reality or that one's surroundings have altered. Usually seen in schizophrenia, panic attacks, and dissociative disorders.

dereism Mental activity that follows a totally subjective and idiosyncratic system of logic and fails to take the facts of reality or experience into consideration. Characteristic of schizophrenia. *See also* **autistic thinking.**

detachment Characterized by distant interpersonal relationships and lack of emotional involvement.

devaluation Defense mechanism in which a person attributes excessively negative qualities to self or others. Seen in depression and paranoid personality disorder.

diminished libido Decreased sexual interest and drive. (Increased libido is often associated with mania.)

dipsomania Compulsion to drink alcoholic beverages.

disinhibition (1) Removal of an inhibitory effect, as in the reduction of the inhibitory function of the cerebral cortex by alcohol. (2) In psychiatry, a greater freedom to act in accordance with inner drives or feelings and with less regard for restraints dictated by cultural norms or one's superego.

disorientation Confusion; impairment of awareness of time, place, and person (the position of the self in relation to other persons). Characteristic of cognitive disorders.

displacement Unconscious defense mechanism by which the emotional component of an unacceptable idea or object is transferred to a more acceptable one. Seen in phobias.

dissociation Unconscious defense mechanism involving the segregation of any group of mental or behavioral processes from the rest of the person's psychic activity; may entail the separation of an idea from its accompanying emotional tone, as seen in dissociative and conversion disorders. Seen in dissociative disorders.

distractibility Inability to focus one's attention; the patient does not respond to the task at hand but attends to irrelevant phenomena in the environment.

doubling The feeling that one has a double who is similar in looks, actions, and feelings. Also known as *Doppelgänger* phenomenon.

dread Massive or pervasive anxiety, usually related to a specific danger.

dreamy state Altered state of consciousness, likened to a dream situation, that develops suddenly and usually lasts a few minutes; accompanied by visual, auditory, and olfactory hallucinations. Commonly associated with temporal lobe lesions.

drowsiness State of impaired awareness associated with a desire or inclination to sleep.

dysarthria Difficulty in articulation—the motor activity of shaping phonated sounds into speech—not in word finding or in grammar.

dyscalculia Difficulty in performing calculations.

dysgeusia Impaired sense of taste.

dysgraphia Difficulty in writing.

dyskinesia Difficulty in performing movements. Seen in extrapyramidal disorders.

dyslalia Faulty articulation caused by structural abnormalities of the articulatory organs or impaired hearing.

dyslexia Specific learning disability syndrome involving an impairment of the previously acquired ability to read; unrelated to the person's intelligence. *Compare with* **alexia.**

dysmetria Impaired ability to gauge distance relative to movements. Seen in neurological deficit.

dysmnesia Impaired memory.

dyspareunia Physical pain in sexual intercourse, usually emotionally caused and more commonly experienced by women; may also result from cystitis, urethritis, or other medical conditions.

dysphagia Difficulty in swallowing.

dysphasia Difficulty in comprehending oral language (*reception dysphasia*) or in trying to express verbal language (*expressive dysphasia*).

dysphonia Difficulty or pain in speaking.

dysphoria Feeling of unpleasantness or discomfort; a mood of general dissatisfaction and restlessness. Occurs in depression and anxiety.

dysprosody Loss of normal speech melody (*prosody*). Common in depression.

dystonia Extrapyramidal motor disturbance consisting of slow, sustained contractions of the axial or appendicular musculature; one movement often predominates, leading to relatively sustained postural deviations; acute dystonic reactions (facial grimacing and torticollis) are occasionally seen with the initiation of antipsychotic drug therapy.

echolalia Psychopathological repeating of words or phrases of one person by another; tends to be repetitive and persistent. Seen in certain kinds of schizophrenia, particularly the catatonic types.

echopraxia The person imitates the clinician's actions even when asked not to do so.

ego-alien Denoting aspects of a person's personality that are viewed as repugnant, unacceptable, or inconsistent with the rest of the personality. Also called *ego-dystonia. Compare with* **ego-syntonic.**

egocentric Self-centered; selfishly preoccupied with one's own needs; lacking interest in others.

ego-dystonic *See* **ego-alien.**

egomania Morbid self-preoccupation or self-centeredness. *See also* **narcissism.**

ego-syntonic Denoting aspects of a personality that are viewed as acceptable and consistent with that person's total personality. Personality traits are usually ego-syntonic. *Compare with* **ego-alien.**

eidetic image Unusually vivid or exact mental image of objects previously seen or imagined.

elation Mood consisting of feelings of joy, euphoria, triumph, and intense self-satisfaction or optimism. Occurs in mania when not grounded in reality.

elevated mood Air of confidence and enjoyment; a mood more cheerful than normal but not necessarily pathological.

emotion Complex feeling state with psychic, somatic, and behavioral components; external manifestation of emotion is *affect.*

emotional insight A level of understanding or awareness that one has emotional problems. It facilitates positive changes in personality and behavior when present.

emotional lability Excessive emotional responsiveness characterized by unstable and rapidly changing emotions.

encopresis Involuntary passage of feces, usually occurring at night or during sleep.

enuresis Incontinence of urine during sleep.

erotomania Delusional belief, more common in women than in men, that someone is deeply in love with them (also known as *de Clérambault syndrome*).

erythrophobia Abnormal fear of blushing.

euphoria Exaggerated feeling of well-being that is inappropriate to real events. Can occur with drugs such as opiates, amphetamines, and alcohol.

euthymia Normal range of mood, implying absence of depressed or elevated mood.

evasion Act of not facing up to, or strategically eluding, something; consists of suppressing an idea that is next in a thought series and replacing it with another idea closely related to it. Also called *paralogia* and *perverted logic.*

exaltation Feeling of intense elation and grandeur.

excited Agitated, purposeless motor activity uninfluenced by external stimuli.

expansive mood Expression of feelings without restraint, frequently with an overestimation of their significance or importance. Seen in mania and grandiose delusional disorder.

expressive aphasia Disturbance of speech in which understanding remains, but the ability to speak is grossly impaired; halting, laborious, and inaccurate speech (also known as *Broca's, nonfluent,* and *motor aphasias*).

expressive dysphasia Difficulty in expressing verbal language; the ability to understand language is intact.

externalization More general term than *projection* that refers to the tendency to perceive in the external world and in external objects elements of one's personality, including instinctual impulses, conflicts, moods, attitudes, and styles of thinking.

extroversion State of one's energies being directed outside oneself. *Compare with* **introversion.**

false memory The recollection and belief by the patient of an event that did not actually occur. In *false memory syndrome,* persons erroneously believe that they sustained an emotional or physical (e.g., sexual) trauma in early life.

fantasy Daydream; fabricated mental picture of a situation or chain of events. A normal form of thinking dominated by unconscious material that seeks wish fulfillment and solutions to conflicts; may serve as the matrix for creativity. The content of the fantasy may indicate mental illness.

fatigue A feeling of weariness, sleepiness, or irritability after a period of mental or bodily activity. Seen in depression, anxiety, neurasthenia, and somatoform disorders.

fausse reconnaissance False recognition, a feature of paramnesia. Can occur in delusional disorders.

fear Unpleasurable emotional state consisting of psychophysiological changes in response to a realistic threat or danger. *Compare with* **anxiety.**

flat affect Absence or near absence of any signs of affective expression.

flight of ideas Rapid succession of fragmentary thoughts or speech in which content changes abruptly and speech may be incoherent. Seen in mania.

floccillation Aimless plucking or picking, usually at bedclothes or clothing, commonly seen in dementia and delirium.

fluent aphasia Aphasia characterized by inability to understand the spoken word; fluent but incoherent speech is present. Also called *Wernicke's, sensory,* and *receptive aphasias.*

folie à deux Mental illness shared by two persons, usually involving a common delusional system; if it involves three persons, it is referred to as *folie à trois,* etc. Also called *shared psychotic disorder.*

formal thought disorder Disturbance in the form of thought rather than the content of thought; thinking characterized by loosened associations, neologisms, and illogical constructs; thought process is disordered, and the person is defined as psychotic. Characteristic of schizophrenia.

formication Tactile hallucination involving the sensation that tiny insects are crawling over the skin. Seen in cocaine addiction and delirium tremens.

free-floating anxiety Severe, pervasive, generalized anxiety that is not attached to any particular idea, object, or event. Observed particularly in anxiety disorders, although it may be seen in some cases of schizophrenia.

fugue Dissociative disorder characterized by a period of almost complete amnesia, during which a person actually flees from an immediate life situation and begins a different life pattern; apart from the amnesia, mental faculties and skills are usually unimpaired.

galactorrhea Abnormal discharge of milk from the breast; may result from the endocrine influence (e.g., prolactin) of dopamine receptor antagonists, such as phenothiazines.

generalized tonic-clonic seizure Generalized onset of tonic-clonic movements of the limbs, tongue biting, and incontinence followed by slow, gradual recovery of consciousness and cognition; also called *grand mal seizure.*

global aphasia Combination of grossly nonfluent aphasia and severe fluent aphasia.

glossolalia Unintelligible jargon that has meaning to the speaker but not to the listener. Occurs in schizophrenia.

grandiosity Exaggerated feelings of one's importance, power, knowledge, or identity. Occurs in delusional disorder and manic states.

grief Alteration in mood and affect consisting of sadness appropriate to a real loss; normally, it is self-limited. *See also* **depression** *and* **mourning.**

guilt Emotional state associated with self-reproach and the need for punishment. In psychoanalysis, refers to a feeling of culpability that stems from a conflict between the ego and the superego (conscience). Guilt has normal psychological and social functions, but special intensity or absence of guilt characterizes many mental disorders, such as depression and antisocial personality disorder, respectively. Psychiatrists distinguish shame as a less internalized form of guilt that relates more to others than to the self. *See also* **shame.**

gustatory hallucination Hallucination primarily involving taste.

gynecomastia Female-like development of the male breasts; may occur as an adverse effect of antipsychotic and antidepressant drugs because of increased prolactin levels or anabolic-androgenic steroid abuse.

hallucination False sensory perception occurring in the absence of any relevant external stimulation of the sensory modality involved. For types of hallucinations, see the specific term.

hallucinosis State in which a person experiences hallucinations without any impairment of consciousness.

haptic hallucination Hallucination of touch.

hebephrenia Complex of symptoms, considered a form of schizophrenia, characterized by wild or silly behavior or mannerisms, inappropriate affect, and delusions and hallucinations that are transient and unsystematized. Hebephrenic schizophrenia is now called *disorganized schizophrenia.*

holophrastic Using a single word to express a combination of ideas. Seen in schizophrenia.

hyperacusis Increased sensitivity to sound.

hyperactivity Increased muscular activity. The term is commonly used to describe a disturbance found in children that is manifested by constant restlessness, overactivity, distractibility, and difficulties in learning. Seen in *attention-deficit/hyperactivity disorder* (ADHD).

hyperalgesia Excessive sensitivity to pain. Seen in somatoform disorder.

hyperesthesia Increased sensitivity to tactile stimulation.

hypermnesia Exaggerated degree of retention and recall. It can be elicited by hypnosis and may be seen in certain prodigies; also may be a feature of OCD, some cases of schizophrenia, and manic episodes of bipolar I disorder.

hyperphagia Increase in appetite and intake of food.

hyperpragia Excessive thinking and mental activity. Generally associated with manic episodes of bipolar I disorder.

hypersomnia Excessive time spent asleep. May be associated with underlying medical or psychiatric disorder or narcolepsy, may be part of the Kleine-Levin syndrome, or may be primary.

hyperventilation Excessive breathing, generally associated with anxiety, which can reduce blood carbon dioxide concentration and can produce lightheadedness, palpitations, numbness, tingling periorally and in the extremities, and, occasionally, syncope.

hypervigilance Excessive attention to and focus on all internal and external stimuli; usually seen in delusional or paranoid states.

hypesthesia Diminished sensitivity to tactile stimulation.

hypnagogic hallucination Hallucination occurring while falling asleep, not ordinarily considered pathological.

hypnopompic hallucination Hallucination occurring while awakening from sleep, not ordinarily considered pathological.

hypnosis Artificially induced alteration of consciousness characterized by increased suggestibility and receptivity to direction.

hypoactivity Decreased motor and cognitive activity, as in psychomotor retardation; visible slowing of thought, speech, and movements. Also called *hypokinesis.*

hypochondria Exaggerated concern about health that is based not on real medical pathology, but on unrealistic interpretations of physical signs or sensations as abnormal.

hypomania Mood abnormality with the qualitative characteristics of mania but somewhat less intense. Seen in cyclothymic disorder.

idea of reference Misinterpretation of incidents and events in the outside world as having direct personal reference to oneself; occasionally observed in normal persons, but frequently seen in paranoid patients. If present with sufficient frequency or intensity or if organized and systematized, these misinterpretations constitute delusions of reference.

illogical thinking Thinking containing erroneous conclusions or internal contradictions; psychopathological only when it is marked and not caused by cultural values or intellectual deficit.

illusion Perceptual misinterpretation of a real external stimulus. *Compare with* **hallucination.**

immediate memory Reproduction, recognition, or recall of perceived material within seconds after presentation. *Compare with* **long-term memory** *and* **short-term memory.**

impaired insight Diminished ability to understand the objective reality of a situation.

impaired judgment Diminished ability to understand a situation correctly and to act appropriately.

impulse control Ability to resist an impulse, drive, or temptation to perform some action.

inappropriate affect Emotional tone out of harmony with the idea, thought, or speech accompanying it. Seen in schizophrenia.

incoherence Communication that is disconnected, disorganized, or incomprehensible. *See also* **word salad.**

incorporation Primitive unconscious defense mechanism in which the psychic representation of another person or aspects of another person are assimilated into oneself through a figurative process of symbolic oral ingestion; represents a special form of introjection and is the earliest mechanism of identification.

increased libido Increase in sexual interest and drive.

ineffability Ecstatic state in which persons insist that their experience is inexpressible and indescribable and that it is impossible to convey what it is like to one who never experienced it.

initial insomnia Falling asleep with difficulty; usually seen in anxiety disorder. *Compare with* **middle insomnia** *and* **terminal insomnia.**

insight Conscious recognition of one's condition. In psychiatry, it refers to the conscious awareness and understanding of one's psychodynamics and symptoms of maladaptive behavior; highly important in effecting changes in the personality and behavior of a person.

insomnia Difficulty in falling asleep or difficulty in staying asleep. It can be related to a mental disorder, can be related to a physical disorder or an adverse effect of medication, or can be primary (not related to a known medical factor or another mental disorder). *See also* **initial insomnia, middle insomnia,** *and* **terminal insomnia.**

intellectual insight Knowledge of the reality of a situation without the ability to use that knowledge successfully to effect an adaptive change in behavior or to master the situation. *Compare with* **true insight.**

intelligence Capacity for learning and ability to recall, to integrate constructively, and to apply what one has learned; the capacity to understand and to think rationally.

intoxication Mental disorder caused by recent ingestion or presence in the body of an exogenous substance producing maladaptive behavior by virtue of its effects on the central nervous system (CNS). The most common psychiatric changes involve disturbances of perception, wakefulness, attention, thinking, judgment, emotional control, and psychomotor behavior; the specific clinical picture depends on the substance ingested.

intropunitive Turning anger inward toward oneself. Commonly observed in depressed patients.

introspection Contemplating one's mental processes to achieve insight.

introversion State in which a person's energies are directed inward toward the self, with little or no interest in the external world.

irrelevant answer Answer that is not responsive to the question.

irritability Abnormal or excessive excitability, with easily triggered anger, annoyance, or impatience.

irritable mood State in which one is easily annoyed and provoked to anger. *See also* **irritability.**

jamais vu Paramnestic phenomenon characterized by a false feeling of unfamiliarity with a real situation that one has previously experienced.

jargon aphasia Aphasia in which the words produced are neologistic, that is, nonsense words created by the patient.

judgment Mental act of comparing or evaluating choices within the framework of a given set of values for the purpose of electing a course of action. If the course of action chosen is consonant with reality or with mature adult standards of behavior, judgment is said to be *intact* or *normal*; judgment is said to be *impaired* if the chosen course of action is frankly maladaptive, results from impulsive decisions based on the need for immediate gratification, or is otherwise not consistent with reality as measured by mature adult standards.

kleptomania Pathological compulsion to steal.

la belle indifférence Inappropriate attitude of calm or lack of concern about one's disability. May be seen in patients with conversion disorder.

labile affect Affective expression characterized by rapid and abrupt changes unrelated to external stimuli.

labile mood Oscillations in mood between euphoria and depression or anxiety.

laconic speech Condition characterized by a reduction in the quantity of spontaneous speech; replies to questions are brief and unelaborated, and little or no unprompted additional information is provided. Occurs in major depression, schizophrenia, and organic mental disorders. Also called *poverty of speech.*

lethologica Momentary forgetting of a name or proper noun. *See* **blocking.**

lilliputian hallucination Visual sensation that persons or objects are reduced in size; more properly regarded as an illusion. *See also* **micropsia.**

localized amnesia Partial loss of memory; amnesia restricted to specific or isolated experiences. Also called *lacunar amnesia* and *patch amnesia.*

logorrhea Copious, pressured, coherent speech; uncontrollable, excessive talking; observed in manic episodes of bipolar disorder. Also called *tachylogia, verbomania,* and *volubility.*

long-term memory Reproduction, recognition, or recall of experiences or information that was experienced in the distant past. Also called remote memory. *Compare with* **immediate memory** *and* **short-term memory.**

loosening of associations Characteristic schizophrenic thinking or speech disturbance involving a disorder in the logical progression of thoughts, manifested as a failure adequately to communicate verbally; unrelated and unconnected ideas shift from one subject to another. *See also* **tangentiality.**

macropsia False perception that objects are larger than they really are. *Compare with* **micropsia.**

magical thinking A form of dereistic thought; thinking similar to that of the preoperational phase in children (Jean Piaget), in which thoughts, words, or actions assume power (e.g., to cause or to prevent events).

malingering Feigning disease to achieve a specific goal, for example, to avoid an unpleasant responsibility.

mania Mood state characterized by elation, agitation, hyperactivity, hypersexuality, and accelerated thinking and speaking (flight of ideas). Seen in bipolar I disorder. *See also* **hypomania.**

manipulation Maneuvering by patients to get their own way; characteristic of antisocial personalities.

mannerism Ingrained, habitual involuntary movement.

melancholia Severe depressive state. Used in the term *involutional melancholia* as a descriptive term and also in reference to a distinct diagnostic entity.

memory Process whereby what is experienced or learned is established as a record in the CNS (registration), where it persists with a variable degree of permanence (retention) and can be recollected or retrieved from storage at will (recall). For types of memory, see **immediate memory, long-term memory,** and **short-term memory.**

mental disorder Psychiatric illness or disease whose manifestations are primarily characterized by behavioral or psychological impairment of function, measured in terms of deviation from some normative concept; associated with distress or disease, not just an expected response to a particular event or limited to relations between a person and society.

mental retardation Subaverage general intellectual functioning that originates in the developmental period and is associated with impaired maturation and learning and social maladjustment. Retardation is commonly defined in terms of intelligence quotient (IQ): mild (between 50 and 55 to 70), moderate (between 35 and 40 to between 50 and 55), severe (between 20 and 25 to between 35 and 40), and profound (below 20 to 25).

metonymy Speech disturbance common in schizophrenia in which the affected person uses a word or phrase that is re- lated to the proper one but is not the one ordinarily used; for example, the patient speaks of consuming a *menu* rather than a *meal*, or refers to losing the *piece of string* of the conversation, rather than the thread of the conversation. *See also* **paraphasia** *and* **word approximation.**

microcephaly Condition in which the head is unusually small as a result of defective brain development and premature ossification of the skull.

micropsia False perception that objects are smaller than they really are. Sometimes called *lilliputian hallucination. Compare with* **macropsia.**

middle insomnia Waking up after falling asleep without difficulty and then having difficulty in falling asleep again. *Compare with* **initial insomnia** *and* **terminal insomnia.**

mimicry Simple, imitative motion activity of childhood.

monomania Mental state characterized by preoccupation with one subject.

mood Pervasive and sustained feeling tone that is experienced internally and that, in the extreme, can markedly influence virtually all aspects of a person's behavior and perception of the world. Distinguished from affect, the external expression of the internal feeling tone. For types of mood, see the specific term.

mood-congruent delusion Delusion with content that is mood appropriate (e.g., depressed patients who believe that they are responsible for the destruction of the world).

mood-congruent hallucination Hallucination with content that is consistent with a depressed or manic mood (e.g., depressed patients hearing voices telling them that they are bad persons and manic patients hearing voices telling them that they have inflated worth, power, or knowledge).

mood-incongruent delusion Delusion based on incorrect reference about external reality, with content that has no association to mood or is mood inappropriate (e.g., depressed patients who believe that they are the new Messiah).

mood-incongruent hallucination Hallucination not associated with real external stimuli, with content that is not consistent with depressed or manic mood (e.g., in depression, hallucinations not involving such themes as guilt, deserved punishment, or inadequacy; in mania, not involving such themes as inflated worth or power).

mood swings Oscillation of a person's emotional feeling tone between periods of elation and periods of depression.

motor aphasia Aphasia in which understanding is intact, but the ability to speak is lost. Also called *Broca's, expressive,* and *nonfluent aphasias.*

mourning Syndrome following loss of a loved one, consisting of preoccupation with the lost individual, weeping, sadness, and repeated reliving of memories. *See also* **bereavement** *and* **grief.**

muscle rigidity State in which the muscles remain immovable; seen in schizophrenia.

mutism Organic or functional absence of the faculty of speech. *See also* **stupor.**

mydriasis Dilation of the pupil; sometimes occurs as an autonomic (anticholinergic) or atropine-like adverse effect of some antipsychotic and antidepressant drugs.

narcissism In psychoanalytic theory, divided into primary and secondary types: *primary narcissism,* the early infantile phase of object relationship development, when the child has not differentiated the self from the outside world, and all sources of pleasure are unrealistically recognized as coming from within the self, giving the child a false sense of omnipotence; *secondary narcissism*, when the libido, once attached to external love objects, is redirected back to the self. *See also* **autistic thinking.**

needle phobia The persistent, intense, pathological fear of receiving an injection.

negative signs In schizophrenia: flat affect, alogia, abulia, and apathy.

negativism Verbal or nonverbal opposition or resistance to outside suggestions and advice; commonly seen in catatonic schizophrenia in which the patient resists any effort to be moved or does the opposite of what is asked.

neologism New word or phrase whose derivation cannot be understood; often seen in schizophrenia. It has also been used to mean a word that has been incorrectly constructed but whose origins are nonetheless understandable (e.g., *headshoe* to mean *hat*), but such constructions are more properly referred to as *word approximations.*

neurological amnesia (1) Auditory amnesia: loss of ability to comprehend sounds or speech. (2) Tactile amnesia: loss of ability to judge the shape of objects by touch. *See also* **astereognosis.** (3) Verbal amnesia: loss of ability to remember words. (4) Visual amnesia: loss of ability to recall or to recognize familiar objects or printed words.

nihilism Delusion of the nonexistence of the self or part of the self; also refers to an attitude of total rejection of established values or extreme skepticism regarding moral and value judgments.

nihilistic delusion Depressive delusion that the world and everything related to it have ceased to exist.

noeisis Revelation in which immense illumination occurs in association with a sense that one has been chosen to lead and command. Can occur in manic or dissociative states.

nominal aphasia Aphasia characterized by difficulty in giving the correct name of an object. *See also* **anomia** *and* **amnestic aphasia.**

nymphomania Abnormal, excessive, insatiable desire in a woman for sexual intercourse. *Compare with* **satyriasis.**

obsession Persistent and recurrent idea, thought, or impulse that cannot be eliminated from consciousness by logic or reasoning; obsessions are involuntary and ego-dystonic. *See also* **compulsion.**

olfactory hallucination Hallucination primarily involving smell or odors; most common in medical disorders, especially in the temporal lobe.

orientation State of awareness of oneself and one's surroundings in terms of time, place, and person.

overactivity Abnormality in motor behavior that can manifest itself as psychomotor agitation, hyperactivity (hyperkinesis), tics, sleepwalking, or compulsions.

overvalued idea False or unreasonable belief or idea that is sustained beyond the bounds of reason. It is held with less intensity or duration than a delusion but is usually associated with mental illness.

panic Acute, intense attack of anxiety associated with personality disorganization; the anxiety is overwhelming and accompanied by feelings of impending doom.

panphobia Overwhelming fear of everything.

pantomime Gesticulation; psychodrama without the use of words.

paramnesia Disturbance of memory in which reality and fantasy are confused. It is observed in dreams and in certain types of schizophrenia and organic mental disorders; it includes phenomena such as *déjà vu* and *déjà entendu,* which may occur occasionally in normal persons.

paranoia Rare psychiatric syndrome marked by the gradual development of a highly elaborate and complex delusional system, generally involving persecutory or grandiose delusions, with few other signs of personality disorganization or thought disorder.

paranoid delusions Includes persecutory delusions and delusions of reference, control, and grandeur.

paranoid ideation Thinking dominated by suspicious, persecutory, or grandiose content of less than delusional proportions.

paraphasia Abnormal speech in which one word is substituted for another, the irrelevant word generally resembling the required one in morphology, meaning, or phonetic composition; the inappropriate word may be a legitimate one used incorrectly, such as *clover* instead of *hand,* or a bizarre nonsense expression, such as *treen* instead of *train.* Paraphasic speech may be seen in organic aphasias and in mental disorders such as schizophrenia. *See also* **metonymy** *and* **word approximation.**

parapraxis Faulty act, such as a slip of the tongue or the misplacement of an article. Freud ascribed parapraxes to unconscious motives.

paresis Weakness or partial paralysis of organic origin.

paresthesia Abnormal spontaneous tactile sensation, such as a burning, tingling, or pins-and-needles sensation.

perception Conscious awareness of elements in the environment by the mental processing of sensory stimuli; sometimes used in a broader sense to refer to the mental process by which all kinds of data—intellectual, emotional, and sensory—are meaningfully organized. *See also* **apperception.**

perseveration (1) Pathological repetition of the same response to different stimuli, as in a repetition of the same verbal response to different questions. (2) Persistent repetition of specific words or concepts in the process of speaking. Seen in cognitive disorders, schizophrenia, and other mental illness. *See also* **verbigeration.**

phantom limb False sensation that an extremity that has been lost is, in fact, present.

phobia Persistent, pathological, unrealistic, intense fear of an object or situation; the phobic person may realize that the fear is irrational but, nonetheless, cannot dispel it. For types of phobias, see the specific term.

pica Craving and eating of nonfood substances, such as paint and clay.

polyphagia Pathological overeating.

positive signs In schizophrenia: hallucinations, delusions, and thought disorder.

posturing Strange, fixed, and bizarre bodily positions held by a patient for an extended time. *See also* **catatonia.**

poverty of content of speech Speech that is adequate in amount but conveys little information because of vagueness, emptiness, or stereotyped phrases.

poverty of speech Restriction in the amount of speech used; replies may be monosyllabic. *See also* **laconic speech.**

preoccupation of thought Centering of thought content on a particular idea, associated with a strong affective tone, such as a paranoid trend or a suicidal or homicidal preoccupation.

pressured speech Increase in the amount of spontaneous speech; rapid, loud, accelerated speech, as occurs in mania, schizophrenia, and cognitive disorders.

primary process thinking In psychoanalysis, the mental activity directly related to the functions of the id and characteristic of unconscious mental processes; marked by primitive, prelogical thinking and by the tendency to seek immediate discharge and gratification of instinctual demands. Includes thinking that is dereistic, illogical, magical; normally found in dreams, abnormally in psychosis. *Compare with* **secondary process thinking.**

projection Unconscious defense mechanism in which persons attribute to another those generally unconscious ideas, thoughts, feelings, and impulses that are in themselves undesirable or unacceptable, as a form of protection from anxiety arising from an inner conflict; by externalizing whatever is unacceptable, they deal with it as a situation apart from themselves.

prosopagnosia Inability to recognize familiar faces that is not due to impaired visual acuity or level of consciousness.

pseudocyesis Rare condition in which a nonpregnant patient has the signs and symptoms of pregnancy, such as abdominal distention, breast enlargement, pigmentation, cessation of menses, and morning sickness.

pseudodementia (1) Dementia-like disorder that can be reversed by appropriate treatment and is not caused by organic brain disease. (2) Condition in which patients show exaggerated indifference to their surroundings in the absence of a mental disorder; also occurs in depression and factitious disorders.

pseudologia phantastica Disorder characterized by uncontrollable lying in which patients elaborate extensive fantasies that they freely communicate and act on.

psychomotor agitation Physical and mental overactivity that is usually nonproductive and is associated with a feeling of inner turmoil, as seen in agitated depression.

psychosis Mental disorder in which the thoughts, affective response, ability to recognize reality, and ability to communicate and relate to others are sufficiently impaired to interfere grossly with the capacity to deal with reality; the classical characteristics of psychosis are impaired reality testing, hallucinations, delusions, and illusions.

psychotic (1) Person experiencing psychosis. (2) Denoting or characteristic of psychosis.

rationalization An unconscious defense mechanism in which irrational or unacceptable behavior, motives, or feelings are logically justified or made consciously tolerable by plausible means.

reaction formation Unconscious defense mechanism in which a person develops a socialized attitude or interest that is the direct antithesis of some infantile wish or impulse that is harbored consciously or unconsciously. One of the earliest and most unstable defense mechanisms, closely related to repression; both are defenses against impulses or urges that are unacceptable to the ego.

reality testing Fundamental ego function that consists of tentative actions that test and objectively evaluate the nature and limits of the environment; includes the ability to differentiate between the external world and the internal world and accurately to judge the relation between the self and the environment.

recall Process of bringing stored memories into consciousness. *See also* **memory.**

recent memory Recall of events over the past few days.

recent past memory Recall of events over the past few months.

receptive aphasia Organic loss of ability to comprehend the meaning of words; fluid and spontaneous, but incoherent and nonsensical, speech. *See also* **fluent aphasia** *and* **sensory aphasia.**

receptive dysphasia Difficulty in comprehending oral language; the impairment involves comprehension and production of language.

regression Unconscious defense mechanism in which a person undergoes a partial or total return to earlier patterns of adaptation; observed in many psychiatric conditions, particularly schizophrenia.

remote memory Recall of events in the distant past.

repression Freud's term for an unconscious defense mechanism in which unacceptable mental contents are banished or kept out of consciousness; important in normal psychological development and in neurotic and psychotic symptom formation. Freud recognized two kinds of repression: (1) repression proper, in which the repressed material was once in the conscious domain, and (2) primal repression, in which the repressed material was never in the conscious realm. *Compare with* **suppression.**

restricted affect Reduction in intensity of feeling tone that is less severe than in blunted affect but clearly reduced. *See also* **constricted affect.**

retrograde amnesia Loss of memory for events preceding the onset of the amnesia. *Compare with* **anterograde amnesia.**

retrospective falsification Memory becomes unintentionally (unconsciously) distorted by being filtered through a person's present emotional, cognitive, and experiential state.

rigidity In psychiatry, a person's resistance to change, a personality trait.

ritual (1) Formalized activity practiced by a person to reduce anxiety, as in OCD. (2) Ceremonial activity of cultural origin.

rumination Constant preoccupation with thinking about a single idea or theme, as in OCD.

satyriasis Morbid, insatiable sexual need or desire in a man. *Compare with* **nymphomania.**

scotoma (1) In psychiatry, a figurative blind spot in a person's psychological awareness. (2) In neurology, a localized visual field defect.

secondary process thinking In psychoanalysis, the form of thinking that is logical, organized, reality oriented, and influenced by the demands of the environment; characterizes the mental activity of the ego. *Compare with* **primary process thinking.**

seizure An attack or sudden onset of certain symptoms, such as convulsions, loss of consciousness, and psychic or sensory disturbances; seen in epilepsy and can be substance induced. For types of seizures, see the specific term.

sensorium Hypothetical sensory center in the brain that is involved with clarity of awareness about oneself and one's surroundings, including the ability to perceive and to process ongoing events in light of past experiences, future options, and current circumstances; sometimes used interchangeably with *consciousness.*

sensory aphasia Organic loss of ability to comprehend the meaning of words; fluid and spontaneous, but incoherent and nonsensical, speech. *See also* **fluent aphasia** *and* **receptive aphasia.**

sensory extinction Neurological sign operationally defined as failure to report one of two simultaneously presented sensory stimuli, despite the fact that either stimulus alone is correctly reported. Also called *sensory inattention.*

shame Failure to live up to self-expectations; often associated with a fantasy of how the person will be seen by others. *See also* **guilt.**

short-term memory Reproduction, recognition, or recall of perceived material within minutes after the initial presentation. *Compare with* **immediate memory** *and* **long-term memory.**

simultanagnosia Impairment in the perception or integration of visual stimuli appearing simultaneously.

somatic delusion Delusion pertaining to the functioning of one's body.

somatic hallucination Hallucination involving the perception of a physical experience localized within the body.

somatopagnosia Inability to recognize a part of one's body as one's own (also called *ignorance of the body* and *autotopagnosia*).

somnolence Pathological sleepiness or drowsiness from which one can be aroused to a normal state of consciousness.

spatial agnosia Inability to recognize spatial relations.

speaking in tongues Expression of a revelatory message through unintelligible words; not considered a disorder of thought if associated with practices of specific Pentecostal religions. *See also* **glossolalia.**

stereotypy Continuous mechanical repetition of speech or physical activities; observed in catatonic schizophrenia.

stupor (1) State of decreased reactivity to stimuli and less than full awareness of one's surroundings; as a disturbance of consciousness, it indicates a condition of partial coma or semicoma. (2) In psychiatry, it is used synonymously with *mutism* and does not necessarily imply a disturbance of consciousness; in *catatonic stupor,* patients are ordinarily aware of their surroundings.

stuttering Frequent repetition or prolongation of a sound or syllable, leading to markedly impaired speech fluency.

sublimation Unconscious defense mechanism in which the energy associated with unacceptable impulses or drives is diverted into personally and socially acceptable channels; unlike other defense mechanisms, it offers some minimal gratification of the instinctual drive or impulse.

substitution Unconscious defense mechanism in which a person replaces an unacceptable wish, drive, emotion, or goal with one that is more acceptable.

suggestibility State of uncritical compliance with influence or of uncritical acceptance of an idea, belief, or attitude; commonly observed among persons with hysterical traits.

suicidal ideation Thoughts or act of taking one's life.

suppression Conscious act of controlling and inhibiting an unacceptable impulse, emotion, or idea; differentiated from repression in that repression is an unconscious process.

symbolization Unconscious defense mechanism in which one idea or object comes to stand for another because of some common aspect or quality in both; based on similarity and association; the symbols formed protect the person from the anxiety that may be attached to the original idea or object.

synesthesia Condition in which the stimulation of one sensory modality is perceived as sensation in a different modality, as when a sound produces a sensation of color.

syntactical aphasia Aphasia characterized by difficulty in understanding spoken speech, associated with gross disorder of thought and expression.

systematized delusion Group of elaborate delusions related to a single event or theme.

tactile hallucination Hallucination primarily involving the sense of touch. Also called *haptic hallucination.*

tangentiality Oblique, digressive, or even irrelevant manner of speech in which the central idea is not communicated.

tension Physiological or psychic arousal, uneasiness, or pressure toward action; an unpleasurable alteration in mental or physical state that seeks relief through action.

terminal insomnia Early morning awakening or waking up at least 2 hours before planning to wake up. *Compare with* **initial insomnia** *and* **middle insomnia.**

thought broadcasting Feeling that one's thoughts are being broadcast or projected into the environment. *See also* **thought withdrawal.**

thought disorder Any disturbance of thinking that affects language, communication, or thought content; the hallmark feature of schizophrenia. Manifestations range from simple blocking and mild circumstantiality to profound loosening of associations, incoherence, and delusions; characterized by a failure to follow semantic and syntactic rules that is inconsistent with the person's education, intelligence, or cultural background.

thought insertion Delusion that thoughts are being implanted in one's mind by other people or forces.

thought latency The period of time between a thought and its verbal expression. Increased in schizophrenia (*see* **blocking**) and decreased in mania (*see* **pressured speech**).

thought withdrawal Delusion that one's thoughts are being removed from one's mind by other people or forces. *See also* **thought broadcasting.**

tic disorders Predominantly psychogenic disorders characterized by involuntary, spasmodic, stereotyped movement of small groups of muscles; seen most predominantly in moments of stress or anxiety, rarely as a result of organic disease.

tinnitus Noises in one or both ears, such as ringing, buzzing, or clicking; an adverse effect of some psychotropic drugs.

tonic convulsion Convulsion in which the muscle contraction is sustained.

trailing phenomenon Perceptual abnormality associated with hallucinogenic drugs in which moving objects are seen as a series of discrete and discontinuous images.

trance Sleep-like state of reduced consciousness and activity.

tremor Rhythmical alteration in movement, which is usually faster than one beat a second; typically, tremors decrease during periods of relaxation and sleep and increase during periods of anger and increased tension.

true insight Understanding of the objective reality of a situation coupled with the motivational and emotional impetus to master the situation or change behavior.

twilight state Disturbed consciousness with hallucinations.

twirling Sign present in autistic children who continually rotate in the direction in which their head is turned.

unconscious (1) One of three divisions of Freud's topographic theory of the mind (the others being the conscious and the preconscious) in which the psychic material is not readily accessible to conscious awareness by ordinary means; its existence may be manifest in symptom formation, in dreams, or under the influence of drugs. (2) In popular (but more ambiguous) usage, any mental material not in the immediate field of awareness. (3) Denoting a state of unawareness, with lack of response to external stimuli, as in a coma.

undoing Unconscious primitive defense mechanism, repetitive in nature, by which a person symbolically acts out in reverse something unacceptable that has already been done or against which the ego must defend itself; a form of magical expiatory action, commonly observed in OCD.

unio mystica Feeling of mystic unity with an infinite power.

vegetative signs In depression, denoting characteristic symptoms such as sleep disturbance (especially early-morning awakening), decreased appetite, constipation, weight loss, and loss of sexual response.

verbigeration Meaningless and stereotyped repetition of words or phrases, as seen in schizophrenia. Also called *cataphasia*. *See also* **perseveration.**

vertigo Sensation that one or the world around one is spinning or revolving; a hallmark of vestibular dysfunction, not to be confused with dizziness.

visual agnosia Inability to recognize objects or persons.

visual amnesia *See* **neurological amnesia.**

visual hallucination Hallucination primarily involving the sense of sight.

waxy flexibility Condition in which a person maintains the body position into which he or she is placed. Also called *catalepsy*.

word approximation Use of conventional words in an unconventional or inappropriate way (metonymy or of new words that are developed by conventional rules of word formation) (e.g., *handshoes* for *gloves* and *time measure* for *clock*); distinguished from a *neologism*, which is a new word whose derivation cannot be understood. *See also* **paraphasia.**

word salad Incoherent, essentially incomprehensible mixture of words and phrases commonly seen in far-advanced cases of schizophrenia. *See also* **incoherence.**

xenophobia Abnormal fear of strangers.

zoophobia Abnormal fear of animals.

5

Classification in Psychiatry

Systems of classification for psychiatric diagnoses have several purposes: to distinguish one psychiatric diagnosis from another, so that clinicians can offer the most effective treatment; to provide a common language among health care professionals; and to explore the still unknown causes of many mental disorders. The two most important psychiatric classifications are the *Diagnostic and Statistical Manual of Mental Disorders* (DSM), developed by the American Psychiatric Association in collaboration with other groups of mental health professionals, and the *International Classification of Diseases* (ICD), developed by the World Health Organization.

DSM-IV-TR's RELATION TO ICD-10

The text revision of the fourth edition of the DSM (DSM-IV-TR) was designed to correspond to the tenth revision of the *International Statistical Classification of Diseases and Related Health Problems* (ICD-10), developed in 1992. This was done to ensure uniform reporting of national and international health statistics. In addition, Medicare requires that billing codes for reimbursement follow ICD-10. ICD-10 is the official classification system used in Europe and many other parts of the world. All categories used in DSM-IV-TR are found in ICD-10, but not all ICD-10 categories are in DSM-IV-TR.

DSM-IV-TR

The DSM-IV-TR is the official psychiatric coding system used in the United States. Although some psychiatrists have been critical of the many versions of DSM that have appeared since 1952, DSM-IV-TR is the official U.S. nomenclature. All terminology used in this textbook conforms to DSM-IV-TR nomenclature. Table 5-1 lists DSM-IV-TR diagnostic categories and the corresponding DSM-IV-TR numerical codes.

Basic Features

Descriptive Approach. The approach to DSM-IV-TR is atheoretical with regard to causes. Thus, DSM-IV-TR attempts to describe the manifestations of the mental disorders and only rarely attempts to account for how the disturbances come about. The definitions of the disorders usually consist of descriptions of clinical features.

Diagnostic Criteria. Specified diagnostic criteria are provided for each specific mental disorder. These criteria include a list of features that must be present for the diagnosis to be made. Such criteria increase the reliability of the diagnostic process.

Systematic Description. DSM-IV-TR also systematically describes each disorder in terms of its associated features: specific age-, culture-, and gender-related features; prevalence, incidence, and risk; course; complications; predisposing factors; familial pattern; and differential diagnosis. In some instances, when many specific disorders share common features, this information is included in the introduction to the entire section. Laboratory findings and associated physical examination signs and symptoms are described when relevant. DSM-IV-TR is not, and does not purport to be, a textbook: No mention is made of theories of causes, management, or treatment, and the controversial issues surrounding a particular diagnostic category are not discussed.

Multiaxial Evaluation

DSM-IV-TR is a multiaxial system that evaluates patients along several variables and contains five axes. Axis I and Axis II make up the entire classification of mental disorder: 17 major classifications (Table 5–1) and more than 300 specific disorders. In many instances, patients have a disorder on both axes. For example, a patient may have major depressive disorder noted on Axis I and obsessive-compulsive personality disorder on Axis II.

Axis I. Axis I consists of clinical disorders and other conditions that may be a focus of clinical attention.

Axis II. Axis II consists of personality disorders and mental retardation. The habitual use of a particular defense mechanism can be indicated on Axis II.

Axis III. Axis III lists any physical disorder or general medical condition that is present in addition to the mental disorder. The physical condition may be causative (e.g., kidney failure causing delirium), the result of a mental disorder (e.g., alcohol gastritis secondary to alcohol dependence), or unrelated to the mental disorder. When a medical condition is causative or causally related to a mental disorder, a mental disorder due to a general condition is listed on Axis I, and the general medical condition is listed on both Axis I and Axis III. In DSM-IV-TR's example—a case in which hypothyroidism is a direct cause of major depressive disorder—the designation on Axis I is mood disorder due to hypothyroidism with depressive features, and hypothyroidism is listed again on Axis III.

Table 5–1
Alphabetical Listing of DSM-IV-TR Diagnoses and DSM-IV-TR Codes

NOS = Not Otherwise Specified.		296.52	Moderate
		296.53	Severe Without Psychotic Features
V62.3	Academic Problem	296.54	Severe With Psychotic Features
V62.4	Acculturation Problem	296.50	Unspecified
308.3	Acute Stress Disorder	296.40	Bipolar I Disorder, Most Recent Episode Hypomanic
	Adjustment Disorders		Bipolar I Disorder, Most Recent Episode Manic
309.9	Unspecified	296.46	In Full Remission
309.24	With Anxiety	296.45	In Partial Remission
309.0	With Depressed Mood	296.41	Mild
309.3	With Disturbance of Conduct	296.42	Moderate
309.28	With Mixed Anxiety and Depressed Mood	296.43	Severe Without Psychotic Features
309.4	With Mixed Disturbance of Emotions and Conduct	296.44	Severe With Psychotic Features
V71.01	Adult Antisocial Behavior	296.40	Unspecified
995.2	Adverse Effects of Medication NOS		Bipolar I Disorder, Most Recent Episode Mixed
780.9	Age-Related Cognitive Decline	296.66	In Full Remission
300.22	Agoraphobia Without History of Panic Disorder	296.65	In Partial Remission
	Alcohol	296.61	Mild
305.00	Abuse	296.62	Moderate
303.90	Dependence	296.63	Severe Without Psychotic Features
291.89	-Induced Anxiety Disorder	296.64	Severe With Psychotic Features
291.89	-Induced Mood Disorder	296.60	Unspecified
291.1	-Induced Persisting Amnestic Disorder	296.7	Bipolar I Disorder, Most Recent Episode Unspecified
291.2	-Induced Persisting Dementia		Bipolar I Disorder, Single Manic Episode
	-Induced Psychotic Disorder	296.06	In Full Remission
291.5	With Delusions	296.05	In Partial Remission
291.3	With Hallucinations	296.01	Mild
291.89	-Induced Sexual Dysfunction	296.02	Moderate
291.89	-Induced Sleep Disorder	296.03	Severe Without Psychotic Features
303.00	Intoxication	296.04	Severe With Psychotic Features
291.0	Intoxication Delirium	296.00	Unspecified
291.9	-Related Disorder NOS	296.89	Bipolar II Disorder
291.81	Withdrawal	300.7	Body Dysmorphic Disorder
291.0	Withdrawal Delirium	V62.89	Borderline Intellectual Functioning
294.0	Amnestic Disorder Due to . . . [Indicate the General Medical Condition]	301.83	Borderline Personality Disorder
		780.59	Breathing-Related Sleep Disorder
294.8	Amnestic Disorder NOS	298.8	Brief Psychotic Disorder
	Amphetamine (or Amphetamine-Like)	307.51	Bulimia Nervosa
305.70	Abuse		Caffeine
304.40	Dependence	292.89	-Induced Anxiety Disorder
292.89	-Induced Anxiety Disorder	292.89	-Induced Sleep Disorder
292.84	-Induced Mood Disorder	305.90	Intoxication
	-Induced Psychotic Disorder	292.9	-Related Disorder NOS
292.11	With Delusions		Cannabis
292.12	With Hallucinations	305.20	Abuse
292.89	-Induced Sexual Dysfunction	304.30	Dependence
292.89	-Induced Sleep Disorder	292.89	-Induced Anxiety Disorder
292.89	Intoxication		-Induced Psychotic Disorder
292.81	Intoxication Delirium	292.11	With Delusions
292.9	-Related Disorder NOS	292.12	With Hallucinations
292.0	Withdrawal	292.89	Intoxication
307.1	Anorexia Nervosa	292.81	Intoxication Delirium
301.7	Antisocial Personality Disorder	292.9	-Related Disorder NOS
293.84	Anxiety Disorder Due to . . . [Indicate the General Medical Condition]	293.89	Catatonic Disorder Due to . . . [Indicate the General Medical Condition]
300.00	Anxiety Disorder NOS	299.10	Childhood Disintegrative Disorder
299.80	Asperger's Disorder	V71.02	Child or Adolescent Antisocial Behavior
	Attention-Deficit/Hyperactivity Disorder	307.22	Chronic Motor or Vocal Tic Disorder
314.01	Combined Type	307.45	Circadian Rhythm Sleep Disorder
314.01	Predominantly Hyperactive-Impulsive Type		Cocaine
314.00	Predominantly Inattentive Type	305.60	Abuse
314.9	Attention-Deficit/Hyperactivity Disorder NOS	304.20	Dependence
299.00	Autistic Disorder	292.89	-Induced Anxiety Disorder
301.82	Avoidant Personality Disorder	292.84	-Induced Mood Disorder
V62.82	Bereavement		-Induced Psychotic Disorder
296.80	Bipolar Disorder NOS	292.11	With Delusions
	Bipolar I Disorder, Most Recent Episode Depressed	292.12	With Hallucinations
296.56	In Full Remission	292.89	-Induced Sexual Dysfunction
296.55	In Partial Remission	292.89	-Induced Sleep Disorder
296.51	Mild		

(continued)

Table 5–1
(Continued)

292.89	Intoxication		315.31	Expressive Language Disorder
292.81	Intoxication Delirium			Factitious Disorder
292.9	-Related Disorder NOS		300.19	With Combined Psychological and Physical Signs and Symptoms
292.0	Withdrawal			
294.9	Cognitive Disorder NOS		300.19	With Predominantly Physical Signs and Symptoms
307.9	Communication Disorder NOS		300.16	With Predominantly Psychological Signs and Symptoms
	Conduct Disorder			
312.81	Childhood-Onset Type		300.19	Factitious Disorder NOS
312.82	Adolescent-Onset Type		307.59	Feeding Disorder of Infancy or Early Childhood
312.89	Unspecified Type		625.0	Female Dyspareunia Due to... *[Indicate the General Medical Condition]*
300.11	Conversion Disorder			
301.13	Cyclothymic Disorder		625.8	Female Hypoactive Sexual Desire Disorder Due to ... *[Indicate the General Medical Condition]*
293.0	Delirium Due to ... *[Indicate the General Medical Condition]*			
780.09	Delirium NOS		302.73	Female Orgasmic Disorder
297.1	Delusional Disorder		302.72	Female Sexual Arousal Disorder
	Dementia Due to Creutzfeldt-Jakob Disease		302.81	Fetishism
294.10*	Without Behavioral Disturbance		302.89	Frotteurism
294.11*	With Behavioral Disturbance			Gender Identity Disorder
	Dementia Due to Head Trauma		302.85	in Adolescents or Adults
294.10*	Without Behavioral Disturbance		302.6	in Children
294.11*	With Behavioral Disturbance		302.6	Gender Identity Disorder NOS
	Dementia Due to HIV Disease		300.02	Generalized Anxiety Disorder
294.10*	Without Behavioral Disturbance			Hallucinogen
294.11*	With Behavioral Disturbance		305.30	Abuse
	Dementia Due to Huntington's Disease		304.50	Dependence
294.10*	Without Behavioral Disturbance		292.89	-Induced Anxiety Disorder
294.11*	With Behavioral Disturbance		292.84	-Induced Mood Disorder
	Dementia Due to Parkinson's Disease			-Induced Psychotic Disorder
294.10*	Without Behavioral Disturbance		292.11	With Delusions
294.11*	With Behavioral Disturbance		292.12	With Hallucinations
	Dementia Due to Pick's Disease		292.89	Intoxication
294.10*	Without Behavioral Disturbance		292.81	Intoxication Delirium
294.11*	With Behavioral Disturbance		292.89	Persisting Perception Disorder
	Dementia Due to ... *[Indicate Other General Medical Condition]*		292.9	-Related Disorder NOS
			301.50	Histrionic Personality Disorder
294.10*	Without Behavioral Disturbance		307.44	Hypersomnia Related to ... *[Indicate the Axis I or Axis II Disorder]*
294.11*	With Behavioral Disturbance			
294.8	Dementia NOS		302.71	Hypoactive Sexual Desire Disorder
	Dementia of the Alzheimer's Type, With Early Onset		300.7	Hypochondriasis
294.10*	Without Behavioral Disturbance		313.82	Identity Problem
294.11*	With Behavioral Disturbance		312.30	Impulse-Control Disorder NOS
	Dementia of the Alzheimer's Type, With Late Onset			Inhalant
294.10*	Without Behavioral Disturbance		305.90	Abuse
294.11*	With Behavioral Disturbance		304.60	Dependence
301.6	Dependent Personality Disorder		292.89	-Induced Anxiety Disorder
300.6	Depersonalization Disorder		292.84	-Induced Mood Disorder
311	Depressive Disorder NOS		292.82	-Induced Persisting Dementia
315.4	Developmental Coordination Disorder			-Induced Psychotic Disorder
799.9	Diagnosis Deferred on Axis II		292.11	With Delusions
799.9	Diagnosis or Condition Deferred on Axis I		292.12	With Hallucinations
313.9	Disorder of Infancy, Childhood, or Adolescence NOS		292.89	Intoxication
315.2	Disorder of Written Expression		292.81	Intoxication Delirium
312.9	Disruptive Behavior Disorder NOS		292.9	-Related Disorder NOS
300.12	Dissociative Amnesia		307.42	Insomnia Related to ... *[Indicate the Axis I or Axis II Disorder]*
300.15	Dissociative Disorder NOS			
300.13	Dissociative Fugue		312.34	Intermittent Explosive Disorder
300.14	Dissociative Identity Disorder		312.32	Kleptomania
302.76	Dyspareunia (Not Due to a General Medical Condition)		315.9	Learning Disorder NOS
				Major Depressive Disorder, Recurrent
307.47	Dyssomnia NOS		296.36	In Full Remission
300.4	Dysthymic Disorder		296.35	In Partial Remission
307.50	Eating Disorder NOS		296.31	Mild
787.6	Encopresis, With Constipation and Overflow Incontinence		296.32	Moderate
			296.33	Severe Without Psychotic Features
307.7	Encopresis, Without Constipation and Overflow Incontinence		296.34	Severe With Psychotic Features
			296.30	Unspecified
307.6	Enuresis (Not Due to a General Medical Condition)			Major Depressive Disorder, Single Episode
			296.26	In Full Remission
302.4	Exhibitionism		296.25	In Partial Remission
			296.21	Mild

(continued)

Table 5–1
(Continued)

296.22	Moderate
296.23	Severe Without Psychotic Features
296.24	Severe With Psychotic Features
296.20	Unspecified
608.89	Male Dyspareunia Due to ...*[Indicate the General Medical Condition]*
302.72	Male Erectile Disorder
607.84	Male Erectile Disorder Due to ... *[Indicate the General Medical Condition]*
608.89	Male Hypoactive Sexual Desire Disorder Due to ... *[Indicate the General Medical Condition]*
302.74	Male Orgasmic Disorder
V65.2	Malingering
315.1	Mathematics Disorder
	Medication-Induced
333.90	Movement Disorder NOS
333.1	Postural Tremor
293.9	Mental Disorder NOS Due to ... *[Indicate the General Medical Condition]*
319	Mental Retardation, Severity Unspecified
317	Mild Mental Retardation
315.32	Mixed Receptive-Expressive Language Disorder
318.0	Moderate Mental Retardation
293.83	Mood Disorder Due to ... *[Indicate the General Medical Condition]*
296.90	Mood Disorder NOS
301.81	Narcissistic Personality Disorder
347	Narcolepsy
V61.21	Neglect of Child
995.52	Neglect of Child *(if focus of attention is on victim)*
	Neuroleptic-Induced
333.99	Acute Akathisia
333.7	Acute Dystonia
332.1	Parkinsonism
333.82	Tardive Dyskinesia
333.92	Neuroleptic Malignant Syndrome
	Nicotine
305.1	Dependence
292.9	-Related Disorder NOS
292.0	Withdrawal
307.47	Nightmare Disorder
V71.09	No Diagnosis on Axis II
V71.09	No Diagnosis or Condition on Axis I
V15.81	Noncompliance With Treatment
300.3	Obsessive-Compulsive Disorder
301.4	Obsessive-Compulsive Personality Disorder
V62.2	Occupational Problem
	Opioid
305.50	Abuse
304.00	Dependence
292.84	-Induced Mood Disorder
	-Induced Psychotic Disorder
292.11	With Delusions
292.12	With Hallucinations
292.89	-Induced Sexual Dysfunction
292.89	-Induced Sleep Disorder
292.89	Intoxication
292.81	Intoxication Delirium
292.9	-Related Disorder NOS
292.0	Withdrawal
313.81	Oppositional Defiant Disorder
625.8	Other Female Sexual Dysfunction Due to ... *[Indicate the General Medical Condition]*
608.89	Other Male Sexual Dysfunction Due to ... *[Indicate the General Medical Condition]*
	Other (or Unknown) Substance
305.90	Abuse
304.90	Dependence
292.89	-Induced Anxiety Disorder
292.81	-Induced Delirium
292.84	-Induced Mood Disorder

292.83	-Induced Persisting Amnestic Disorder
292.82	-Induced Persisting Dementia
	-Induced Psychotic Disorder
292.11	With Delusions
292.12	With Hallucinations
292.89	-Induced Sexual Dysfunction
292.89	-Induced Sleep Disorder
292.89	Intoxication
292.9	-Related Disorder NOS
292.0	Withdrawal
	Pain Disorder
307.89	Associated With Both Psychological Factors and a General Medical Condition
307.80	Associated With Psychological Factors
	Panic Disorder
300.21	With Agoraphobia
300.01	Without Agoraphobia
301.0	Paranoid Personality Disorder
302.9	Paraphilia NOS
307.47	Parasomnia NOS
V61.20	Parent-Child Relational Problem
V61.10	Partner Relational Problem
312.31	Pathological Gambling
302.2	Pedophilia
310.1	Personality Change Due to ... *[Indicate the General Medical Condition]*
301.9	Personality Disorder NOS
299.80	Pervasive Developmental Disorder NOS
V62.89	Phase of Life Problem
	Phencyclidine (or Phencyclidine-Like)
305.90	Abuse
304.60	Dependence
292.89	-Induced Anxiety Disorder
292.84	-Induced Mood Disorder
	-Induced Psychotic Disorder
292.11	With Delusions
292.12	With Hallucinations
292.89	Intoxication
292.81	Intoxication Delirium
292.9	-Related Disorder NOS
315.39	Phonological Disorder
V61.12	Physical Abuse of Adult (if by partner)
V62.83	Physical Abuse of Adult (if by person other than partner)
995.81	Physical Abuse of Adult *(if focus of attention is on victim)*
V61.21	Physical Abuse of Child
995.54	Physical Abuse of Child *(if focus of attention is on victim)*
307.52	Pica
304.80	Polysubstance Dependence
309.81	Posttraumatic Stress Disorder
302.75	Premature Ejaculation
307.44	Primary Hypersomnia
307.42	Primary Insomnia
318.2	Profound Mental Retardation
316	Psychological Factor Affecting Medical Condition
	Psychotic Disorder Due to ... *[Indicate the General Medical Condition]*
293.81	With Delusions
293.82	With Hallucinations
298.9	Psychotic Disorder NOS
312.33	Pyromania
313.89	Reactive Attachment Disorder of Infancy or Early Childhood
315.00	Reading Disorder
V62.81	Relational Problem NOS
V61.9	Relational Problem Related to a Mental Disorder or General Medical Condition
V62.89	Religious or Spiritual Problem
299.80	Rett's Disorder

(continued)

Table 5–1
(Continued)

307.53	Rumination Disorder		302.79	Sexual Aversion Disorder
295.70	Schizoaffective Disorder		302.9	Sexual Disorder NOS
301.20	Schizoid Personality Disorder Schizophrenia		302.70	Sexual Dysfunction NOS
295.20	Catatonic Type		302.83	Sexual Masochism
295.10	Disorganized Type		302.84	Sexual Sadism
295.30	Paranoid Type		297.3	Shared Psychotic Disorder
295.60	Residual Type		V61.8	Sibling Relational Problem
295.90	Undifferentiated Type			Sleep Disorder Due to . . . *[Indicate the General Medical Condition]*
295.40	Schizophreniform Disorder		780.54	Hypersomnia Type
301.22	Schizotypal Personality Disorder		780.52	Insomnia Type
	Sedative, Hypnotic, or Anxiolytic		780.59	Mixed Type
305.40	Abuse		780.59	Parasomnia Type
304.10	Dependence		307.46	Sleep Terror Disorder
292.89	-Induced Anxiety Disorder		307.46	Sleepwalking Disorder
292.84	-Induced Mood Disorder		300.23	Social Phobia
292.83	-Induced Persisting Amnestic Disorder		300.81	Somatization Disorder
292.82	-Induced Persisting Dementia		300.82	Somatoform Disorder NOS
	-Induced Psychotic Disorder		300.29	Specific Phobia
292.11	With Delusions		307.3	Stereotypic Movement Disorder
292.12	With Hallucinations		307.0	Stuttering
292.89	-Induced Sexual Dysfunction		307.20	Tic Disorder NOS
292.89	-Induced Sleep Disorder		307.23	Tourette's Disorder
292.89	Intoxication		307.21	Transient Tic Disorder
292.81	Intoxication Delirium		302.3	Transvestic Fetishism
292.9	-Related Disorder NOS		312.39	Trichotillomania
292.0	Withdrawal		300.82	Undifferentiated Somatoform Disorder
292.81	Withdrawal Delirium		300.9	Unspecified Mental Disorder (nonpsychotic)
313.23	Selective Mutism		306.51	Vaginismus (Not Due to a General Medical Condition)
309.21	Separation Anxiety Disorder			Vascular Dementia
318.1	Severe Mental Retardation		290.40	Uncomplicated
V61.12	Sexual Abuse of Adult (if by partner)		290.41	With Delirium
V62.83	Sexual Abuse of Adult (if by person other than partner)		290.42	With Delusions
995.83	Sexual Abuse of Adult *(if focus of attention is on victim)*		290.43	With Depressed Mood
V61.21	Sexual Abuse of Child		302.82	Voyeurism
995.53	Sexual Abuse of Child *(if focus of attention is on victim)*			

*ICD-9-CM code valid after October 1, 2000.

Axis IV.   Axis IV is used to code the psychosocial and environmental problems that contribute significantly to the development or exacerbation of the current disorder. The evaluation of stressors is based on a clinician's assessment of the stress that an average person with similar sociocultural values and circumstances would experience from the psychosocial stressors. This judgment is based on the amount of change that the stressor causes in the person's life, the degree to which the event is desired and under the person's control, and the number of stressors. Stressors may be positive (such as a job promotion) or negative (such as the loss of a loved one). Information about stressors may be important in formulating a treatment plan that includes attempts to remove the psychosocial stressors or to help the patient cope with them.

Axis V.   Axis V is a global assessment of functioning (GAF) scale in which clinicians judge patients' overall levels of functioning during a particular time (e.g., at the time of the evaluation, or the patient's highest level of functioning for at least a few months during the past year). Functioning is considered a composite of three major areas: social functioning, occupational functioning, and psychological functioning. The GAF

scale, based on a continuum of mental health and mental illness, is a 100-point scale, 100 representing the highest level of functioning in all areas. Persons who had a high level of functioning before an episode of illness generally have a better prognosis than do those who had a low level of functioning.

Multiaxial Evaluation Report Form.   Table 5–2 shows the DSM-IV-TR Multiaxial Evaluation Report form. Examples of how to record the results of a DSM-IV-TR multiaxial evaluation are given in Table 5–3.

Nonaxial Format.   DSM-IV-TR also allows clinicians who do not wish to use the multiaxial format to list the diagnoses serially, with the principal diagnosis listed first (Table 5–4).

Severity of Disorder.   Depending on the clinical picture and the presence or absence of signs and symptoms and their intensity, the severity of a disorder may be mild, moderate, or severe, and the disorder may be in partial or full remission. The following guidelines are used by DSM-IV-TR.

Table 5–2
DSM-IV-TR Multiaxial Evaluation Report Form

The following form is offered as one possibility for reporting multiaxial evaluations. In some settings, this form may be used exactly as is; in other settings, the form may be adapted to satisfy special needs.

AXIS I: Clinical Disorders
Other Conditions That May Be a Focus of Clinical Attention
Diagnostic code   DSM-IV name

___ ___   _____
___ ___   _____
___ ___   _____

AXIS II: Personality Disorders
    Mental Retardation
Diagnostic code   DSM-IV name

___ ___   _____
___ ___   _____

AXIS III: General Medical Conditions
ICD-9-CM code   ICD-9-CM name

___ ___   _____
___ ___   _____
___ ___   _____

AXIS IV: Psychosocial and Environmental Problems
Check:
❑ Problems with primary support group
    Specify: _____
❑ Problems related to the social environment
    Specify: _____
❑ Educational problems Specify: _____
❑ Occupational problems Specify: _____
❑ Housing problems Specify: _____
❑ Economic problems Specify: _____
❑ Problems with access to health care services
    Specify: _____
❑ Problems related to interaction with the legal system/crime
    Specify: _____
❑ Other psychosocial and environmental problems
    Specify: _____

AXIS V: Global Assessment of Functioning Scale
                    Score: _____
                    Time Frame: _____

From American Psychiatric Association. *Diagnostic and Statistical Manual of Mental Disorders.* 4th ed. Text rev. Washington, DC: American Psychiatric Association; copyright 2000, with permission.

Table 5–3
DSM-IV Examples of How to Record the Results of a DSM-IV Multiaxial Evaluation

Example 1:		
Axis I	296.23	Major depressive disorder, single episode, severe without psychotic features
	305.00	Alcohol abuse
Axis II	301.6	Dependent personality disorder Frequent use of denial
Axis III		None
Axis IV		Threat of job loss
Axis V	GAF = 35	(current)
Example 2:		
Axis I	300.4	Dysthymic disorder
	315.00	Reading disorder
Axis II	V71.09	No diagnosis
Axis III	382.9	Otitis media, recurrent
Axis IV		Victim of child neglect
Axis V	GAF = 53	(current)
Example 3:		
Axis I	293.83	Mood disorder due to hypothyroidism, with depressive features
Axis II	V71.09	No diagnosis, histrionic personality features
Axis III	244.9	Hypothyroidism
	365.23	Chronic angle-closure glaucoma
Axis IV		None
Axis V	GAF = 45	(on admission)
	GAF = 65	(at discharge)
Example 4:		
Axis I	V61.1	Partner relational problem
Axis II	V71.09	No diagnosis
Axis III		None
Axis IV		Unemployment
Axis V	GAF = 83	(highest level past year)

From American Psychiatric Association. *Diagnostic and Statistical Manual of Mental Disorders.* 4th ed. Text rev. Washington, DC: American Psychiatric Association; copyright 2000, with permission.

the disturbance, and the need for continued evaluation or prophylactic treatment.

Other Criteria

Multiple Diagnoses.   When a person has more than one Axis I disorder, the principal diagnosis is indicated by listing it first. According to DSM-IV-TR, the *principal diagnosis* is the condition chiefly responsible for the signs and symptoms of the individual. It may be difficult in situations of "dual diagnosis" (a substance-related diagnosis such as amphetamine dependence accompanied by a non–substance-related diagnosis such as schizophrenia) to say which is the principal diagnosis. DSM-IV-TR states, "For example, it may be unclear which diagnosis should be considered "principal" for an individual hospitalized with both Schizophrenia and Amphetamine Intoxication, because each condition may have contributed equally to the need for admission and treatment."

Provisional Diagnosis.   If there is diagnostic uncertainty, the clinician can write "(Provisional)" following the diagnosis.

MILD.   Few, if any, symptoms in excess of those required to make the diagnosis are present, and symptoms result in no more than minor impairment in social or occupational functioning.

MODERATE.   Symptoms or functional impairment between "mild" and "severe" are present.

SEVERE.   Many symptoms in excess of those required to make the diagnosis or several symptoms that are particularly severe are present, or the symptoms result in marked impairment in social or occupational functioning.

IN PARTIAL REMISSION.   The full criteria for the disorder were previously met, but currently only some of the symptoms or signs of the disorder remain.

IN FULL REMISSION.   There are no longer any symptoms or signs of the disorder, but it is still clinically relevant to note the disorder. The differentiation of In Full Remission from Recovered requires consideration of many factors, including the characteristic course of the disorder, the length of time since the last period of disturbance, the total duration of

Table 5–4
DSM-IV-TR Nonaxial Format

Clinicians who do not wish to use the multiaxial format may simply list the appropriate diagnoses. Those choosing this option should follow the general rule of recording as many coexisting mental disorders, general medical conditions, and other factors that are relevant to the care and treatment of the individual. The principal diagnosis or the reason for visit should be listed first.

The examples below illustrate the reporting of diagnoses in a format that does not use the multiaxial system.

Example 1:

296.23	Major depressive disorder, single episode, severe without psychotic features
305.00	Alcohol abuse
301.6	Dependent personality disorder
	Frequent use of denial

Example 2:

300.4	Dysthymic disorder
315.00	Reading disorder
382.9	Otitis media, recurrent

Example 3:

293.83	Mood disorder due to hypothyroidism with depressive features
244.9	Hypothyroidism
365.23	Chronic angle-closure glaucoma
	Histrionic personality features

Example 4:

V61.1	Partner relational problem

From American Psychiatric Association. *Diagnostic and Statistical Manual of Mental Disorders.* 4th ed. Text rev. Washington, DC: American Psychiatric Association; copyright 2000, with permission.

A person may appear to have major depressive disorder but be unable to give an adequate history to establish that the full criteria are met. The differential diagnosis depends on the duration of illness. For example, DSM-IV-TR states, "a diagnosis of Schizophreniform Disorder requires a duration of less than 6 months and can only be given provisionally if assigned before remission has occurred."

Prior History.   For some purposes, noting a prior history of a disorder may be useful. DSM-IV-TR states that a past diagnosis of mental disorder can "be indicated by using the specifier Prior History (e.g., Separation Anxiety Disorder, Prior History, for an individual with a history of Separation Anxiety Disorder who has no current disorder or who currently meets criteria for Panic Disorder)."

Not Otherwise Specified Categories.   Each diagnosis has a "not otherwise specified" (NOS) category. According to DSM-IV-TR, an NOS diagnosis may be appropriate (1) either when the symptoms are below the diagnostic threshold for one of the specific disorders or when there is an atypical or mixed presentation, (2) the symptom pattern has not been included in the DSM-IV-TR classification, but it causes clinically significant distress or impairment (research criteria for some of these symptom patterns have been included in an appendix), or (3) the cause is uncertain (i.e., whether it is primary or secondary).

6

Psychiatric Rating Scales

Many different questionnaires, interviews, checklists, outcome assessments, and other instruments are used by psychiatrists and mental health professionals to aid in treatment planning by helping to establish a diagnosis, identify comorbid conditions, and assess levels of functioning. They are collectively called psychiatric rating scales or rating instruments and hundreds of them have been developed, some better than others.

It is important to realize that rating scales are not a panacea. They can provide erroneous measurements because of difficulties in administration or limitations in the construct of the scale itself. Ideally, they aid clinicians by helping them to confirm their diagnoses or clarify their thinking in ambiguous situations. They also can provide a baseline for follow-up of the progress of an illness over time or in response to specific interventions. This is particularly useful in the conduct of psychiatric research.

RATING SCALES USED IN DSM-IV-TR

Rating scales form an integral part of the text revision of the fourth edition of the *Diagnostic and Statistical Manual of Mental Disorders* (DSM-IV-TR). The rating scales used are broad and measure the overall severity of a patient's illness.

Global Assessment of Functioning Scale (GAF)

Axis V in DSM-IV-TR uses the GAF scale (Table 6–1). This axis is used to report a clinician's judgment of a patient's overall level of functioning. The information is used to decide on a treatment plan and later to measure the plan's effect.

Social and Occupational Functioning Assessment Scale (SOFAS)

This scale can be used to track a patient's progress in social and occupational areas (Table 6–2). It is independent of the psychiatric diagnosis and the severity of the patient's psychological symptoms.

Global Assessment of Relational Functioning (GARF)

This scale measures the overall functioning of a family or other ongoing relationship. It is an important measurement because the development of mental illness is higher in dysfunctional families, and recovery is slower in the absence of a supportive social network (Table 6–3).

Defensive Functioning Scale (DFS)

This scale covers the defense mechanisms used by the patient to cope with stressors. Humor, suppression, anticipation, and sublimation are among the healthiest defense mechanisms. Denial, acting-out, projection, and projective identification are some of the most pathological (Table 6–4).

OTHER SCALES

Brief Psychiatric Rating Scale (BPRS)

This is a short scale used to measure the severity of psychiatric symptomatology. It has been used for decades as an outcome measure in treatment studies of schizophrenia. It is most useful for patients with fairly significant impairment.

Hamilton Rating Scales for Depression and Anxiety (HAM-D and HAM-A, respectively)

These rating scales are used to monitor the severity of depression and anxiety and are scored from 0 to 4, with total scored of greater than 9 considered the borderline of pathology. The scales are useful for measuring the effects of treatment, particularly with pharmacologic agents.

Scales for the Assessment of Positive Symptoms (SAPS) and Assessment of Negative Symptoms (SANS)

These scales are designed to measure negative and positive symptoms in schizophrenia. They are primarily used in research to measure change induced by psychopharmacologic agents over the course of treatment (Tables 6–5 and 6–6).

Positive and Negative Syndrome Scale (PANSS)

This scale also measures negative and positive symptoms of schizophrenia and other psychotic disorders. It has become the standard tool for assessing clinical outcome in treatment studies of schizophrenia.

Rating scales have been developed for almost every diagnostic group and are central to psychiatric research, but they may also be used in clinical practice. They tend to be rather long, however, especially with individuals reporting many symptoms. Access to instruments via the World Wide Web is increasing rapidly, and many of these tests are available for purchase or download by using a search engine such as Google Scholar.

Table 6–1
Global Assessment of Functioning (GAF) Scale

Consider psychological, social, and occupational functioning on a hypothetical continuum of mental health–illness. Do not include impairment in functioning due to physical (or environmental) limitations.

Code   (**Note:** Use intermediate codes when appropriate, e.g., 45, 68, 72.)

100–91   Superior functioning in a wide range of activities, life's problems never seem to get out of hand, is sought out by others because of his or her many positive qualities. No symptoms.

90–81   Absent or minimal symptoms (e.g., mild anxiety before an exam), good functioning in all areas, interested and involved in a wide range of activities, socially effective, generally satisfied with life, no more than everyday problems or concerns (e.g., an occasional argument with family members).

80–71   If symptoms are present, they are transient and expectable reactions to psychosocial stressors (e.g., difficulty concentrating after family argument): no more than slight impairment in social, occupational, or school functioning (e.g., temporarily falling behind in schoolwork).

70–61   Some mild symptoms (e.g., depressed mood and mild insomnia) OR some difficulty in social, occupational, or school functioning (e.g., occasional truancy, or theft within the household), but generally functioning pretty well, has some meaningful interpersonal relationships.

60–51   Moderate symptoms (e.g., flat affect and circumstantial speech, occasional panic attacks) OR moderate difficulty in social, occupational, or school functioning (e.g., few friends, conflicts with peers or coworkers).

50–41   Serious symptoms (e.g., suicidal ideation, severe obsessional rituals, frequent shoplifting) OR any serious impairment in social, occupational, or school functioning (e.g., no friends, unable to keep a job).

40–31   Some impairment in reality testing or communication (e.g., speech is at times illogical, obscure, or irrelevant) OR major impairment in several areas, such as work or school, family relations, judgment, thinking, or mood (e.g., depressed man avoids friends, neglects family, and is unable to work; child frequently beats up younger children, is defiant at home, and is failing at school).

30–21   Behavior is considerably influenced by delusions or hallucinations OR serious impairment in communication or judgment (e.g., sometimes incoherent, acts grossly inappropriately, suicidal preoccupation) OR inability to function in almost all areas (e.g., stays in bed all day; no job, home, or friends).

20–11   Some danger of hurting self or others (e.g., suicide attempts without clear expectation of death, frequently violent, manic excitement) OR occasionally fails to maintain minimal personal hygiene (e.g., smears feces) OR gross impairment in communication (e.g., largely incoherent or mute).

10–1   Persistent danger of severely hurting self or others (e.g., recurrent violence) OR persistent inability to maintain minimal personal hygiene OR serious suicidal act with clear expectation of death.

0   Inadequate information.

The GAF Scale is a revision of the GAS (Endicott J, Spitzer RL, Fleiss JL, Cohen I. The Global Assessment Scale: a procedure for measuring overall severity of psychiatric disturbance. *Arch Gen Psychiatry.* 1976;33:766) and CGAS (Shaffer D, Gould MS, Brasio J, et al. Children's Global Assessment Scale (CGAS). *Arch Gen Psychiatry.* 1983;40:1228). They are revisions of the Global Scale of the Health-Sickness Rating Scale (Luborsky I. Clinicians' judgments of mental health. *Arch Gen Psychiatry.* 1962;7:407).
From American Psychiatric Association. *Diagnostic and Statistical Manual of Mental Disorders,* 4th ed. Text rev. Washington, DC: American Psychiatric Association; copyright 2000, with permission.

Table 6–2
Social and Occupational Functioning Assessment Scale (SOFAS)

Consider social and occupational functioning on a continuum from excellent functioning to grossly impaired functioning. Include impairments in functioning due to physical limitations, as well as those due to mental impairments. To be counted, impairment must be a direct consequence of mental and physical health problems; the effects of lack of opportunity and other environmental limitations are not to be considered.

Code   (**Note:** Use intermediate codes when appropriate, e.g., 45, 68, 72.)

100	Superior functioning in a wide range of activities.	50	Serious impairment in social, occupational, or school functioning (e.g., no friends, unable to keep a job).
91		41	
90	Good functioning in all areas, occupationally and socially effective.	40	Major impairment in several areas, such as work or school, family relations (e.g., depressed man avoids friends, neglects family, and is unable to work; child frequently beats up younger children, is defiant at home, and is failing at school).
81		31	
80	No more than a slight impairment in social, occupational, or school functioning (e.g., infrequent interpersonal conflict, temporarily falling behind in schoolwork).	30	Inability to function in almost all areas (e.g., stays in bed all day; no job, home, or friends).
71		21	
70	Some difficulty in social, occupational, or school functioning, but generally functioning well, has some meaningful interpersonal relationships.	20	Occasionally fails to maintain minimal personal hygiene; unable to function independently.
61		11	
60	Moderate difficulty in social, occupational, or school functioning (e.g., few friends, conflicts with peers or coworkers).	10	Persistent inability to maintain minimal personal hygiene. Unable to function without harming self or others or without considerable external support (e.g., nursing care and supervision).
51		1	
		0	Inadequate information.

Note: The rating of overall psychological functioning on a scale of 0–100 was operationalized by Luborsky in the Health-Sickness Rating Scale. (Luborsky L. Clinicians' judgments of mental health. *Arch Gen Psychiatry*. 1962;7:407). Spitzer and colleagues developed a revision of the Health-Sickness Rating Scale called the Global Assessment Scale (GAS) (Endicott J, Spitzer RL, Fleiss JL, et al. The Global Assessment Scale: a procedure for measuring overall severity of psychiatric disturbance. *Arch Gen Psychiatry*. 1976;33:766). The SOFAS is derived from the GAS and its development is described in Goldman HH, Skodol AE, Lave TR. Revising Axis V for DSM-IV: a review of measures of social functioning. *Am J Psychiatry*. 1992;149:1148.
From American Psychiatric Association. *Diagnostic and Statistical Manual of Mental Disorders*. 4th ed. Text rev. Washington, DC: American Psychiatric Association; copyright 2000, with permission.

Table 6–3
Global Assessment of Relational Functioning (GARF)

INSTRUCTIONS: The GARF Scale can be used to indicate an overall judgment of the functioning of a family or other ongoing relationship on a hypothetical continuum ranging from competent, optimal relational functioning to a disrupted, dysfunctional relationship. It is analogous to Axis V (Global Assessment of Functioning Scale) provided for individuals in DSM-IV. The GARF Scale permits the clinician to rate the degree to which a family or other ongoing relational unit meets the affective and/or instrumental needs of its members in the following areas:

A. *Problem solving*—skills in negotiating goals, rules, and routines: adaptability to stress; communication skills; ability to resolve conflict.

B. *Organization*—maintenance of interpersonal roles and subsystem boundaries; hierarchical functioning, coalitions and distribution of power, control and responsibility.

C. *Emotional climate*—tone and range of feelings; quality of caring, empathy, involvement and attachment/commitment; sharing of values; mutual affective responsiveness, respect, and regard; quality of sexual functioning.

In most instances, the GARF Scale should be used to rate functioning during the current period (i.e., the level of relational functioning at the time of the evaluation). In some settings, the GARF Scale may also be used to rate functioning for other time periods (i.e., the highest level of relational functioning for at least a few months during the past year). **Note:** Use specific, intermediate codes when possible, for example, 45, 68, 72. If detailed information is not adequate to make specific ratings, use midpoints of the five ranges, that is, 90, 70, 50, 30, or 10. **(81–100) Overall:** Relational unit is functioning satisfactorily from self-report of participants and from perspectives of observers.

Agreed-on patterns or routines exist that help meet the usual needs of each family/couple member; there is flexibility for change in response to unusual demands or events; occasional conflicts and stressful transitions are resolved through problem-solving communication and negotiation.

There is a shared understanding and agreement about roles and appropriate tasks; decision making is established for each functional area, and there is recognition of the unique characteristics and merit of each subsystem (e.g., parents/spouses, siblings, and individuals).

There is a situationally appropriate, optimistic atmosphere in the family; a wide range of feelings is freely expressed and managed within the family; there is a general atmosphere of warmth, caring, and sharing of values among all family members. Sexual relations of adult members are satisfactory.

(61–80) Overall: Functioning of relational unit is somewhat unsatisfactory. Over a period of time, many but not all difficulties are resolved without complaints.

Daily routines are present but there is some pain and difficulty in responding to the unusual. Some conflicts remain unresolved, but do not disrupt family functioning.

(continued)

Table 6–3
(Continued)

Decision making is usually competent, but efforts at control of one another quite often are greater than necessary or are ineffective. Individuals and relationships are clearly demarcated but sometimes a specific subsystem is depreciated or scapegoated.

A range of feeling is expressed, but instances of emotional blocking or tension are evident. Warmth and caring are present but are marred by a family member's irritability and frustrations. Sexual activity of adult members may be reduced or problematic.

(41–60) Overall: Relational unit has occasional times of satisfying and competent functioning together, but clearly dysfunctional, unsatisfying relationships tend to predominate.

Communication is frequently inhibited by unresolved conflicts that often interfere with daily routines; there is significant difficulty in adapting to family stress and transitional change.

Decision making is only intermittently competent and effective; either excessive rigidity or significant lack of structure is evident at these times. Individual needs are quite often submerged by a partner or coalition.

Pain or ineffective anger or emotional deadness interferes with family enjoyment. Although there is some warmth and support for members, it is usually unequally distributed. Troublesome sexual difficulties between adults are often present.

(21–40) Overall: Relational unit is obviously and seriously dysfunctional; forms and time periods of satisfactory relating are rare.

Family/couple routines do not meet the needs of members; they are grimly adhered to or blithely ignored. Life cycle changes, such as departures or entries into the relational unit, generate painful conflict and obviously frustrating failures of problem solving.

Decision making is tyrannical or quite ineffective. The unique characteristics of individuals are unappreciated or ignored by either rigid or confusingly fluid coalitions.

There are infrequent periods of enjoyment of life together; frequent distancing or open hostility reflect significant conflicts that remain unresolved and quite painful. Sexual dysfunction among adult members is commonplace.

(1–20) Overall: Relational unit has become too dysfunctional to retain continuity of contact and attachment.

Family/couple routines are negligible (e.g., no mealtime, sleeping, or waking schedule); family members often do not know where others are or when they will be in or out; there is little effective communication among family members.

Family/couple members are not organized in such a way that personal or generational responsibilities are recognized. Boundaries of relational unit as a whole and subsystems cannot be identified or agreed upon. Family members are physically endangered or injured or sexually attacked.

Despair and cynicism are pervasive; there is little attention to the emotional needs of others; there is almost no sense of attachment, commitment, or concern about one another's welfare.

0 Inadequate information.

Table 6–4
Defensive Functioning Scale

High adaptive level. This level of defensive functioning results in optimal adaptation in the handling of stressors. These defenses usually maximize gratification and allow the conscious awareness of feelings, ideas, and their consequences. They also promote an optimum balance among conflicting motives. Examples of defenses characteristically at this level are
- anticipation
- affiliation
- altruism
- humor
- self-assertion
- self-observation
- sublimation
- suppression

Mental inhibitions (compromise formation) level. Defensive functioning at this level keeps potentially threatening ideas, feelings, memories, wishes, or fears out of awareness. Examples are
- displacement
- dissociation
- intellectualization
- isolation of affect
- reaction formation
- repression
- undoing

Minor image-distorting level. This level is characterized by distortions in the image of the self, body, or others that may be employed to regulate self-esteem. Examples are
- devaluation
- idealization
- omnipotence

Disavowal level. This level is characterized by keeping unpleasant or unacceptable stressors, impulses, ideas, affect, or responsibility out of awareness with or without a misattribution of these to external causes. Examples are
- denial
- projection
- rationalization

Major image-distorting level. This level is characterized by gross distortion or misattribution of the image of self or others. Examples are
- autistic fantasy
- projective identification
- splitting of self-image or image of others

Action level. This level is characterized by defensive functioning that deals with internal or external stressors by action or withdrawal. Examples are
- acting out
- apathetic withdrawal
- help-rejecting complaining
- passive aggression

Level of defensive dysregulation. This level is characterized by failure of defensive regulation to contain the individual's reaction to stressors, leading to a pronounced break with objective reality. Examples are
- delusional projection
- psychotic denial
- psychotic distortion

Table 6–5
Scale for the Assessment of Negative Symptoms (SANS)

0 = None   1 = Questionable   2 = Mild   3 = Moderate   4 = Marked   5 = Severe

Affective flattening or blunting

1 *Unchanging facial expression*   0 1 2 3 4 5
The patient's face appears wooden,
changes less than expected as
emotional content of discourse changes.

2 *Decreased spontaneous movements*   0 1 2 3 4 5
The patient shows few or no
spontaneous movements, does not shift
position, move extremities, etc.

3 *Paucity of expressive gestures*   0 1 2 3 4 5
The patient does not use hand gestures,
body position, etc., as an aid to
expressing his ideas.

4 *Poor eye contact*   0 1 2 3 4 5
The patient avoids eye contact or
"stares through" interviewer even when
speaking.

5 *Affective nonresponsivity*   0 1 2 3 4 5
The patient fails to smile or laugh when
prompted.

6 *Lack of vocal inflections*   0 1 2 3 4 5
The patient fails to show normal vocal
emphasis patterns, is often monotonic.

7 *Global rating of affective flattening*   0 1 2 3 4 5
This rating should focus on overall
severity of symptoms, especially
unresponsiveness, eye contact, facial
expression, and vocal inflections.

Alogia

8 *Poverty of speech*   0 1 2 3 4 5
The patient's replies to questions are
restricted in *amount* tend to be brief,
concrete, and unelaborated.

9 *Poverty of content of speech*   0 1 2 3 4 5
The patient's replies are adequate in
amount but tend to be vague,
overconcrete, or over-generalized, and
convey little information.

10 *Blocking*   0 1 2 3 4 5
The patient indicates, either
spontaneously or with prompting, that
his [her] train of thought was
interrupted.

11 *Increased latency of response*   0 1 2 3 4 5
The patient takes a long time to reply to
questions; prompting indicates the
patient is aware of the question.

12 *Global rating of alogia*   0 1 2 3 4 5
The core features of alogia are poverty
of speech and poverty of content.

Avolition-apathy

13 *Grooming and hygiene*   0 1 2 3 4 5
The patient's clothes may be sloppy or
soiled, and he [she] may have greasy
hair, body odor, etc.

14 *Impersistence at work or school*   0 1 2 3 4 5
The patient has difficulty seeking or
maintaining employment, completing
school work, keeping house, etc. If an
inpatient, cannot persist at ward
activities, such as occupational therapy,
playing cards, etc.

15 *Physical anergia*   0 1 2 3 4 5
The patient tends to be physically inert.
He [she] may sit for hours and does not
initiate spontaneous activity.

16 *Global rating of avolition-apathy*   0 1 2 3 4 5
Strong weight may be given to one or
two prominent symptoms if particularly
striking.

Anhedonia-asociality

17 *Recreational interests and activities*   0 1 2 3 4 5
The patient may have few or no
interests. Both the quality and quantity
of interests should be taken into
account.

18 *Sexual activity*   0 1 2 3 4 5
The patient may show a decrease in
sexual interest and activity, or
enjoyment when active.

19 *Ability to feel intimacy and closeness*   0 1 2 3 4 5
The patient may display an inability to
form close or intimate relationships,
especially with the opposite sex and
family.

20 *Relationships with friends and peers*   0 1 2 3 4 5
The patient may have few or no friends
and may prefer to spend all of his [her]
time isolated.

21 *Global rating of anhedonia-asociality*   0 1 2 3 4 5
This rating should reflect overall
severity, taking into account the
patient's age, family status, etc.

Attention

22 *Social inattentiveness*   0 1 2 3 4 5
The patient appears uninvolved or
unengaged. He [she] may seem spacey.

23 *Inattentiveness during mental status*   0 1 2 3 4 5
testing
Tests of "serial 7s" (at least five
subtractions) and spelling *world*
backwards: Score: 2 = 1 error; 3 = 2
errors; 4 = 3 errors.

24 *Global rating of attention*   0 1 2 3 4 5
This rating should assess the patient's
overall concentration, clinically and on
tests.

From Nancy C. Andreasen, M.D., Ph.D., Department of Psychiatry, College of Medicine, The University of Iowa, Iowa City, IA 52242. with permission.

Table 6–6
Scale for the Assessment of Positive Symptoms (SAPS)

0 = None   1 = Questionable   2 = Mild   3 = Moderate   4 = Marked   5 = Severe

Hallucinations

1 *Auditory hallucinations*   0 1 2 3 4 5
The patient reports voices, noises, or other
sounds that no one else hears.

2 *Voices commenting*   0 1 2 3 4 5
The patient reports a voice which makes a
running commentary on his [her] behavior or
thoughts.

3 *Voices conversing*   0 1 2 3 4 5
The patient reports hearing two or more
voices conversing.

4 *Somatic or tactile hallucinations*   0 1 2 3 4 5
The patient reports experiencing peculiar
physical sensations in the body.

5 *Olfactory hallucinations*   0 1 2 3 4 5
The patient reports experiencing unusual smells
which no one else notices.

6 *Visual hallucinations*   0 1 2 3 4 5
The patient sees shapes or people that are not
actually present.

7 *Global rating of hallucinations*   0 1 2 3 4 5
This rating should be based on the duration and
severity of the hallucinations and their effects
on the patient's life.

Delusions

8 *Persecutory delusions*   0 1 2 3 4 5
The patient believes he [she] is being conspired
against or persecuted in some way.

9 *Delusions of jealousy*   0 1 2 3 4 5
The patient believes his [her] spouse is having
an affair with someone.

10 *Delusions of guilt or sin*   0 1 2 3 4 5
The patient believes that he [she] has
committed some terrible sin or done something
unforgivable.

11 *Grandiose delusions*   0 1 2 3 4 5
The patient believes he [she] has special
powers or abilities.

12 *Religious delusions*   0 1 2 3 4 5
The patient is preoccupied with false beliefs of
a religious nature.

13 *Somatic delusions*   0 1 2 3 4 5
The patient believes that somehow his [her]
body is diseased, abnormal, or changed.

14 *Delusions of reference*   0 1 2 3 4 5
The patient believes that insignificant remarks
or events refer to him [her] or have some
special meaning.

15 *Delusions of being controlled*   0 1 2 3 4 5
The patient feels that his [her] feelings or
actions are controlled by some outside force.

16 *Delusions of mind reading*   0 1 2 3 4 5
The patient feels that people can read his [her]
mind or know his [her] thoughts.

17 *Thought broadcasting*   0 1 2 3 4 5
The patient believes that his [her] thoughts are
broadcast so that he himself [she herself] or
others can hear them.

18 *Thought insertion*   0 1 2 3 4 5
The patient believes that thoughts that are not
his [her] own have been inserted into his [her]
mind.

19 *Thought withdrawal*   0 1 2 3 4 5
The patient believes that thoughts have been
taken away from his [her] mind.

20 *Global rating of delusions*   0 1 2 3 4 5
This rating should be based on the duration and
persistence of the delusions and their effect on
the patient's life.

Bizarre behavior

21 *Clothing and appearance*   0 1 2 3 4 5
The patient dresses in an unusual manner or
does other strange things to alter his [her]
appearance.

22 *Social and sexual behavior*   0 1 2 3 4 5
The patient may do things considered
inappropriate according to usual social norms
(e.g., masturbating in public).

23 *Aggressive and agitated behavior*   0 1 2 3 4 5
The patient may behave in an aggressive,
agitated manner, often unpredictably.

24 *Repetitive or stereotyped behavior*   0 1 2 3 4 5
The patient develops a set of repetitive actions
or rituals that he [she] must perform over and
over.

25 *Global rating of bizarre behavior*   0 1 2 3 4 5
This rating should reflect the type of behavior
and the extent to which it deviates from social
norms.

Positive formal thought disorder

26 *Derailment*   0 1 2 3 4 5
A pattern of speech in which ideas slip off track
onto ideas obliquely related or unrelated.

27 *Tangentiality*   0 1 2 3 4 5
Replying to a question in an oblique or
irrelevant manner.

28 *Incoherence*   0 1 2 3 4 5
A pattern of speech which is essentially
incomprehensible at times.

29 *Illogicality*   0 1 2 3 4 5
A pattern of speech in which conclusions are
reached which do not follow logically.

30 *Circumstantiality*   0 1 2 3 4 5
A pattern of speech which is very indirect and
delayed in reaching its goal idea.

31 *Pressure of speech*   0 1 2 3 4 5
The patient's speech is rapid and difficult to
interrupt; the amount of speech produced is
greater than that considered normal.

32 *Distractible speech*   0 1 2 3 4 5
The patient is distracted by nearby stimuli
which interrupt his [her] flow of speech.

33 *Clanging*   0 1 2 3 4 5
A pattern of speech in which sounds rather than
meaningful relationships govern word choice.

34 *Global rating of positive formal thought disorder*   0 1 2 3 4 5
This rating should reflect the frequency of
abnormality and degree to which it affects the
patient's ability to communicate.

Inappropriate affect

35 *Inappropriate affect*   0 1 2 3 4 5
The patient's affect is inappropriate or
incongruous, not simply flat or blunted.

7

Delirium, Dementia, and Amnestic and Other Cognitive Disorders and Mental Disorders Due to a General Medical Condition

▲ 7.1 Overview

Cognition includes memory, language, orientation, judgment, conducting of interpersonal relationships, performance of actions (praxis), and problem solving. Cognitive disorders reflect disruption in one or more of these domains, and are also frequently complicated by behavioral symptoms. Cognitive disorders exemplify the complex interfaces among neurology, medicine, and psychiatry, in that medical or neurological conditions often lead to cognitive disorders that, in turn, are associated with behavioral symptoms. It can be argued that of all psychiatric conditions, cognitive disorders best demonstrate how biological insults result in behavioral symptomatology. The clinician must carefully assess the history and context of the presentation of these disorders before arriving at a diagnosis and treatment plan. Advances in molecular biology, diagnostic techniques, and medication management have significantly improved the ability to recognize and treat cognitive disorders.

In the text revision of the fourth edition of the *Diagnostic Statistical Manual of Mental Disorders* (DSM-IV-TR), three groups of disorders—delirium, dementia, and the amnestic disorders—are characterized by the primary symptom common to all the disorders, which is an impairment in cognition (as in memory, language, or attention). Although DSM-IV-TR acknowledges that other psychiatric disorders can exhibit some cognitive impairment as a symptom, cognitive impairment is the cardinal symptom in delirium, dementia, and the amnestic disorders. Within each of these diagnostic categories, DSM-IV-TR delimits specific types (Table 7.1–1).

In the past, these conditions were classified under the heading "organic mental disorders" or "organic brain disorders." Traditionally, those disorders had an identifiable pathological condition such as brain tumor, cerebrovascular disease, or drug intoxication. Those brain disorders with no generally accepted organic basis (e.g., depression) were called *functional disorders*.

This century-old distinction between organic and functional disorders is outdated and has been deleted from the nomenclature. Every psychiatric disorder has an organic (i.e., biological or chemical) component. Because of this reassessment, the concept of functional disorders has been determined to be misleading, and the term *functional* and its historical opposite, *organic*, are not used in DSM-IV-TR.

A further indication that the dichotomy is no longer valid is the revival of the term *neuropsychiatry*, which emphasizes the somatic substructure on which mental operations and emotions are based; it is concerned with the psychopathological accompaniments of brain dysfunction as observed in seizure disorders, for example. Neuropsychiatry focuses on the psychiatric aspects of neurological disorders and the role of brain dysfunction in psychiatric disorders.

CLASSIFICATION

For each of the three major groups—delirium, dementia, and amnestic disorders—there are subcategories based on etiology. They are defined and summarized as follows.

Delirium

Delirium is marked by short-term confusion and changes in cognition. There are four subcategories, based on several causes: (1) general medical condition (e.g., infection), (2) substance induced (e.g., cocaine, opioids, phencyclidine [PCP]), (3) multiple causes (e.g., head trauma and kidney disease), and (4) delirium not otherwise specified (e.g., sleep deprivation).

Dementia

Dementia is marked by severe impairment in memory, judgment, orientation, and cognition. There are six subcategories: (1) dementia of the Alzheimer's type, which usually occurs in persons older than 65 years of age and is manifested by progressive intellectual disorientation and dementia, delusions, or depression; (2) vascular dementia, caused by vessel thrombosis or hemorrhage; (3) other medical conditions (e.g., human immunodeficiency virus disease, head trauma, Pick's disease, and Creutzfeldt-Jakob disease, which is caused by a slow-growing, transmittable virus); (4) substance induced, caused by toxin or

Table 7.1–1
DSM-IV-TR Cognitive Disorders

Delirium
    Delirium due to a general medical condition
    Substance-induced delirium
    Delirium due to multiple etiologies
    Delirium not otherwise specified
Dementia
    Dementia of the Alzheimer's type
    Vascular dementia
    Dementia due to other general medical conditions
        Dementia due to human immunodeficiency virus
          (HIV) disease
        Dementia due to head trauma
        Dementia due to Parkinson's disease
        Dementia due to Huntington's disease
        Dementia due to Pick's disease
        Dementia due to Creutzfeldt-Jakob disease
        Dementia due to other general medical conditions
    Substance-induced persisting dementia
    Dementia due to multiple etiologies
    Dementia not otherwise specified
Amnestic disorders
    Amnestic disorder due to a general medical condition
    Substance-induced persisting amnestic disorder
    Amnestic disorder not otherwise specified
    Cognitive disorder not otherwise specified

DSM-IV-TR, text revision of the fourth edition of the *Diagnostic Statistical Manual of Mental Disorders.*

Table 7.1–2
DSM-IV-TR Diagnostic Criteria for Cognitive Disorder Not Otherwise Specified

This category is for disorders that are characterized by cognitive dysfunction presumed to be due to the direct physiological effect of a general medical condition that do not meet criteria for any of the specific deliriums, dementias, or amnestic disorders listed in this section and that are not better classified as delirium not otherwise specified, dementia not otherwise specified, or amnestic disorder not otherwise specified. For cognitive dysfunction due to a specific or unknown substance, the specific substance-related disorder not otherwise specified category should be used.

Examples include

1. Mild neurocognitive disorder: impairment in cognitive functioning as evidenced by neuropsychological testing or quantified clinical assessment, accompanied by objective evidence of a systemic general medical condition or central nervous system dysfunction
2. Postconcussional disorder: following a head trauma, impairment in memory or attention with associated symptoms

From American Psychiatric Association. *Diagnostic and Statistical Manual of Mental Disorders.* 4th ed. Text rev. Washington, DC: American Psychiatric Association; copyright 2000, with permission.

medication (e.g., gasoline fumes, atropine); (5) multiple etiologies; and (6) not otherwise specified (if cause is unknown).

Amnestic Disorder

Amnestic disorder is marked by memory impairment and forgetfulness. The three subcategories are (1) caused by medical condition (hypoxia), (2) caused by toxin or medication (e.g., marijuana, diazepam), and (3) not otherwise specified.

Cognitive Disorder Not Otherwise Specified

Cognitive disorder not otherwise specified is a DSM-IV-TR category that allows for the diagnosis of a cognitive disorder that does not meet the criteria for delirium, dementia, or amnestic disorders (Table 7.1–2). The cause of these syndromes is presumed to involve a specific general medical condition, a pharmacologically active agent, or possibly both.

CLINICAL EVALUATION

During the history taking, the clinician seeks to elicit the development of the illness. Subtle cognitive disorders, fluctuating symptoms, and progressing disease processes may be tracked effectively. The clinician should obtain a detailed rendition of changes in the patient's daily routine involving such factors as self-care, job responsibilities, and work habits; meal preparation; shopping and personal support; interactions with friends; hobbies and sports; reading interests; religious, social, and recreational activities; and ability to maintain personal finances. Understanding the life history of each patient provides an invaluable source of baseline data regarding changes in function, such as attention and concentration, intellectual abilities, personality,

motor skills, and mood and perception. The examiner seeks to find the particular pursuits that the patient considers most important, or central, to his or her lifestyle and attempts to discern how those pursuits have been affected by the emerging clinical condition. Such a method provides the opportunity to appraise both the impact of the illness and the patient-specific baseline for monitoring the effects of future therapies.

Mental Status Examination

After taking a thorough history, the clinician's primary tool is the assessment of the patient's mental status. As with the physical examination, the mental status examination is a means of surveying functions and abilities to allow a definition of personal strengths and weaknesses. It is a repeatable, structured assessment of symptoms and signs that promotes effective communication between clinicians. It also establishes the basis for future comparison, essential for documenting therapeutic effectiveness, and it allows comparisons between different patients, with a generalization of findings from one patient to another.

Cognition

When testing cognitive functions, the clinician should evaluate memory, visuospatial and constructional abilities, and reading, writing, and mathematical abilities. Assessment of abstraction ability is also valuable; however, whereas a patient's performance on tasks such as proverb interpretation may be a useful bedside projective test in some patients, the specific interpretation may result from a variety of factors, such as poor education, low intelligence, and failure to understand the concept of proverbs, as well as from a broad array of primary and secondary psychopathological disturbances.

PATHOLOGY AND LABORATORY EXAMINATION

As with all medical tests, psychiatric evaluations such as the mental status examination must be interpreted in the overall context of thorough clinical and laboratory assessment. Psychiatric and neuropsychiatric patients require careful physical examination, especially when issues exist involving etiologically related or comorbid medical conditions. When consulting internists and other medical specialists, the clinician must ask specific questions to focus the differential diagnostic process and use the consultation most effectively. In particular, most systemic medical or primary cerebral diseases that lead to psychopathological disturbances also manifest with a variety of peripheral or central abnormalities.

A screening laboratory evaluation is sought initially and may be followed by a variety of ancillary tests to increase the diagnostic specificity. Table 7.1–3 lists such procedures, some of which are described in subsequent sections.

Table 7.1–3
Screening Laboratory Tests

General Tests
   Complete blood cell count
   Erythrocyte sedimentation rate
   Electrolytes
   Glucose
   Blood urea nitrogen and serum creatinine
   Liver function tests
   Serum calcium and phosphorus
   Thyroid function tests
   Serum protein
   Levels of all drugs
   Urinalysis
   Pregnancy test for women of childbearing age
   Electrocardiography
Ancillary Laboratory Tests
Blood
   Blood cultures
   Rapid plasma reagin test
   Human immunodeficiency virus testing (enzyme-linked
      immunosorbent assay [ELISA] and Western blot)
   Serum heavy metals
   Serum copper
   Ceruloplasmin
   Serum B_{12}, red blood cell (RBC) folate levels
Urine
   Culture
   Toxicology
   Heavy metal screen
Electrography
   Electroencephalography
   Evoked potentials
   Polysomnography
   Nocturnal penile tumescence
Cerebrospinal fluid
   Glucose, protein
   Cell count
   Cultures (bacterial, viral, fungal)
   Cryptococcal antigen
   Venereal Disease Research Laboratory test
Radiography
   Computed tomography
   Magnetic resonance imaging
   Positron emission tomography
   Single photon emission computed tomography

Courtesy of Eric D. Caine, M.D., and Jeffrey M. Lyness, M.D.

▲ 7.2 Delirium

Delirium is defined by the acute onset of fluctuating cognitive impairment and a disturbance of consciousness with reduced ability to attend. Delirium is a syndrome, not a disease, and it has many causes, all of which result in a similar pattern of signs and symptoms relating to the patient's level of consciousness and cognitive impairment. Delirium is underrecognized by health care workers. Part of the problem is that the syndrome has a variety of other names. The intent of the text revision of the fourth edition of the *Diagnostic and Statistical Manual of Mental Disorders* (DSM-IV-TR) was to help consolidate the myriad of terms into a single diagnostic label.

In DSM-IV-TR, delirium is "characterized by a disturbance of consciousness and a change in cognition that develop over a short ... time." The hallmark symptom of delirium is an impairment of consciousness, usually occurring in association with global impairments of cognitive functions. Abnormalities of mood, perception, and behavior are common psychiatric symptoms; tremor, asterixis, nystagmus, incoordination, and urinary incontinence are common neurological symptoms. Classically, delirium has a sudden onset (hours or days), a brief and fluctuating course, and rapid improvement when the causative factor is identified and eliminated, but each of these characteristic features can vary in individual patients. Physicians must recognize delirium to identify and treat the underlying cause and avert the development of delirium-related complications such as accidental injury because of the patient's clouded consciousness.

EPIDEMIOLOGY

Delirium is a common disorder. According to DSM-IV-TR, the point prevalence of delirium in the general population is 0.4 percent for people 18 years of age and older and 1.1 percent for people 55 and older. Approximately 10 to 30 percent of medically ill patients who are hospitalized exhibit delirium. Approximately 30 percent of patients in surgical intensive care units and cardiac intensive care units and 40 to 50 percent of patients who are recovering from surgery for hip fractures have an episode of delirium. The highest rate of delirium is found in postcardiotomy patients—more than 90 percent in some studies. An estimated 20 percent of patients with severe burns and 30 to 40 percent of patients with acquired immune deficiency syndrome (AIDS) have episodes of delirium while they are hospitalized. Delirium develops in 80 percent of terminally ill patients. The causes of postoperative delirium include the stress of surgery, postoperative pain, insomnia, pain medication, electrolyte imbalances, infection, fever, and blood loss.

Numerous factors can increase a patient's risk for delirium. These range from extremes of age to the number of medications taken. Advanced age is a major risk factor for the development of delirium. Approximately 30 to 40 percent of hospitalized patients older than age 65 years have an episode of delirium, and another 10 to 15 percent of elderly persons exhibit delirium on admission to the hospital. Of nursing home residents older than age 75 years, 60 percent have repeated episodes of delirium. Other predisposing factors for the development of delirium are preexisting brain damage (e.g., dementia, cerebrovascular disease, tumor), a history of delirium, alcohol dependence, diabetes, cancer, sensory impairment (e.g., blindness), and malnutrition. Male gender is an independent risk factor for delirium according to DSM-IV-TR.

Delirium is a poor prognostic sign. Rates of institutionalization are increased threefold for patients 65 years and older who exhibit delirium while in the hospital. The 3-month mortality rate of patients who have an episode of delirium is estimated to be 23 to 33 percent. The 1-year mortality rate for patients who have an episode of delirium may be as high as 50 percent. Elderly patients who experience delirium while hospitalized have a 20 to 75 percent mortality rate during that hospitalization. After discharge, up to 15 percent of these persons die within a 1-month period, and 25 percent die within 6 months.

ETIOLOGY

The major causes of delirium are central nervous system disease (e.g., epilepsy), systemic disease (e.g., cardiac failure), and either intoxication or withdrawal from pharmacological or toxic agents. When evaluating patients with delirium, clinicians should assume that any drug that a patient has taken may be etiologically relevant to the delirium.

DIAGNOSIS AND CLINICAL FEATURES

The syndrome of delirium is almost always caused by one or more systemic or cerebral derangements that affect brain function.

The DSM-IV-TR gives separate diagnostic criteria for each type of delirium: (1) delirium due to a general medical condition (Table 7.2–1), (2) substance intoxication delirium (Table 7.2–2), (3) substance withdrawal delirium (Table 7.2–3), (4) delirium

Table 7.2–2
DSM-IV-TR Diagnostic Criteria for Substance Intoxication Delirium

A. Disturbance of consciousness (i.e., reduced clarity of awareness of the environment) with reduced ability to focus, sustain, or shift attention.
B. A change in cognition (such as memory deficit, disorientation, language disturbance) or the development of a perceptual disturbance that is not better accounted for by a preexisting, established, or evolving dementia.
C. The disturbance develops over a short period of time (usually hours to days) and tends to fluctuate during the course of the day.
D. There is evidence from the history, physical examination, or laboratory findings of either (1) or (2):
  (1) the symptoms in Criteria A and B developed during substance intoxication
  (2) medication use is etiologically related to the disturbance*

Note: This diagnosis should be made instead of a diagnosis of substance intoxication only when the cognitive symptoms are in excess of those usually associated with the intoxication syndrome and when the symptoms are sufficiently severe to warrant independent clinical attention.
*Note: The diagnosis should be recorded as substance-induced delirium if related to medication use.

Code (Specific substance) intoxication delirium:
(Alcohol; Amphetamine [or amphetamine-like substance]; Cannabis; Cocaine; Hallucinogen; Inhalant; Opioid; Phencyclidine [or phencyclidine-like substance]; Sedative, hypnotic, or anxiolytic; Other [or unknown] substance [e.g., cimetidine, digitalis, benztropine])

From American Psychiatric Association. *Diagnostic and Statistical Manual of Mental Disorders.* 4th ed. Text rev. Washington, DC: American Psychiatric Association; copyright 2000, with permission.

Table 7.2–1
DSM-IV-TR Diagnostic Criteria for 293.0 Delirium Due to General Medical Condition

A. Disturbance of consciousness (i.e., reduced clarity of awareness of the environment) with reduced ability to focus, sustain, or shift attention.
B. A change in cognition (such as memory deficit, disorientation, language disturbance) or the development of a perceptual disturbance that is not better accounted for by a preexisting, established, or evolving dementia.
C. The disturbance develops over a short period of time (usually hours to days) and tends to fluctuate during the course of the day.
D. There is evidence from the history, physical examination, or laboratory findings that the disturbance is caused by the direct physiological consequences of a general medical condition.
Coding note: If delirium is superimposed on a preexisting vascular dementia, indicate the delirium by coding vascular dementia, with delirium.
Coding note: Include the name of the general medical condition on Axis I, e.g., Delirium due to hepatic encephalopathy; also code the general medical condition on Axis III.

From American Psychiatric Association. *Diagnostic and Statistical Manual of Mental Disorders.* 4th ed. Text rev. Washington, DC: American Psychiatric Association; copyright 2000, with permission.

Table 7.2–3
DSM-IV-TR Diagnostic Criteria for Substance Withdrawal Delirium

A. Disturbance of consciousness (i.e., reduced clarity of awareness of the environment) with reduced ability to focus, sustain, or shift attention.
B. A change in cognition (such as memory deficit, disorientation, language disturbance) or the development of a perceptual disturbance that is not better accounted for by a preexisting, established, or evolving dementia.
C. The disturbance develops over a short period of time (usually hours to days) and tends to fluctuate during the course of the day.
D. There is evidence from the history, physical examination, or laboratory findings that the symptoms in Criteria A and B developed during, or shortly after, a withdrawal syndrome.
Note: This diagnosis should be made instead of a diagnosis of substance withdrawal only when the cognitive symptoms are in excess of those usually associated with the withdrawal syndrome and when the symptoms are sufficiently severe to warrant independent clinical attention.

Code (Specific substance) withdrawal delirium:
(Alcohol; Sedative, hypnotic, or anxiolytic; Other [or unknown] substance)

From American Psychiatric Association. *Diagnostic and Statistical Manual of Mental Disorders.* 4th ed. Text rev. Washington, DC: American Psychiatric Association; copyright 2000, with permission.

Table 7.2–4
DSM-IV-TR Diagnostic Criteria for Delirium Due to Multiple Etiologies

A. Disturbance of consciousness (i.e., reduced clarity of awareness of the environment) with reduced ability to focus, sustain, or shift attention.
B. A change in cognition (such as memory deficit, disorientation, language disturbance) or the development of a perceptual disturbance that is not better accounted for by a preexisting, established, or evolving dementia.
C. The disturbance develops over a short period of time (usually hours to days) and tends to fluctuate during the course of the day.
D. There is evidence from the history, physical examination, or laboratory findings that the delirium has more than one etiology (e.g., more than one etiological general medical condition, a general medical condition plus substance intoxication or medication side effect).

Coding note: Use multiple codes reflecting specific delirium and specific etiologies, e.g., Delirium due to viral encephalitis; Alcohol withdrawal delirium.

From American Psychiatric Association. *Diagnostic and Statistical Manual of Mental Disorders.* 4th ed. Text rev. Washington, DC: American Psychiatric Association; copyright 2000, with permission.

due to multiple etiologies (Table 7.2–4), and (5) delirium not otherwise specified (Table 7.2–5) for a delirium of unknown cause or of causes not listed, such as sensory deprivation. The syndrome, however, is the same, regardless of cause.

The core features of delirium include altered consciousness, such as decreased level of consciousness; altered attention, which can include diminished ability to focus, sustain, or shift attention; impairment in other realms of cognitive function, which can manifest as disorientation (especially to time and space) and decreased memory; relatively rapid onset (usually hours to days); brief duration (usually days to weeks); and often marked, unpredictable fluctuations in severity and other clinical manifestations during the course of the day, sometimes worse at night (sundowning), which may range from periods of lucidity to quite severe cognitive impairment and disorganization.

Associated clinical features are often present and may be prominent. They may include disorganization of thought processes (ranging from mild tangentiality to frank incoherence), perceptual disturbances such as illusions and hallucinations, psychomotor hyperactivity and hypoactivity, disruption of the sleep-

Table 7.2–5
DSM-IV-TR Diagnostic Criteria for Delirium Not Otherwise Specified

This category should be used to diagnose a delirium that does not meet criteria for any of the specific types of delirium described in this section.

Examples include

1. A clinical presentation of delirium that is suspected to be due to a general medical condition or substance use but for which there is insufficient evidence to establish a specific etiology.
2. Delirium due to causes not listed in this section (e.g., sensory deprivation).

From American Psychiatric Association. *Diagnostic and Statistical Manual of Mental Disorders.* 4th ed. Text rev. Washington, DC: American Psychiatric Association; copyright 2000, with permission.

wake cycle (often manifested as fragmented sleep at night, with or without daytime drowsiness), mood alterations (from subtle irritability to obvious dysphoria, anxiety, or even euphoria), and other manifestations of altered neurological function (e.g., autonomic hyperactivity or instability, myoclonic jerking, and dysarthria). The electroencephalogram (EEG) usually shows diffuse slowing of background activity, although patients with delirium caused by alcohol or sedative-hypnotic withdrawal have low-voltage fast activity.

The major neurotransmitter hypothesized to be involved in delirium is acetylcholine, and the major neuroanatomical area is the reticular formation. The reticular formation of the brainstem is the principal area regulating attention and arousal; the major pathway implicated in delirium is the dorsal tegmental pathway, which projects from the mesencephalic reticular formation to the tectum and thalamus. Several studies have reported that a variety of delirium-inducing factors result in decreased acetylcholine activity in the brain. One of the most common causes of delirium is toxicity from too many prescribed medications with anticholinergic activity. In addition to the anticholinergic drugs themselves, many drugs used in psychiatry have similar effects (e.g., atropine, amitriptyline [Elavil], doxepin [Sinequan], nortriptyline [Aventyl], imipramine [Tofranil], and the phenothiazine class). Researchers have suggested other pathophysiological mechanisms for delirium. In particular, the delirium associated with alcohol withdrawal has been associated with hyperactivity of the locus ceruleus and its noradrenergic neurons. Other neurotransmitters that have been implicated are serotonin and glutamate.

PHYSICAL AND LABORATORY EXAMINATIONS

Delirium is usually diagnosed at the bedside and is characterized by the sudden onset of symptoms. A bedside mental status examination—such as the Mini-Mental State Examination, the mental status examination, or neurologic signs—can be used to document the cognitive impairment and provide a baseline from which to measure the patient's clinical course. The physical examination often reveals clues to the cause of the delirium. The presence of a known physical illness or a history of head trauma or alcohol or other substance dependence increases the likelihood of the diagnosis.

The laboratory workup of a patient with delirium should include standard tests and additional studies indicated by the clinical situation. In delirium, the EEG characteristically shows a generalized slowing of activity and may be useful in differentiating delirium from depression or psychosis. The EEG of a delirious patient sometimes shows focal areas of hyperactivity. In rare cases, it may be difficult to differentiate delirium related to epilepsy from delirium related to other causes.

DIFFERENTIAL DIAGNOSIS

Delirium versus Dementia

A number of clinical features help distinguish delirium from dementia. The major differential points between dementia and delirium are the time to development of the condition and the fluctuation in level of attention in delirium compared with relatively consistent attention in dementia. The time to development of symptoms is usually short in delirium, and, except for vascular dementia caused by stroke, it is usually gradual and insidious in dementia. Although both conditions include cognitive impairment, the changes in dementia are more stable over time and, for example, usually do not fluctuate over the course of a day. A patient with dementia is usually alert; a patient with delirium has episodes of decreased consciousness. Occasionally, delirium occurs in a patient with dementia, a condition known as *beclouded dementia*. A dual diagnosis of delirium can be made when there is a definite history of preexisting dementia.

Delirium versus Schizophrenia or Depression

Delirium must also be differentiated from schizophrenia and depressive disorder. Some patients with psychotic disorders, usually schizophrenia or manic episodes, can have periods of extremely disorganized behavior difficult to distinguish from delirium. In general, however, the hallucinations and delusions of patients with schizophrenia are more constant and better organized than those of patients with delirium. Patients with schizophrenia usually experience no change in their level of consciousness or in their orientation. Patients with hypoactive symptoms of delirium may appear somewhat similar to severely depressed patients, but they can be distinguished on the basis of an EEG. Other psychiatric diagnoses to consider in the differential diagnosis of delirium are brief psychotic disorder, schizophreniform disorder, and dissociative disorders. Patients with factitious disorders may attempt to simulate the symptoms of delirium but usually reveal the factitious nature of their symptoms by inconsistencies on their mental status examinations, and an EEG can easily separate the two diagnoses.

COURSE AND PROGNOSIS

Although the onset of delirium is usually sudden, prodromal symptoms (e.g., restlessness and fearfulness) can occur in the days preceding the onset of florid symptoms. The symptoms of delirium usually persist as long as the causally relevant factors are present, although delirium generally lasts less than a week. After identification and removal of the causative factors, the symptoms of delirium usually recede over a 3- to 7-day period, although some symptoms may take up to 2 weeks to resolve completely. The older the patient and the longer the patient has been delirious, the longer does the delirium take to resolve. Recall of what occurred during a delirium, once it is over, is characteristically spotty; a patient may refer to the episode as a bad dream or a nightmare only vaguely remembered. As stated in the discussion on epidemiology, the occurrence of delirium is associated with a high mortality rate in the ensuing year, primarily because of the serious nature of the associated medical conditions that lead to delirium.

Whether delirium progresses to dementia has not been demonstrated in carefully controlled studies, although many clinicians believe that they have seen such a progression. A clinical observation that has been validated by some studies, however, is that periods of delirium are sometimes followed by depression or posttraumatic stress disorder.

TREATMENT

In treating delirium, the primary goal is to treat the underlying cause. When the underlying condition is anticholinergic toxic-ity, the use of physostigmine salicylate (Antilirium), 1 to 2 mg intravenously or intramuscularly, with repeated doses in 15 to 30 minutes may be indicated. The other important goal of treatment is to provide physical, sensory, and environmental support. Physical support is necessary so that delirious patients do not get into situations in which they may have accidents. Patients with delirium should be neither sensory deprived nor overly stimulated by the environment. They are usually helped by having a friend or relative in the room or by the presence of a regular sitter. Familiar pictures and decorations, the presence of a clock or a calendar, and regular orientations to person, place, and time help make patients with delirium comfortable. Delirium can sometimes occur in older patients wearing eye patches after cataract surgery ("black-patch delirium"). Such patients can be helped by placing pinholes in the patches to let in some stimuli or by occasionally removing one patch at a time during recovery.

Pharmacotherapy

The two major symptoms of delirium that may require pharmacological treatment are psychosis and insomnia. A commonly used drug for psychosis is haloperidol (Haldol), a butyrophenone antipsychotic drug. Depending on a patient's age, weight, and physical condition, the initial dose may range from 2 to 6 mg intramuscularly, repeated in an hour if the patient remains agitated. As soon as the patient is calm, oral medication in liquid concentrate or tablet form should begin. Two daily oral doses should suffice, with two thirds of the dose being given at bedtime. To achieve the same therapeutic effect, the oral dose should be approximately 1.5 times the parenteral dose. The effective total daily dose of haloperidol may range from 5 to 40 mg for most patients with delirium. Droperidol (Inapsine) is a butyrophenone available as an alternative intravenous formulation, although careful monitoring of the electrocardiogram may be prudent with this treatment. Phenothiazines should be avoided in delirious patients because these drugs are associated with significant anticholinergic activity.

Use of second-generation antipsychotics, such as risperidone (Risperdal), clozapine (Clozaril), olanzapine (Zyprexa), quetiapine (Seroquel), ziprasidone (Geodon), and aripiprazole (Abilify), may be considered for delirium management, but clinical trial experience with these agents for delirium is limited. Ziprasidone appears to have an activating effect and may not be appropriate in delirium management. Olanzapine is available for intramuscular (IM) use and as a rapidly disintegrating oral preparation. These routes of administration may be preferable for some patients with delirium who are poorly compliant with medications or who are too sedated to safely swallow medications. For patients with Parkinson's disease and delirium who require antipsychotic medications, clozapine and quetiapine have some support in the literature and are less likely to exacerbate parkinsonian symptoms.

Insomnia is best treated with benzodiazepines with short or intermediate half-lives (e.g., lorazepam [Ativan] 1 to 2 mg at bedtime). Benzodiazepines with long half-lives and barbiturates should be avoided unless they are being used as part of the treatment for the underlying disorder (e.g., alcohol withdrawal). There have been case reports of improvement in or remission of delirious states caused by intractable medical illnesses with electroconvulsive therapy (ECT); however, routine consideration of

ECT for delirium is not advised. If delirium is caused by severe pain or dyspnea, a physician should not hesitate to prescribe opioids for both their analgesic and sedative effects.

▲ 7.3 Dementia

Dementia is defined as a progressive impairment of cognitive functions occurring in clear consciousness (e.g., in the absence of delirium). Dementia consists of a variety of symptoms that suggest chronic and widespread dysfunction. Global impairment of intellect is the essential feature, manifested as difficulty with memory, attention, thinking, and comprehension. Other mental functions can often be affected, including mood, personality, judgment, and social behavior. Although specific diagnostic criteria are found for various dementias, such as Alzheimer's disease or vascular dementia, all dementias have certain common elements that result in significant impairment in social or occupational functioning and cause a significant decline from a previous level of functioning.

The critical clinical points of dementia are the identification of the syndrome and the clinical workup of its cause. The disorder may be progressive or static, permanent or reversible. An underlying cause is always assumed, although, in rare cases, it is impossible to determine a specific cause. The potential reversibility of dementia is related to the underlying pathological condition and to the availability and application of effective treatment. Approximately 15 percent of people with dementia have reversible illnesses if treatment is initiated before irreversible damage takes place.

EPIDEMIOLOGY

With the aging population, the prevalence of dementia is rising. The prevalence of moderate to severe dementia in different population groups is approximately 5 percent in the general population older than 65 years of age, 20 to 40 percent in the general population older than 85 years of age, 15 to 20 percent in outpatient general medical practices, and 50 percent in chronic care facilities.

Of all patients with dementia, 50 to 60 percent have the most common type of dementia, dementia of the Alzheimer's type (Alzheimer's disease). Dementia of the Alzheimer's type increases in prevalence with increasing age. For persons aged 65 years, men have a prevalence rate of 0.6 percent and women of 0.8 percent. At age 90 years, rates are 21 percent. For all these figures, 40 to 60 percent of cases are moderate to severe. The respective rates of prevalence for males and females are 11 and 14 percent at age 85 years, 21 and 25 percent at age 90 years, and 36 and 41 percent at age 95 years. Patients with dementia of the Alzheimer's type occupy more than 50 percent of nursing home beds. More than 2 million persons with dementia are cared for in these homes. By 2050, current predictions suggest that there will be 14 million Americans with Alzheimer's disease and, therefore, more than 18 million people with dementia.

The second most common type of dementia is vascular dementia, which is causally related to cerebrovascular diseases. Hypertension predisposes a person to the disease. Vascular dementias account for 15 to 30 percent of all dementia cases. Vascular dementia is most common in persons between the ages of 60 and 70 years and is more common in men than in women. Approximately 10 to 15 percent of patients have coexisting vascular dementia and dementia of the Alzheimer's type.

Other common causes of dementia, each representing 1 to 5 percent of all cases, include head trauma, alcohol-related dementias, and various movement disorder–related dementias, such as Huntington's disease and Parkinson's disease. Because dementia is a fairly general syndrome, it has many causes, and clinicians must embark on a careful clinical workup of a patient with dementia to establish its cause.

ETIOLOGY

The most common causes of dementia in individuals older than 65 years of age are (1) Alzheimer's disease, (2) vascular dementia, and (3) mixed vascular and Alzheimer's dementia. Other illnesses that account for approximately 10 percent include Lewy body dementia; Pick's disease; frontotemporal dementias; normal pressure hydrocephalus (NPH); alcoholic dementia; infectious dementia, such as that due to infection with human immunodeficiency virus (HIV) or syphilis; and Parkinson's disease. Many types of dementias evaluated in clinical settings can be attributable to reversible causes, such as metabolic abnormalities (e.g., hypothyroidism), nutritional deficiencies (e.g., vitamin B_{12} or folate deficiencies), or dementia syndrome due to depression.

Dementia of the Alzheimer's Type

In 1907, Alois Alzheimer first described the condition that later assumed his name. He described a 51-year-old woman with a $4\frac{1}{2}$-year course of progressive dementia. The final diagnosis of Alzheimer's disease requires a neuropathological examination of the brain; nevertheless, dementia of the Alzheimer's type is commonly diagnosed in the clinical setting after other causes of dementia have been excluded from diagnostic consideration.

Genetic Factors. Although the cause of dementia of the Alzheimer's type remains unknown, progress has been made in understanding the molecular basis of the amyloid deposits that are a hallmark of the disorder's neuropathology. Some studies have indicated that as many as 40 percent of patients have a family history of dementia of the Alzheimer's type; thus, genetic factors are presumed to play a part in the development of the disorder, at least in some cases. Additional support for a genetic influence is the concordance rate for monozygotic twins, which is higher than the rate for dizygotic twins (43 percent vs. 8 percent, respectively). In several well-documented cases, the disorder has been transmitted in families through an autosomal dominant gene, although such transmission is rare. Alzheimer's type dementia has shown linkage to chromosomes 1, 14, and 21.

AMYLOID PRECURSOR PROTEIN. The gene for amyloid precursor protein is on the long arm of chromosome 21. The process of differential splicing yields four forms of amyloid precursor protein. The $\beta/A4$ protein, the major constituent of senile plaques, is a 42-amino acid peptide that is a breakdown product of amyloid precursor protein. In Down syndrome (trisomy 21), three copies of the amyloid precursor protein gene are found, and in a disease in which a mutation is found at codon 717 in the amyloid precursor protein gene, a pathological process results in the excessive deposition of $\beta/A4$ protein. Whether the processing of abnormal amyloid precursor protein is of primary causative significance in Alzheimer's disease is unknown, but many research groups are studying both the normal metabolic processing of amyloid precursor protein and its processing in patients with dementia of the Alzheimer's type in an attempt to answer this question.

MULTIPLE E4 GENES. One study implicated gene E4 in the origin of Alzheimer's disease. People with one copy of the gene have Alzheimer's disease three times more frequently than do those with no E4 gene, and people with two E4 genes have the disease eight times more frequently than do those with no E4 gene. Diagnostic testing for this gene is not currently recommended because it is found in persons without dementia and not found in all cases of dementia.

Neuropathology. The classic gross neuroanatomical observation of a brain from a patient with Alzheimer's disease is diffuse atrophy with flattened cortical sulci and enlarged cerebral ventricles. The classic and pathognomonic microscopic findings are senile plaques, neurofibrillary tangles, neuronal loss (particularly in the cortex and the hippocampus), synaptic loss (perhaps as much as 50 percent in the cortex), and granulovascular degeneration of the neurons. Neurofibrillary tangles are composed of cytoskeletal elements, primarily phosphorylated tau protein, although other cytoskeletal proteins are also present. Neurofibrillary tangles are not unique to Alzheimer's disease; they also occur in Down syndrome, dementia pugilistica (punch-drunk syndrome), Parkinson-dementia complex of Guam, Hallervorden-Spatz disease, and the brains of normal people as they age. Neurofibrillary tangles are commonly found in the cortex, the hippocampus, the substantia nigra, and the locus ceruleus.

Senile plaques, also referred to as *amyloid plaques*, more strongly indicate Alzheimer's disease, although they are also seen in Down syndrome and, to some extent, in normal aging. Senile plaques are composed of a particular protein, β/A4, and astrocytes, dystrophic neuronal processes, and microglia. The number and the density of senile plaques present in postmortem brains have been correlated with the severity of the disease that affected the persons.

Neurotransmitters. The neurotransmitters that are most often implicated in the pathophysiological condition of Alzheimer's disease are acetylcholine and norepinephrine, both of which are hypothesized to be hypoactive in Alzheimer's disease. Several studies have reported data consistent with the hypothesis that specific degeneration of cholinergic neurons is present in the nucleus basalis of Meynert in persons with Alzheimer's disease. Other data supporting a cholinergic deficit in Alzheimer's disease demonstrate decreased acetylcholine and choline acetyltransferase concentrations in the brain. Choline acetyltransferase is the key enzyme for the synthesis of acetylcholine, and a reduction in choline acetyltransferase concentration suggests a decrease in the number of cholinergic neurons present. Additional support for the cholinergic deficit hypothesis comes from the observation that cholinergic antagonists, such as scopolamine and atropine, impair cognitive abilities, whereas cholinergic agonists, such as physostigmine and arecoline, enhance cognitive abilities. Decreased norepinephrine activity in Alzheimer's disease is suggested by the decrease in norepinephrine-containing neurons in the locus ceruleus found in some pathological examinations of brains from persons with Alzheimer's disease. Two other neurotransmitters implicated

in the pathophysiological condition of Alzheimer's disease are the neuroactive peptides somatostatin and corticotropin; decreased concentrations of both have been reported in persons with Alzheimer's disease.

Other Causes. Another theory to explain the development of Alzheimer's disease is that an abnormality in the regulation of membrane phospholipid metabolism results in membranes that are less fluid—that is, more rigid—than normal. Several investigators are using molecular resonance spectroscopic imaging to assess this hypothesis directly in patients with dementia of the Alzheimer's type. Aluminum toxicity has also been hypothesized to be a causative factor because high levels of aluminum have been found in the brains of some patients with Alzheimer's disease, but this is no longer considered a significant etiological factor. Excessive stimulation by the transmitter glutamate that may damage neurons is another theory of causation.

Familial Multiple System Taupathy with Presenile Dementia

A recently discovered type of dementia, familial multiple system taupathy, shares some brain abnormalities found in people with Alzheimer's disease. The gene that causes the disorder is thought to be carried on chromosome 17. The symptoms of the disorder include short-term memory problems and difficulty maintaining balance and walking. The onset of disease occurs in the 40s and 50s, and persons with the disease live an average of 11 years after the onset of symptoms.

As in patients with Alzheimer's disease, tau protein builds up in neurons and glial cells of persons with familial multiple system taupathy. Eventually, the protein buildup kills brain cells. The disorder is not associated with the senile plaques associated with Alzheimer's disease.

Vascular Dementia

The primary cause of vascular dementia, formerly referred to as *multi-infarct dementia*, is presumed to be multiple areas of cerebral vascular disease, resulting in a symptom pattern of dementia. Vascular dementia is most commonly seen in men, especially those with preexisting hypertension or other cardiovascular risk factors. The disorder affects primarily small- and medium-sized cerebral vessels, which undergo infarction and produce multiple parenchymal lesions spread over wide areas of the brain. The causes of the infarctions may include occlusion of the vessels by arteriosclerotic plaques or thromboemboli from distant origins (e.g., heart valves). An examination of a patient may reveal carotid bruits, funduscopic abnormalities, or enlarged cardiac chambers.

Binswanger's Disease

Binswanger's disease, also known as *subcortical arteriosclerotic encephalopathy*, is characterized by the presence of many small infarctions of the white matter that spare the cortical regions. Although Binswanger's disease was previously considered a rare condition, the advent of sophisticated and powerful imaging techniques, such as magnetic resonance imaging (MRI), has revealed that the condition is more common than previously thought.

Pick's Disease

In contrast to the parietal-temporal distribution of pathological findings in Alzheimer's disease, Pick's disease is characterized by a preponderance of atrophy in the frontotemporal regions. These regions also have neuronal loss, gliosis, and neuronal Pick's bodies, which are masses of cytoskeletal elements. Pick's bodies are seen in some postmortem specimens but are not necessary for the diagnosis. The cause of Pick's disease is unknown, but the disease constitutes approximately 5 percent of all irreversible dementias. It is most common in men, especially those who have a first-degree relative with the condition. Pick's disease is difficult to distinguish from dementia of the Alzheimer's type, although the early stages of Pick's disease are more often characterized by personality and behavioral changes with relative preservation of other cognitive functions, and it typically begins before 75 years of age. Familial cases may have an earlier onset, and some studies have shown that approximately one half of the cases of Pick's disease are familial. Features of Klüver-Bucy syndrome (e.g., hypersexuality, placidity, and hyperorality) are much more common in Pick's disease than in Alzheimer's disease.

Lewy Body Disease

Lewy body disease is a dementia clinically similar to Alzheimer's disease and is often characterized by hallucinations, parkinsonian features, and extrapyramidal signs. Lewy inclusion bodies are found in the cerebral cortex. The exact incidence is unknown. These patients show marked adverse effects when given antipsychotic medications.

Huntington's Disease

Huntington's disease is classically associated with the development of dementia. The dementia seen in this disease is the subcortical type of dementia, characterized by more motor abnormalities and fewer language abnormalities than in the cortical type of dementia. The dementia of Huntington's disease exhibits psychomotor slowing and difficulty with complex tasks, but memory, language, and insight remain relatively intact in the early and middle stages of the illness. As the disease progresses, however, the dementia becomes complete; the features distinguishing it from dementia of the Alzheimer's type are the high incidence of depression and psychosis, in addition to the classic choreoathetoid movement disorder.

Parkinson's Disease

As with Huntington's disease, parkinsonism is a disease of the basal ganglia commonly associated with dementia and depression. An estimated 20 to 30 percent of patients with Parkinson's disease have dementia, and an additional 30 to 40 percent have measurable impairment in cognitive abilities. The slow movements of persons with Parkinson's disease are paralleled in the slow thinking of some affected patients, a feature that clinicians may refer to as *bradyphrenia*.

HIV-Related Dementia

Encephalopathy in HIV infection is associated with dementia and is termed *acquired immune deficiency syndrome* (AIDS) *dementia complex,* or *HIV dementia*. Patients infected with HIV experience dementia at an annual rate of approximately 14 percent. An estimated 75 percent of patients with AIDS have involvement of the central nervous system (CNS) at the time of autopsy. The development of dementia in people infected with HIV is often paralleled by the appearance of parenchymal abnormalities in MRI scans. Other infectious dementias are caused by *Cryptococcus* or *Treponema pallidum*.

The diagnosis of AIDS dementia complex is made by confirmation of HIV infection and exclusion of alternative pathology to explain cognitive impairment. The American Academy of Neurology AIDS Task Force developed research criteria for the clinical diagnosis of CNS disorders in adults and adolescents. The AIDS Task Force criteria for AIDS dementia complex require laboratory evidence for systemic HIV, at least two cognitive deficits, and the presence of motor abnormalities or personality changes. Personality changes may be manifested by apathy, emotional lability, or behavioral disinhibition. As with the text revision of the fourth edition of *Diagnostic and Statistical Manual of Mental Disorders* (DSM-IV-TR), the AIDS Task Force criteria also require the absence of clouding of consciousness or evidence of another etiology that could produce the cognitive impairment. Cognitive, motor, and behavioral changes are assessed using physical, neurological, and psychiatric examinations, in addition to neuropsychological testing.

Head Trauma–Related Dementia

Dementia can be a sequela of head trauma. The so-called punch-drunk syndrome (dementia pugilistica) occurs in boxers after repeated head trauma over many years. It is characterized by emotional lability, dysarthria, and impulsivity.

DIAGNOSIS AND CLINICAL FEATURES

The dementia diagnoses in DSM-IV-TR are dementia of the Alzheimer's type (Table 7.3–1), vascular dementia (Table 7.3–2), dementia due to other general medical conditions (Table 7.3–3), substance-induced persisting dementia (Table 7.3–4), dementia due to multiple etiologies (Table 7.3–5), and dementia not otherwise specified (Table 7.3–6).

The diagnosis of dementia is based on the clinical examination, including a mental status examination, and on information from the patient's family, friends, and employers. Complaints of a personality change in a patient older than age 40 years suggest that a diagnosis of dementia should be carefully considered.

Clinicians should note patients' complaints about intellectual impairment and forgetfulness as well as evidence of patients' evasion, denial, or rationalization aimed at concealing cognitive deficits. Excessive orderliness, social withdrawal, or a tendency to relate events in minute detail can be characteristic, and sudden outbursts of anger or sarcasm can occur. Patients' appearance and behavior should be observed. Lability of emotions, sloppy grooming, uninhibited remarks, silly jokes, or a dull, apathetic, or vacuous facial expression and manner suggest the presence of dementia, especially when coupled with memory impairment.

Memory impairment is typically an early and prominent feature in dementia, especially in dementias involving the cortex, such as dementia of the Alzheimer's type. Early in the course of

Table 7.3–1
DSM-IV-TR Diagnostic Criteria for Dementia of the Alzheimer's Type

A. The development of multiple cognitive deficits manifested by both
   (1) memory impairment (impaired ability to learn new information or to recall previously learned information)
   (2) one (or more) of the following cognitive disturbances:
      (a) aphasia (language disturbance)
      (b) apraxia (impaired ability to carry out motor activities despite intact motor function)
      (c) agnosia (failure to recognize or identify objects despite intact sensory function)
      (d) disturbance in executive functioning (i.e., planning, organizing, sequencing, abstracting)
B. The cognitive deficits in Criteria A1 and A2 each cause significant impairment in social or occupational functioning and represent a significant decline from a previous level of functioning.
C. The course is characterized by gradual onset and continuing cognitive decline.
D. The cognitive deficits in Criteria A1 and A2 are not due to any of the following:
   (1) other central nervous system conditions that cause progressive deficits in memory and cognition (e.g., cerebrovascular disease, Parkinson's disease, Huntington's disease, subdural hematoma, normal pressure hydrocephalus, brain tumor)
   (2) systemic conditions that are known to cause dementia (e.g., hypothyroidism, vitamin B_{12} or folic acid deficiency, niacin deficiency, hypercalcemia, neurosyphilis, HIV infection)
   (3) substance-induced conditions
E. The deficits do not occur exclusively during the course of a delirium.
F. The disturbance is not better accounted for by another Axis I disorder (e.g., major depressive disorder, schizophrenia).

Code based on presence or absence of a clinically significant behavioral disturbance:
Without behavioral disturbance: if the cognitive disturbance is not accompanied by any clinically significant behavioral disturbance.
With behavioral disturbance: if the cognitive disturbance is accompanied by a clinically significant behavioral disturbance (e.g., wandering, agitation).

Specify subtype:
With early onset: if onset is at age 65 years or below
With late onset: if onset is after age 65 years
Coding note: Also code Alzheimer's disease on Axis III. Indicate other prominent clinical features related to the Alzheimer's disease on Axis I (e.g., Mood disorder due to Alzheimer's disease, with depressive features, and Personality change due to Alzheimer's disease, aggressive type).

HIV, human immunodeficiency virus.
From American Psychiatric Association. *Diagnostic and Statistical Manual of Mental Disorders.* 4th ed. Text rev. Washington, DC: American Psychiatric Association; copyright 2000, with permission.

Table 7.3–2
DSM-IV-TR Diagnostic Criteria for Vascular Dementia

A. The development of multiple cognitive deficits manifested by both
   (1) memory impairment (impaired ability to learn new information or to recall previously learned information)
   (2) one (or more) of the following cognitive disturbances:
      (a) aphasia (language disturbance)
      (b) apraxia (impaired ability to carry out motor activities despite intact motor function)
      (c) agnosia (failure to recognize or identify objects despite intact sensory function)
      (d) disturbance in executive functioning (i.e., planning, organizing, sequencing, abstracting)
B. The cognitive deficits in Criteria A1 and A2 each cause significant impairment in social or occupational functioning and represent a significant decline from a previous level of functioning.
C. Focal neurological signs and symptoms (e.g., exaggeration of deep tendon reflexes, extensor plantar response, pseudobulbar palsy, gait abnormalities, weakness of an extremity) or laboratory evidence indicative of cerebrovascular disease (e.g., multiple infarctions involving cortex and underlying white matter) that are judged to be etiologically related to the disturbance.
D. The deficits do not occur exclusively during the course of a delirium.

Code based on predominant features:
With delirium: if delirium is superimposed on the dementia
With delusions: if delusions are the predominant feature
With depressed mood: if depressed mood (including presentations that meet full symptom criteria for a major depressive episode) is the predominant feature. A separate diagnosis of mood disorder due to a general medical condition is not given.
Uncomplicated: if none of the above predominates in the current clinical presentation

Specify if:
With behavioral disturbance
Coding note: Also code cerebrovascular condition on Axis III.

From American Psychiatric Association. *Diagnostic and Statistical Manual of Mental Disorders.* 4th ed. Text rev. Washington, DC: American Psychiatric Association; copyright 2000, with permission.

the course of a dementing illness. For example, patients with dementia may forget how to get back to their rooms after going to the bathroom. No matter how severe the disorientation seems, however, patients show no impairment in their level of consciousness.

Dementing processes that affect the cortex, primarily dementia of the Alzheimer's type and vascular dementia, can affect patients' language abilities. DSM-IV-TR includes aphasia as one of the diagnostic criteria. The language difficulty may be characterized by a vague, stereotyped, imprecise, or circumstantial locution, and patients may also have difficulty naming objects.

Psychiatric and Neurological Changes

Personality. Changes in the personality of a person with dementia are especially disturbing for their families. Preexisting personality traits may be accentuated during the development of a dementia. Patients with dementia may also become introverted and seem to be less concerned than they previously were about the effects of their behavior on others. Persons with

dementia, memory impairment is mild and usually most marked for recent events; people forget telephone numbers, conversations, and events of the day. As the course of dementia progresses, memory impairment becomes severe, and only the earliest learned information (e.g., a person's place of birth) is retained.

Inasmuch as memory is important for orientation to person, place, and time, orientation can be progressively affected during

Table 7.3–3
DSM-IV-TR Diagnostic Criteria for Dementia Due to Other General Medical Conditions

A. The development of multiple cognitive deficits manifested by both
   (1) memory impairment (impaired ability to learn new information or to recall previously learned information)
   (2) one (or more) of the following cognitive disturbances:
       (a) aphasia (language disturbance)
       (b) apraxia (impaired ability to carry out motor activities despite intact motor function)
       (c) agnosia (failure to recognize or identify objects despite intact sensory function)
       (d) disturbance in executive functioning (i.e., planning, organizing, sequencing, abstracting)
B. The cognitive deficits in Criteria A1 and A2 each cause significant impairment in social or occupational functioning and represent a significant decline from a previous level of functioning.
C. There is evidence from the history, physical examination, or laboratory findings that the disturbance is the direct physiological consequence of a general medical condition other than Alzheimer's disease or cerebrovascular disease (e.g., HIV infection, traumatic brain injury, Parkinson's disease, Huntington's disease, Pick's disease, Creutzfeldt-Jakob disease, normal-pressure hydrocephalus, hypothyroidism, brain tumor, or vitamin B_{12} deficiency).
D. The deficits do not occur exclusively during the course of a delirium.

Code based on presence or absence of a clinically significant behavioral disturbance:

Without behavioral disturbance: if the cognitive disturbance is not accompanied by any clinically significant behavioral disturbance.
With behavioral disturbance: if the cognitive disturbance is accompanied by a clinically significant behavioral disturbance (e.g., wandering, agitation).
Coding note: Also code the general medical condition on Axis III (e.g., HIV infection, head injury, Parkinson's disease, Huntington's disease, Pick's disease, Creutzfeldt-Jakob disease).

HIV, human immunodeficiency virus.
From American Psychiatric Association. *Diagnostic and Statistical Manual of Mental Disorders.* 4th ed. Text rev. Washington, DC: American Psychiatric Association; copyright 2000, with permission.

Table 7.3–4
DSM-IV-TR Diagnostic Criteria for Substance-Induced Persisting Dementia

A. The development of multiple cognitive deficits manifested by both
   (1) memory impairment (impaired ability to learn new information or to recall previously learned information)
   (2) one (or more) of the following cognitive disturbances:
       (a) aphasia (language disturbance)
       (b) apraxia (impaired ability to carry out motor activities despite intact motor function)
       (c) agnosia (failure to recognize or identify objects despite intact sensory function)
       (d) disturbance in executive functioning (i.e., planning, organizing, sequencing, abstracting)
B. The cognitive deficits in Criteria A1 and A2 each cause significant impairment in social or occupational functioning and represent a significant decline from a previous level of functioning.
C. The deficits do not occur exclusively during the course of a delirium and persist beyond the usual duration of substance intoxication or withdrawal.
D. There is evidence from the history, physical examination, or laboratory findings that the deficits are etiologically related to the persisting effects of substance use (e.g., a drug of abuse, a medication).

Code (Specific substance)-induced persisting dementia:
(Alcohol; Inhalant; Sedative, hypnotic, or anxiolytic; Other [or unknown] substance)

From American Psychiatric Association. *Diagnostic and Statistical Manual of Mental Disorders.* 4th ed. Text rev. Washington, DC: American Psychiatric Association; copyright 2000, with permission.

Table 7.3–5
DSM-IV-TR Diagnostic Criteria for Dementia Due to Multiple Etiologies

A. The development of multiple cognitive deficits manifested by both
   (1) memory impairment (impaired ability to learn new information or to recall previously learned information)
   (2) one (or more) of the following cognitive disturbances:
       (a) aphasia (language disturbance)
       (b) apraxia (impaired ability to carry out motor activities despite intact motor function)
       (c) agnosia (failure to recognize or identify objects despite intact sensory function)
       (d) disturbance in executive functioning (i.e., planning, organizing, sequencing, abstracting)
B. The cognitive deficits in Criteria A1 and A2 each cause significant impairment in social or occupational functioning and represent a significant decline from a previous level of functioning.
C. There is evidence from the history, physical examination, or laboratory findings that the disturbance has more than one etiology (e.g., head trauma plus chronic alcohol use, dementia of the Alzheimer's type with the subsequent development of vascular dementia).
D. The deficits do not occur exclusively during the course of a delirium.
Coding note: Use multiple codes based on specific dementias and specific etiologies, e.g., Dementia of the Alzheimer's type, with late onset, without behavioral disturbance; Vascular dementia, uncomplicated.

From American Psychiatric Association. *Diagnostic and Statistical Manual of Mental Disorders.* 4th ed. Text rev. Washington, DC: American Psychiatric Association; copyright 2000, with permission.

dementia who have paranoid delusions are generally hostile to family members and caretakers. Patients with frontal and temporal involvement are likely to have marked personality changes and may be irritable and explosive.

Hallucinations and Delusions. An estimated 20 to 30 percent of patients with dementia (primarily patients with dementia of the Alzheimer's type) have hallucinations, and 30 to 40 percent have delusions, primarily of a paranoid or persecutory and unsystematized nature, although complex, sustained, and well-systematized delusions are also reported by these patients. Physical aggression and other forms of violence are common in demented patients who also have psychotic symptoms.

Mood. In addition to psychosis and personality changes, depression and anxiety are major symptoms in an estimated 40 to 50 percent of patients with dementia, although the full syndrome of depressive disorder may be present in only 10 to 20 percent.

Table 7.3–6
DSM-IV-TR Diagnostic Criteria for Dementia Not Otherwise Specified

This category should be used to diagnose a dementia that does not meet criteria for any of the specific types described in this section.
An example is a clinical presentation of dementia for which there is insufficient evidence to establish a specific etiology.

From American Psychiatric Association. *Diagnostic and Statistical Manual of Mental Disorders.* 4th ed. Text rev. Washington, DC: American Psychiatric Association; copyright 2000, with permission.

Patients with dementia may also exhibit pathological laughter or crying—that is, extremes of emotions—with no apparent provocation.

Cognitive Change.   In addition to the aphasias in patients with dementia, apraxias and agnosias are common, and they are included as potential diagnostic criteria in DSM-IV-TR. Other neurological signs that can be associated with dementia are seizures, seen in approximately 10 percent of patients with dementia of the Alzheimer's type and in 20 percent of patients with vascular dementia, and atypical neurological presentations, such as nondominant parietal lobe syndromes. Primitive reflexes—such as the grasp, snout, suck, tonic-foot, and palmomental reflexes—may be present on neurological examination, and myoclonic jerks are present in 5 to 10 percent of patients.

Patients with vascular dementia may have additional neurological symptoms, such as headaches, dizziness, faintness, weakness, focal neurological signs, and sleep disturbances, possibly attributable to the location of the cerebrovascular disease. Pseudobulbar palsy, dysarthria, and dysphagia are also more common in vascular dementia than in other dementing conditions.

Catastrophic Reaction.   Patients with dementia also exhibit a reduced ability to apply what Kurt Goldstein called the "abstract attitude." Patients have difficulty generalizing from a single instance, forming concepts, and grasping similarities and differences among concepts. Furthermore, the ability to solve problems, to reason logically, and to make sound judgments is compromised. Goldstein also described a catastrophic reaction marked by agitation secondary to the subjective awareness of intellectual deficits under stressful circumstances. Persons usually attempt to compensate for defects by using strategies to avoid demonstrating failures in intellectual performance; they may change the subject, make jokes, or otherwise divert the interviewer. Lack of judgment and poor impulse control appear commonly, particularly in dementias that primarily affect the frontal lobes. Examples of these impairments include coarse language, inappropriate jokes, neglect of personal appearance and hygiene, and a general disregard for the conventional rules of social conduct.

Sundowner Syndrome.   Sundowner syndrome is characterized by drowsiness, confusion, ataxia, and accidental falls. It occurs in older people who are overly sedated and in patients with dementia who react adversely to even a small dose of a psychoactive drug. The syndrome also occurs in demented patients when external stimuli, such as light and interpersonal orienting cues, are diminished.

Dementia of the Alzheimer's Type

The DSM-IV-TR diagnostic criteria for dementia of the Alzheimer's type emphasize the presence of memory impairment and the associated presence of at least one other symptom of cognitive decline (aphasia, apraxia, agnosia, or abnormal executive functioning). The diagnostic criteria also require a continuing and gradual decline in functioning, impairment in social or occupational functioning, and the exclusion of other causes of dementia. According to DSM-IV-TR, the age of onset can be characterized as early (at age 65 years or younger) or late (after age 65 years), and any predominant behavioral symptom should be coded with the diagnosis, if appropriate.

A 61-year-old high school science department head, an experienced and enthusiastic camper and hiker, became extremely fearful while on a trek in the mountains. Gradually, over the next few months, he lost interest in his usual hobbies. Formerly a voracious reader, he stopped reading. He had difficulty doing computations and made gross errors in home financial management. On several occasions, he became lost while driving in areas that were formerly familiar to him. He began to write notes to himself so that he would not forget to do errands. Very abruptly, and in uncharacteristic fashion, he decided to retire from work, without discussing his plans with his wife. Intellectual deterioration gradually progressed. He spent most of the day piling miscellaneous objects in one place and then transporting them to another spot in the house. He became stubborn and querulous. Eventually, he required assistance in shaving and dressing.

When examined 6 years after the first symptoms had developed, the patient was alert and cooperative. He was disoriented with respect to place and time. He could not recall the names of four or five objects after a 5-minute interval of distraction. He could not remember the names of his college and graduate school or the subject in which he had majored. He could describe his job by title only. In 1978 he thought that Kennedy was president of the United States. He did not know Stalin's nationality. His speech was fluent and well articulated, but he had considerable difficulty finding words and used many long, essentially meaningless phrases. He called a cup a vase and identified the rims of his glasses as the "the holders." He did simple calculations poorly. He could not copy a cube or draw a house. His interpretation of proverbs was concrete, and he had no insight into the nature of his disturbance.

An elementary neurological examination revealed nothing abnormal, and routine laboratory tests were also negative. A computed tomography scan, however, showed marked cortical atrophy. (Reprinted with permission from *DSM-IV-TR Casebook.*)

Vascular Dementia

The general symptoms of vascular dementia are the same as those for dementia of the Alzheimer's type, but the diagnosis of vascular dementia requires either clinical or laboratory evidence in support of a vascular cause of the dementia. Vascular dementia

emotional support for the patients and their families, and pharmacological treatment for specific symptoms, including disruptive behavior.

Psychosocial Therapies

The deterioration of mental faculties has significant psychological meaning for patients with dementia. The experience of a sense of continuity over time depends on memory. Recent memory is lost before remote memory in most cases of dementia, and many patients are highly distressed by clearly recalling how they used to function while observing their obvious deterioration. At the most fundamental level, the self is a product of brain functioning. Patients' identities begin to fade as the illness progresses, and they can recall less and less of their past. Emotional reactions ranging from depression to severe anxiety to catastrophic terror can stem from the realization that the sense of self is disappearing.

Patients often benefit from a supportive and educational psychotherapy in which the nature and course of their illness are clearly explained. They may also benefit from assistance in grieving and accepting the extent of their disability and from attention to self-esteem issues. Any areas of intact functioning should be maximized by helping patients identify activities in which successful functioning is possible. A psychodynamic assessment of defective ego functions and cognitive limitations can also be useful. Clinicians can help patients find ways to deal with the defective ego functions, such as keeping calendars for orientation problems, making schedules to help structure activities, and taking notes for memory problems.

Psychodynamic interventions with family members of patients with dementia may be of great assistance. Those who take care of a patient struggle with feelings of guilt, grief, anger, and exhaustion as they watch a family member gradually deteriorate. A common problem that develops among caregivers involves their self-sacrifice in caring for a patient. The gradually developing resentment from this self-sacrifice is often suppressed because of the guilt feelings it produces. Clinicians can help caregivers understand the complex mixture of feelings associated with seeing a loved one decline and can provide understanding as well as permission to express these feelings. Clinicians must also be aware of the caregivers' tendencies to blame themselves or others for patients' illnesses and must appreciate the role that patients with dementia play in the lives of family members.

Pharmacotherapy

Clinicians may prescribe benzodiazepines for insomnia and anxiety, antidepressants for depression, and antipsychotic drugs for delusions and hallucinations, but they should be aware of possible idiosyncratic drug effects in older people (e.g., paradoxical excitement, confusion, and increased sedation). In general, drugs with high anticholinergic activity should be avoided.

Donepezil (Aricept), rivastigmine (Exelon), galantamine (Remiryl), and tacrine (Cognex) are cholinesterase inhibitors used to treat mild to moderate cognitive impairment in Alzheimer's disease. They reduce the inactivation of the neurotransmitter acetylcholine and, thus, potentiate the cholinergic neurotransmitter, which in turn produces a modest improvement in memory and goal-directed thought. These drugs are most useful for persons with mild to moderate memory loss who have sufficient preservation of their basal forebrain cholinergic neurons to benefit from augmentation of cholinergic neurotransmission.

Donepezil is well tolerated and widely used. Tacrine is rarely used because of its potential for hepatotoxicity. Fewer clinical data are available for rivastigmine and galantamine, which appear more likely to cause gastrointestinal and neuropsychiatric adverse effects than does donepezil. None of these medications prevents the progressive neuronal degeneration of the disorder. Prescribing information for anticholinesterase inhibitors can be found in Section 32.14.

Memantine (Namenda) protects neurons from excessive amounts of glutamate, which may be neurotoxic. The drug is sometimes combined with donepezil. It has been known to improve dementia.

Other Treatment Approaches. Other drugs that are being tested for cognitive-enhancing activity include general cerebral metabolic enhancers, calcium channel inhibitors, and serotonergic agents. Some studies have shown that selegiline (Eldepryl), a selective type B monoamine oxidase (MAO_B) inhibitor, may slow the advance of this disease. Ondansetron (Zofran), a 5-HT_3 receptor antagonist, is under investigation.

Estrogen replacement therapy may reduce the risk of cognitive decline in postmenopausal women; however, more studies are needed to confirm this effect. Complementary and alternative medicine studies of ginkgo biloba and other phytomedicinals are being studied to see if they have a positive effect on cognition. Reports have appeared of patients using nonsteroidal antiinflammatory agents having a lower risk of developing Alzheimer's disease. Vitamin E has not been shown to be of value in preventing the disease.

▲ 7.4 Amnestic Disorders

The amnestic disorders are a broad category that includes a variety of diseases and conditions that present with an amnestic syndrome. The syndrome is defined primarily by impairment in the ability to create new memories. Three variations of the amnestic disorder diagnosis, differing in etiology, are offered: amnestic disorder due to a general medical condition (such as head trauma), substance-induced persisting amnestic disorder (such as that due to carbon monoxide poisoning or chronic alcohol consumption), and amnestic disorder not otherwise specified for cases in which the etiology is unclear. There are two modifiers: (1) transient, for duration less than 1 month, and (2) chronic, for conditions extending beyond 1 month.

EPIDEMIOLOGY

No adequate studies have reported on the incidence or prevalence of amnestic disorders. Amnesia is most commonly found in alcohol use disorders and in head injury. In general practice and hospital settings, the frequency of amnesia related to chronic alcohol abuse has decreased, and the frequency of amnesia related to head trauma has increased.

ETIOLOGY

The major neuroanatomical structures involved in memory and in the development of an amnestic disorder are particular diencephalic structures such as the dorsomedial and midline nuclei of the thalamus and midtemporal lobe structures such as the hippocampus, the mamillary bodies, and the amygdala. Although amnesia is usually the result of bilateral damage to these structures, some cases of unilateral damage result in an amnestic disorder, and evidence indicates that the left hemisphere may be more critical than the right hemisphere in the development of memory disorders. Many studies of memory and amnesia in animals have suggested that other brain areas may also be involved in the symptoms accompanying amnesia. Frontal lobe involvement can result in such symptoms as confabulation and apathy, which can be seen in patients with amnestic disorders.

Amnestic disorders have many potential causes. Thiamine deficiency, hypoglycemia, hypoxia (including carbon monoxide poisoning), and herpes simplex encephalitis all have a predilection to damage the temporal lobes, particularly the hippocampi, and thus can be associated with the development of amnestic disorders. Similarly, when tumors, cerebrovascular diseases, surgical procedures, or multiple sclerosis plaques involve the diencephalic or temporal regions of the brain, the symptoms of an amnestic disorder may develop. General insults to the brain, such as seizures, electroconvulsive therapy (ECT), and head trauma, can also result in memory impairment. Transient global amnesia is presumed to be a cerebrovascular disorder involving transient impairment in blood flow through the vertebrobasilar arteries.

Many drugs have been associated with the development of amnesia, and clinicians should review all drugs taken, including nonprescription drugs, in the diagnostic workup of a patient with amnesia. The benzodiazepines are the most commonly used prescription drugs associated with amnesia. All benzodiazepines can be associated with amnesia, especially if combined with alcohol. When triazolam (Halcion) is used in doses of 0.25 mg or less, which are generally equivalent to standard doses of other benzodiazepines, amnesia is no more often associated with triazolam than with other benzodiazepines. With alcohol and higher doses, anterograde amnesia has been reported.

DIAGNOSIS

For the diagnosis of amnestic disorder, the text revision of the fourth edition of *Diagnostic and Statistical Manual of Mental Disorders* (DSM-IV-TR) requires the "development of memory impairment as manifested by impairment in the ability to learn new information or the inability to recall previously learned information," and the "memory disturbance [must cause] ... significant impairment in social or occupational functioning." A diagnosis of amnestic disorder due to a general medical condition (Table 7.4–1) is made when evidence exists of a causatively relevant specific medical condition (including physical trauma). DSM-IV-TR further categorizes the diagnosis as transient or chronic. A diagnosis of substance-induced persisting amnestic disorder is made when evidence suggests that the symptoms are causatively related to the use of a substance (Table 7.4–2). DSM-IV-TR refers clinicians to specific diagnoses within substance-related disorders: alcohol-induced persisting amnestic disorder; sedative, hypnotic, or anxiolytic-induced persisting

Table 7.4–1
DSM-IV-TR Diagnostic Criteria for Amnestic Disorder Due to a General Medical Condition

A. The development of memory impairment as manifested by impairment in the ability to learn new information or the inability to recall previously learned information.
B. The memory disturbance causes significant impairment in social or occupational functioning and represents a significant decline from a previous level of functioning.
C. The memory disturbance does not occur exclusively during the course of a delirium or a dementia.
D. There is evidence from the history, physical examination, or laboratory findings that the disturbance is the direct physiological consequence of a general medical condition (including physical trauma).

Specify if:
Transient: if memory impairment lasts for 1 month or less
Chronic: if memory impairment lasts for more than 1 month
Coding note: Include the name of the general medical condition on Axis I, e.g., Amnestic disorder due to head trauma; also code the general medical condition on Axis III.

From American Psychiatric Association. *Diagnostic and Statistical Manual of Mental Disorders.* 4th ed. Text rev. Washington, DC: American Psychiatric Association; copyright 2000, with permission.

amnestic disorder; and other (or unknown) substance-induced persisting amnestic disorder. DSM-IV-TR also provides the diagnosis of amnestic disorder not otherwise specified (Table 7.4–3).

CLINICAL FEATURES AND SUBTYPES

The central symptom of amnestic disorders is the development of a memory disorder characterized by impairment in the ability to learn new information (anterograde amnesia) and the inability to recall previously remembered knowledge (retrograde amnesia). The symptom must result in significant problems for patients in their social or occupational functioning. The time in which a patient is amnestic can begin directly at the point of trauma or include a period before the trauma. Memory for the time during

Table 7.4–2
DSM-IV-TR Diagnostic Criteria for Substance-Induced Persisting Amnestic Disorder

A. The development of memory impairment as manifested by impairment in the ability to learn new information or the inability to recall previously learned information.
B. The memory disturbance causes significant impairment in social or occupational functioning and represents a significant decline from a previous level of functioning.
C. The memory disturbance does not occur exclusively during the course of a delirium or a dementia and persists beyond the usual duration of substance intoxication or withdrawal.
D. There is evidence from the history, physical examination, or laboratory findings that the memory disturbance is etiologically related to the persisting effects of substance use (e.g., a drug of abuse, a medication).

Code (Specific substance)-induced persisting amnestic disorder:

(Alcohol; Sedative, hypnotic, or anxiolytic; Other [or unknown] substance)

From American Psychiatric Association. *Diagnostic and Statistical Manual of Mental Disorders.* 4th ed. Text rev. Washington, DC: American Psychiatric Association; copyright 2000, with permission.

Table 7.4–3
DSM-IV-TR Diagnostic Criteria for Amnestic Disorder Not Otherwise Specified

This category should be used to diagnose an amnestic disorder that does not meet criteria for any of the specific types described in this section.

An example is a clinical presentation of amnesia for which there is insufficient evidence to establish a specific etiology (i.e., dissociative, substance induced, or due to a general medical condition).

From American Psychiatric Association. *Diagnostic and Statistical Manual of Mental Disorders.* 4th ed. Text rev. Washington, DC: American Psychiatric Association; copyright 2000, with permission.

the physical insult (e.g., during a cerebrovascular event) may also be lost.

Short-term and recent memory are usually impaired. Patients cannot remember what they had for breakfast or lunch, the name of the hospital, or their doctors. In some patients, the amnesia is so profound that the patient cannot orient himself or herself to city and time, although orientation to person is seldom lost in amnestic disorders. Memory for overlearned information or events from the remote past, such as childhood experiences, is good; but memory for events from the less remote past (over the past decade) is impaired. Immediate memory (tested, for example, by asking a patient to repeat six numbers) remains intact. With improvement, patients may experience a gradual shrinking of the time for which memory has been lost, although some patients experience a gradual improvement in memory for the entire period.

The onset of symptoms can be sudden, as in trauma, cerebrovascular events, and neurotoxic chemical assaults, or gradual, as in nutritional deficiency and cerebral tumors. The amnesia can be of short duration (specified by DSM-IV-TR as transient if lasting 1 month or less) or of long duration (specified by DSM-IV-TR as persistent if lasting more than 1 month).

A variety of other symptoms can be associated with amnestic disorders. For patients with other cognitive impairments, a diagnosis of dementia or delirium is more appropriate than a diagnosis of an amnestic disorder. Both subtle and gross changes in personality can accompany the symptoms of memory impairment in amnestic disorders. Patients may be apathetic, lack initiative, have unprovoked episodes of agitation, or appear to be overly friendly or agreeable. Patients with amnestic disorders can also appear bewildered and confused and may attempt to cover their confusion with confabulatory answers to questions. Characteristically, patients with amnestic disorders do not have good insight into their neuropsychiatric conditions.

A 73-year-old survivor of the Holocaust was admitted to the psychiatric unit from a local nursing home. She was born in Germany to a middle-class family. Her education was truncated due to internment in a concentration camp. She immigrated to Israel after liberation from the concentration camp and later to the United States, where she married and raised a family. Premorbidly, she was described as a quiet, intelligent, and loving woman who spoke several languages. At 55 years of age, she had a significant carbon monoxide exposure when a gas line leaked while she and her husband

slept. Her husband died of carbon monoxide poisoning, but the patient survived after a period of coma. Once stabilized, she displayed significant cognitive and behavioral problems. She had difficulty with learning new information and making appropriate plans. She retained the abilities to perform activities of daily living but could not be relied on to pay bills, buy food, cook, or clean, despite appearing to have retained the intellectual ability to do these tasks. She was admitted to a nursing home after several difficult years at home or in the homes of relatives. In the nursing home, she was able to learn her way about the facility. She displayed little interest in scheduled group activities, hobbies, reading, or television. She had frequent behavioral problems. She repeatedly pressed staff to get her sweets and snacks and cursed them vociferously with racial epithets and disparaging comments on their weight and dress. On one occasion, she scratched the cars of several staff with a key. Neuropsychological testing demonstrated severe deficits in delayed recall, intact performance on language and general knowledge measures, and moderate deficits on domains of executive function, such as concept formation and cognitive flexibility. She was noted to respond immediately to firmly set limits and rewards, but deficits in memory prevented long-term incorporation of these boundaries. Management involved development of a behavioral plan that could be implemented at the nursing home and empirical trials of medications aimed at amelioration of irritability. (Courtesy of Hillel Grossman, M.D.)

Cerebrovascular Diseases

Cerebrovascular diseases affecting the hippocampus involve the posterior cerebral and basilar arteries and their branches. Infarctions are rarely limited to the hippocampus; they often involve the occipital or parietal lobes. Thus, common accompanying symptoms of cerebrovascular diseases in this region are focal neurological signs involving vision or sensory modalities. Cerebrovascular diseases affecting the bilateral medial thalamus, particularly the anterior portions, are often associated with symptoms of amnestic disorders. A few case studies report amnestic disorders from rupture of an aneurysm of the anterior communicating artery, resulting in infarction of the basal forebrain region.

Multiple Sclerosis

The pathophysiological process of multiple sclerosis involves the seemingly random formation of plaques within the brain parenchyma. When the plaques occur in the temporal lobe and the diencephalic regions, symptoms of memory impairment can occur. In fact, the most common cognitive complaints in patients with multiple sclerosis involve impaired memory, which occurs in 40 to 60 percent of patients. Characteristically, digit span memory is normal, but immediate recall and delayed recall of information are impaired. The memory impairment can affect both verbal and nonverbal material.

Korsakoff's Syndrome

Korsakoff's syndrome is an amnestic syndrome caused by thiamine deficiency, most commonly associated with the poor nutritional habits of people with chronic alcohol abuse. Other causes of poor nutrition (e.g., starvation), gastric carcinoma, hemodialysis, hyperemesis gravidarum, prolonged intravenous hyperalimentation, and gastric plication can also result in thiamine deficiency. Korsakoff's syndrome is often associated with Wernicke's encephalopathy, which is the associated syndrome of confusion, ataxia, and ophthalmoplegia. In patients with these thiamine deficiency–related symptoms, the neuropathological findings include hyperplasia of the small blood vessels with occasional hemorrhages, hypertrophy of astrocytes, and subtle changes in neuronal axons. Although the delirium clears up within a month or so, the amnestic syndrome either accompanies or follows untreated Wernicke's encephalopathy in approximately 85 percent of all cases.

Patients with Korsakoff's syndrome typically demonstrate a change in personality as well, such that they display a lack of initiative, diminished spontaneity, and a lack of interest or concern. These changes appear frontal lobe–like, similar to the personality change ascribed to patients with frontal lobe lesions or degeneration. Indeed, such patients often demonstrate *executive function* deficits on neuropsychological tasks involving attention, planning, set shifting, and inferential reasoning consistent with frontal pattern injuries. For this reason, Korsakoff's syndrome is not a pure memory disorder, although it certainly is a good paradigm of the more common clinical presentations for the amnestic syndrome.

The onset of Korsakoff's syndrome can be gradual. Recent memory tends to be affected more than is remote memory, but this feature is variable. Confabulation, apathy, and passivity are often prominent symptoms in the syndrome. With treatment, patients may remain amnestic for up to 3 months and then gradually improve over the ensuing year. Administration of thiamine may prevent the development of additional amnestic symptoms, but the treatment seldom reverses severe amnestic symptoms once they are present. Approximately one third to one fourth of all patients recover completely, and approximately one fourth of all patients have no improvement of their symptoms.

Alcoholic Blackouts

Some persons with severe alcohol abuse may exhibit the syndrome commonly referred to as an alcoholic blackout. Characteristically, these persons awake in the morning with a conscious awareness of being unable to remember a period the night before during which they were intoxicated. Sometimes, specific behaviors (hiding money in a secret place and provoking fights) are associated with the blackouts.

Electroconvulsive Therapy

ECT treatments are usually associated with retrograde amnesia for a period of several minutes before the treatment and anterograde amnesia after the treatment. The anterograde amnesia usually resolves within 5 hours. Mild memory deficits may remain for 1 to 2 months after a course of ECT treatments, but the symptoms are completely resolved 6 to 9 months after treatment.

Head Injury

Head injuries (both closed and penetrating) can result in a wide range of neuropsychiatric symptoms, including dementia, depression, personality changes, and amnestic disorders. Amnestic disorders caused by head injuries are commonly associated with a period of retrograde amnesia leading up to the traumatic incident and amnesia for the traumatic incident itself. The severity of the brain injury correlates somewhat with the duration and severity of the amnestic syndrome, but the best correlate of eventual improvement is the degree of clinical improvement in the amnesia during the first week after the patient regains consciousness.

Transient Global Amnesia

Transient global amnesia is characterized by the abrupt loss of the ability to recall recent events or to remember new information. The syndrome is often characterized by mild confusion and a lack of insight into the problem, a clear sensorium, and, occasionally, the inability to perform some well-learned complex tasks. Episodes last from 6 to 24 hours. Studies suggest that transient global amnesia occurs in 5 to 10 cases per 100,000 persons per year, although for patients older than age 50 years, the rate may be as high as 30 cases per 100,000 persons per year. The pathophysiology is unknown, but it likely involves ischemia of the temporal lobe and the diencephalic brain regions. Several studies of patients with single photon emission computed tomography (SPECT) have shown decreased blood flow in the temporal and parietotemporal regions, particularly in the left hemisphere. Patients with transient global amnesia almost universally experience complete improvement, although one study found that approximately 20 percent of patients may have recurrence of the episode, and another study found that approximately 7 percent of patients may have epilepsy. Patients with transient global amnesia have been differentiated from patients with transient ischemic attacks in that fewer of the former patients have diabetes, hypercholesterolemia, and hypertriglyceridemia but more have hypertension and migrainous episodes.

PATHOLOGY AND LABORATORY EXAMINATION

Laboratory findings diagnostic of amnestic disorder may be obtained using quantitative neuropsychological testing. Standardized tests also are available to assess recall of well-known historical events or public figures to characterize an individual's inability to remember previously learned information. Performance on such tests varies among individuals with amnestic disorder. Subtle deficits in other cognitive functions may be noted in individuals with amnestic disorder. Memory deficits, however, constitute the predominant feature of the mental status examination and account largely for any functional deficits. No specific or diagnostic features are detectable on imaging studies such as magnetic resonance imaging (MRI) or computed tomography (CT). Damage of midtemporal lobe structures is common, however, and may be reflected in enlargement of third ventricle or temporal horns or in structural atrophy detected by MRI.

DIFFERENTIAL DIAGNOSIS

To make the diagnosis, clinicians must obtain a patient's history, conduct a complete physical examination, and order all appropriate laboratory tests. Other diagnoses, however, can be confused with the amnestic disorders.

Dementia and Delirium

Amnestic disorders can be distinguished from delirium because they occur in the absence of a disturbance of consciousness and are striking for the relative preservation of other cognitive domains.

Both Alzheimer's dementia and the amnestic disorders can have an insidious onset with slow progression, as in a Korsakoff's psychosis in a chronic drinker. Amnestic disorders, however, can also develop precipitously, as in Wernicke's encephalopathy, transient global amnesia, or anoxic insults. Although Alzheimer's dementia progresses relentlessly, amnestic disorders tend to remain static or even improve once the offending cause has been removed. In terms of the actual memory deficits, the amnestic disorder and Alzheimer's disease still differ. Alzheimer's disease has an impact on retrieval, in addition to encoding and consolidation. The deficits in Alzheimer's disease extend beyond memory to general knowledge (semantic memory), language, praxis, and general function. These are spared in amnestic disorders. The dementias associated with Parkinson's disease, acquired immune deficiency syndrome (AIDS), and other subcortical disorders demonstrate disproportionate impairment of retrieval but relatively intact encoding and consolidation and, thus, can be distinguished from amnestic disorders. The subcortical pattern dementias are also likely to display motor symptoms, such as bradykinesia, chorea, or tremor, that are not components of the amnestic disorders.

Normal Aging

Some minor impairment in memory may accompany normal aging, but the DSM-IV-TR requirement that the memory impairment cause significant impairment in social or occupational functioning should exclude normal aging from the diagnosis.

Dissociative Disorders

The dissociative disorders can sometimes be difficult to differentiate from the amnestic disorders. Patients with dissociative disorders, however, are more likely to have lost their orientation to self and may have more selective memory deficits than do patients with amnestic disorders. For example, patients with dissociative disorders may not know their names or home addresses, but they are still able to learn new information and remember selected past memories. Dissociative disorders are also often associated with emotionally stressful life events involving money, the legal system, or troubled relationships.

Factitious Disorders

Patients with factitious disorders who are mimicking an amnestic disorder often have inconsistent results on memory tests and have no evidence of an identifiable cause. These findings, coupled with evidence of primary or secondary gain for a patient, should suggest a factitious disorder.

COURSE AND PROGNOSIS

The course of an amnestic disorder depends on its etiology and treatment, particularly acute treatment. Generally, the amnestic disorder has a static course. Little improvement is seen over time, but also no progression of the disorder occurs. The exceptions are the acute amnesias, such as transient global amnesia, which resolves entirely over hours to days, and the amnestic disorder associated with head trauma, which improves steadily in the months subsequent to the trauma. Amnesia secondary to processes that destroy brain tissue, such as stroke, tumor, and infection, are irreversible, although, again, static, once the acute infection or ischemia has been staunched.

TREATMENT

The primary approach to treating amnestic disorders is to treat the underlying cause. Although a patient is amnestic, supportive prompts about the date, the time, and the patient's location can be helpful and can reduce the patient's anxiety. After resolution of the amnestic episode, psychotherapy of some type (cognitive, psychodynamic, or supportive) may help patients incorporate the amnestic experience into their lives.

Psychotherapy

Psychodynamic interventions may be of considerable value for patients who have amnestic disorders that result from insults to the brain. Understanding the course of recovery in such patients helps clinicians to be sensitive to the narcissistic injury inherent in damage to the central nervous system.

The first phase of recovery, in which patients are incapable of processing what happened because the ego defenses are overwhelmed, requires clinicians to serve as a supportive auxiliary ego who explains to a patient what is happening and provides missing ego functions. In the second phase of recovery, as the realization of the injury sets in, patients may become angry and feel victimized by the malevolent hand of fate. They may view others, including the clinician, as bad or destructive, and clinicians must contain these projections without becoming punitive or retaliatory. Clinicians can build a therapeutic alliance with patients by explaining slowly and clearly what happened and by offering an explanation for a patient's internal experience. The third phase of recovery is integrative. As a patient accepts what happened, a clinician can help the patient form a new identity by connecting current experiences of the self with past experiences. Grieving over the lost faculties may be an important feature of the third phase.

Most patients who are amnestic because of brain injury engage in denial. Clinicians must respect and empathize with the patient's need to deny the reality of what has happened. Insensitive and blunt confrontations destroy any developing therapeutic alliance and can cause patients to feel attacked. In a sensitive approach, clinicians help patients accept their cognitive limitations by exposing them to these deficits bit by bit over time. When patients fully accept what has happened, they may need assistance in forgiving themselves and any others involved so that they can get on with their lives. Clinicians must also be wary of being seduced into thinking that all of the patient's symptoms are directly related to the brain insult. An evaluation of preexisting personality disorders, such as borderline, antisocial, and narcissistic personality disorders, must be part of the overall assessment; many patients with personality disorders place themselves in situations that predispose them to injuries. These personality features may become a crucial part of the psychodynamic psychotherapy.

Recently, centers for cognitive rehabilitation have been established whose rehabilitation-oriented therapeutic milieu is intended to promote recovery from brain injury, especially that from traumatic causes. Despite the high cost of extended care at these sites, which provide both long-term institutional and daytime services, no data have been developed to define therapeutic effectiveness for the heterogeneous groups of patients who participate in such tasks as memory retaining.

▲ 7.5 Mental Disorders Due to a General Medical Condition

Increasingly, scientific views of mental illness recognize that, whether caused by an identifiable anomaly (e.g., brain tumor), a neurotransmitter disturbance of unclear origin (e.g., schizophrenia), or a consequence of deranged upbringing or environment (e.g., personality disorder), all mental disorders ultimately share one common underlying theme: aberration in brain function. Treatments for those conditions, whether psychological or biological, attempt to restore normal brain chemistry. The differential diagnosis for a mental syndrome in a patient should always include consideration of (1) any general medical condition that a patient may have and (2) any prescription, nonprescription, or illegal substances that a patient may be taking. Although some specific medical conditions have classically been associated with mental syndromes, a much larger number of general medical conditions have been associated with mental syndromes in case reports and small studies.

In the text revision of the fourth edition of *Diagnostic and Statistical Manual of Mental Disorders* (DSM-IV-TR), each mental disorder due to a general medical condition is classified within the category that most resembles the symptoms. For example, the diagnosis of psychotic disorder due to general medical condition is found in the DSM-IV-TR section on schizophrenia and other psychotic disorders. A clinician evaluating a patient with depression can refer to the DSM-IV-TR section on mood disorders and find mood disorder due to a general medical condition as one of the diagnoses.

MOOD DISORDER DUE TO A GENERAL MEDICAL CONDITION

Mood disorders, particularly depression, accompany a range of medical problems. Also known as *secondary mood disorders*, these conditions are characterized by a prominent mood alteration thought to be the direct physiological effect of a specific medical illness or agent. These disorders are often difficult to define and have not been extensively researched; however, the key feature is prominent, persistent, distressing, or functionally impairing depressed mood (anhedonia) or elevated, expansive, or irritable mood, judged to be caused either by medical or surgical illness or by substance intoxication or withdrawal. Cognitive impairment is not the predominant clinical feature; otherwise, the mood disturbance would be viewed as part of delirium, dementia, or other cognitive deficit disorder. The diagnostician is asked to specify if the mood syndrome is manic, depressed, or mixed and if criteria for a fully symptomatic major depressive or manic syndrome are fulfilled.

Epidemiology

Mood disorder due to a general medical condition, with depressive features, appears to affect men and women equally, in contrast to major depressive disorder, which predominates in women. As much as 50 percent of all poststroke patients experience depressive illness. A similar prevalence pertains to individuals with pancreatic cancer. Forty percent of patients with Parkinson's disease are depressed. Major and minor depressive episodes are common after certain illnesses such as Huntington's disease, human immunodeficiency virus (HIV) infection, and multiple sclerosis (MS). Secondary mania is less prevalent in neurological disease than is depression; however, many experienced clinicians report a high rate of euphoria in patients with MS. Depressive disorders associated with terminal or painful conditions carry the greatest risk of suicide.

Diagnosis and Clinical Features

Patients with depression may experience psychological symptoms (e.g., sad mood, lack of pleasure or interest in usual activities, tearfulness, concentration disturbance, and suicidal ideation) or somatic symptoms (e.g., fatigue, sleep disturbance, and appetite disturbance), or both psychological and somatic symptoms. Diagnosis in the medically ill can be confounded by the presence of somatic symptoms related purely to medical illness, not to depression. In an effort to overcome the underdiagnosis of depression in the medically ill, most practitioners favor including somatic symptoms in identifying mood syndromes.

The DSM-IV-TR provides diagnostic criteria for mood disorder due to a general medical condition *with (1) depressive features, (2) major depressive–like episode, (3) manic features*, or *(4) mixed features*. In general, these criteria are less strict than for corresponding primary mood disorders. The subtype *with major depressive–like episode* is not available for substance-induced mood disorder (Table 7.5–1).

> A 45-year-old toy designer was admitted to the hospital after a series of suicidal gestures culminating in an attempt to strangle himself with a piece of wire. Four months before admission, his family had observed that he was becoming depressed: when at home, he spent long periods sitting in a chair; he slept more than usual; and he had given up his habits of reading the evening paper and puttering around the house. Within 1 month, he was unable to get out of bed in the morning to go to work. He expressed considerable guilt but could not make up his mind to seek help until forced to do so by his family. He had not responded to 2 months of outpatient antidepressant drug therapy and had made several half-hearted attempts to cut his wrists before the serious attempt that precipitated the admission.
>
> Physical examination revealed signs of increased intracranial pressure, and a computed tomography (CT) scan showed a large frontal-lobe tumor. (Reprinted with permission from *DSM-IV-TR Casebook.*)

Differential Diagnosis

Mood changes occurring during the course of delirium are acute and fluctuating and should be attributed to that disorder, not to mood disorder due to a general medical condition or to substance-induced mood disorder. Pain syndromes can depress mood, but do so through psychological, not physiological means, and may appropriately lead to a diagnosis of primary mood disorder. In the medically ill, somatic complaints, such as sleep disturbance,

Table 7.5–1
DSM-IV-TR Criteria for Mood Disorder Due to a General Medical Condition

A. A prominent and persistent disturbance in mood predominates in the clinical picture and is characterized by either (or both) of the following:
   (1) Depressed mood or markedly diminished pleasure in all, or almost all, activities
   (2) Elevated, expansive, or irritable mood.
B. There is evidence from the history, physical examination, or laboratory findings that the disturbance is the direct physiological consequence of a general medical condition.
C. The disturbance is not better accounted for by another mental disorder (e.g., adjustment disorder with depressed mood in response to the stress of having a general medical condition).
D. The disturbance does not occur exclusively during the course of a delirium.
E. The symptoms cause clinically significant distress or impairment in social, occupational, or other important areas of functioning.

Specify:
With depressive features: if the predominant mood is depressed, but the full criteria are not met for a major depressive disorder
With major depressive–like episode: if all criteria for major depressive episode are met, except, clearly, for the criterion that the symptoms are not due to the physiological effects of a substance or a general medical condition
With manic features: if the predominant mood is elevated, euphoric, or irritable
With mixed features: if the symptoms of mania and depression are present, but neither predominates

From American Psychiatric Association. *Diagnostic and Statistical Manual of Mental Disorders.* 4th ed. Text rev. Washington, DC; American Psychiatric Association; 2000, with permission.

anorexia, and fatigue, may be counted toward a diagnosis of major depressive episode or mood disorder due to a general medical condition, unless those complaints are purely attributable to the medical illness.

Mood disorder due to a general medical condition can be distinguished from substance-induced mood disorder by examination of time course of symptoms, response to correction of suspect medical conditions or discontinuation of substances, and, occasionally, urine or blood toxicology results.

Course and Prognosis

The course of mood disorder due to a general medical condition largely depends on the course of the underlying medical state, as well as the extent of concurrent psychiatric intervention. Similar considerations apply to substance-induced mood disorder. Prognosis for mood symptoms is best when etiological medical illnesses or medications are most susceptible to correction (e.g., treatment of hypothyroidism and cessation of alcohol use).

When such intervention is not possible (e.g., halting immunosuppressant use in an individual after kidney transplant) or fails to lead to prompt remission of mood symptoms, formal psychiatric treatment is indicated.

Treatment

Standard antidepressant medications, including tricyclic drugs, monoamine oxidase inhibitors (MAOIs), selective serotonin re-

uptake inhibitors (SSRIs), and psychostimulants, are effective in many depressed patients with medical and neurological illnesses or substance use disorders. Electroconvulsive therapy (ECT) may be useful in patients who do not respond to medication.

The clinician treating a patient with a secondary mood disorder should treat the underlying medical cause as effectively as possible. Standard treatment approaches for the corresponding primary mood disorder should be used, although the risk of toxic effects from psychotropic drugs may require more gradual dose increases. At a minimum, psychotherapy should focus on psychoeducational issues. The concept of a behavioral disturbance secondary to medical illness may be new or difficult for many patients and families to understand. Specific intrapsychic, interpersonal, and family issues are addressed as indicated in psychotherapy.

PSYCHOTIC DISORDER DUE TO A GENERAL MEDICAL CONDITION

To establish the diagnosis of psychotic disorder due to a general medical condition, the clinician first must exclude syndromes in which psychotic symptoms may be present in association with cognitive impairment (e.g., delirium and dementia of the Alzheimer's type). Disorders in this category are not associated usually with changes in the sensorium.

Epidemiology

The incidence and prevalence of secondary psychotic disorders in the general population are unknown. As much as 40 percent of individuals with temporal lobe epilepsy experience psychosis. The prevalence of psychotic symptoms is increased in selected clinical populations, such as nursing home residents, but it is unclear how to extrapolate these findings to other patient groups.

Etiology

Virtually any cerebral or systemic disease that affects brain function can produce psychotic symptoms. Degenerative disorders, such as Alzheimer's disease or Huntington's disease, can present initially with new-onset psychosis, with minimal evidence of cognitive impairment at the earliest stages.

Diagnosis and Clinical Features

Two DSM-IV-TR subtypes exist for psychotic disorder due to a general medical condition: *with delusions*, to be used if the predominant psychotic symptoms are delusional, and *with hallucinations*, to be used if hallucinations of any form comprise the primary psychotic symptoms (Table 7.5–2).

To establish the diagnosis of a secondary psychotic syndrome, the clinician first determines that the patient is not delirious, as evidenced by a stable level of consciousness. A careful mental status assessment is conducted to exclude significant cognitive impairments, such as those encountered in dementia or amnestic disorder. The next step is to search for systemic or cerebral diseases that might be causally related to the psychosis.

Table 7.5–2
DSM-IV-TR Criteria for Psychotic Disorder Due to a General Medical Condition

A. Prominent hallucinations or delusions.
B. There is evidence from the history, physical examination, or laboratory findings that the disturbance is the direct physiological consequence of a general medical condition.
C. The disturbance is not better accounted for by another mental disorder.
D. The disturbance does not occur exclusively during the course of a delirium.

Specify:
With delusions, if delusions are the predominant symptom
With hallucinations, if hallucinations are the predominant symptom

From American Psychiatric Association. *Diagnostic and Statistical Manual of Mental Disorders.* 4th ed. Text rev. Washington, DC; American Psychiatric Association; 2000, with permission.

Psychotic symptomatology per se is not helpful in distinguishing a secondary from a primary (idiopathic) cause.

A systematic physical and neurological examination should be performed. The examiner should bear in mind, however, that nonlocalizing, soft neurological signs and a variety of dyskinesias can be present in schizophrenia. An evaluation with magnetic resonance imaging (MRI) for any new-onset psychosis is recommended, irrespective of patient age. The detection of a systemic or cerebral abnormality (e.g., a brain tumor) may lead to the determination of secondary psychosis; however, establishing a diagnosis of secondary psychotic syndrome requires thoughtful clinical reasoning.

Differential Diagnosis

Primary psychotic disorders, such as schizophrenia, and primary mood disorders with psychotic features may present with symptoms identical or similar to psychotic disorder due to a general medical condition; however, in primary disorders, no medical or substance cause is identifiable, despite laboratory workup. Delirium may present with psychotic symptoms, but, in contrast to psychotic disorder due to a general medical condition, delirium-related psychosis is acute and fluctuating, commonly associated with disturbance in consciousness and cognitive defects. Psychosis resulting from dementia may be diagnosed as psychotic disorder due to a general medical condition, except in the case of vascular dementia, which, according to the International Classification of Disease (ICD) coding requirements, should be diagnosed as vascular dementia with delusions.

Unique characteristics may assist in differentiating primary from induced psychoses. Most cases of nonauditory hallucinosis are due to medical conditions, substances, or both. The converse is not true: Auditory hallucinations can occur in primary and induced psychoses. Stimulant (e.g., amphetamine and cocaine) intoxication psychosis may involve a perception of bugs crawling under the skin (formication). Temporal lobe epilepsy often is associated with olfactory hallucinations and religious delusions. Right parietal lobe lesions can induce a contralateral neglect state of delusional nature in which individuals disown parts of their bodies. Occipital lesions, whether caused by tumor or cerebrovascular accident, can produce visual hallucinations.

When the clinician is considering the relative roles of medical conditions and substances in a patient with psychosis, diagnosis may be assisted by chronology of symptoms, response to removal of suspect substances or alleviation of medical illnesses, and toxicology results.

Course and Prognosis

The course of the underlying medical illness or substance use commonly dictates the course of psychosis due to a general medical condition or substance, with several notable exceptions. Psychosis caused by certain medications (e.g., immunosuppressants) gradually may subside even when use of those medications is continued. Minimizing doses of such medications consistent with therapeutic efficacy often facilitates resolution of psychosis. Certain degenerative brain disorders (e.g., Parkinson's disease) can be characterized by episodic lapses into psychosis, even as the underlying medical condition advances. If abuse of substances persists over a lengthy period, psychosis (e.g., hallucinations from alcohol) may fail to remit even during extended intervals of abstinence.

Treatment

The principles of treatment for a secondary psychotic disorder are similar to those for any secondary neuropsychiatric disorder, namely, rapid identification of the etiological agent and treatment of the underlying cause. Antipsychotic medication may provide symptomatic relief.

ANXIETY DISORDER DUE TO A GENERAL MEDICAL CONDITION

Definition

In *anxiety disorder due to a general medical condition*, the individual experiences anxiety that causes clinically significant distress or impairment in functioning. This anxiety must represent a direct physiological, not emotional, consequence of a general medical condition. In *substance-induced anxiety disorder*, the anxiety symptoms are the product of a prescribed medication or stem from intoxication or withdrawal from a nonprescribed substance, typically a drug of abuse.

Epidemiology

Few data exist by which to estimate the prevalence of anxiety disorder due to a general medical condition. It is believed that medically ill individuals in general have higher rates of anxiety disorder than do the general population. Rates of panic and generalized anxiety are especially high in neurological, endocrine, and cardiology patients, although this finding does not necessarily prove a physiological link. Approximately one third of patients with hypothyroidism and two thirds of patients with hyperthyroidism may experience anxiety symptoms. As much as 40 percent of patients with Parkinson's disease have anxiety disorders. Prevalence of most anxiety disorders is higher in women than in men.

Etiology

Causes most commonly described in anxiety syndromes include substance-related states (intoxication with caffeine, cocaine, amphetamines, and other sympathomimetic agents; withdrawal from nicotine, sedative-hypnotics, and alcohol), endocrinopathies (especially pheochromocytoma, hyperthyroidism, hypercortisolemic states, and hyperparathyroidism), metabolic derangements (e.g., hypoxemia, hypercalcemia, and hypoglycemia), and neurological disorders (including vascular, trauma, and degenerative types). Many of these conditions are either inherently transient or easily remediable. Whether that reflects the pathophysiology of secondary anxiety or is an artifact of reporting (e.g., anxiety with subacute onset and complete resolution after removal of a pheochromocytoma is more likely to be reported as an example of anxiety due to a medical illness than is chronic anxiety in the context of chronic obstructive pulmonary disease) is not known. Much attention has been paid to the association of panic attacks and mitral valve prolapse. The nature of that association is unknown, and therefore the diagnosis of panic attacks secondary to mitral valve prolapse currently is premature. Of interest, several recent reports have sought to tie obsessive-compulsive symptoms to the development of pathology in the basal ganglia.

Diagnosis and Clinical Features

Anxiety stemming from a general medical condition or substance may present with physical complaints (e.g., chest pain, palpitation, abdominal distress, diaphoresis, dizziness, tremulousness, and urinary frequency), generalized symptoms of fear and excessive worry, outright panic attacks associated with fear of dying or losing control, recurrent obsessive thoughts or ritualistic compulsive behaviors, or phobia with associated avoidant behavior (Table 7.5–3).

Table 7.5–3
DSM-IV-TR Criteria for Anxiety Disorder Due to a General Medical Condition

A. Prominent anxiety, panic attacks, or obsessions or compulsions predominate in the clinical picture.
B. There is evidence from the history, physical examination, or laboratory findings that the disturbance is the direct physiological consequence of a general medical condition.
C. The disturbance is not better accounted for by another mental disorder (e.g., adjustment disorder with anxiety in which the stressor is a serious general medical condition).
D. The disturbance does not occur exclusively during the course of a delirium.
E. The disturbance causes clinical significant distress or impairment in social, occupational, or other important areas of functioning.
Specify:
With generalized anxiety: if excessive anxiety or worry about a number of events or activities predominates in the clinical presentation
With panic attacks: if panic attacks predominate in the clinical presentation
With obsessive-compulsive symptoms: if obsessions or compulsions predominate in the clinical presentation

From American Psychiatric Association. *Diagnostic and Statistical Manual of Mental Disorders*. 4th ed. Text rev. Washington, DC; American Psychiatric Association; 2000, with permission.

A 78-year-old retired lumber company president sought help for the onset of a series of attacks in which he experienced marked apprehension, restlessness, and the need to be outdoors to relieve his sense of discomfort. He described the most recent event as having occurred at 3 AM a week earlier: He awoke from sleep and felt "the walls were caving in" on him. He denied that this was related to dreaming and said that he was fully awake at the time. He arose, dressed, and went outside in subzero weather; once outside, he noted gradual improvement (but not full resolution) of his symptoms. Complete resolution took a full day.

In response to pointed questioning, the patient denied dyspnea, palpitations, choking sensations, paresthesias, or nausea. He reported trembling and some sweating, together with intermittent dizziness. He imagined that he would die (or lose consciousness) if he could not "escape" from his house. He spoke of a need "to be active."

On questioning, the patient recalled a similar series of attacks almost 30 years earlier after eye surgery for an injury. He described bilateral patching of his eyes and being confined to bed for days, with his head sandbagged to preclude movement. Once ambulatory, he had experienced these attacks for more than 1 year.

The patient denied recent sleep dysfunction, change in appetite or weight, crying spells, or decreased energy. He had been taking diazepam for approximately 2 months for feelings of increased nervousness and tension. He had noted mild memory problems of late.

Further inquiry established a problem with balance and intermittent pain in the right arm and a complaint of indigestion and intermittent diarrhea. The patient had stopped gardening the past summer because of his balance problem. On examination, he was found to have a "beefy" red tongue (which he said was painful), difficulty with tandem gait and rapid alternating motion, and a mild intention tremor. He denied urinary incontinence.

Laboratory studies revealed a macrocytic anemia and vitamin B_{12} deficiency. The patient was given vitamin B_{12} replacement, and his attacks did not recur. (Reprinted with permission from *DSM-IV-TR Casebook*.)

Differential Diagnosis

Anxiety disorder due to a general medical condition symptomatically can resemble corresponding primary anxiety disorders. Acute onset, lack of family history, and occurrence within the context of acute medical illness or introduction of new medications or substances suggest a nonprimary cause.

Individuals with delirium commonly experience anxiety and panic symptoms, but these fluctuate and are accompanied by other delirium symptoms such as cognitive loss and inattentiveness; furthermore, anxiety symptoms diminish as delirium subsides. Patients with psychosis of any origin can experience anxiety commonly related to delusions or hallucinations. Depressive disorders often present with anxiety symptoms, mandating that the clinician inquire broadly about depressive symptoms in any patient whose primary complaint is anxiety. Dementia often is associated with agitation or anxiety, especially at night (called *sundowning*), but an independent anxiety diagnosis is warranted only if it becomes a source of prominent clinical attention. Adjustment disorders with anxiety arising within the context of reaction to medical or other life stressors should not be diagnosed as anxiety disorder due to a general medical condition.

Course and Prognosis

Anxiety disorder due to a general medical condition usually fluctuates in direct relation to the course of the provoking factor. Medical conditions responsive to treatment or cure (e.g., correction of hypothyroidism and reduction in caffeine consumption) often provide concomitant relief of anxiety symptoms, although such relief may lag the rate or extent of improvement in the underlying medical condition. Chronic, incurable medical conditions associated with persistent physiological insult (e.g., chronic obstructive pulmonary disease) or recurrent relapse to substance use can contribute to seeming refractoriness of associated anxiety symptoms. In medication-induced anxiety, if complete cessation of the offending factor (e.g., immunosuppressant therapy) is not possible, dose reduction, when clinically feasible, often brings substantial relief.

Treatment

Aside from treating the underlying causes, clinicians have found benzodiazepines helpful in decreasing anxiety symptoms; supportive psychotherapy (including psychoeducational issues focusing on the diagnosis and prognosis) may also be useful. The efficacy of other, more specific therapies in secondary syndromes (e.g., antidepressant medications for panic attacks, SSRIs for obsessive-compulsive symptoms, behavior therapy for simple phobias) is unknown, but they may be of use.

SLEEP DISORDER DUE TO A GENERAL MEDICAL CONDITION

Diagnosis

Sleep disorders can manifest in four ways: by an excess of sleep (hypersomnia), by a deficiency of sleep (insomnia), by abnormal behavior or activity during sleep (parasomnia), and by a disturbance in the timing of sleep (circadian rhythm sleep disorders). Primary sleep disorders occur unrelated to any other medical or psychiatric illness (Table 7.5–4).

Mr. Thompson, a 62-year-old married man, has diabetic neuropathy, which contributes to bilateral leg pain and resultant middle-of-the-night awakening. Recently, after undergoing surgical resection of pancreatic cancer, Mr. Thompson began to experience difficulty falling asleep as well.

At the time of interview, Mr. Thompson reported that he was depressed and worried about his cancer diagnosis. He had concentration difficulties and loss of pleasure in usual activities. Furthermore, as bedtime approached, he acknowledged becoming extremely anxious in anticipation of sleep difficulties. Mr. Thompson slept into the late morning hours and took daytime naps to compensate for nocturnal sleep difficulties. To promote sleep, his general practitioner had

prescribed diazepam, and then temazepam (Restoril), with limited success.

A trial of nortriptyline, 25 mg at bedtime, was initiated to foster pain relief and to promote sleep. When this proved only partially efficacious, trazodone, 50 mg at bedtime, was added. Mr. Thompson was instructed to establish a standard time for lying down at night and arising in the morning. Evening relaxation strategies also were identified. Nortriptyline dosing was gradually raised until an antidepressant therapeutic blood level was achieved. Psychotherapy was used to assist Mr. Thompson in coping with his medical problems and his fears of death related to his cancer diagnosis. With this regimen, pain, mood, and sleep symptoms gradually subsided. (Courtesy of Martin Allan Drooker M.D.)

Treatment

The diagnosis of a secondary sleep disorder hinges on the identification of an active disease process known to exert the observed effect on sleep. Treatment first addresses the underlying neurological or medical disease. Symptomatic treatments focus on behavior modification, such as improvement of sleep hygiene. Pharmacological options can also be used, such as benzodiazepines for restless legs syndrome or nocturnal myoclonus, stimulants for hypersomnia, and tricyclic antidepressant medications for manipulation of rapid eye movement (REM) sleep.

SEXUAL DYSFUNCTION DUE TO A GENERAL MEDICAL CONDITION

Sexual dysfunction often has psychological and physical underpinnings. *Sexual dysfunction due to a general medical condition*

**Table 7.5–4
DSM-IV-TR Criteria for Sleep Disorder Due to a General Medical Condition**

A. A prominent disturbance in sleep that is sufficiently severe to warrant independent clinical attention.
B. There is evidence from the history, physical examination, or laboratory findings that the sleep disturbance is the direct physiological consequence of a general medical condition.
C. The disturbance is not better accounted for by another mental disorder (e.g., an adjustment disorder in which the stressor is a serious medical illness).
D. The disturbance does not occur exclusively during the course of a delirium.
E. The disturbance does not meet the criteria for breathing-related sleep disorder or narcolepsy.
F. The sleep disturbance causes clinically significant distress or impairment in social, occupational, or other important areas of functioning.

Specify type:
Insomnia type: if the predominant sleep disturbance is insomnia
Hypersomnia type: if the predominant sleep disturbance is hypersomnia
Parasomnia type: if the predominant sleep disturbance is a parasomnia
Mixed type: if more than one sleep disturbance is present and none predominate of comparable sexual dysfunction that was not substance-induced

From American Psychiatric Association. *Diagnostic and Statistical Manual of Mental Disorders.* 4th ed. Text rev. Washington, DC; American Psychiatric Association; 2000, with permission.

Table 7.5–5
DSM-IV-TR Criteria for Sexual Dysfunction Due to a General Medical Condition

A. Clinically significant sexual dysfunction that results in marked distress or interpersonal difficulty predominates in the clinical picture.
B. There is evidence from the history, physical examination, or laboratory findings that the sexual dysfunction is fully explained by the direct physiological effects of a general medical condition.
C. The disturbance is not better accounted for by another mental disorder (e.g., major depressive disorder).

Select code and term based on the predominant sexual dysfunction:

Female hypoactive sexual desire disorder due to . . . [insert general medical condition here]: if deficient or absent sexual desire is the predominant feature.
Male hypoactive sexual desire disorder due to . . . [insert general medical condition here]: if deficient or absent sexual desire is the predominant feature.
Male erectile disorder due to . . . [insert general medical condition here]: if male erectile dysfunction is the predominant feature.
Female dyspareunia due to . . . [insert general medical condition here]: if pain associated with intercourse is the predominant feature.
Male dyspareunia due to . . . [insert general medical condition here]: if pain associated with intercourse is the predominant feature.
Other female sexual dysfunction due to . . . [insert general medical condition here]: if some other feature is predominant (e.g., orgasmic disorder) or if no feature predominates.
Other male sexual dysfunction due to . . . [insert general medical condition here]: if some other feature is predominant (e.g., orgasmic disorder) or if no feature predominates.

From American Psychiatric Association. *Diagnostic and Statistical Manual of Mental Disorders.* 4th ed. Text rev. Washington, DC; American Psychiatric Association; 2000, with permission.

subsumes multiple forms of medically induced sexual disturbance, including erectile dysfunction, pain during sexual intercourse, low sexual desire, and orgasmic disorders. The DSM-IV-TR criteria for sexual dysfunction due to a general medical condition are listed in Table 7.5–5.

Epidemiology

Little is known regarding the prevalence of sexual dysfunction due to general medical illness. In general, prevalence rates for sexual complaints are highest for female hypoactive sexual desire and orgasm problems and for premature ejaculation in men. High rates of sexual dysfunction are described in patients with cardiac conditions, cancer, diabetes, and HIV. Forty to 50 percent of individuals with MS describe sexual dysfunction. Cerebrovascular accident impairs sexual functioning, with the possibility that, in men, greater impairment follows right-hemispheric cerebrovascular injury than left-hemispheric injury. Delayed orgasm can affect as much as 50 percent of individuals taking SSRIs.

Etiology

The type of sexual dysfunction is affected by the cause, but specificity is rare; that is, a given cause can manifest as one

(or more than one) of several syndromes. General categories include medications and drugs of abuse, local disease processes that affect the primary or secondary sexual organs, and systemic illnesses that affect sexual organs via neurological, vascular, or endocrinological routes.

Course and Prognosis

The course and prognosis of secondary sexual dysfunctions vary widely, depending on the cause. Drug-induced syndromes generally remit with discontinuation (or dose reduction) of the offending agent. Endocrine-based dysfunctions also generally improve with restoration of normal physiology. By contrast, dysfunctions caused by neurological disease can run protracted, even progressive, courses.

Treatment

The treatment approach varies widely, depending on the etiology. When reversal of the underlying cause is not possible, supportive and behaviorally oriented psychotherapy with the patient (and perhaps the partner) may minimize distress and increase sexual satisfaction (e.g., by developing sexual interactions that are not limited by the specific dysfunction). Support groups for people with specific types of dysfunctions are available. Other symptom-based treatments can be used in certain conditions; for example, sildenafil (Viagra) administration or surgical implantation of a penile prosthesis may be used in the treatment of male erectile dysfunction.

MENTAL DISORDERS DUE TO A GENERAL MEDICAL CONDITION NOT ELSEWHERE CLASSIFIED

The DSM-IV-TR has three additional diagnostic categories for clinical presentations of mental disorders due to a general medical condition that do not meet the diagnostic criteria for specific diagnoses. The first of the diagnoses is catatonic disorder due to a general medical condition (Table 7.5–6). The second is personality change due to a general medical condition. The third diagnosis is mental disorder not otherwise specified due to a general medical condition (Table 7.5–7).

Catatonia Due to a Medical Condition

Catatonia can be caused by a variety of medical or surgical conditions. It is characterized usually by fixed posture and waxy flexibility. Mutism, negativism, and echolalia may be associated features.

Epidemiology. Catatonia is an uncommon condition. It is mostly seen in advanced primary mood or psychotic illnesses. Among inpatients with catatonia, 25 to 50 percent are related to mood disorders (e.g., major depressive episode, recurrent, with catatonic features), and approximately 10 percent are associated with schizophrenia. Data are scant on catatonia's rate of occurrence due to medical conditions or substances.

Table 7.5–6
DSM-IV-TR Diagnostic Criteria for Catatonic Disorder Due to a General Medical Condition

A. The presence of catatonia as manifested by motoric immobility, excessive motor activity (that is apparently purposeless and not influenced by external stimuli), extreme negativism or mutism, peculiarities of voluntary movement, or echolalia or echopraxia.
B. There is evidence from the history, physical examination, or laboratory findings that the disturbance is the direct physiological consequence of a general medical condition.
C. The disturbance is not better accounted for by another mental disorder (e.g., a manic episode).
D. The disturbance does not occur exclusively during the course of a delirium.
Coding note: Include the name of the general medical condition on Axis I, e.g., Catatonic disorder due to hepatic encephalopathy; also code the general medical condition on Axis III.

From American Psychiatric Association. *Diagnostic and Statistical Manual of Mental Disorders.* 4th ed. Text rev. Washington, DC: American Psychiatric Association; copyright 2000, with permission.

Diagnosis and Clinical Features. Peculiarities of movement are the most characteristic feature, usually rigidity. Hyperactivity and psychomotor agitation can also occur (Table 7.5–6). A thorough medical workup is necessary to confirm the diagnosis.

Course and Prognosis. The course and prognosis are intimately related to the cause. Neoplasms, encephalitis, head trauma, diabetes, and other metabolic disorders can manifest with catatonic features. If the underlying disorder is treatable, the catatonic syndrome will resolve.

Treatment. Treatment must be directed to the underlying cause. Antipsychotic medications may improve postural abnormalities even though they have no effect on the underlying disorder. Schizophrenia must always be ruled out in patients who present with catatonic symptoms. ECT has been shown to be a useful first-choice method of treatment.

Table 7.5–7
DSM-IV-TR Diagnostic Criteria for Mental Disorder Not Otherwise Specified Due to a General Medical Condition

This residual category should be used for situations in which it has been established that the disturbance is caused by the direct physiological effects of a general medical condition but the criteria are not met for a specific mental disorder due to a general medical condition (e.g., dissociative symptoms due to complex partial seizures).
Coding note: Include the name of the general medical condition on Axis I, e.g., Mental disorder not otherwise specified due to HIV disease; also code the general medical condition on Axis III.

HIV, human immunodeficiency virus.
From American Psychiatric Association. *Diagnostic and Statistical Manual of Mental Disorders.* 4th ed. Text rev. Washington, DC: American Psychiatric Association; copyright 2000, with permission.

Personality Change Due to a General Medical Condition

Personality change means that the person's fundamental means of interacting and behaving have been altered. When a true personality change occurs in adulthood, the clinician should always suspect brain injury. Almost every medical disorder can be accompanied by personality change, however.

Epidemiology. No reliable epidemiological data exist on personality trait changes in medical conditions. Specific personality trait changes for particular brain diseases—for example, passive and self-centered behaviors in patients with dementia of the Alzheimer's type—have been reported. Similarly, apathy has been described in patients with frontal lobe lesions.

Etiology. Diseases that preferentially affect the frontal lobes or subcortical structures are more likely to manifest with prominent personality change. Head trauma is a common cause. Frontal lobe tumors, such as meningiomas and gliomas, can grow to considerable size before coming to medical attention because they can be neurologically silent (i.e., without focal signs). Progressive dementia syndromes, especially those with a subcortical pattern of degeneration, such as acquired immune deficiency syndrome (AIDS) dementia complex, Huntington's disease, or progressive supranuclear palsy, often cause significant personality disturbance. MS can impinge on the personality, reflecting subcortical white matter degeneration. Exposure to toxins with a predilection for white matter, such as irradiation, can also produce significant personality change disproportionate to the cognitive or motor impairment.

Diagnosis and Clinical Features. The DSM-IV-TR diagnostic criteria for personality change due to a general medical condition are listed in Table 7.5–8.

Mr. Davis is a 49-year-old married man without a psychiatric history who was admitted to the hospital with sudden onset of severe headache. Workup revealed subarachnoid hemorrhage caused by the rupture of an intracranial aneurysm. Cerebral vasospasm, obstructive hydrocephalus, and coma ensued. Neurosurgical intervention was undertaken to clip the aneurysm and to install a ventriculoperitoneal shunt.

After a lengthy course of inpatient rehabilitation, Mr. Davis experienced outbursts of anger, episodic depressed mood, off-color remarks that verged on offensive, and impairment in his appreciation for subtlety in humor and conversation. No evidence of psychosis was observed. Family members reported that Mr. Davis always had been one to "speak his mind" and to react defensively when he felt criticized.

Brain imaging demonstrated encephalomalacia in the right frontal lobe. Mild cognitive dysfunction not rising to the level of dementia was diagnosed on neuropsychological testing. (Courtesy of Martin Allan Drooker M.D.)

Course and Prognosis. Course depends on the nature of the medical or neurological insult. Personality changes resulting

Table 7.5–8
DSM-IV-TR Diagnostic Criteria for Personality Change Due to a General Medical Condition

A. A persistent personality disturbance that represents a change from the individual's previous characteristic personality pattern. (In children, the disturbance involves a marked deviation from normal development or a significant change in the child's usual behavior patterns lasting at least 1 year.)
B. There is evidence from the history, physical examination, or laboratory findings that the disturbance is the direct physiological consequence of a general medical condition.
C. The disturbance is not better accounted for by another mental disorder (including other mental disorders due to a general medical condition).
D. The disturbance does not occur exclusively during the course of a delirium.
E. The disturbance causes clinically significant distress or impairment in social, occupational, or other important areas of functioning.

Specify type:
Labile type: if the predominant feature is affective lability
Disinhibited type: if the predominant feature is poor impulse control as evidenced by sexual indiscretions, etc.
Aggressive type: if the predominant feature is aggressive behavior
Apathetic type: if the predominant feature is marked apathy and indifference
Paranoid type: if the predominant feature is suspiciousness or paranoid ideation
Other type: if the presentation is not characterized by any of the above subtypes
Combined type: if more than one feature predominates in the clinical picture
Unspecified type
Coding note: Include the name of the general medical condition on Axis I, e.g., Personality change due to temporal lobe epilepsy; also code the general medical condition on Axis III.

From American Psychiatric Association. *Diagnostic and Statistical Manual of Mental Disorders.* 4th ed. Text rev. Washington, DC: American Psychiatric Association; copyright 2000, with permission.

from medical conditions likely to yield to intervention (e.g., correction of hypothyroidism) are more amenable to improvement than are personality changes due to medical conditions that are static (e.g., brain injury after head trauma) or progressive in nature (e.g., Huntington's disease).

Treatment.   Treatment of secondary personality syndromes is first directed toward correcting the underlying cause. Lithium carbonate (Eskalith), carbamazepine (Tegretol), and valproic acid (Depakote) have been used for the control of affective lability and impulsivity. Aggression or explosiveness can be treated with lithium, anticonvulsant medications, or a combination of lithium and an anticonvulsant agent. Centrally active β-adrenergic receptor antagonists, such as propranolol (Inderal), have some efficacy as well. Apathy and inertia have occasionally improved with psychostimulant agents. Because cognition and verbal skills may be preserved in patients with secondary personality changes, they may be candidates for psychotherapy. Families should be involved in the therapy process, with a focus on education and understanding the origins of the patient's inappropriate behaviors. Issues such as competency, disability, and advocacy are frequently of clinical concern with these patients in light of the unpredictable and pervasive behavior change.

SPECIFIC DISORDERS

Epilepsy

Epilepsy is the most common chronic neurological disease in the general population and affects approximately 1 percent of the population in the United States. For psychiatrists, the major concerns about epilepsy are consideration of an epileptic diagnosis in psychiatric patients, the psychosocial ramifications of a diagnosis of epilepsy for a patient, and the psychological and cognitive effects of commonly used anticonvulsant drugs. With regard to the first of these concerns, 30 to 50 percent of all persons with epilepsy have psychiatric difficulties sometime during the course of their illness. The most common behavioral symptom of epilepsy is a change in personality. Psychosis and violence occur much less commonly than was previously believed.

Definitions.   A seizure is a transient paroxysmal pathophysiological disturbance of cerebral function caused by a spontaneous, excessive discharge of neurons. Patients are said to have epilepsy if they have a chronic condition characterized by recurrent seizure. The ictus, or ictal event, is the seizure itself. The nonictal periods are categorized as preictal, postictal, and interictal. The symptoms during the ictal event are determined primarily by the site of origin in the brain for the seizure and by the pattern of the spread of seizure activity through the brain. Interictal symptoms are influenced by the ictal event and other neuropsychiatric and psychosocial factors, such as coexisting psychiatric or neurological disorders, the presence of psychosocial stressors, and premorbid personality traits.

Classification.   The two major categories of seizures are partial and generalized. Partial seizures involve epileptiform activity in localized brain regions. Generalized seizures involve the entire brain. A classification system for seizures is outlined in Table 7.5–9.

GENERALIZED SEIZURES.   Generalized tonic-clonic seizures exhibit the classic symptoms of loss of consciousness, generalized tonic-clonic movements of the limbs, tongue biting, and incontinence. Although the diagnosis of the ictal events of the seizure is relatively straightforward, the postictal state, characterized by a slow, gradual recovery of consciousness and cognition, occasionally presents a diagnostic dilemma for a psychiatrist in an emergency room. The recovery period from a generalized tonic-clonic seizure ranges from a few minutes to many hours, and the clinical picture is that of a gradually clearing delirium. The most common psychiatric problems associated with generalized seizures involve helping patients adjust to a chronic neurological disorder and assessing the cognitive or behavioral effects of anticonvulsant drugs.

Absence Seizure (Petit Mal).   A difficult type of generalized seizure for a psychiatrist to diagnose is an absence, or petit mal, seizure. The epileptic nature of the episodes may go unrecognized because the characteristic motor or sensory manifestations of epilepsy may be absent or so slight that they do not arouse suspicion. Petit mal epilepsy usually begins in childhood between the ages of 5 and 7 years and ceases by puberty. Brief disruptions of consciousness, during which the patient suddenly loses contact with the environment, are characteristic of petit mal epilepsy, but the patient has no true loss of consciousness and no convulsive movements during the episodes. The electroencephalogram

Table 7.5–9
International Classification of Epileptic Seizures

I. Partial seizures (seizures beginning locally)
  A. Partial seizures with elementary symptoms (generally without impairment of consciousness)
    1. With motor symptoms
    2. With sensory symptoms
    3. With autonomic symptoms
    4. Compound forms
  B. Partial seizures with complex symptoms (generally with impairment of consciousness; temporal lobe or psychomotor seizures)
    1. With impairment of consciousness only
    2. With cognitive symptoms
    3. With affective symptoms
    4. With psychosensory symptoms
    5. With psychosensory symptoms (automatisms)
    6. Compound forms
  C. Partial seizures secondarily generalized
II. Generalized seizures (bilaterally symmetrical and without local onset)
  A. Absences (petit mal)
  B. Myoclonus
  C. Infantile spasms
  D. Clonic seizures
  E. Tonic seizures
  F. Tonic-clonic seizures (grand mal)
  G. Atonic seizures
  H. Akinetic seizures
III. Unilateral seizures
IV. Unclassified seizures (because of incomplete data)

Adapted from Gastaut H. Clinical and electroencephalographical classification of epileptic seizures. *Epilepsia.* 1970;11:102.

(EEG) produces a characteristic pattern of three-per-second spike-and-wave activity. In rare instances, petit mal epilepsy begins in adulthood. Adult-onset petit mal epilepsy can be characterized by sudden, recurrent psychotic episodes or deliriums that appear and disappear abruptly. The symptoms may be accompanied by a history of falling or fainting spells.

PARTIAL SEIZURES. Partial seizures are classified as either simple (without alterations in consciousness) or complex (with an alteration in consciousness). Somewhat more than half of all patients with partial seizures have complex partial seizures. Other terms used for complex partial seizures are temporal lobe epilepsy, psychomotor seizures, and limbic epilepsy; these terms, however, are not accurate descriptions of the clinical situation. Complex partial epilepsy, the most common form of epilepsy in adults, affects approximately 3 in 1,000 persons. About 30 percent of patients with complex partial seizures have major mental illness such as depression.

Symptoms

PREICTAL SYMPTOMS. Preictal events (auras) in complex partial epilepsy include autonomic sensations (e.g., fullness in the stomach, blushing, and changes in respiration), cognitive sensations (e.g., *déjà vu*, *jamais vu*, forced thinking, dreamy states), affective states (e.g., fear, panic, depression, elation), and, classically, automatisms (e.g., lip smacking, rubbing, chewing).

ICTAL SYMPTOMS. Brief, disorganized, and uninhibited behavior characterizes the ictal event. Although some defense attorneys may claim otherwise, rarely does a person exhibit organized, directed violent behavior during an epileptic episode. The

cognitive symptoms include amnesia for the time during the seizure and a period of resolving delirium after the seizure. A seizure focus can be found on an EEG in 25 to 50 percent of all patients with complex partial epilepsy. The use of sphenoidal or anterior temporal electrodes and sleep-deprived EEGs may increase the likelihood of finding an EEG abnormality. Multiple normal EEGs are often obtained for a patient with complex partial epilepsy; therefore, normal EEGs cannot be used to exclude a diagnosis of complex partial epilepsy. The use of long-term EEG recordings (usually 24 to 72 hours) can help clinicians detect a seizure focus in some patients. Most studies show that the use of nasopharyngeal leads does not add much to the sensitivity of an EEG, but they do add to the discomfort of the procedure for the patient.

INTERICTAL SYMPTOMS

Personality Disturbances. The most frequent psychiatric abnormalities reported in patients with epilepsy are personality disorders, and they are especially likely to occur in patients with epilepsy of temporal lobe origin. The most common features are religiosity, a heightened experience of emotions—a quality usually called *viscosity of personality*—and changes in sexual behavior. The syndrome in its complete form is relatively rare, even in those with complex partial seizures of temporal lobe origin. Many patients are not affected by personality disturbances; others suffer from a variety of disturbances that differ strikingly from the classic syndrome.

Changes in sexual behavior may be manifested by hypersexuality; deviations in sexual interest, such as fetishism and transvestism; and, most commonly, hyposexuality. The hyposexuality is characterized both by a lack of interest in sexual matters and by reduced sexual arousal. Some patients with the onset of complex partial epilepsy before puberty may fail to reach a normal level of sexual interest after puberty, although this characteristic may not disturb the patient. For patients with the onset of complex partial epilepsy after puberty, the change in sexual interest may be bothersome and worrisome.

Psychotic Symptoms. Interictal psychotic states are more common than ictal psychoses. Schizophrenia-like interictal episodes can occur in patients with epilepsy, particularly those with temporal lobe origins. An estimated 10 percent of all patients with complex partial epilepsy have psychotic symptoms. Risk factors for the symptoms include female gender, left-handedness, the onset of seizures during puberty, and a left-sided lesion.

The onset of psychotic symptoms in epilepsy is variable. Classically, psychotic symptoms appear in patients who have had epilepsy for a long time, and the onset of psychotic symptoms is preceded by the development of personality changes related to the epileptic brain activity. The most characteristic symptoms of the psychoses are hallucinations and paranoid delusions. Patients usually remain warm and appropriate in affect, in contrast to the abnormalities of affect commonly seen in patients with schizophrenia. The thought disorder symptoms in patients with psychotic epilepsy are most commonly those involving conceptualization and circumstantiality, rather than the classic schizophrenic symptoms of blocking and looseness.

Violence. Episodic violence has been a problem in some patients with epilepsy, especially epilepsy of temporal and frontal lobe origin. Whether the violence is a manifestation of the seizure itself or is of interictal psychopathological origin is uncertain. Most evidence points to the extreme rarity of violence as an ictal phenomenon. Only in rare cases should violence in the patient with epilepsy be attributed to the seizure itself.

Mood Disorder Symptoms. Mood disorder symptoms, such as depression and mania, are seen less often in epilepsy than are schizophrenia-like symptoms. The mood disorder symptoms that do occur tend to be episodic and appear most often when the epileptic foci affect the temporal lobe of the nondominant cerebral hemisphere. The importance of mood disorder symptoms may be attested to by the increased incidence of attempted suicide in people with epilepsy.

Diagnosis.   A correct diagnosis of epilepsy can be particularly difficult when the ictal and interictal symptoms of epilepsy are severe manifestations of psychiatric symptoms in the absence of significant changes in consciousness and cognitive abilities. Psychiatrists, therefore, must maintain a high level of suspicion during the evaluation of a new patient and must consider the possibility of an epileptic disorder, even in the absence of the classic signs and symptoms. Another differential diagnosis to consider is pseudoseizure, in which a patient has some conscious control over mimicking the symptoms of a seizure.

For patients who have previously received a diagnosis of epilepsy, the appearance of new psychiatric symptoms should be considered as possibly representing an evolution in their epileptic symptoms. The appearance of psychotic symptoms, mood disorder symptoms, personality changes, or symptoms of anxiety (e.g., panic attacks) should cause a clinician to evaluate the control of the patient's epilepsy and to assess the patient for the presence of an independent mental disorder. In such circumstances, the clinician should evaluate the patient's compliance with the anticonvulsant drug regimen and should consider whether the psychiatric symptoms could be adverse effects from the antiepileptic drugs themselves. When psychiatric symptoms appear in a patient who has had epilepsy diagnosed or considered as a diagnosis in the past, the clinician should obtain results of one or more EEG examinations.

Treatment.   First-line drugs for generalized tonic-clonic seizures are valproate and phenytoin (Dilantin). First-line drugs for partial seizures include carbamazepine, oxcarbazepine (Trileptal), and phenytoin. Ethosuximide (Zarontin) and valproate are first-line drugs for absence (petit mal) seizures. Carbamazepine and valproic acid may be helpful in controlling the symptoms of irritability and outbursts of aggression, as are the typical antipsychotic drugs. Psychotherapy, family counseling, and group therapy may be useful in addressing the psychosocial issues associated with epilepsy. In addition, clinicians should be aware that many antiepileptic drugs cause mild to moderate cognitive impairment, and an adjustment of the dosage or a change in medications should be considered if symptoms of cognitive impairment are a problem in a patient.

Brain Tumors

Brain tumors and cerebrovascular diseases can cause virtually any psychiatric symptom or syndrome, but cerebrovascular diseases, by the nature of their onset and symptom pattern, are rarely misdiagnosed as mental disorders. In general, tumors are associated with fewer psychopathological signs and symptoms than are cerebrovascular diseases affecting a similar volume of brain tissue. The two key approaches to the diagnosis of either condition are a comprehensive clinical history and a complete neurological examination. Performance of the appropriate brain imaging technique is usually the final diagnostic procedure; the imaging should confirm the clinical diagnosis.

Clinical Features, Course, and Prognosis.   Mental symptoms are experienced at some time during the course of illness in approximately 50 percent of patients with brain tumors. In approximately 80 percent of these patients with mental symptoms, the tumors are located in frontal or limbic brain regions rather than in parietal or temporal regions. Meningiomas are likely to cause focal symptoms by compressing a limited region of the cortex, whereas gliomas are likely to cause diffuse symptoms. Delirium is most often a component of rapidly growing, large, or metastatic tumors. If a patient's history and a physical examination reveal bowel or bladder incontinence, a frontal lobe tumor should be suspected; if the history and examination reveal abnormalities in memory and speech, a temporal lobe tumor should be suspected.

COGNITION.   Impaired intellectual functioning often accompanies the presence of a brain tumor, regardless of its type or location.

LANGUAGE SKILLS.   Disorders of language function may be severe, particularly if tumor growth is rapid. In fact, defects of language function often obscure all other mental symptoms.

MEMORY.   Loss of memory is a frequent symptom of brain tumors. Patients with brain tumors exhibit Korsakoff's syndrome and retain no memory of events that occurred since the illness began. Events of the immediate past, even painful ones, are lost. Patients, however, retain old memories and are unaware of their loss of recent memory.

PERCEPTION.   Prominent perceptual defects are often associated with behavioral disorders, especially because patients must integrate tactile, auditory, and visual perceptions to function normally.

AWARENESS.   Alterations of consciousness are common late symptoms of increased intracranial pressure caused by a brain tumor. Tumors arising in the upper part of the brainstem can produce a unique symptom called *akinetic mutism*, or *vigilant coma*. The patient is immobile and mute, yet alert.

Head Trauma

Head trauma can result in an array of mental symptoms and lead to a diagnosis of dementia due to head trauma or to mental disorder not otherwise specified due to a general medical condition (e.g., postconcussional disorder). The postconcussive syndrome remains controversial, because it focuses on the wide range of psychiatric symptoms, some serious, that can follow what seems to be minor head trauma. DSM-IV-TR includes a set of research criteria for postconcussional disorder in an appendix (Table 7.5–10).

Pathophysiology.   Head trauma is a common clinical situation; an estimated 2 million incidents involve head trauma each year. Head trauma most commonly occurs in people 15 to 25 years of age and has a male-to-female predominance of approximately 3 to 1. Gross estimates based on the severity of the head trauma suggest that virtually all patients with serious head trauma, more than half of patients with moderate head trauma, and about 10 percent of patients with mild head trauma have ongoing neuropsychiatric sequelae resulting from the head trauma. Head trauma can be divided grossly into penetrating head trauma (e.g., trauma produced by a bullet) and blunt trauma, in which there is no physical penetration of the skull. Blunt trauma is far more common than penetrating head trauma. Motor

Table 7.5–10
DSM-IV-TR Research Criteria for Postconcussional Disorder

A. A history of head trauma that has caused significant cerebral concussion.
  Note: The manifestations of concussion include loss of consciousness, posttraumatic amnesia, and, less commonly, posttraumatic onset of seizures. The specific method of defining this criterion needs to be established by further research.
B. Evidence from neuropsychological testing or quantified cognitive assessment of difficulty in attention (concentrating, shifting focus of attention, performing simultaneous cognitive tasks) or memory (learning or recalling information).
C. Three (or more) of the following occur shortly after the trauma and last at least 3 months:
  (1) becoming fatigued easily
  (2) disordered sleep
  (3) headache
  (4) vertigo or dizziness
  (5) irritability or aggression on little or no provocation
  (6) anxiety, depression, or affective lability
  (7) changes in personality (e.g., social or sexual inappropriateness)
  (8) apathy or lack of spontaneity
D. The symptoms in Criteria B and C have their onset following head trauma or else represent a substantial worsening of preexisting symptoms.
E. The disturbance causes significant impairment in social or occupational functioning and represents a significant decline from a previous level of functioning. In school-age children, the impairment may be manifested by a significant worsening in school or academic performance dating from the trauma.
F. The symptoms do not meet criteria for dementia due to head trauma and are not better accounted for by another mental disorder (e.g., amnestic disorder due to head trauma, personality change due to head trauma).

From American Psychiatric Association. *Diagnostic and Statistical Manual of Mental Disorders.* 4th ed. Text rev. Washington, DC: American Psychiatric Association; copyright 2000, with permission.

vehicle accidents account for more than half of all the incidents of blunt central nervous system (CNS) trauma; falls, violence, and sports-related head trauma account for most of the remaining cases.

Symptoms. The two major clusters of symptoms related to head trauma are those of cognitive impairment and of behavioral sequelae. After a period of posttraumatic amnesia, there is usually a 6- to 12-month period of recovery, after which the remaining symptoms are likely to be permanent. The most common cognitive problems are decreased speed in information processing, decreased attention, increased distractibility, deficits in problem-solving and in the ability to sustain effort, and problems with memory and learning new information. A variety of language disabilities can also occur.

Behaviorally, the major symptoms involve depression, increased impulsivity, increased aggression, and changes in personality. These symptoms can be further exacerbated by the use of alcohol, which is often involved in the head trauma event itself. A debate has ensued about how preexisting character and personality traits affect the development of behavioral symptoms after head trauma. The critical studies needed to answer the question definitively have not yet been done, but the weight of opinion is leaning toward a biologically and neuroanatomically based association between the head trauma and the behavioral sequelae.

Treatment. The treatment of the cognitive and behavioral disorders in head trauma patients is basically similar to the treatment approaches used in other patients with these symptoms. One difference is that patients with head trauma may be particularly susceptible to the side effects associated with psychotropic drugs; therefore, treatment with these agents should be initiated in lower dosages than usual, and they should be titrated upward more slowly than usual. Standard antidepressants can be used to treat depression, and either anticonvulsants or antipsychotics can be used to treat aggression and impulsivity. Other approaches to the symptoms include lithium, calcium channel blockers, and β-adrenergic receptor antagonists.

Clinicians must support patients through individual or group psychotherapy and should support the major caretakers through couples and family therapy. Patients with minor and moderate head trauma often rejoin their families and restart their jobs; therefore, all involved parties need help to adjust to any changes in the patient's personality and mental abilities.

Demyelinating Disorders

Multiple Sclerosis. MS is characterized by multiple episodes of symptoms, pathophysiologically related to multifocal lesions in the white matter of the CNS. The cause remains unknown, but studies have focused on slow viral infections and disturbances in the immune system. The estimated prevalence of MS in the Western Hemisphere is 50 per 100,000 people. The disease is much more frequent in cold and temperate climates than in the tropics and subtropics and more common in women than in men; it is predominantly a disease of young adults. In most patients, the onset occurs between the ages of 20 and 40 years.

The neuropsychiatric symptoms of MS can be divided into cognitive and behavioral types. Research reports have found that 30 to 50 percent of patients with MS have mild cognitive impairment and that 20 to 30 percent of them have serious cognitive impairments. Although evidence indicates that patients with MS experience a decline in their general intelligence, memory is the most commonly affected cognitive function. The severity of the memory impairment does not seem to be correlated with the severity of the neurological symptoms or the duration of the illness.

The behavioral symptoms associated with MS are varied and can include euphoria, depression, and personality changes. Psychosis is a rare complication. Approximately 25 percent of persons with MS exhibit a euphoric mood that is not hypomanic, but somewhat more cheerful than their situation warrants and not necessarily in character with their disposition before the onset of MS. Only 10 percent of patients with MS have a sustained and elevated mood, although it is still not truly hypomanic. Depression, however, is common; it affects 25 to 50 percent of patients with MS and results in a higher rate of suicide than is seen in the general population. Risk factors for suicide in patients with MS are male sex, onset of MS before age 30, and a relatively recent diagnosis of the disorder. Personality changes are also common in patients with MS; they affect 20 to 40 percent of patients and are often characterized by increased irritability or apathy.

Amyotrophic Lateral Sclerosis (ALS). ALS is a progressive, noninherited disease of asymmetrical muscle atrophy. It begins in adult life and progresses over months or years to involve all the striated muscles except the cardiac and ocular muscles. In addition to muscle atrophy, patients have signs of pyramidal tract involvement. The illness is rare and occurs in approximately 1.6 persons per 100,000 annually. A few patients have concomitant dementia. The disease progresses rapidly, and death generally occurs within 4 years of onset.

Infectious Diseases

Herpes Simplex Encephalitis. Herpes simplex encephalitis, the most common type of focal encephalitis, most commonly affects the frontal and temporal lobes. The symptoms often include anosmia, olfactory and gustatory hallucinations, and personality changes and can also involve bizarre or psychotic behaviors. Complex partial epilepsy may also develop in patients with herpes simplex encephalitis. Although the mortality rate for the infection has decreased, many patients exhibit personality changes, symptoms of memory loss, and psychotic symptoms.

Rabies Encephalitis. The incubation period for rabies ranges from 10 days to 1 year, after which symptoms of restlessness, overactivity, and agitation can develop. Hydrophobia, present in up to 50 percent of patients, is characterized by an intense fear of drinking water. The fear develops from the severe laryngeal and diaphragmatic spasms that the patients experience when they drink water. Once rabies encephalitis develops, the disease is fatal within days or weeks.

Neurosyphilis. Neurosyphilis (also known as general paresis) appears 10 to 15 years after the primary *Treponema* infection. Since the advent of penicillin, neurosyphilis has become a rare disorder, although AIDS is associated with reintroducing neurosyphilis into medical practice in some urban settings. Neurosyphilis generally affects the frontal lobes and results in personality changes, development of poor judgment, irritability, and decreased care for self. Delusions of grandeur develop in 10 to 20 percent of affected patients. The disease progresses with the development of dementia and tremor, until patients are paretic. The neurological symptoms include Argyll-Robertson pupils, which are small, irregular, and unequal and have light-near reflex dissociation, tremor, dysarthria, and hyperreflexia. Cerebrospinal fluid (CSF) examination shows lymphocytosis, increased protein, and a positive result on a Venereal Disease Research Laboratory (VDRL) test.

Chronic Meningitis. Chronic meningitis is now seen more often than in the recent past because of the immunocompromised condition of people with AIDS. The usual causative agents are *Mycobacterium tuberculosis*, *Cryptococcus*, and *Coccidioides*. The usual symptoms are headache, memory impairment, confusion, and fever.

Lyme Disease. Lyme disease is caused by infection with the spirochete *Borrelia burgdorferi* transmitted through the bite of the deer tick (*Ixodes scapularis*), which feed on infected deer and mice. About 16,000 cases are reported annually in the United States.

A characteristic bull's-eye rash is found at the site of the tick bite, followed shortly thereafter by flu-like symptoms. Impaired cognitive functioning and mood changes are associated with the illness and may be the presenting complaint. These include memory lapses, difficulty concentrating, irritability, and depression.

No clear-cut diagnostic test is available. About 50 percent of patients become seropositive to *B. burgdorferi*. Prophylaxis vaccine is not always effective and is controversial. Treatment consists of a 14- to 21-day course of doxycycline (Vibramycin), which results in a 90 percent cure rate. Specific psychotropic drugs can be targeted to treat the psychiatric sign or symptom (e.g., diazepam [Valium] for anxiety). Left untreated, about 60 percent of persons develop a chronic condition. Such patients may be given an erroneous diagnosis of a primary depression rather than one secondary to the medical condition. Support groups for patients with chronic Lyme disease are important. Group members provide each other with emotional support that helps improve their quality of life.

Prion Disease. Prion disease is a group of related disorders caused by a transmissible infectious protein known as a *prion*. Included in this group are Creutzfeldt-Jakob disease (CJD), Gerstmann-Straussler syndrome (GSS), fatal familial insomnia (FFI), and kuru. A variant of CJD (vCJD), also called "mad cow disease," appeared in 1995 in the United Kingdom and is attributed to the transmission of bovine spongiform encephalopathy (BSE) from cattle to humans. Collectively, these disorders are also known as *subacute spongiform encephalopathy* because of shared neuropathological changes that consist of (1) spongiform vacuolization, (2) neuronal loss, and (3) astrocyte proliferation in the cerebral cortex. Amyloid plaques may or may not be present.

ETIOLOGY. Prions are transmissible agents, but differ from viruses in that they lack nucleic acid. Prions are mutated proteins generated from the human prion protein gene (PrP), which is located on the short arm of chromosome 20. No direct link exists between prion disease and Alzheimer's disease, which has been traced to chromosome 21.

The PrP mutates into a disease-related isoform PrP-Super-C (PrP^{Sc}) that can replicate and is infectious. The neuropathological changes that occur in prion disease are presumed to be caused by direct neurotoxic effects of PrP^{Sc}.

The specific prion disease that develops depends on the mutation of PrP that occurs. Mutations at PrP 178N/129V cause CJD; mutations at 178N/129M cause FFI; and mutations at 102L/129M cause GSS and kuru. Other mutations of PrP have been described, and research continues in this important area of genomic identification. Some mutations are both fully penetrant and autosomal dominant and account for inherited forms of prion disease. For example, both GSS and FFI are inherited disorders, and about 10 percent of cases of CJD are also inherited. Prenatal testing for the abnormal PrP gene is available; whether or not such testing should be routinely done is open to question at this time.

CREUTZFELDT-JAKOB DISEASE. First described in 1920, CJD is an invariably fatal, rapidly progressive disorder that occurs mainly in middle-aged or older adults. It manifests initially with fatigue, flu-like symptoms, and cognitive impairment. As the disease progresses, focal neurological findings such as aphasia and apraxia occur.

Psychiatric manifestations are protean and include emotional lability, anxiety, euphoria, depression, delusions, hallucinations, or marked personality changes. The disease progresses over months, leading to dementia, akinetic mutism, coma, and death.

The rates of CJD range from 1 to 2 cases per 1 million persons a year, worldwide. The infectious agent self-replicates and can be transmitted to humans by inoculation with infected tissue and sometimes by ingestion of contaminated food. Iatrogenic transmission has been reported via transplantation of contaminated cornea or dura mater or to children via contaminated supplies of human growth hormone derived from infected persons. Neurosurgical transmission has also been reported. Household contacts are not at greater risk for developing the disease than the general population, unless there is direct inoculation.

Diagnosis requires pathological examination of the cortex, which reveals the classic triad of spongiform vacuolation, loss of neurons, and astrocyte cell proliferation. The cortex and basal ganglia are most affected. An immunoassay test for CJD in the CSF shows promise in supporting the diagnosis; however, this needs to be tested more extensively. Although not specific for CJD, EEG abnormalities are present in nearly all patients, consisting of a slow and irregular background rhythm with periodic complex discharges. Computed tomography (CT) and MRI studies may reveal cortical atrophy later in the course of disease. Single photon emission computed tomography (SPECT) and positron emission tomography (PET) reveal heterogeneously decreased uptake throughout the cortex.

No known treatment exists for CJD. Death usually occurs within 6 months after diagnosis.

VARIANT CJD. In 1995 a variant of CJD (vCJD) appeared in the United Kingdom. The patients affected all died; they were young (under 40 years of age), and none had risk factors of CJD. At autopsy, prion disease was found. The disease was attributed to the transmission in the United Kingdom of BSE between cattle and from cattle to humans in the 1980s. BSE appears to have originated from sheep scrapie-contaminated feed given to cattle. Scrapie is a spongiform encephalopathy found in sheep and goats that has not been shown to cause human disease; however, it is transmissible to other animal species.

The mean age of onset is 29 years and about 150 people worldwide had been infected as of 2006. Clinicians must be alert to the diagnosis in young people with behavioral and psychiatric abnormalities in association with cerebellar signs such as ataxia or myoclonus. The psychiatric presentation of vCJD is not specific. Most patients reported depression, withdrawal, anxiety, and sleep disturbance. Paranoid delusions have occurred. Neuropathological changes are similar to those in vCJD, with the addition of amyloid plaques.

Epidemiological data are still being gathered. The incubation period for vCJD and the amount of infected meat product required to cause infection are unknown. One patient was reported to have been a vegetarian for 5 years before his disease was diagnosed. vCJD can be diagnosed antemortem by examining the tonsils with Western blot immunostains to detect PrP^{Sc} in lymphoid tissue. Diagnosis relies on the development of progressive neurodegenerative features in persons who have ingested contaminated meat or brains. No cure exists, and death usually occurs within 2 to 3 years after diagnosis. Prevention is dependent on careful monitoring of cattle for disease and feeding them grain instead of meat by-products.

KURU. Kuru is an epidemic prion disease found in New Guinea that is caused by cannibalistic funeral rituals in which the brains of the deceased are eaten. Women are more affected by the disorder than men, presumably because they participate in the ceremony to a greater extent. Death usually occurs within 2 years after symptoms develop. Neuropsychiatric signs and symptoms consist of ataxia, chorea, strabismus, delirium, and dementia. Pathological changes are similar to those with other prion disease: neuronal loss, spongiform lesions, and astrocytic proliferation. The cerebellum is most affected. Iatrogenic transmission of kuru has

occurred when cadaveric material such as dura mater and cornea was transplanted into normal recipients. Since the cessation of cannibalism in New Guinea, the incidence of the disease has decreased drastically.

GERSTMANN-STRAUSSLER-SCHEINKER DISEASE. First described in 1928, GSS is a neurodegenerative syndrome characterized by ataxia, chorea, and cognitive decline leading to dementia. It is caused by a mutation in the PrP gene that is fully penetrant and autosomal dominant; thus the disease is inherited, and affected families have been identified over several generations. Genetic testing can confirm the presence of the abnormal genes before onset. Pathological changes characteristic of prion disease are present: spongiform lesions, neuronal loss, and astrocyte proliferation. Amyloid plaques have been found in the cerebellum. Onset of the disease occurs between 30 and 40 years of age. The disease is fatal within 5 years of onset.

FATAL FAMILIAL INSOMNIA. FFI is an inherited prion disease that primarily affects the thalamus. A syndrome of insomnia and autonomic nervous system dysfunction consisting of fever, sweating, labile blood pressure, and tachycardia occurs that is debilitating. Onset is in middle adulthood, and death usually occurs in 1 year. No treatment currently exists.

Immune Disorders

The major immune disorder in contemporary society is AIDS, but other immune disorders can also present diagnostic and treatment challenges to mental health clinicians.

Systemic Lupus Erythematosus.
Systemic lupus erythematosus (SLE) is an autoimmune disease that involves inflammation of multiple organ systems. The officially accepted diagnosis of SLE requires a patient to have 4 of 11 criteria that have been defined by the American Rheumatism Association. Between 5 and 50 percent of patients with SLE have mental symptoms at the initial presentation, and approximately 50 percent eventually show neuropsychiatric manifestations. The major symptoms are depression, insomnia, emotional lability, nervousness, and confusion. Treatment with steroids commonly induces further psychiatric complications, including mania and psychosis.

Endocrine Disorders

Thyroid Disorders.
Hyperthyroidism is characterized by confusion, anxiety, and an agitated, depressive syndrome. Patients may also complain of being easily fatigued and of feeling generally weak. Insomnia, weight loss despite increased appetite, tremulousness, palpitations, and increased perspiration are also common symptoms. Serious psychiatric symptoms include impairments in memory, orientation, and judgment; manic excitement; delusions; and hallucinations.

Parathyroid Disorders.
Dysfunction of the parathyroid gland results in the abnormal regulation of calcium metabolism. Excessive secretion of parathyroid hormone causes hypercalcemia, which can result in delirium, personality changes, and apathy in 50 to 60 percent of patients and cognitive impairments in approximately 25 percent of patients. Neuromuscular excitability, which depends on proper calcium ion concentration, is reduced, and muscle weakness may appear.

Hypocalcemia can occur with hypoparathyroid disorders and can result in neuropsychiatric symptoms of delirium and

The most common coinfection in persons infected with HIV who have AIDS is *Pneumocystis carinii* pneumonia, which is characterized by a chronic, nonproductive cough and dyspnea, sometimes sufficiently severe to result in hypoxemia and its resultant cognitive effects. Diagnosis is made with fiberoptic bronchoscopy and alveolar lavage. The pneumonia is usually treatable with trimethoprim and sulfamethoxazole (Bactrim, Septra) or pentamidine isethionate (Pentam), which can also be used for prophylaxis against the pneumonia. The other disease that was initially associated with the development of AIDS is Kaposi's sarcoma, a previously rare, blue-purple–tinted skin lesion. For unknown reasons, Kaposi's sarcoma is less commonly associated with cases of recently diagnosed AIDS.

Although *Pneumocystis carinii* pneumonia and Kaposi's sarcoma are the two classic AIDS-related infectious and neoplastic disorders, the severely disabled cellular immune system of patients infected with HIV permits the development of a staggering array of infections and neoplasms. The most common infections are from protozoa such as *Toxoplasma gondii*, fungi such as *Cryptococcus neoformans* and *Candida albicans*, bacteria such as *Mycobacterium avium-intracellulare*, and viruses such as cytomegalovirus and herpes simplex virus.

For psychiatrists, the importance of these nonneurological, nonpsychiatric complications lies in their biological effects on patients' brain functions (e.g., hypoxia with *Pneumocystis carinii* pneumonia) and their psychological effects on patients' moods and anxiety states. Furthermore, because each of the conditions is usually treated by an additional drug, psychiatrists need to be aware of the adverse CNS effects of many medications.

Neurological Factors

An extensive array of disease processes can affect the brain of a patient infected with HIV. The most important diseases for mental health workers to be aware of are *HIV mild neurocognitive disorder* and *HIV-associated dementia*. The latter is a cortical or subcortical type of dementia that can affect 50 percent of patients infected with HIV to some degree. Other diseases and complications of treatment must also be considered in the differential diagnosis of a patient who is HIV infected and has neuropsychiatric symptoms. Symptoms such as photophobia, headache, stiff neck, motor weakness, sensory loss, and changes in level of consciousness should alert a mental health worker that the patient should be examined for possible development of a CNS opportunistic infection or a CNS neoplasm. HIV infection can also result in a variety of peripheral neuropathies that should prompt mental health clinicians to reconsider the extent of CNS involvement.

Psychiatric Syndromes

HIV-Associated Dementia.   The text revision of the fourth edition of the *Diagnostic and Statistical Manual of Mental Disorders* (DSM-IV-TR) allows the diagnosis of dementia due to HIV disease when there is "the presence of a dementia that is judged to be the direct pathophysiological consequence of human immunodeficiency virus (HIV) disease." (See Table 7.3–3 in Chapter 7.)

Although HIV-associated dementia is found in a large proportion of patients infected with HIV, other causes of dementia in these patients must be considered. These causes include CNS infections, CNS neoplasms, CNS abnormalities caused by systemic disorders and endocrinopathies, and adverse CNS responses to drugs. The development of dementia is generally a poor prognostic sign, and 50 to 75 percent of patients with dementia die within 6 months.

Mild Neurocognitive Disorder.   A less severe form of brain involvement is called *HIV-associated neurocognitive disorder*, also known as *HIV encephalopathy*. It is characterized by impaired cognitive functioning and reduced mental activity that interferes with work, homemaking, or social functioning. No laboratory findings are specific to the disorder, and it occurs independent of depression and anxiety. Progression to HIV-associated dementia usually occurs but may be prevented by early treatment.

Delirium.   Delirium can result from the same causes that lead to dementia in patients infected with HIV. Clinicians have classified delirious states characterized by both increased and decreased activity. Delirium in patients infected with HIV is probably underdiagnosed, but it should always precipitate a medical workup of a patient infected with HIV to determine whether a new CNS-related process has begun.

Anxiety Disorders.   Patients with HIV infection may have any of the anxiety disorders, but generalized anxiety disorder, posttraumatic stress disorder, and obsessive-compulsive disorder are particularly common.

Adjustment Disorder.   Adjustment disorder with anxiety or depressed mood has been reported to occur in 5 to 20 percent of patients infected with HIV. The incidence of adjustment disorder in persons infected with HIV is higher than usual in some special populations, such as military recruits and prison inmates.

Depressive Disorders.   From 4 to 40 percent of those infected with HIV are reported to meet the diagnostic criteria for depressive disorders. The pre–HIV infection prevalence of depressive disorders may be higher than usual in some groups who are at risk for contracting HIV. Another reason for the reported variation in prevalence rates is the variable application of the diagnostic criteria; some of the criteria for depressive disorders (poor sleep and weight loss) can also be caused by the HIV infection itself. Depression is higher in women than in men.

Mania.   Mood disorder with manic features, with or without hallucinations, delusions, or a disorder of thought process, can complicate any stage of HIV infection, but most commonly occurs in late-stage disease complicated by neurocognitive impairment.

Substance Abuse.   Substance abuse is a problem not only for IV substance abusers who contract HIV-related diseases, but also for other patients with HIV, who may have used illegal substances only occasionally in the past but may now be tempted to use them regularly to deal with depression or anxiety.

Suicide.   Suicidal ideation and suicide attempts may increase in patients with HIV infection and AIDS. The risk factors for suicide among persons infected with HIV are having friends who died from AIDS, recent notification of HIV seropositivity, relapses, difficult social issues relating to homosexuality, inadequate social and financial support, and the presence of dementia or delirium.

Psychotic Disorder.   Psychotic symptoms are usually later-stage complications of HIV infection. They require immediate medical and neurological evaluation and often require management with antipsychotic medications.

Worried Well.   The so-called worried well are those in high-risk groups who, although they are seronegative and disease free, are anxious about contracting the virus. Some are reassured by repeated negative serum test results, but others cannot be reassured. Their worried well status can progress quickly to generalized anxiety disorder, panic attacks, obsessive-compulsive disorder, and hypochondriasis.

TREATMENT

Prevention is the primary approach to HIV infection. Primary prevention involves protecting persons from getting the disease; secondary prevention involves modification of the disease's course. All persons with any risk of HIV infection should be informed about safe-sex practices and about the necessity to avoid sharing contaminated hypodermic needles. Preventive strategies, however, are complicated by the complex societal values surrounding sexual acts, sexual orientation, birth control, and substance abuse. Many public health officials have advocated condom distribution in schools and the distribution of clean needles to drug addicts. These issues remain controversial, although condom use has been shown to be a fairly (although not completely) safe and effective preventive strategy against HIV infection. Those who are conservative and religious argue that the educational message should be sexual abstinence. Many university laboratories and pharmaceutical companies are attempting to develop a vaccine to protect persons from infection by HIV.

The assessment of patients infected with HIV should include a complete sexual and substance abuse history, a psychiatric history, and an evaluation of the support systems available to them. Clinicians must understand a patient's history with regard to sexual orientation and substance abuse, and the patient must feel that the therapist is not judging past or present behaviors. A therapist can often encourage a sense of trust and empathy in the patient by asking specific, well-informed, straightforward questions about the homosexual or substance-using culture. The therapist must also determine the patient's knowledge about HIV and AIDS.

The homosexual community has provided a significant support system for those infected with HIV, particularly for persons who are gay and bisexual. Public education campaigns within this community have resulted in significant (more than 50 percent) reductions in the highest-risk sexual practices, although some gay men still practice high-risk sex. Homosexual men are likely to practice safe sex if they know the safe-sex guidelines, have access to a support group, are in a steady relationship, and have a close relationship with a person with AIDS. Partly because of the many biases against them, IV substance users with AIDS have received little support, and little progress has been made in educating these persons, who are a major reservoir for spread of the virus to women, heterosexual men, and children.

Pharmacotherapy

A growing list of agents that act at different points in viral replication has raised for the first time the hope that HIV might be permanently suppressed or actually eradicated from the body. At the time of this writing, the active agents are in two general classes: reverse transcriptase inhibitors and protease inhibitors. The reverse transcriptase inhibitors are further subdivided into the nucleoside reverse transcriptase inhibitor group and the non-nucleoside reverse transcriptase inhibitors. In addition to the new nucleoside reverse transcriptase inhibitors, nonnucleoside reverse transcriptase inhibitors, and protease inhibitors, other classes of drugs are under investigation. These include agents that interfere with HIV cell binding and fusion inhibitors (e.g.,

enfurvitide [Fuzeon]), the action of HIV integrase, and certain HIV genes such as *gag*, among others.

The antiretroviral agents have many adverse effects. Of importance to psychiatrists is that protease inhibitors are metabolized by the hepatic cytochrome P450 oxidase system and, therefore, can increase levels of certain psychotropic drugs that are similarly metabolized. These include bupropion (Wellbutrin), meperidine (Demerol), various benzodiazepines, and selective serotonin reuptake inhibitors (SSRIs). Therefore, caution must be exercised in prescribing psychotropic drugs to persons taking protease inhibitors.

Beyond treatment directed specifically against HIV, many interventions are available to prevent and treat various complications of immunodeficiency caused by opportunistic viral, bacterial, fungal, and protozoan infections. Both survival and quality of life have improved substantially because of early diagnosis and treatment of these opportunistic conditions.

The use of combination antiretroviral regimens in conjunction with more specific treatments of complications has prolonged the survival of both asymptomatic and symptomatic HIV-infected persons. Despite progress in maintaining patients longer and in better states of health, the ultimate outcome, however, is still uncertain; that is, it is unclear whether any person who is HIV infected can expect to escape developing AIDS and ultimately dying from it. Those who are HIV infected are keenly aware of this prognosis, and their concern sometimes takes the form of psychiatric disturbances.

Novel treatments may also be useful. Neuronal excitotoxicity, mediated through the activation of glutamatergic receptors by the HIV envelope protein gp120, is a potentially important mechanism by which brain dysfunction might occur in HIV infection. Memantine is an open-channel antagonist of N-methyl-D-aspartate (NMDA)–type glutamate receptors that is generally well tolerated. It is being used as a treatment for dementia of the Alzheimer's type in Europe. On the assumption that an agent that could dislodge gp120 from neural receptor sites might be useful, an octapeptide called D-ala-peptide-T-amide (DAPTA; Peptide T) has been used in phase II clinical trials. Compared with placebo, peptide T was associated with neuropsychological improvement in cognitively impaired individuals (with CD4 counts less than 200) and a reduced likelihood of progression of impairment on 6-month follow-up. Calcium channel inhibitors, which theoretically seemed potentially useful, have not proven successful.

The remaining forms of treatment are principally supportive. The most important step is to exclude other potentially treatable conditions, such as secondary infections or neoplasia, metabolic abnormalities with low-grade delirium, or other psychiatric disorders (e.g., major depressive disorder). Once the diagnosis is clear, then the usual supportive measures for neurocognitively impaired persons should be used. These include identifying areas of cognitive strength and deficit, reducing emphasis on areas that are now impaired (e.g., divided attention, speeded processing), emphasizing efforts to maintain good orientation and reality testing, and avoiding medications that might further compromise cognitive function, in particular, benzodiazepine drugs. If they must be used, such medications should be given at lower-than-usual doses. Antidepressant and antipsychotic agents, if indicated, may also have to be prescribed in much lower doses (e.g., 25 percent of the usual recommended dose).

Psychotherapy

Approaches.   Major psychodynamic themes for patients infected with HIV involve self-blame, self-esteem, and issues regarding death. The psychiatrist can help patients deal with feelings of guilt regarding behaviors that contributed to infection or AIDS. Some patients with HIV and AIDS feel that they are being punished. Difficult health care decisions, such as whether to initiate or continue taking antiretroviral medication and terminal care and life-support systems, should be explored, and here denial of illness may be evident. Major practical themes involve employment, medical benefits, life insurance, career plans, dating and sex, and relationships with families and friends. The entire range of psychotherapeutic approaches may be appropriate for patients with HIV-related disorders. Both individual and group therapy can be effective. Individual therapy may be either short-term or long-term and may be supportive, cognitive, behavioral, or psychodynamic. Group therapy techniques can range from psychodynamic to completely supportive in nature.

Among the fears that must be confronted is the concern that once the individual's serostatus has been revealed, he or she has lost control of who next learns of the seroconversion. In deciding whether to tell others, patients must also address the sense of betrayal that others might feel if they are not told but somehow otherwise find out. The same issues apply to the person's work environment. As a practical matter, the individual may need to decide whether to tell a trusted colleague in case of a job-related accident that might put others at risk of infection. Similarly, parents must decide when or whether to tell their children. Some parents want to tell very young children as soon as possible, whereas other parents prefer to withhold this information until their child's teenage years, for fear of "taking away their childhood." The question of custody of children after the parent's death must be considered. The same question of timing will arise about when to tell children that they are seropositive. The parent must balance fears that telling the child's school will lead to discrimination with the desire to guard their child's and others' safety in case of an accident.

The psychiatrist may have a special role regarding HIV treatment. The advent of protease inhibitors and the promise of additional, increasingly effective therapies have brought hopes of a "cure" to patients and physicians alike. Even patients who have failed one or more rounds of combination therapies may find that family, friends, and physicians continue to be optimistic. The psychiatrist may be the only "safe" person to whom the patient can express discouragement, weariness, fear of treatment failure, and fury or guilt for not being able to tolerate successful therapy or for not responding to regimens that have benefited others. The psychiatrist also may be the only one confronting unrealistic expectations of cure or the assumption that safe-sex practices are no longer relevant. Paradoxically, the therapeutic task also may be to examine the patient's reaction to a reprieve from certain death—the so-called second-life agenda.

Direct counseling regarding substance use and its potential adverse effects on the health of the patient who is HIV infected is indicated. Specific treatments for particular substance-related disorders should be initiated if necessary for the total well-being of the patient.

Therapist-Related Issues.   Countertransference issues and burnout of therapists who treat many patients infected with HIV must be evaluated regularly. Therapists must acknowledge to themselves their predetermined attitudes toward sexual orientation and substance use so that those attitudes do not interfere with the treatment of the patient. Issues regarding the therapist's own sexual identity, past behaviors, and eventual death may also give rise to countertransference issues. Psychotherapists who have practices with many patients infected with HIV can begin to have their effectiveness impaired by professional burnout. Some studies have found that seeing many such patients in a short time seems to be more stressful to therapists than seeing a smaller number of those infected with HIV over a longer period.

Involvement of Significant Others.   The patient's family, lover, and close friends are often important allies in treatment. The patient's spouse or lover may have guilt feelings about possibly having infected the patient or may experience anger at the patient for possibly infecting him or her. The involvement of members of the patient's support group can help the therapist assess the patient's cognitive function and can also aid in planning financial and living arrangements for the patient. The patient's significant others may themselves benefit from the attention of the therapist in helping them cope with the illness and the impending loss of a friend or family member.

Partner Notification.   Although no clear consensus has been reached, recommendations are that patients who are sexually active and infected with HIV should be counseled about potential risk to their sexual partners. In addition, known partners should be notified of exposure risk and potential infection as well. Partner notification has been an extremely hotly debated topic; however, many states have developed legislation requiring or allowing either physicians or health department officials to notify partners of patients who are HIV infected of their risk. The current standard, despite the controversy, appears to be an obligation on the part of health care professionals to notify anyone who could be construed as clearly at risk and clearly identifiable and who may be unaware of his or her risk.

A particularly difficult situation is that of sex-industry workers known to be HIV infected and known to be working actively as prostitutes. Public health issues exist that pose a risk both for these patients and, depending on the politics of the circumstances, their potential partners, clients, customers, victims, or victimizers. The response to this problem has ranged from a sense that sex-industry workers and their clients can make their own decisions and should be responsible for their own behavior all the way to the sentiment that such people should be arrested and jailed for attempted murder. It has also been noted that some sex-industry workers are impaired by a variety of psychiatric conditions, including cognitive impairment, major mental illness, personality disorder, and substance abuse disorders. These may further contribute to the sense that some sex-industry workers may be less than fully responsible for their behavior. Recommendations have been made for voluntary and involuntary interventions regarding these patients. Specific psychiatric interventions regarding competency, ability to consent, capacity, and, most important, treatment for the conditions that impair such people are critical to the mental health needs of patients with HIV.

9 ▲

Substance-Related Disorders

▲ 9.1 Introduction and Overview

This section covers substance dependence and substance abuse, with descriptions of the clinical phenomena associated with the use of 11 designated classes of pharmacological agents: alcohol; amphetamines or similarly acting agents; caffeine; cannabis; cocaine; hallucinogens; inhalants; nicotine; opioids; phencyclidine (PCP) or similar agents; and a group that includes sedatives, hypnotics, and anxiolytics. A residual 12th category includes a variety of agents not in the 11 designated classes, such as anabolic steroids and nitrous oxide.

A perennial debate in the United States relates to the most effective way to handle drug problems. In the past few years, a small but growing number of government officials, commentators, and academics have argued that the present policy of aggressively prosecuting drug sellers and users should be reconsidered. They have compared the current drug policy with the prohibition of alcohol from 1920 to 1934 and have argued that abolishing drug laws would eliminate the profit motive, the gangs, and the drug dealers. Although she stopped short of endorsing such a radical reversal of the nation's drug policy, former U.S. Surgeon General Joycelyn Elders, M.D. (served from 1993 to 1994), recommended that the government study the possibility of legalizing drugs of abuse and suggested that doing so might reduce the incidence of violent crimes.

TERMINOLOGY

The concept of substance dependence has had many officially recognized and commonly used meanings over the decades. Two concepts have been used to define aspects of dependence: behavioral and physical. In *behavioral dependence*, substance-seeking activities and related evidence of pathological use patterns are emphasized, whereas *physical dependence* refers to the physical (physiological) effects of multiple episodes of substance use. In definitions stressing physical dependence, ideas of tolerance or withdrawal appear in the classification criteria (Table 9.1–1). The term *intoxication* is used for a reversible, nondependent experience with a substance that produces impairment (Table 9.1–2).

Somewhat related to dependence are the words *addiction* and *addict*. The word *addict* has acquired a distinctive, unseemly, and pejorative connotation that ignores the concept of substance abuse as a medical disorder. Addiction has also been trivialized in popular usage, as in the phrases *TV addiction* and *money addiction*. Although these connotations have helped the officially sanctioned nomenclature to avoid use of the word addiction,

common neurochemical and neuroanatomical substrates may be found among all the addictions, whether to substances or to gambling, sex, stealing, or eating. These various addictions may have similar effects on the activities of specific reward areas of the brain, such as the ventral tegmental area, the locus ceruleus, and the nucleus accumbens.

Psychological dependence, also referred to as habituation, is characterized by a continuous or intermittent craving for the substance to avoid a dysphoric state.

When making a diagnosis, clinicians should specify whether symptoms of physiological abuse or dependence are present (Tables 9.1–3 and 9.1–4) and also determine whether the disorder is in full or partial remission. The text revision of the fourth edition of the *Diagnostic and Statistical Manual of Mental Disorders* (DSM-IV-TR) allows clinicians to record the current state of the substance dependence by providing a list of course modifiers. A summary of key terms related to dependence and abuse is provided in Table 9.1–5.

EPIDEMIOLOGY

The National Institute of Drug Abuse (NIDA) and other agencies, such as the National Survey of Drug Use and Heath (NSDUH), conduct periodic surveys of the use of illicit drugs in the United States. As of 2004 an estimated 22.5 million persons over the age of 12 years (about 10 percent of the total U.S. population) were classified as suffering from a substance-related disorder. Of this group, about 15 million were dependent on or abused alcohol.

In 2004, 67.8 percent (0.3 million) persons were dependent on or abused heroin; 17.6 percent (4.5 million) abused marijuana; 27.8 percent (1.6 million) abused cocaine; and 12.3 percent (1.4 million) were classified with dependence on, or abuse of, pain relievers.

With regard to age at first use, those who started to use drugs at an earlier age (14 years or younger) were more likely to become addicted than those who started at a later age. This applied to all substances of abuse, but particularly alcohol. Among adults aged 18 years or older who first tried alcohol at age 14 years or younger, 17.9 percent were classified as alcoholics compared with only 4.1 percent who first used alcohol at age 18 years or older.

Rates of abuse also varied according to age. The rate for dependence or abuse was 1.3 percent at age 12 years, and rates generally increased until the highest rate was reached (25.4 percent) at age 21 years. After age 21 years, a general decline occurred with age. By age 65 years, only about 1 percent of persons had used an illicit substance within the past year, which lends

Table 9.1–1
DSM-IV-TR Criteria for Substance Withdrawal

A. The development of a substance-specific syndrome due to the cessation of (or reduction in) substance use that has been heavy and prolonged.
B. The substance-specific syndrome causes clinically significant distress or impairment in social, occupational, or other important areas of functioning.
C. The symptoms are not due to a general medical condition and are not better accounted for by another mental disorder.

From American Psychiatric Association. *Diagnostic and Statistical Manual of Mental Disorders.* 4th ed. Text rev. Washington, DC: American Psychiatric Association; copyright 2000, with permission.

credence to the clinical observation that addicts tend to "burn out" as they age.

More men than women used drugs; the highest lifetime rate was among American Indian or Alaska Natives; whites were more affected than blacks; those with some college education used more substances than those with less education; and the unemployed had higher rates than those with either part-time or full-time employment.

Rates of substance dependence or abuse varied by region in the United States. Rates were higher in the Midwest and West than in the Northeast and South. Rates were also higher in large metropolitan counties than in small metropolitan counties and were lowest in completely rural counties. Rates were also higher among persons on parole or on supervised release from jail (40.8 percent vs. 9.2 percent). A continued need exists for programs to reduce the number of persons driving while under the influence of drugs or alcohol. The percentage of drivers who admitted driving under the influence of alcohol at some time during the past year increased from 10 percent in 2000 to 13.5 percent in 2004, and those driving under the influence of drugs increased from 3.1 percent to 6 percent during the same period. A comprehensive survey of drug use and trends in the United States is available at http://www.samhasa.gov.

ETIOLOGY

The model of drug dependence conceptualizes dependence as a result of a process in which multiple interacting factors influence

Table 9.1–2
DSM-IV-TR Criteria for Substance Intoxication

A. The development of a reversible substance-specific syndrome due to recent ingestion of (or exposure to) a substance. Note: Different substances may produce similar or identical syndromes.
B. Clinically significant maladaptive behavioral or psychological changes that are due to the effect of the substance on the central nervous system (e.g., belligerence, mood lability, cognitive impairment, impaired judgment, impaired social or occupational functioning) and develop during or shortly after use of the substance.
C. The symptoms are not due to a general medical condition and are not better accounted for by another mental disorder.

From American Psychiatric Association. *Diagnostic and Statistical Manual of Mental Disorders.* 4th ed. Text rev. Washington, DC: American Psychiatric Association; copyright 2000, with permission.

Table 9.1–3
DSM-IV-TR Criteria for Substance Abuse

A. A maladaptive pattern of substance use leading to clinically significant impairment or distress, as manifested by one (or more) of the following, occurring within a 12-month period:
   (1) recurrent substance use resulting in a failure to fulfill major role obligations at work, school, or home (e.g., repeated absences or poor work performance related to substance use; substance-related absences, suspensions, or expulsions from school; neglect of children or household)
   (2) recurrent substance use in situations in which it is physically hazardous (e.g., driving an automobile or operating a machine when impaired by substance use)
   (3) recurrent substance-related legal problems (e.g., arrests for substance-related disorderly conduct)
   (4) continued substance use despite having persistent or recurrent social or interpersonal problems caused or exacerbated by the effects of the substance (e.g., arguments with spouse about consequences of intoxication, physical fights)
B. The symptoms have never met the criteria for Substance Dependence for this class of substance.

From American Psychiatric Association. *Diagnostic and Statistical Manual of Mental Disorders.* 4th ed. Text rev. Washington, DC: American Psychiatric Association; copyright 2000, with permission.

drug-using behavior and the loss of flexibility with respect to decisions about using a given drug. Although the actions of a given drug are critical in the process, it is not assumed that all people who become dependent on the same drug experience its effects in the same way or are motivated by the same set of factors. Furthermore, it is postulated that different factors may be more or less important at different stages of the process. Thus, drug availability, social acceptability, and peer pressures may be the major determinants of initial experimentation with a drug, but other factors, such as personality and individual biology, probably are more important in how the effects of a given drug are perceived and the degree to which repeated drug use produces changes in the central nervous system (CNS). Other factors, including the particular actions of the drug, may be primary determinants of whether drug use progresses to drug dependence, whereas still others may be important influences on the likelihood that drug use leads to (1) adverse effects or (2) successful recovery from dependence.

It has been asserted that addiction is a "brain disease," that the critical processes that transform voluntary drug-using behavior to compulsive drug use are changes in the structure and neurochemistry of the brain of the drug user. Sufficient evidence now indicates that such changes in relevant parts of the brain do occur. The perplexing and unanswered question is whether these changes are both necessary and sufficient to account for the drug-using behavior. Many argue that they are not, that the capacity of drug-dependent individuals to modify their drug-using behavior in response to positive reinforcers or aversive contingencies indicates that the nature of addiction is more complex and requires the interaction of multiple factors.

Psychodynamic Factors

The range of psychodynamic theories about substance abuse reflects the various popular theories during the past 100 years.

**Table 9.1–4
DSM-IV-TR Diagnostic Criteria for Substance Dependence**

A maladaptive pattern of substance use, leading to clinically significant impairment or distress, as manifested by three (or more) of the following, occurring at any time in the same 12-month period:

(1) tolerance, as defined by either of the following:

    (a) a need for markedly increased amounts of the substance to achieve intoxication or desired effect

    (b) markedly diminished effect with continued use of the same amount of the substance

(2) withdrawal, as manifested by either of the following:

    (a) the characteristic withdrawal syndrome for the substance (refer to Criteria A and B of the criteria sets for Withdrawal from the specific substances)

    (b) the same (or a closely related) substance is taken to relieve or avoid withdrawal symptoms

(3) the substance is often taken in larger amounts or over a longer period than was intended

(4) there is a persistent desire or unsuccessful efforts to cut down or control substance use

(5) a great deal of time is spent in activities necessary to obtain the substance (e.g., visiting multiple doctors or driving long distances), use the substance (e.g., chain-smoking), or recover from its effects

(6) important social, occupational, or recreational activities are given up or reduced because of substance use

(7) the substance use is continued despite knowledge of having a persistent or recurrent physical or psychological problem that is likely to have been caused or exacerbated by the substance (e.g., current cocaine use despite recognition of cocaine-induced depression, or continued drinking despite recognition that an ulcer was made worse by alcohol consumption)

Specify if:

    With Physiological Dependence: evidence of tolerance or withdrawal (i.e., either Item 1 or 2 is present)

    Without Physiological Dependence: no evidence of tolerance or withdrawal (i.e., neither Item 1 nor 2 is present)

Course specifiers:

    Early Full Remission
    Early Partial Remission
    Sustained Full Remission
    Sustained Partial Remission
    On Agonist Therapy
    In a Controlled Environment

From American Psychiatric Association. *Diagnostic and Statistical Manual of Mental Disorders.* 4th ed. Text rev. Washington, DC: American Psychiatric Association; copyright 2000, with permission.

**Table 9.1–5
Terms Used in Dependence and Abuse**

Dependence The repeated use of a drug or chemical substance, with or without physical dependence. Physical dependence indicates an altered physiological state due to repeated administration of a drug, the cessation of which results in a specific syndrome.

Abuse Use of any drug, usually by self-administration, in a manner that deviates from approved social or medical patterns.

Misuse Similar to abuse but usually applies to drugs prescribed by physicians that are not used properly.

Addiction The repeated and increased use of a substance, the deprivation of which gives rise to symptoms of distress and an irresistible urge to use the agent again and which leads also to physical and mental deterioration. The term is no longer included in the official nomenclature, having been replaced by the term dependence, but it is a useful term in common usage.

Intoxication A reversible syndrome caused by a specific substance (e.g., alcohol) that affects one or more of the following mental functions: memory, orientation, mood, judgment, and behavioral, social, or occupational functioning.

Withdrawal A substance-specific syndrome that occurs after stopping or reducing the amount of the drug or substance that has been used regularly over a prolonged period of time. The syndrome is characterized by physiological signs and symptoms in addition to psychological changes such as disturbances in thinking, feeling, and behavior. Also called *abstinence syndrome* or *discontinuation syndrome.*

Tolerance Phenomenon in which, after repeated administration, a given dose of drug produces a decreased effect or increasingly larger doses must be administered to obtain the effect observed with the original dose. *Behavioral tolerance* reflects the ability of the person to perform tasks despite the effects of the drug.

Cross-tolerance Refers to the ability of one drug to be substituted for another, each usually producing the same physiological and psychological effect (e.g., diazepam and barbiturates). Also known as *cross-dependence.*

Neuroadaptation Neurochemical or neurophysiological changes in the body that result from the repeated administration of a drug. Neuroadaptation accounts for the phenomenon of tolerance. *Pharmacokinetic adaptation* refers to adaptation of the metabolizing system in the body. *Cellular* or *pharmacodynamic adaptation* refers to the ability of the nervous system to function despite high blood levels of the offending substance.

Co-dependence Term used to refer to family members affected by or influencing the behavior of the substance abuser. Related to the term *enabler*, which is a person who facilitates the abuser's addictive behavior (e.g., providing drugs directly or money to by drugs). Enabling also includes the unwillingness of a family member to accept addiction as a medical-psychiatric disorder or to deny that person is abusing a substance.

From American Psychiatric Association. *Diagnostic and Statistical Manual of Mental Disorders.* 4th ed. Text rev. Washington, DC: American Psychiatric Association; copyright 2000, with permission.

According to classic theories, substance abuse is a masturbatory equivalent (some heroin users describe the initial "rush" as similar to a prolonged sexual orgasm), a defense against anxious impulses, or a manifestation of oral regression (i.e., dependency). Recent psychodynamic formulations relate substance use as a reflection of disturbed ego functions (i.e., the inability to deal with reality). As a form of self-medication, alcohol may be used to control panic, opioids to diminish anger, and amphetamines to alleviate depression. Some addicts have great difficulty recognizing their inner emotional states, a condition called *alexithymia* (being unable to find words to describe their feelings).

Learning and Conditioning. Drug use, whether occasional or compulsive, can be viewed as behavior maintained by its consequences. Drugs can reinforce antecedent behaviors by terminating some noxious or aversive state such as pain, anxiety, or depression. In some social situations, the drug use, apart from its pharmacological effects, can be reinforcing if it results in special status or the approval of friends. Each use of the drug evokes rapid positive reinforcement, either as a result of the rush (the drug-induced euphoria), alleviation of disturbed affects, alleviation of withdrawal symptoms, or any combination of these effects. In addition, some drugs may sensitize neural systems to the reinforcing effects of the drug. Eventually, the paraphernalia (needles, bottles, cigarette packs) and behaviors associated with substance use can become secondary reinforcers, as well as cues signaling availability of the substance, and in their presence, craving or a desire to experience the effects increases.

Drug users respond to the drug-related stimuli with increased activity in limbic regions, including the amygdala and the anterior cingulate. Such drug-related activation of limbic areas has been demonstrated with a variety of drugs, including cocaine, opioids, and cigarettes (nicotine). Of interest, the same regions activated by cocaine-related stimuli in cocaine users are activated by sexual stimuli in both normal controls and cocaine users.

In addition to the operant reinforcement of drug-using and drug-seeking behaviors, other learning mechanisms probably play a role in dependence and relapse. Opioid and alcohol withdrawal phenomena can be conditioned (in the Pavlovian or classic sense) to environmental or interoceptive stimuli. For a long time after withdrawal (from opioids, nicotine, or alcohol), the addict exposed to environmental stimuli previously linked with substance use or withdrawal may experience conditioned withdrawal, conditioned craving, or both. The increased feelings of craving are not necessarily accompanied by symptoms of withdrawal. The most intense craving is elicited by conditions associated with the availability or use of the substance, such as watching someone else use heroin or light a cigarette or being offered some drug by a friend. Those learning and conditioning phenomena can be superimposed on any preexisting psychopathology, but preexisting difficulties are not required for the development of powerfully reinforced substance-seeking behavior.

Genetic Factors

Strong evidence from studies of twins, adoptees, and siblings brought up separately indicates that the cause of alcohol abuse has a genetic component. Many less-conclusive data show that other types of substance abuse or substance dependence have a genetic pattern in their development. Researchers recently have used restriction fragment length polymorphism (RFLP) in the study of substance abuse and substance dependence, and associations to genes that affect dopamine production have been postulated.

Neurochemical Factors

Receptors and Receptor Systems.   With the exception of alcohol, researchers have identified particular neurotransmitters or neurotransmitter receptors involved with most substances of abuse. Some researchers base their studies on such hypotheses. The opioids, for example, act on opioid receptors. A person with too little endogenous opioid activity (e.g., low concentrations of endorphins) or with too much activity of an endogenous opioid antagonist may be at risk for developing opioid dependence. Even in a person with completely normal endogenous receptor function and neurotransmitter concentration, the long-term use of a particular substance of abuse may eventually modulate receptor systems in the brain so that the presence of the exogenous substance is needed to maintain homeostasis. Such a receptor-

level process may be the mechanism for developing tolerance within the CNS. Demonstrating modulation of neurotransmitter release and neurotransmitter receptor function has proved difficult, however, and recent research focuses on the effects of substances on the second-messenger system and on gene regulation.

Pathways and Neurotransmitters

The major neurotransmitters possibly involved in developing substance abuse and substance dependence are the opioid, catecholamine (particularly dopamine), and γ-aminobutyric acid (GABA) systems. The dopaminergic neurons in the ventral tegmental area are particularly important. These neurons project to the cortical and limbic regions, especially the nucleus accumbens. This pathway is probably involved in the sensation of reward and may be the major mediator of the effects of such substances as amphetamine and cocaine. The locus ceruleus, the largest group of adrenergic neurons, probably mediates the effects of the opiates and the opioids. These pathways have collectively been called the *brain-reward circuitry*.

COMORBIDITY

Comorbidity is the occurrence of two or more psychiatric disorders in a single patient at the same time. A high prevalence of additional psychiatric disorders is found among persons seeking treatment for alcohol, cocaine, or opioid dependence; some studies have shown that up to 50 percent of addicts have a comorbid psychiatric disorder. Although opioid, cocaine, and alcohol abusers with current psychiatric problems are more likely to seek treatment, those who do not seek treatment are not necessarily free of comorbid psychiatric problems; such persons may have social supports that enable them to deny the impact that drug use is having on their lives. Two large epidemiological studies have shown that even among representative samples of the population, those who meet the criteria for alcohol or drug abuse and dependence (excluding tobacco dependence) are far more likely to meet the criteria for other psychiatric disorders also.

Antisocial Personality Disorder.   In various studies, 35 to 60 percent of patients with substance abuse or substance dependence also meet the diagnostic criteria for antisocial personality disorder. The number is even higher when investigators include persons who meet all the antisocial personality disorder diagnostic criteria except the requirement that the symptoms started at an early age. That is, a high percentage of patients with substance abuse or substance dependence diagnoses have a pattern of antisocial behavior, whether it was present before the substance use started or developed during the course of the substance use. Patients with substance abuse or substance dependence diagnoses who have antisocial personality disorder are likely to use more illegal substances, have more psychopathology, be less satisfied with their lives, and be more impulsive, isolated, and depressed than patients with antisocial personality disorders alone.

Depression and Suicide.   Depressive symptoms are common among persons diagnosed with substance abuse or substance dependence. About one third to one half of all those with opioid abuse or opioid dependence and about 40 percent of those with alcohol abuse or alcohol dependence meet the criteria for major depressive disorder sometime during their lives. Substance use is also a major precipitating factor for suicide. Persons who abuse substances are about 20 times more likely to die by suicide than the general population. About 15 percent of persons with alcohol abuse or alcohol dependence have been reported to commit suicide. This frequency of suicide is second only to the frequency in patients with major depressive disorder.

TREATMENT AND REHABILITATION

Some persons who develop substance-related problems recover without formal treatment, especially as they age. For those patients with less severe disorders, such as nicotine addiction, relatively brief interventions are often as effective as more intensive treatments. Because these brief interventions do not change the environment, alter drug-induced brain changes, or provide new skills, a change in the patient's motivation (cognitive change) probably has the best impact on the drug-using behavior. For those individuals who do not respond or whose dependence is more severe, a variety of interventions appear to be effective.

It is useful to distinguish among specific procedures or techniques (e.g., individual therapy, family therapy, group therapy, relapse prevention, and pharmacotherapy) and treatment programs. Most programs use a number of specific procedures and involve several professional disciplines as well as nonprofessionals who have special skills or personal experience with the substance problem being treated. The best treatment programs combine specific procedures and disciplines to meet the needs of the individual patient after a careful assessment.

No classification is generally accepted for either the specific procedures used in treatment or programs using various combinations of procedures. This lack of standardized terminology for categorizing procedures and programs presents a problem, even when the field of interest is narrowed from substance problems in general to treatment for a single substance, such as alcohol, tobacco, or cocaine. Except in carefully monitored research projects, even the definitions of specific procedures (e.g., individual counseling, group therapy, and methadone maintenance) tend to be so imprecise that one usually cannot infer just what transactions are supposed to occur. Nevertheless, for descriptive purposes, programs are often broadly grouped on the basis of one or more of their salient characteristics: whether the program is aimed at merely controlling acute withdrawal and consequences of recent drug use (detoxification) or is focused on longer-term behavioral change; whether the program makes extensive use of pharmacological interventions; and the degree to which the program is based on individual psychotherapy, Alcoholics Anonymous (AA) or other 12-step principles, or therapeutic community principles. For example, government agencies recently categorized publicly funded treatment programs for drug dependence as (1) methadone maintenance (mostly outpatient), (2) outpatient drug-free programs, (3) therapeutic communities, or (4) short-term inpatient programs.

Selecting a Treatment

Not all interventions are applicable to all varieties of substance use or dependence, and some of the more coercive interventions used for illicit drugs are not applicable to substances that are legally available, such as tobacco. Addictive behaviors do not change abruptly but through a series of stages. Five stages in this gradual process have been proposed: precontemplation, contemplation, preparation, action, and maintenance. For some types of addictions the therapeutic alliance is enhanced when the treatment approach is tailored to the patient's stage of readiness to change. Interventions for some drug use disorders may have a specific pharmacological agent as an important component; for example, disulfiram, naltrexone (ReVia), or acamprosate for alcoholism; methadone (Dolophine), levomethadyl acetate (ORLAAM), or buprenorphine (Buprenex) for heroin addiction; and nicotine delivery devices or bupropion (Zyban) for tobacco dependence. Not all interventions are likely to be useful to health care professionals. For example, many youthful offenders with histories of drug use or dependence are now remanded to special facilities (boot camps); other programs for offenders (and sometimes for employees) rely almost exclusively on the deterrent effect of frequent urine testing; and a third group of programs is built around religious conversion or rededication in a specific religious sect or denomination. In contrast to the numerous studies suggesting some value for brief interventions for smoking and for problem drinking, few controlled studies are conducted of brief interventions for those seeking treatment for dependence on illicit drugs.

In general, brief interventions (such as a few weeks of detoxification, whether in or out of a hospital) used for persons who are severely dependent on illicit opioids have limited effect on outcome measured a few months later. Substantial reductions in illicit drug use, antisocial behaviors, and psychiatric distress among patients dependent on cocaine or heroin are much more likely following treatment lasting at least 3 months. Such a time-in-treatment effect is seen across very different modalities, from residential therapeutic communities to ambulatory methadone maintenance programs. Although some patients appear to benefit from a few days or weeks of treatment, a substantial percentage of users of illicit drugs drop out (or are dropped) from treatment before they have achieved significant benefits.

Some of the variance in treatment outcomes can be attributed to differences in the characteristics of patients entering treatment and by events and conditions following treatment. Programs based on similar philosophical principles and using what seem to be similar therapeutic procedures vary greatly in effectiveness, however. Some of the differences among programs that seem to be similar reflect the range and intensity of services offered. Programs with professionally trained staffs that provide more comprehensive services to patients with more severe psychiatric difficulties are more likely to be able to retain those patients in treatment and help them make positive changes. Differences in the skills of individual counselors and professionals can strongly affect outcomes.

Such generalizations concerning programs serving illicit drug users may not hold for programs dealing with those seeking treatment for alcohol, tobacco, or even cannabis problems uncomplicated by heavy use of illicit drugs. In such cases, relatively brief periods of individual or group counseling can produce long-lasting reductions in drug use. The outcomes usually considered in programs dealing with illicit drugs have typically included measures of social functioning, employment, and criminal activity, as well as decreased drug-using behavior.

▲ 9.2 Alcohol-Related Disorders

Alcohol use disorders are common lethal conditions that often masquerade as other psychiatric syndromes. The average alcohol-dependent person decreases his or her life span by 10 to 15 years, and alcohol contributes to 22,000 deaths and 2 million nonfatal injuries each year. Recent years have witnessed a blossoming of clinically relevant research regarding alcohol abuse and dependence, including information on specific genetic influences, the clinical course of these conditions, and the development of new and helpful treatments.

An understanding of the effects of alcohol and the clinical importance of alcohol-related disorders is essential for the practice of psychiatry. Alcohol intoxication can cause irritability, violent behavior, feelings of depression, and, in rare instances, hallucinations and delusions. Longer-term, escalating levels of alcohol consumption can produce tolerance as well as such intense adaptation of the body that cessation of use can precipitate a withdrawal syndrome usually marked by insomnia, evidence of hyperactivity of the autonomic nervous system, and feelings of anxiety. Thus, in an adequate evaluation of life problems and psychiatric symptoms in a patient, the clinician must consider the possibility that the clinical situation reflects the effects of alcohol.

Although alcohol abuse and dependency are commonly called alcoholism, the text revision of the fourth edition of the *Diagnostic and Statistical Manual of Mental Disorders* (DSM-IV-TR) does not use the term because it lacks a precise definition. The term remains in common use, however.

EPIDEMIOLOGY

PREVALENCE OF DRINKING

At some time during life, 90 percent of the population in the United States drinks, with most people beginning their alcohol intake in the early to middle teens. By the end of high school, 80 percent of students have consumed alcohol, and more than 60 percent have been intoxicated. At any time, two out of three men are drinkers, with a ratio of persisting alcohol intake of approximately 1.3 men to 1.0 woman, and the highest prevalence of drinking is from the middle or late teens to the mid-20s.

Different groups in the United States have different rates of drinkers. Generally, groups with high education and high socioeconomic status have the highest proportion of people who currently imbibe. Among religious groups, Jews have the highest proportion of individuals who consume alcohol but the lowest number of people with alcohol dependence. Conservative Protestants and Catholics are less likely to use alcohol than liberal Protestants and Catholics. Other groups, such as the Irish, have higher rates of severe alcohol problems, but they also have significantly higher rates of abstention. Very high rates of alcohol problems are found among most, but not all, American Indian and Inuit tribes.

In the United States in the mid-1990s, the average person older than 14 years of age consumed 2.2 gallons of absolute alcohol a year. This amount sounds substantial, but it is considerably less than the more than 5 gallons of absolute ethanol consumed each year at the time of the American Revolution. The current figure also represents a significant decrease from the amounts consumed during the mid-1970s and the 2.7 gallons per capita in 1981.

Drinking alcohol-containing beverages is generally considered an acceptable and common habit in the United States. About 90 percent of all U.S. residents have had an alcohol-containing drink at least once in their lives, and about 51 percent of all U.S. adults are current users of alcohol. After heart disease and cancer, alcohol-related disorders constitute the third-most-significant health problem in the United States today; beer accounts for about one half of all alcohol consumption, liquor for about one third, and wine for about one sixth. About 30 to 45 percent of all adults in the United States have had at least one transient episode of an alcohol-related problem, usually an alcohol-induced amnestic episode (e.g., a blackout), driving a motor vehicle while intoxicated, or missing school or work because of excessive drinking. About 10 percent of women and 20 percent of men have met the diagnostic criteria for alcohol abuse during their lifetime, and 3 to 5 percent of women and 10 percent of men have met the diagnostic criteria for the more serious diagnosis of alcohol dependence during their lifetime. About 200,000 deaths each year are directly related to alcohol abuse. The common causes of death among persons with the alcohol-related disorders are suicide, cancer, heart disease, and hepatic disease. Although persons involved in automotive fatalities do not always meet the diagnostic criteria for an alcohol-related disorder, drunken drivers are involved in about 50 percent of all automotive fatalities, and this percentage increases to about 75 percent when only accidents occurring in the late evening are considered. Alcohol use and alcohol-related disorders are also associated with about 50 percent of all homicides and 25 percent of all suicides. Alcohol abuse reduces life expectancy by about 10 years, and alcohol leads all other substances in substance-related deaths.

COMORBIDITY /Relatedness

The psychiatric diagnoses most commonly associated with the alcohol-related disorders are other substance-related disorders, antisocial personality disorder, mood disorders, and anxiety disorders. Although the data are somewhat controversial, most suggest that persons with alcohol-related disorders have a markedly higher suicide rate than the general population.

Antisocial Personality Disorder

A relation between antisocial personality disorder and alcohol-related disorders has frequently been reported. Some studies suggest that antisocial personality disorder is particularly common in men with an alcohol-related disorder and can precede the development of the alcohol-related disorder. Other studies, however, suggest that antisocial personality disorder and alcohol-related disorders are completely distinct entities that are not causally related.

Mood Disorders

About 30 to 40 percent of persons with an alcohol-related disorder meet the diagnostic criteria for major depressive disorder sometime during their lifetime. Depression is more common in women than in men with these disorders. Several studies reported that depression is likely to occur in patients with alcohol-related disorders who have a high daily consumption of alcohol and a family history of alcohol abuse. Persons with alcohol-related disorders and major depressive disorder are at great risk for attempting suicide and are likely to have other substance-related disorder diagnoses. Some clinicians recommend antidepressant drug therapy for depressive symptoms that remain after 2 to 3 weeks of sobriety. Patients with bipolar I disorder are thought to be at risk for developing an alcohol-related disorder; they may use alcohol to self-medicate their manic episodes. Some studies have shown that persons with both alcohol-related disorder and depressive disorder diagnoses have concentrations of dopamine metabolites (homovanillic acid) and γ-aminobutyric acid (GABA) in their cerebrospinal fluid.

Anxiety Disorders

Many persons use alcohol for its efficacy in alleviating anxiety. Although the comorbidity between alcohol-related disorders and mood disorders is fairly widely recognized, it is less well known that perhaps 25 to 50 percent of all persons with alcohol-related disorders also meet the diagnostic criteria for an anxiety disorder. Phobias and panic disorder are particularly frequent comorbid diagnoses in these patients. Some data indicate that alcohol may be used in an attempt to self-medicate symptoms of agoraphobia or social phobia, but an alcohol-related disorder is likely to precede the development of panic disorder or generalized anxiety disorder.

Suicide

Most estimates of the prevalence of suicide among persons with alcohol-related disorders range from 10 to 15 percent, although alcohol use itself may be involved in a much higher percentage of suicides. Some investigators have questioned whether the suicide rate among persons with alcohol-related disorders is as high as the numbers suggest. Factors that have been associated with suicide among persons with alcohol-related disorders include the presence of a major depressive episode, weak psychosocial support systems, a serious coexisting medical condition, unemployment, and living alone.

ETIOLOGY

Many factors affect the decision to drink, the development of temporary alcohol-related difficulties in the teenage years and the 20s, and the development of alcohol dependence. The initiation of alcohol intake probably depends largely on social, religious, and psychological factors, although genetic characteristics might also contribute. The factors that influence the decision to drink or those that contribute to temporary problems might differ, however, from those that add to the risk for the severe, recurring problems of alcohol dependence.

A similar interplay between genetic and environmental influences contributes to many medical and psychiatric conditions, and, thus, a review of these factors in alcoholism offers information about complex genetic disorders overall. Dominant or recessive genes, although important, only explain relatively rare conditions. Most disorders have some level of genetic predisposition that usually relates to a series of different genetically influenced characteristics, each of which increases or decreases the risk for the disorder.

It is likely that a series of genetic influences combines to explain approximately 60 percent of the proportion of risk for alcoholism, with environment responsible for the remaining proportion of the variance. The divisions offered in this section, therefore, are more heuristic than real because it is the combination of a series of psychological, sociocultural, biological, and other factors that are responsible for the development of severe, repetitive alcohol-related life problems.

Psychological Theories

A variety of theories relate to the use of alcohol to reduce tension, increase feelings of power, and decrease the effects of psychological pain. Perhaps the greatest interest has been paid to the observation that people with alcohol-related problems often report that alcohol decreases their feelings of nervousness and helps them cope with the day-to-day stresses of life. The psychological theories are built, in part, on the observation among nonalcoholic people that the intake of low doses of alcohol in a tense social setting or after a difficult day can be associated with an enhanced feeling of well-being and an improved ease of interactions. In high doses, especially at falling blood alcohol levels, however, most measures of muscle tension and psychological feelings of nervousness and tension are increased. Thus, tension-reducing effects of this drug might have an impact mostly on light to moderate drinkers or add to the relief of withdrawal symptoms but play a minor role in causing alcoholism. It is difficult definitively to evaluate theories that focus on alcohol's potential to enhance feelings of being powerful and sexually attractive and to decrease the effects of psychological pain.

Psychodynamic Theories

Perhaps related to the disinhibiting or anxiety-lowering effects of lower doses of alcohol is the hypothesis that some people may use this drug to help them deal with self-punitive harsh superegos and to decrease unconscious stress levels. In addition, classic psychoanalytical theory hypothesizes that at least some alcoholic people may have become fixated at the oral stage of development and use alcohol to relieve their frustrations by taking the substance by mouth. Hypotheses regarding arrested phases of psychosexual development, although heuristically useful, have had little effect on the usual treatment approaches and are not the focus of extensive ongoing research. Similarly, most studies have not been able to document an "addictive personality" present in most alcoholics and associated with a propensity to lack control of intake of a wide range of substances and foods. Although pathological scores on personality tests are often seen during intoxication, withdrawal, and early recovery, many of these characteristics are not found to predate alcoholism, and most disappear with abstinence. Similarly, prospective studies of children of alcoholics who themselves have no cooccurring disorders usually document high risks mostly for alcoholism. As will be described, one partial exception to these comments occurs with the extreme levels of impulsivity seen in the 15 to 20 percent of alcoholic men with antisocial personality disorder, because they have high risks for criminality, violence, and multiple substance dependencies.

Behavioral Theories

Expectations about the rewarding effects of drinking, cognitive attitudes toward responsibility for one's behavior, and subsequent reinforcement after alcohol intake all contribute to the decision to drink again after the first experience with alcohol and to continue to imbibe despite problems. These issues are important in efforts to modify drinking behaviors in the general population, and they contribute to some important aspects of alcoholic rehabilitation.

Sociocultural Theories

Sociocultural theories are often based on extrapolations from social groups that have high or low rates of alcoholism. Theorists hypothesize that ethnic groups, such as Jews, who introduce children to modest levels of drinking in a family atmosphere and eschew drunkenness have low rates of alcoholism. Some other groups, such as Irish men or some American Indian tribes with high rates of abstention but a tradition of drinking to the point of drunkenness among drinkers, are believed to have high rates of alcoholism. These theories, however, often depend on stereotypes that tend to be erroneous, and prominent exceptions to these rules exist. For example, some theories based on observations of the Irish and the French have incorrectly predicted high rates of alcoholism among the Italians.

Nonetheless, environmental events, presumably including cultural factors, account for as much as 40 percent of the alcoholism risk. Thus, although these are difficult to study, it is likely that cultural attitudes toward drinking, drunkenness, and personal responsibility for consequences are important contributors to the rates of alcohol-related problems in a society. In the final analysis, social and psychological theories are probably highly relevant because they outline factors that contribute to the onset of drinking, the development of temporary alcohol-related life difficulties, and even alcoholism. The problem is how to gather relatively definitive data to support or refute the theories.

Childhood History

Researchers have identified several factors in the childhood histories of persons with later alcohol-related disorders and in children at high risk for having an alcohol-related disorder because one or both of their parents are affected. In experimental studies, children at high risk for alcohol-related disorders have been found to possess, on average, a range of deficits on neurocognitive testing, low amplitude of the P300 wave on evoked potential testing, and a variety of abnormalities on electroencephalogram (EEG) recordings. Studies of high-risk offspring in their 20s have also shown a generally blunted effect of alcohol compared with that seen in persons whose parents have not been diagnosed with alcohol-related disorder. These findings suggest that a heritable biological brain function may predispose a person to an alcohol-related disorder. A childhood history of attention-deficit/hyperactivity disorder (ADHD), conduct disorder, or both increases a child's risk for an alcohol-related disorder as an adult. Personality disorders, especially antisocial personality disorder, as noted previously, also predispose a person to an alcohol-related disorder.

Genetic Theories

Importance of Genetic Influences.   Four lines of evidence support the conclusion that alcoholism is genetically influenced. First, a three- to fourfold increased risk for severe alcohol problems is seen in close relatives of alcoholic people. The rate of alcohol problems increases with the number of alcoholic relatives, the severity of their illness, and the closeness of their genetic relationship to the person under study. The family investigations do little to separate the importance of genetics and environment, and the second approach, twin studies, takes the data a step further. The rate of similarity, or concordance, for severe alcohol-related problems is significantly higher in identical twins of alcoholic individuals than in fraternal twins in most investigations, which estimate that genes explain 60 percent of the variance, with the remainder relating to nonshared, probably adult environmental influences. Third, the adoption-type studies have all revealed a significantly enhanced risk for alcoholism in the offspring of alcoholic parents, even when the children had been separated from their biological parents close to birth and raised without any knowledge of the problems within the biological family. The risk for severe alcohol-related difficulties is not further enhanced by being raised by an alcoholic adoptive family. Finally, studies in animals support the importance of a variety of yet-to-be-identified genes in the free-choice use of alcohol, subsequent levels of intoxication, and some consequences.

EFFECTS OF ALCOHOL

The term *alcohol* refers to a large group of organic molecules that have a hydroxyl group ($-OH$) attached to a saturated carbon atom. Ethyl alcohol, also called *ethanol*, is the common form of alcohol; sometimes referred to as *beverage alcohol*, ethyl alcohol is used for drinking. The chemical formula for ethanol is CH_3-CH_2-OH.

The characteristic tastes and flavors of alcohol-containing beverages result from their methods of production, which produce various congeners in the final product, including methanol, butanol, aldehydes, phenols, tannins, and trace amounts of various metals. Although the congeners may confer some differential psychoactive effects on the various alcohol-containing beverages, these differences are minimal compared with the effects of ethanol itself. A single drink is usually considered to contain about 12 g of ethanol, which is the content of 12 ounces of beer (7.2 proof, 3.6 percent ethanol in the United States), one 4-ounce glass of nonfortified wine, or 1 to 1.5 ounces of an 80-proof (40 percent ethanol) liquor (e.g., whiskey or gin). In calculating patients' alcohol intake, however, clinicians should be aware that beers vary in their alcohol content, that beers are available in small and large cans and mugs, that glasses of wine range from 2 to 6 ounces, and that mixed drinks at some bars and in most homes contain 2 to 3 ounces of liquor. Nonetheless, using the moderate sizes of drinks, clinicians can estimate that a single drink increases the blood alcohol level of a 150-pound man by 15 to 20 mg/dL, which is about the concentration of alcohol that an average person can metabolize in 1 hour.

The possible beneficial effects of alcohol have been publicized, especially by its makers and distributors. Most attention has focused on some epidemiological data that suggest that one or two glasses of red wine each day lower the incidence of cardiovascular disease; these findings, however, are highly controversial.

Absorption

About 10 percent of consumed alcohol is absorbed from the stomach, the remainder from the small intestine. Peak blood concentration of alcohol is reached in 30 to 90 minutes and usually in 45 to 60 minutes, depending on whether the alcohol was taken on an empty stomach (which enhances absorption) or with food (which delays absorption). The time to peak blood concentration also depends on the time during which the alcohol was consumed; rapid drinking reduces the time to peak concentration, whereas slower drinking increases it. Absorption is most rapid with beverages containing 15 to 30 percent alcohol (30 to 60 proof). There is some dispute about whether carbonation (e.g., in champagne and in drinks mixed with seltzer) enhances the absorption of alcohol.

The body has protective devices against inundation by alcohol. For example, if the concentration of alcohol in the stomach becomes too high, mucus is secreted, and the pyloric valve closes. These actions slow the absorption and keep the alcohol from passing into the small intestine, where there are no significant restraints to absorption. Thus, a large amount of alcohol can remain unabsorbed in the stomach for hours. Furthermore, pylorospasm often results in nausea and vomiting.

Once alcohol is absorbed into the bloodstream, it is distributed to all body tissues. Because alcohol is uniformly dissolved in the body's water, tissues containing a high proportion of water receive a high concentration of alcohol. The intoxicating effects are greater when the blood alcohol concentration is rising than when it is falling (the Mellanby effects). For this reason, the rate of absorption bears directly on the intoxication response.

Metabolism

About 90 percent of absorbed alcohol is metabolized through oxidation in the liver; the remaining 10 percent is excreted unchanged by the kidneys and lungs. The rate of oxidation by the liver is constant and independent of the body's energy requirements. The body can metabolize about 15 mg/dL per hour, with a range of 10 to 34 mg/dL per hour. That is, the average person oxidizes three fourths of an ounce of 40 percent (80 proof) alcohol in an hour. In persons with a history of excessive alcohol consumption, upregulation of the necessary enzymes results in rapid alcohol metabolism.

Alcohol is metabolized by two enzymes: alcohol dehydrogenase (ADH) and aldehyde dehydrogenase. ADH catalyzes the conversion of alcohol into acetaldehyde, which is a toxic compound; aldehyde dehydrogenase catalyzes the conversion of acetaldehyde into acetic acid. Aldehyde dehydrogenase is inhibited by disulfiram (Antabuse), often used in the treatment of alcohol-related disorders. Some studies have shown that women have a lower ADH blood content than men; this fact may account for women's tendency to become more intoxicated than men after drinking the same amount of alcohol. The decreased function of alcohol-metabolizing enzymes in some Asian persons can also lead to easy intoxication and toxic symptoms.

Effects on the Brain

Biochemistry.   In contrast to most other substances of abuse with identified receptor targets—such as the N-methyl-D-aspartate (NMDA) receptor of phencyclidine (PCP)—no single molecular target has been identified as the mediator for the effects of alcohol. The long-standing theory about the biochemical effects of alcohol concerns its effects on the membranes of neurons. Data support the hypothesis that alcohol produces its effects by intercalating itself into membranes and, thus, increasing fluidity of the membranes with short-term use. With long-term use, however, the theory hypothesizes that the membranes become rigid or stiff. The fluidity of the membranes is critical to normal functioning of receptors, ion channels, and other membrane-bound functional proteins. In recent studies, researchers have attempted to identify specific molecular targets for the effects of alcohol. Most attention has been focused on the effects of alcohol at ion channels. Specifically, studies have found that alcohol ion channel activities associated with the nicotinic acetylcholine, serotonin 5-hydroxytryptamine 3 (5-HT$_3$), and GABA type A (GABA$_A$) receptors are enhanced by alcohol, whereas ion channel activities associated with glutamate receptors and voltage-gated calcium channels are inhibited.

Behavioral Effects.   As the net result of the molecular activities, alcohol functions as a depressant much as do the barbiturates and the benzodiazepines, with which alcohol has some cross-tolerance and cross-dependence. At a level of 0.05 percent alcohol in the blood, thought, judgment, and restraint are loosened and sometimes disrupted. At a concentration of 0.1 percent, voluntary motor actions usually become perceptibly clumsy. In most states, legal intoxication ranges from 0.1 to 0.15 percent blood alcohol level. At 0.2 percent, the function of the entire motor area of the brain is measurably depressed, and the parts of the brain that control emotional behavior are also affected. At 0.3 percent, a person is commonly confused or may become stuporous; at 0.4 to 0.5 percent, the person falls into a coma. At higher levels, the primitive centers of the brain that control breathing and heart rate are affected, and death ensues secondary to direct respiratory depression or the aspiration of vomitus. Persons with long-term histories of alcohol abuse, however, can tolerate much higher concentrations of alcohol than can alcohol-naive persons; their alcohol tolerance may cause them falsely to appear less intoxicated than they really are.

Sleep Effects.   Although alcohol consumed in the evening usually increases the ease of falling asleep (decreased sleep latency), alcohol also has adverse effects on sleep architecture. Specifically, alcohol use is associated with a decrease in rapid eye movement sleep (REM or dream sleep) and deep sleep (stage 4) and more sleep fragmentation, with more and longer episodes of awakening. Therefore, the idea that drinking alcohol helps persons fall asleep is a myth.

Other Physiological Effects

Liver.   The major adverse effects of alcohol use are related to liver damage. Alcohol use, even as short as week-long episodes of increased drinking, can result in an accumulation of fats and proteins, which produce the appearance of a fatty liver, sometimes found on physical examination as an enlarged liver. The association between fatty infiltration of the liver and serious liver damage remains unclear. Alcohol use, however, is associated with the development of alcoholic hepatitis and hepatic cirrhosis.

Gastrointestinal System.   Long-term heavy drinking is associated with developing esophagitis, gastritis, achlorhydria, and gastric ulcers. The development of esophageal varices can accompany particularly heavy alcohol abuse; the rupture of the varices is a medical emergency often resulting in death by exsanguination. Disorders of the small intestine occasionally occur, and pancreatitis, pancreatic insufficiency, and pancreatic cancer are also associated with heavy alcohol use. Heavy alcohol intake may interfere with the normal processes of food digestion and absorption; as a result, consumed food is inadequately digested. Alcohol abuse also appears to inhibit the intestine's capacity to absorb various nutrients, such as vitamins and amino acids. This effect, coupled with the often poor dietary habits of those with alcohol-related disorders, can cause serious vitamin deficiencies, particularly of the B vitamins.

Other Bodily Systems. Significant intake of alcohol has been associated with increased blood pressure, dysregulation of lipoprotein and triglyceride metabolism, and increased risk for myocardial infarctions and cerebrovascular diseases. Alcohol has been shown to affect the hearts of nonalcoholic persons who do not usually drink, increasing the resting cardiac output, the heart rate, and the myocardial oxygen consumption. Evidence indicates that alcohol intake can adversely affect the hematopoietic system and can increase the incidence of cancer, particularly head, neck, esophageal, stomach, hepatic, colonic, and lung cancer. Acute intoxication may also be associated with hypoglycemia, which, when unrecognized, may be responsible for some of the sudden deaths of persons who are intoxicated. Muscle weakness is another side effect of alcoholism. Recent evidence shows that alcohol intake raises the blood concentration of estradiol in women. The increase in estradiol correlates with the blood alcohol level.

Laboratory Tests. The adverse effects of alcohol appear in common laboratory tests, which can be useful diagnostic aids in identifying persons with alcohol-related disorders. The γ-glutamyl transpeptidase levels are high in about 80 percent of those with alcohol-related disorders, and the mean corpuscular volume (MCV) is high in about 60 percent, more so in women than in men. Other laboratory test values that may be high in association with alcohol abuse are those of uric acid, triglycerides, aspartate aminotransferase (AST), and alanine aminotransferase (ALT).

Drug Interactions

The interaction between alcohol and other substances can be dangerous, even fatal. Certain substances, such as alcohol and phenobarbital (Luminal), are metabolized by the liver, and their prolonged use can lead to acceleration of their metabolism. When persons with alcohol-related disorders are sober, this accelerated metabolism makes them unusually tolerant to many drugs such as sedatives and hypnotics; when they are intoxicated, however, these drugs compete with the alcohol for the same detoxification mechanisms, and potentially toxic concentrations of all involved substances can accumulate in the blood.

The effects of alcohol and other central nervous system (CNS) depressants are usually synergistic. Sedatives, hypnotics, and drugs that relieve pain, motion sickness, head colds, and allergy symptoms must be used with caution by persons with alcohol-related disorders. Narcotics depress the sensory areas of the cerebral cortex and can produce pain relief, sedation, apathy, drowsiness, and sleep; high doses can result in respiratory failure and death. Increasing the doses of sedative-hypnotic drugs, such as chloral hydrate (Noctec) and benzodiazepines, especially when they are combined with alcohol, produces a range of effects from sedation to motor and intellectual impairment to stupor, coma, and death. Because sedatives and other psychotropic drugs can potentiate the effects of alcohol, patients should be instructed about the dangers of combining CNS depressants and alcohol, particularly when they are driving or operating machinery.

DISORDERS

DSM-IV-TR lists the alcohol-related disorders (Table 9.2–1) and specifies the diagnostic criteria for alcohol intoxication (Table 9.2–2) and alcohol withdrawal (Table 9.2–3). The diagnostic criteria for the other alcohol-related disorders are listed in DSM-IV-TR under the major symptom. For example, the diagnostic criteria for alcohol-induced anxiety disorder are found in the

Table 9.2–1
DSM-IV-TR Alcohol-Related Disorders

Alcohol use disorders
Alcohol dependence
Alcohol abuse
Alcohol-induced disorders
Alcohol intoxication
Alcohol withdrawal
   Specify if:
      With perceptual disturbances
Alcohol intoxication delirium
Alcohol withdrawal delirium
Alcohol-induced persisting dementia
Alcohol-induced persisting amnestic disorder
Alcohol-induced psychotic disorder, with delusions
   Specify if:
      With onset during intoxication
      With onset during withdrawal
Alcohol-induced psychotic disorder, with hallucinations
   Specify if:
      With onset during intoxication
      With onset during withdrawal
Alcohol-induced mood disorder
   Specify if:
      With onset during intoxication
      With onset during withdrawal
Alcohol-induced anxiety disorder
   Specify if:
      With onset during intoxication
      With onset during withdrawal
Alcohol-induced sexual dysfunction
   Specify if:
      With onset during intoxication
Alcohol-induced sleep disorder
   Specify if:
      With onset during intoxication
      With onset during withdrawal
Alcohol disorder not otherwise specified

From American Psychiatric Association. *Diagnostic and Statistical Manual of Mental Disorders*. 4th ed. Text rev. Washington, DC: American Psychiatric Association; copyright 2000, with permission.

Table 9.2–2
DSM-IV-TR Diagnostic Criteria for Alcohol Intoxication

A. Recent ingestion of alcohol.
B. Clinically significant maladaptive behavioral or psychological changes (e.g., inappropriate sexual or aggressive behavior, mood lability, impaired judgment, impaired social or occupational functioning) that developed during, or shortly after, alcohol ingestion.
C. One (or more) of the following signs, developing during, or shortly after, alcohol use:
   (1) slurred speech
   (2) incoordination
   (3) unsteady gait
   (4) nystagmus
   (5) impairment in attention or memory
   (6) stupor or coma
D. The symptoms are not due to a general medical condition and are not better accounted for by another mental disorder.

From American Psychiatric Association. *Diagnostic and Statistical Manual of Mental Disorders*. 4th ed. Text rev. Washington, DC: American Psychiatric Association; copyright 2000, with permission.

Table 9.2–3
DSM-IV-TR Diagnostic Criteria for Alcohol Withdrawal

A. Cessation of (or reduction in) alcohol use that has been heavy and prolonged.

B. Two (or more) of the following, developing within several hours to a few days after Criterion A:

   (1) autonomic hyperactivity (e.g., sweating or pulse rate greater than 100)

   (2) increased hand tremor

   (3) insomnia

   (4) nausea or vomiting

   (5) transient visual, tactile, or auditory hallucinations or illusions

   (6) psychomotor agitation

   (7) anxiety

   (8) grand mal seizures

C. The symptoms in Criterion B cause clinically significant distress or impairment in social, occupational, or other important areas of functioning.

D. The symptoms are not due to a general medical condition and are not better accounted for by another mental disorder.

Specify if:

With perceptual disturbances

From American Psychiatric Association. *Diagnostic and Statistical Manual of Mental Disorders.* 4th ed. Text rev. Washington, DC: American Psychiatric Association; copyright 2000, with permission.

anxiety disorders category under the heading Substance-Induced Anxiety Disorder.

Alcohol Dependence and Alcohol Abuse

Diagnosis and Clinical Features. In DSM-IV-TR, all substance-related disorders use the same criteria for dependence and abuse (see Tables 9.1–3 and 9.1–4). A need for daily use of large amounts of alcohol for adequate functioning, a regular pattern of heavy drinking limited to weekends, and long periods of sobriety interspersed with binges of heavy alcohol intake lasting for weeks or months strongly suggest alcohol dependence and alcohol abuse. The drinking patterns are often associated with certain behaviors: the inability to cut down or stop drinking; repeated efforts to control or reduce excessive drinking by "going on the wagon" (periods of temporary abstinence) or by restricting drinking to certain times of the day; binges (remaining intoxicated throughout the day for at least 2 days); occasional consumption of a fifth of spirits (or its equivalent in wine or beer); amnestic periods for events occurring while intoxicated (blackouts); the continuation of drinking despite a serious physical disorder that the person knows is exacerbated by alcohol use; and drinking nonbeverage alcohol, such as fuel and commercial products containing alcohol. In addition, persons with alcohol dependence and alcohol abuse show impaired social or occupational functioning because of alcohol use (e.g., violence while intoxicated, absence from work, job loss), legal difficulties (e.g., arrest for intoxicated behavior and traffic accidents while intoxicated), and arguments or difficulties with family members or friends about excessive alcohol consumption. According to DSM-IV-TR, the current rate of alcohol dependence is 5 percent.

A 39-year-old prominent businessman, Mr. G, was referred for evaluation by a clinician who was concerned that he was making little progress with the patient's mood swings and somatic complaints. Therapy, primarily using a cognitive and behavioral approach, had been instituted 6 months previously for a condition that involved depressive symptoms and irritability present most, but not all, days for the prior several years. Mr. G had recently had a routine physical examination at work and was noted to have mild hypertension (blood pressure of 145/95) along with a blood test that revealed an MCV of 92.5 μm^3 and a γ-glutamyltransferase level of 43 U/L.

On interview, the patient admitted that his wife had been complaining for several years about his drinking pattern of one to two bottles of wine (i.e., 6 to 12 standard drinks) per day. She noted that the mornings after drinking he was more irritable than usual, and she complained about his restless sleep. Mr. G had recognized potential problems and tried on several occasions to cut back on his drinking. These efforts usually resulted in periods of abstinence of between 2 and 4 weeks, followed by several months of establishing clear rules that set limits on his intake that always gave way to increased drinking as part of a celebration, business trip, vacation, or in the context of daily stresses. Mr. G noted that once ad-lib drinking began, he slowly increased the amount consumed per day to maintain the desired effects. He denied ever experiencing full-blown alcohol withdrawal, although he did report "hangovers" lasting 6 to 12 hours but rarely going into the second day. (Courtesy of Marc A. Schuckit, M.D.)

Subtypes of Alcohol Dependence. Various researchers have attempted to divide alcohol dependence into subtypes based primarily on phenomenological characteristics. One recent classification notes that type A alcohol dependence is characterized by late onset, few childhood risk factors, relatively mild dependence, few alcohol-related problems, and little psychopathology. Type B alcohol dependence is characterized by many childhood risk factors, severe dependence, an early onset of alcohol-related problems, much psychopathology, a strong family history of alcohol abuse, frequent polysubstance abuse, a long history of alcohol treatment, and a high number of severe life stresses. Some researchers have found that type A persons who are alcohol dependent may respond to interactional psychotherapies, whereas type B persons who are alcohol dependent may respond to training in coping skills.

Other subtyping schemes of alcohol dependence have received fairly wide recognition in the literature. One group of investigators proposed three subtypes: early-stage problem drinkers, who do not yet have complete alcohol dependence syndromes; affiliative drinkers, who tend to drink daily in moderate amounts in social settings; and schizoid-isolated drinkers, who have severe dependence and tend to drink in binges and often alone.

Another investigator described gamma alcohol dependence, which is thought to be common in the United States and represents the alcohol dependence seen in those who are active in Alcoholics Anonymous (AA). This variant concerns control problems in which persons are unable to stop drinking once they start. When drinking is terminated as a result of ill health or lack of money, these persons can abstain for varying periods. In delta alcohol dependence, perhaps more common in Europe than in the United States, persons who are alcohol dependent must drink a certain amount each day but are unaware of a lack of control. The alcohol use disorder may not be discovered until a person who must stop drinking for some reason exhibits withdrawal symptoms.

Another researcher has suggested a *type I, male-limited* variety of alcohol dependence, characterized by late onset, more evidence of psychological than of physical dependence, and the presence of guilt feelings. *Type II, male-limited* alcohol dependence is characterized by onset at an early age, spontaneous seeking of alcohol for consumption, and a socially disruptive set of behaviors when intoxicated.

Four subtypes of alcoholism were postulated by still another investigator. The first is *antisocial alcoholism*, typically with a predominance in men, a poor prognosis, early onset of alcohol-related problems, and a close association with antisocial personality disorder. The second is *developmentally cumulative alcoholism*, with a primary tendency for alcohol abuse that is exacerbated with time as cultural expectations foster increased opportunities to drink. The third is *negative-affect alcoholism*, which is more common in women than in men; according to this hypothesis, women are likely to use alcohol for mood regulation and to help ease social relationships. The fourth is *developmentally limited alcoholism*, with frequent bouts of consuming large amounts of alcohol; the bouts become less frequent as persons age and respond to the increased expectations of society about their jobs and families.

Alcohol Intoxication

The DSM-IV-TR diagnostic criteria for alcohol intoxication are based on evidence of recent ingestion of ethanol, maladaptive behavior, and at least one of six possible physiological correlates of intoxication (Table 9.2–1).

As a conservative approach to identifying blood levels that are likely to have major effects on driving abilities, the legal definition of intoxication in most states in the United States requires a blood concentration of 80 or 100 mg ethanol per dL of blood (mg/dL), which is the same as 0.08 to 0.10 g/dL. For most people, a rough estimate of the levels of impairment likely to be seen at various blood alcohol concentrations can be outlined. Evidence of behavioral changes, a slowing in motor performance, and a decrease in the ability to think clearly occurs at doses as low as 20 to 30 mg/dL. Blood concentrations between 100 and 200 mg/dL are likely to increase the impairment in coordination and judgment to severe problems with coordination (ataxia), increasing lability of mood, and progressively greater levels of cognitive deterioration. Anyone who does not show significant levels of impairment in motor and mental performance at approximately 150 mg/dL probably has significant pharmacodynamic tolerance. In that range, most people without significant tolerance also experience relatively severe nausea and vomiting. With blood alcohol concentrations in the 200 to 300 mg/dL range, the slurring of speech is likely to become more intense, and memory impairment (*anterograde amnesia* or *alcoholic blackouts*) becomes pronounced. Further increases in blood

alcohol concentration result in the first level of anesthesia, and the nontolerant person who reaches 400 mg/dL or more risks respiratory failure, coma, and death.

Alcohol Withdrawal

Alcohol withdrawal, even without delirium, can be serious; it can include seizures and autonomic hyperactivity. Conditions that may predispose to, or aggravate, withdrawal symptoms include fatigue, malnutrition, physical illness, and depression. The DSM-IV-TR criteria for alcohol withdrawal (Table 9.2–3) require the cessation or reduction of alcohol use that was heavy and prolonged as well as the presence of specific physical or neuropsychiatric symptoms. The diagnosis also allows for the specification "with perceptual disturbances." One recent positron emission tomographic (PET) study of blood flow during alcohol withdrawal in otherwise healthy persons with alcohol dependence reported a globally low rate of metabolic activity, although, with further inspection of the data, the authors concluded that activity was especially low in the left parietal and right frontal areas.

The classic sign of alcohol withdrawal is tremulousness, although the spectrum of symptoms can expand to include psychotic and perceptual symptoms (e.g., delusions and hallucinations), seizures, and the symptoms of delirium tremens (DTs), called alcohol withdrawal delirium in DSM-IV-TR. Tremulousness (commonly called the "shakes" or the "jitters") develops 6 to 8 hours after the cessation of drinking, the psychotic and perceptual symptoms begin in 8 to 12 hours, seizures in 12 to 24 hours, and DTs during 72 hours, although physicians should watch for the development of DTs for the first week of withdrawal. The syndrome of withdrawal sometimes skips the usual progression and, for example, goes directly to DTs.

The tremor of alcohol withdrawal can be similar to either physiological tremor, with a continuous tremor of great amplitude and of more than 8 Hz, or familial tremor, with bursts of tremor activity slower than 8 Hz. Other symptoms of withdrawal include general irritability, gastrointestinal symptoms (e.g., nausea and vomiting), and sympathetic autonomic hyperactivity, including anxiety, arousal, sweating, facial flushing, mydriasis, tachycardia, and mild hypertension. Patients experiencing alcohol withdrawal are generally alert but may startle easily.

Mr. T is a 64-year-old lawyer with a 35-year history of alcohol dependence. Alcohol-related problems have included tolerance, spending a great deal of time using alcohol (despite a relatively successful career), repeatedly giving up important business and family events because he was too intoxicated or hung over, and significant interference with his relationship with his wife. She complained about his sarcastic wit and lack of care about her areas of interest.

Mr. T had been able to stop drinking on multiple occasions in the past, at which times he experienced a tremor, anxiety, and problems sleeping. He typically self-medicated these symptoms with five or more 10-mg capsules of chlordiazepoxide per day, using pills that had been prescribed for him by his general practitioner in response to his complaints of anxiety and insomnia. Recently, Mr. T was diagnosed with moderate hypertension and adult-onset diabetes, with the result that his family practitioner urged him to stop drinking. In recognition of his age and his associated medical problems, it was believed that withdrawal would be best treated in a medical setting.

An examination confirmed the medical diagnoses along with a mildly decreased hematocrit (38 percent). The evaluation, carried out approximately 12 hours after his most recent drink, also revealed the smell of alcohol remaining on his breath, with a blood alcohol level of 50 mg/dL. The patient demonstrated a prominent tremor of both hands along with a pulse of 110 beats per minute, a respiratory rate of 25 breaths per minute, and a blood pressure of 150/96. Mr. T complained of feeling agitated, noted that he felt very tired but was unable to sleep, but was otherwise alert and oriented. (Courtesy of Marc A. Schuckit, M.D.)

Withdrawal Seizures. Seizures associated with alcohol withdrawal are stereotyped, generalized, and tonic-clonic in character. Patients often have more than one seizure 3 to 6 hours after the first seizure. Status epilepticus is relatively rare and occurs in less than 3 percent of patients. Although anticonvulsant medications are not required in the management of alcohol withdrawal seizures, the cause of the seizures is difficult to establish when a patient is first assessed in the emergency room; thus, many patients with withdrawal seizures receive anticonvulsant medications, which are then discontinued once the cause of the seizures is recognized. Seizure activity in patients with known alcohol abuse histories should still prompt clinicians to consider other causative factors, such as head injuries, CNS infections, CNS neoplasms, and other cerebrovascular diseases; long-term severe alcohol abuse can result in hypoglycemia, hyponatremia, and hypomagnesaemia—all of which can also be associated with seizures.

Treatment. The primary medications for the control of alcohol withdrawal symptoms are the benzodiazepines. Many studies have found that benzodiazepines help control seizure activity, delirium, anxiety, tachycardia, hypertension, diaphoresis, and tremor associated with alcohol withdrawal. Benzodiazepines can be given either orally or parenterally; neither diazepam (Valium) nor chlordiazepoxide (Librium), however, should be given intramuscularly (IM) because of their erratic absorption by this route. Clinicians must titrate the dose of the benzodiazepine, starting with a high dose and lowering the dose as the patient recovers. Sufficient benzodiazepines should be given to keep patients calm and sedated but not so sedated that they cannot be aroused for clinicians to perform appropriate procedures, including neurological examinations.

Although benzodiazepines are the standard treatment for alcohol withdrawal, studies have shown that carbamazepine (Tegretol) in daily doses of 800 mg is as effective as benzodiazepines and has the added benefit of minimal abuse liability. Carbamazepine use is gradually becoming common in the United States and Europe. The β-adrenergic receptor antagonists and clonidine (Catapres) have also been used to block the symptoms of sympathetic hyperactivity, but neither drug is an effective treatment for seizures or delirium.

Delirium

Diagnosis and Clinical Features. The DSM-IV-TR contains the diagnostic criteria for alcohol intoxication delirium in the category of substance intoxication delirium and the diagnostic criteria for alcohol withdrawal delirium in the category of substance withdrawal delirium (see Tables 7.2–2 and 7.2–3 in Chapter 7, Section 7.2). Patients with recognized alcohol withdrawal symptoms should be carefully monitored to prevent progression to alcohol withdrawal delirium, the most severe form of the withdrawal syndrome, also known as DTs. Alcohol withdrawal delirium is a medical emergency that can result in significant morbidity and mortality. Patients with delirium are a danger to themselves and to others. Because of the unpredictability of their behavior, patients with delirium may be assaultive or suicidal or may act on hallucinations or delusional thoughts as if they were genuine dangers. Untreated, DTs has a mortality rate of 20 percent, usually as a result of an intercurrent medical illness such as pneumonia, renal disease, hepatic insufficiency, or heart failure. Although withdrawal seizures commonly precede the development of alcohol withdrawal delirium, delirium can also appear unheralded. The essential feature of the syndrome is delirium occurring within 1 week after a person stops drinking or reduces the intake of alcohol. In addition to the symptoms of delirium, the features of alcohol intoxication delirium include autonomic hyperactivity such as tachycardia, diaphoresis, fever, anxiety, insomnia, and hypertension; perceptual distortions, most frequently visual or tactile hallucinations; and fluctuating levels of psychomotor activity, ranging from hyperexcitability to lethargy.

About 5 percent of persons with alcohol-related disorders who are hospitalized have DTs. Because the syndrome usually develops on the third hospital day, a patient admitted for an unrelated condition may unexpectedly have an episode of delirium, the first sign of a previously undiagnosed alcohol-related disorder. Episodes of DTs usually begin in a patient's 30s or 40s after 5 to 15 years of heavy drinking, typically of the binge type. Physical illness (e.g., hepatitis or pancreatitis) predisposes to the syndrome; a person in good physical health rarely has DTs during alcohol withdrawal.

A 73-year-old professor emeritus at a university was believed to be in good health when he entered the hospital for an elective hernia repair. Perhaps reflecting his status in the community, the relatively brief history contained no detailed notes of his drinking pattern and made no mention of his γ-glutamyltransferase value of 55 U/L along with the MCV of 93.5 μm^3. Eight hours postsurgery, the nursing staff noted a sharp increase in the pulse rate to 110, an increase in blood pressure to 150/100, prominent diaphoresis, and a tremor to both hands, after which the patient demonstrated a brief but intense grand mal convulsion. He awoke extremely agitated and disoriented to time, place, and person. A reevaluation of the history and an interview with the wife documented alcohol dependence with a consumption of approximately six standard drinks per night. Over the following 4 days, the patient's autonomic nervous system dysfunction decreased as his cognitive impairment disappeared. His condition is classified as alcohol withdrawal delirium in DSM-IV-TR.

Treatment.   The best treatment for DTs is prevention. Patients withdrawing from alcohol who exhibit withdrawal phenomena should receive a benzodiazepine, such as 25 to 50 mg of chlordiazepoxide, every 2 to 4 hours until they seem to be out of danger. Once the delirium appears, however, 50 to 100 mg of chlordiazepoxide should be given every 4 hours orally, or lorazepam (Ativan) should be given intravenously (IV) if oral medication is not possible. Antipsychotic medications that may reduce the seizure threshold in patients should be avoided. A high-calorie, high-carbohydrate diet supplemented by multivitamins is also important.

Physically restraining patients with the DTs is risky; they may fight against the restraints to a dangerous level of exhaustion. When patients are disorderly and uncontrollable, a seclusion room can be used. Dehydration, often exacerbated by diaphoresis and fever, can be corrected with fluids given by mouth or IV. Anorexia, vomiting, and diarrhea often occur during withdrawal. Antipsychotic medications should be avoided because they may reduce the seizure threshold in the patient. The emergence of focal neurological symptoms, lateralizing seizures, increased intracranial pressure, or evidence of skull fractures or other indications of CNS pathology should prompt clinicians to examine a patient for additional neurological disease. Nonbenzodiazepine anticonvulsant medication is not useful in preventing or treating alcohol withdrawal convulsions, although benzodiazepines are generally effective.

Warm, supportive psychotherapy in the treatment of DTs is essential. Patients are often bewildered, frightened, and anxious because of their tumultuous symptoms, and skillful verbal support is imperative.

Alcohol-Induced Persisting Dementia

The legitimacy of the concept of alcohol-induced persisting dementia remains controversial; some clinicians and researchers believe that it is difficult to separate the toxic effects of alcohol abuse from the CNS damage done by poor nutrition and multiple trauma and that following the malfunctioning of other bodily organs such as the liver, the pancreas, and the kidneys. Although several studies have found enlarged ventricles and cortical atrophy in persons with dementia and a history of alcohol dependence, the studies do not help clarify the cause of the dementia. Nonetheless, DSM-IV-TR includes the diagnosis of alcohol-induced persisting dementia (Table 7.3–4). The controversy about the diagnosis should encourage clinicians to complete a diagnostic assessment of the dementia before concluding that it was caused by alcohol.

Alcohol-Induced Persisting Amnestic Disorder

Diagnosis and Clinical Features.   The diagnostic criteria of alcohol-induced persisting amnestic disorder are contained in the DSM-IV-TR category of substance-induced persisting amnestic disorder (Table 7.4–2). The essential feature of alcohol-induced persisting amnestic disorder is a disturbance in short-term memory caused by prolonged heavy use of alcohol. Because the disorder usually occurs in persons who have been drinking heavily for many years, the disorder is rare in persons younger than age 35 years.

Wernicke-Korsakoff Syndrome.   The classic names for alcohol-induced persisting amnestic disorder are Wernicke's encephalopathy (a set of acute symptoms) and Korsakoff's syndrome (a chronic condition). Whereas Wernicke's encephalopathy is completely reversible with treatment, only about 20 percent of patients with Korsakoff's syndrome recover. The pathophysiological connection between the two syndromes is thiamine deficiency, caused either by poor nutritional habits or by malabsorption problems. Thiamine is a cofactor for several important enzymes and may also be involved in conduction of the axon potential along the axon and in synaptic transmission. The neuropathological lesions are symmetrical and paraventricular, involving the mammillary bodies, the thalamus, the hypothalamus, the midbrain, the pons, the medulla, the fornix, and the cerebellum.

Wernicke's encephalopathy, also called *alcoholic encephalopathy*, is an acute neurological disorder characterized by ataxia (affecting primarily the gait), vestibular dysfunction, confusion, and a variety of ocular motility abnormalities, including horizontal nystagmus, lateral orbital palsy, and gaze palsy. These eye signs are usually bilateral but not necessarily symmetrical. Other eye signs may include a sluggish reaction to light and anisocoria. Wernicke's encephalopathy may clear spontaneously in a few days or weeks or may progress into Korsakoff's syndrome.

Treatment.   In the early stages, Wernicke's encephalopathy responds rapidly to large doses of parenteral thiamine, which is believed to be effective in preventing the progression into Korsakoff's syndrome. The dose of thiamine is usually initiated at 100 mg by mouth two to three times daily and is continued for 1 to 2 weeks. In patients with alcohol-related disorders who are receiving IV administration of glucose solution, it is good practice to include 100 mg of thiamine in each liter of the glucose solution.

Korsakoff's syndrome is the chronic amnestic syndrome that can follow Wernicke's encephalopathy, and the two syndromes are believed to be pathophysiologically related. The cardinal features of Korsakoff's syndrome are impaired mental syndrome (especially recent memory) and anterograde amnesia in an alert and responsive patient. The patient may or may not have the symptom of confabulation. Treatment of Korsakoff's syndrome is also thiamine given 100 mg by mouth two to three times daily; the treatment regimen should continue for 3 to 12 months. Few patients who progress to Korsakoff's syndrome ever fully recover, although many have some improvement in their cognitive abilities with thiamine and nutritional support.

Blackouts.   Alcohol-related blackouts are not included in DSM-IV-TR's diagnostic classification, although the symptom of alcohol intoxication is common. Blackouts are similar to episodes of transient global amnesia (see Chapter 7, Section 7.4) in that they are discrete episodes of anterograde amnesia that occur in association with alcohol intoxication. The periods of amnesia can be particularly distressing when persons fear that they have unknowingly harmed someone or behaved imprudently while intoxicated. During a blackout, persons have relatively intact remote memory but experience a specific short-term memory deficit in which they are unable to recall events that happened in the previous 5 or 10 minutes. Because their other intellectual faculties are well preserved, they can perform complicated tasks and appear normal to casual observers. The neurobiological mechanisms for alcoholic blackouts are now known at the molecular level; alcohol blocks the consolidation of new memories into old memories, a process that is thought to involve the hippocampus and related temporal lobe structures.

Alcohol-Induced Psychotic Disorder

Diagnosis and Clinical Features.   The diagnostic criteria for alcohol-induced psychotic disorders, such as delusions and hallucinations, are found in the DSM-IV-TR category of substance-induced psychotic disorder (see Table 11.4–5). DSM-IV-TR further allows the specification of onset (during intoxication or withdrawal) and whether hallucinations or delusions are present. The most common hallucinations are auditory, usually voices, but they are often unstructured. The voices are characteristically maligning, reproachful, or threatening, although some patients report that the voices are pleasant and nondisruptive. The hallucinations usually last less than a week, but during that week impaired reality testing is common. After the episode, most patients realize the hallucinatory nature of the symptoms.

Hallucinations after alcohol withdrawal are considered rare, and the syndrome is distinct from alcohol withdrawal delirium. The hallucinations can occur at any age, but usually appear in persons abusing alcohol for a long time. Although the hallucinations usually resolve within a week, some may linger; in these cases, clinicians must consider other psychotic disorders in the differential diagnosis. Alcohol withdrawal–related hallucinations are differentiated from the hallucinations of schizophrenia by the temporal association with alcohol withdrawal, the absence of a classic history of schizophrenia, and their usually short-lived duration. Alcohol withdrawal–related hallucinations are differentiated from the DTs by the presence of a clear sensorium in patients.

A 39-year-old male letter carrier was brought to an emergency room by the police after he behaved in an unusual fashion at home and complained that his neighbors were trying to kill him. The history obtained from the patient and his wife revealed that his psychotic thinking developed slowly over the preceding 3 weeks; he began with feelings that persons were looking at him at work, progressed to vague feelings that persons were against him, and went on to frank auditory hallucinations that persons at work and in the neighboring houses were talking about their plans to kill him. He had no insight into those paranoid delusions and auditory hallucinations. The relatively abrupt onset of the syndrome—he was in his late 30s—pointed to a potential organic cause, and further probing documented that he had been drinking between 6 and 18 beers daily for at least the preceding 10 weeks. A diagnosis of alcohol-induced psychotic disorder with onset during intoxication was made, and both hallucinations and delusions disappeared after 3 weeks of abstinence. After alcohol treatment, the man stayed sober for the next 8 months. He later resumed heavy drinking, however, and had a recurrence of both hallucinations and delusions. (Courtesy of Marc A. Schuckit, M.D.)

Treatment.   The treatment of alcohol withdrawal–related hallucinations is much like the treatment of DTs—benzodiazepines, adequate nutrition, and fluids if necessary. If this regimen fails or for long-term cases, antipsychotics may be used.

Alcohol-Induced Mood Disorder

The DSM-IV-TR allows for the diagnosis of alcohol-induced mood disorder with manic, depressive, or mixed features (see Table 12.3–8) and also for the specification of onset during either intoxication or withdrawal. As with all the secondary and substance-induced disorders, clinicians must consider whether the abused substance and the symptoms have a causal relation.

A consultation was requested on a 42-year-old woman with alcohol dependence who complained of persisting severe depressive symptoms despite 5 days of abstinence. In the initial stage of the interview she noted that she had "always been depressed" and felt that she "drank to cope with the depressive symptoms." Her current complaint included a prominent sadness that had persisted for several weeks, difficulties concentrating, initial and terminal insomnia, and a feeling of hopelessness and guilt. In an effort to distinguish between an alcohol-induced mood disorder and an independent major depressive episode, a time-line–based history was obtained. This focused on the age of onset of alcohol dependence, periods of abstinence that extended for several months or more since the onset of dependence, and the ages of occurrence of clear major depressive episodes lasting several weeks or more at a time. Despite this patient's original complaints, it became clear that there had been no major depressive episodes prior to her mid-20s, when alcohol dependence began, and that during a 1-year period of abstinence related to the gestation and neonatal period of her son, her mood had significantly improved. A provisional diagnosis of an alcohol-induced mood disorder was made. The patient was offered education, reassurance, and cognitive therapy to help her to deal with the depressive symptoms, but no antidepressant medications were prescribed. The depressive symptoms remained at their original intensity for several additional days and then began to improve. By approximately 3 weeks abstinence the patient no longer met criteria for a major depressive episode, although she demonstrated mood swings similar to dysphemia for several additional weeks. This case is a fairly typical example of an alcohol-induced mood disorder in an individual with alcohol dependence. (Courtesy of Marc A. Schuckit, M.D.)

Alcohol-Induced Anxiety Disorder

The DSM-IV-TR allows for the diagnosis of alcohol-induced anxiety disorder (see Table 13.7–2) and suggests that the diagnosis specify whether the symptoms are those of generalized anxiety, panic attacks, obsessive-compulsive symptoms, or phobic symptoms and whether the onset was during intoxication or during withdrawal. The association between alcohol use and anxiety symptoms was discussed previously; deciding whether the anxiety symptoms are primary or secondary can be difficult.

A 48-year-old woman was referred for evaluation and treatment of her recent onset of panic attacks. These episodes occurred two to three times per week over the past 6 months, with each lasting typically between 10 and 20 minutes. Panic symptoms occurred regardless of levels of life stress and could not be explained by current medications or medical conditions. The workup included an evaluation of her laboratory test values, which revealed a carbohydrate-deficient transferrin (CDT) level of 28 U/L, a uric acid level of 7.1 mg, and a γ-glutamyltransferase value of 47. All other blood tests were within normal limits.

The atypical age of onset of the panic attacks, along with the blood results, encouraged the clinician to probe further regarding the pattern of alcohol-related life problems with both the patient and, separately, her spouse. This step documented a history of alcohol dependence with an onset at approximately 35 years of age, with no evidence of panic disorder before that date. Nor did the patient have repetitive panic attacks beyond 2 weeks of abstinence during her frequent periods of nondrinking, which often lasted for 3 or 4 months. A working diagnosis of alcohol dependence with an alcohol-induced anxiety disorder characterized by panic attacks was made, and the patient was encouraged to abstain and was appropriately treated for possible withdrawal symptoms. Over the subsequent 3 weeks after a taper of benzodiazepines used for the treatment of withdrawal, the panic symptoms diminished in intensity and subsequently disappeared. (Courtesy of Marc A. Schuckit, M.D.)

Alcohol-Induced Sexual Dysfunction

In DSM-IV-TR, the formal diagnosis of symptoms of sexual dysfunction associated with alcohol intoxication is alcohol-induced sexual dysfunction (see Table 17.2–11).

Alcohol-Induced Sleep Disorder

In DSM-IV-TR, the diagnostic criteria for alcohol-induced sleep disorders with an onset during either alcohol intoxication or alcohol withdrawal are found in the sleep disorders section (see Table 20.2–14).

Alcohol-Related Use Disorder Not Otherwise Specified

The DSM-IV-TR allows for the diagnosis of alcohol-related disorder not otherwise specified for alcohol-related disorders that do not meet the diagnostic criteria for any of the other diagnoses (Table 9.2–4).

Idiosyncratic Alcohol Intoxication. Whether there is such a diagnostic entity as idiosyncratic alcohol intoxication is under debate; DSM-IV-TR does not recognize this category

Table 9.2–4
DSM-IV-TR Diagnostic Criteria for Alcohol-Related Disorder Not Otherwise Specified

The alcohol-related disorder not otherwise specified category is for disorders associated with the use of alcohol that are not classifiable as alcohol dependence, alcohol abuse, alcohol intoxication, alcohol withdrawal, alcohol intoxication delirium, alcohol withdrawal delirium, alcohol-induced persisting dementia, alcohol-induced persisting amnestic disorder, alcohol-induced psychotic disorder, alcohol-induced mood disorder, alcohol-induced anxiety disorder, alcohol-induced sexual dysfunction, or alcohol-induced sleep disorder.

From American Psychiatric Association. *Diagnostic and Statistical Manual of Mental Disorders.* 4th ed. Text rev. Washington, DC: American Psychiatric Association; copyright 2000, with permission.

as an official diagnosis. Several well-controlled studies of persons who supposedly have the disorder have raised questions about the validity of the designation. The condition has been variously called pathologic, complicated, atypical, and paranoid alcohol intoxication; all of these terms indicate that a severe behavioral syndrome develops rapidly after a person consumes a small amount of alcohol that would have minimal behavioral effects on most persons. The diagnosis is important in the forensic arena because alcohol intoxication is not generally accepted as a reason for judging persons not responsible for their activities. Idiosyncratic alcohol intoxication, however, can be used in a person's defense if a defense lawyer can argue successfully that the defendant has an unexpected, idiosyncratic, pathological reaction to a minimal amount of alcohol.

In anecdotal reports, persons with idiosyncratic alcohol intoxication have been described as confused and disoriented and as experiencing illusions, transitory delusions, and visual hallucinations. Persons may display greatly increased psychomotor activity and impulsive, aggressive behavior. They may be dangerous to others and may also exhibit suicidal ideation and make suicide attempts. The disorder, usually described as lasting for a few hours, terminates in prolonged sleep, and those affected cannot recall the episodes on awakening. The cause of the condition is unknown, but it is reported to be most common in persons with high levels of anxiety. According to one hypothesis, alcohol causes sufficient disorganization and loss of control to release aggressive impulses. Another suggestion is that brain damage, particularly encephalitic or traumatic damage, predisposes some persons to an intolerance for alcohol and thus to abnormal behavior after they ingest only small amounts. Other predisposing factors may include advancing age, use of sedative-hypnotic drugs, and a feeling of fatigue. A person's behavior while intoxicated tends to be atypical; after one weak drink, a quiet, shy person becomes belligerent and aggressive.

In treating idiosyncratic alcohol intoxication, clinicians must help protect patients from harming themselves and others. Physical restraint may be necessary but is difficult because of the abrupt onset of the condition. Once a patient has been restrained, injection of an antipsychotic drug, such as haloperidol (Haldol), is useful for controlling assaultiveness. This condition must be differentiated from other causes of abrupt behavioral change, such as complex partial epilepsy. Some persons with the disorder reportedly showed temporal lobe spiking on an EEG after ingesting small amounts of alcohol.

Other Alcohol-Related Neurological Disorders

Only the major neuropsychiatric syndromes associated with alcohol use have been discussed here. The complete list of neurological syndromes is lengthy. Alcoholic pellagra encephalopathy is one diagnosis of potential interest to psychiatrists presented with a patient who appears to be afflicted with Wernicke-Korsakoff syndrome but does not respond to thiamine treatment. The symptoms of alcoholic pellagra encephalopathy include confusion, clouding of consciousness, myoclonus, oppositional hypertonias, fatigue, apathy, irritability, anorexia, insomnia, and sometimes delirium. Patients suffer from a deficiency of niacin (nicotinic acid), and the specific treatment is 50 mg of niacin by mouth four times daily or 25 mg parenterally two to three times daily.

Fetal Alcohol Syndrome

Data indicate that women who are pregnant or are breast-feeding should not drink alcohol. Fetal alcohol syndrome, the leading cause of mental retardation in the United States, occurs when mothers drinking alcohol expose fetuses to alcohol in utero. The alcohol inhibits intrauterine growth and postnatal development. Microcephaly, craniofacial malformations, and limb and heart defects are common in affected infants. Short adult stature and development of a range of adult maladaptive behaviors have also been associated with fetal alcohol syndrome.

Women with alcohol-related disorders have a 35 percent risk of having a child with defects. Although the precise mechanism of the damage to the fetus is unknown, the damage seems to result from exposure in utero to ethanol or to its metabolites; alcohol may also cause hormone imbalances that increase the risk of abnormalities.

PROGNOSIS

Between 10 and 40 percent of alcoholic persons enter some kind of formal treatment program during the course of their alcohol problems. A number of prognostic signs are favorable. First is the absence of preexisting antisocial personality disorder or a diagnosis of other substance abuse or dependence. Second, evidence of general life stability with a job, continuing close family contacts, and the absence of severe legal problems also bodes well for the patient. Third, if the patient stays for the full course of the initial rehabilitation (perhaps 2 to 4 weeks), the chances of maintaining abstinence are good. The combination of these three attributes predicts at least a 60 percent chance for 1 or more years of abstinence. Few studies have documented the long-term course, but researchers agree that 1 year of abstinence is associated with a good chance for continued abstinence over an extended period. Alcoholic persons with severe drug problems (especially IV drug use or cocaine or amphetamine dependence) and those who are homeless may have only a 10 to 15 percent or so chance of achieving 1 year of abstinence, however.

Accurately predicting whether any specific person will achieve or maintain abstinence is impossible, but the prognostic factors just listed are associated with an increased likelihood of abstinence. The factors reflecting life stability, however, probably explain only 20 percent or less of the course of alcohol use disorders. Many forces that are difficult to measure affect the clinical course significantly; they are likely to include such intangibles as motivational level and the quality of the patient's social support system.

In general, alcoholic persons with preexisting independent major psychiatric disorders—such as antisocial personality disorder, schizophrenia, and bipolar I disorder—are likely to run the course of their independent psychiatric illness. Thus, for example, clinicians must treat the patient with bipolar I disorder who has secondary alcoholism with appropriate psychotherapy and lithium (Eskalith), use relevant psychological and behavioral techniques for the patient with antisocial personality disorder, and offer appropriate antipsychotic medications on a long-term basis to the patient with schizophrenia. The goal is to minimize the symptoms of the independent psychiatric disorder in the hope that greater life stability will be associated with a better prognosis for the patient's alcohol problems.

TREATMENT AND REHABILITATION

Three general steps are involved in treating the alcoholic person after the disorder has been diagnosed: intervention, detoxification, and rehabilitation. These approaches assume that all possible efforts have been made to optimize medical functioning and to address psychiatric emergencies. Thus, for example, an alcoholic person with symptoms of depression sufficiently severe to be suicidal requires inpatient hospitalization for at least several days until the suicidal ideation disappears. Similarly, a person presenting with cardiomyopathy, liver difficulties, or gastrointestinal bleeding first needs adequate treatment of the medical emergency.

The patient with alcohol abuse or dependence must then be brought face-to-face with the reality of the disorder (intervention), be detoxified if needed, and begin rehabilitation. The essentials of these three steps for an alcoholic person with independent psychiatric syndromes closely resemble the approaches used for the primary alcoholic person without independent psychiatric syndromes. In the former case, however, the treatments are applied after the psychiatric disorder has been stabilized as much as possible.

Intervention

The goal in the intervention step, which has also been called *confrontation*, is to break through feelings of denial and help the patient recognize the adverse consequences likely to occur if the disorder is not treated. Intervention is a process aimed at maximizing the motivation for treatment and continued abstinence.

This step often involves convincing patients that they are responsible for their own actions while reminding them of how alcohol has created significant life impairments. The psychiatrist often finds it useful to take advantage of the person's chief presenting complaint, whether it is insomnia, difficulties with sexual performance, an inability to cope with life stresses, depression, anxiety, or psychotic symptoms. The psychiatrist can then explain how alcohol has either created or contributed to these problems and can reassure the patient that abstinence can be achieved with a minimum of discomfort.

A physician was consulted by a 43-year-old businessman who was concerned about his wife. He had recently been confronted by their 21-year-old daughter, who felt that her mother was an alcoholic. The daughter noted her mother's slurred speech on several recent occasions when she had called home, noted times during the day when the mother was apparently home but did not answer the telephone, and observed high levels of alcohol consumption. A more detailed history revealed that the husband had been concerned about the wife's drinking pattern for at least 5 years; he related her practice of staying up after he went to bed and retiring later with alcohol on her breath. He also noted her consumption of 10 to 12 drinks at parties, with the resulting tendency to isolate herself from the remaining guests, her panic-like behavior regarding the need to pack liquor when they went on trips where alcohol might not be readily available, and what he observed to be a tremor of her hands some mornings during breakfast. The husband was given several potential courses of action, including the possibility of referring his wife for treatment with the physician. He was advised to share his concern with his wife when she was not actively intoxicated, emphasizing specific times and events when her impairment with alcohol was noted. He was also asked to consider whether a close friend of many years and the adult daughter might be included in this intervention, and it was suggested that a tentative appointment might be made with the clinician (or with an alcohol and drug treatment program) so that a next step could be established if the intervention was successful. (Courtesy of Marc A. Schuckit, M.D.)

Family

The family can be of great help in the intervention. Family members must learn not to protect the patient from the problems caused by alcohol; otherwise, the patient may not be able to gather the energy and the motivation necessary to stop drinking. During the intervention stage, the family can also suggest that the patient meet with persons who are recovering from alcoholism, perhaps through AA, and they can meet with groups, such as Al-Anon, that reach out to family members. Those support groups for families meet many times a week and help family members and friends see that they are not alone in their fears, worry, and feelings of guilt. Members share coping strategies and help each other find community resources. The groups can be most useful in helping family members rebuild their lives, even if the alcoholic person refuses to seek help.

Detoxification

Most persons with alcohol dependence have relatively mild symptoms when they stop drinking. If the patient is in relatively good health, is adequately nourished, and has a good social support system, the depressant withdrawal syndrome usually resembles a mild case of the flu. Even intense withdrawal syndromes rarely approach the severity of symptoms described by some early textbooks in the field.

The essential first step in detoxification is a thorough physical examination. In the absence of a serious medical disorder or combined drug abuse, severe alcohol withdrawal is unlikely. The second step is to offer rest, adequate nutrition, and multiple vitamins, especially those containing thiamine.

Mild or Moderate Withdrawal

Withdrawal develops because the brain has physically adapted to the presence of a brain depressant and cannot function adequately in the absence of the drug. Giving sufficient brain depressant on the first day to diminish symptoms and then weaning the patient off the drug over the next 5 days offers most patients optimal relief and minimizes the possibility that severe withdrawal will develop. Any depressant—including alcohol, barbiturates, or any of the benzodiazepines—can work, but most clinicians choose a benzodiazepine for its relative safety. Adequate treatment can be given with either short-acting drugs (e.g., lorazepam), or long-acting substances (e.g., chlordiazepoxide and diazepam).

An example of treatment is the administration of 25 mg of chlordiazepoxide by mouth three or four times a day on the first day, with a notation to skip a dose if the patient is asleep or feeling sleepy. An additional one or two 25-mg doses can be given during the first 24 hours if the patient is jittery or shows signs of increasing tremor or autonomic dysfunction. Whatever benzodiazepine dose is required on the first day can be decreased by 20 percent each subsequent day, with a resulting need for no further medication after 4 or 5 days. When giving a long-acting agent, such as chlordiazepoxide, the clinician must avoid producing excessive sleepiness through overmedication; if the patient is sleepy, the next scheduled dose should be omitted. When taking a short-acting drug, such as lorazepam, the patient must not miss any dose because rapid changes in benzodiazepine concentrations in the blood can precipitate severe withdrawal.

A social model program of detoxification saves money by avoiding medications while using social supports. This less-expensive regimen can be helpful for mild or moderate withdrawal syndromes. Some clinicians have also recommended β-adrenergic receptor antagonists (e.g., propranolol [Inderal]) or α-adrenergic receptor agonists (e.g., clonidine), although these medications do not appear to be superior to the benzodiazepines. Unlike the brain depressants, these other agents do little to decrease the risk of seizures or delirium.

Severe Withdrawal

For the approximately 1 to 3 percent of alcoholic patients with extreme autonomic dysfunction, agitation, and confusion—that is, those with alcoholic withdrawal delirium, or DTs—no optimal treatment has yet been developed. The first step is to ask why such a severe and relatively uncommon withdrawal syndrome has occurred; the answer often relates to a severe concomitant medical problem that needs immediate treatment. The withdrawal symptoms can then be minimized through the use of either benzodiazepines (in which case high doses are sometimes required) or antipsychotic agents, such as haloperidol. Once again, on the first or second day, doses are used to control behavior, and the patient can be weaned off the medication by about the fifth day.

Another 1 to 3 percent of patients may have a single grand mal convulsion; the rare person has multiple fits, with the peak incidence on the second day of withdrawal. Such patients require neurological evaluation, but in the absence of evidence of a seizure disorder, they do not benefit from anticonvulsant drugs.

Rehabilitation

For most patients, rehabilitation includes three major components: (1) continued efforts to increase and maintain high levels of motivation for abstinence, (2) work to help the patient readjust to a lifestyle free of alcohol, and (3) relapse prevention.

Because these steps are carried out in the context of acute and protracted withdrawal syndromes and life crises, treatment requires repeated presentations of similar materials that remind the patient how important abstinence is and that help the patient develop new day-to-day support systems and coping styles.

No single major life event, traumatic life period, or identifiable psychiatric disorder is known to be a unique cause of alcoholism. In addition, the effects of any causes of alcoholism are likely to have been diluted by the effects of alcohol on the brain and the years of an altered lifestyle, so that the alcoholism has developed a life of its own. This is true even though many alcoholic persons believe that the cause was depression, anxiety, life stress, or pain syndromes. Research, data from records, and resource persons usually reveal that alcohol contributed to the mood disorder, accident, or life stress, not vice versa.

The same general treatment approach is used in inpatient and outpatient settings. Selection of the more expensive and intensive inpatient mode often depends on evidence of additional severe medical or psychiatric syndromes, the absence of appropriate nearby outpatient groups and facilities, and the patient's history of having failed in outpatient care. The treatment process in either setting involves intervention, optimizing physical and psychological functioning, enhancing motivation, reaching out to family, and using the first 2 to 4 weeks of care as an intensive period of help. Those efforts must be followed by at least 3 to 6 months of less frequent outpatient care. Outpatient care uses a combination of individual and group counseling, judicious avoidance of psychotropic medications unless needed for independent disorders, and involvement in such self-help groups as AA.

Counseling

Counseling efforts in the first several months should focus on day-to-day life issues to help patients maintain a high level of motivation for abstinence and to enhance their functioning. Psychotherapy techniques that provoke anxiety or that require deep insights have not been shown to be of benefit during the early months of recovery and, at least theoretically, may actually impair efforts at maintaining abstinence. Thus, this discussion focuses on the efforts likely to characterize the first 3 to 6 months of care.

Counseling or therapy can be carried out in an individual or group setting; few data indicate that either approach is superior. The technique used is not likely to matter greatly and usually boils down to simple day-to-day counseling or almost any behavioral or psychotherapeutic approach focusing on the here and now. To optimize motivation, treatment sessions should explore the consequences of drinking, the likely future course of alcohol-related life problems, and the marked improvement that can be expected with abstinence. Whether in an inpatient or an outpatient setting, individual or group counseling is usually offered a minimum of three times a week for the first 2 to 4 weeks, followed by less intense efforts, perhaps once a week, for the subsequent 3 to 6 months.

Much time in counseling deals with how to build a lifestyle free of alcohol. Discussions cover the need for a sober peer group, a plan for social and recreational events without drinking, and approaches for reestablishing communication with family members and friends.

The third major component, relapse prevention, first identifies situations in which the risk for relapse is high. The counselor must help the patient develop modes of coping to be used when the craving for alcohol increases or when any event or emotional state makes a return to drinking likely. An important part of relapse prevention is reminding the patient about the appropriate attitude toward slips. Short-term experiences with alcohol can never be used as an excuse for returning to regular drinking. The efforts to achieve and maintain a sober lifestyle are not a game in which all benefits are lost with that first sip. Rather, recovery is a process of trial and error; patients use slips that occur to identify high-risk situations and to develop more appropriate coping techniques.

Most treatment efforts recognize the effects that alcoholism has on the significant persons in the patient's life, and an important aspect of recovery involves helping family members and close friends understand alcoholism and realize that rehabilitation is an ongoing process that lasts for 6 to 12 or more months. Couples and family counseling and support groups for relatives and friends help the persons involved to rebuild relationships, to learn how to avoid protecting the patient from the consequences of any drinking in the future, and to be as supportive as possible of the alcoholic patient's recovery program.

Medications

If detoxification has been completed and the patient is not one of the 10 to 15 percent of alcoholic persons who have an independent mood disorder, schizophrenia, or anxiety disorder, little evidence favors prescribing psychotropic medications for the treatment of alcoholism. Lingering levels of anxiety and insomnia as part of a reaction to life stresses and protracted abstinence should be treated with behavior modification approaches and reassurance. Medications for these symptoms (including benzodiazepines) are likely to lose their effectiveness much faster than the insomnia disappears; thus, the patient may increase the dose and have subsequent problems. Similarly, sadness and mood swings can linger at low levels for several months. Controlled clinical trials, however, indicate no benefit in prescribing antidepressant medications or lithium to treat the average alcoholic person who has no independent or long-lasting psychiatric disorder. The mood disorder will clear before the medications can take effect, and patients who resume drinking while on the medications face significant potential dangers. With little or no evidence that the medications are effective, the dangers significantly outweigh any potential benefits from their routine use.

One possible exception to the proscription against the use of medications is the alcohol-sensitizing agent disulfiram. Disulfiram is given in daily doses of 250 mg before the patient is discharged from the intensive first phase of outpatient rehabilitation or from inpatient care. The goal is to place the patient in a condition in which drinking alcohol precipitates an uncomfortable physical reaction, including nausea, vomiting, and a burning sensation in the face and stomach. Few data prove that disulfiram is more effective than a placebo, however, probably because most persons stop taking the disulfiram when they resume drinking. Many clinicians have stopped routinely prescribing the agent, partly in recognition of the dangers associated with the drug itself: mood swings, rare instances of psychosis, the possibility of increased peripheral neuropathies, the relatively rare occurrence

Table 9.2–5
Medications for Treating Alcohol Dependence

	Disulfiram (Antabuse)	Naltrexone (ReVia)	Acamprosate (Campral)
Action	Inhibits intermediate metabolism of alcohol, causing a buildup of acetaldehyde and a reaction of flushing, sweating, nausea, and tachycardia if a patient drinks alcohol	Blocks opioid receptors, resulting in reduced craving and reduced reward in response to drinking	Affects glutamate and GABA neurotransmitter systems, but its alcohol-related action is unclear
Contraindications	Concomitant use of alcohol or alcohol-containing preparations or metronidazole; coronary artery disease; severe myocardial disease	Currently using opioids or in acute opioid withdrawal; anticipated need for opioid analgesics; acute hepatitis or liver failure	Severe renal impairment (CrCl ≤30 mL/min)
Precautions	High impulsivity—likely to drink while using it; psychoses (current or history); diabetes mellitus; epilepsy; hepatic dysfunction; hypothyroidism; renal impairment; rubber contact dermatitis	Other hepatic disease; renal impairment; history of suicide attempts; if opioid analgesia is required, larger doses may be required, and respiratory depression may be deeper and more prolonged	Moderate renal impairment (dose adjustment for CrCl 30–50 mL/min); depression or suicidality
Serious adverse reactions	Hepatitis; optic neuritis; peripheral neuropathy; psychotic reactions Pregnancy Category C	Will precipitate severe withdrawal if patient is dependent on opioids; hepatoxicity (uncommon at usual doses) Pregnancy Category C	Anxiety; depression; rare events include the following: suicide attempt, acute kidney failure, heart failure, mesenteric arterial occlusion, cardiomyopathy, deep thrombophlebitits, and shock Pregnancy Category C
Common side effects	Metallic aftertaste; dermatitis	Nausea; abdominal pain; constipation; dizziness; headache; anxiety; fatigue	Diarrhea; flatulence; nausea; abdominal pain; headache; back pain; infection; flu syndrome; chills; somnolence; decreased libido; amnesia; confusion
Examples of drug interactions	Amitriptyline; anticoagulants such as warfarin; diazepam; isoniazid; metronidazole; phenytoin; theophylline; warfarin; any nonprescription drug containing alcohol	Opioid analgesics (blocks action); yohimbine (use with naltrexone increases negative drug effects)	No clinically relevant interactions known
Usual adult dose	*Oral dose*: 250 mg daily (range 125–500 mg) *Before prescribing*: (1) warn that the patient should not take disulfiram for at least 12 hrs after drinking and that a disulfiram–alcohol reaction can occur up to 2 wks after the last dose; and (2) warn about alcohol in the diet (e.g., sauces and vinegars) and in medications and toiletries *Follow-up*: Monitor liver function tests periodically	*Oral dose*: 50 mg daily *Before prescribing*: Evaluate for possible current opioid use; consider a urine toxicology screen for opioids, including synthetic opioids; obtain liver function tests *Follow-up*: Monitor liver function tests periodically	*Oral dose*: 666 mg (two 333-mg tablets) three times daily *or*, for patients with moderate renal impairment (CrCl 30–50 mL/min), reduce to 333 mg (one tablet) three times daily *Before prescribing*: Establish abstinence

CrCl, creatinine clearance; GABA, γ-aminobutyric acid.

of other significant neuropathies, and potentially fatal hepatitis. Moreover, patients with preexisting heart disease, cerebral thrombosis, diabetes, and a number of other conditions cannot be given disulfiram because an alcohol reaction to the disulfiram could be fatal.

Two additional promising pharmacological interventions have recently been studied. The first involves the opioid antago- nist naltrexone (ReVia), which at least theoretically is believed possibly to decrease the craving for alcohol or blunt the reward- ing effects of drinking. In any event, two relatively small (ap- proximately 90 patients on the active drug across the studies) and short-term (3 months of active treatment) investigations using 50 mg per day of this drug had potentially promising results. Eval- uating the full impact of this medication, however, will require longer-term studies of relatively large groups of more diverse patients.

The second medication of interest, acamprosate (Campral), has been tested in over 5,000 alcohol-dependent patients in Europe. This drug is not yet available in the United States. Used in doses of approximately 2,000 mg per day, this medication was associated with approximately 10 to 20 percent more positive outcomes than placebo when used in the context of the usual psychological and behavioral treatment regimens for alcoholism. The mechanism of action of acamprosate is not known, but it may act directly or indirectly at GABA receptors or at NMDA sites, the effects of which alter the development of tolerance or physical dependence on alcohol. A summary of medications used for alcohol dependence is given in Table 9.2–5.

Another medication with potential promise in the treatment of alcoholism is the nonbenzodiazepine antianxiety drug buspirone (BuSpar), although the effect of this drug on alcohol rehabilitation is inconsistent between studies. No evidence exists that antidepressant medications such as the selective serotonin reuptake inhibitors (SSRIs), lithium, or antipsychotic medications are significantly effective in the treatment of alcoholism.

Alcoholics Anonymous

Clinicians must recognize the potential importance of self-help groups such as AA. Members of AA have help available 24 hours a day, associate with a sober peer group, learn that it is possible to participate in social functions without drinking, and are given a model of recovery by observing the accomplishments of sober members of the group.

Learning about AA usually begins during inpatient or outpatient rehabilitation. The clinician can play a major role in helping patients understand the differences between specific groups. Some are comprised only of men or women, and others are mixed; some meetings are comprised mostly of blue-collar men and women, whereas others are mostly for professionals; some groups place great emphasis on religion, and others are eclectic. Patients with coexisting psychiatric disorders may need some additional education about AA. The clinician should remind them that some members of AA may not understand their special need for medications and should arm the patients with ways of coping when group members inappropriately suggest that the required medications be stopped. Although difficult to evaluate using double-blind controls, most studies indicate that participation in AA is associated with improved outcomes, and incorporation into treatment programs saves money.

▲ 9.3 Amphetamine (or Amphetamine-Like)–Related Disorders

Amphetamines and amphetamine-like drugs are the most widely used illicit substances, second only to cannabis, in the United States, Asia, Great Britain, Australia, and several other Western European countries. Methamphetamine, a con-gener of amphetamine, has become even more popular in recent years.

The racemate amphetamine sulfate (Benzedrine) was first synthesized in 1887 and was introduced to clinical practice in 1932 as an over-the-counter inhaler for the treatment of nasal congestion and asthma. In 1937, amphetamine sulfate tablets were introduced for the treatment of narcolepsy, postencephalitic parkinsonism, depression, and lethargy. In the 1970s, a variety of social and regulatory factors began to curb widespread amphetamine distribution. The current U.S. Food and Drug Administration (FDA)–approved indications for amphetamine are limited to attention-deficit/hyperactivity disorder (ADHD) and narcolepsy; however, amphetamines are also used in the treatment of obesity, depression, dysthymia, chronic fatigue syndrome, acquired immune deficiency syndrome (AIDS), dementia, and neurasthenia.

PREPARATIONS

The major amphetamines currently available and used in the United States are dextroamphetamine (Dexedrine), methamphetamine (Desoxyn), a mixed dextroamphetamine-amphetamine salt (Adderall), and the amphetamine-like compound methylphenidate (Ritalin). These drugs go by such street names as ice, crystal, crystal meth, and speed. As a general class, the amphetamines are referred to as analeptics, sympathomimetics, stimulants, and psychostimulants. The typical amphetamines are used to increase performance and to induce a euphoric feeling, for example, by students studying for examinations, by long-distance truck drivers on trips, by business people with important deadlines, by athletes in competition, and by soldiers during wartime. Although not as addictive as cocaine, amphetamines are nonetheless addictive drugs.

Other amphetamine-like substances are ephedrine, pseudoephedrine, and phenylpropanolamine (PPA). These drugs, PPA in particular, can dangerously exacerbate hypertension, precipitate a toxic psychosis, cause intestinal infarction, or result in death. The safety margin for PPA is particularly narrow, and three to four times the normal dose can result in life-threatening hypertension. In 2005, medications containing PPA were recalled by the FDA, and in 2006, the FDA prohibited the sale of over-the-counter medications containing ephedrine and regulated the sale of over-the-counter medications containing pseudoephedrine, which was being used illegally to make methamphetamine.

Amphetamine-type drugs with abuse potential also include phendimetrazine (Preludin), which is included in Schedule II of the Controlled Substance Act (CSA), and diethylpropion (Tenuate), benzphetamine (Didrex), and phentermine (Ionamin), which are included in Schedule III or IV of the CSA. It is presumed that all of these drugs are capable of producing all of the listed amphetamine-induced disorders. Modafinil (Provigil), used in the treatment of narcolepsy, also has stimulant and euphorigenic effects in humans, but its toxicity and likelihood of producing amphetamine-induced disorders are unknown.

Methamphetamine is a potent form of amphetamine that abusers of the substance inhale, smoke, or inject intravenously (IV). Its psychological effects last for hours and are described as particularly powerful. Unlike cocaine (see Section 9.6), which must be imported, methamphetamine is a synthetic drug that can be manufactured domestically in illicit laboratories.

Other agents called *substituted* or *designer amphetamines* are discussed separately later in this section.

EPIDEMIOLOGY

The National Household Survey on Drug Abuse (NHSDA) conducted in 2001 found that 7.1 percent of persons 12 years of age and older reported lifetime nonmedical use of stimulants, a significant increase since the 4.5 percent found in the 1997 survey. The highest rates of use in the past year (1.5 percent) were among 18- to 25-year-olds, followed by 12- to 17-year-olds. The treatment admission rate for primary amphetamine abuse in the United States is about 30 per 100,000 people 12 years of age or older. Thirteen states had amphetamine admission rates of at least 55 per 100,000, and eight of these had rates of 100 per 100,000 or more. A strong association of methamphetamine abuse and crime exists.

Amphetamine use occurs in all socioeconomic groups and is increasing among white professionals. Because amphetamines are available by prescription for specific indications, prescribing physicians must be aware of the risk of amphetamine abuse by others, including friends and family members of the patient receiving the amphetamine. No reliable data are available on the epidemiology of designer amphetamine use, but they are greatly abused. According to the text revision of the fourth edition of *Diagnostic and Statistical Manual of Mental Disorders* (DSM-IV-TR), the lifetime prevalence of amphetamine dependence and abuse is 1.5 percent, and the male to female ratio is 1.

According to NHSDA, methamphetamine abuse continues to spread geographically and to different populations. In addition to the "super labs" in California and trafficking from Mexico, a proliferation of small "mom and pop" laboratories has occurred throughout the country, especially in rural areas. Methamphetamine abuse and production levels are high in Hawaii, West Coast areas, and some Southwestern areas, and abuse and manufacture continue to move eastward. New populations of methamphetamine users include Hispanics, young people in Denver, club goers in Boston, and African-Americans in Texas. One half of women arrested in Honolulu tested positive in 2002, as did nearly 42 percent in Phoenix and 37 percent in San Diego. Not only methamphetamine users, but also children exposed to methamphetamine laboratories are in danger of serious health consequences.

NEUROPHARMACOLOGY

All of the amphetamines are rapidly absorbed orally and have a rapid onset of action, usually within 1 hour when taken orally. The classic amphetamines are also taken IV and have an almost immediate effect by this route. Nonprescribed amphetamines and designer amphetamines are also inhaled ("snorting"). Tolerance develops with both classic and designer amphetamines, although amphetamine users often overcome the tolerance by taking more of the drug. Amphetamine is less addictive than cocaine, as evidenced by experiments on rats in which not all animals spontaneously self-administered low doses of amphetamine.

The classic amphetamines (i.e., dextroamphetamine, methamphetamine, and methylphenidate) produce their primary effects by causing the release of catecholamines, particularly dopamine, from presynaptic terminals. The effects are particularly potent for the dopaminergic neurons projecting from the ventral tegmental area to the cerebral cortex and the limbic areas. This pathway has been termed the *reward circuit pathway*, and its activation is probably the major addicting mechanism for the amphetamines. The designer amphetamines cause the release of catecholamines (dopamine and norepinephrine) and of serotonin, the neurotransmitter implicated as the major neurochemical pathway for hallucinogens. Therefore, the clinical effects of designer amphetamines are a blend of the effects of classic amphetamines and those of hallucinogens.

DIAGNOSIS

The DSM-IV-TR lists many amphetamine (or amphetamine-like)–related disorders (Table 9.3–1), but specifies diagnostic criteria only for amphetamine intoxication (Table 9.3–2), amphetamine withdrawal (Table 9.3–3), and amphetamine-related disorder not otherwise specified (Table 9.3–4) in the section on amphetamine (or amphetamine-like)–related disorders. The diagnostic criteria for the other amphetamine (or amphetamine-like)–related disorders are contained in the DSM-IV-TR sections dealing with the primary phenomenological symptom (e.g., psychosis).

Amphetamine Dependence and Amphetamine Abuse

The DSM-IV-TR criteria for dependence and abuse are applied to amphetamine and its related substances (see Tables 9.1–3 to 9.1–5 in Section 9.1). Amphetamine dependence can result in a rapid downward spiral of a person's abilities to cope with

Table 9.3–1
DSM-IV-TR Amphetamine (or Amphetamine-Like)–Related Disorders

Amphetamine use disorders
Amphetamine dependence
Amphetamine abuse
Amphetamine-induced disorders
Amphetamine intoxication
   Specify if:
      With perceptual disturbances
Amphetamine withdrawal
Amphetamine intoxication delirium
Amphetamine-induced psychotic disorder, with delusions
   Specify if:
      With onset during intoxication
Amphetamine-induced psychotic disorder, with hallucinations
   Specify if:
      With onset during intoxication
Amphetamine-induced mood disorder
   Specify if:
      With onset during intoxication
      With onset during withdrawal
Amphetamine-induced anxiety disorder
   Specify if:
      With onset during intoxication
Amphetamine-induced sexual dysfunction
   Specify if:
      With onset during intoxication
Amphetamine-induced sleep disorder
   Specify if:
      With onset during intoxication
      With onset during withdrawal
Amphetamine-related disorder not otherwise specified

From American Psychiatric Association. *Diagnostic and Statistical Manual of Mental Disorders.* 4th ed. Text rev. Washington, DC: American Psychiatric Association; copyright 2000, with permission.

Table 9.3–2
DSM-IV-TR Diagnostic Criteria for Amphetamine Intoxication

A. Recent use of amphetamine or a related substance (e.g., methylphenidate).
B. Clinically significant maladaptive behavioral or psychological changes (e.g., euphoria or affective blunting; changes in sociability; hypervigilance; interpersonal sensitivity; anxiety, tension, or anger; stereotyped behaviors; impaired judgment; or impaired social or occupational functioning) that developed during, or shortly after, use of amphetamine or a related substance.
C. Two (or more) of the following developing during, or shortly after, use of amphetamine or a related substance:

(1) tachycardia or bradycardia
(2) capillary dilation
(3) elevated or lowered blood pressure
(4) perspiration or chills
(5) nausea or vomiting
(6) evidence of weight loss
(7) psychomotor agitation or retardation
(8) muscular weakness, respiratory depression, chest pain, or cardiac arrhythmias
(9) confusion, seizures, dyskinesias, dystonias, or coma

D. The symptoms are not due to a general medical condition and are not better accounted for by another mental disorder.
Specify if:
With perceptual disturbances

From American Psychiatric Association. *Diagnostic and Statistical Manual of Mental Disorders.* 4th ed. Text rev. Washington, DC: American Psychiatric Association; copyright 2000, with permission.

work- and family-related obligations and stresses. A person who abuses amphetamines requires increasingly high doses of amphetamine to obtain the usual high, and physical signs of amphetamine abuse (e.g., decreased weight and paranoid ideas) almost always develop with continued abuse.

Amphetamine Intoxication

The intoxication syndromes of cocaine (which blocks dopamine reuptake) and amphetamines (which cause the release of

Table 9.3–3
DSM-IV-TR Diagnostic Criteria for Amphetamine Withdrawal

A. Cessation of (or reduction in) amphetamine (or a related substance) use that has been heavy and prolonged.
B. Dysphoric mood and two (or more) of the following physiological changes, developing within a few hours to several days after Criterion A:

(1) fatigue
(2) vivid, unpleasant dreams
(3) insomnia or hypersomnia
(4) increased appetite
(5) psychomotor retardation or agitation

C. The symptoms in Criterion B cause clinically significant distress or impairment in social, occupational, or other important areas of functioning.
D. The symptoms are not due to a general medical condition and are not better accounted for by another mental disorder.

From American Psychiatric Association. *Diagnostic and Statistical Manual of Mental Disorders.* 4th ed. Text rev. Washington, DC: American Psychiatric Association; copyright 2000, with permission.

Table 9.3–4
DSM-IV-TR Diagnostic Criteria for Amphetamine-Related Disorder Not Otherwise Specified

The amphetamine-related disorder not otherwise specified category is for disorders associated with the use of amphetamine (or a related substance) that are not classifiable as amphetamine dependence, amphetamine abuse, amphetamine intoxication, amphetamine withdrawal, amphetamine intoxication delirium, amphetamine-induced psychotic disorder, amphetamine-induced mood disorder, amphetamine-induced anxiety disorder, amphetamine-induced sexual dysfunction, or amphetamine-induced sleep disorder.

From American Psychiatric Association. *Diagnostic and Statistical Manual of Mental Disorders.* 4th ed. Text rev. Washington, DC: American Psychiatric Association; copyright 2000, with permission.

dopamine) are similar. Because more rigorous, in-depth research has been done on cocaine abuse and intoxication than on amphetamines, the clinical literature on amphetamines has been strongly influenced by the clinical findings of cocaine abuse. In DSM-IV-TR, the diagnostic criteria for amphetamine intoxication (Table 9.3–2) and cocaine intoxication (see Table 9.6–2) are separated but are virtually the same. DSM-IV-TR specifies perceptual disturbances as a symptom of amphetamine intoxication. If intact reality testing is absent, a diagnosis of amphetamine-induced psychotic disorder with onset during intoxication is indicated. The symptoms of amphetamine intoxication are mostly resolved after 24 hours and are generally completely resolved after 48 hours.

An 18-year-old high school senior was brought to the emergency room by police after being picked up wandering in traffic on the Triborough Bridge. He was angry, agitated, and aggressive and talked of various people who were deliberately trying to "confuse" him by giving him misleading directions. His story was rambling and disjointed, but he admitted to the police officer that he had been using "speed." In the emergency room he had difficulty focusing his attention and had to ask that questions be repeated. He was disoriented as to time and place and was unable to repeat the names of three objects after five minutes. The family gave a history of the patient's regular use of "pep pills" over the past two years, during which time he was frequently "high" and did very poorly in school. (Reprinted with permission from *DSM-III-R Casebook*.)

Amphetamine Withdrawal

After amphetamine intoxication, a crash occurs, with symptoms of anxiety, tremulousness, dysphoric mood, lethargy, fatigue, nightmares (accompanied by rebound rapid eye movement [REM] sleep), headache, profuse sweating, muscle cramps, stomach cramps, and insatiable hunger. The withdrawal symptoms generally peak in 2 to 4 days and are resolved in 1 week. The most serious withdrawal symptom is depression, which can be particularly severe after the sustained use of high doses of amphetamine and can be associated with suicidal ideation or behavior. The DSM-IV-TR diagnostic criteria for amphetamine withdrawal (Table 9.3–3) specify that a dysphoric mood and physiological changes are necessary for the diagnosis.

Amphetamine Intoxication Delirium

Under substance-related disorder, DSM-IV-TR includes a diagnosis of amphetamine intoxication delirium (see Table 7.2–2). Delirium associated with amphetamine use generally results from high doses of amphetamine or from sustained use, and so sleep deprivation affects the clinical presentation. The combination of amphetamines with other substances and the use of amphetamines by a person with preexisting brain damage can also cause development of delirium. It is not uncommon for university students using amphetamines to cram for examinations to exhibit this type of delirium.

Amphetamine-Induced Psychotic Disorder

The clinical similarity of amphetamine-induced psychosis to paranoid schizophrenia has prompted extensive study of the neurochemistry of amphetamine-induced psychosis to elucidate the pathophysiology of paranoid schizophrenia. The hallmark of amphetamine-induced psychotic disorder is the presence of paranoia. Amphetamine-induced psychotic disorder can be distinguished from paranoid schizophrenia by several differentiating characteristics associated with the former, including a predominance of visual hallucinations, generally appropriate affects, hyperactivity, hypersexuality, confusion and incoherence, and little evidence of disordered thinking (e.g., looseness of associations). In several studies, investigators also noted that, although the positive symptoms of amphetamine-induced psychotic disorder and schizophrenia are similar, amphetamine-induced psychotic disorder generally lacks the affective flattening and alogia of schizophrenia. Clinically, however, acute amphetamine-induced psychotic disorder can be completely indistinguishable from schizophrenia, and only the resolution of the symptoms in a few days or a positive finding in a urine drug screen test eventually reveals the correct diagnosis.

The treatment of choice for amphetamine-induced psychotic disorder is the short-term use of an antipsychotic medication such as haloperidol (Haldol). DSM-IV-TR lists the diagnostic criteria for amphetamine-induced psychotic disorder with the other psychotic disorders (see Table 11.4–5) and allows clinicians to specify whether delusions or hallucinations are the predominant symptoms.

Amphetamine-Induced Mood Disorder

According to DSM-IV-TR, the onset of amphetamine-induced mood disorder can occur during intoxication or withdrawal (see Table 12.3–8). In general, intoxication is associated with manic or mixed mood features, whereas withdrawal is associated with depressive mood features.

Amphetamine-Induced Anxiety Disorder

In DSM-IV-TR, the onset of amphetamine-induced anxiety disorder can also occur during intoxication or withdrawal (see Table 13.7–2). Amphetamine, like cocaine, can induce symptoms similar to those seen in obsessive-compulsive disorder, panic disorder, and phobic disorders, in particular.

Amphetamine-Induced Sexual Dysfunction

Amphetamines may be prescribed as an antidote to the sexual side effects of serotonergic agents such as fluoxetine (Prozac), but they are often misused by persons to enhance sexual experiences. High doses and long-term use are associated with erectile disorder and other sexual dysfunctions. These dysfunctions are classified in DSM-IV-TR as amphetamine-induced sexual dysfunction with onset during intoxication (see Table 17.2–11).

Amphetamine-Induced Sleep Disorder

The diagnostic criteria for amphetamine-induced sleep disorder with onset during intoxication or withdrawal are found in the DSM-IV-TR section on sleep disorders (see Table 20.2–14). Amphetamine intoxication can produce insomnia and sleep deprivation, whereas persons undergoing amphetamine withdrawal can experience hypersomnolence and nightmares.

Disorder Not Otherwise Specified

If an amphetamine (or amphetamine-like)–related disorder does not meet the criteria of one or more of the categories discussed previously, it can be diagnosed as an amphetamine-related disorder not otherwise specified (Table 9.3–4).

CLINICAL FEATURES

In persons who have not previously used amphetamines, a single 5-mg dose increases the sense of well-being and induces elation, euphoria, and friendliness. Small doses generally improve attention and increase performance on written, oral, and performance tasks. An associated decrease in fatigue, induction of anorexia, and heightening of the pain threshold are also seen. Undesirable effects result from the use of high doses for long periods.

Adverse Effects

Amphetamines

PHYSICAL.   Amphetamine abuse can produce adverse effects, the most serious of which include cerebrovascular, cardiac, and gastrointestinal effects. Among the specific life-threatening conditions are myocardial infarction, severe hypertension, cerebrovascular disease, and ischemic colitis. A continuum of neurological symptoms, from twitching, to tetany, to seizures, to coma and death, is associated with increasingly high amphetamine doses. Intravenous use of amphetamines can transmit human immunodeficiency virus (HIV) and hepatitis and further the development of lung abscesses, endocarditis, and necrotizing angiitis. Several studies have shown that abusers of amphetamines knew little—or did not care—about safe-sex practices and the use of condoms. The non–life-threatening adverse effects of amphetamine abuse include flushing, pallor, cyanosis, fever, headache, tachycardia, palpitations, nausea, vomiting, bruxism (teeth grinding), shortness of breath, tremor, and ataxia. Pregnant women who use amphetamines often have babies with low birthweight, small head circumference, early gestational age, and growth retardation.

PSYCHOLOGICAL.   The adverse psychological effects associated with amphetamine use include restlessness, dysphoria, insomnia, irritability, hostility, and confusion. Amphetamine use can also induce symptoms of anxiety disorders, such as generalized anxiety disorder and panic disorder, as well as ideas of reference, paranoid delusions, and hallucinations.

Other Agents

SUBSTITUTED AMPHETAMINES.   MDMA (3,4-methylene-dioxymethamphetamine) is one of a series of substituted amphetamines that also includes MDEA (3,4-methylenedioxy-*N*-ethylamphetamine), MDA (3,4-methylene-dioxyamphetamine), DOB (2,5-dimethoxy-4-bromoamphetamine), PMA (para-methoxyamphetamine), and others. These drugs produce subjective effects resembling those of amphetamine and LSD (lysergic acid diethylamide), and in that sense, MDMA and similar analogues may represent a distinct category of drugs.

A methamphetamine derivative that came into use in the 1980s, MDMA was not technically subject to legal regulation at the time. Although it has been labeled a "designer drug" in the belief that it was deliberately synthesized to evade legal regulation, it was actually synthesized and patented in 1914. Several psychiatrists used it as an adjunct to psychotherapy and concluded that it had value. At one time, it was advertised as legal and was used in psychotherapy for its subjective effects. It was never approved by the FDA, however. Its use raised questions of both safety and legality because the related amphetamine derivatives MDA, DOB, and PMA had caused a number of overdose deaths, and MDA was known to cause extensive destruction of serotonergic nerve terminals in the central nervous system (CNS). Using emergency scheduling authority, the Drug Enforcement Agency made MDMA a Schedule I drug under the CSA, along with LSD, heroin, and marijuana. Despite its illegal status, MDMA continues to be manufactured, distributed, and used in the United States, Europe, and Australia. Its use is common in Australia and Great Britain at extended dances ("raves") popular with adolescents and young adults.

Mechanisms of Action.   The unusual properties of the drugs may be a consequence of the different actions of the optical isomers: the $R(-)$ isomers produce LSD-like effects, and the amphetamine-like properties are linked to $S(+)$ isomers. The LSD-like actions, in turn, may be linked to the capacity to release serotonin. The various derivatives may exhibit significant differences in subjective effects and toxicity. Animals in laboratory experiments will self-administer the drugs, suggesting prominent amphetamine-like effects.

Subjective Effects.   After taking usual doses (100 to 150 mg), MDMA users experience elevated mood and, according to various reports, increased self-confidence and sensory sensitivity; peaceful feelings coupled with insight, empathy, and closeness to persons; and decreased appetite. Difficulty concentrating and an increased capacity to focus have both been reported. Dysphoric reactions, psychotomimetic effects, and psychosis have also been reported. Higher doses seem more likely to produce psychotomimetic effects. Sympathomimetic effects of tachycardia, palpitation, increased blood pressure, sweating, and bruxism are common. The subjective effects are reported to be prominent for about 4 to 8 hours, but they may not last as long or may last longer, depending on the dose and route of administration. The drug is usually taken orally but is also snorted and injected. Both tachyphylaxis and some tolerance are reported by users.

Toxicity.   Although it is not as toxic as MDA, various somatic toxicities have been attributed to MDMA use, as well as fatal overdoses. It does not appear to be neurotoxic when injected into the brains of animals, but it is metabolized to MDA in both animals and humans. In animals, MDMA produces selective, long-lasting damage to serotonergic nerve terminals. It is not certain if the levels of the MDA metabolite reached in humans after the usual doses of MDMA suffice to produce lasting damage. Users of MDMA show differences in neuroendocrine responses to serotonergic probes, and studies of former MDMA users show global and regional decreases in serotonin transporter binding, as measured by positron emission tomography.

Currently, no established clinical uses exist for MDMA, although before its regulation, there were several reports of its beneficial effects as an adjunct to psychotherapy.

KHAT.   The fresh leaves of *Catha edulis*, a bush native to East Africa, have been used as a stimulant in the Middle East, Africa, and the Arabian Peninsula for at least 1,000 years. Khat is still widely used in Ethiopia, Kenya, Somalia, and Yemen. The amphetamine-like effects of khat have long been recognized, and, although efforts to isolate the active ingredient were first undertaken in the 19th century, only since the 1970s has cathinone ($S[-]\alpha$-aminopropiophenone or $S[-]$2-amino-1-phenyl-1-propanone) been identified as the substance responsible. Cathinone is a precursor moiety that is nonenzymatically converted in the plant to the less-active entities norephedrine and cathine (norpseudoephedrine), which explains why only the fresh leaves of the plant are valued for their stimulant effects. Cathinone has most of the CNS and peripheral actions of amphetamine and appears to have the same mechanism of action. In humans, it elevates mood, decreases hunger, and alleviates fatigue. At high doses, it can induce an amphetamine-like psychosis in humans. Because it is typically absorbed buccally after chewing the leaf and because the alkaloid is metabolized relatively rapidly, high toxic blood levels are rarely reached. Concern about khat use is linked to its dependence-producing properties rather than to its acute toxicity. It is estimated that five million doses are consumed each day, despite prohibition of its use in a number of African and Arab countries.

In the 1990s, several clandestine laboratories began synthesizing methcathinone, a drug with actions similar to those of cathinone. Known by a number of street names (e.g., "CAT," "goob," and "crank"), its popularity is primarily owing to its ease of synthesis from ephedrine or pseudoephedrine, which were readily available until they were placed under special controls. Methcathinone has been moved to Schedule I of the CSA. The patterns of use, adverse effects, and complications closely resemble those reported for amphetamine.

CLUB DRUGS.   The use of a certain group of substances popularly called *club drugs* is often associated with dance clubs, bars, and all-night dance parties (raves). The group includes LSD, γ-hydroxybutyrate (GHB), ketamine, methamphetamine, MDMA ("ecstasy"), and Rohypnol or "roofies" (flunitrazepam). These substances are not all in the same drug class, nor do they produce the same physical or subjective effects. GHB, ketamine, and Rohypnol have been called *date rape drugs* because they produce disorienting and sedating effects, and often users cannot recall what occurred during all or part of an episode under the influence of the drug. Hence, it is alleged that these drugs might be surreptitiously placed in a beverage, or a person might be convinced to take the drug and then not recall clearly what occurred after ingestion.

Emergency department mentions of GHB, ketamine, and Rohypnol are relatively few. Of the club drugs, methamphetamine is the substance that accounts for the largest share of treatment admissions.

TREATMENT AND REHABILITATION

The treatment of amphetamine (or amphetamine-like)–related disorders shares with cocaine-related disorders the difficulty of helping patients remain abstinent from the drug, which is powerfully reinforcing and induces craving. An inpatient setting and the use of multiple therapeutic methods (individual, family, and group psychotherapy) are usually necessary to achieve lasting abstinence. The treatment of specific amphetamine-induced disorders (e.g., amphetamine-induced psychotic disorder and amphetamine-induced anxiety disorder) with specific drugs (e.g., antipsychotic and anxiolytics) may be necessary on a short-term basis. Antipsychotics may be prescribed for the first few days. In the absence of psychosis, diazepam (Valium) is useful to treat patients' agitation and hyperactivity.

Physicians should establish a therapeutic alliance with patients to deal with the underlying depression, personality disorder, or both. Because many patients are heavily dependent on the drug, however, psychotherapy may be especially difficult.

Comorbid conditions, such as depression, may respond to antidepressant medication. Bupropion (Wellbutrin) may be of use after patients have withdrawn from amphetamine. It has the effect of producing feelings of well-being as these patients cope with the dysphoria that may accompany abstinence.

▲ 9.4 Caffeine-Related Disorders

Caffeine is the most widely consumed psychoactive substance in the world. Although numerous studies have documented the safety of caffeine when used in typical daily doses, psychiatric symptoms and disorders can be associated with its use. Although rates for these disorders are not well established, even a low prevalence could still result in a considerable number of people with these disorders because of the widespread use of caffeine. Hence, it is important for the clinician to be familiar with caffeine, its effects, and problems that can be associated with its use.

The text revision of the fourth edition of the *Diagnostic and Statistical Manual of Mental Disorders* (DSM-IV-TR) recognizes several caffeine-related disorders (e.g., caffeine intoxication, caffeine-induced anxiety disorder, and caffeine-induced sleep disorder). Other caffeine-related disorders, such as caffeine withdrawal and caffeine dependence, are not official diagnoses in DSM-IV-TR, but they can also be of clinical interest.

EPIDEMIOLOGY

Caffeine is contained in drinks, foods, prescription medicines, and over-the-counter medicines. An adult in the United States consumes about 200 mg of caffeine per day on average, although 20 to 30 percent of all adults consume more than 500 mg per day. The per capita use of coffee in the United States is 10.2 pounds per year. A cup of coffee generally contains 100 to 150 mg of caffeine; tea contains about one third as much. Many over-the-counter medications contain one third to one half as much caffeine as a cup of coffee, and some migraine medications and over-the-counter stimulants contain more caffeine than a cup of coffee. Cocoa, chocolate, and soft drinks contain significant amounts of caffeine, enough to cause some symptoms of caffeine intoxication in small children when they ingest a candy bar and a 12-ounce cola drink.

Caffeine consumption also varies by age. The average daily caffeine consumption of caffeine consumers of all ages is 2.79 mg/kg of body weight in the United States. A substantial amount of caffeine is consumed even by young children (i.e., more than 1 mg/kg for children between the ages of 1 and 5 years). Worldwide, estimates place the average daily per capita caffeine consumption at about 70 mg. According to DSM-IV-TR, the actual prevalence of caffeine-related disorders is unknown, but up to 85 percent of adults consume caffeine in any given year.

COMORBIDITY

Persons with caffeine-related disorders are more likely to have additional substance-related disorders than are those without diagnoses of caffeine-related disorders. About two thirds of those who consume large amounts of caffeine daily also use sedative and hypnotic drugs.

ETIOLOGY

After exposure to caffeine, continued caffeine consumption can be influenced by several factors, such as the pharmacological effects of caffeine, caffeine's reinforcing effects, genetic predispositions to caffeine use, and personal attributes of the consumer.

NEUROPHARMACOLOGY

Caffeine, a methylxanthine, is more potent than another commonly used methylxanthine, theophylline (Primatene). The half-life of caffeine in the human body is 3 to 10 hours, and the time of peak concentration is 30 to 60 minutes. Caffeine readily crosses the blood–brain barrier. Caffeine acts primarily as an antagonist of the adenosine receptors. Adenosine receptors activate an inhibitory G protein (Gi) and, thus, inhibit the formation of the second-messenger cyclic adenosine monophosphate (cAMP). Caffeine intake, therefore, results in an increase in intraneuronal cAMP concentrations in neurons with adenosine receptors. Three cups of coffee are estimated to deliver so much caffeine to the brain that about 50 percent of the adenosine receptors are occupied by caffeine. Several experiments indicate that caffeine, especially at high doses or concentrations, can affect dopamine and noradrenergic neurons. Specifically, dopamine activity may be enhanced by caffeine, a hypothesis that could explain clinical reports associating caffeine intake with an exacerbation of psychotic symptoms in patients with schizophrenia. Activation of noradrenergic neurons has been hypothesized to be involved in the mediation of some symptoms of caffeine withdrawal.

Subjective Effects and Reinforcement

Single low to moderate doses of caffeine (i.e., 20 to 200 mg) can produce a profile of subjective effects in humans that is generally identified as pleasurable. Thus, studies have shown that such doses of caffeine result in increased ratings on measures such as well-being, energy and concentration, and motivation to work. In addition, these doses of caffeine produce decreases in ratings of feeling sleepy or tired. Doses of caffeine in the range of 300 to 800 mg (the equivalent of several cups of brewed coffee ingested at once) produce effects that are often rated as being unpleasant, such as anxiety and nervousness. Although animal studies have generally found it difficult to demonstrate that caffeine functions as a reinforcer, well-controlled studies in humans have shown that people choose caffeine over placebo when given the choice under controlled experimental conditions. In habitual users, the reinforcing effects of caffeine are potentiated by the ability to suppress low-grade withdrawal symptoms after overnight abstinence. Thus, the profile of caffeine's subjective effects and its ability to function as a reinforcer contribute to the regular use of caffeine.

Genetics and Caffeine Use

Some genetic predisposition may exist to continued coffee use after exposure to coffee. Investigations comparing coffee or caffeine use in monozygotic and dizygotic twins have shown higher concordance rates for monozygotic twins for total caffeine consumption, heavy use, caffeine tolerance, caffeine withdrawal, and caffeine intoxication, with heritabilities ranging between 35 and 77 percent. Multivariate structural equation modeling of caffeine use, cigarette smoking, and alcohol use suggests that a common genetic factor—polysubstance use—underlines use of these three substances.

Age, Sex, and Race

The relationship between long-term chronic caffeine use and demographical features, such as age, sex, and race, has not been widely studied. Some evidence suggests that middle-aged people may use more caffeine, although caffeine use in adolescents is not uncommon. No evidence indicates that caffeine use differs between men and women, and no data specifically address caffeine use for different races. Some evidence suggests that, for both children and adults in the United States, whites consume more caffeine than blacks.

Special Populations

Cigarette smokers consume more caffeine than nonsmokers. This observation may reflect a common genetic vulnerability to caffeine use and cigarette smoking. It may also be related to increased rates of caffeine elimination in cigarette smokers. Preclinical and clinical studies indicate that regular caffeine use can potentiate the reinforcing effects of nicotine.

Heavy use and clinical dependence on alcohol is associated with heavy use and clinical dependence on caffeine as well. Individuals with anxiety disorders tend to report lower levels of caffeine use, although one study showed that a greater proportion of heavy caffeine consumers also use benzodiazepines. Several studies have also shown high daily amounts of caffeine use in psychiatric patients. For example, several studies have found that such patients consume the equivalent of an average of five or more cups of brewed coffee each day. Finally, high daily caffeine consumption has also been noted in prisoners.

Personality

Although attempts have been made to link preferential use of caffeine to particular personality types, results from these studies do not suggest that any particular personality type is especially linked to caffeine use.

Effects on Cerebral Blood Flow

Most studies have found that caffeine results in global cerebral vasoconstriction, with a resultant decrease in cerebral blood flow (CBF), although this effect may not occur in persons over 65 years of age. According to one recent study, tolerance does not develop to these vasoconstrictive effects, and the CBF shows a rebound increase after withdrawal from caffeine. Some clinicians believe that caffeine use can cause a similar constriction in the coronary arteries and produce angina in the absence of atherosclerosis.

DIAGNOSIS

The diagnosis of caffeine intoxication or other caffeine-related disorders depends primarily on a comprehensive history of a patient's intake of caffeine-containing products. The history should cover whether a patient has experienced any symptoms of caffeine withdrawal during periods when caffeine consumption was either stopped or severely reduced. The differential diagnosis for caffeine-related disorders should include the following psychiatric diagnoses: generalized anxiety disorder, panic disorder with or without agoraphobia, bipolar II disorder, attention-deficit/hyperactivity disorder, and sleep disorders. The differential diagnosis should include the abuse of caffeine-containing over-the-counter medications, anabolic steroids, and other stimulants, such as amphetamines and cocaine. A urine sample may be needed to screen for these substances. The differential diagnosis should also include hyperthyroidism and pheochromocytoma.

The DSM-IV-TR lists the caffeine-related disorders (Table 9.4–1) and provides diagnostic criteria for caffeine intoxication (Table 9.4–2), but it does not formally recognize a diagnosis of caffeine withdrawal, which is classified as a caffeine-related disorder not otherwise specified (Table 9.4–3). The diagnostic criteria for other caffeine-related disorders are contained in the sections specific for the principal symptom (e.g., as a substance-induced anxiety disorder for caffeine-induced anxiety disorder).

Caffeine Intoxication

The DSM-IV-TR specifies the diagnostic criteria for caffeine intoxication (Table 9.4–2), including the recent consumption of caffeine, usually in excess of 250 mg. The annual incidence of caffeine intoxication is an estimated 10 percent, although some clinicians and investigators suspect that the actual incidence is much higher. The common symptoms associated with caffeine intoxication include anxiety, psychomotor agitation, restlessness, irritability, and psychophysiological complaints such as muscle twitching, flushed face, nausea, diuresis, gastrointestinal distress, excessive perspiration, tingling in the fingers and toes, and insomnia. Consumption of more than 1 g of caffeine can produce rambling speech, confused thinking, cardiac arrhythmias, inexhaustibleness, marked agitation, tinnitus, and mild visual hallucinations (light flashes). Consumption of more than 10 g of caffeine can cause generalized tonic-clonic seizures, respiratory failure, and death.

Table 9.4–1
DSM-IV-TR Caffeine-Related Disorders

Caffeine-induced disorders
Caffeine intoxication
Caffeine-induced anxiety disorder
   Specify if:
      With onset during intoxication
Caffeine-induced sleep disorder
   Specify if:
      With onset during intoxication
Caffeine-related disorder not otherwise specified

From American Psychiatric Association. *Diagnostic and Statistical Manual of Mental Disorders.* 4th ed. Text rev. Washington, DC: American Psychiatric Association; copyright 2000, with permission.

Table 9.4–2
DSM-IV-TR Diagnostic Criteria for Caffeine Intoxication

A. Recent consumption of caffeine, usually in excess of 250 mg (e.g., more than 2–3 cups of brewed coffee).
B. Five (or more) of the following signs, developing during, or shortly after, caffeine use:
    (1) restlessness
    (2) nervousness
    (3) excitement
    (4) insomnia
    (5) flushed face
    (6) diuresis
    (7) gastrointestinal disturbance
    (8) muscle twitching
    (9) rambling flow of thought and speech
    (10) tachycardia or cardiac arrhythmia
    (11) periods of inexhaustibility
    (12) psychomotor agitation
C. The symptoms in Criterion B cause clinically significant distress or impairment in social, occupational, or other important areas of functioning.
D. The symptoms are not due to a general medical condition and are not better accounted for by another mental disorder (e.g., an Anxiety Disorder).

From American Psychiatric Association. *Diagnostic and Statistical Manual of Mental Disorders*. 4th ed. Text rev. Washington, DC: American Psychiatric Association; copyright 2000, with permission.

Caffeine Withdrawal

Despite the fact that the DSM-IV-TR does not include a diagnosis of caffeine withdrawal, several well-controlled studies indicate that caffeine withdrawal is a real phenomenon, and DSM-IV-TR gives research criteria for caffeine withdrawal (Table 9.4–4). The appearance of withdrawal symptoms reflects the tolerance and physiological dependence that develop with continued caffeine use. Several epidemiological studies have reported symptoms of caffeine withdrawal in 50 to 75 percent of all caffeine users studied. The most common symptoms are headache and fatigue; other symptoms include anxiety, irritability, mild depressive symptoms, impaired psychomotor performance, nausea, vomiting, craving for caffeine, and muscle pain and stiffness. The number and severity of the withdrawal symptoms are correlated with the amount of caffeine ingested and the abruptness of the withdrawal. Caffeine withdrawal symptoms have their onset 12 to 24 hours after the last dose; the symptoms peak in 24 to 48 hours and resolve within 1 week.

Table 9.4–3
DSM-IV-TR Diagnostic Criteria for Caffeine-Related Disorder Not Otherwise Specified

The caffeine-related disorder not otherwise specified category is for disorders associated with the use of caffeine that are not classifiable as caffeine intoxication, caffeine-induced anxiety disorder, or caffeine-induced sleep disorder. An example is caffeine withdrawal.

From American Psychiatric Association. *Diagnostic and Statistical Manual of Mental Disorders*. 4th ed. Text rev. Washington, DC: American Psychiatric Association; copyright 2000, with permission.

Table 9.4–4
DSM-IV-TR Research Criteria for Caffeine Withdrawal

A. Prolonged daily use of caffeine.
B. Abrupt cessation of caffeine use, or reduction in the amount of caffeine used, closely followed by headache and one (or more) of the following symptoms:
    (1) marked fatigue or drowsiness
    (2) marked anxiety or depression
    (3) nausea or vomiting
C. The symptoms in Criterion B cause clinically significant distress or impairment in social, occupational, or other important areas of functioning.
D. The symptoms are not due to the direct physiological effects of a general medical condition (e.g., migraine, viral illness) and are not better accounted for by another mental disorder.

From American Psychiatric Association. *Diagnostic and Statistical Manual of Mental Disorders*. 4th ed. Text rev. Washington, DC: American Psychiatric Association; copyright 2000, with permission.

The induction of caffeine withdrawal can sometimes be iatrogenic. Physicians often ask their patients to discontinue caffeine intake before certain medical procedures, such as endoscopy, colonoscopy, and cardiac catheterization. Physicians also often recommend that patients with anxiety symptoms, cardiac arrhythmias, esophagitis, hiatal hernias, fibrocystic disease of the breast, and insomnia stop caffeine intake. Some persons simply decide that it would be good for them to stop using caffeine-containing products. In all these situations, caffeine users should taper the use of caffeine-containing products over a 7- to 14-day period rather than stop abruptly.

Caffeine-Induced Anxiety Disorder

Caffeine-induced anxiety disorder, which can occur during caffeine intoxication, is a DSM-IV-TR diagnosis (see Table 13.7–2). The anxiety related to caffeine use can resemble that of generalized anxiety disorder. Patients with the disorder may be perceived as "wired," overly talkative, and irritable; they may complain of not sleeping well and of having energy to burn. Caffeine can induce and exacerbate panic attacks in persons with a panic disorder, and although a causative association between caffeine and a panic disorder has not been demonstrated, patients with panic disorder should avoid caffeine.

Caffeine-Induced Sleep Disorder

Caffeine-induced sleep disorder, which can occur during caffeine intoxication, is a DSM-IV-TR diagnosis (see Table 20.2–14). Caffeine is associated with delay in falling asleep, inability to remain asleep, and early-morning awakening.

Caffeine Dependence

Caffeine dependence is not included in DSM-IV-TR, which explicitly states, "A diagnosis of Substance Dependence can be applied to every class of substance except caffeine." Despite the absence of caffeine dependence in DSM-IV-TR, evidence supports a diagnosis of caffeine dependence in some people with problematic caffeine consumption. No studies have examined the course and prognosis for patients with a diagnosis of caffeine dependence. Persons with caffeine dependence have reported continued use of caffeine despite repeated efforts to discontinue their caffeine use.

> Mrs. G was a 35-year-old married, white homemaker with three children, aged 8, 6, and 2. She took no prescription medications, took a multivitamin and vitamins C and E on a daily basis, did not smoke, and had no history of psychiatric problems. She drank moderate amounts of alcohol on the weekends, had smoked marijuana in college but had not used it since, and had no other history of illicit drug use.
>
> She had started consuming caffeinated beverages while in college, and her current beverage of choice was caffeinated diet cola. Mrs. G had her first soft drink early in the morning, shortly after getting out of bed, and she jokingly called it her "morning hit." She spaced out her bottles of soft drinks over the course of the day, with her last bottle at dinnertime. She typically drank four to five 20-oz bottles of caffeinated diet cola each day.
>
> She and her husband had argued about her caffeinated soft drink use in the past, and her husband had believed she should not drink caffeinated soft drinks while pregnant. However, she had continued to do so during each of her pregnancies. Despite a desire to stop drinking caffeinated soft drinks, she was unable to do so. She described having a strong desire to drink caffeinated soft drinks, and if she resisted this desire, she found that she could not think of anything else. She drank caffeinated soft drinks in her car, which had a manual transmission, and noted that she fumbled while shifting and holding the soft drink and spilled it in the car. She also noted that her teeth had become yellowed, and she suspected this was related to her tendency to swish the soft drink in her mouth before swallowing it. When asked to describe a time when she stopped using soft drinks, she reported that she had run out of it on the day one of her children was to have a birthday party, and she did not have time to leave her home to buy more. In the early afternoon of that day, a few hours before the scheduled start of the party, she felt extreme lethargy, a severe headache, irritability, and craving for a soft drink. She called her husband and told him she planned to cancel the party. She then went to the grocery store to buy soft drinks, and after drinking two bottles, she felt well enough to host the party.
>
> Although initially expressing interest in decreasing or stopping her caffeinated soft drink use, Mrs. G did not attend scheduled follow-up appointments after her first evaluation. When finally contacted at home, she reported she had only sought help initially at her husband's request, and she had decided to try to cut down on her caffeine use on her own. (Courtesy of Eric Strain, M.D. and Roland R. Griffiths, Ph.D.)

Caffeine-Related Disorder Not Otherwise Specified

The DSM-IV-TR contains a residual category for caffeine-related disorders that do not meet the criteria for caffeine intoxication, caffeine-induced anxiety disorder, or caffeine-induced sleep disorder (Table 9.4–3).

CLINICAL FEATURES

Signs and Symptoms

After the ingestion of 50 to 100 mg of caffeine, common symptoms include increased alertness, a mild sense of well-being, and a sense of improved verbal and motor performance. Caffeine ingestion is also associated with diuresis, cardiac muscle stimulation, increased intestinal peristalsis, increased gastric acid secretion, and (usually mildly) increased blood pressure.

Caffeine Use and Nonpsychiatric Illnesses.   Despite numerous studies examining the relationship between caffeine use and physical illness, significant health risk from nonreversible pathological consequences of caffeine use, such as cancer, heart disease, and human reproduction, has not been conclusively demonstrated. Nonetheless, caffeine use is often considered to be contraindicated for various conditions, including generalized anxiety disorder, panic disorder, primary insomnia, gastroesophageal reflux, and pregnancy. In addition, the modest ability of caffeine to increase blood pressure and the documented cholesterol-elevating compounds of unfiltered coffee have raised the issue of the relationship of caffeine and coffee use to cardiovascular disease. Finally, there may be a mild association between higher daily caffeine use in women and delayed conception and slightly lower birth weight. Studies, however, have not found such associations, and effects, when found, are usually with relatively high daily doses of caffeine (e.g., the equivalent of five cups of brewed coffee per day). For a woman who is considering pregnancy, especially if there is some difficulty in conceiving, it may be useful to counsel eliminating caffeine use. Similarly, for a woman who becomes pregnant and has moderate to high daily caffeine consumption, a discussion about decreasing her daily caffeine use may be warranted.

TREATMENT

Analgesics, such as aspirin, almost always can control the headaches and muscle aches that may accompany caffeine withdrawal. Rarely do patients require benzodiazepines to relieve withdrawal symptoms. If benzodiazepines are used for this purpose, they should be used in small doses for a brief time, about 7 to 10 days at the longest.

The first step in reducing or eliminating caffeine use is to have patients determine their daily consumption of caffeine. This can best be accomplished by having the patient keep a daily food diary. The patient must recognize all sources of caffeine in the diet, including forms of caffeine (e.g., beverages, medications), and accurately record the amount consumed. After several days of keeping such a diary, the clinician can meet with the patient, review the diary, and determine the average daily caffeine dose in milligrams.

The patient and clinician should then decide on a fading schedule for caffeine consumption. Such a schedule could involve a decrease in increments of 10 percent every few days. Because caffeine is typically consumed in beverage form, the patient can use a substitution procedure in which a decaffeinated beverage is gradually used in place of the caffeinated beverage. The diary should be maintained during this time, so that the patient's progress can be monitored. The fading should be individualized for each patient so that the rate of decrease in caffeine consumption minimizes withdrawal symptoms. The patient should probably avoid stopping all caffeine use abruptly, because withdrawal symptoms are likely to develop with sudden discontinuation of all caffeine use.

▲ 9.5 Cannabis-Related Disorders

Cannabis preparations are obtained from the Indian hemp plant *Cannabis sativa*, a hardy, aromatic annual herb. The cannabis plant has been used in China, India, and the Middle East for approximately 8,000 years for its fiber and as a medicinal agent. It is the most commonly used illicit drug in the United States and, by most estimates, around the world as well.

CANNABIS PREPARATIONS

All parts of *Cannabis sativa* contain psychoactive cannabinoids, of which (−)-Δ9-tetrahydrocannabinol (Δ9-THC) is most abundant. The most potent forms of cannabis come from the flowering tops of the plants or from the dried, black-brown, resinous exudate from the leaves, which is referred to as hashish or hash. The cannabis plant is usually cut, dried, chopped, and rolled into cigarettes (commonly called "joints"), which are then smoked. The common names for cannabis are marijuana, grass, pot, weed, tea, and Mary Jane. Other names, which describe cannabis types of various strengths, are hemp, chasra, bhang, ganja, dagga, and sinsemilla. The potency of marijuana preparations has increased in recent years because of improved agricultural techniques used in cultivation, so that plants may contain up to 15 or 20 percent THC.

EPIDEMIOLOGY

Prevalence and Recent Trends

Based on the 2003 National Surveys on Drug Use and Health (NSDUH), an estimated 90.8 million adults (42.9 percent) aged 18 years or older had used marijuana at least once in their lifetime. Among this group, about 2 percent used the drug before age 12 years, about 53 percent between 12 and 17 years, and about 45 percent after age 18 years.

The *Monitoring the Future* survey of adolescents in school indicates recent increases in lifetime, annual, current (within the past 30 days), and daily use of marijuana by eighth and tenth graders, continuing a trend that began in the early 1990s. In 1996, about 23 percent of eighth-graders and about 40 percent of tenth-graders reported having used marijuana, and, in 1998 and 1999, more than one fourth of marijuana initiates were aged 14 years or younger. The average age was 17 years.

According to the text revision of the fourth edition of *Diagnostic and Statistical Manual of Mental Disorders* (DSM-IV-TR), there is a 5 percent lifetime rate of cannabis abuse or dependence, but that figure may be too low according to NSDUH surveys.

Demographic Correlates

The rate of past-year and current marijuana use by males was almost twice the rate for females overall among those aged 26 years and older. This gap between the sexes narrows with younger users; at ages 12 to 17 years, there are no significant differences.

Race and ethnicity were also related to marijuana use, but the relationships varied by age group. Among those aged 12 to 17 years, whites had higher rates of lifetime and past-year marijuana use than blacks. Among those 17 to 34 years of age, whites reported higher levels of lifetime use than blacks and Hispanics. But among those 35 years and older, whites and blacks reported the same levels of use. The lifetime rates for black adults were significantly higher than those for Hispanics.

NEUROPHARMACOLOGY

As stated previously, the principal component of cannabis is Δ 9-THC; however, the cannabis plant contains more than 400 chemicals, of which about 60 are chemically related to Δ 9-THC. In humans, Δ 9-THC is rapidly converted into 11-hydroxy-Δ9-THC, the metabolite that is active in the central nervous system (CNS).

A specific receptor for the cannabinols has been identified, cloned, and characterized. The cannabinoid receptor, a member of the G-protein-linked family of receptors, is linked to the inhibitory G protein (Gi), which is linked to adenylyl cyclase in an inhibitory fashion. The cannabinoid receptor is found in highest concentrations in the basal ganglia, the hippocampus, and the cerebellum, with lower concentrations in the cerebral cortex. It is not found in the brainstem, a fact consistent with cannabis' minimal effects on respiratory and cardiac functions. Studies in animals have shown that the cannabinoids affect the monoamine and γ-aminobutyric acid (GABA) neurons.

According to most studies, animals do not self-administer cannabinoids as they do most other substances of abuse. Moreover, there is some debate about whether the cannabinoids stimulate the so-called reward centers of the brain, such as the dopaminergic neurons of the ventral tegmental area. Tolerance to cannabis does develop, however, and psychological dependence has been found, although the evidence for physiological dependence is not strong. Withdrawal symptoms in humans are limited to modest increases in irritability, restlessness, insomnia, and anorexia and mild nausea; all of these symptoms appear only when a person abruptly stops taking high doses of cannabis.

When cannabis is smoked, the euphoric effects appear within minutes, peak in about 30 minutes, and last 2 to 4 hours. Some motor and cognitive effects last 5 to 12 hours. Cannabis can also be taken orally when it is prepared in food, such as brownies and cakes. About two to three times as much cannabis must be taken orally to be as potent as cannabis taken by inhaling its smoke. Many variables affect the psychoactive properties of cannabis, including the potency of the cannabis used, the route of administration, the smoking technique, the effects of pyrolysis on the cannabinoid content, the dose, the setting, and the user's past experience, expectations, and unique biological vulnerability to the effects of cannabinoids.

DIAGNOSIS AND CLINICAL FEATURES

The most common physical effects of cannabis are dilation of the conjunctival blood vessels (red eye) and mild tachycardia. At high doses, orthostatic hypotension may appear. Increased appetite—often referred to as "the munchies"—and dry mouth are common effects of cannabis intoxication. That no clearly

Table 9.5–1
DSM-IV-TR Cannabis-Related Disorders

Cannabis use disorders
Cannabis dependence
Cannabis abuse
Cannabis-induced disorders
Cannabis intoxication
  Specify if:
    With perceptual disturbances
Cannabis intoxication delirium
Cannabis-induced psychotic disorder, with delusions
  Specify if:
    With onset during intoxication
Cannabis-induced psychotic disorder, with hallucinations
  Specify if:
    With onset during intoxication
Cannabis-induced anxiety disorder
  Specify if:
    With onset during intoxication
Cannabis-related disorder not otherwise specified

From American Psychiatric Association. *Diagnostic and Statistical Manual of Mental Disorders.* 4th ed. Text rev. Washington, DC: American Psychiatric Association; copyright 2000, with permission.

Table 9.5–2
DSM-IV-TR Diagnostic Criteria for Cannabis Intoxication

A. Recent use of cannabis.
B. Clinically significant maladaptive behavioral or psychological changes (e.g., impaired motor coordination, euphoria, anxiety, sensation of slowed time, impaired judgment, social withdrawal) that developed during, or shortly after, cannabis use.
C. Two (or more) of the following signs, developing within 2 hours of cannabis use:
  (1) conjunctival injection
  (2) increased appetite
  (3) dry mouth
  (4) tachycardia
D. The symptoms are not due to a general medical condition and are not better accounted for by another mental disorder.
Specify if:
  With perceptual disturbances

From American Psychiatric Association. *Diagnostic and Statistical Manual of Mental Disorders.* 4th ed. Text rev. Washington, DC: American Psychiatric Association; copyright 2000, with permission.

documented case of death caused by cannabis intoxication alone reflects the substance's lack of effect on the respiratory rate. The most serious potential adverse effects of cannabis use are those caused by inhaling the same carcinogenic hydrocarbons present in conventional tobacco, and some data indicate that heavy cannabis users are at risk for chronic respiratory disease and lung cancer. The practice of smoking cannabis-containing cigarettes to their very ends, so-called "roaches," further increases the intake of tar (particulate matter). Many reports indicate that long-term cannabis use is associated with cerebral atrophy, seizure susceptibility, chromosomal damage, birth defects, impaired immune reactivity, alterations in testosterone concentrations, and dysregulation of menstrual cycles; these reports, however, have not been conclusively replicated, and the association between these findings and cannabis use is uncertain.

The DSM-IV-TR lists the cannabis-related disorders (Table 9.5–1) but has specific criteria within the cannabis-related disorders section only for cannabis intoxication (Table 9.5–2). The diagnostic criteria for the other cannabis-related disorders are contained in those DSM-IV-TR sections that focus on the major phenomenological symptom—for example, cannabis-induced psychotic disorder, with delusions, in the DSM-IV-TR section on substance-induced psychotic disorder (see Table 11.4–5).

Cannabis Dependence and Cannabis Abuse

The DSM-IV-TR includes the diagnoses of cannabis dependence and cannabis abuse (see Tables 9.1–3, 9.1–4, and 9.1–5). The experimental data clearly show tolerance to many of the effects of cannabis, but the data are less supportive of the existence of physical dependence. Psychological dependence on cannabis use does develop in long-term users.

Cannabis Intoxication

The DSM-IV-TR formalizes the diagnostic criteria for cannabis intoxication (Table 9.5–2). These criteria state that the diagnosis can be augmented with the phrase "with perceptual distur-

bances." If intact reality testing is not present, the diagnosis is cannabis-induced psychotic disorder.

Cannabis intoxication commonly heightens users' sensitivities to external stimuli, reveals new details, makes colors seem brighter and richer than in the past, and subjectively slows the appreciation of time. In high doses, users may experience depersonalization and derealization. Motor skills are impaired by cannabis use, and the impairment in motor skills remains after the subjective, euphoriant effects have resolved. For 8 to 12 hours after using cannabis, users' impaired motor skills interfere with the operation of motor vehicles and other heavy machinery. Moreover, these effects are additive to those of alcohol, which is commonly used in combination with cannabis.

Cannabis Intoxication Delirium

Cannabis intoxication delirium is a DSM-IV-TR diagnosis (see Table 7.2–2). The delirium associated with cannabis intoxication is characterized by marked impairment on cognition and performance tasks. Even modest doses of cannabis impair memory, reaction time, perception, motor coordination, and attention. High doses that also impair users' levels of consciousness have marked effects on cognitive measures.

Cannabis-Induced Psychotic Disorder

Cannabis-induced psychotic disorder (see Table 11.4–5) is diagnosed in the presence of a cannabis-induced psychosis. Cannabis-induced psychotic disorder is rare; transient paranoid ideation is more common.

A 35-year-old white married male who was naïve to cannabis use was given two "joints" by a friend. He smoked the first of the two in the same manner that he normally smoked a cigarette (in about 3 to 5 minutes). Noting no major effects, he proceeded immediately to smoke the second in the same amount of time. Within 30 minutes, he began to experience rapid heartbeat, dry mouth, mounting anxiety and the delusional belief that his throat was closing up and that he was going to die. That belief induced further panic and the patient was brought to the emergency room in the midst of a psychotic experience. Reassurance that he would not die had no effect. He was sedated with diazepam and some of his anxiety diminished. He eventually went to sleep and on awakening in about 5 hours he was asymptomatic with full recall of previous events.

Florid psychosis is somewhat common in countries in which some persons have long-term access to cannabis of particularly high potency. The psychotic episodes are sometimes referred to as "hemp insanity." Cannabis use rarely causes a "bad-trip" experience, which is often associated with hallucinogen intoxication. When cannabis-induced psychotic disorder does occur, it may be correlated with a preexisting personality disorder in the affected person.

Cannabis-Induced Anxiety Disorder

Cannabis-induced anxiety disorder (see Table 13.7–2) is a common diagnosis for acute cannabis intoxication, which in many persons induces short-lived anxiety states often provoked by paranoid thoughts. In such circumstances, panic attacks may be induced, based on ill-defined and disorganized fears. The appearance of anxiety symptoms is correlated with the dose and is the most frequent adverse reaction to the moderate use of smoked cannabis. Inexperienced users are much more likely to experience anxiety symptoms than are experienced users.

Cannabis-Related Disorder Not Otherwise Specified

The DSM-IV-TR does not formally recognize cannabis-induced mood disorders; therefore, such disorders are classified as cannabis-related disorders not otherwise specified (Table 9.5–3). Cannabis intoxication can be associated with depressive symptoms, although such symptoms may suggest long-term cannabis use. Hypomania, however, is a common symptom in cannabis intoxication.

The DSM-IV-TR also does not formally recognize cannabis-induced sleep disorders or cannabis-induced sexual dysfunction; therefore, both are classified as cannabis-related disorders

Table 9.5–3
DSM-IV-TR Diagnostic Criteria for Cannabis-Related Disorder Not Otherwise Specified

The cannabis-related disorder not otherwise specified category is for disorders associated with the use of cannabis that are not classifiable as cannabis dependence, cannabis abuse, cannabis intoxication, cannabis intoxication delirium, cannabis-induced psychotic disorder, or cannabis-induced anxiety disorder.

From American Psychiatric Association. *Diagnostic and Statistical Manual of Mental Disorders.* 4th ed. Text rev. Washington, DC: American Psychiatric Association; copyright 2000, with permission.

not otherwise specified. When either sleep disorder or sexual dysfunction symptoms are related to cannabis use, they almost always resolve within days or a week after cessation of cannabis use.

Flashbacks.   Persisting perceptual abnormalities after cannabis use are not formally classified in DSM-IV-TR, although there are case reports of persons who have experienced—at times significantly—sensations related to cannabis intoxication after the short-term effects of the substance have disappeared. Continued debate concerns whether flashbacks are related to cannabis use alone or to the concomitant use of hallucinogens or of cannabis tainted with phencyclidine (PCP).

Cognitive Impairment.   Clinical and experimental evidence indicates that the long-term use of cannabis may produce subtle forms of cognitive impairment in the higher cognitive functions of memory, attention, and organization and in the integration of complex information. This evidence suggests that the longer the period of heavy cannabis use, the more pronounced is the cognitive impairment. Nonetheless, because the impairments in performance are subtle, it remains to be determined how significant they are for everyday functioning. It also remains to be investigated whether these impairments can be reversed after an extended period of abstinence from cannabis.

Amotivational Syndrome.   A controversial cannabis-related syndrome is *amotivational syndrome.* Whether the syndrome is related to cannabis use or reflects characterological traits in a subgroup of persons regardless of cannabis use is under debate. Traditionally, the amotivational syndrome has been associated with long-term heavy use and has been characterized by a person's unwillingness to persist in a task—be it at school, at work, or in any setting that requires prolonged attention or tenacity. Persons are described as becoming apathetic and anergic, usually gaining weight, and appearing slothful.

TREATMENT AND REHABILITATION

Treatment of cannabis use rests on the same principles as treatment of other substances of abuse—abstinence and support. Abstinence can be achieved through direct interventions, such as hospitalization, or through careful monitoring on an outpatient basis by the use of urine drug screens, which can detect cannabis for up to 4 weeks after use. Support can be achieved through the use of individual, family, and group psychotherapies. Education should be a cornerstone for both abstinence and support programs. A patient who does not understand the intellectual reasons for addressing a substance-abuse problem has little motivation to stop. For some patients, an antianxiety drug may be useful for short-term relief of withdrawal symptoms. For other patients, cannabis use may be related to an underlying depressive disorder that may respond to specific antidepressant treatment.

MEDICAL USE OF MARIJUANA

Marijuana has been used as a medicinal herb for centuries, and cannabis was listed in the U.S. Pharmacopoeia until the end of the 19th century as a remedy for anxiety, depression, and gastrointestinal disorders, among others. Currently, cannabis is a controlled substance with a high potential for abuse and no medical use recognized by the Drug Enforcement Agency

(DEA); however, it is used to treat various disorders, such as the nausea secondary to chemotherapy, multiple sclerosis (MS), chronic pain, acquired immune deficiency syndrome (AIDS), epilepsy, and glaucoma. In 1996, California residents approved the California Compensation Use Act that allowed state residents to grow and use marijuana for these disorders: in 2001, however, the U.S. Supreme Court ruled 8 to 0 that the manufacture and distribution of marijuana are illegal under any circumstances. In addition, the Court held that patients using marijuana for medical purposes can be prosecuted; however, as of 2006, 11 states— Alaska, California, Colorado, Hawaii, Maine, Maryland, Montana, Nevada, Oregon, Vermont, and Washington—have passed laws exempting patients who use cannabis under a physician's supervision from state criminal penalties.

In addition to the Supreme Court ruling, periodically the federal government attempts to prosecute doctors who prescribe the drug for medical use with the threat of loss of licensure or jail sentences. In a strongly worded editorial, the *New England Journal of Medicine* urged that "Federal authorities should rescind their prohibition of the medical use of marijuana for seriously ill patients and allow physicians to decide which patients to treat." The editorial concluded by commenting on the role of the physician: "Some physicians will have the courage to challenge the continued proscription of marijuana for the sick. Eventually, their actions will force the courts to adjudicate between the rights of those at death's door and the absolute power of bureaucrats whose decisions are based more on reflexive ideology and political correctness than on compassion."

Dronabinol, a synthetic form of THC, has been approved by the U.S. Food and Drug Administration (FDA); some researchers believe, however, that when taken orally, it is not as effective as smoking the entire plant product. In 2006, regulatory officials authorized the first U.S. clinical trial investigating the efficacy of Sativex, an oral spray consisting of natural cannabis extracts, for the treatment of cancer pain. Sativex is currently available by prescription in Canada and on a limited basis in Spain and Great Britain for patients suffering from neuropathic pain, MS, and other conditions.

▲ 9.6 Cocaine-Related Disorders

Few public health issues attracted as much media attention in the United States during the 1980s and early 1990s as the problems resulting from the use of cocaine and crack, a highly potent form of cocaine. Although the intranasal use of cocaine hydrochloride during that time was associated with high-income, "jet-set" users, since the beginning of the 21st century, smokable crack cocaine has become an endemic drug problem in the inner cities across the United States and around the world.

Cocaine is an alkaloid derived from the shrub *Erythroxylon coca*, which is indigenous to South America, where the leaves of the shrub are chewed by local inhabitants to obtain the stimulating effects. The cocaine alkaloid was first isolated in 1860 and first used as a local anesthetic in 1880. It is still used as a local anesthetic, especially for eye, nose, and throat surgery, for which its vasoconstrictive and analgesic effects are helpful. In 1884, Sigmund Freud made a study of cocaine's general

pharmacological effects and, for a period of time, according to his biographers, was addicted to the drug. In the 1880s and 1890s, cocaine was widely touted as a cure for many ills and was listed in the 1899 *Merck Manual*. It was the active ingredient in the beverage Coca-Cola until 1902. In 1914, however, once its addictive and adverse effects had been recognized, cocaine was classified as a narcotic, along with morphine and heroin.

DEFINITIONS

Substance use can be associated with a number of distinct disorders of which dependence and abuse are but two; the text revision of the fourth edition of *Diagnostic and Statistical Manual of Mental Disorders* (DSM-IV-TR) describes ten others for cocaine. Cocaine dependence is defined in DSM-IV-TR as a cluster of physiological, behavioral, and cognitive symptoms that, taken together, indicate that the person continues to use cocaine despite significant problems related to such use. It is defined in the tenth revision of *International Statistical Classification of Diseases and Related Health Problems* (ICD-10) as a cluster of physiological, behavioral, and cognitive phenomena in which a person gives much higher priority to cocaine use than to other behaviors that once had a greater value. Central to these definitions is the emphasis placed on the drug-using behavior, its maladaptive nature, and how over time the voluntary choice to engage in that behavior shifts and becomes constrained as a result of interactions with the drug.

EPIDEMIOLOGY

Cocaine Use

In 2002 and 2003, 5.9 million (2.5 percent) persons aged 12 years or older had used cocaine in the past year, and more than 2.1 million (0.9 percent) persons had used cocaine in the past month. Persons aged 18 to 25 years (6.7 percent) had a higher rate of past-year cocaine use than persons aged 26 years or older (1.9 percent) and youths aged 12 to 17 years (1.9 percent). Males (3.4 percent) were more than twice as likely as females (1.6 percent) to have used cocaine in the past year. Asians had the lowest rate of past-year cocaine use (0.7 percent) compared with other racial or ethnic groups.

Cocaine Abuse and Dependence

In 2002 and 2003, more than 1.5 million (0.6 percent) persons aged 12 years or older met the criteria for abuse of, or dependence on, cocaine in the past year. Persons aged 18 to 25 years (1.2 percent) had the highest rate of past-year cocaine abuse or dependence, followed by persons aged 26 years or older (0.6 percent) and youths aged 12 to 17 years (0.4 percent). Males (0.9 percent) were more than twice as likely as females (0.4 percent) to have met the criteria for cocaine abuse or dependence. Blacks (1.1 percent) and Hispanics (0.9 percent) had higher rates of cocaine abuse or dependence than whites (0.5 percent), and the rate for Asians (0.1 percent) was lower than that for blacks, Hispanics, whites, American Indians or Alaskan Natives (1.2 percent), and non-Hispanic persons who identified themselves with two or more races (0.9 percent).

Crack Cocaine

An estimated 1.5 million (0.6 percent) persons aged 12 years or older had used crack cocaine in the past year, and 586,000 (0.2 percent) persons had used crack cocaine in the past month. Persons aged 18 to 25 years (0.9 percent) had the highest rate of past-year crack use, followed by persons aged 26 years or older (0.6 percent) and youths aged 12 to 17 years (0.4 percent). Males (0.9 percent) were more than twice as likely as females (0.4 percent) to have used crack cocaine in the past year. Asians had the lowest rate of past-year crack cocaine use (0.1 percent) compared with other racial or ethnic groups. Blacks (1.6 percent), American Indians or Alaska Natives (1.3 percent), Native Hawaiians or Other Pacific Islanders (1.2 percent), and persons who identified themselves with two or more non-Hispanic races (1.5 percent) had higher rates of past-year crack cocaine use than whites (0.5 percent) and Hispanics or Latinos (0.5 percent).

Current cocaine use is on the decline, primarily because of increased awareness of cocaine's risks as well as a comprehensive public campaign about cocaine and its effects. The societal effects of the decrease in cocaine use, however, have been somewhat offset by the frequent use in recent years of crack.

COMORBIDITY

As with other substance-related disorders, cocaine-related disorders are often accompanied by additional psychiatric disorders. The development of mood disorders and alcohol-related disorders usually follows the onset of cocaine-related disorders, whereas anxiety disorders, antisocial personality disorder, and attention-deficit/hyperactivity disorder (ADHD) are thought to precede the development of cocaine-related disorders. Most studies of comorbidity in patients with cocaine-related disorders have shown that major depressive disorder, bipolar II disorder, cyclothymic disorder, anxiety disorders, and antisocial personality disorder are the most commonly associated psychiatric diagnoses.

ETIOLOGY

Genetic Factors

The most convincing evidence of a genetic influence on cocaine dependence comes from studies of twins. Monozygotic twins have higher concordance rates for stimulant dependence (cocaine, amphetamines, and amphetamine-like drugs) than dizygotic twins. The analyses indicate that genetic factors and unique (unshared) environmental factors contribute about equally to the development of stimulant dependence.

Sociocultural Factors

Social, cultural, and economic factors are powerful determinants of initial use, continuing use, and relapse. Excessive use is far more likely in countries where cocaine is readily available. Different economic opportunities may influence certain groups more than others to engage in selling illicit drugs, and selling is more likely to be carried out in familiar communities than in those where the seller runs a high risk of arrest.

Learning and Conditioning

Learning and conditioning are also considered important in perpetuating cocaine use. Each inhalation or injection of cocaine yields a "rush" and a euphoric experience that reinforce the antecedent drug-taking behavior. In addition, the environmental cues associated with substance use become associated with the euphoric state so that long after a period of cessation, such cues (e.g., white powder and paraphernalia) can elicit memories of the euphoric state and reawaken craving for cocaine.

In cocaine abusers (but not in normal controls), cocaine-related stimuli activate brain regions subserving episodic and working memory and produce electroencephalographic (EEG) arousal (desynchronization). Increased metabolic activity in the limbic-related regions, such as the amygdala, parahippocampal gyrus, and dorsolateral prefrontal cortex, reportedly correlates with reports of craving for cocaine, but the degree of EEG arousal does not.

Pharmacological Factors

As a result of actions in the central nervous system (CNS), cocaine can produce a sense of alertness, euphoria, and well-being. Users may experience decreased hunger and less need for sleep. Performance impaired by fatigue is usually improved. Some users believe that cocaine enhances sexual performance.

NEUROPHARMACOLOGY

Cocaine's primary pharmacodynamic action related to its behavioral effects is competitive blockade of dopamine reuptake by the dopamine transporter. This blockade increases the concentration of dopamine in the synaptic cleft and results in increased activation of both dopamine type 1 (D_1) and type 2 (D_2) receptors. The effects of cocaine on the activity mediated by D_3, D_4, and D_5 receptors are not yet well understood, but at least one preclinical study has implicated the D_3 receptor. Although the behavioral effects are attributed primarily to the blockade of dopamine reuptake, cocaine also blocks the reuptake of norepinephrine and serotonin. The behavioral effects related to these activities are receiving increased attention in the scientific literature. The effects of cocaine on cerebral blood flow and cerebral glucose use have also been studied. Results in most studies generally show that cocaine is associated with decreased cerebral blood flow and possibly with the development of patchy areas of decreased glucose use.

The behavioral effects of cocaine are felt almost immediately and last for a relatively brief time (30 to 60 minutes); thus, users require repeated doses of the drug to maintain the feelings of intoxication. Despite the short-lived behavioral effects, metabolites of cocaine can be present in the blood and urine for up to 10 days.

Cocaine has powerful addictive qualities. Because of its potency as a positive reinforcer of behavior, psychological dependence on cocaine can develop after a single use. With repeated administration, both tolerance and sensitivity to various effects of cocaine can arise, although the development of tolerance or sensitivity is apparently caused by many factors and is not easily predicted. Physiological dependence on cocaine does occur, although cocaine withdrawal is mild compared with withdrawal from opiates and opioids.

Researchers recently reported that positron emission tomography (PET) scans of the brains of patients being treated for cocaine addiction show high activation in the mesolimbic dopamine system when addicts profoundly crave a drug. Researchers exposed patients to cues that had previously caused them to crave cocaine, and patients described feelings of intense cravings for the drug while PET scans showed activation in areas from the amygdala and the anterior cingulate to the tip of both temporal lobes. Some researchers claim that the mesolimbic dopamine system is also active in patients with nicotine addiction, and the same system has been linked to cravings for heroin, morphine, amphetamines, marijuana, and alcohol.

The D_2 receptors in the mesolimbic dopamine system have been held responsible for the heightened activity during periods of craving. PET scans of patients recovering from cocaine addiction are reported to show a drop in neuronal activity consistent with a lessened ability to receive dopamine, and the reduction in this ability, although it decreases over time, is apparent as long as $1^1/_2$ years after withdrawal. The pattern of reduced brain activity reflects the course of the craving; between the third and fourth weeks of withdrawal, the activity is at its lowest level, and the risk of patient relapse is highest. After about 1 year, the brains of former addicts are almost back to normal, although whether the dopamine cells ever return to a completely normal state is debatable.

METHODS OF USE

Because drug dealers often dilute cocaine powder with sugar or procaine, street cocaine varies greatly in purity. Cocaine is sometimes cut with amphetamine. The most common method of using cocaine is inhaling the finely chopped powder into the nose, a practice referred to as "snorting" or "tooting." Other methods of ingesting cocaine are subcutaneous or intravenous (IV) injection and smoking (freebasing). Freebasing involves mixing street cocaine with chemically extracted pure cocaine alkaloid (the freebase) to get an increased effect. Smoking is also the method used to ingest crack cocaine. Inhaling is the least dangerous method of cocaine use; IV injection and smoking are the most dangerous. The most direct methods of ingestion are often associated with cerebrovascular diseases, cardiac abnormalities, and death. Although cocaine can be taken orally, it is rarely ingested via this, the least effective, route.

Crack

Crack, a freebase form of cocaine, is extremely potent. It is sold in small, ready-to-smoke amounts, often called "rocks." Crack cocaine is highly addictive; even one or two experiences with the drug can cause intense craving for more. Users have been known to resort to extremes of behavior to obtain the money to buy more crack. Reports from urban emergency rooms have also associated extremes of violence with crack abuse.

DIAGNOSIS AND CLINICAL FEATURES

The DSM-IV-TR lists many cocaine-related disorders (Table 9.6–1) but only specifies the diagnostic criteria for cocaine intoxication (Table 9.6–2) and cocaine withdrawal (Table 9.6–3) within the cocaine-related disorders section. The diagnostic criteria for the other cocaine-related disorders are in the DSM-IV-TR sections that focus on the principal symptom—for example, cocaine-induced mood disorder in the mood disorders section (see Table 12.3–8).

Cocaine Dependence and Abuse

The DSM-IV-TR uses the general guidelines for substance dependence and substance abuse to diagnose cocaine dependence and cocaine abuse (see Tables 9.1–3 to 9.1–5). Clinically and practically, cocaine dependence or cocaine abuse can be

Table 9.6–1
DSM-IV-TR Cocaine-Related Disorders

Cocaine use disorders
Cocaine dependence
Cocaine abuse
Cocaine-induced disorders
Cocaine intoxication
Specify if:
    With perceptual disturbances
Cocaine withdrawal
Cocaine intoxication delirium
Cocaine-induced psychotic disorder, with delusions
Specify if:
    With onset during intoxication
Cocaine-induced psychotic disorder, with hallucinations
Specify if:
    With onset during intoxication
Cocaine-induced mood disorder
Specify if:
    With onset during intoxication
    With onset during withdrawal
Cocaine-induced anxiety disorder
Specify if:
    With onset during intoxication
    With onset during withdrawal
Cocaine-induced sexual dysfunction
Specify if:
    With onset during intoxication
Cocaine-induced sleep disorder
Specify if:
    With onset during intoxication
    With onset during withdrawal
Cocaine-related disorder not otherwise specified

From American Psychiatric Association. *Diagnostic and Statistical Manual of Mental Disorders.* 4th ed. Text rev. Washington, DC: American Psychiatric Association; copyright 2000, with permission.

Table 9.6–2
DSM-IV-TR Diagnostic Criteria for Cocaine Intoxication

A. Recent use of cocaine.
B. Clinically significant maladaptive behavioral or psychological changes (e.g., euphoria or affective blunting; changes in sociability; hypervigilance; interpersonal sensitivity; anxiety, tension, or anger; stereotyped behaviors; impaired judgment; or impaired social or occupational functioning) that developed during, or shortly after, use of cocaine.
C. Two (or more) of the following, developing during, or shortly after, cocaine use:

    (1) tachycardia or bradycardia
    (2) pupillary dilation
    (3) elevated or lowered blood pressure
    (4) perspiration or chills
    (5) nausea or vomiting
    (6) evidence of weight loss
    (7) psychomotor agitation or retardation
    (8) muscular weakness, respiratory depression, chest pain, or cardiac arrhythmias
    (9) confusion, seizures, dyskinesias, dystonias, or coma

D. The symptoms are not due to a general medical condition and are not better accounted for by another mental disorder.

Specify if:
With perceptual disturbances

From American Psychiatric Association. *Diagnostic and Statistical Manual of Mental Disorders.* 4th ed. Text rev. Washington, DC: American Psychiatric Association; copyright 2000, with permission.

Table 9.6–3
DSM-IV-TR Diagnostic Criteria for Cocaine Withdrawal

A. Cessation of (or reduction in) cocaine use that has been heavy and prolonged.

B. Dysphoric mood and two (or more) of the following physiological changes, developing within a few hours to several days after Criterion A:
   (1) fatigue
   (2) vivid, unpleasant dreams
   (3) insomnia or hypersomnia
   (4) increased appetite
   (5) psychomotor retardation or agitation

C. The symptoms in Criterion B cause clinically significant distress or impairment in social, occupational, or other important areas of functioning.

D. The symptoms are not due to a general medical condition and are not better accounted for by another mental disorder.

From American Psychiatric Association. *Diagnostic and Statistical Manual of Mental Disorders.* 4th ed. Text rev. Washington, DC: American Psychiatric Association; copyright 2000, with permission.

suspected in patients who evidence unexplained changes in personality. Common changes associated with cocaine use are irritability, impaired ability to concentrate, compulsive behavior, severe insomnia, and weight loss. Colleagues at work and family members may notice a person's general and increasing inability to perform the expected tasks associated with work and family life. The patient may show new evidence of increased debt or inability to pay bills on time because of the large sums used to buy cocaine. Cocaine abusers often excuse themselves from work or social situations every 30 to 60 minutes to find a secluded place to inhale more cocaine. Because of the vasoconstricting effects of cocaine, users almost always develop nasal congestion, which they may attempt to self-medicate with decongestant sprays.

T. Taylor was a separated, 39-year-old African-American man who was admitted to a psychiatric day program in the shelter where he lived when he complained of sudden impulses to stab other residents. The staff in the shelter described him variously as "manipulative" and "charming." He gives a long history of abuse of alcohol, heroin, and cocaine, but says he has been "clean" for 3 weeks. He reports several arrests for felonies, including armed robbery and kidnapping, for which he always seems to have an explanation that minimizes his own responsibility.

Mr. Taylor entered the city shelter system 2 years earlier when the woman he was living with threw him out because she couldn't tolerate his temper and substance abuse. During his marriage to another woman 20 years ago, he was able to work briefly in blue-collar jobs in between prison and hospital stays. He has not worked for the past 7 years and has never paid child support to his wife.

Life did not begin easily for Mr. Taylor. His father left home before he was born, leaving behind a family scandal. The family story is that his father impregnated his wife's sister, causing Mr. Taylor to be treated like an outcast by the family. His mother had nine children, each with a different father. She had chronic depression and had received extensive

psychiatric treatment. All of her children have psychiatric or substance abuse problems.

When Mr. Taylor was 3, his mother turned him over to a succession of reluctant caregivers on both sides of the family. He was physically abused by some of his mother's boyfriends, being whipped with belts and electric cords. He dropped out of school in seventh grade because "a teacher embarrassed me." He began drinking when he entered the Job Corps at age 16. In his late teens and early 20s, he used nasal cocaine and heroin, then intravenous heroin for about a year. He stopped using drugs in his mid-20s, but continued to binge on alcohol every few weeks.

At age 19, after an argument with his wife, he cut his wrists and was hospitalized for 6 months. He was given an antidepressant, an unknown tranquilizer, and psychotherapy following his discharge, but stopped treatment when he felt better. Over the ensuing 20 years there were multiple hospitalizations when he was suicidal or had violent impulses. At one point he jumped off a bridge, sustaining multiple fractures. He has never exhibited manic symptoms, nor has he ever had delusions or hallucinations.

The one psychiatric chart that was available outlined an extensive criminal record and gives the patient the diagnosis of Antisocial Personality Disorder. His criminal history included charges for multiple armed robberies, desertion and neglect of a minor, and kidnapping of a 20-year-old man. With reference to the last crime, he said that he held the man at bay with a machete while his friends stole the man's car.

Follow-up.   Over a 10-month treatment period, Mr. Taylor exhibited an intense attachment to his female caseworker. He often demanded immediate attention. When frustrated, he would occasionally become intoxicated and verbally abusive. This was especially the case when his caseworker left the program for another job. However, he did refrain from violent behavior and enrolled in a group for drug abusers who also have other psychiatric problems. An anticonvulsant drug helped him control his aggressive impulses. He also received individual and group counseling and social skills training and took part in a work and money-management program.

Mr. Taylor was accepted into a community residence and has been able to maintain his housing and his outpatient treatment in a day program during a 9-month period. He is monitored closely by his shelter caseworker, who intervenes when problems arise. (Reprinted with permission from *DSM-IV-TR Casebook.*)

Cocaine Intoxication

The DSM-IV-TR specifies the diagnostic criteria for cocaine intoxication (Table 9.6–2), which emphasizes the behavioral and physical signs and symptoms of cocaine use. The DSM-IV-TR diagnostic criteria allow for specification of the presence of perceptual disturbances. If hallucinations are present in the absence of intact reality testing, the appropriate diagnosis is cocaine-induced psychotic disorder, with hallucinations.

drug and direct energies in different directions. This approach can be used on an outpatient basis.

Network Therapy.   Network therapy was developed as a specialized type of combined individual and group therapy to ensure greater success in the office-based treatment of addicted patients. Network therapy uses both psychodynamic and cognitive-behavioral approaches to individual therapy while engaging the patient in a group support network. The group, composed of the patient's family and peers, is used as a therapeutic network joining the patient and therapist at intervals in therapy sessions. The approach promotes group cohesiveness as a vehicle for engaging patients in this treatment. This network is managed by the therapist to provide cohesiveness and support and to promote compliance with treatment. Although network therapy has not received systematic controlled evaluation, it is frequently applied in the psychiatric practice because it is one of the few manualized approaches that has been designed for use by individual practitioners in an office setting.

Pharmacological Adjuncts

No current pharmacological treatments produce decreases in cocaine use comparable to the decreases in opioid use seen when heroin users are treated with methadone, levomethadyl acetate (ORLAAM) (commonly called L-α-acetylmethadol [LAAM]), or buprenorphine (Buprenex). A variety of pharmacological agents, most of which are approved for other uses, have been, and are being, tested clinically for the treatment of cocaine dependence and relapse.

Cocaine users presumed to have preexisting ADHD or mood disorders have been treated with methylphenidate (Ritalin) and lithium (Eskalith), respectively. Those drugs are of little or no benefit in patients without the disorders, and clinicians should adhere strictly to maximal diagnostic criteria before using either of them in the treatment of cocaine dependence. In patients with ADHD, slow-release forms of methylphenidate may be less likely to trigger cocaine craving, but the impact of such pharmacotherapy on cocaine use remains to be demonstrated.

Many pharmacological agents have been explored on the premise that chronic cocaine use alters the function of multiple neurotransmitter systems, especially the dopaminergic and serotonergic transmitters regulating hedonic tone, and that cocaine induces a state of relative dopaminergic deficiency. Although the evidence for such alterations in dopaminergic function has been growing, it has been difficult to demonstrate that agents theoretically capable of modifying dopamine function can alter the course of treatment.

Tricyclic antidepressant drugs yielded some positive results when used early in treatment with minimally drug-dependent patients; however, they are of little or no use for inducing abstinence in moderate or severe cases.

Also tried but not confirmed effective in controlled studies are other antidepressants, such as bupropion, monoamine oxidase inhibitors (MAOIs), selective serotonin reuptake inhibitors (SSRIs), antipsychotics, lithium, several different calcium channel inhibitors, and anticonvulsants. One study found that 300 mg a day of phenytoin (Dilantin) reduced cocaine use; this study requires replication.

Several agents are being developed that have not been tried in human studies. These include agents that would selectively block or stimulate dopamine receptor subtypes (e.g., selective D_1 agonists) and drugs that can selectively block the access of cocaine to the dopamine transporters but still permit the transporters to remove cocaine from the synapse. Another approach is aimed at preventing cocaine from reaching the brain by using antibodies to bind cocaine in the bloodstream (a so-called "cocaine vaccine"). Such cocaine-binding antibodies do reduce the reinforcing ef-

fects of cocaine in animal models. Also under study are catalytic antibodies that accelerate the hydrolysis of cocaine, and butyrylcholinesterase (pseudocholinesterase), which appears to hydrolyze cocaine selectively and is normally present in the body.

Vigabatrin is a drug that has been used as a treatment for refractory pediatric epilepsy that appears to function by significantly elevating brain γ-aminobutyric acid levels. In animals, it was also noted to attenuate cocaine-, nicotine-, heroin-, alcohol-, and methamphetamine-induced increases in extracellular nucleus accumbens dopamine as well as drug-seeking behaviors associated with these biochemical changes. Preliminary clinical studies suggest efficacy for the treatment of cocaine and methamphetamine dependence. Large-scale clinical trials for this indication are underway.

▲ 9.7 Hallucinogen-Related Disorders

Hallucinogenic drugs have been used for thousands of years. Historically, drug-induced hallucinogenic states were usually part of social and religious rituals. Recognition of the profound effects of lysergic acid diethylamide (LSD) on mental functioning in 1943 markedly changed things. Unlike plant-based hallucinogens, such as psilocybin mushrooms and peyote cacti, more potent chemically synthesized hallucinogenic compounds such as LSD could be more readily researched, distributed, and used, leading to continued fascination with this heterogeneous group of drugs and to many thousands of scientific reports of hallucinogenic drug effects, speculations about mechanisms of action, and discussions of medical and societal problems resulting from hallucinogen distribution, use, and consequences.

PREPARATIONS

Hallucinogens are natural and synthetic substances that are variously called *psychedelics* or *psychotomimetics* because, besides inducing hallucinations, they produce a loss of contact with reality and an experience of expanded and heightened consciousness. The hallucinogens are classified as Schedule I drugs; the U.S. Food and Drug Administration (FDA) has decreed that they have no medical use and a high abuse potential.

The classic, naturally occurring hallucinogens are psilocybin (from some mushrooms) and mescaline (from peyote cactus); others are harmine, harmaline, ibogaine, and N,N-dimethyltryptamine (DMT). The classic synthetic hallucinogen is LSD, synthesized in 1938 by Albert Hoffman, who later accidentally ingested some of the drug and experienced the first LSD-induced hallucinogenic episode. Some researchers classify the substituted or so-called designer amphetamines, such as 3,4-methylenedioxyamphetamine (MDMA), as hallucinogens. Because these drugs are structurally related to amphetamines, this textbook classifies them as amphetamine-like substances, and they are covered in Section 9.3.

EPIDEMIOLOGY

The incidence of hallucinogen use has exhibited two notable periods of increase. Between 1965 and 1969, there was a tenfold increase in the estimated annual number of initiates. This increase was driven primarily by the use of LSD. The second period of increase in first-time hallucinogen use occurred from around 1992 until 2000, fueled mainly by increases in use of "ecstasy" (i.e., MDMA). Decreases in initiation of both LSD and ecstasy were evident between 2001 and 2002, coinciding with an overall drop in hallucinogen incidence from 1.6 million to 1.1 million.

According to the text revision of the fourth edition of *Diagnostic and Statistical Manual of Mental Disorders* (DSM-IV-TR), 10 percent of persons in the United States had used a hallucinogen at least once. Hallucinogen use is most common among young (15 to 35 years of age) white men. The ratio of whites to blacks who have used a hallucinogen is 2 to 1, and the white-to-Hispanic ratio is about 1.5 to 1. Men represent 62 percent of those who have used a hallucinogen at some time and 75 percent of those who have used a hallucinogen in the preceding month. Persons 26 to 34 years of age show the highest use of hallucinogens, with 15.5 percent having used a hallucinogen at least once. Persons 18 to 25 years of age have the highest recent use of a hallucinogen.

Cultural factors influence the use of hallucinogens; their use in the western United States is significantly higher than in the southern United States. Hallucinogen use is associated with less morbidity and less mortality than that of some other substances. For example, one study found that only 1 percent of substance-related emergency room visits were related to hallucinogens, compared with 40 percent for cocaine-related problems. Of persons visiting the emergency room for hallucinogen-related reasons, however, more than 50 percent were younger than 20 years of age. A resurgence in the popularity of hallucinogens has been reported. According to DSM-IV-TR, the lifetime rate of hallucinogen abuse is about 0.6 percent, with a 12-month prevalence of about 0.1 percent.

NEUROPHARMACOLOGY

Although most hallucinogenic substances vary in their pharmacological effects, LSD can serve as a hallucinogenic prototype. The pharmacodynamic effect of LSD remains controversial, although it is generally agreed that the drug acts on the serotonergic system, either as an antagonist or as an agonist. Data suggest that LSD acts as a partial agonist at postsynaptic serotonin receptors.

Most hallucinogens are well absorbed after oral ingestion, although some are ingested by inhalation, smoking, or intravenous injection. Tolerance for LSD and other hallucinogens develops rapidly and is virtually complete after 3 or 4 days of continuous use. Tolerance also reverses quickly, usually in 4 to 7 days. Neither physical dependence nor withdrawal symptoms occur with hallucinogens, but a user can develop a psychological dependence on the insight-inducing experiences of episodes of hallucinogen use.

DIAGNOSIS

The DSM-IV-TR lists a number of hallucinogen-related disorders (Table 9.7–1) but contains specific diagnostic criteria only for hallucinogen intoxication (Table 9.7–2) and hallucinogen persisting perception disorder (flashbacks) (Table 9.7–3). The diagnostic criteria for the other hallucinogen use disorders are contained in the DSM-IV-TR sections that are specific to each

**Table 9.7–1
DSM-IV-TR Hallucinogen-Related Disorders**

Hallucinogen use disorders
Hallucinogen dependence
Hallucinogen abuse
Hallucinogen-induced disorders
Hallucinogen intoxication
Hallucinogen persisting perception disorder (flashbacks)
Hallucinogen intoxication delirium
Hallucinogen-induced psychotic disorder, with delusions
  Specify if:
    With onset during intoxication
Hallucinogen-induced psychotic disorder, with hallucinations
  Specify if:
    With onset during intoxication
Hallucinogen-induced mood disorder
  Specify if:
    With onset during intoxication
Hallucinogen-induced anxiety disorder
  Specify if:
    With onset during intoxication
Hallucinogen-related disorder not otherwise specified

From American Psychiatric Association. *Diagnostic and Statistical Manual of Mental Disorders.* 4th ed. Text rev. Washington, DC: American Psychiatric Association; copyright 2000, with permission.

symptom—for example, hallucinogen-induced mood disorder (see Table 12.3–8).

Hallucinogen Dependence and Hallucinogen Abuse

Long-term hallucinogen use is not common. As stated previously, no physical addiction occurs. Although psychological

**Table 9.7–2
DSM-IV-TR Diagnostic Criteria for Hallucinogen Intoxication**

A. Recent use of a hallucinogen.
B. Clinically significant maladaptive behavioral or psychological changes (e.g., marked anxiety or depression, ideas of reference, fear of losing one's mind, paranoid ideation, impaired judgment, or impaired social or occupational functioning) that developed during, or shortly after, hallucinogen use.
C. Perceptual changes occurring in a state of full wakefulness and alertness (e.g., subjective intensification of perceptions, depersonalization, derealization, illusions, hallucinations, synesthesias) that developed during, or shortly after, hallucinogen use.
D. Two (or more) of the following signs, developing during, or shortly after, hallucinogen use:
  (1) pupillary dilation
  (2) tachycardia
  (3) sweating
  (4) palpitations
  (5) blurring of vision
  (6) tremors
  (7) incoordination
E. The symptoms are not due to a general medical condition and are not better accounted for by another mental disorder.

From American Psychiatric Association. *Diagnostic and Statistical Manual of Mental Disorders.* 4th ed. Text rev. Washington, DC: American Psychiatric Association; copyright 2000, with permission.

Table 9.7–3
DSM-IV-TR Diagnostic Criteria for Hallucinogen Persisting Perception Disorder (Flashbacks)

A. The reexperiencing, following cessation of use of a hallucinogen, of one or more of the perceptual symptoms that were experienced while intoxicated with the hallucinogen (e.g., geometric hallucinations, false perceptions of movement in the peripheral visual fields, flashes of color, intensified colors, trails of images of moving objects, positive afterimages, halos around objects, macropsia, and micropsia).

B. The symptoms in Criterion A cause clinically significant distress or impairment in social, occupational, or other important areas of functioning.

C. The symptoms are not due to a general medical condition (e.g., anatomical lesions and infections of the brain, visual epilepsies) and are not better accounted for by another mental disorder (e.g., delirium, dementia, schizophrenia) or hypnopompic hallucinations.

From American Psychiatric Association. *Diagnostic and Statistical Manual of Mental Disorders.* 4th ed. Text rev. Washington, DC: American Psychiatric Association; copyright 2000, with permission.

dependence occurs, it is rare, in part because each LSD experience is different and in part because there is no reliable euphoria. Nonetheless, hallucinogen dependence and hallucinogen abuse are genuine syndromes, defined by DSM-IV-TR criteria (see Tables 9.1–3 to 9.1–5).

Hallucinogen Intoxication

Intoxication with hallucinogens is defined in DSM-IV-TR as characterized by maladaptive behavioral and perceptual changes and by certain physiological signs (Table 9.7–2). The differential diagnosis for hallucinogen intoxication includes anticholinergic and amphetamine intoxication and alcohol withdrawal. The preferred treatment for hallucinogen intoxication is talking down the patient; during this process, guides can reassure patients that the symptoms are drug induced, that they are not going crazy, and that the symptoms will resolve shortly. In the most severe cases, dopaminergic antagonists—for example, haloperidol (Haldol)— or benzodiazepines—for example, diazepam (Valium)—can be used for a limited time. Hallucinogen intoxication usually lacks a withdrawal syndrome.

Hallucinogen Persisting Perception Disorder

Long after ingesting a hallucinogen, a person can experience a flashback of hallucinogenic symptoms. This syndrome is diagnosed as *hallucinogen persisting perception disorder* (Table 9.7–3) in DSM-IV-TR. According to studies, from 15 to 80 percent of users of hallucinogens report having experienced flashbacks. The differential diagnosis for flashbacks includes migraine, seizures, visual system abnormalities, and posttraumatic stress disorder. The following can trigger a flashback: emotional stress; sensory deprivation, such as monotonous driving; or use of another psychoactive substance, such as alcohol or marijuana.

Flashbacks are spontaneous, transitory recurrences of the substance-induced experience. Most flashbacks are episodes of visual distortion, geometric hallucinations, hallucinations of sounds or voices, false perceptions of movement in peripheral fields, flashes of color, trails of images from moving objects,

positive afterimages and halos, macropsia, micropsia, time expansion, physical symptoms, or relived intense emotion. The episodes usually last a few seconds to a few minutes, but they sometimes last longer. Most often, even in the presence of distinct perceptual disturbances, the person has insight into the pathological nature of the disturbance. Suicidal behavior, major depressive disorder, and panic disorders are potential complications.

A 20-year-old undergraduate presented with a chief complaint of seeing the air. The visual disturbance consisted of perception of white pinpoint specks in both the central and peripheral visual fields too numerous to count. They were constantly present and were accompanied by the perception of trails of moving objects left behind as they passed through the patient's visual field. Attending a hockey game was difficult, as the brightly dressed players left streaks of their own images against the white of the ice for seconds at a time. The patient also described the false perception of movement in stable objects, usually in his peripheral visual fields; halos around objects; and positive and negative afterimages. Other symptoms included mild depression, daily bitemporal headache, and a loss of concentration in the last year.

The visual syndrome had gradually emerged over the past 3 months following experimentation with the hallucinogenic drug LCD-25 on three separate occasions in the preceding 3 months. He feared he had sustained some kind of "brain damage" from the drug experience. He denied use of any other agents, including amphetamines, phencyclidine, narcotics, or alcohol, to excess. He had smoked marijuana twice a week for a period of 7 months at age 17.

The patient had consulted two ophthalmologists, both of whom confirmed that the white pinpoint specks were not vitreous floaters (diagnostically insignificant particulate matter floating in the vitreous humor of the eye that can cause the perception of "specks"). A neurologist's examination also proved negative. A therapeutic trial of an anticonvulsant medication resulted in a 50 percent improvement in the patient's visual symptoms and remission of his depression. (Reprinted with permission from *DSM-IV-TR Casebook.*)

Hallucinogen Intoxication Delirium

The DSM-IV-TR allows for the diagnosis of hallucinogen intoxication delirium (see Table 7.2–2), a relatively rare disorder beginning during intoxication in those who have ingested pure hallucinogens. Hallucinogens are often mixed with other substances, however, and the other components or their interactions with the hallucinogens can produce clinical delirium.

Hallucinogen-Induced Psychotic Disorders

If psychotic symptoms are present in the absence of retained reality testing, a diagnosis of hallucinogen-induced psychotic disorder may be warranted (see Table 11.4–5). DSM-IV-TR also allows clinicians to specify whether hallucinations or delusions are the prominent symptoms. The most common adverse effect of LSD and related substances is a "bad trip," an experience resembling the acute panic reaction to cannabis but sometimes more severe; a bad trip can occasionally produce true psychotic symptoms. The bad trip generally ends when the immediate effects of the hallucinogen wear off, but its course is variable. Occasionally, a protracted psychotic episode is difficult to distinguish from a nonorganic psychotic disorder. Whether a chronic psychosis after drug ingestion is the result of the drug ingestion, is unrelated to the drug ingestion, or is a combination of both the drug ingestion and predisposing factors is currently unanswerable.

Occasionally, the psychotic disorder is prolonged, a reaction thought to be most common in persons with preexisting schizoid personality disorder and prepsychotic personalities, an unstable ego balance, or much anxiety. Such persons cannot cope with the perceptual changes, body-image distortions, and symbolic unconscious material stimulated by the hallucinogen. The rate of previous mental instability in persons hospitalized for LSD reactions is high. Adverse reactions occurred in the late 1960s when LSD was being promoted as a self-prescribed psychotherapy for emotional crises in the lives of seriously disturbed persons. Now that this practice is less frequent, prolonged adverse reactions are less common.

A 22-year-old female photography student presented to the hospital with inappropriate mood and bizarre thinking. She had no prior psychiatric history. Nine days before admission, she ingested one or two psilocybin mushrooms. Following the immediate ingestion, the patient began to giggle. She then described euphoria, which progressed to auditory hallucinations and belief in the ability to broadcast her thoughts on the media. Two days later she repeated the ingestion, and continued to exhibit psychotic symptoms to the day of admission. When examined she heard voices telling her she could be president, and reported the sounds of "lambs crying." She continued to giggle inappropriately, bizarrely turning her head from side to side ritualistically. She continued to describe euphoria, but with an intermittent sense of hopelessness in a context of thought blocking. Her self-description was "feeling lucky." She was given haloperidol, 10 mg twice a day, along with benztropine (Cogentin) 1 mg three times a day and lithium carbonate (Eskalith) 300 mg twice a day. On this regimen her psychosis abated after 5 days.

Hallucinogen-Induced Mood Disorder

The DSM-IV-TR provides a diagnostic category for hallucinogen-induced mood disorder (see Table 12.3–8). Unlike cocaine-induced mood disorder and amphetamine-induced mood disorder, in which the symptoms are somewhat predictable, mood disorder symptoms accompanying hallucinogen abuse can vary. Abusers may experience manic-like symptoms with grandiose delusions or depression-like feelings and ideas or mixed symptoms. As with the hallucinogen-induced psychotic disorder symptoms, the symptoms of hallucinogen-induced mood disorder usually resolve once the drug has been eliminated from the person's body.

Hallucinogen-Induced Anxiety Disorder

Hallucinogen-induced anxiety disorder (see Table 13.7–2) also varies in its symptom pattern, but few data about symptom patterns are available. Anecdotally, emergency room physicians who treat patients with hallucinogen-related disorders frequently report panic disorder with agoraphobia.

A 20-year-old man had a 7-year history of polysubstance abuse, including having used LSD an estimated 400 times. While driving with his girlfriend, he ingested an unknown quantity of LSD and became intoxicated; he reported using no other drugs at this time. Within minutes after ingestion, he began to experience visual hallucinations that intensified as he drove. When he attempted to speak to his girlfriend, he saw that she had become a giant lizard. He became terrified and attempted to kill her by crashing the car, injuring himself and his passenger. By the time of discharge from the hospital 3 days later, his panic had resolved.

Hallucinogen-Related Disorder Not Otherwise Specified

When a patient with a hallucinogen-related disorder does not meet the diagnostic criteria for any of the standard hallucinogen-related disorders, the patient may be classified as having hallucinogen-related disorder not otherwise specified (Table 9.7–4). DSM-IV-TR does not have a diagnostic category of hallucinogen withdrawal, but some clinicians anecdotally report a syndrome with depression and anxiety after cessation of frequent hallucinogen use. Such a syndrome may best fit the diagnosis of hallucinogen-related disorder not otherwise specified.

CLINICAL FEATURES
Lysergic Acid Diethylamide

A large class of hallucinogenic compounds with well-studied structure–activity relationships is represented by the prototype LSD. LSD is a synthetic base derived from the lysergic acid nucleus from the ergot alkaloids. That family of compounds was discovered in rye fungus and was responsible for lethal

Table 9.7–4
DSM-IV-TR Diagnostic Criteria for Hallucinogen-Related Disorder Not Otherwise Specified

The hallucinogen-related disorder not otherwise specified category is for disorders associated with the use of hallucinogens that are not classifiable as hallucinogen dependence, hallucinogen abuse, hallucinogen intoxication, hallucinogen persisting perception disorder, hallucinogen intoxication delirium, hallucinogen-induced psychotic disorder, hallucinogen-induced mood disorder, or hallucinogen-induced anxiety disorder.

From American Psychiatric Association. *Diagnostic and Statistical Manual of Mental Disorders.* 4th ed. Text rev. Washington, DC: American Psychiatric Association; copyright 2000, with permission.

outbreaks of so-called St. Anthony's fire in the Middle Ages. The compounds are also present in morning glory seeds in low concentrations. Many homologs and analogs of LSD have been studied. None of them has potency exceeding that of LSD.

Physiological symptoms from LSD are typically few and relatively mild. Dilated pupils, increased deep tendon motor reflexes and muscle tension, and mild motor incoordination and ataxia are common. Increased heart rate, respiration, and blood pressure are modest in degree and variable, as are nausea, decreased appetite, and salivation.

The usual sequence of changes follows a pattern of somatic symptoms appearing first, then mood and perceptual changes, and, finally, psychological changes, although effects overlap and, depending on the particular hallucinogen, the time of onset and offset varies. The intensity of LSD effects in a nontolerant user generally is proportional to dose, with 25 μg as an approximate threshold dose.

The syndrome produced by LSD resembles that produced by mescaline, psilocybin, and some of the amphetamine analogs. The major difference among LSD, psilocybin, and mescaline is potency. A 1.5-μg/kg dose of LSD is roughly equivalent to 225 μg/kg of psilocybin, which is equivalent to 5 mg/kg of mescaline. With mescaline, onset of symptoms is slower, and more nausea and vomiting occur, but in general, the perceptual effects are more similar than different.

Tolerance, particularly to the sensory and other psychological effects, is evident as soon as the second or third day of successive LSD use. Four to 6 days free of LSD is necessary to lose significant tolerance. Tolerance is associated with frequent use of any of the hallucinogens. Cross-tolerance among mescaline, psilocybin, and LSD occurs, but not between amphetamine and LSD, despite the chemical similarity of amphetamine and mescaline.

Previously distributed as tablets, liquid, powder, and gelatin squares, in recent years, LSD has been commonly distributed as "blotter acid." Sheets of paper are soaked with LSD, dried, and perforated into small squares. Popular designs are stamped on the paper. Each sheet contains as many as a few hundred squares; one square containing 30 to 75 μg of LSD is one chewed dose, more or less. Planned massive ingestion is uncommon, but massive ingestion does happen by accident.

The onset of action of LSD occurs within 1 hour, peaks in 2 to 4 hours, and lasts 8 to 12 hours. The sympathomimetic effects of LSD include tremors, tachycardia, hypertension, hyperthermia, sweating, blurring of vision, and mydriasis. Death caused by cardiac or cerebrovascular pathology related to hypertension or hyperthermia can occur with hallucinogenic use. A syndrome similar to neuroleptic malignant syndrome has reportedly been associated with LSD. Death can also be caused by a physical injury when LSD use impairs judgment about motor vehicle traffic or a person's supposed ability to fly, for example. The psychological effects are usually well tolerated, but when persons cannot recall experiences or appreciate that the experiences are substance induced, they may fear the onset of insanity.

With hallucinogen use, perceptions become unusually brilliant and intense. Colors and textures seem to be richer than in the past, contours sharpened, music more emotionally profound, and smells and tastes heightened. Synesthesia is common; colors may be heard or sounds seen. Changes in body image and alterations of time and space perception also occur. Hallucinations are usually visual, often of geometric forms and figures, but auditory and tactile hallucinations are sometimes experienced. Emotions become unusually intense and may change abruptly and often; two seemingly incompatible feelings may be experienced at the same time. Suggestibility is greatly heightened, and sensitivity or detachment from other persons may arise. Other common features are a seeming awareness of internal organs, the recovery of lost early memories, the release of unconscious material in symbolic form, and regression and the apparent reliving of past events, including birth. Introspective reflection and feelings of religious and philosophical insight are common. The sense of self is greatly changed, sometimes to the point of depersonalization, merging with the external world, separation of self from body, or total dissolution of the ego in mystical ecstasy.

No clear evidence indicates a drastic personality change or chronic psychosis produced by long-term LSD use by moderate users not otherwise predisposed to these conditions. Some heavy users of hallucinogens, however, may experience chronic anxiety or depression and may benefit from a psychological or pharmacological approach that addresses the underlying problem.

Many persons maintain that a single experience with LSD has given them increased creative capacity, new psychological insight, relief from neurotic or psychosomatic symptoms, or a desirable change in personality. In the 1950s and 1960s, psychiatrists showed great interest in LSD and related substances, both as potential models for functional psychosis and as possible pharmacotherapeutic agents. The availability of these compounds to researchers in the basic neurosciences has led to many scientific advances.

Phenethylamines

Phenethylamines are compounds with simple chemical structures and structural similarity to the neurotransmitters dopamine and norepinephrine. Mescaline (3,4,5-trimethoxyphenethylamine), a classic hallucinogen in every sense of the term, was the first hallucinogen isolated from the peyote cactus that grows in the southwestern United States and northern Mexico. Mescaline human pharmacology was characterized in 1896 and its structure verified by synthesis 23 years later. Although many psychoactive plants have been recognized dating to before recorded history, mescaline was the only structurally identified hallucinogen until LSD was described in 1943.

Mescaline

Mescaline is usually consumed as peyote "buttons" picked from the small blue-green cacti *Lophophora williamsii* and *Lophophora diffusa*. The buttons are the dried, round, fleshy cactus tops. Mescaline is the active hallucinogenic alkaloid in the buttons. Use of peyote is legal for members of the Native American Church in some states. Adverse reactions to peyote are rare during structured religious use. Peyote usually is not consumed casually because of its bitter taste and sometimes severe nausea and vomiting preceding the hallucinogenic effects.

Many structural variations of mescaline have been investigated and structure–activity relationships fairly well characterized. One analog, 2,5-dimethoxy-4-methylamphetamine (DOM), also known as STP, an unusually potent amphetamine with hallucinogen properties, had a relatively brief period of illicit popularity and notoriety in the 1960s.

Another series of phenethylamine analogs with hallucinogenic properties comprises the 3,4-methylenedioxyamphetamine (MDA)–related amphetamines. The currently most popular and, to society, most troublesome member of this large family of drugs is MDMA, or ecstasy, more a relatively mild stimulant than a hallucinogen. MDMA produces an altered state of consciousness with sensory changes and, most important for some users, a feeling of enhanced personal interactions. MDMA is discussed in more detail in Section 9.3 on amphetamine-related disorders.

Many plants contain N,N-dimethyltryptamine (DMT), which is also found normally in human biofluids at very low concentrations. When DMT is taken parenterally or by sniffing, a brief, intense hallucinogenic episode can result. As with mescaline in the phenethylamine group, DMT is one of the oldest, best documented, but least potent of the tryptamine hallucinogens. Synthesized homologs of DMT have been evaluated in humans and structure–activity relationships reasonably well described.

Psilocybin Analogs

An unusual collection of tryptamines has its origin in the world of fungi. The natural prototype is psilocybin itself. That and related homologs have been found in as many as 100 species of mushroom, largely of the *Psilocybe* genus.

Psilocybin is usually ingested as mushrooms. Many species of psilocybin-containing mushrooms are found worldwide. In the United States, large *Psilocybe cubensis* (gold caps) grow in Florida and Texas and are easily grown with cultivation kits advertised in drug-oriented magazines and on the Internet. The tiny *Psilocybe semilanceata* (liberty cap) grows in lawns and pastures in the Pacific Northwest. Psilocybin remains active when the mushrooms are dried or cooked into omelets or other foods.

Psilocybin mushrooms are used in religious activities by Mexican Indians. They are valued in Western society by users who prefer to ingest a mushroom instead of a synthetic chemical. Of course, one danger of eating wild mushrooms is misidentification and ingestion of a poisonous variety. At a large American university, 24 percent of students reported using psychedelic mushrooms or mescaline, compared with 17 percent who reported LSD use. Psilocybin sold as pills or capsules usually contains phencyclidine (PCP) or LSD instead.

ADDITIONAL HALLUCINOGENS
Ibogaine

Ibogaine is a complex alkaloid found in the African shrub *Tabernanthe iboga*. Ibogaine is a hallucinogen at the 400-mg dose range. The plant originates in Africa and traditionally is used in sacramental initiation ceremonies. Although it has not been a popular hallucinogen because of its unpleasant somatic effects when taken at hallucinogenic doses, patients exposed to ibogaine may be encountered by a psychiatrist because of the therapeutic claims.

Ayahuasca

Ayahuasca, much discussed on Internet hallucinogen Web sites, originally referred to a decoction from one or more South American plants. The substance contains the alkaloids harmaline and harmine. Both of those β-carboline alkaloids have hallucinogenic properties, but the resulting visual sensory alterations are accompanied by considerable nausea.

Salvia divinorum

American Indians in northern Oaxaca, Mexico, have used *Salvia divinorum* as a medicine and as a sacred sacrament, which is now widely discussed, advertised, and sold on the Internet. When the plant is chewed or dried leaves smoked, it produces hallucinogen effects. Salvinorin-A, an active component in the plant, is parenterally potent, active at 250-μg doses when smoked, and of scientific and potential medical interest because it binds to the opioid κ-receptor.

TREATMENT
Hallucinogen Intoxication

Persons have historically been treated for hallucinogen intoxication by psychological support for the remainder of the trip, so-called "talking down." This is a time-consuming and potentially hazardous undertaking, given the lability of a patient with hallucinogen-related delusions. Accordingly, treatment of hallucinogen intoxication is the oral administration of 20 mg of diazepam. This medication brings the LSD experience and any associated panic to a halt within 20 minutes and should be considered superior to "talking down" the patient over a period of hours or to administering antipsychotic agents. The marketing of lower doses of LSD and a more sophisticated approach to treatment of casualties by drug users themselves have combined to reduce the appearance of this once-common disorder in psychiatric treatment facilities.

Hallucinogen Persisting Disorder

Treatment for hallucinogen persisting perception disorder is palliative. The first step in the process is correct identification of the disorder; it is not uncommon for the patient to consult a number of specialists before the diagnosis is made. Pharmacological approaches include long-lasting benzodiazepines, such as clonazepam (Klonopin) and, to a lesser extent, anticonvulsants, including valproic acid (Depakene) and carbamazepine (Tegretol). Currently, no drug is completely effective in ablating symptoms. Antipsychotic agents should only be used in the treatment of hallucinogen-induced psychoses because they may have a paradoxical effect and exacerbate symptoms. A second dimension of treatment is behavioral. The patient must be instructed to avoid gratuitous stimulation in the form of over-the-counter drugs, caffeine, and alcohol and avoidable physical and emotional stressors. Marijuana smoke is a particularly strong intensifier of the disorder, even when passively inhaled. Finally, three comorbid conditions are associated with hallucinogen persisting perception disorder: panic disorder, major depression, and alcohol dependence. All of these conditions require primary prevention and early intervention.

Hallucinogen-Induced Psychosis

Treatment of hallucinogen-induced psychosis does not differ from conventional treatment for other psychoses. In addition to antipsychotic medications, a number of agents are reportedly effective, including lithium carbonate, carbamazepine, and electroconvulsive therapy. Antidepressant drugs, benzodiazepines, and anticonvulsant agents may each have a role in treatment as well. One hallmark of this disorder is that, as opposed to schizophrenia, in which negative symptoms and poor interpersonal relatedness may commonly be found, patients with hallucinogen-induced psychosis exhibit the positive symptoms of hallucinations and delusions while retaining the ability to relate to the psychiatrist. Medical therapies are best applied in a context of supportive, educational, and family therapies. The goals of treatment are the control of symptoms, a minimal use of hospitals, daily work, the development and preservation of social relationships, and the management of comorbid illnesses such as alcohol dependence.

▲ 9.8 Inhalant-Related Disorders

Inhalant drugs (also called *inhalants* or *volatile substances*) are volatile hydrocarbons such as toluene, *n*-hexane, methyl butyl ketone, trichloroethylene, trichloroethane, dichloromethane, gasoline, and butane. These chemicals are sold in four commercial classes: (1) solvents for glues and adhesives; (2) propellants for aerosol paint sprays, hair sprays, frying pan sprays, and shaving cream; (3) thinners (e.g., for paint products and typing correction fluids); and (4) fuels. At room temperature, these compounds volatilize to gaseous fumes that can be inhaled through the nose or mouth, entering the bloodstream by the transpulmonary route. Despite their chemical differences, it is generally believed, although not proved, that these compounds share certain pharmacological properties.

The text revision of the fourth edition of *Diagnostic and Statistical Manual of Mental Disorders* (DSM-IV-TR) specifically excludes anesthetic gases (e.g., nitrous oxide and ether) and short-acting vasodilators (e.g., amyl nitrite) from the inhalant-related disorders, which are classified as other (or unknown) substance-related disorders and are discussed in Section 9.14.

EPIDEMIOLOGY

Inhalant substances are easily available, legal, and inexpensive. These three factors contribute to the high use of inhalants among poor persons and young persons. According to DSM-IV-TR, about 6 percent of persons in the United States had used inhalants at least once, and about 1 percent of persons are current users. Among young adults 18 to 25 years of age, 11 percent had used inhalants at least once, and 2 percent were current users. Among adolescents 12 to 17 years of age, 7 percent had used inhalants at least once, and 2 percent were current users. In one study of high school seniors, 18 percent reported having used inhalants at least once, and 2.7 percent reported having used inhalants within the preceding month. White users of inhalants are more common than either black or Hispanic users. Most users (up to 80 percent) are male. Some data suggest that inhalant use may be more common in suburban communities in the United States than in urban communities.

Inhalant use accounts for 1 percent of all substance-related deaths and less than 0.5 percent of all substance-related emergency room visits. About 20 percent of the emergency room visits for inhalant use involve persons younger than 18 years of age. Inhalant use among adolescents may be most common in those whose parents or older siblings use illegal substances. Inhalant use among adolescents is also associated with an increased likelihood of conduct disorder or antisocial personality disorder. Between 1994 and 2000, the number of new inhalant users increased more than 50 percent, from 618,000 new users in 1994 to 979,000 in 2000. These estimates were higher than a previous peak in 1978 (662,000 new users).

NEUROPHARMACOLOGY

Inhalants most used by American adolescents are (in descending order) gasoline, glue (which usually contains toluene), spray paint, solvents, cleaning fluids, and assorted other aerosols. Sniffing vapor through the nose or huffing (taking deep breaths) through the mouth leads to transpulmonary absorption with very rapid drug access to the brain. Breathing through a solvent-soaked cloth, inhaling fumes from a glue-containing bag, huffing vapor sprayed into a plastic bag, or breathing vapor from a gasoline can are common. Approximately 15 to 20 breaths of 1 percent gasoline vapor produce several hours of intoxication. Inhaled toluene concentrations from a glue-containing bag may reach 10,000 ppm, and vapors from several tubes of glue may be inhaled each day. By comparison, one study of just 100 ppm of toluene showed that a 6-hour exposure produced a temporary neuropsychological performance decrement of approximately 10 percent.

Inhalants generally act as a central nervous system (CNS) depressant. Tolerance for inhalants can develop, although withdrawal symptoms are usually fairly mild and are not classified as a disorder in DSM-IV-TR.

Inhalants are rapidly absorbed through the lungs and rapidly delivered to the brain. The effects appear within 5 minutes and can last for 30 minutes to several hours, depending on the inhalant substance and the dose. The concentrations of many inhalant substances in blood are increased when used in combination with alcohol, perhaps because of competition for hepatic enzymes. Although about one fifth of an inhalant substance is excreted unchanged by the lungs, the remainder is metabolized by the liver. Inhalants are detectable in the blood for 4 to 10 hours after use, and blood samples should be taken in the emergency room when inhalant use is suspected.

Much like alcohol, inhalants have specific pharmacodynamic effects that are not well understood. Because their effects are generally similar and additive to the effects of other CNS depressants (e.g., ethanol, barbiturates, and benzodiazepines), some investigators have suggested that inhalants operate by enhancing the γ-aminobutyric acid (GABA) system. Other investigators have suggested that inhalants work through membrane fluidization, which has also been hypothesized to be a pharmacodynamic effect of ethanol.

DIAGNOSIS

The DSM-IV-TR lists a number of inhalant-related disorders (Table 9.8–1) but contains specific diagnostic criteria only for inhalant intoxication (Table 9.8–2) within the inhalant-related disorders section. The diagnostic criteria of other inhalant-related disorders are specified in the DSM-IV-TR sections that specifically address the major symptoms—for example, inhalant-induced psychotic disorders (see Table 11.4–5).

Table 9.8–1
DSM-IV-TR Inhalant-Related Disorders

Inhalant use disorders
Inhalant dependence
Inhalant abuse
Inhalant-induced disorders
Inhalant intoxication
Inhalant intoxication delirium
Inhalant-induced persisting dementia
Inhalant-induced psychotic disorder, with delusions
  Specify if:
    With onset during intoxication
Inhalant-induced psychotic disorder, with hallucinations
  Specify if:
    With onset during intoxication
Inhalant-induced mood disorder
  Specify if:
    With onset during intoxication
Inhalant-induced anxiety disorder
  Specify if:
    With onset during intoxication
Inhalant-related disorder not otherwise specified

From American Psychiatric Association. *Diagnostic and Statistical Manual of Mental Disorders.* 4th ed. Text rev. Washington, DC: American Psychiatric Association; copyright 2000, with permission.

Inhalant Dependence and Inhalant Abuse

Most persons probably use inhalants for a short time without developing a pattern of long-term use resulting in dependence and abuse. Nonetheless, dependence and abuse of inhalants occur and are diagnosed according to the standard DSM-IV-TR criteria for substance abuse and dependence (see Tables 9.1–3 to 9.1–5).

Table 9.8–2
DSM-IV-TR Diagnostic Criteria for Inhalant Intoxication

A. Recent intentional use or short-term, high-dose exposure to volatile inhalants (excluding anesthetic gases and short-acting vasodilators).
B. Clinically significant maladaptive behavioral or psychological changes (e.g., belligerence, assaultiveness, apathy, impaired judgment, impaired social or occupational functioning) that developed during, or shortly after, use of or exposure to volatile inhalants.
C. Two (or more) of the following signs, developing during, or shortly after, inhalant use or exposure:
  (1) dizziness
  (2) nystagmus
  (3) incoordination
  (4) slurred speech
  (5) unsteady gait
  (6) lethargy
  (7) depressed reflexes
  (8) psychomotor retardation
  (9) tremor
  (10) generalized muscle weakness
  (11) blurred vision or diplopia
  (12) stupor or coma
  (13) euphoria
D. The symptoms are not due to a general medical condition and are not better accounted for by another mental disorder.

From American Psychiatric Association. *Diagnostic and Statistical Manual of Mental Disorders.* 4th ed. Text rev. Washington, DC: American Psychiatric Association; copyright 2000, with permission.

Inhalant Intoxication

The DSM-IV-TR diagnostic criteria for inhalant intoxication (Table 9.8–2) specify the presence of maladaptive behavioral changes and at least two physical symptoms. The intoxicated state is often characterized by apathy, diminished social and occupational functioning, impaired judgment, and impulsive or aggressive behavior, and it can be accompanied by nausea, anorexia, nystagmus, depressed reflexes, and diplopia. With high doses and long exposures, a user's neurological status can progress to stupor and unconsciousness, and a person may later be amnestic for the period of intoxication. Clinicians can sometimes identify a recent user of inhalants by rashes around the patient's nose and mouth; unusual breath odors; the residue of the inhalant substances on the patient's face, hands, or clothing; and irritation of the patient's eyes, throat, lungs, and nose. The disorder can be chronic as in the following case.

> A 16-year-old single Hispanic female was referred to a university substance-treatment program for evaluation. The patient had been convicted for auto theft, menacing with a weapon, and being out of control by her family. By age 15, she had regularly been using inhalants and drinking alcohol heavily. She had tried typewriter-erasing fluid, bleach, tile cleaner, hairspray, nail polish, glue, and gasoline, but preferred spray paint. She had sniffed paint many times each day for about 6 months at age 15, using a maximum of eight paint cans per day. The patient said, "It blacks out everything." Sometimes she had lost consciousness, and she believed that the paint had impaired her memory and made her "dumb." (Courtesy of Thomas J. Crowley, M.D.)

Inhalant Intoxication Delirium

The DSM-IV-TR provides a diagnostic category for inhalant intoxication delirium (see Table 7.2–2). Delirium can be induced by the effects of the inhalants themselves, by pharmacodynamic interactions with other substances, and by the hypoxia that may be associated with either the inhalant or its method of inhalation. If the delirium results in severe behavioral disturbances, short-term treatment with a dopamine receptor antagonist, such as haloperidol (Haldol), may be necessary. Benzodiazepines should be avoided because of the possibility of increasing the patient's respiratory depression.

Inhalant-Induced Persisting Dementia

Inhalant-induced persisting dementia (see Table 7.3–4), as with delirium, may result from the neurotoxic effects of the inhalants themselves; the neurotoxic effects of the metals (e.g., lead) commonly used in inhalants; or the effects of frequent and prolonged periods of hypoxia. The dementia caused by inhalants is likely to be irreversible in all but the mildest cases.

Inhalant-Induced Psychotic Disorder

Inhalant-induced psychotic disorder is a DSM-IV-TR diagnosis (see Table 11.4–5). Clinicians can specify hallucinations or

Table 9.8–3
DSM-IV-TR Diagnostic Criteria for Inhalant-Related Disorder Not Otherwise Specified

The inhalant-related disorder not otherwise specified category is for disorders associated with the use of inhalants that are not classifiable as inhalant dependence, inhalant abuse, inhalant intoxication, inhalant intoxication delirium, inhalant-induced persisting dementia, inhalant-induced psychotic disorder, inhalant-induced mood disorder, or inhalant-induced anxiety disorder.

From American Psychiatric Association. *Diagnostic and Statistical Manual of Mental Disorders.* 4th ed. Text rev. Washington, DC: American Psychiatric Association; copyright 2000, with permission.

delusions as the predominant symptoms. Paranoid states are probably the most common psychotic syndromes during inhalant intoxication.

Inhalant-Induced Mood Disorder and Inhalant-Induced Anxiety Disorder

Inhalant-induced mood disorder (see Table 12.3–8) and inhalant-induced anxiety disorder (see Table 13.7–2) are DSM-IV-TR diagnoses that allow the classification of inhalant-related disorders characterized by prominent mood and anxiety symptoms. Depressive disorders are the most common mood disorders associated with inhalant use, and panic disorders and generalized anxiety disorder are the most common anxiety disorders.

Inhalant-Related Disorder Not Otherwise Specified

Inhalant-related disorder not otherwise specified is the recommended DSM-IV-TR diagnosis for inhalant-related disorders that do not fit into one of the diagnostic categories discussed previously (Table 9.8–3).

CLINICAL FEATURES

In small initial doses, inhalants can be disinhibiting and produce feelings of euphoria and excitement and pleasant floating sensations, the effects for which persons presumably use the drugs. High doses of inhalants can cause psychological symptoms of fearfulness, sensory illusions, auditory and visual hallucinations, and distortions of body size. The neurological symptoms can include slurred speech, decreased speed of talking, and ataxia. Long-term use can be associated with irritability, emotional lability, and impaired memory.

Tolerance for the inhalants does develop; although not recognized by DSM-IV-TR, a withdrawal syndrome can accompany the cessation of inhalant use. The withdrawal syndrome does not occur frequently; when it does, it can be characterized by sleep disturbances, irritability, jitteriness, sweating, nausea, vomiting, tachycardia, and (sometimes) delusions and hallucinations.

Organ Pathology and Neurological Effects

Inhalants are associated with many potentially serious adverse effects. The most serious of these is death, which can result from respiratory depression, cardiac arrhythmias, asphyxiation, aspiration of vomitus, or accident or injury (e.g., driving while intoxicated with inhalants). Placing an inhalant-soaked rag and one's head into a plastic bag, a common procedure, can cause coma and suffocation.

Chronic inhalant users may have numerous neurological problems. Computed tomography (CT) and magnetic resonance imaging (MRI) reveal diffuse cerebral, cerebellar, and brainstem atrophy with white matter disease, a leukoencephalopathy. Single photon CT of former solvent-abusing adolescents showed both increases and decreases of blood flow in different cerebral areas. Several studies of house painters and factory workers who have been exposed to solvents for long periods also have found evidence of brain atrophy on CT scans, with decreased cerebral blood flow.

Neurological and behavioral signs and symptoms can include hearing loss, peripheral neuropathy, headache, paresthesias, cerebellar signs, persisting motor impairment, parkinsonism, apathy, poor concentration, memory loss, visual-spatial dysfunction, impaired processing of linguistic material, and lead encephalopathy. White matter changes, or pontine atrophy on MRI, have been associated with worse intelligence quotient (IQ) test results. The combination of organic solvents with high concentrations of copper, zinc, and heavy metals has been associated with the development of brain atrophy, temporal lobe epilepsy, decreased IQ, and a variety of electroencephalographic (EEG) changes.

Other serious adverse effects associated with long-term inhalant use include irreversible hepatic disease or renal damage (tubular acidosis) and permanent muscle damage associated with rhabdomyolysis. Additional adverse effects include cardiovascular and pulmonary symptoms (e.g., chest pain and bronchospasm) as well as gastrointestinal (GI) symptoms (e.g., pain, nausea, vomiting, and hematemesis). There are several clinical reports of toluene embryopathy, with signs such as those of fetal alcohol syndrome. These include low birthweight, microcephaly, shortened palpebral fissures, small face, low-set ears, and other dysmorphic signs. These babies reportedly develop slowly, show hyperactivity, and have cerebellar dysfunction. No convincing evidence indicates, however, that toluene, the best-studied inhalant, produces genetic damage in somatic cells.

TREATMENT

Inhalant intoxication, as with alcohol intoxication, usually requires no medical attention and resolves spontaneously. Effects of the intoxication, such as coma, bronchospasm, laryngospasm, cardiac arrhythmias, trauma, or burns, need treatment, however. Otherwise, care primarily involves reassurance, quiet support, and attention to vital signs and level of consciousness. Sedative drugs, including benzodiazepines, are contraindicated because they worsen inhalant intoxication.

No established treatment exists for the cognitive and memory problems of inhalant-induced persisting dementia. Street outreach and extensive social service support have been offered to severely deteriorated, inhalant-dependent, homeless adults. Patients may require extensive support within their families or in foster or domiciliary care.

The course and treatment of inhalant-induced psychotic disorder are like those of inhalant intoxication. The disorder is brief, lasting a few hours to (at most) a very few weeks beyond the intoxication. Vigorous treatment of such life-threatening complications as respiratory or cardiac arrest, together with conservative management of the intoxication itself, is appropriate.

Confusion, panic, and psychosis mandate special attention to patient safety. Severe agitation may require cautious control with haloperidol (5 mg intramuscularly per 70 kg of body weight). Sedative drugs should be avoided because they may aggravate the psychosis. Inhalant-induced anxiety and mood disorders may precipitate suicidal ideation, and patients should be carefully evaluated for that possibility. Antianxiety medications and antidepressants are not useful in the acute phase of the disorder; they may be of use in cases of a coexisting anxiety or depressive illness.

Day Treatment and Residential Programs

Day treatment and residential programs have been used successfully, especially for adolescent abusers with combined substance dependence and other psychiatric disorders. Treatment addresses the comorbid state, which, in most cases, is conduct disorder or, in other instances, may be attention-deficit/hyperactivity disorder (ADHD), major depressive disorder, dysthymic disorder, or posttraumatic stress disorder (PTSD). Attention is also directed to experiences of abuse or neglect, which is very common in these patients. Both group and individual therapies are used that are behaviorally oriented, with immediate rewards for progress toward objectively defined goals in treatment and punishments for lapses to previous behaviors. Patients attend on-site schools with special education teachers, together with planned recreational activities, and the programs provide birth control consultations. The patients' families, often very chaotic, are engaged in modifications of structural family therapy or multisystemic therapy, both of which have good empirical support. Participation in 12-step programs is required. Treatment interventions are coordinated closely with interventions by community social workers and probation officers. Progress is monitored with urine and breath samples analyzed for alcohol and other drugs at intake and frequently during treatment.

Treatment usually lasts 3 to 12 months. Termination is considered successful if the youth has practiced a plan to stay abstinent; is showing fewer antisocial behaviors; has a plan to continue any needed psychiatric treatment (e.g., treatment for comorbid depression); has a plan to live in a supportive, drug-free environment; is interacting with the family in a more productive way; is working or attending school; and is associating with drug-free, nondelinquent peers.

▲ 9.9 Nicotine-Related Disorders

Nicotine is one of the most highly addictive and heavily used drugs in the United States and around the world. It causes lung cancer, emphysema, and cardiovascular disease, and secondhand smoke is associated with lung cancer in adults and respiratory illness in children.

The landmark 1988 publication of *The Surgeon General's Report on the Health Consequences of Smoking: Nicotine Addiction* increased the awareness of the hazards of smoking to the American public. However, the fact that about 30 percent of the population continue to smoke despite the mountain of data showing how dangerous the habit is to their health is testament to the powerfully addictive properties of nicotine. The ill effects of cigarette and cigar smoking are reflected in the estimate that 60 percent of the direct health care costs in the United States go to treat tobacco-related illnesses and amount to an estimated $1 billion a day.

EPIDEMIOLOGY

The *2004 Monitoring the Future Survey* concluded that, despite the demonstrated health risk associated with cigarette smoking, young Americans continue to smoke. However, 30-day smoking rates among high school students declined from peaks reached in 1996 for eighth-graders (21.0 percent) and tenth-graders (30.4 percent) and in 1997 for seniors (36.5 percent). In 2004, 30-day rates reached the lowest levels ever reported by Monitoring the Future surveys for eighth-graders (9.2 percent) and 10th-graders (16.0 percent). Of high school seniors, 25 percent reported smoking during the month preceding their responses to the survey.

Lifetime cigarette use among tenth-graders decreased significantly, from 43.0 percent in 2003 to 40.7 percent in 2004. Among tenth-graders, a significantly decreased number of students reported that they smoke one-half pack or more cigarettes per day.

The decrease in smoking rates among young Americans corresponds to several years in which increased proportions of teens said they believe a "great" health risk is associated with cigarette smoking and expressed disapproval of smoking one or more packs of cigarettes a day. Students' personal disapproval of smoking had risen for some years but showed no further increase in 2004. In 2004, 85.7 percent of 8th-graders, 82.7 percent of 10th-graders, and 76.2 percent of 12th-graders stated that they "disapprove" or "strongly disapprove" of people smoking one or more packs of cigarettes per day. In addition, 8th- and 10th-graders reported significant increases in the perceived harmfulness of smoking one or more packs of cigarettes per day.

The World Health Organization (WHO) estimates there are 1 billion smokers worldwide, and they smoke 6 trillion cigarettes a year. The WHO also estimates that tobacco kills more than 3 million persons each year. Although the number of persons in the United States who smoke is decreasing, the number of persons smoking in developing countries is increasing. The rate of quitting smoking has been highest among well-educated white men and lowest among women, blacks, teenagers, and those with low levels of education.

Tobacco is the most common form of nicotine. It most commonly is smoked in cigarettes, then, in descending order, smoked in cigars, used as snuff, used as chewing tobacco, and smoked in pipes. About 3 percent of all persons in the United States currently use snuff or chewing tobacco, and about 6 percent of young adults aged 18 to 25 years use those forms of tobacco.

Currently, about 25 percent of Americans smoke, 25 percent are former smokers, and 50 percent have never smoked cigarettes. The mean age of onset of smoking is 16 years, and few persons start smoking after 20 years. Dependence features appear to develop quickly. Classroom and other programs to prevent initiation are only mildly effective, but increased taxation does decrease initiation.

More than 75 percent of smokers have tried to quit, and about 40 percent try to quit each year. On a given attempt, only 30 percent remain abstinent for even 2 days, and only 5 to 10 percent stop permanently. Most smokers make 5 to 10 attempts, however, so eventually 50 percent of "ever smokers" quit. In the past, 90 percent of successful attempts to quit involved no treatment. With the advent of over-the-counter (OTC) and nonnicotine medications in 1998, about one third of all attempts involved the use of medication.

In terms of the diagnosis of nicotine dependence per se, about 20 percent of the population develops nicotine dependence at some point, making it one of the most prevalent psychiatric disorders. According to the text revision of the fourth edition of *Diagnostic and Statistical Manual of Mental Disorders* (DSM-IV-TR), approximately 85 percent of current daily smokers are nicotine dependent. Nicotine withdrawal occurs in about 50 percent of smokers who try to quit.

According to the Centers for Disease Control and Prevention, regional differences exist in smoking throughout the United States. The 12 areas with the highest prevalence of current smoking are Kentucky, Nevada, Missouri, Indiana, Ohio, West Virginia, North Carolina, Tennessee, New Hampshire, Alabama, Arkansas, and Alaska. The 12 areas with lowest prevalence are Utah, Puerto Rico, California, Arizona, Montana, Hawaii, Minnesota, Connecticut, Massachusetts, Colorado, Maryland, and Washington. Utah had the lowest prevalence for men (14.5 percent), and Puerto Rico had the lowest for women (9.9 percent).

Education

Level of education attainment correlated with tobacco use. Of adults who had not completed high school, 37 percent smoked cigarettes, whereas only 17 percent of college graduates smoked.

Psychiatric Patients

Psychiatrists must be particularly concerned and knowledgeable about nicotine dependence because of the high proportion of psychiatric patients who smoke. Approximately 50 percent of all psychiatric outpatients, 70 percent of outpatients with bipolar I disorder, almost 90 percent of outpatients with schizophrenia, and 70 percent of substance use disorder patients smoke. Moreover, data indicate that patients with depressive disorders or anxiety disorders are less successful in their attempts to quit smoking than other persons; thus, a holistic health approach for these patients probably includes helping them address their smoking habits in addition to the primary mental disorder. The high percentage of patients with schizophrenia who smoke has been attributed to nicotine's ability to reduce their extraordinary sensitivity to outside sensory stimuli and to increase their concentration. In that sense, such patients are self-monitoring to relieve distress.

Death

Death is the primary adverse effect of cigarette smoking. Tobacco use is associated with approximately 400,000 premature deaths each year in the United States—25 percent of all deaths. The causes of death include chronic bronchitis and emphysema (51,000 deaths), bronchogenic cancer (106,000 deaths), 35 percent of fatal myocardial infarctions (115,000 deaths), cerebrovascular disease, cardiovascular disease, and almost all cases of chronic obstructive pulmonary disease and lung cancer. The increased use of chewing tobacco and snuff (smokeless tobacco) has been associated with the development of oropharyngeal cancer, and the resurgence of cigar smoking is likely to lead to an increase in the occurrence of this type of cancer.

Researchers have found that 30 percent of cancer deaths in the United States are caused by tobacco smoke, the most lethal carcinogen in the United States. Smoking (mainly cigarette smoking) causes cancer of the lung, upper respiratory tract, esophagus, bladder, and pancreas and probably of the stomach, liver, and kidney. Smokers are eight times more likely than nonsmokers to develop lung cancer, and lung cancer has surpassed breast cancer as the leading cause of cancer-related deaths in women. Even secondhand smoke (discussed later) causes a few thousand cancer deaths each year in the United States, about the same number as are caused by radon exposure. Despite these staggering statistics, smokers can dramatically lower their chances of developing smoke-related cancers simply by quitting.

NEUROPHARMACOLOGY

The psychoactive component of tobacco is nicotine, which affects the central nervous system (CNS) by acting as an agonist at the nicotinic subtype of acetylcholine receptors. About 25 percent of the nicotine inhaled during smoking reaches the bloodstream, through which nicotine reaches the brain within 15 seconds. The half-life of nicotine is about 2 hours. Nicotine is believed to produce its positive-reinforcing and addictive properties by activating the dopaminergic pathway projecting from the ventral tegmental area to the cerebral cortex and the limbic system. In addition to activating this dopamine reward system, nicotine causes an increase in the concentrations of circulating norepinephrine and epinephrine and an increase in the release of vasopressin, β-endorphin, adrenocorticotropic hormone (ACTH), and cortisol. These hormones are thought to contribute to the basic stimulatory effects of nicotine on the CNS.

DIAGNOSIS

The DSM-IV-TR lists three nicotine-related disorders (Table 9.9–1) but contains specific diagnostic criteria for only nicotine withdrawal (Table 9.9–2) in the nicotine-related disorders section. The other nicotine-related disorders recognized by

Table 9.9–1
DSM-IV-TR Nicotine-Related Disorders

Nicotine use disorder
Nicotine dependence
Nicotine-induced disorder
Nicotine withdrawal
Nicotine-related disorder not otherwise specified

From American Psychiatric Association. *Diagnostic and Statistical Manual of Mental Disorders.* 4th ed. Text rev. Washington, DC: American Psychiatric Association; copyright 2000, with permission.

Table 9.9–2
DSM-IV-TR Diagnostic Criteria for Nicotine Withdrawal

A. Daily use of nicotine for at least several weeks.
B. Abrupt cessation of nicotine use, or reduction in the amount of nicotine used, followed within 24 hours by four (or more) of the following signs:
(1) dysphoric or depressed mood
(2) insomnia
(3) irritability, frustration, or anger
(4) anxiety
(5) difficulty concentrating
(6) restlessness
(7) decreased heart rate
(8) increased appetite or weight gain
C. The symptoms in Criterion B cause clinically significant distress or impairment in social, occupational, or other important areas of functioning.
D. The symptoms are not due to a general medical condition and are not better accounted for by another mental disorder.

From American Psychiatric Association. *Diagnostic and Statistical Manual of Mental Disorders.* 4th ed. Text rev. Washington, DC: American Psychiatric Association; copyright 2000, with permission.

DSM-IV-TR are nicotine dependence and nicotine-related disorder not otherwise specified.

Nicotine Dependence

The DSM-IV-TR does have a diagnosis of nicotine dependence (see Tables 9.1–4 and 9.1–5) but not nicotine abuse. Dependence on nicotine develops quickly, probably because nicotine activates the ventral tegmental area dopaminergic system, the same system affected by cocaine and amphetamine. The development of dependence is enhanced by strong social factors that encourage smoking in some settings and by the powerful effects of tobacco company advertising. Persons are likely to smoke if their parents or siblings smoke and serve as role models. Several recent studies have also suggested a genetic diathesis toward nicotine dependence. Most persons who smoke want to quit and have tried many times to quit but have been unsuccessful.

Nicotine Withdrawal

The DSM-IV-TR does not have a diagnostic category for nicotine intoxication but does have a diagnostic category for nicotine withdrawal (Table 9.9–2). Withdrawal symptoms can develop within 2 hours of smoking the last cigarette; they generally peak in the first 24 to 48 hours and can last for weeks or months. The common symptoms include an intense craving for nicotine, tension, irritability, difficulty concentrating, drowsiness and paradoxical trouble sleeping, decreased heart rate and blood pressure, increased appetite and weight gain, decreased motor performance, and increased muscle tension. A mild syndrome of nicotine withdrawal can appear when a smoker switches from regular to low-nicotine cigarettes.

Nicotine-Related Disorder Not Otherwise Specified

Nicotine-related disorder not otherwise specified is a diagnostic category for nicotine-related disorders that do not fit into one

Table 9.9–3
DSM-IV-TR Diagnostic Criteria for Nicotine-Related Disorder Not Otherwise Specified

The nicotine-related disorder not otherwise specified category is for disorders associated with the use of nicotine that are not classifiable as nicotine dependence or nicotine withdrawal.

From American Psychiatric Association. *Diagnostic and Statistical Manual of Mental Disorders.* 4th ed. Text rev. Washington, DC: American Psychiatric Association; copyright 2000, with permission.

of the categories discussed previously (Table 9.9–3). Such diagnoses may include nicotine intoxication, nicotine abuse, and mood disorders and anxiety disorders associated with nicotine use.

CLINICAL FEATURES

Behaviorally, the stimulatory effects of nicotine produce improved attention, learning, reaction time, and problem-solving ability. Tobacco users also report that cigarette smoking lifts their mood, decreases tension, and lessens depressive feelings. Results of studies of the effects of nicotine on cerebral blood flow (CBF) suggest that short-term nicotine exposure increases CBF without changing cerebral oxygen metabolism, but long-term nicotine exposure decreases CBF. In contrast to its stimulatory CNS effects, nicotine acts as a skeletal muscle relaxant.

Adverse Effects

Nicotine is a highly toxic alkaloid. Doses of 60 mg in an adult are fatal secondary to respiratory paralysis; doses of 0.5 mg are delivered by smoking an average cigarette. In low doses the signs and symptoms of nicotine toxicity include nausea, vomiting, salivation, pallor (caused by peripheral vasoconstriction), weakness, abdominal pain (caused by increased peristalsis), diarrhea, dizziness, headache, increased blood pressure, tachycardia, tremor, and cold sweats. Toxicity is also associated with an inability to concentrate, confusion, and sensory disturbances. Nicotine is further associated with a decrease in the user's amount of rapid eye movement (REM) sleep. Tobacco use during pregnancy has been associated with an increased incidence of low-birthweight babies and an increased incidence of newborns with persistent pulmonary hypertension.

Health Benefits of Smoking Cessation

Smoking cessation has major and immediate health benefits for persons of all ages and provides benefits for persons with and without smoking-related diseases. Former smokers live longer than those who continue to smoke. Smoking cessation decreases the risk for lung cancer and other cancers, myocardial infarction, cerebrovascular diseases, and chronic lung diseases. Women who stop smoking before pregnancy or during the first 3 to 4 months of pregnancy reduce their risk for having low-birthweight infants to that of women who never smoked. The health benefits of smoking cessation substantially exceed any risks from the average 5-pound (2.3 kg) weight gain or any adverse psychological effects after quitting.

TREATMENT

Psychiatrists should advise all patients to quit smoking. For patients who are ready to stop smoking, it is best to set a "quit date." Most clinicians and smokers prefer abrupt cessation, but because no good data indicate that abrupt cessation is better than gradual cessation, patient preference for gradual cessation should be respected. Brief advice should focus on the need for medication or group therapy, weight gain concerns, high-risk situations, making cigarettes unavailable, and so forth. Because relapse is often rapid, the first follow-up phone call or visit should be 2 to 3 days after the quit date. These strategies have been shown to double self-initiated quit rates.

Psychosocial Therapies

Behavior therapy is the most widely accepted and well-proved psychological therapy for smoking. Skills training and relapse prevention identify high-risk situations and plan and practice behavioral or cognitive coping skills for those situations in which smoking occurs. Stimulus control involves eliminating cues for smoking in the environment. Aversive therapy has smokers smoke repeatedly and rapidly to the point of nausea, which associates smoking with unpleasant, rather than pleasant, sensations. Aversive therapy appears to be effective but requires a good therapeutic alliance and patient compliance.

Hypnosis.   Some patients benefit from a series of hypnotic sessions. Suggestions about the benefits of not smoking are offered and assimilated into the patient's cognitive framework as a result. Posthypnotic suggestions that cause cigarettes to taste bad or to produce nausea when smoked are also used.

Psychopharmacological Therapies

Nicotine Replacement Therapies.   All nicotine replacement therapies double cessation rates, presumably because they reduce nicotine withdrawal. These therapies can also be used to reduce withdrawal in patients on smoke-free wards. Replacement therapies use a short period of maintenance of 6 to 12 weeks often followed by a gradual reduction period of another 6 to 12 weeks.

Nicotine polacrilex gum (Nicorette) is an OTC product that releases nicotine via chewing and buccal absorption. A 2-mg variety for those who smoke fewer than 25 cigarettes a day and a 4-mg variety for those who smoke more than 25 cigarettes a day are available. Smokers are directed to use one to two pieces of gum per hour up to a maximum of 24 pieces per day after abrupt cessation. Venous blood concentrations from the gum are one third to one half of the between-cigarette levels. Acidic beverages (coffee, tea, soda, and juice) should not be used before, during, or after gum use because they decrease absorption. Compliance with the gum has often been a problem. Adverse effects are minor and include bad taste and sore jaws. About 20 percent of those who quit use the gum for long periods, but 2 percent use gum for longer than 1 year; long-term use does not appear to be harmful. The major advantage of nicotine gum is its ability to provide relief in high-risk situations.

Nicotine lozenges (Commit) deliver nicotine and are also available in 2- and 4-mg forms; they are useful especially for patients who smoke a cigarette immediately on awakening. Generally, 9 to 20 lozenges a day are used during the first 6 weeks, with decrease in dose thereafter. Lozenges offer the highest level of nicotine of all nicotine replacement products. Users must suck the lozenge until it is dissolved and not swallow it. Side effects include insomnia, nausea, heartburn, headache, and hiccups.

Nicotine patches, also sold OTC, are available in a 16-hour, no-taper preparation (Nicotrol) and a 24- or 16-hour tapering preparation (Nicoderm CQ). Patches are administered each morning and produce blood concentrations that are about half of those from smoking. Compliance is high, and the only major adverse effects are rashes and, with 24-hour wear, insomnia. Using gum and patches in high-risk situations increases quit rates by another 5 to 10 percent. No studies have been done to determine the relative efficacies of 24- or 16-hour patches or of taper and no-taper patches. After 6 to 12 weeks, the patch is discontinued because it is not for long-term use.

Nicotine nasal spray (Nicotrol), available only by prescription, produces nicotine concentrations in the blood that are more similar to those from smoking a cigarette, and it appears to be especially helpful for heavily dependent smokers. The spray, however, causes rhinitis, watering eyes, and coughing in more than 70 percent of patients. Although initial data suggested abuse liability, further trials have not found this.

The nicotine inhaler, a prescription product, was designed to deliver nicotine to the lungs, but the nicotine is actually absorbed in the upper throat. It delivers 4 mg per cartridge, and resultant nicotine levels are low. The major asset of the inhaler is that it provides a behavioral substitute for smoking. The inhaler doubles quit rates. These devices require frequent puffing—about 20 minutes to extract 4 mg of nicotine—and have minor adverse effects.

Nonnicotine Medications.   Nonnicotine therapy may help smokers who object philosophically to the notion of replacement therapy and smokers who fail replacement therapy. Bupropion (Zyban) (marketed as Wellbutrin for depression) is an antidepressant medication that has both dopaminergic and adrenergic actions. Bupropion is started at 150 mg per day for 3 days and increased to 150 mg twice a day for 6 to 12 weeks. Daily doses of 300 mg double quit rates in smokers with and without a history of depression. In one study, combined bupropion and nicotine patch had higher quit rates than either alone. Adverse effects include insomnia and nausea, but these are rarely significant. Seizures have not occurred in smoking trials. Of interest, nortriptyline (Pamelor) appears to be effective for smoking cessation and is recommended as a second-line drug.

Clonidine (Catapres) decreases sympathetic activity from the locus ceruleus and, thus, is thought to abate withdrawal symptoms. Whether given as a patch or orally, 0.2 to 0.4 mg a day of clonidine appears to double quit rates; however, the scientific database for the efficacy of clonidine is neither as extensive nor as reliable as that for nicotine replacement; in addition, clonidine can cause drowsiness and hypotension. Some patients benefit from benzodiazepine therapy (10 to 30 mg per day) for the first 2 to 3 weeks of abstinence.

A nicotine vaccine that produces nicotine-specific antibodies in the brain is under investigation at the National Institute on Drug Abuse (NIDA).

Combined Psychosocial and Pharmacological Therapy

Several studies have shown that combining nicotine replacement and behavior therapy increases quit rates over either therapy alone.

Smoke-Free Environment

Secondhand smoke can contribute to lung cancer death and coronary heart disease in adult nonsmokers. Each year, an estimated 3,000 lung cancer deaths and 62,000 deaths from coronary artery disease in adult nonsmokers are attributed to secondhand smoke. Among children, secondhand smoke is implicated in sudden infant death syndrome, low birthweight, chronic middle ear infections, and respiratory illnesses (e.g., asthma, bronchitis, and pneumonia). Two national health objectives for 2010 are to reduce cigarette smoking among adults to 12 percent and the proportion of nonsmokers exposed to environmental tobacco smoke to 45 percent.

Involuntary exposure to secondhand smoke remains a common public health hazard that is preventable by appropriate regulatory policies. Bans on smoking in public places reduce exposure to secondhand smoke and the number of cigarettes smoked by smokers. Support is nearly universal for bans in schools and day-care centers and strong for bans in indoor work areas and restaurants. Clean indoor air policies are one way to change social norms about smoking and reduce tobacco consumption. Bans on outdoor smoking in areas such as public parks are increasing, and in 2006 one municipality in California banned smoking entirely within city limits except in one's home or car, and windows had to remain closed.

▲ 9.10 Opioid-Related Disorders

More than 20 chemically distinct opioid drugs are in clinical use throughout the world. In the developed countries, the opioid drug most frequently associated with abuse and dependence is heroin—a drug that is not approved for therapeutic purposes in the United States. These drugs are all prototypical μ-opioid receptor agonists, and all produce similar subjective effects. The patterns of use and some aspects of opioid toxicity are powerfully influenced, however, by the route of administration and the metabolism of the specific opioid, as well as by the social conditions that determine its price and purity and the sanctions attached to nonmedical use.

Opioids have been used for at least 3,500 years, mostly in the form of crude opium or in alcoholic solutions of opium. Morphine was first isolated in 1806 and codeine in 1832. Over the next century, pure morphine and codeine gradually replaced crude opium for medicinal purposes, although nonmedical use of opium (as for smoking) persists in some parts of the world.

The text revision of the fourth edition of *Diagnostic and Statistical Manual of Mental Disorders* (DSM-IV-TR) divides opioid-related disorders into opioid use disorders (opioid abuse and opioid dependence) and nine other opioid-induced disorders (e.g., intoxication, withdrawal).

Opioid dependence is a cluster of physiological, behavioral, and cognitive symptoms, which together indicates repeated and continuing use of opioid drugs, despite significant problems related to such use. Drug dependence, in general, has also been defined by the World Health Organization (WHO) as a syndrome in which the use of a drug or class of drugs takes on a much higher priority for a given person than other behaviors that once had a higher value. These brief definitions each has as its central feature an emphasis on the drug-using behavior itself, its maladaptive nature, and how the choice to engage in that behavior shifts and becomes constrained as a result of interaction with the drug over time.

Opioid abuse is a term used to designate a pattern of maladaptive use of an opioid drug leading to clinically significant impairment or distress and occurring within a 12-month period, but one in which the symptoms have never met the criteria for opioid dependence.

The opioid-induced disorders as defined by DSM-IV-TR include such common phenomena as opioid intoxication, opioid withdrawal, opioid-induced sleep disorder, and opioid-induced sexual dysfunction. Opioid intoxication delirium is occasionally seen in hospitalized patients. Opioid-induced psychotic disorder, opioid-induced mood disorder, and opioid-induced anxiety disorder, by contrast, are quite uncommon with μ-agonist opioids but have been seen with certain mixed agonist-antagonist opioids acting at other receptors. DSM-IV-TR also includes opioid-related disorder not otherwise specified for situations that do not meet the criteria for any of the other opioid-related disorders.

In addition to the morbidity and mortality associated directly with the opioid-related disorders, the association between the transmission of the human immunodeficiency virus (HIV) and intravenous opioid and opiate use is now recognized as a leading national health concern. The words *opiate* and *opioid* come from the word opium, the juice of the opium poppy, *Papaver somniferum*, which contains approximately 20 opium alkaloids, including morphine.

Many synthetic opioids have been manufactured, including meperidine (Demerol), methadone (Dolophine), pentazocine (Talwin), and propoxyphene (Darvon). Methadone is the current gold standard in the treatment of opioid dependence. Opioid antagonists have been synthesized to treat opioid overdose and opioid dependence. This class of drugs includes naloxone (Narcan), naltrexone (ReVia), nalorphine, levallorphan, and apomorphine. Compounds with mixed agonist and antagonist activity at opioid receptors have been synthesized and include pentazocine, butorphanol (Stadol), and buprenorphine (Buprenex). Studies have found buprenorphine to be an effective treatment for opioid dependence.

EPIDEMIOLOGY

The use and dependence rates derived from national surveys do not accurately reflect fluctuations in drug use among opioid-dependent and previously opioid-dependent populations. When the supply of illicit heroin increases in purity or decreases in price, use among that vulnerable population tends to increase, with subsequent increases in adverse consequences (emergency room visits) and requests for treatment. The number of current heroin users in the United States has been estimated to be between 600,000 and 800,000. The number of people estimated to have used heroin at any time in their lives (lifetime users) is estimated at approximately 3 million.

In 2004, an estimated 118,000 persons had used heroin for the first time within the past previous 12 months. The average age of first use among recent initiates was 24.4 years in 2004. No significant changes were seen in the number of initiates or in the average age of first use from 2002 to 2004. Opioid use in the United States experienced a resurgence in the 1990s, with emergency department visits related to heroin abuse doubling between 1990 and 1995. This increase in heroin use was associated with an increase in heroin purity and a decrease in its street price. In the late 1990s, heroin use increased among people who were 18 to 25 years of age, and a brief upsurge was seen in the use of oxycodone (OxyContin) from pharmaceutical sources. Methods of administration other than injecting, such as smoking and snorting, increased in popularity. In 2004, the number of new nonmedical users of OxyContin was 615,000, with an average age at first use of 24.5 years. Comparable data on past-year OxyContin initiation are not available for prior years, but calendar year estimates of OxyContin initiation show a steady increase in the number of initiates from 1995, the year this drug was first available, through 2003. The male-to-female ratio of persons with heroin dependence is about 3 to 1. Users of opioids typically started to use substances in their teens and early 20s; currently, most persons with opioid dependence are in their 30s and 40s. According to DSM-IV-TR, the tendency for dependence to remit generally begins after age 40 years and has been called "maturing out." Many persons, however, have remained opioid dependent for 50 years or longer. In the United States, persons tend to experience their first opioid-induced experience in their early teens or even as young as 10 years of age. Early induction into the drug culture is likely in communities in which substance abuse is rampant and in families in which the parents are substance abusers. A heroin habit can cost a person hundreds of dollars a day; thus, a person with opioid dependence needs to obtain money through criminal activities, including prostitution. The involvement of persons with opioid dependence in prostitution accounts for much of the spread of HIV. According to DSM-IV-TR, the lifetime prevalence for heroin use is about 1 percent, with 0.2 percent having taken the drug during the prior year.

NEUROPHARMACOLOGY

The primary effects of the opioids are mediated through the opioid receptors, which were discovered in the second half of the 1970s. The μ-opioid receptors are involved in the regulation and mediation of analgesia, respiratory depression, constipation, and dependence; the κ-opioid receptors, with analgesia, diuresis, and sedation; and the Δ-opioid receptors, possibly with analgesia.

In 1974, enkephalin, an endogenous pentapeptide with opioid-like actions, was identified. This discovery led to the identification of three classes of endogenous opioids within the brain, including the endorphins and the enkephalins. Endorphins are involved in neural transmission and pain suppression. They are released naturally in the body when a person is physically hurt and account, in part, for the absence of pain during acute injuries.

The opioids also have significant effects on the dopaminergic and noradrenergic neurotransmitter systems. Several types of data indicate that the addictive rewarding properties of opioids are mediated through activation of the ventral tegmental area dopaminergic neurons that project to the cerebral cortex and the limbic system.

Heroin, the most commonly abused opioid, is more potent and lipid soluble than morphine. Because of those properties, heroin crosses the blood–brain barrier faster and has a more rapid onset than morphine. Heroin was first introduced as a treatment for morphine addiction, but heroin, in fact, is more dependence producing than morphine. Codeine, which occurs naturally as about 0.5 percent of the opiate alkaloids in opium, is absorbed easily through the gastrointestinal tract and is subsequently transformed into morphine in the body. Results of at least one study using positron emission tomography (PET) suggested that one effect of all opioids is decreased cerebral blood flow in selected brain regions in persons with opioid dependence.

Tolerance and Dependence

Tolerance does not develop uniformly to all actions of opioid drugs. Tolerance to some actions of opioids can be so high that a 100-fold increase in dose is required to produce the original effect. For example, terminally ill cancer patients may need 200 to 300 mg a day of morphine, whereas a dose of 60 mg can easily be fatal to an opioid-naïve person. The symptoms of opioid withdrawal do not appear unless a person has been using opioids for a long time or when cessation is particularly abrupt, as occurs functionally when an opioid antagonist is given. The long-term use of opioids results in changes in the number and sensitivity of opioid receptors, which mediate at least some of the effects of tolerance and withdrawal. Although long-term use is associated with increased sensitivity of the dopaminergic, cholinergic, and serotonergic neurons, the effect of opioids on the noradrenergic neurons is probably the primary mediator of the symptoms of opioid withdrawal. Short-term use of opioids apparently decreases the activity of the noradrenergic neurons in the locus ceruleus; long-term use activates a compensatory homeostatic mechanism within the neurons, and opioid withdrawal results in rebound hyperactivity. This hypothesis also provides an explanation for why clonidine (Catapres), an α_2-adrenergic receptor agonist that decreases the release of norepinephrine, is useful in the treatment of opioid withdrawal symptoms.

COMORBIDITY

About 90 percent of persons with opioid dependence have an additional psychiatric disorder. The most common comorbid psychiatric diagnoses are major depressive disorder, alcohol use disorders, antisocial personality disorder, and anxiety disorders. About 15 percent of persons with opioid dependence attempt to commit suicide at least once. The high prevalence of comorbidity with other psychiatric diagnoses highlights the need to develop a broad-based treatment program that also addresses patients' associated psychiatric disorders.

ETIOLOGY

Psychosocial Factors

Opioid dependence is not limited to low socioeconomic classes, although the incidence of opioid dependence is greater in these groups than in higher socioeconomic classes. Social factors associated with urban poverty probably contribute to opioid dependence. About 50 percent of urban heroin users are children of single parents or divorced parents and are from families in which at least one other member has a substance-related disorder. Children from such settings are at high risk for opioid dependence, especially if they also evidence behavioral problems in school or other signs of conduct disorder.

Some consistent behavior patterns seem to be especially pronounced in adolescents with opioid dependence. These patterns have been called the *heroin behavior syndrome*: underlying depression, often of an agitated type and frequently accompanied by anxiety symptoms; impulsiveness expressed by a passive-aggressive orientation; fear of failure; use of heroin as an antianxiety agent to mask feelings of low self-esteem, hopelessness, and aggression; limited coping strategies and low frustration tolerance accompanied by the need for immediate gratification; sensitivity to drug contingencies, with a keen awareness of the relation between good feelings and the act of drug taking; feelings of behavioral impotence counteracted by momentary control over the life situation by means of substances; and disturbances in social and interpersonal relationships with peers maintained by mutual substance experiences.

Biological and Genetic Factors

Evidence exists for common and drug-specific, genetically transmitted vulnerability factors that increase the likelihood of developing drug dependence. Individuals who abuse a substance from any category are more likely to abuse substances from other categories. Monozygotic twins are more likely than dizygotic twins to be concordant for opioid dependence. Multivariate modeling techniques indicated that not only was the genetic contribution high for heroin abuse in this group, but also that a higher proportion of the variance because of genetic factors was not shared with the common vulnerability factor—that is, it was specific for opioids.

A person with an opioid-related disorder may have had genetically determined hypoactivity of the opiate system. Researchers are investigating the possibility that such hypoactivity may be caused by too few, or less-sensitive, opioid receptors, by release of too little endogenous opioid, or by overly high concentrations of a hypothesized endogenous opioid antagonist. A biological predisposition to an opioid-related disorder may also be associated with abnormal functioning in either the dopaminergic or the noradrenergic neurotransmitter system.

Psychodynamic Theory

In psychoanalytic literature, the behavior of persons addicted to narcotics has been described in terms of libidinal fixation, with regression to pregenital, oral, or even more archaic levels of psychosexual development. The need to explain the relation of drug abuse, defense mechanisms, impulse control, affective disturbances, and adaptive mechanisms led to the shift from psychosexual formulations to formulations emphasizing ego psychology. Serious ego pathology, often thought to be associated with substance abuse, is considered to indicate profound developmental disturbances. Problems of the relation between the ego and affects emerge as a key area of difficulty.

**Table 9.10–1
DSM-IV-TR Opioid-Related Disorders**

Opioid use disorders
Opioid dependence
Opioid abuse
Opioid-induced disorders
Opioid intoxication
   Specify if:
       With perceptual disturbances
Opioid withdrawal
Opioid intoxication delirium
Opioid-induced psychotic disorder, with delusions
   Specify if:
       With onset during intoxication
Opioid-induced psychotic disorder, with hallucinations
   Specify if:
       With onset during intoxication
Opioid-induced mood disorder
   Specify if:
       With onset during intoxication
Opioid-induced sexual dysfunction
   Specify if:
       With onset during intoxication
Opioid-induced sleep disorder
   Specify if:
       With onset during intoxication
       With onset during withdrawal
Opioid-related disorder not otherwise specified

From American Psychiatric Association. *Diagnostic and Statistical Manual of Mental Disorders.* 4th ed. Text rev. Washington, DC: American Psychiatric Association; copyright 2000, with permission.

DIAGNOSIS

The DSM-IV-TR lists several opioid-related disorders (Table 9.10–1) but contains specific diagnostic criteria only for opioid intoxication (Table 9.10–2) and opioid withdrawal (Table 9.10–3) within the section on opioid-related disorders. The diagnostic criteria for the other opioid-related disorders are

**Table 9.10–2
DSM-IV-TR Diagnostic Criteria for Opioid Intoxication**

A. Recent use of an opioid.
B. Clinically significant maladaptive behavioral or psychological changes (e.g., initial euphoria followed by apathy, dysphoria, psychomotor agitation or retardation, impaired judgment, or impaired social or occupational functioning) that developed during, or shortly after, opioid use.
C. Pupillary constriction (or pupillary dilation due to anoxia from severe overdose) and one (or more) of the following signs, developing during, or shortly after, opioid use:
   (1) drowsiness or coma
   (2) slurred speech
   (3) impairment in attention or memory
D. The symptoms are not due to a general medical condition and are not better accounted for by another mental disorder.
Specify if:
   With perceptual disturbances

From American Psychiatric Association. *Diagnostic and Statistical Manual of Mental Disorders.* 4th ed. Text rev. Washington, DC: American Psychiatric Association; copyright 2000, with permission.

Table 9.10–3
DSM-IV-TR Diagnostic Criteria for Opioid Withdrawal

A. Either of the following:
  (1) cessation of (or reduction in) opioid use that has been heavy and prolonged (several weeks or longer)
  (2) administration of an opioid antagonist after a period of opioid use
B. Three (or more) of the following, developing within minutes to several days after Criterion A:
  (1) dysphoric mood
  (2) nausea or vomiting
  (3) muscle aches
  (4) lacrimation or rhinorrhea
  (5) pupillary dilation, piloerection, or sweating
  (6) diarrhea
  (7) yawning
  (8) fever
  (9) insomnia
C. The symptoms in Criterion B cause clinically significant distress or impairment in social, occupational, or other important areas of functioning.
D. The symptoms are not due to a general medical condition and are not better accounted for by another mental disorder.

From American Psychiatric Association. *Diagnostic and Statistical Manual of Mental Disorders.* 4th ed. Text rev. Washington, DC: American Psychiatric Association; copyright 2000, with permission.

contained within the DSM-IV-TR sections that deal specifically with the predominant symptom—for example, opioid-induced mood disorder (see Table 12.3–8).

Opioid Dependence and Opioid Abuse

Opioid dependence and opioid abuse are defined in DSM-IV-TR according to the general criteria for these disorders (see Tables 9.1–3 to 9.1–5).

A 42-year-old executive in a public relations firm was referred for psychiatric consultation by his surgeon, who discovered him sneaking large quantities of a codeine-containing cough medicine into the hospital. The patient had been a heavy cigarette smoker for 20 years and had a chronic, hacking cough. He had come into the hospital for a hernia repair and found the pain for the incision unbearable when he coughed.

An operation on his back 5 years previously had led his doctors to prescribe codeine to help relieve the incisional pain at that time. Over the intervening 5 years, however, the patient had continued to use codeine-containing tablets and had increased his intake to 60 90-mg tablets daily. He stated that he often "just took them by the handful—not to feel good, you understand, just to get by." He spent considerable time and effort developing a circle of physicians and pharmacists to whom he would "make the rounds" at least three times a week to obtain new supplies of pills. He had tried several times to stop using codeine, but had failed. During this period he lost two jobs because of lax work habits and was divorced by his wife of 11 years. (Reprinted with permission from *DSM-IV-TR Casebook.*)

Opioid Intoxication

The DSM-IV-TR defines opioid intoxication as including maladaptive behavioral changes and some specific physical symptoms of opioid use (Table 9.10–2). In general, altered mood, psychomotor retardation, drowsiness, slurred speech, and impaired memory and attention in the presence of other indicators of recent opioid use strongly suggest a diagnosis of opioid intoxication. DSM-IV-TR allows for the specification of "with perceptual disturbances."

Opioid Withdrawal

The general rule about the onset and duration of withdrawal symptoms is that substances with short durations of action tend to produce short, intense withdrawal syndromes and substances with long durations of action produce prolonged, but mild, withdrawal syndromes. An exception to the rule, narcotic antagonist–precipitated withdrawal after long-acting opioid dependence can be severe.

An abstinence syndrome can be precipitated by administration of an opioid antagonist. The symptoms can begin within seconds of such an intravenous injection and peak in about 1 hour. Opioid craving rarely occurs in the context of analgesic administration for pain from physical disorders or surgery. The full withdrawal syndrome, including intense craving for opioids, usually occurs only secondary to abrupt cessation of use in persons with opioid dependence.

Morphine and Heroin.   The morphine and heroin withdrawal syndrome begins 6 to 8 hours after the last dose, usually after a 1- to 2-week period of continuous use or after the administration of a narcotic antagonist. The withdrawal syndrome reaches its peak intensity during the second or third day and subsides during the next 7 to 10 days, but some symptoms may persist for 6 months or longer.

Meperidine.   The withdrawal syndrome from meperidine begins quickly, reaches a peak in 8 to 12 hours, and ends in 4 to 5 days.

Methadone.   Methadone withdrawal usually begins 1 to 3 days after the last dose and ends in 10 to 14 days.

Symptoms.   Opioid withdrawal symptoms (Table 9.10–3) consist of severe muscle cramps and bone aches, profuse diarrhea, abdominal cramps, rhinorrhea, lacrimation, piloerection or gooseflesh (from which comes the term *cold turkey* for the abstinence syndrome), yawning, fever, pupillary dilation, hypertension, tachycardia, and temperature dysregulation, including hypothermia and hyperthermia. Persons with opioid dependence seldom die from opioid withdrawal, unless they have a severe preexisting physical illness such as cardiac disease. Residual symptoms—such as insomnia, bradycardia, temperature dysregulation, and a craving for opioids—can persist for months after withdrawal. Associated features of opioid withdrawal include restlessness, irritability, depression, tremor, weakness, nausea, and vomiting. At any time during the abstinence syndrome, a single injection of morphine or heroin eliminates all of the symptoms.

Opioid Intoxication Delirium

Opioid intoxication delirium (see Table 7.2–2) is most likely to happen when opioids are used in high doses, are mixed with other psychoactive compounds, or are used by a person with preexisting brain damage or a central nervous system (CNS) disorder (e.g., epilepsy).

Opioid-Induced Psychotic Disorder

Opioid-induced psychotic disorder can begin during opioid intoxication. The DSM-IV-TR diagnostic criteria are contained in the section on schizophrenia and other psychotic disorders (see Table 11.4–5). Clinicians can specify whether hallucinations or delusions are the predominant symptoms.

Opioid-Induced Mood Disorder

Opioid-induced mood disorder can begin during opioid intoxication (see Table 12.3–8). Opioid-induced mood disorder symptoms can have a manic, depressed, or mixed nature, depending on a person's response to opioids. A person coming to psychiatric attention with opioid-induced mood disorder usually has mixed symptoms, combining irritability, expansiveness, and depression.

Opioid-Induced Sleep Disorder and Opioid-Induced Sexual Dysfunction

Opioid-induced sleep disorder (see Table 20.2–14) and opioid-induced sexual dysfunction (see Table 17.2–11) are diagnostic categories in DSM-IV-TR. Hypersomnia is likely to be more common with opioids than insomnia. The most common sexual dysfunction is likely to be impotence.

Opioid-Related Disorder Not Otherwise Specified

The DSM-IV-TR includes diagnoses for opioid-related disorders with symptoms of delirium, abnormal mood, psychosis, abnormal sleep, and sexual dysfunction. Clinical situations that do not fit into these categories exemplify appropriate cases for the use of the DSM-IV-TR diagnosis of opioid-related disorder not otherwise specified (Table 9.10–4).

Table 9.10–4
DSM-IV-TR Diagnostic Criteria for Opioid-Related Disorder Not Otherwise Specified

The opioid-related disorder not otherwise specified category is for disorders associated with the use of opioids that are not classifiable as opioid dependence, opioid abuse, opioid intoxication, opioid withdrawal, opioid intoxication delirium, opioid-induced psychotic disorder, opioid-induced mood disorder, opioid-induced sexual dysfunction, or opioid-induced sleep disorder.

From American Psychiatric Association. *Diagnostic and Statistical Manual of Mental Disorders.* 4th ed. Text rev. Washington, DC: American Psychiatric Association; copyright 2000, with permission.

CLINICAL FEATURES

Opioids can be taken orally, snorted intranasally, and injected intravenously (IV) or subcutaneously. Opioids are subjectively addictive because of the euphoric high (the rush) that users experience, especially those who take the substances IV. The associated symptoms include a feeling of warmth, heaviness of the extremities, dry mouth, itchy face (especially the nose), and facial flushing. The initial euphoria is followed by a period of sedation, known in street parlance as "nodding off." Opioid use can induce dysphoria, nausea, and vomiting in opioid-naïve persons.

The physical effects of opioids include respiratory depression, pupillary constriction, smooth muscle contraction (including the ureters and the bile ducts), constipation, and changes in blood pressure, heart rate, and body temperature. The respiratory depressant effects are mediated at the level of the brainstem.

Adverse Effects

The most common and most serious adverse effect associated with the opioid-related disorders is the potential transmission of hepatitis and HIV through the use of contaminated needles by more than one person. Persons can experience idiosyncratic allergic reactions to opioids, which result in anaphylactic shock, pulmonary edema, and death if they do not receive prompt and adequate treatment. Another serious adverse effect is an idiosyncratic drug interaction between meperidine and monoamine oxidase inhibitors (MAOIs), which can produce gross autonomic instability, severe behavioral agitation, coma, seizures, and death. Opioids and MAOIs should not be given together for this reason.

Opioid Overdose

Death from an overdose of an opioid is usually attributable to respiratory arrest from the respiratory depressant effect of the drug. The symptoms of overdose include marked unresponsiveness, coma, slow respiration, hypothermia, hypotension, and bradycardia. When presented with the clinical triad of coma, pinpoint pupils, and respiratory depression, clinicians should consider opioid overdose as a primary diagnosis. They can also inspect the patient's body for needle tracks in the arms, legs, ankles, groin, and even the dorsal vein of the penis.

MPTP-Induced Parkinsonism

In 1976, after ingesting an opioid contaminated with methylphenyltetrahydropyridine (MPTP), several persons developed a syndrome of irreversible parkinsonism. The mechanism for the neurotoxic effect is as follows: MPTP is converted into 1-methyl-4-phenylpyridinium (MPP+) by the enzyme monoamine oxidase and is then taken up by dopaminergic neurons. Because MPP+ binds to melanin in substantia nigra neurons, MPP+ is concentrated in these neurons and eventually kills the cells. PET studies of persons who ingested MPTP but remained asymptomatic have shown a decreased number of dopamine-binding sites in the substantia nigra. This decrease reflects a loss in the number of dopaminergic neurons in that region.

TREATMENT AND REHABILITATION

Overdose Treatment

The first task in overdose treatment is to ensure an adequate airway. Tracheopharyngeal secretions should be aspirated; an airway may be inserted. The patient should be ventilated mechanically until naloxone, a specific opioid antagonist, can be given. Naloxone is administered IV at a slow rate—initially about 0.8 mg per 70 kg of body weight. Signs of improvement (increased respiratory rate and pupillary dilation) should occur promptly. In opioid-dependent patients, too much naloxone may produce signs of withdrawal as well as reversal of overdose. If no response to the initial dose occurs, naloxone administration may be repeated after intervals of a few minutes. Previously, it was thought that if no response was observed after 4 to 5 mg, the CNS depression was probably not caused solely by opioids. The duration of action of naloxone is short compared with that of many opioids, such as methadone and levomethadyl acetate, and repeated administration may be required to prevent recurrence of opioid toxicity.

Medically Supervised Withdrawal and Detoxification

Opioid Agents for Treating Opioid Withdrawal

METHADONE.   Methadone is a synthetic narcotic (an opioid) that substitutes for heroin and can be taken orally. When given to addicts to replace their usual substance of abuse, the drug suppresses withdrawal symptoms. A daily dose of 20 to 80 mg suffices to stabilize a patient, although daily doses of up to 120 mg have been used. The duration of action for methadone exceeds 24 hours; thus, once-daily dosing is adequate. Methadone maintenance is continued until the patient can be withdrawn from methadone, which itself causes dependence. An abstinence syndrome occurs with methadone withdrawal, but patients are detoxified from methadone more easily than from heroin. Clonidine (0.1 to 0.3 mg three to four times a day) is usually given during the detoxification period.

Methadone maintenance has several advantages. First, it frees persons with opioid dependence from using injectable heroin and, thus, reduces the chance of spreading HIV through contaminated needles. Second, methadone produces minimal euphoria and rarely causes drowsiness or depression when taken for a long time. Third, methadone allows patients to engage in gainful employment instead of criminal activity. The major disadvantage of methadone use is that patients remain dependent on a narcotic.

Other Opioid Substitutes

LEVOMETHADYL (LAAM).   LAAM is an opioid agonist that suppresses opioid withdrawal. It is no longer used, however, because some patients developed prolonged QT intervals associated with potentially fatal arrhythmias (torsades de pointes).

BUPRENORPHINE.   As with methadone and LAAM, buprenorphine is an opioid agonist approved for opioid dependence in 2002. It can be dispensed on an outpatient basis, but prescribing physicians must demonstrate that they have received special training in its use. Buprenorphine in a daily dose of 8 to 10 mg appears to reduce heroin use. Buprenorphine also is effective

in thrice-weekly dosing because of its slow dissociation from opioid receptors. After repeated administration, it attenuates or blocks the subjective effects of parenterally administered opioids such as heroin or morphine. A mild opioid withdrawal syndrome occurs if the drug is abruptly discontinued after chronic administrations.

Opioid Antagonists.   Opioid antagonists block or antagonize the effects of opioids. Unlike methadone, they do not exert narcotic effects and do not cause dependence. Opioid antagonists include naloxone, which is used in the treatment of opioid overdose because it reverses the effects of narcotics, and naltrexone, the longest-acting (72 hours) antagonist. The theory for using an antagonist for opioid-related disorders is that blocking opioid agonist effects, particularly euphoria, discourages persons with opioid dependence from substance-seeking behavior and, thus, deconditions this behavior. The major weakness of the antagonist treatment model is the lack of any mechanism that compels a person to continue to take the antagonist.

Pregnant Women with Opioid Dependence

Neonatal addiction is a significant problem. About three fourths of all infants born to addicted mothers experience the withdrawal syndrome.

Neonatal Withdrawal.   Although opioid withdrawal rarely is fatal for the otherwise healthy adult, it is hazardous to the fetus and can lead to miscarriage or fetal death. Maintaining a pregnant woman with opioid dependence on a low dose of methadone (10 to 40 mg daily) may be the least hazardous course to follow. At this dose, neonatal withdrawal is usually mild and can be managed with low doses of paregoric. If pregnancy begins while a woman is taking high doses of methadone, the dose should be reduced slowly (e.g., 1 mg every 3 days), and fetal movements should be monitored. If withdrawal is necessary or desired, it is least hazardous during the second trimester.

Fetal AIDS Transmission.   Acquired immune deficiency syndrome (AIDS) is the other major risk to the fetus of a woman with opioid dependence. Pregnant women can pass HIV, the causative agent of AIDS, to the fetus through the placental circulation. An HIV-infected mother can also pass HIV to the infant through breast-feeding. The use of zidovudine (Retrovir) alone or in combination with other anti-HIV medications in infected women can decrease the incidence of HIV in newborns.

Psychotherapy

The entire range of psychotherapeutic modalities is appropriate for treating opioid-related disorders. Individual psychotherapy, behavioral therapy, cognitive-behavioral therapy, family therapy, support groups (e.g., Narcotics Anonymous [NA]), and social skills training may all prove effective for specific patients. Social skills training should be particularly emphasized for patients with few social skills. Family therapy is usually indicated when the patient lives with family members.

Therapeutic Communities

Therapeutic communities are residences in which all members have a substance abuse problem. Abstinence is the rule; to be admitted to such a community, a person must show a high level of motivation. The goals are to effect a complete change of lifestyle, including abstinence from substances; to develop personal honesty, responsibility, and useful social skills; and to eliminate antisocial attitudes and criminal behavior.

The staff members of most therapeutic communities are persons with former substance dependence who often put prospective candidates through a rigorous screening process to test their motivation. Self-help through the use of confrontational groups and isolation from the outside world and from friends associated with the drug life are emphasized. The prototypical community for persons with substance dependence is Phoenix House, where the residents live for long periods (usually 12 to 18 months) while receiving treatment. They are allowed to return to their old environments only when they have demonstrated their ability to handle increased responsibility within the therapeutic community. Therapeutic communities can be effective but require large staffs and extensive facilities. Moreover, dropout rates are high; up to 75 percent of those who enter therapeutic communities leave within the first month.

Education and Needle Exchange

Although the essential treatment of opioid use disorders is encouraging persons to abstain from opioids, education about the transmission of HIV must receive equal attention. Persons with opioid dependence who use IV or subcutaneous routes of administration must be taught available safe-sex practices. Free needle-exchange programs are often subject to intense political and societal pressures but, where allowed, should be made available to persons with opioid dependence. Several studies have indicated that unsafe needle sharing is common when it is difficult to obtain enough clean needles and is also common in persons with legal difficulties, severe substance problems, and psychiatric symptoms. These are just the persons most likely to be involved in transmitting HIV.

Narcotics Anonymous

Narcotics Anonymous is a self-help group of abstinent drug addicts modeled on the 12-step principles of Alcoholics Anonymous (AA). Such groups exist in most large cities and can provide useful group support. The outcome for patients treated in 12-step programs is generally good, but the anonymity that is at the core of the 12-step model has made detailed evaluation of its efficacy in treating opioid dependence difficult.

▲ 9.11 Phencyclidine (or Phencyclidine-Like)-Related Disorders

Phencyclidine (PCP; 1-1 [phenylcyclohexyl] piperidine), also known as *angel dust*, was first developed as a novel anesthetic in the late 1950s. This drug and the closely related compound ketamine were termed *dissociative anesthetics* because they produced a condition in which subjects were awake but apparently insensitive to, or dissociated from, the environment. The symptoms induced by PCP and ketamine closely resemble those observed in schizophrenia. As early as 1959, therefore, it was proposed that PCP psychosis might serve as a heuristically valuable model for schizophrenia. PCP entered the illicit street market in 1965. In the late 1970s, it was one of the leading drugs of abuse in the United States. Although its popularity has subsequently declined, the popularity of ketamine has been steadily increasing.

Phencyclidine and ketamine exert their unique behavioral effects by blocking N-methyl-D-aspartate (NMDA)–type receptors for the excitatory neurotransmitter glutamate. PCP and ketamine intoxication can present with a variety of symptoms, from anxiety to psychosis. Treatment remains largely symptomatic and supportive. Few studies have assessed medication effects on PCP or ketamine intoxication effects directly. PCP and ketamine induce psychotic symptoms that closely resemble those of schizophrenia. As such, these drugs have been frequently used in challenge studies to investigate brain mechanisms in schizophrenia. Although PCP is no longer used in controlled human studies, ketamine challenge studies are ongoing and continue to provide critical insights into schizophrenia.

Phencyclidine was first used illicitly in San Francisco in the late 1960s. Since then, about 30 chemical analogs have been produced and are intermittently available on the streets of major U.S. cities. The effects of PCP are similar to those of such hallucinogens as lysergic acid diethylamide (LSD). Because of differing pharmacology and some difference in clinical effects, however, the text revision of the fourth edition of the *Diagnostic and Statistical Manual of Mental Disorders* (DSM-IV-TR) classifies the arylcyclohexylamines as a separate category. PCP has also been of interest to schizophrenia researchers, who have used PCP-induced chemical and behavioral changes in animals as a possible model of schizophrenia.

EPIDEMIOLOGY

Phencyclidine and some related substances are relatively easy to synthesize in illegal laboratories and relatively inexpensive to buy on the street. The variable quality of the laboratories, however, results in a range of potency and purity. PCP use varies most markedly with geography. Most users of PCP also use other substances, particularly alcohol, but also opiates, opioids, marijuana, amphetamines, and cocaine. PCP is frequently added to marijuana, with severe untoward effects on users. According to DSM-IV-TR, the actual rate of PCP dependence and abuse is not known, but PCP is associated with 3 percent of substance abuse deaths and 32 percent of substance-related emergency room visits nationally.

Some areas of some cities have a tenfold higher use rate of PCP than other areas. The highest PCP use in the United States is in Washington, D.C., where PCP accounts for 18 percent of all substance-related deaths and more than 1,000 emergency room visits per year. In Los Angeles, Chicago, and Baltimore, the comparable figure is 6 percent. Overall, most users are between 18 and 25 years of age, and they account for 50 percent of cases. Patients are more likely to be male than female, especially those who visit emergency rooms. Twice as many whites as blacks are users, although blacks account for more visits to hospitals for PCP-related disorders than do whites. PCP use appears to be rising, with some reports showing a 50 percent increase, particularly in urban areas.

NEUROPHARMACOLOGY

Phencyclidine and its related compounds are variously sold as a crystalline powder, paste, liquid, or drug-soaked paper (blotter). PCP is most commonly used as an additive to a cannabis- or parsley-containing cigarette. Experienced users report that the effects of 2 to 3 mg of smoked PCP occur in about 5 minutes and plateau in 30 minutes. The bioavailability of PCP is about 75 percent when taken by intravenous administration and about 30 percent when smoked. The half-life of PCP in humans is about 20 hours, and the half-life of ketamine in humans is about 2 hours.

The primary pharmacodynamic effect of PCP and ketamine is as an antagonist at the NMDA subtype of glutamate receptors. PCP binds to a site within the NMDA-associated calcium channel and prevents the influx of calcium ions. PCP also activates the dopaminergic neurons of the ventral tegmental area, which project to the cerebral cortex and the limbic system. Activation of these neurons is usually involved in mediating the reinforcing qualities of PCP.

Tolerance for the effects of PCP occurs in humans, although physical dependence generally does not occur. In animals that are administered more PCP per pound for longer times than virtually any humans, PCP does induce physical dependence, however, with marked withdrawal symptoms of lethargy, depression, and craving. Physical symptoms of withdrawal in humans are rare, probably as a function of dose and duration of use. Although physical dependence on PCP is rare in humans, psychological dependence on both PCP and ketamine is common, and some users become psychologically dependent on the PCP-induced psychological state.

That PCP is made in illicit laboratories contributes to the increased likelihood of impurities in the final product. One such contaminant is 1-piperidenocyclohexane carbonitrite, which releases hydrogen cyanide in small quantities when ingested. Another contaminant is piperidine, which can be recognized by its strong, fishy odor.

DIAGNOSIS

The DSM-IV-TR lists a number of PCP (or PCP-like)–related disorders (Table 9.11–1) but outlines the specific diagnostic criteria for only PCP intoxication (Table 9.11–2) within the PCP (or PCP-like)–related disorders section. The diagnostic criteria for other PCP (or PCP-like)–related disorders are listed in the sections that deal with specific symptoms—for example, PCP-induced anxiety disorder is in the anxiety disorders section.

PCP Dependence and PCP Abuse

The DSM-IV-TR uses the general criteria for PCP dependence and PCP abuse (see Tables 9.1–3 to 9.1–5). Some long-term users of PCP are said to be "crystallized," a syndrome characterized by dulled thinking, decreased reflexes, loss of memory, loss of

Table 9.11–1
DSM-IV-TR Phencyclidine-Related Disorders

Phencyclidine use disorders
Phencyclidine dependence
Phencyclidine abuse
Phencyclidine-induced disorders
Phencyclidine intoxication
  Specify if:
    With perceptual disturbances
Phencyclidine intoxication delirium
Phencyclidine-induced psychotic disorder, with delusions
  Specify if:
    With onset during intoxication
Phencyclidine-induced psychotic disorder, with hallucination
  Specify if:
    With onset during intoxication
Phencyclidine-induced mood disorder
  Specify if:
    With onset during intoxication
Phencyclidine-induced anxiety disorder
  Specify if:
    With onset during intoxication
Phencyclidine-related disorder not otherwise specified

From American Psychiatric Association. *Diagnostic and Statistical Manual of Mental Disorders.* 4th ed. Text rev. Washington, DC: American Psychiatric Association; copyright 2000, with permission.

impulse control, depression, lethargy, and impaired concentration.

According to DSM-IV-TR, in the United States, more than 3 percent of those age 12 years and older acknowledged ever using PCP, with 0.2 percent reporting use in the prior year. The highest lifetime prevalence was in those aged 26 to 34 years (4 percent), whereas the highest proportion using PCP in the prior year (0.7 percent) was in those aged 12 to 17 years.

Table 9.11–2
DSM-IV-TR Diagnostic Criteria for Phencyclidine Intoxication

A. Recent use of phencyclidine (or a related substance).
B. Clinically significant maladaptive behavioral changes (e.g., belligerence, assaultiveness, impulsiveness, unpredictability, psychomotor agitation, impaired judgment, or impaired social or occupational functioning) that developed during, or shortly after, phencyclidine use.
C. Within an hour (less when smoked, "snorted," or used intravenously), two (or more) of the following signs:
  (1) vertical or horizontal nystagmus
  (2) hypertension or tachycardia
  (3) numbness or diminished responsiveness to pain
  (4) ataxia
  (5) dysarthria
  (6) muscle rigidity
  (7) seizures or coma
  (8) hyperacusis
D. The symptoms are not due to a general medical condition and are not better accounted for by another mental disorder.
Specify if:
With perceptual disturbances

From American Psychiatric Association. *Diagnostic and Statistical Manual of Mental Disorders.* 4th ed. Text rev. Washington, DC: American Psychiatric Association; copyright 2000, with permission.

PCP Intoxication

Short-term PCP intoxication can have potentially severe complications and must often be considered a psychiatric emergency. DSM-IV-TR gives specific criteria for PCP intoxication (Table 9.11–2). Clinicians can specify the presence of perceptual disturbances.

Some patients may be brought to psychiatric attention within hours of ingesting PCP, but often 2 to 3 days elapse before psychiatric help is sought. The long interval between drug ingestion and the appearance of the patient in a clinic usually reflects the attempts of friends to deal with the psychosis by "talking down" the patient. Persons who lose consciousness are brought for help earlier than those who remain conscious. Most patients recover completely within a day or two, but some remain psychotic for as long as 2 weeks. Patients who are first seen in a coma often exhibit disorientation, hallucinations, confusion, and difficulty communicating on regaining consciousness. These symptoms may also be seen in noncomatose patients, but their symptoms appear to be less severe than those of comatose patients. Behavioral disturbances sometimes are severe; they can include public masturbation, stripping off clothes, violence, urinary incontinence, crying, and inappropriate laughing. Patients frequently have amnesia for the entire period of the psychosis.

PCP Intoxication Delirium

Phencyclidine intoxication delirium is included as a diagnostic category in DSM-IV-TR (see Table 7.2–2). An estimated 25 percent of all PCP-related emergency room patients may meet the criteria for the disorder, which can be characterized by agitated, violent, and bizarre behavior.

PCP-Induced Psychotic Disorder

Phencyclidine-induced psychotic disorder is included as a diagnostic category in DSM-IV-TR (see Table 11.4–5). Clinicians can further specify whether the predominant symptoms are delusions or hallucinations. An estimated 6 percent of PCP-related emergency room patients may meet the criteria for the disorder. About 40 percent of these patients have physical signs of hypertension and nystagmus, and 10 percent have been injured accidentally during the psychosis. The psychosis can last from 1 to 30 days, with an average of 4 to 5 days.

PCP-Induced Mood Disorder

Phencyclidine-induced mood disorder is included as a diagnostic category in DSM-IV-TR (see Table 12.3–8). An estimated 3 percent of PCP-related emergency room patients meet the criteria for the disorder, with most fitting the criteria for a manic-like episode. About 40 to 50 percent have been accidentally injured during the course of their manic symptoms.

PCP-Induced Anxiety Disorder

Phencyclidine-induced anxiety disorder is included as a diagnostic category in DSM-IV-TR (see Table 13.7–2). Anxiety is probably the most common symptom causing a PCP-intoxicated person to seek help in an emergency room.

Table 9.11–3
DSM-IV-TR Diagnostic Criteria for Phencyclidine-Related Disorder Not Otherwise Specified

The phencyclidine-related disorder not otherwise specified category is for disorders associated with the use of phencyclidine that are not classifiable as phencyclidine dependence, phencyclidine abuse, phencyclidine intoxication, phencyclidine intoxication delirium, phencyclidine-induced psychotic disorder, phencyclidine-induced mood disorder, or phencyclidine-induced anxiety disorder.

From American Psychiatric Association. *Diagnostic and Statistical Manual of Mental Disorders.* 4th ed. Text rev. Washington, DC: American Psychiatric Association; copyright 2000, with permission.

PCP-Related Disorder Not Otherwise Specified

The diagnosis of PCP-related disorder not otherwise specified is the appropriate diagnosis for a patient who does not fit into any of the previously described diagnoses (Table 9.11–3).

CLINICAL FEATURES

The amount of PCP varies greatly from PCP-laced cigarette to cigarette; 1 g may be used to make as few as four or as many as several dozen cigarettes. Less than 5 mg of PCP is considered a low dose, and doses above 10 mg are considered high. Dose variability makes it difficult to predict the effect, although smoking PCP is the easiest and most reliable way for users to titrate the dose.

Persons who have just taken PCP are frequently uncommunicative, appear to be oblivious, and report active fantasy production. They experience speedy feelings, euphoria, bodily warmth, tingling, peaceful floating sensations, and, occasionally, feelings of depersonalization, isolation, and estrangement. Sometimes, they have auditory and visual hallucinations. They often have striking alterations of body image, distortions of space and time perception, and delusions. They may experience intensified dependence feelings, confusion, and disorganization of thought. Users may be sympathetic, sociable, and talkative at one moment but hostile and negative at another. Anxiety is sometimes reported; it is often the most prominent presenting symptom during an adverse reaction. Nystagmus, hypertension, and hyperthermia are common effects of PCP. Head-rolling movements, stroking, grimacing, muscle rigidity on stimulation, repeated episodes of vomiting, and repetitive chanting speech are sometimes observed.

The short-term effects last 3 to 6 hours and sometimes give way to a mild depression in which the user becomes irritable, somewhat paranoid, and occasionally belligerent, irrationally assaultive, suicidal, or homicidal. The effects can last for several days. Users sometimes find that it takes 1 to 2 days to recover completely; laboratory tests show that PCP can remain in the patient's blood and urine for more than a week.

DIFFERENTIAL DIAGNOSIS

Depending on a patient's status at the time of admission, the differential diagnosis may include sedative or narcotic overdose, psychotic disorder as a consequence of the use of psychedelic drugs, and brief psychotic disorder. Laboratory analysis may help to establish the diagnosis, particularly in the many cases in which the substance history is unreliable or unattainable.

TREATMENT

Treatment of PCP intoxication aims to reduce systemic PCP levels and to address significant medical, behavioral, and psychiatric issues. For intoxication and PCP-induced psychotic disorder, although resolution of current symptoms and signs is paramount, the long-term goal of treatment is to prevent relapse to PCP use. PCP levels can fluctuate over many hours or even days, especially after oral administration. A prolonged period of clinical observation is therefore mandatory before concluding that no serious or life-threatening complications will ensue.

Trapping of ionized PCP in the stomach has led to the suggestion of continuous nasogastric suction as a treatment for PCP intoxication. This strategy, however, can be needlessly intrusive and can induce electrolyte imbalances. Administration of activated charcoal is safer, and it binds PCP and diminishes toxic effects of PCP in animals.

Trapping of ionized PCP in urine has led to the suggestion of urinary acidification as an aid to drug elimination. This strategy, however, may be ineffective and is potentially dangerous. Only a small portion of PCP is excreted in urine, metabolic acidosis itself carries significant risks, and acidic urine can increase the risk of renal failure secondary to rhabdomyolysis. Because of the extremely large volume of distribution of PCP, neither hemodialysis nor hemoperfusion can significantly promote drug clearance.

No drug is known to function as a direct PCP antagonist. Any compound binding to the PCP receptor, which is located within the ion channel of the NMDA receptor, would block NMDA receptor–mediated ion fluxes as does PCP itself. NMDA receptor mechanisms predict that pharmacological strategies promoting NMDA receptor activation (e.g., administration of a glycine-site agonist drug) would promote rapid dissociation of PCP from its binding sites. No clinical trials of NMDA agonists for PCP or ketamine intoxication in humans have been carried out. Treatment must therefore be supportive and directed at specific symptoms and signs of toxicity. Classic measures should be used for medical crises, including seizures, hypothermia, and hypertensive crisis.

Because PCP disrupts sensory input, environmental stimuli can cause unpredictable, exaggerated, distorted, or violent reactions. A cornerstone of treatment, therefore, is minimization of sensory inputs to PCP-intoxicated patients. Patients should be evaluated and treated in as quiet and isolated an environment as possible. Precautionary physical restraint is recommended by some authorities, with the risk of rhabdomyolysis from struggle against the restraints balanced by the avoidance of violent or disruptive behavior. Pharmacological sedation can be accomplished with oral or intramuscular (IM) antipsychotics or benzodiazepines; no convincing evidence indicates that either class of compounds is clinically superior. Because of the anticholinergic actions of PCP at high doses, neuroleptics with potent intrinsic anticholinergic properties should be avoided.

COURSE AND PROGNOSIS

Complete recovery from PCP intoxication is the rule in the absence of major medical complications. Many patients, however, relapse to PCP use immediately after discharge from treatment, even for severe PCP-related complications. Intoxication usually occurs in the context of abuse, dependence, or both. No specific behavioral treatments for PCP abuse and dependence have been described, however. Case reports indicate successful responses to residential and intensive outpatient treatment regimens with long-term follow-up, including urine monitoring with or without contingency contracting.

Ketamine

Ketamine is a dissociative anesthetic agent, originally derived from PCP, that is available for use in human and veterinary medicine. It has become a drug of abuse, with sources exclusively from stolen supplies. It is available as a powder or in solution for intranasal, oral, inhalational, or (rarely) intravenous use. Ketamine functions by working at the NMDA receptor and, as with PCP, can cause hallucinations and a dissociated state in which the patient has an altered sense of the body and reality and little concern for the environment.

Ketamine causes cardiovascular stimulation and no respiratory depression. On physical examination, the patient may be hypertensive and tachycardic, and have increased salivation and bidirectional or rotary nystagmus, or both. The onset of action is within seconds when used intravenously, and analgesia lasting 40 minutes and dissociative effects lasting for hours have been described. Cardiovascular status should be monitored and supportive care administered. A dystonic reaction has been described, as have flashbacks, but a more common complication is related to a lack of concern for the environment or personal safety.

Ketamine has a briefer duration of effect than PCP. Peak ketamine levels occur approximately 20 minutes after IM injection. After intranasal administration, the duration of effect is approximately 1 hour. Ketamine is N-demethylated by liver microsomal cytochrome P450, especially CYP3A, into norketamine. Ketamine, norketamine, and dehydronorketamine can be detected in urine, with half-lives of 3, 4, and 7 hours, respectively. Urinary ketamine and norketamine levels vary widely from individual to individual and can range from 10 to 7,000 ng/mL after intoxication. The relationship between serum ketamine levels and clinical symptoms has not been formally studied. Ketamine is often used in combination with other drugs of abuse, especially cocaine. Ketamine does not appear to interfere with, and may enhance, cocaine metabolism.

▲ 9.12 Sedative-, Hypnotic-, or Anxiolytic-Related Disorders

The drugs discussed in this section are referred to as *anxiolytic* or *sedative-hypnotic* drugs. The terminology is ambiguous for several reasons: (1) sedatives are drugs that reduce subjective tension and induce mental calmness; however, the same can be said of anxiolytics; (2) hypnotics are drugs used to induce sleep, but sedatives and anxiolytics given in sufficiently high doses also produce sleep; and (3) hypnotics in low doses, instead of inducing sleep, produce daytime sedation just as do sedatives and anxiolytics. Finally, in the older literature, all of these drugs are sometimes called *minor tranquillizers*, a term that is vague, poorly defined, and, therefore, best avoided.

The three groups of drugs associated with this class of substance-related disorders are benzodiazepines, barbiturates, and barbiturate-like substances. Each group is discussed in this section.

In addition to their psychiatric indications, these drugs are also used as antiepileptics, muscle relaxants, anesthetics, and anesthetic adjuvants. Alcohol and all drugs of this class are cross-tolerant, and their effects are additive. Physical and psychological dependence develops to these drugs, and all are associated with withdrawal symptoms.

BENZODIAZEPINES

Many benzodiazepines, differing primarily in their half-lives, are available in the United States. Examples of benzodiazepines are diazepam, flurazepam (Dalmane), oxazepam (Serax), and chlordiazepoxide (Librium). Benzodiazepines are used primarily as anxiolytics, hypnotics, antiepileptics, and anesthetics, as well as for alcohol withdrawal. After their introduction in the United States in the 1960s, benzodiazepines rapidly became the most prescribed drugs; about 15 percent of all persons in the United States have had a benzodiazepine prescribed by a physician. Increasing awareness of the risks for dependence on benzodiazepines and increased regulatory requirements, however, have decreased the number of benzodiazepine prescriptions. The Drug Enforcement Agency (DEA) classifies all benzodiazepines as Schedule IV controlled substances.

Flunitrazepam (Rohypnol), a benzodiazepine used in Mexico, South America, and Europe but not available in the United States, has become a drug of abuse. When taken with alcohol, it has been associated with promiscuous sexual behavior and rape. It is illegal to bring flunitrazepam into the United States. Although misused in the United States, it remains a standard anxiolytic in many countries.

Nonbenzodiazepine sedatives such as zolpidem (Ambien), zalepon (Sonata), and esczopiclone (Lunesta)—the so-called Z drugs—have clinical effects similar to the benzodiapines and are also subject to misuse and dependence.

BARBITURATES

Before the introduction of benzodiazepines, barbiturates were frequently prescribed, but because of their high abuse potential, their use is much rarer today. Secobarbital (popularly known as "reds," "red devils," "seggies," and "downers"), pentobarbital (Nembutal) (known as "yellow jackets," "yellows," and "nembies"), and a secobarbital-amobarbital combination (known as "reds and blues," "rainbows," "double-trouble," and "tooies") are easily available on the street from drug dealers. Pentobarbital, secobarbital, and amobarbital (Amytal) are now under the same federal legal controls as morphine.

The first barbiturate, barbital (Veronal), was introduced in the United States in 1903. Barbital and phenobarbital (Solfoton, Luminal), which were introduced shortly thereafter, are long-acting drugs with half-lives of 12 to 24 hours. Amobarbital is an intermediate-acting barbiturate with a half-life of 6 to 12 hours. Pentobarbital and secobarbital are short-acting barbiturates with half-lives of 3 to 6 hours. Although barbiturates are useful and

effective sedatives, they are highly lethal, with only ten times the normal dose producing coma and death.

BARBITURATE-LIKE SUBSTANCES

The most commonly abused barbiturate-like substance is methaqualone, which is no longer manufactured in the United States. It is often used by young persons who believe that the substance heightens the pleasure of sexual activity. Abusers of methaqualone commonly take one or two standard tablets (usually 300 mg per tablet) to obtain the desired effects. The street names for methaqualone include "mandrakes" (from the U. K. preparation Mandrax) and "soapers" (from the brand name Sopor). "Luding out" (from the brand name Quaalude) means getting high on methaqualone, which is often combined with excessive alcohol intake.

Other barbiturate-like substances include meprobamate (Equanil), a carbamate derivative that has weak efficacy as an antianxiety agent but has muscle-relaxant effects and is used for that purpose; chloral hydrate, a hypnotic that is highly toxic to the gastrointestinal (GI) system and, when combined with alcohol, is known as a "Mickey Finn"; and ethchlorvynol, a rapidly acting sedative agent with anticonvulsant and muscle-relaxing properties. All are subject to abuse.

EPIDEMIOLOGY

According to the text revision of the fourth edition of the *Diagnostic and Statistical Manual of Mental Disorders* (DSM-IV-TR), about 6 percent of individuals have used either sedatives or tranquilizers illicitly, including 0.3 percent who reported illicit use of sedatives in the prior year and 0.1 percent who reported use of sedatives in the prior month. The age group with the highest lifetime prevalence of sedative (3 percent) or tranquilizer (6 percent) use was 26 to 34 years of age, and those aged 18 to 25 years were most likely to have used them in the prior year. About one fourth to one third of all substance-related emergency room visits involve substances of this class. The patients have a female-to-male ratio of 3 to 1 and a white-to-black ratio of 2 to 1. Some persons use benzodiazepines alone, but persons who use cocaine often use benzodiazepines to reduce withdrawal symptoms, and opioid abusers use them to enhance the euphoric effects of opioids. Because they are easily obtained, benzodiazepines are also used by abusers of stimulants, hallucinogens, and phencyclidine (PCP) to help reduce the anxiety that can be caused by those substances.

Whereas barbiturate abuse is common among mature adults who have long histories of abuse of these substances, benzodiazepines are abused by a younger age group, usually those younger than 40 years of age. This group may have a slight male predominance and has a white-to-black ratio of about 2 to 1. Benzodiazepines are probably not abused as frequently as other substances for the purpose of getting "high," or inducing a euphoric feeling. Rather, they are used when a person wishes to experience a general relaxed feeling.

NEUROPHARMACOLOGY

The benzodiazepines, barbiturates, and barbiturate-like substances all have their primary effects on the γ-aminobutyric acid

(GABA) type A (GABA$_A$) receptor complex, which contains a chloride ion channel, a binding site for GABA, and a well-defined binding site for benzodiazepines. The barbiturates and barbiturate-like substances are also believed to bind somewhere on the GABA$_A$ receptor complex. When a benzodiazepine, barbiturate, or barbiturate-like substance does bind to the complex, the effect is to increase the affinity of the receptor for its endogenous neurotransmitter, GABA, and to increase the flow of chloride ions through the channel into the neuron. The influx of negatively charged chloride ions into the neuron is inhibitory and hyperpolarizes the neuron relative to the extracellular space.

Although all the substances in this class induce tolerance and physical dependence, the mechanisms behind these effects are best understood for the benzodiazepines. After long-term benzodiazepine use, the receptor effects caused by the agonist are attenuated. Specifically, GABA stimulation of the GABA$_A$ receptors results in less chloride influx than was caused by GABA stimulation before the benzodiazepine administration. This downregulation of receptor response is not caused by a decrease in receptor number or by decreased affinity of the receptor for GABA. The basis for the downregulation seems to be in the coupling between the GABA-binding site and the activation of the chloride ion channel. This decreased efficiency in coupling may be regulated within the GABA$_A$ receptor complex itself or by other neuronal mechanisms.

DIAGNOSIS

The DSM-IV-TR lists a number of sedative-, hypnotic-, or anxiolytic-related disorders (Table 9.12–1) but includes specific diagnostic criteria only for sedative, hypnotic, or anxiolytic intoxication (Table 9.12–2) and sedative, hypnotic, or anxiolytic withdrawal (Table 9.12–3). The diagnostic criteria for other sedative-, hypnotic-, or anxiolytic-related disorders are outlined in the DSM-IV-TR sections that are specific for the major symptom—for example, sedative-, hypnotic-, or anxiolytic-induced psychotic disorder (see Table 11.4–5).

Dependence and Abuse

Sedative, hypnotic, or anxiolytic dependence and sedative, hypnotic, or anxiolytic abuse are diagnosed according to the general criteria in DSM-IV-TR for substance dependence and substance abuse (see Tables 9.1–3 to 9.1–5).

Intoxication

The DSM-IV-TR contains a single set of diagnostic criteria for intoxication by any sedative, hypnotic, or anxiolytic substance (Table 9.12–2). Although the intoxication syndromes induced by all these drugs are similar, subtle clinical differences are observable, especially with intoxications that involve low doses. The diagnosis of intoxication by one of this class of substances is best confirmed by obtaining a blood sample for substance screening.

Benzodiazepines. Benzodiazepine intoxication can be associated with behavioral disinhibition, potentially resulting in hostile or aggressive behavior in some persons. The effect is

Table 9.12–1
DSM-IV-TR Sedative-, Hypnotic-, or Anxiolytic-Related Disorders

Sedative, hypnotic, or anxiolytic use disorders
Sedative, hypnotic, or anxiolytic dependence
Sedative, hypnotic, or anxiolytic abuse
Sedative-, hypnotic-, or anxiolytic-induced disorders
Sedative, hypnotic, or anxiolytic intoxication
Sedative, hypnotic, or anxiolytic withdrawal
 Specify if:
  With perceptual disturbances
Sedative, hypnotic, or anxiolytic intoxication delirium
Sedative, hypnotic, or anxiolytic withdrawal delirium
Sedative-, hypnotic-, or anxiolytic-induced persisting dementia
Sedative-, hypnotic-, or anxiolytic-induced psychotic disorder, with delusions
 Specify if:
  With onset during intoxication
  With onset during withdrawal
Sedative-, hypnotic-, or anxiolytic-induced psychotic disorder, with hallucinations
 Specify if:
  With onset during intoxication
  With onset during withdrawal
Sedative-, hypnotic-, or anxiolytic-induced mood disorder
 Specify if:
  With onset during intoxication
  With onset during withdrawal
Sedative-, hypnotic-, or anxiolytic-induced anxiety disorder
 Specify if:
  With onset during withdrawal
Sedative-, hypnotic-, or anxiolytic-induced sexual dysfunction
 Specify if:
  With onset during intoxication
Sedative-, hypnotic-, or anxiolytic-induced sleep disorder
 Specify if:
  With onset during intoxication
  With onset during withdrawal
Sedative-, hypnotic-, or anxiolytic-related disorder not otherwise specified

From American Psychiatric Association. *Diagnostic and Statistical Manual of Mental Disorders.* 4th ed. Text rev. Washington, DC: American Psychiatric Association; copyright 2000, with permission.

perhaps most common when benzodiazepines are taken in combination with alcohol. Benzodiazepine intoxication is associated with less euphoria than is intoxication by other drugs in this class. This characteristic is the basis for the lower abuse and dependence potential of benzodiazepines than of barbiturates.

Barbiturates and Barbiturate-Like Substances. When barbiturates and barbiturate-like substances are taken in relatively low doses, the clinical syndrome of intoxication is indistinguishable from that associated with alcohol intoxication. The symptoms include sluggishness, incoordination, difficulty thinking, poor memory, slow speech and comprehension, faulty judgment, disinhibited sexual aggressive impulses, narrowed range of attention, emotional lability, and exaggerated basic personality traits. The sluggishness usually resolves after a few hours, but depending primarily on the half-life of the abused substance, impaired judgment, distorted mood, and impaired motor skills may remain for 12 to 24 hours. Other potential symptoms are hostility, argumentativeness, moroseness, and, occasionally, paranoid and suicidal ideation. The neurological effects include

Table 9.12–2
DSM-IV-TR Diagnostic Criteria for Sedative, Hypnotic, or Anxiolytic Intoxication

A. Recent use of a sedative, hypnotic, or anxiolytic.

B. Clinically significant maladaptive behavioral or psychological changes (e.g., inappropriate sexual or aggressive behavior, mood lability, impaired judgment, impaired social or occupational functioning) that developed during, or shortly after, sedative, hypnotic, or anxiolytic use.

C. One (or more) of the following signs, developing during, or shortly after, sedative, hypnotic, or anxiolytic use:

  (1) slurred speech
  (2) incoordination
  (3) unsteady gait
  (4) nystagmus
  (5) impairment in attention or memory
  (6) stupor or coma

D. The symptoms are not due to a general medical condition and are not better accounted for by another mental disorder.

From American Psychiatric Association. *Diagnostic and Statistical Manual of Mental Disorders.* 4th ed. Text rev. Washington, DC: American Psychiatric Association; copyright 2000, with permission.

nystagmus, diplopia, strabismus, ataxic gait, positive Romberg's sign, hypotonia, and decreased superficial reflexes.

Withdrawal

The DSM-IV-TR contains a single set of diagnostic criteria for withdrawal from any sedative, hypnotic, or anxiolytic substance (Table 9.12–3). Clinicians can specify "with perceptual disturbances" if illusions, altered perceptions, or hallucinations are present but accompanied by intact reality testing. It needs to be kept in mind that benzodiazepines are associated with a withdrawal syndrome and that withdrawal from barbiturates can be

Table 9.12–3
DSM-IV-TR Diagnostic Criteria for Sedative, Hypnotic, or Anxiolytic Withdrawal

A. Cessation of (or reduction in) sedative, hypnotic, or anxiolytic use that has been heavy and prolonged.

B. Two (or more) of the following, developing within several hours to a few days after Criterion A:

  (1) autonomic hyperactivity (e.g., sweating or pulse rate greater than 100)
  (2) increased hand tremor
  (3) insomnia
  (4) nausea or vomiting
  (5) transient visual, tactile, or auditory hallucinations or illusions
  (6) psychomotor agitation
  (7) anxiety
  (8) grand mal seizures

C. The symptoms in Criterion B cause clinically significant distress or impairment in social, occupational, or other important areas of functioning.

D. The symptoms are not due to a general medical condition and are not better accounted for by another mental disorder.

Specify if:
  With perceptual disturbances

From American Psychiatric Association. *Diagnostic and Statistical Manual of Mental Disorders.* 4th ed. Text rev. Washington, DC: American Psychiatric Association; copyright 2000, with permission.

life threatening. Withdrawal from benzodiazepines can also result in serious medical complications, such as seizures.

Benzodiazepines.   The severity of the withdrawal syndrome associated with the benzodiazepines varies significantly depending on the average dose and the duration of use, but a mild withdrawal syndrome can follow even short-term use of relatively low doses of benzodiazepines. A significant withdrawal syndrome is likely to occur at cessation of doses in the range of 40 mg a day for diazepam, for example, although 10 to 20 mg a day taken for a month can also result in a withdrawal syndrome when drug administration is stopped. The onset of withdrawal symptoms usually occurs 2 to 3 days after the cessation of use, but with long-acting drugs, such as diazepam, the latency before onset can be 5 or 6 days. The symptoms include anxiety, dysphoria, intolerance for bright lights and loud noises, nausea, sweating, muscle twitching, and sometimes seizures (generally at doses of 50 mg a day or more of diazepam).

Barbiturates and Barbiturate-Like Substances.   The withdrawal syndrome for barbiturate and barbiturate-like substances ranges from mild symptoms (e.g., anxiety, weakness, sweating, and insomnia) to severe symptoms (e.g., seizures, delirium, cardiovascular collapse, and death). Persons who have been abusing phenobarbital in the range of 400 mg a day may experience mild withdrawal symptoms; those who have been abusing the substance in the range of 800 mg a day can experience orthostatic hypotension, weakness, tremor, and severe anxiety. About 75 percent of these persons have withdrawal-related seizures. Users of doses higher than 800 mg a day may experience anorexia, delirium, hallucinations, and repeated seizures.

Most symptoms appear in the first 3 days of abstinence, and seizures generally occur on the second or third day, when the symptoms are worst. If seizures do occur, they always precede the development of delirium. The symptoms rarely occur more than 1 week after stopping the substance. A psychotic disorder, if it develops, starts on the third to eighth day. The various associated symptoms generally run their course within 2 to 3 days but can last as long as 2 weeks. The first episode of the syndrome usually occurs after 5 to 15 years of heavy substance use.

Delirium

The DSM-IV-TR allows for the diagnosis of sedative, hypnotic, or anxiolytic intoxication delirium and sedative, hypnotic, or anxiolytic withdrawal delirium (see Tables 7.2–2 and 7.2–3). Delirium that is indistinguishable from delirium tremens associated with alcohol withdrawal is seen more commonly with barbiturate withdrawal than with benzodiazepine withdrawal. Delirium associated with intoxication can be seen with either barbiturates or benzodiazepines if the dosages are sufficiently high.

Persisting Dementia

The DSM-IV-TR allows for the diagnosis of sedative-, hypnotic-, or anxiolytic-induced persisting dementia (see Table 7.3–4). The existence of the disorder is controversial because uncertainty exists whether a persisting dementia is caused by the substance use itself or by associated features of the substance use. The diagnosis must be further evaluated by using DSM-IV-TR criteria to ascertain validity.

Persisting Amnestic Disorder

The DSM-IV-TR allows for the diagnosis of sedative-, hypnotic-, or anxiolytic-induced persisting amnestic disorder (see Table 7.4–2). Amnestic disorders associated with sedatives, hypnotics, and anxiolytics may be underdiagnosed. One exception is the increased number of reports of amnestic episodes associated with short-term use of benzodiazepines with short half-lives (e.g., triazolam [Halcion]).

Psychotic Disorders

The psychotic symptoms of barbiturate withdrawal can be indistinguishable from those of alcohol-associated delirium tremens. Agitation, delusions, and hallucinations are usually visual, but sometimes tactile or auditory features develop after about 1 week of abstinence. Psychotic symptoms associated with intoxication or withdrawal are more common with barbiturates than with benzodiazepines and are diagnosed as sedative-, hypnotic-, or anxiolytic-induced psychotic disorders (see Table 11.4–5). Clinicians can further specify whether delusions or hallucinations are the predominant symptoms.

Other Disorders

Sedative, hypnotic, and anxiolytic use has also been associated with mood disorders (see Table 12.3–8), anxiety disorders (see Table 13.7–2), sleep disorders (see Table 20.2–14), and sexual dysfunctions (see Table 17.2–11). When none of the previously discussed diagnostic categories is appropriate for a person with a sedative, hypnotic, or anxiolytic use disorder, the appropriate diagnosis is sedative-, hypnotic-, or anxiolytic-related disorder not otherwise specified (Table 9.12–4).

CLINICAL FEATURES

Patterns of Abuse

Oral Use.   Sedatives, hypnotics, and anxiolytics can all be taken orally, either occasionally to achieve a time-limited specific effect or regularly to obtain a constant, usually mild, intoxication state. The occasional use pattern is associated with young persons

Table 9.12–4
DSM-IV-TR Diagnostic Criteria for Sedative-, Hypnotic-, or Anxiolytic-Related Disorder Not Otherwise Specified

The sedative-, hypnotic-, or anxiolytic-related disorder not otherwise specified category is for disorders associated with the use of sedatives, hypnotics, or anxiolytics that are not classifiable as sedative, hypnotic, or anxiolytic dependence; sedative, hypnotic, or anxiolytic abuse; sedative, hypnotic, or anxiolytic intoxication; sedative, hypnotic, or anxiolytic withdrawal; sedative, hypnotic, or anxiolytic intoxication delirium; sedative, hypnotic, or anxiolytic withdrawal delirium; sedative-, hypnotic-, or anxiolytic-induced persisting dementia; sedative-, hypnotic-, or anxiolytic-induced persisting amnestic disorder; sedative-, hypnotic-, or anxiolytic-induced psychotic disorder; sedative-, hypnotic-, or anxiolytic-induced mood disorder; sedative-, hypnotic-, or anxiolytic-induced anxiety disorder; sedative-, hypnotic-, or anxiolytic-induced sexual dysfunction; or sedative-, hypnotic-, or anxiolytic-induced sleep disorder.

From American Psychiatric Association. *Diagnostic and Statistical Manual of Mental Disorders.* 4th ed. Text rev. Washington, DC: American Psychiatric Association; copyright 2000, with permission.

who take the substance to achieve specific effects—relaxation for an evening, intensification of sexual activities, and a short-lived period of mild euphoria. The user's personality and expectations about the substance's effects and the setting in which the substance is taken also affect the substance-induced experience. The regular use pattern is associated with middle-aged, middle-class persons who usually obtain the substance from a family physician as a prescription for insomnia or anxiety. Abusers of this type may have prescriptions from several physicians, and the pattern of abuse may go undetected until obvious signs of abuse or dependence are noticed by the person's family, coworkers, or physicians.

Intravenous Use.   A severe form of abuse involves the intravenous use of this class of substances. The users are mainly young adults intimately involved with illegal substances. Intravenous barbiturate use is associated with a pleasant, warm, drowsy feeling, and users may be inclined to use barbiturates more than opioids because barbiturates are less costly. The physical dangers of injection include transmission of the human immunodeficiency virus (HIV), cellulitis, vascular complications from accidental injection into an artery, infections, and allergic reactions to contaminants. Intravenous use is associated with rapid and profound tolerance and dependence and a severe withdrawal syndrome.

Overdose

Benzodiazepines.   In contrast to the barbiturates and the barbiturate-like substances, the benzodiazepines have a large margin of safety when taken in overdoses, a feature that has contributed significantly to their rapid acceptance. The ratio of lethal dose to effective dose is about 200 to 1 or higher because of the minimal degree of respiratory depression associated with the benzodiazepines. Even when grossly excessive amounts (more than 2 g) are taken in suicide attempts, the symptoms include only drowsiness, lethargy, ataxia, some confusion, and mild depression of the user's vital signs. A much more serious condition prevails when benzodiazepines are taken in overdose in combination with other sedative-hypnotic substances, such as alcohol. In such cases, small doses of benzodiazepines can cause death. The availability of flumazenil (Romazicon), a specific benzodiazepine antagonist, has reduced the lethality of the benzodiazepines. Flumazenil can be used in emergency rooms to reverse the effects of the benzodiazepines.

Barbiturates.   Barbiturates are lethal when taken in overdose because they induce respiratory depression. In addition to intentional suicide attempts, accidental or unintentional overdoses are common. Barbiturates in home medicine cabinets are a common cause of fatal drug overdoses in children. As with benzodiazepines, the lethal effects of the barbiturates are additive to those of other sedatives or hypnotics, including alcohol and benzodiazepines. Barbiturate overdose is characterized by the induction of coma, respiratory arrest, cardiovascular failure, and death.

The lethal dose varies with the route of administration and the degree of tolerance for the substance after a history of long-term abuse. For the most commonly abused barbiturates, the ratio of lethal dose to effective dose ranges between 3 to 1 and 30 to 1.

Dependent users often take an average daily dose of 1.5 g of a short-acting barbiturate, and some have been reported to take as much as 2.5 g a day for months.

The lethal dose is not much greater for the long-term abuser than for the neophyte. Tolerance develops quickly to the point at which withdrawal in a hospital becomes necessary to prevent accidental death from overdose.

Barbiturate-Like Substances.   The barbiturate-like substances vary in their lethality and are usually intermediate between the relative safety of the benzodiazepines and the high lethality of the barbiturates. An overdose of methaqualone, for example, can result in restlessness, delirium, hypertonia, muscle spasms, convulsions, and, in very high doses, death. Unlike barbiturates, methaqualone rarely causes severe cardiovascular or respiratory depression, and most fatalities result from combining methaqualone with alcohol.

TREATMENT AND REHABILITATION

Withdrawal

Benzodiazepines.   Because some benzodiazepines are eliminated from the body slowly, symptoms of withdrawal can continue to develop for several weeks. To prevent seizures and other withdrawal symptoms, clinicians should gradually reduce the dosage. Several reports indicate that carbamazepine (Tegretol) may be useful in the treatment of benzodiazepine withdrawal.

Barbiturates.   To avoid sudden death during barbiturate withdrawal, clinicians must follow conservative clinical guidelines. Clinicians should not give barbiturates to a comatose or grossly intoxicated patient. A clinician should attempt to determine a patient's usual daily dose of barbiturates and then verify the dose clinically. For example, a clinician can give a test dose of 200 mg of pentobarbital every hour until a mild intoxication occurs but withdrawal symptoms are absent. The clinician can then taper the total daily dose at a rate of about 10 percent of the total daily dose. Once the correct dose is determined, a long-acting barbiturate can be used for the detoxification period. During this process, the patient may begin to experience withdrawal symptoms, in which case the clinician should halve the daily decrement.

In the withdrawal procedure, phenobarbital can be substituted for the more commonly abused short-acting barbiturates. The effects of phenobarbital last longer, and because barbiturate blood levels fluctuate less, phenobarbital does not cause observable toxic signs or a serious overdose. An adequate dose is 30 mg of phenobarbital for every 100 mg of the short-acting substance. The user should be maintained for at least 2 days at that level before the dose is reduced further. The regimen is analogous to the substitution of methadone for heroin.

After withdrawal is complete, the patient must overcome the desire to start taking the substance again. Although substitution of nonbarbiturate sedatives or hypnotics for barbiturates has been suggested as a preventive therapeutic measure, this often results in replacing one substance dependence with another. If a user is to remain substance free, follow-up treatment, usually with psychiatric help and community support, is vital. Otherwise, a patient will almost certainly return to barbiturates or a substance with similar hazards.

Overdose

The treatment of overdose of this class of substances involves gastric lavage, activated charcoal, and careful monitoring of vital signs and central nervous system (CNS) activity. Patients who overdose and come to medical attention while awake should be kept from slipping into unconsciousness. Vomiting should be induced, and activated charcoal should be administered to delay gastric absorption. If a patient is comatose, the clinician must establish an intravenous fluid line, monitor the patient's vital signs, insert an endotracheal tube to maintain a patent airway, and provide mechanical ventilation, if necessary. Hospitalization of a comatose patient in an intensive care unit is usually required during the early stages of recovery from such overdoses.

▲ 9.13 Anabolic-Androgenic Steroid Abuse

Anabolic steroids are a family of drugs composed of the natural male hormone testosterone and a group of more than 50 synthetic analogs of testosterone synthesized over the last 60 years. These drugs all exhibit various degrees of anabolic (muscle building) and androgenic (masculinizing) effects. It is important not to confuse the anabolic-androgenic steroids (AAS) (testosterone-like hormones) with corticosteroids (cortisol-like hormones such as hydrocortisone and prednisone). Corticosteroids have no muscle-building properties and, hence, little abuse potential; they are widely prescribed to treat numerous inflammatory conditions such as poison ivy or asthma. AAS, by contrast, have only limited legitimate medical applications, such as in the treatment of hypogonadal men, the wasting syndrome associated with human immunodeficiency virus (HIV) infection, and a few specific diseases such as hereditary angioedema and Fanconi's anemia. AAS, however, are widely used illicitly, especially by boys and young men seeking to gain increased muscle mass and strength, either for athletic purposes or simply to improve personal appearance.

EPIDEMIOLOGY

Use of AAS is widespread among men in the United States, but is much less frequent among women. Approximately 890,000 American men and approximately 190,000 American women reported having used AAS at some time during their lives. Approximately 286,000 men and 26,000 women are estimated to use steroids each year. Among this number, nearly one third, or 98,000, were between 12 and 17 years of age. Various studies of high school students in the United States have produced even higher estimates of the prevalence of anabolic steroid use among adolescents. Across studies of high school students, it is estimated that 3 to 12 percent of males and 0.5 to 2.0 percent of females have used AAS during their lifetimes.

The current high rates of steroid use among younger individuals appear to represent an important shift in the epidemiology of steroid use. In the 1970s, use of these drugs was largely confined to competition bodybuilders, other elite weight-training athletes, and elite athletes in other sports. Since then, however, it appears that an increasing number of young men, and occasionally even young women, may be using these drugs purely to enhance personal appearance rather than for any athletic purpose.

PHARMACOLOGY

All steroid drugs—including AAS, estrogens, and corticosteroids—are synthesized in vivo from cholesterol and resemble cholesterol in their chemical structure. Testosterone has a four-ring chemical structure containing 19 carbon atoms.

Normal testosterone plasma concentrations for men range from 300 to 1,000 ng/dL. Generally, 200 mg of testosterone cypionate taken every 2 weeks restores physiological testosterone concentrations in a hypogonadal male. A eugonadal male who initiates physiological doses of testosterone has no net gain in testosterone concentrations because exogenously administered AAS shut down endogenous testosterone production via feedback inhibition of the hypothalamic-pituitary-gonadal axis. Consequently, illicit users take higher-than-therapeutic dosages to achieve supraphysiological effects. The dose–response curve for anabolic effects may be logarithmic, which could explain why illicit users generally take 10 to 100 times the therapeutic doses. Doses in this range are most easily achieved by taking combinations of oral and injected AAS, which illicit AAS users often do. Transdermal testosterone, available by prescription for testosterone replacement therapy, may also be used.

Therapeutic Indications

The AAS are primarily indicated for testosterone deficiency (male hypogonadism), hereditary angioedema (a congenital skin disorder), and some uncommon forms of anemia caused by bone marrow or renal failure. In women, they are given, although not as first-choice agents, for metastatic breast cancer, osteoporosis, endometriosis, and adjunctive treatment of menopausal symptoms. In men, they have been used experimentally as a male contraceptive and for treating major depressive disorder and sexual disorders in eugonadal men. Recently, they have been used to treat wasting syndromes associated with acquired immune deficiency syndrome (AIDS). Controlled studies have also suggested that testosterone has antidepressant effects in some men infected with HIV with major depressive disorder, and it is also a supplementary (augmentation) treatment in some depressed men with low endogenous testosterone levels who are refractory to conventional antidepressants.

Adverse Reactions

The most common adverse medical effects of AAS involve the cardiovascular, hepatic, reproductive, and dermatological systems.

The AAS produce an adverse cholesterol profile by increasing levels of low-density-lipoprotein cholesterol and decreasing levels of high-density-lipoprotein cholesterol. High-dose use of AAS can also activate hemostasis and increase blood pressure. Isolated case reports of myocardial infarction, cardiomyopathy,

left ventricular hypertrophy, and stroke among users of AAS, including fatalities, have appeared,

Among the AAS-induced endocrine effects in men are testicular atrophy and sterility, both usually reversible after discontinuing AAS, and gynecomastia, which may persist until surgical removal. In women, shrinkage of breast tissue, irregular menses (diminution or cessation), and masculinization (clitoral hypertrophy, hirsutism, and deepened voice) can occur. Masculinizing effects in women may be irreversible. Androgens taken during pregnancy could cause masculinization of a female fetus. Dermatological effects include acne and male pattern baldness. Abuse of AAS by children has led to concerns that AAS-induced premature closure of bony epiphyses could cause shortened stature. Other uncommon adverse effects include edema of the extremities caused by water retention, exacerbation of tic disorders, sleep apnea, and polycythemia.

ETIOLOGY

The major reason for taking illicit AAS is to enhance either athletic performance or physical appearance. Taking AAS is reinforced because they can produce the athletic and physical effects that users desire, especially when combined with proper diet and training. Further reinforcement derives from winning competitions and from social admiration for physical appearance. AAS users also perceive that they can train more intensively for longer durations with less fatigue and with decreased recovery times between workouts.

Although the anabolic or muscle-building properties of AAS are clearly important to those seeking to enhance athletic performance and physical appearance, psychoactive effects may also be important in the persistent and dependent use of AAS. Anecdotally, some AAS users report feelings of power, aggressiveness, and euphoria, which become associated with, and can, reinforce AAS taking.

In general, males are more likely to take AAS than females, and athletes are more likely to take AAS than nonathletes. Some male and female weight lifters may have muscle dysmorphia, a form of body dysmorphic disorder in which the individual feels that he or she is not sufficiently muscular and lean.

DIAGNOSIS AND CLINICAL FEATURES

Steroids may initially induce euphoria and hyperactivity. After relatively short periods, however, their use can become associated with increased anger, arousal, irritability, hostility, anxiety, somatization, and depression (especially during times when steroids are not used). Several studies have demonstrated that 2 to 15 percent of anabolic steroid abusers experience hypomanic or manic episodes, and a smaller percentage may have clearly psychotic symptoms. Also disturbing is a correlation between steroid abuse and violence ("roid rage" in the parlance of users). Steroid abusers with no record of antisocial behavior or violence have committed murders and other violent crimes.

Steroids are addictive substances. When abusers stop taking steroids, they can become depressed, anxious, and concerned about their bodies' physical state. Some similarities have been noted between athletes' views of their muscles and the views of patients with anorexia nervosa about their bodies; to an observer, both groups seem to distort realistic assessment of the body.

Iatrogenic addiction is a consideration in view of the increasing number of geriatric patients who are receiving testosterone from their physicians in an attempt to increase libido and reverse some aspects of aging.

TREATMENT

Abstinence is the treatment goal of choice for patients manifesting AAS abuse or dependence. To the extent that users of AAS abuse other addictive substances (including alcohol), traditional treatment approaches for substance-related disorders may be used. Nevertheless, AAS users may differ from other addicted patients in several ways that have implications for treatment. First, the euphorigenic and reinforcing effects of AAS may only become apparent after weeks or months of use in conjunction with intensive exercising. When compared with immediately and passively reinforcing drugs, such as cocaine, heroin, and alcohol, AAS use may entail more delayed gratification. Second, AAS users may manifest greater commitment to culturally endorsed values of physical fitness, success, victory, and goal directness than users of other illicit drugs. Finally, AAS users are often preoccupied with their physical attributes and may rely excessively on these attributes for self-esteem. Treatment therefore depends on a therapeutic alliance that is based on a thorough and nonjudgmental understanding of the patient's values and motivations for using AAS.

AAS Withdrawal

Supportive therapy and monitoring are essential for treating AAS withdrawal because suicidal depressions can occur. Hospitalization may be required when suicidal ideation is severe. Patients should be educated about the possible course of withdrawal and reassured that symptoms are time limited and manageable. Antidepressant agents are best reserved for patients whose depressive symptomatology persists for several weeks after AAS discontinuation and who meet criteria for major depressive disorder. Selective serotonin reuptake inhibitors (SSRIs) are the preferred agents because of their favorable adverse effect profile and their effectiveness in the only reported case series of treated AAS users with major depressive disorder. Physical withdrawal symptoms are not life threatening and do not ordinarily require pharmacotherapy. Nonsteroidal antiinflammatory drugs (NSAIDs) may be useful to treat musculoskeletal pain and headaches.

ANABOLIC STEROID–INDUCED MOOD DISORDERS

Irritability, aggressiveness, hypomania, and frank mania associated with anabolic steroid use probably represent the most important public health issues associated with these drugs. Although athletes using these drugs have long recognized that syndromes of anger and irritability could be associated with AAS use, these syndromes were little recognized in the scientific literature until the late 1980s and 1990s. Since then, a series of observational field studies of athletes has suggested that some AAS users develop prominent hypomanic or even manic symptoms during AAS use.

A possible serious consequence of AAS-induced mood disorders may be violent or even homicidal behavior. Several published reports have anecdotally described individuals with no apparent history of psychiatric disorder, no criminal record, and no history of violence who committed violent crimes, including murder, while under the influence of AAS. In a number of cases, AAS use has been cited in criminal trials as a possible mitigating factor in the defense of such individuals. Although a causal link is difficult to establish in these cases, evidence of AAS use has frequently been presented in forensic settings as a possible mitigating factor in criminal behavior.

Depressive syndromes induced by AAS have occurred, and suicide is a risk. A brief and self-limited syndrome of depression occurs on AAS withdrawal, probably as a result of the depression of the hypothalamic-pituitary-gonadal axis after exogenous AAS administration.

ANABOLIC STEROID–INDUCED PSYCHOTIC DISORDER

Psychotic symptoms are rare in association with anabolic steroid use, but they have been described in a few cases, primarily in individuals who were using the equivalent of more than 1,000 mg of testosterone a week. Usually, these symptoms have consisted of grandiose or paranoid delusions, generally occurring in the context of a manic episode, although occasionally occurring in the absence of a frank manic syndrome. In most cases reported, psychotic symptoms have disappeared promptly (within a few weeks) after the discontinuation of the offending agent, although temporary treatment with antipsychotic agents was sometimes required.

ANABOLIC STEROID–RELATED DISORDER NOT OTHERWISE SPECIFIED

Symptoms of anxiety disorders, such as panic disorder and social phobia, can occur during AAS use. AAS use may serve as a gateway to the use of opioid agonist or antagonists, such as nalbuphine, or to use of frank opioid agonists, such as heroin. A study of men admitted for substance dependence treatment in Massachusetts produced similar findings.

DEHYDROEPIANDROSTERONE AND ANDRO-STENEDIONE

Dehydroepiandrosterone (DHEA), a precursor hormone for both estrogens and androgens, is available over the counter. Recent years have seen an interest in DHEA for improving cognition, depression, sex drive, and general well-being in elderly adults. Some reports suggest that DHEA in doses of 50 to 100 mg per day increases the sense of physical and social well-being in women aged 40 to 70 years. Reports also exist of androgenic effects, including irreversible hirsutism, hair loss, voice deepening, and other undesirable sequelae. In addition, DHEA has at least a theoretical potential of enhancing tumor growth in persons with latent, hormone-sensitive malignancies, such as prostate, cervical, and breast cancer. Despite its significant popularity, few controlled data exist on the safety or efficacy of DHEA.

▲ 9.14 Other Substance-Related Disorders

This section deals with a diverse group of drugs not covered in the previous sections that cannot be easily grouped together. The text revision of the fourth edition of *Diagnostic and Statistical Manual of Mental Disorders* (DSM-IV-TR) includes a diagnostic category for these substances called other (or unknown) substance-related disorders (Table 9.14–1). Some of these substances are discussed here.

Table 9.13–1
DSM-IV-TR Criteria for Other (or Unknown) Substance-Related Disorders

The other or (unknown) substance-related disorders category is for classifying substance-related disorders associated with substances not listed above. Examples of these substances, which are described in more detail below, include anabolic steroids, nitrite inhalants ("poppers"), nitrous oxide, over-the-counter and prescription medications not otherwise covered by the 11 categories (e.g., cortisol, antihistamines, benztropine), and other substances that have psychoactive effects. In addition, this category may be used when the specific substance is unknown (e.g., an intoxication after taking a bottle of unlabeled pills).	*Other (or unknown) substance use disorders* **Other (or unknown) substance use dependence** **Other (or unknown) substance abuse** *Other (or unknown) substance-induced disorders* **Other (or unknown) substance intoxication** *Specify* if: With perceptual disturbances **Other (or unknown) substance withdrawal** *Specify* if: With perceptual disturbances **Other (or unknown) substance-induced delirium** **Other (or unknown) substance-induced persisting dementia** **Other (or unknown) substance-induced persisting amnestic disorder** **Other (or unknown) substance psychotic disorder, with delusions** *Specify* if: With onset during intoxication With onset during withdrawal

Anabolic steroids sometimes produce an initial sense of enhanced well-being (or even euphoria), which is replaced after repeated use by lack of energy, irritability, and other forms of dysphoria. Continued use of these substances may lead to more severe symptoms (e.g., depressive symptomatology) and general medical conditions (liver disease).

Nitrite inhalants ("poppers" forms of amyl, butyl, and isobutyl nitrite) produce an intoxication that is characterized by a feeling of fullness in the head, mild euphoria, a change in the perception of time, relaxation of smooth muscles, and a possible increase in sexual feelings. In addition to possible compulsive use, these substances carry dangers of potential impairment of immune functioning, irritation of the respiratory system, a decrease in the oxygen-carrying capacity of the blood, and a toxic reaction that can include vomiting, severe headache, hypotension, and dizziness.

Nitrous Oxide ("laughing gas") causes rapid onset of an intoxication that is characterized by lightheadedness and a floating sensation that clears in a matter of minutes after administration is stopped. There are reports of temporary but clinically relevant confusion and reversible paranoid states when nitrous oxide is used regularly.

Other substances that are capable of producing mild intoxication include **catnip**, which can produce states similar to those observed with marijuana and which in high doses is reported to result in LSD-type perceptions; **betel nut**, which is chewed in many cultures to produce a mild euphoria and floating sensation; and **kava** (a substance derived from the South Pacific pepper plant), which produces sedation, incoordination, weight loss, mild forms of hepatitis, and lung abnormalities. In addition, individuals can develop dependence and impairment through repeated self-administration of **over-the-counter** and **prescription drugs**, including **cortisol, antiparkinsonian agents** that have anticholinergic properties, and **antihistamines.**

Texts and criteria sets have already been provided to define the generic aspects of substance dependence, substance abuse, substance intoxication, and substance withdrawal that are applicable across classes of substances. The other (or unknown) substance-induced disorders are described in the sections of the manual with disorders with which they share phenomenology (e.g., other for unknown); substance-induced mood disorder is included in the mood disorders section. Listed below are the other (or unknown) substance use disorders and the other (or unknown) substance-induced disorders.

Other (or unknown) substance-induced psychotic disorder, with hallucinations
Specify if:
With onset during intoxication
With onset during withdrawal
Other (or unknown) substance-induced mood disorder
Specify if:
With onset during intoxication
With onset during withdrawal
Other (or unknown) substance-induced anxiety disorder
Specify if:
With onset during intoxication
With onset during withdrawal
Other (or unknown) substance-induced sexual dysfunction
Specify if:
With onset during intoxication
Other (or unknown) substance-induced sleep disorder
Specify if:
With onset during intoxication
Other (or unknown) substance-related disorder not otherwise specified

From American Psychiatric Association. *Diagnostic and Statistical Manual of Mental Disorders.* 4th ed. Text rev. Washington, DC: American Psychiatric Association; copyright 2000, with permission.

GAMMA HYDROXYBUTYRATE

Gamma hydroxybutyrate (GHB) is a naturally occurring transmitter in the brain that is related to sleep regulation. GHB increases dopamine levels in the brain. In general, GHB is a central nervous system (CNS) depressant with effects through the endogenous opioid system. It is used to induce anesthesia and long-term sedation, but its unpredictable duration of action limits its use. It has recently been studied for the treatment of alcohol and opioid withdrawal and narcolepsy.

Until 1990, GHB was sold in U.S. health food stores, and body builders used it as a steroid alternative. Reports indicate, however, that GHB is abused for its intoxicating effects and consciousness-altering properties. It is variously referred to as "GBH" and "liquid ecstasy" and is sold illicitly in various forms (e.g., powder and liquid). Similar chemicals, which the body converts to GBH, include γ-butyrolactone (GBL) and 1,4-butanediol. Adverse effects include nausea, vomiting, respiratory problems, seizures, coma, and death. In some reports, GHB abuse has been linked to a syndrome similar to Wernicke-Korsakoff syndrome.

NITRITE INHALANTS

The nitrite inhalants include amyl, butyl, and isobutyl nitrites, all of which are called "poppers" in popular jargon. The intoxication syndromes seen with nitrites can differ markedly from the syndromes seen with the standard inhalant substances, such as lighter fluid and airplane glue. Nitrite inhalants are used by persons seeking the associated mild euphoria, altered sense of time, feeling of fullness in the head, and, possibly, increased sexual feelings. The nitrite compounds are used by some gay men and users of other drugs to heighten sexual stimulation during orgasm and, in some cases, to relax the anal sphincter for penile penetration. Under such circumstances, a person may use the substance for a few or a dozen times within several hours.

Adverse reactions include a toxic syndrome characterized by nausea, vomiting, headache, hypotension, drowsiness, and irritation of the respiratory tract. Some evidence indicates that nitrite inhalants can adversely affect immune function. Because sildenafil (Viagra) and its congeners are lethal when combined with nitrite compounds, persons at risk should be cautioned never to use the two together.

NITROUS OXIDE

Nitrous oxide, commonly known as "laughing gas," is a widely available anesthetic agent that is subject to abuse because of its ability to produce feelings of lightheadedness and of floating, sometimes experienced as pleasurable or specifically as sexual. With long-term abuse patterns, nitrous oxide use has been associated with delirium and paranoia. Female dental assistants exposed to high levels of nitrous oxide have reportedly experienced reduced fertility.

A 35-year-old male dentist with no history of other substance problems complained of problems with nitrous oxide abuse for 10 years. This had begun as experimentation with what he had considered a harmless substance. His rate of use increased over several years, however, eventually becoming almost daily for months at a time. He felt a craving before sessions of use. Then, using the gas while alone in his office, he immediately felt numbness, a change in his temperature and heart rate, and alleviation of depressed feelings. "Things would go through my mind. Time was erased." He sometimes fell asleep. Sessions might last a few minutes or up to 8 hours. They ended when the craving and euphoria ended. He had often tried to stop or cut down, sometimes consulting a professional about the problem.

OTHER SUBSTANCES

Nutmeg.   Nutmeg can be ingested in a number of preparations. When nutmeg is taken in sufficiently high doses, it can induce depersonalization, derealization, and a feeling of heaviness in the limbs. In sufficiently high doses, morning glory seeds can produce a syndrome resembling that seen with lysergic acid diethylamide (LSD), characterized by altered sensory perceptions and mild visual hallucinations.

Catnip.   Catnip can produce cannabis-like intoxication in low doses and LSD-like intoxication in high doses.

Betel Nuts.   Betel nuts, when chewed, can produce a mild euphoria and a feeling of floating in space.

Kava.   Kava, derived from a pepper plant native to the South Pacific, produces sedation and incoordination and is associated with hepatitis, lung abnormalities, and weight loss.

Over-the-Counter Drugs.   Some persons abuse over-the-counter and prescription medications, such as cortisol, antiparkinsonian agents, and antihistamines.

Ephedra.   Ephedra, a natural substance found in herbal tea, acts like epinephrine and, when abused, produces cardiac arrhythmia and fatalities.

Chocolate.   A controversial possible substance of abuse is chocolate derived from the cacao bean. Anandamide, an ingredient in chocolate, stimulates the same receptors as marijuana. Other compounds in chocolate include tryptophan, the precursor of serotonin, and phenylalanine, an amphetamine-like substance, both of which improve mood. So-called chocoholics may be self-medicating because of a depressive diathesis.

POLYSUBSTANCE-RELATED DISORDER

Substance users often abuse more than one substance. In DSM-IV-TR, a diagnosis of polysubstance dependence is appropriate if, for a period of at least 12 months, a person has repeatedly used substances from at least three categories (not including nicotine and caffeine), even if the diagnostic criteria for a substance-related disorder are not met for any single substance, as long as, during this period, the criteria for substance dependence have been met for the substances considered as a group (Table 9.14–2).

    Table 9.14–2
DSM-IV-TR Criteria for Polysubstance Dependence

This diagnosis is reserved for behavior during the same 12-month period in which the person was repeatedly using at least three groups of substances (not including caffeine and nicotine), but no single substance has predominated. Further, during this period, the dependence criteria were met for substances as a group but not for any specific substance.

From American Psychiatric Association. *Diagnostic and Statistical Manual of Mental Disorders.* 4th ed. Text rev. Washington, DC: American Psychiatric Association; copyright 2000, with permission.

TREATMENT AND REHABILITATION

Treatment approaches for the substances covered in this section vary according to substances, patterns of abuse, availability of psychosocial support systems, and patients' individual features. Two major treatment goals for substance abuse have been determined: the first is abstinence from the substance, and the second is the physical, psychiatric, and psychosocial well-being of the patient. Significant damage has often been done to a patient's support systems during prolonged periods of substance abuse. For a patient to stop a pattern of substance abuse successfully, adequate psychosocial supports must be in place to foster the difficult change in behavior.

In some rare cases, it may be necessary to initiate treatment on an inpatient unit. Although an outpatient setting is more desirable than an inpatient setting, the temptations available to an outpatient for repeated use may present too high a hurdle for the initiation of treatment. Inpatient treatment is also indicated in the case of severe medical or psychiatric symptoms, a history of failed outpatient treatments, a lack of psychosocial supports, or a particularly severe or long-term history of substance abuse. After an initial period of detoxification, patients need a sustained period of rehabilitation. Throughout treatment, individual, family, and group therapies can be effective. Education about substance abuse and support for patients' efforts are essential factors in treatment.

Schizophrenia is a clinical syndrome of variable but profoundly disruptive psychopathology that involves cognition, emotion, perception, and other aspects of behavior. The expression of these manifestations varies across patients and over time, but the effect of the illness is always severe and is usually long lasting. The disorder usually begins before age 25 years, persists throughout life, and affects persons of all social classes. Both patients and their families often suffer from poor care and social ostracism because of widespread ignorance about the disorder. Although schizophrenia is discussed as if it is a single disease, it probably comprises a group of disorders with heterogeneous etiologies, and it includes patients whose clinical presentations, treatment response, and courses of illness vary. Clinicians should appreciate that the diagnosis of schizophrenia is based entirely on the psychiatric history and mental status examination. There is no laboratory test for schizophrenia.

HISTORY

Written descriptions of symptoms commonly observed today in patients with schizophrenia are found throughout history. Early Greek physicians described delusions of grandeur, paranoia, and deterioration in cognitive functions and personality. It was not until the 19th century, however, that schizophrenia emerged as a medical condition worthy of study and treatment. Two major figures in psychiatry and neurology who studied the disorder were Emil Kraepelin (1856–1926) and Eugen Bleuler (1857–1939). Earlier, Benedict Morel (1809–1873), a French psychiatrist, had used the term *démence précoce* to describe deteriorated patients whose illness began in adolescence.

Emil Kraepelin

Kraepelin translated Morel's *démence précoce* into dementia precox, a term that emphasized the change in cognition (dementia) and early onset (precox) of the disorder. Patients with dementia precox were described as having a long-term deteriorating course and the clinical symptoms of hallucinations and delusions. Kraepelin distinguished these patients from those who underwent distinct episodes of illness alternating with periods of normal functioning, which he classified as having manic-depressive psychosis. Another condition, called *paranoia*, was characterized by persistent persecutory delusions. These patients lacked the deteriorating course of dementia precox and the intermittent symptoms of manic-depressive psychosis.

Eugen Bleuler

Bleuler coined the term *schizophrenia*, which replaced dementia precox in the literature. He chose the term to express the presence of schisms between thought, emotion, and behavior in patients with the disorder.

Bleuler stressed that, unlike Kraepelin's concept of dementia precox, schizophrenia need not have a deteriorating course. This term is often misconstrued, especially by lay people, to mean split personality. Split personality, called dissociative identity disorder in the text revision of the fourth edition of *Diagnostic and Statistical Manual of Mental Disorders* (DSM-IV-TR), differs completely from schizophrenia (see Chapter 16).

The Four As. Bleuler identified specific fundamental (or primary) symptoms of schizophrenia to develop his theory about the internal mental schisms of patients. These symptoms included associational disturbances of thought, especially looseness, affective disturbances, autism, and ambivalence, summarized as the four As: associations, affect, autism, and ambivalence. Bleuler also identified accessory (secondary) symptoms, which included those symptoms that Kraepelin saw as major indicators of dementia precox: hallucinations and delusions.

Other Theorists

Ernst Kretschmer (1888–1926).
Kretschmer compiled data to support the idea that schizophrenia occurred more often among persons with asthenic (i.e., slender, lightly muscled physiques), athletic, or dysplastic body types rather than among persons with pyknic (i.e., short, stocky physiques) body types. He thought the latter were more likely to incur bipolar disorders. His observations may seem strange, but they are not inconsistent with a superficial impression of the body types in many persons with schizophrenia.

Kurt Schneider (1887–1967).
Schneider contributed a description of first-rank symptoms (e.g., hallucinations, delusions), which, he stressed, were not specific for schizophrenia and were not to be rigidly applied but were useful for making diagnoses. He emphasized that in patients who showed no first-rank symptoms, the disorder could be diagnosed exclusively on the basis of second-rank symptoms and an otherwise typical clinical appearance. Clinicians frequently ignore his warnings and sometimes see the absence of first-rank symptoms during a single interview as evidence that a person does not have schizophrenia.

Karl Jaspers (1883–1969).
Jaspers, a psychiatrist and philosopher, played a major role in developing existential psychoanalysis. He was interested in the phenomenology of mental illness and the subjective feelings of patients with mental illness. His work paved the way toward trying to understand the psychological meaning of schizophrenic signs and symptoms such as delusions and hallucinations.

Adolf Meyer (1866–1950).
Meyer, the founder of psychobiology, saw schizophrenia as a reaction to life stresses. It was a maladaptation that was understandable in terms of the patient's life experiences. Meyer's view was represented in the nomenclature of the 1950s, which referred to the schizophrenic reaction. In later editions of DSM the term reaction was dropped.

EPIDEMIOLOGY

In the United States, the lifetime prevalence of schizophrenia is about 1 percent, which means that about 1 person in 100 will develop schizophrenia during his or her lifetime. The Epidemiologic Catchment Area (ECA) study sponsored by the National Institute of Mental Health reported a lifetime prevalence of 0.6 to 1.9 percent. According to DSM-IV-TR, the annual incidence of schizophrenia ranges from 0.5 to 5.0 per 10,000, with some geographic variation (e.g., the incidence is higher for persons born in urban areas of industrialized nations). Schizophrenia is found in all societies and geographical areas, and incidence and prevalence rates are roughly equal worldwide. In the United States about 0.05 percent of the total population is treated for schizophrenia in any single year, and only about half of all patients with schizophrenia obtain treatment, in spite of the severity of the disorder.

Gender and Age

Schizophrenia is equally prevalent in men and women. The two genders differ, however, in the onset and course of illness. Onset is earlier in men than in women. More than one half of all male schizophrenia patients but only one third of all female schizophrenia patients are first admitted to a psychiatric hospital before age 25 years. The peak ages of onset are 10 to 25 years for men and 25 to 35 years for women. Unlike men, women display a bimodal age distribution, with a second peak occurring in middle age. Approximately 3 to 10 percent of women with schizophrenia present with disease onset after age 40 years. About 90 percent of patients in treatment for schizophrenia are between 15 and 55 years old. Onset of schizophrenia before age 10 years or after age 60 years is extremely rare. Some studies have indicated that men are more likely to be impaired by negative symptoms (described in what follows) than are women and that women are more likely to have better social functioning than are men prior to disease onset. In general, the outcome for female schizophrenia patients is better than that for male schizophrenia patients. When onset occurs after age 45 years, the disorder is characterized as late-onset schizophrenia.

Reproductive Factors

The use of psychopharmacologic drugs, open-door policies in hospitals, deinstitutionalization in state hospitals, emphasis on rehabilitation, and community-based care for patients have all led to an increase in the marriage and fertility rates among persons with schizophrenia. Because of these factors, the number of children born to parents with schizophrenia is continually increasing. The fertility rate for persons with schizophrenia is close to that for the general population. First-degree biological relatives of persons with schizophrenia have a ten-times-greater risk for developing the disease than the general population.

Medical Illness

Persons with schizophrenia have a higher mortality rate from accidents and natural causes than the general population. Institution- or treatment-related variables do not explain the increased mortality rate, but the higher rate may be related to the fact that the diagnosis and treatment of medical and surgical conditions in schizophrenia patients can be clinical challenges. Several studies have shown that up to 80 percent of all schizophrenia patients have significant concurrent medical illnesses and that up to 50 percent of these conditions may be undiagnosed.

Infection and Birth Season

Persons who develop schizophrenia are more likely to have been born in the winter and early spring and less likely to have been born in late spring and summer. In the Northern Hemisphere, including the United States, persons with schizophrenia are more often born in the months from January to April. In the Southern Hemisphere, persons with schizophrenia are more often born in the months from July to September. Season-specific risk factors, such as a virus or a seasonal change in diet, may be operative. Another hypothesis is that persons with a genetic predisposition for schizophrenia have a decreased biological advantage to survive season-specific insults.

Studies have pointed to gestational and birth complications, exposure to influenza epidemics or maternal starvation during pregnancy, Rhesus factor incompatibility, and an excess of winter births in the etiology of schizophrenia. The nature of these factors suggests a neurodevelopmental pathological process in schizophrenia, but the exact pathophysiological mechanism associated with these risk factors is not known.

Evidence that prenatal malnutrition may play a role in schizophrenia was derived from the studies of the Dutch "Hunger Winter" of 1944 to 1945. Severe caloric restriction in the western Netherlands was associated with substantially decreased fertility, increased mortality, and diminished birthweight. Unlike most other famines, it was time limited, and the extent and timing of caloric restriction and psychiatric outcomes were well documented. Exposure to the peak of the famine during the periconceptional period was associated with a significant, twofold increased risk of schizophrenia. In a subsequent study, this cohort exposed to famine in early gestation also showed an increase in risk of schizoid personality disorders.

Epidemiological data show a high incidence of schizophrenia after prenatal exposure to influenza during several epidemics of the disease. Some studies show that the frequency of schizophrenia is increased following exposure to influenza—which occurs in the winter—during the second trimester of pregnancy. Other data supporting a viral hypothesis are an increased number of physical anomalies at birth, an increased rate of pregnancy and birth complications, seasonality of birth consistent with viral infection, geographical clusters of adult cases, and seasonality of hospitalizations.

Viral theories stem from the fact that several specific such theories have the power to explain the particular localization of pathology necessary to account for a range of manifestations in schizophrenia without overt febrile encephalitis.

Substance Abuse

Substance abuse is common in schizophrenia. The lifetime prevalence of any drug abuse (other than tobacco) is often much greater than 50 percent. For all drugs of abuse (other than tobacco), abuse is associated with poorer function. In one population-based study, the lifetime prevalence of alcohol within schizophrenia was 40 percent. Alcohol abuse increases risk of hospitalization and, in some patients, may increase psychotic symptoms. People with schizophrenia have an increased prevalence of abuse of common street drugs. There has been particular interest in the association between cannabis and schizophrenia. Those reporting high levels of cannabis use (more than 50 occasions) were at sixfold-increased risk of schizophrenia compared to nonusers. The use of amphetamines, cocaine, and similar drugs should raise particular concern because of their marked ability to increase psychotic symptoms.

Nicotine.

Up to 90 percent of schizophrenic patients may be dependent on nicotine. Apart from smoking-associated mortality, nicotine decreases the blood concentrations of some antipsychotics. There are suggestions that the increased prevalence in smoking is due, at least in part, to brain abnormalities in nicotinic receptors. A specific polymorphism in a nicotinic receptor has been linked to genetic risk for schizophrenia. Nicotine administration appears to improve some cognitive impairments and parkinsonism in schizophrenia, possibly because of nicotine-dependent activation of dopamine neurons. Recent studies have also demonstrated that nicotine may decrease positive symptoms such as hallucinations in schizophrenia patients by its effect on nicotine receptors in the brain that reduce the perception of outside stimuli, especially noise. In that sense, smoking is a form of self-medication.

Population Density

The prevalence of schizophrenia has been correlated with local population density in cities with populations of more than 1 million people. The correlation is weaker in cities of 100,000 to 500,000 people and is absent in cities with fewer than 10,000 people. The effect of population density is consistent with the observation that the incidence of schizophrenia in children of either one or two parents with schizophrenia is twice as high in cities as in rural communities. These observations suggest that social stressors in urban settings may affect the development of schizophrenia in persons at risk.

Socioeconomic and Cultural Factors

Economics.

Because schizophrenia begins early in life, causes significant and long-lasting impairments, makes heavy demands for hospital care, and requires ongoing clinical care, rehabilitation, and support services, the financial cost of the illness in the United States is estimated to exceed that of all cancers combined. The locus of care has shifted dramatically over the last 50 years from long-term hospital-based care to acute hospital care and community-based services. In 1955, approximately 500,000 hospital beds in the United States were occupied by the mentally ill—the majority of these with a diagnosis of schizophrenia. The figure is now less than 250,000 hospital beds. Deinstitutionalization has dramatically reduced the number of beds in custodial facilities, but an overall evaluation of its consequences is disheartening. Many patients have simply been transferred to alternative forms of custodial care (in contrast to treatment or rehabilitative services), including nursing home care and poorly supervised shelter arrangements. Patients with a diagnosis of schizophrenia are reported to account for 15 to 45 percent of homeless Americans.

Hospitalization.

As mentioned previously, the development of effective antipsychotic drugs and changes in political and popular attitudes toward the treatment and the rights of persons who are mentally ill have dramatically changed the patterns of hospitalization for schizophrenia patients since the mid-1950s. Even with antipsychotic medication, however, the probability of readmission within 2 years after discharge from the first hospitalization is about 40 to 60 percent. Patients with schizophrenia occupy about 50 percent of all mental-hospital beds and account for about 16 percent of all psychiatric patients who receive any treatment.

ETIOLOGY

Genetic Factors

There is a genetic contribution to some, perhaps all, forms of schizophrenia, and a high proportion of the variance in liability to schizophrenia is due to additive genetic effects. For example, schizophrenia and schizophrenia-related disorders (e.g., schizotypal, schizoid, and paranoid personality disorders) occur at an increased rate among the biological relatives of patients with schizophrenia. The likelihood of a person's having schizophrenia is correlated with the closeness of the relationship to an affected relative (e.g., first-degree or second-degree relative). In the case of monozygotic twins, who have identical genetic endowment, there is an approximately 50 percent concordance rate for schizophrenia. This rate is four to five times the concordance rate in dizygotic twins or the rate of occurrence found in other first-degree relatives (i.e., siblings, parents, or offspring). The role of genetic factors is further reflected in the drop-off in the occurrence of schizophrenia among second- and third-degree relatives, in whom one would hypothesize a decreased genetic loading. The finding of a higher rate of schizophrenia among the biological relatives of an adopted-away person who develops schizophrenia, as compared to the adoptive, nonbiological relatives who rear the patient, provides further support to the genetic contribution in the etiology of schizophrenia. Nevertheless, the monozygotic twin data clearly demonstrate the fact that individuals who are genetically vulnerable to schizophrenia do not inevitably develop schizophrenia; other factors (e.g., environment) must be involved in determining a schizophrenia outcome. If a vulnerability-liability model of schizophrenia is correct in its postulation of an environmental influence, then other biological or psychosocial environment factors may prevent or cause schizophrenia in the genetically vulnerable individual.

There is robust data indicating that the age of the father has a direct correlation with the development of schizophrenia. In studies of schizophrenic patients with no history of illness in either the maternal or paternal line, it was found that those born from fathers older the age of 60 years were vulnerable to developing the disorder. Presumably spermatogenesis in older men is subject to greater epigenetic damage than that in younger men.

The modes of genetic transmission in schizophrenia are unknown, but several genes appear to make a contribution to schizophrenia vulnerability. Linkage and association genetic studies have provided strong evidence for nine linkage sites: 1q, 5q, 6p, 6q, 8p, 10p, 13q, 15q, and 22q. Further analyses of these chromosomal sites have led to the identification of specific candidate genes, and the best current candidates are

α7 nicotinic receptor, *DISC 1, GRM 3, COMT, NRG 1, RGS 4*, and *G*72. Recently, mutations of the genes dystrobrevin (DTNBP1) and neureglin 1 have been found to be associated with negative features of schizophrenia.

Biochemical Factors

Dopamine Hypothesis. The simplest formulation of the dopamine hypothesis of schizophrenia posits that schizophrenia results from too much dopaminergic activity. The theory evolved from two observations. First, the efficacy and the potency of many antipsychotic drugs (i.e., the dopamine receptor antagonists [DRAs]) are correlated with their ability to act as antagonists of the dopamine type 2 (D_2) receptor. Second, drugs that increase dopaminergic activity, notably cocaine and amphetamine, are psychotomimetic. The basic theory does not elaborate on whether the dopaminergic hyperactivity is due to too much release of dopamine, too many dopamine receptors, hypersensitivity of the dopamine receptors to dopamine, or a combination of these mechanisms. Which dopamine tracts in the brain are involved is also not specified in the theory, although the mesocortical and mesolimbic tracts are most often implicated. The dopaminergic neurons in these tracts project from their cell bodies in the midbrain to dopaminoceptive neurons in the limbic system and the cerebral cortex.

Excessive dopamine release in patients with schizophrenia has been linked to the severity of positive psychotic symptoms. Positron emission tomography studies of dopamine receptors document an increase in D_2 receptors in the caudate nucleus of drug-free patients with schizophrenia. There have also been reports of increased dopamine concentration in the amygdala, decreased density of the dopamine transporter, and increased numbers of dopamine type 4 receptors in the entorhinal cortex.

Serotonin. Current hypotheses posit serotonin excess as a cause of positive and negative symptoms in schizophrenia. The robust serotonin antagonist activity of clozapine and other second-generation antipsychotics, coupled with the effectiveness of clozapine in decreasing positive symptoms in chronic patients, has contributed to the credibility of this proposition.

Norepinephrine. Anhedonia—the impaired capacity for emotional gratification and the decreased ability to experience pleasure—has long been noted to be a prominent feature of schizophrenia. A selective neuronal degeneration within the norepinephrine reward neural system could account for this aspect of schizophrenic symptomatology. However, biochemical and pharmacological data bearing on this proposal are inconclusive.

GABA. The inhibitory amino acid neurotransmitter γ-aminobutyric acid (GABA) has been implicated in the pathophysiology of schizophrenia based on the finding that some patients with schizophrenia have a loss of GABAergic neurons in the hippocampus. GABA has a regulatory effect on dopamine activity, and the loss of inhibitory GABAergic neurons could lead to the hyperactivity of dopaminergic neurons.

Neuropeptides. Neuropeptides, such as substance P and neurotensin, are localized with the catecholamine and indolamine neurotransmitters and influence the action of these neurotransmitters. Alteration in neuropeptide mechanisms could facilitate, inhibit, or otherwise alter the pattern of firing these neuronal systems.

Glutamate. Glutamate has been implicated because ingestion of phencyclidine (PCP), a glutamate antagonist, produces an acute syndrome similar to schizophrenia. The hypotheses proposed about glutamate include those of hyperactivity, hypoactivity, and glutamate-induced neurotoxicity. New drugs are in development that influence glutamate.

Acetylcholine and Nicotine. Postmortem studies in schizophrenia have demonstrated decreased muscarinic and nicotinic receptors in the caudate-putamen, hippocampus, and selected regions of the prefrontal cortex. These receptors play a role in the regulation of neurotransmitter systems involved in cognition, which is impaired in schizophrenia.

Neuropathology

In the 19th century, neuropathologists failed to find a neuropathological basis for schizophrenia, and thus they classified schizophrenia as a functional disorder. By the end of the 20th century, however, researchers had made significant strides in revealing a potential neuropathological basis for schizophrenia, primarily in the limbic system and the basal ganglia, including neuropathological or neurochemical abnormalities in the cerebral cortex, the thalamus, and the brainstem. The loss of brain volume widely reported in schizophrenic brains appears to result from reduced density of the axons, dendrites, and synapses that mediate associative functions of the brain. Synaptic density is highest at age 1 year, then is pared down to adult values in early adolescence. One theory, based in part on the observation that patients often develop schizophrenic symptoms during adolescence, holds that schizophrenia results from excessive pruning of synapses during this phase of development.

Cerebral Ventricles. Computed tomography (CT) scans of patients with schizophrenia have consistently shown lateral and third ventricular enlargement and some reduction in cortical volume. Reduced volumes of cortical gray matter have been demonstrated during the earliest stages of the disease. Several investigators have attempted to determine whether the abnormalities detected by CT are progressive or static. Some studies have concluded that the lesions observed on CT scan are present at the onset of the illness and do not progress. Other studies, however, have concluded that the pathological process visualized on CT scan continues to progress during the illness. Thus, whether an active pathological process is continuing to evolve in schizophrenia patients is uncertain.

Reduced Symmetry. There is a reduced symmetry in several brain areas in schizophrenia, including the temporal, frontal, and occipital lobes. This reduced symmetry is believed by some investigators to originate during fetal life and to be indicative of a disruption in brain lateralization during neurodevelopment.

Limbic System. Because of its role in controlling emotions, the limbic system has been hypothesized to be involved in the pathophysiology of schizophrenia. Studies of postmortem brain samples from schizophrenic patients have shown a decrease in the size of the region including the amygdala, the hippocampus, and the parahippocampal gyrus. This neuropathological finding agrees with the observation made by magnetic resonance imaging studies of patients with schizophrenia. The hippocampus is not only smaller in size in schizophrenia, but it is also functionally abnormal as indicated by disturbances in glutamate transmission. Disorganization of the neurons within the hippocampus of schizophrenia patients has also been reported.

Prefrontal Cortex.   There is considerable evidence from post-mortem brain studies that supports anatomical abnormalities in the prefrontal cortex in schizophrenia. Functional deficits in the prefrontal brain imaging region have also been demonstrated. It has long been noted that several symptoms of schizophrenia mimic those found in persons with prefrontal lobotomies or *frontal lobe syndromes*.

Thalamus.   Some studies of the thalamus show evidence of volume shrinkage or neuronal loss, in particular subnuclei. The medial dorsal nucleus of the thalamus, which has reciprocal connections with the prefrontal cortex, has been reported to contain a reduced number of neurons. The total number of neurons, oligodendrocytes, and astrocytes is reduced by 30 to 45 percent in schizophrenic subjects. This putative finding does not appear to be due to the effects of antipsychotic drugs, because the volume of the thalamus is similar in size between schizophrenics treated chronically with medication and neuroleptic-naive subjects.

Basal Ganglia and Cerebellum.   The basal ganglia and cerebellum have been of theoretical interest in schizophrenia for at least two reasons. First, many patients with schizophrenia show odd movements, even in the absence of medication-induced movement disorders (e.g., tardive dyskinesia). The odd movements can include an awkward gait, facial grimacing, and stereotypies. Because the basal ganglia and cerebellum are involved in the control of movement, disease in these areas is implicated in the pathophysiology of schizophrenia. Second, the movement disorders involving the basal ganglia (e.g., Huntington's disease, Parkinson's disease) are the ones most commonly associated with psychosis. Neuropathological studies of the basal ganglia have produced variable and inconclusive reports about cell loss or the reduction of volume of the globus pallidus and the substantia nigra. Studies have also shown an increase in the number of D_2 receptors in the caudate, the putamen, and the nucleus accumbens. The question remains, however, whether the increase is secondary to the patient having received antipsychotic medications. Some investigators have begun to study the serotonergic system in the basal ganglia; a role for serotonin in psychotic disorder is suggested by the clinical usefulness of antipsychotic drugs that are serotonin antagonists (e.g., clozapine, risperidone).

Neural Circuits

There has been a gradual evolution from conceptualizing schizophrenia as a disorder that involves discrete areas of the brain to a perspective that views schizophrenia as a disorder of brain neural circuits. For example, as mentioned previously, the basal ganglia and cerebellum are reciprocally connected to the frontal lobes, and the abnormalities in frontal lobe function seen in some brain-imaging studies may be due to disease in either area rather than in the frontal lobes themselves. It is also hypothesized that an early developmental lesion of the dopaminergic tracts to the prefrontal cortex results in the disturbance of prefrontal and limbic system function and leads to the positive and negative symptoms and cognitive impairments observed in patients with schizophrenia.

Brain Metabolism

Studies using magnetic resonance spectroscopy, a technique that measures the concentration of specific molecules in the brain, found that patients with schizophrenia had lower levels of phosphomonoesters and inorganic phosphate and higher levels of phosphodiesters than a control group. Furthermore, concentrations of *N*-acetyl aspartate, a marker of neurons, were lower in the hippocampus and frontal lobes of patients with schizophrenia.

Applied Electrophysiology

Electroencephalographic studies indicate that many schizophrenia patients have abnormal records, increased sensitivity to activation procedures (e.g., frequent spike activity after sleep deprivation), decreased alpha activity, increased theta and delta activity, possibly more epileptiform activity than usual, and possibly more left-sided abnormalities than usual. Schizophrenia patients also exhibit an inability to filter out irrelevant sounds and are extremely sensitive to background noise. The flooding of sound that results makes concentration difficult and may be a factor in the production of auditory hallucinations. This sound sensitivity may be associated with a genetic defect.

Complex Partial Epilepsy.   Schizophrenia-like psychoses have been reported to occur more frequently than expected in patients with complex partial seizures, especially seizures involving the temporal lobes. Factors associated with the development of psychosis in these patients include a left-sided seizure focus, medial temporal location of the lesion, and early onset of seizures. The first-rank symptoms described by Schneider may be similar to symptoms of patients with complex partial epilepsy and may reflect the presence of a temporal lobe disorder when seen in patients with schizophrenia.

Evoked Potentials

A large number of abnormalities in evoked potential among patients with schizophrenia has been described. The P300 has been most studied and is defined as a large, positive evoked-potential wave that occurs about 300 ms after a sensory stimulus is detected. The major source of the P300 wave may be located in the limbic system structures of the medial temporal lobes. In patients with schizophrenia, the P300 has been reported to be statistically smaller than that in comparison groups. Abnormalities in the P300 wave have also been reported to be more common in children who, because they have affected parents, are at high risk for schizophrenia. Whether the characteristics of the P300 represent a state or a trait phenomenon remains controversial. Other evoked potentials reported to be abnormal in patients with schizophrenia are the N100 and the contingent negative variation. The N100 is a negative wave that occurs about 100 ms after a stimulus, and the contingent negative variation is a slowly developing, negative-voltage shift following the presentation of a sensory stimulus that is a warning for an upcoming stimulus. The evoked-potential data have been interpreted as indicating that although patients with schizophrenia are unusually sensitive to a sensory stimulus (larger early evoked potentials), they compensate for the increased sensitivity by blunting the processing of information at higher cortical levels (indicated by smaller late evoked potentials).

Eye Movement Dysfunction

The inability to follow a moving visual target accurately is the defining basis for the disorders of smooth visual pursuit and disinhibition of saccadic eye movements seen in patients with schizophrenia. Eye movement dysfunction may be a trait marker for schizophrenia; it is independent of drug treatment and clinical state and is also seen in first-degree relatives of probands with schizophrenia. Various studies have reported abnormal eye movements in 50 to 85 percent of patients with schizophrenia, compared with about 25 percent in psychiatric patients without schizophrenia and less than 10 percent in non–psychiatrically ill control subjects.

Psychoneuroimmunology

Several immunological abnormalities have been associated with patients who have schizophrenia. The abnormalities include decreased T-cell interleukin-2 production, reduced number and responsiveness of peripheral lymphocytes, abnormal cellular and humoral reactivity to neurons, and the presence of brain-directed (antibrain) antibodies. The data can be interpreted variously as representing the effects of a neurotoxic virus or of an endogenous autoimmune disorder. Most carefully conducted investigations that have searched for evidence of neurotoxic viral infections in schizophrenia have had negative results, although epidemiological data show a high incidence of schizophrenia after prenatal exposure to influenza during several epidemics of the disease. Other data supporting a viral hypothesis are an increased number of physical anomalies at birth, an increased rate of pregnancy and birth complications, seasonality of birth consistent with viral infection, geographical clusters of adult cases, and seasonality of hospitalizations. Nonetheless, the inability to detect genetic evidence of viral infection reduces the significance of all circumstantial data. The possibility of autoimmune brain antibodies has some data to support it; the pathophysiological process, if it exists, however, probably explains only a subset of the population with schizophrenia.

Psychoneuroendocrinology

Many reports describe neuroendocrine differences between groups of patients with schizophrenia and groups of control subjects. For example, results of the dexamethasone-suppression test have been reported to be abnormal in various subgroups of patients with schizophrenia, although the practical or predictive value of the test in schizophrenia has been questioned. One carefully done report, however, has correlated persistent nonsuppression on the dexamethasone-suppression test in schizophrenia with a poor long-term outcome.

Some data suggest decreased concentrations of luteinizing-hormone, follicle-stimulating hormone, perhaps correlated with age of onset and length of illness. Two additional reported abnormalities may be correlated with the presence of negative symptoms: a blunted release of prolactin and growth hormone on gonadotropin-releasing hormone or thyrotropin-releasing hormone stimulation and a blunted release of growth hormone on apomorphine stimulation.

PSYCHOSOCIAL AND PSYCHOANALYTIC THEORIES

If schizophrenia is a disease of the brain, it is likely to parallel diseases of other organs (e.g., myocardial infarctions and diabetes) whose courses are affected by psychosocial stress. Thus, clinicians should consider psychosocial as well as biological factors affecting schizophrenia.

The disorder affects individual patients, each of whom has a unique psychological makeup. Although many psychodynamic theories about the pathogenesis of schizophrenia seem out of date, perceptive clinical observations can help contemporary clinicians understand how the disease may affect a patient's psyche.

Psychoanalytic Theories

Sigmund Freud postulated that schizophrenia resulted from developmental fixations that occurred earlier than those culminating in the development of neuroses. These fixations produce defects in ego development, and Freud postulated that such defects contributed to the symptoms of schizophrenia. Ego disintegration in schizophrenia represents a return to the time when the ego was not yet, or had just begun, to be established. Because the ego affects the interpretation of reality and the control of inner drives, such as sex and aggression, these ego functions are impaired. Thus, intrapsychic conflict arising from the early fixations and the ego

defect, which may have resulted from poor early object relations, fuel the psychotic symptoms.

As described by Margaret Mahler, there are distortions in the reciprocal relationship between the infant and the mother. The child is unable to separate from, and progress beyond, the closeness and complete dependence that characterize the mother–child relationship in the oral phase of development. As a result, the person's identity never becomes secure.

Paul Federn hypothesized that the defect in ego functions permits intense hostility and aggression to distort the mother–infant relationship, which leads to eventual personality disorganization and vulnerability to stress. The onset of symptoms during adolescence occurs when teenagers need a strong ego to function independently, to separate from the parents, to identify tasks, to control increased internal drives, and to cope with intense external stimulation.

Harry Stack Sullivan viewed schizophrenia as a disturbance in interpersonal relatedness. The patient's massive anxiety creates a sense of unrelatedness that is transformed into distortions called parataxic distortions, which are usually, but not always, persecutory. To Sullivan, schizophrenia is an adaptive method to avoid panic, terror, and disintegration of the sense of self. The source of pathological anxiety results from cumulative experimental traumas during development.

Psychoanalytic theory also postulates that the various symptoms of schizophrenia have symbolic meaning for individual patients. For example, fantasies of the world coming to an end may indicate a perception that a person's internal world has broken down. Feelings of inferiority are replaced by delusions of grandeur and omnipotence. Hallucinations may be substitutes for patients' inability to deal with objective reality and may represent their inner wishes or fears. Delusions, like hallucinations, are regressive, restitutive attempts to create a new reality or to express hidden fears or impulses.

Regardless of the theoretical model, all psychodynamic approaches are founded on the premise that psychotic symptoms have meaning in schizophrenia. Patients, for example, may become grandiose after an injury to their self-esteem. Similarly, all theories recognize that human relatedness may be terrifying for persons with schizophrenia. Although research on the efficacy of psychotherapy with schizophrenia shows mixed results, concerned persons who offer compassion and a sanctuary in the confusing world of the schizophrenic must be a cornerstone of any overall treatment plan. Long-term follow-up studies show that some patients who bury psychotic episodes probably do not benefit from exploratory psychotherapy, but those who are able to integrate the psychotic experience into their lives may benefit from some insight-oriented approaches. There is renewed interest in the use of long-term individual psychotherapy in the treatment of schizophrenia, especially when combined with medication.

Learning Theories

According to learning theorists, children who later have schizophrenia learn irrational reactions and ways of thinking by imitating parents who have their own significant emotional problems. In learning theory, the poor interpersonal relationships of persons with schizophrenia develop because of poor models for learning during childhood.

Family Dynamics

In a study of British 4-year-old children, those who had a poor mother–child relationship had a sixfold increase in the risk of developing schizophrenia, and offspring from schizophrenic mothers who were adopted away at birth were more likely to develop the illness if they were reared in adverse circumstances compared to those raised in loving homes by stable adoptive parents. Nevertheless, no well-controlled evidence indicates that a specific family pattern plays a causative role in the development of schizophrenia. Some patients with schizophrenia do come from dysfunctional families, just as many non–psychiatrically ill persons do. It is important, however, not to overlook pathological family behavior that can significantly increase the emotional stress with which a vulnerable patient with schizophrenia must cope.

Double Bind.   The double-bind concept was formulated by Gregory Bateson and Donald Jackson to describe a hypothetical family in which children receive conflicting parental messages about their behavior, attitudes, and feelings. In Bateson's hypothesis, children withdraw into a psychotic state to escape the unsolvable confusion of the double bind. Unfortunately, the family studies that were conducted to validate the theory were seriously flawed methodologically. The theory has value only as a descriptive pattern, not as a causal explanation of schizophrenia. An example of a double bind is the parent who tells the child to provide cookies for his or her friends and then chastises the child for giving away too many cookies to playmates.

Schisms and Skewed Families.   Theodore Lidz described two abnormal patterns of family behavior. In one family type, with a prominent schism between the parents, one parent is overly close to a child of the opposite sex. In the other family type, a skewed relationship between a child and one parent involves a power struggle between the parents and the resulting dominance of one parent. These dynamics stress the tenuous adaptive capacity of the schizophrenic person.

Pseudomutual and Pseudohostile Families.   As described by Lyman Wynne, some families suppress emotional expression by consistently using pseudomutual or pseudohostile verbal communication. In such families, a unique verbal communication develops, and when a child leaves home and must relate to other persons, problems may arise. The child's verbal communication may be incomprehensible to outsiders.

Expressed Emotion.   Parents or other caretakers may behave with overt criticism, hostility, and overinvolvement toward a person with schizophrenia. Many studies have indicated that in families with high levels of expressed emotion (often abbreviated EE), the relapse rate for schizophrenia is high. The assessment of expressed emotion involves analyzing both what is said and the manner in which it is said.

DIAGNOSIS

The DSM-IV-TR diagnostic criteria include course specifiers (i.e., prognosis) that offer clinicians several options and describe actual clinical situations (Table 10–1). The presence of hallucinations or delusions is not necessary for a diagnosis of schizophrenia when the patient exhibits two of the symptoms listed as symptoms 1 through 5 in Criterion A in Table 10-1 (e.g., disorganized speech). Criterion B requires that impaired functioning, although not deteriorations, be present during the active phase of the illness. Symptoms must persist for at least 6 months, and a diagnosis of schizoaffective disorder or mood disorder must be absent.

Subtypes

DSM-IV-TR classifies the subtypes of schizophrenia as paranoid, disorganized, catatonic, undifferentiated, and residual (Table 10–2), based predominantly on clinical presentation. These subtypes are not closely correlated with different prognoses;

Table 10–1
DSM-IV-TR Diagnostic Criteria for Schizophrenia

A. Characteristic symptoms: Two (or more) of the following, each present for a significant portion of time during a 1-month period (or less if successfully treated):
   (1) delusions
   (2) hallucinations
   (3) disorganized speech (e.g., frequent derailment or incoherence)
   (4) grossly disorganized or catatonic behavior
   (5) negative symptoms, i.e., affective flattening, alogia, or avolition

   Note: Only one Criterion A symptom is required if delusions are bizarre or hallucinations consist of a voice keeping up a running commentary on the person's behavior or thoughts, or two or more voices conversing with each other.

B. *Social/occupational dysfunction*: For a significant portion of the time since the onset of the disturbance, one or more major areas of functioning such as work, interpersonal relations, or self-care are markedly below the level achieved prior to the onset (or when the onset is in childhood or adolescence, failure to achieve expected level of interpersonal, academic, or occupational achievement).

C. *Duration*: Continuous signs of the disturbance persist for at least 6 months. This 6-month period must include at least 1 month of symptoms (or less if successfully treated) that meet Criterion A (i.e., active-phase symptoms) and may include periods of prodromal or residual symptoms. During these prodromal or residual periods, the signs of the disturbance may be manifested by only negative symptoms or two or more symptoms listed in Criterion A present in an attenuated form (e.g., odd beliefs, unusual perceptual experiences).

D. *Schizoaffective and mood disorder exclusion*: Schizoaffective disorder and mood disorder with psychotic features have been ruled out because either (1) no major depressive, manic, or mixed episodes have occurred concurrently with the active-phase symptoms; or (2) if mood episodes have occurred during active-phase symptoms, their total duration has been brief relative to the duration of the active and residual periods.

E. *Substance/general medical condition exclusion*: The disturbance is not due to the direct physiological effects of a substance (e.g., a drug of abuse, a medication) or a general medical condition.

F. *Relationship to a pervasive developmental disorder*: If there is a history of autistic disorder or another pervasive developmental disorder, the additional diagnosis of schizophrenia is made only if prominent delusions or hallucinations are also present for at least a month (or less if successfully treated).

Classification of longitudinal course (can be applied only after at least 1 year has elapsed since the initial onset of active-phase symptoms):

   Episodic with interepisode residual symptoms (episodes are defined by the reemergence of prominent psychotic symptoms); also *specify* if: **with prominent negative symptoms**
   Episodic with no interepisode residual symptoms
   Continuous (prominent psychotic symptoms are present throughout the period of observation); also *specify* if: **with prominent negative symptoms**
   Single episode in partial remission: also *specify* if: **with prominent negative symptoms**
   Single episode in full remission
   Other or unspecified pattern

From American Psychiatric Association. *Diagnostic and Statistical Manual of Mental Disorders.* 4th ed. Text rev. Washington, DC: American Psychiatric Association; copyright 2000, with permission.

Table 10–2
DSM-IV-TR Diagnostic Criteria for Schizophrenia Subtypes

Paranoid type

A type of schizophrenia in which the following criteria are met:

A. Preoccupation with one or more delusions or frequent auditory hallucinations.

B. None of the following is prominent: disorganized speech, disorganized or catatonic behavior, or flat or inappropriate affect.

Disorganized type

A type of schizophrenia in which the following criteria are met:

A. All of the following are prominent:

    (1) disorganized speech

    (2) disorganized behavior

    (3) flat or inappropriate affect

B. The criteria are not met for catatonic type.

Catatonic type

A type of schizophrenia in which the clinical picture is dominated by at least two of the following:

(1) motoric immobility as evidenced by catalepsy (including waxy flexibility) or stupor

(2) excessive motor activity (that is apparently purposeless and not influenced by external stimuli)

(3) extreme negativism (an apparently motiveless resistance to all instructions or maintenance of a rigid posture against attempts to be moved) or mutism

(4) peculiarities of voluntary movement as evidenced by posturing (voluntary assumption of inappropriate or bizarre postures), stereotyped movements, prominent mannerisms, or prominent grimacing

(5) echolalia or echopraxia

Undifferentiated type

A type of schizophrenia in which symptoms that meet Criterion A are present, but the criteria are not met for the paranoid, disorganized, or catatonic type.

Residual type

A type of schizophrenia in which the following criteria are met:

A. Absence of prominent delusions, hallucinations, disorganized speech, and grossly disorganized or catatonic behavior.

B. There is continuing evidence of the disturbance, as indicated by the presence of negative symptoms or two or more symptoms listed in Criterion A for schizophrenia, present in an attenuated form (e.g., odd beliefs, unusual perceptual experiences).

From American Psychiatric Association. *Diagnostic and Statistical Manual of Mental Disorders.* 4th ed. Text rev. Washington, DC: American Psychiatric Association; copyright 2000, with permission.

Table 10–3
Features Weighting toward Good to Poor Prognosis in Schizophrenia

Good Prognosis	Poor Prognosis
Late onset	Young onset
Obvious precipitating factors	No precipitating factors
Acute onset	Insidious onset
Good premorbid social, sexual, and work histories	Poor premorbid social, sexual, and work histories
Mood disorder symptoms (especially depressive disorders)	Withdrawn, autistic behavior
Married	Single, divorced, or widowed
Family history of mood disorders	Family history of schizophrenia
Good support systems	Poor support systems
Positive symptoms	Negative symptoms
	Neurological signs and symptoms
	History of perinatal trauma
	No remissions in 3 years
	Many relapses
	History of assaultiveness

of schizophrenia is characterized mainly by the presence of delusions of persecution or grandeur. Patients with paranoid schizophrenia usually have their first episode of illness at an older age than do patients with catatonic or disorganized schizophrenia. Patients in whom schizophrenia occurs in their late 20s or 30s have usually established a social life that may help them through their illness, and the ego resources of paranoid patients tend to be greater than those of patients with catatonic and disorganized schizophrenia. Patients with the paranoid type of schizophrenia show less regression of their mental faculties, emotional responses, and behavior than do patients with other types of schizophrenia.

Patients with paranoid schizophrenia are typically tense, suspicious, guarded, reserved, and sometimes hostile or aggressive, but they can occasionally conduct themselves adequately in social situations. Their intelligence in areas not invaded by their psychosis tends to remain intact.

The following case illustrates ideas of reference and paranoid delusions. A married man, aged 38, with a history of dependable, conscientious work as a bookkeeper, became sleepless, anxious, and unable to concentrate. He developed the belief that his vision was failing because of poisons secretly placed in his food by former neighbors. He found a misprint in a newspaper that he felt was placed there by the editor to shame him publicly. Admitted to the psychiatric service of a general hospital, he said that cars passing up and down the street contained agents who were spying on him. He believed that the electric light bulbs in his room were emanating a purifying radiation to counteract syphilitic germs, which he was supposedly breathing into the atmosphere, although a physical examination was negative for syphilis.

for such differentiation, specific predictors of prognosis are best consulted (Table 10–3). The 10th revision of *International Statistical Classification of Diseases and Related Health Problems* (ICD-10), in contrast, uses nine subtypes: paranoid schizophrenia, hebephrenia, catatonic schizophrenia, undifferentiated schizophrenia, postschizophrenic depression, residual schizophrenia, simple schizophrenia, other schizophrenia, and schizophrenia, unspecified, with eight possibilities for classifying the course of the disorder, ranging from continuous to complete remission.

Paranoid Type. The paranoid type of schizophrenia is characterized by preoccupation with one or more delusions or frequent auditory hallucinations. Classically, the paranoid type

Disorganized Type. The disorganized (formerly called hebephrenic) type of schizophrenia is characterized by a marked regression to primitive, disinhibited, and unorganized behavior and by the absence of symptoms that meet the criteria for the catatonic type. The onset of this subtype is generally early, before age 25 years. Disorganized patients are usually active but in an aimless, nonconstructive manner. Their thought disorder is pronounced, and their contact with reality is poor. Their personal appearance is disheveled, and their social behavior and their emotional responses are inappropriate. They often burst into laughter without any apparent reason. Incongruous grinning and grimacing are common in these patients, whose behavior is best described as silly or fatuous.

The patient AB, a 32 year old woman, began to lose weight and became careless about her work, which deteriorated in quality and quantity. She believed that other women at her place of employment were circulating slanderous stories concerning her and complained that a young man employed in the same plant had put his arm around her and insulted her. Her family demanded that the charge be investigated, which showed not only that the charge was without foundation, but that the man in question had not spoken to her for months. One day she returned from her work, and as she entered the house, laughed loudly, watched her sister-in-law suspiciously, refused to answer questions, and at the sight of her brother began to cry. She refused to go to the bathroom, saying that a man was looking in the windows at her. She ate no food, and the next day she declared that her sisters were "bad women," that everyone was talking about her, and that someone had been having sexual relations with her, and that although she could not see him, he was "always around."

The patient was admitted to a public hospital. As she entered the admitting office, she laughed loudly and repeatedly screamed in a loud tone, "She cannot stay here; she's got to go home!" She grimaced and performed various stereotyped movements of her hands. When seen on the ward an hour later, she paid no attention to questions, although she talked to herself in a childish tone. She moved about constantly, walked on her toes in a dancing manner, pointed aimlessly about, and put out her tongue and sucked her lips in the manner of an infant. At times she moaned and cried like a child but shed no tears. As the months passed, she remained silly, childish, preoccupied, inaccessible, grimacing, gesturing, pointing at objects in a stereotyped way, and usually chattering to herself in a peculiar high-pitched voice, little of what she said being understood. Her condition continued to deteriorate, and she remained unkempt and presented a picture of extreme introversion and regression with no interest either in the activities of the institution or in her relatives who visited her. (Adapted from a case of Arthur P. Noyes, M.D., and Lawrence C. Kolb, M.D.)

Catatonic Type. The catatonic type of schizophrenia, which was common several decades ago, has become rare in Europe and North America. The classic feature of the catatonic type is a marked disturbance in motor function; this disturbance may involve stupor, negativism, rigidity, excitement, or posturing. Sometimes, the patient shows rapid alteration between extremes of excitement and stupor. Associated features include stereotypies, mannerisms, and waxy flexibility. Mutism is particularly common. During catatonic excitement, patients need careful supervision to prevent them from hurting themselves or others. Medical care may be needed because of malnutrition, exhaustion, hyperpyrexia, or self-inflicted injury.

AC, aged 32 years, was admitted to the hospital. On arrival he was noted to be an asthenic, poorly nourished man with dilated pupils, hyperactive tendon reflexes, and a pulse rate of 120 beats per minute. He showed many mannerisms, laid down on the floor, pulled at his foot, made undirected violent striking movements, struck attendants, grimaced, assumed rigid and strange postures, refused to speak, and appeared to be having auditory hallucinations. When seen later in the day, he was found to be in a stuporous state. His face was without expression, he was mute and rigid, and paid no attention to those about him or to their questions. His eyes were closed and the lids could be separated only with effort. There was no response to pinpricks or other painful stimuli.

He gradually became accessible, and when asked concerning himself, he referred to his stuporous period as sleep and maintained that he had no recollection of any events occurring during it. He said, "I didn't know anything. Everything seemed to be dark as far as my mind is concerned. Then I began to see a little light, like the shape of a star. Then my head got through the star gradually. I saw more and more light until I saw everything in a perfect form a few days ago." He explained his mutism by saying that he had been afraid he would "say the wrong thing," also that he "didn't know exactly what to talk about." From his obviously inadequate emotional response and his statement that he was "a scientist and an inventor of the most extraordinary genius of the twentieth century," it was plain that he was still far from well. (Adapted from a case of Arthur P. Noyes, M.D., and Lawrence C. Kolb, M.D.)

Undifferentiated Type. Frequently, patients who are clearly schizophrenic cannot be easily fitted into one or another type. DSM-IV-TR classifies these patients as having schizophrenia of the undifferentiated type.

A 15-year-old girl attended a summer camp, where she had difficulties getting along with the other children and developed animosity towards one of the counselors. On her return home she refused to listen to her parents and she heard the voice of a man talking to her, although she could not see him. She rapidly began to show bizarre behavior, characterized by grimacing, violent outbursts, and inability to take care of herself.

Her school record has always been good, and she was fluent in three languages. Her parents described her as having been a quiet, rather shut-in child with no abnormal traits in childhood. Family relations were reported as having been satisfactory.

On admission to a psychiatric hospital, the patient's speech was incoherent. She showed marked disturbances of formal thinking and blocking of thoughts. She was impulsive and appeared to be hallucinating. She stated that she heard voices in her right ear that a popular singer was running after her with a knife. She also thought that her father was intent on killing her. She thought that she was pregnant because she had hugged one of the residents.

She is often incontinent and most of the time neglects her physical appearance. But occasionally she will spend hours dressing herself, looking in the mirror, and putting on excessive makeup. At times, she has been seen eating her feces. Occasionally she adopted the roles of a singer or dancer. She makes incoherent statements like: "Will I live forever? Nurse, I don't throw my love away. It is my stomach and it hurts." In the dining room she attempted to grasp the genitals of male patients.

Two months of neuroleptic treatment brought no apparent improvement. She was then given a course of electroconvulsive therapy. She remains in the hospital, where her behavior has, for more than a year and a half, continued to be very disturbed.

Residual Type

According to DSM-IV-TR, the residual type of schizophrenia is characterized by continuing evidence of the schizophrenic disturbance in the absence of a complete set of active symptoms or of sufficient symptoms to meet the diagnosis of another type of schizophrenia. Emotional blunting, social withdrawal, eccentric behavior, illogical thinking, and mild loosening of associations commonly appear in the residual type. When delusions or hallucinations occur, they are neither prominent nor accompanied by strong affect.

Other Subtypes

The subtyping of schizophrenia has had a long history; other subtyping schemes appear in the literature, especially literature from countries other than the United States.

Bouffée Délirante (Acute Delusional Psychosis). This French diagnostic concept differs from a diagnosis of schizophrenia primarily on the basis of a symptom duration of less than 3 months. The diagnosis is similar to the DSM-IV-TR diagnosis of schizophreniform disorder. French clinicians report that about 40 percent of patients with a diagnosis of *bouffée délirante* progress in their illness and are eventually classified as having schizophrenia.

Latent. The concept of latent schizophrenia was developed during a time when theorists conceived of the disorder in broad diagnostic terms. Currently, patients must be very mentally ill to warrant a diagnosis of schizophrenia, but with a broad diagnostic concept of schizophrenia, the condition of patients who would not currently be thought of as severely ill could have received a diagnosis of schizophrenia. Latent schizophrenia, for example,

was often the diagnosis used for what are now called borderline, schizoid, and schizotypal personality disorders. These patients may occasionally show peculiar behaviors or thought disorders but do not consistently manifest psychotic symptoms. In the past, the syndrome was also termed borderline schizophrenia.

Oneiroid. The oneiroid state refers to a dream-like state in which patients may be deeply perplexed and not fully oriented in time and place. The term oneiroid schizophrenic has been used for patients who are engaged in their hallucinatory experiences to the exclusion of involvement in the real world. When an oneiroid state is present, clinicians should be particularly careful to examine patients for medical or neurological causes of the symptoms.

After a 20-year-old woman, a college student, had recovered from her schizophrenic breakdown, she wrote the following description of her experiences during the oneiroid phase:

This is how I remember it. The road has changed. It is twisted and it used to be straight. Nothing is constant—all is in motion. The trees are moving. They do not remain at rest. How is it my mother does not bump into the trees that are moving? I follow my mother. I am afraid, but I follow. I have to share my strange thoughts with someone. We are sitting on a bench. The bench seems low. It, too, has moved. "The bench is low," I say, "Yes," says my mother. "This isn't how it used to be. How come there are no people around? There are usually lots of people and it is Sunday and there are no people. This is strange." All these strange questions irritate my mother who then says she must be going soon. While I continue thinking I'm in a kind of nowhere....

There are no days; no nights; sometimes it is darker than other times—that's all. It is never quite black, just dark gray. There is no such thing as time—there is only eternity. There is no such thing as death—nor heaven and hell—there is only a timeless—hateful—spaceless—worsening of things. You can never go forward; you must always regress into this horrific mess....

The outside was moving rather swiftly, everything seemed topsy-turvy—things were flying about. It was very strange. I wanted to get back to the quiet very badly but when I got back I couldn't remember where anything was (e.g., the bathroom)...

(Courtesy of Heinz E. Lehmann, M.D.)

Paraphrenia. The term paraphrenia is sometimes used as a synonym for paranoid schizophrenia or for either a progressively deteriorating course of illness or the presence of a well-systemized delusional system. The multiple meanings of the term render it ineffectual in communicating information.

Pseudoneurotic Schizophrenia. Occasionally, patients who initially have such symptoms as anxiety, phobias, obsessions, and compulsions later reveal symptoms of thought disorder and psychosis. These patients are characterized by symptoms of pananxiety, panphobia, panambivalence, and sometimes chaotic sexuality. Unlike persons with anxiety

Table 10–4
DSM-IV-TR Research Criteria for Simple
Deteriorative Disorder (Simple Schizophrenia)

A. Progressive development over a period of at least a year of
   all of the following:
   (1) marked decline in occupational or academic functioning
   (2) gradual appearance and deepening of negative
       symptoms such as affective flattening, alogia, and
       avolition
   (3) poor interpersonal rapport, social isolation, or social
       withdrawal
B. Criterion A for schizophrenia has never been met.
C. The symptoms are not better accounted for by schizotypal
   or schizoid personality disorder, a psychotic disorder, a
   mood disorder, an anxiety disorder, a dementia, or mental
   retardation and are not due to the direct physiological
   effects of a substance or a general medical condition.

From American Psychiatric Association. *Diagnostic and Statistical
Manual of Mental Disorders.* 4th ed. Text rev. Washington, DC:
American Psychiatric Association; copyright 2000, with permission.

disorders, pseudoneurotic patients have free-floating anxiety that
rarely subsides. In clinical descriptions, the patients seldom become overtly and severely psychotic. This condition is currently
diagnosed in DSM-IV-TR as borderline personality disorder.

**Simple Deteriorative Disorder (Simple Schizophre-
nia).**   Simple deteriorative disorder is characterized by a gradual, insidious loss of drive and ambition. Patients with the
disorder are usually not overtly psychotic and do not experience persistent hallucinations or delusions. Their primary symptom is withdrawal from social and work-related situations. The
syndrome must be differentiated from depression, a phobia, a
dementia, or an exacerbation of personality traits. Clinicians
should be sure that patients truly meet the diagnostic criteria
for schizophrenia before making the diagnosis. Simple deteriorative disorder appears as a diagnostic category in an appendix
of DSM-IV-TR (Table 10–4).

An unmarried man, 27 years old, was brought to the mental
hospital because he had on several occasions become violent toward his father. For a few weeks he had hallucinations
and heard voices. The voices eventually ceased, but he then
adopted a strange way of life. He would sit up all night, sleep
all day, and become very angry when his father tried to get
him out of bed. He did not shave or wash for weeks, smoked
continuously, ate very irregularly, and drank enormous quantities of tea.

In the hospital he adjusted rapidly to the new environment
and was found to be generally cooperative. He showed no
marked abnormalities of mental state or behavior, except for
his lack of concern for just about anything. He kept to himself
as much as possible and conversed little with patients or staff.
His personal hygiene had to be supervised by the nursing
staff; otherwise he would quickly become dirty and very
untidy.

Six years after his admission to the hospital, he is described as shiftless and careless, sullen and unreasonable.

He lies on a couch all day long. Although many efforts have
been made to get the patient to accept therapeutic work assignments, he refuses to consider any kind of regular occupation. In the summer he wanders about the hospital grounds or
lies under a tree. In the winter he wanders through the tunnels
connecting the various hospital buildings and is often seen
stretched out for hours under the warm pipes that carry the
steam through the tunnels. (Courtesy of Heinz E. Lehmann,
M.D.)

Postpsychotic Depressive Disorder of Schizophrenia.
Following an acute schizophrenia episode some patients become
depressed. The symptoms of postpsychotic depressive disorder
of schizophrenia can closely resemble the symptoms of the residual phase of schizophrenia as well as the adverse effects of commonly used antipsychotic medications. The diagnosis should not
be made if they are substance induced or part of a mood disorder
due to a general medical condition. ICD-10 describes a category
called postschizophrenia depression arising in the aftermath of a
schizophrenic illness. These depressive states occur in up to 25
percent of patients with schizophrenia and are associated with
an increased risk of suicide. (Further discussion of the disorder
can be found in Section 12.3.)

Early-Onset Schizophrenia.   A small minority of patients
manifest schizophrenia in childhood. Such children may at first
present diagnostic problems, particularly with differentiation
from mental retardation and autistic disorder. Recent studies have
established that the diagnosis of childhood schizophrenia may
be based on the same symptoms used for adult schizophrenia. Its
onset is usually insidious, its course tends to be chronic, and the
prognosis is mostly unfavorable. (Chapter 47 contains further
discussion of early-onset schizophrenia.)

Late-Onset Schizophrenia.   Late-onset schizophrenia is
clinically indistinguishable from schizophrenia but has an onset
after age 45 years. This condition tends to appear more frequently
in women and also tends to be characterized by a predominance
of paranoid symptoms. The prognosis is favorable, and these
patients usually do well on antipsychotic medication.

Deficit Schizophrenia.   In the 1980s, criteria were promul-
gated for a subtype of schizophrenia characterized by enduring,
idiopathic negative symptoms. These patients were said to exhibit the deficit syndrome. This group of patients is now said
to have deficit schizophrenia. Patients with schizophrenia with
positive symptoms are said to have nondeficit schizophrenia.
The symptoms used to define deficit schizophrenia are strongly
interrelated, although various combinations of the six negative
symptoms in the criteria can be found.

Deficit patients have a more severe course of illness than
nondeficit patients, with a higher prevalence of abnormal involuntary movements before administration of antipsychotic drugs
and poorer social function before the onset of psychotic symptoms. The onset of their first psychotic episode is more often
insidious, and they show less long-term recovery of function
than do nondeficit patients. Deficit patients are also less likely

to marry than are other patients with schizophrenia. However, despite their poorer level of function and greater social isolation, both of which should increase a patient's stress and, therefore, the risk of serious depression, deficit patients appear to have a decreased risk of major depression and probably have a decreased risk of suicide as well.

The risk factors of deficit patients differ from those of non-deficit patients; deficit schizophrenia is associated with an excess of summer births, whereas nondeficit patients have an excess of winter births. Deficit schizophrenia may also be associated with a greater familial risk of schizophrenia and of mild, deficit-like features in the nonpsychotic relatives of deficit probands. Within a family with multiply affected siblings, the deficit-nondeficit categorization tends to be uniform. The deficit group also has a higher prevalence of men.

The psychopathology of deficit patients affects treatment; their lack of motivation, lack of distress, greater cognitive impairment, and asocial nature undermine the efficacy of psychosocial interventions, as well as their adherence to medication regimens. Their cognitive impairment, which is greater than that of non-deficit subjects, also contributes to this lack of efficacy.

Psychological Testing.   Patients with schizophrenia generally perform poorly on a wide range of neuropsychological tests. Vigilance, memory, and concept formation are most affected and consistent with pathological involvement in the frontotemporal cortex.

Objective measures of neuropsychological performance, such as the Halstead-Reitan battery and the Luria-Nebraska battery, often give abnormal findings, such as bilateral frontal and temporal lobe dysfunction, including impairments in attention, retention time, and problem-solving ability. Motor ability is also impaired, possibly related to brain asymmetry.

Intelligence Tests.   When groups of patients with schizophrenia are compared with groups of psychiatric patients without schizophrenia or with the general population, the schizophrenia patients tend to score lower on intelligence tests. Statistically, the evidence suggests that low intelligence is often present at the onset, and intelligence may continue to deteriorate with the progression of the disorder.

Projective and Personality Tests.   Projective tests, such as the Rorschach test and the Thematic Apperception Test, may indicate bizarre ideation. Personality inventories, such as the Minnesota Multiphasic Personality Inventory, often give abnormal results in schizophrenia, but the contribution to diagnosis and treatment planning is minimal.

CLINICAL FEATURES

A discussion of the clinical signs and symptoms of schizophrenia raises three key issues. First, no clinical sign or symptom is pathognomonic for schizophrenia; every sign or symptom seen in schizophrenia occurs in other psychiatric and neurological disorders. This observation is contrary to the often-heard clinical opinion that certain signs and symptoms are diagnostic of schizophrenia. Therefore, a patient's history is essential for its diagnosis; clinicians cannot diagnose the condition simply by results of a mental status examination, which may vary. Second, a patient's symptoms change with time. For example, a patient may have intermittent hallucinations and a varying ability to perform adequately in social situations, or significant symp-

toms of a mood disorder may come and go during the course of schizophrenia. Third, clinicians must take into account the patient's educational level, intellectual ability, and cultural and subcultural membership. An impaired ability to understand abstract concepts, for example, may reflect either the patient's education or his or her intelligence. Religious organizations and cults may have customs that seem strange to outsiders but are normal to those within the cultural setting.

Premorbid Signs and Symptoms

In theoretical formulations of the course of schizophrenia, premorbid signs and symptoms appear before the prodromal phase of the illness. The differentiation implies that premorbid signs and symptoms exist before the disease process evidences itself and that the prodromal signs and symptoms are parts of the evolving disorder. In the typical, but not invariable, premorbid history of schizophrenia, patients had schizoid or schizotypal personalities characterized as quiet, passive, and introverted; as children they had few friends. Preschizophrenic adolescents may have no close friends and no dates and may avoid team sports. They may enjoy watching movies and television or listening to music or playing computer games to the exclusion of social activities. Some adolescent patients may show a sudden onset of obsessive-compulsive behavior as part of the prodromal picture.

The validity of the prodromal signs and symptoms, almost invariably recognized after the diagnosis of schizophrenia has been made, is uncertain; once schizophrenia is diagnosed, the retrospective remembrance of early signs and symptoms is affected. Nevertheless, although the first hospitalization is often thought to mark the beginning of the disorder, signs and symptoms have often been present for months or even years. The signs may have started with complaints about somatic symptoms, such as headache, back and muscle pain, weakness, and digestive problems. The initial diagnosis may be malingering, chronic fatigue syndrome, or somatization disorder. Family and friends may eventually notice that the person has changed and is no longer functioning well in occupational, social, and personal activities. During this stage, a patient may begin to develop an interest in abstract ideas, philosophy, the occult, or religious questions. Additional prodromal signs and symptoms can include markedly peculiar behavior, abnormal affect, unusual speech, bizarre ideas, and strange perceptual experiences.

Mental Status Examination

General Description.   The appearance of a patient with schizophrenia can range from that of a completely disheveled, screaming, agitated person to an obsessively groomed, completely silent, and immobile person. Between these two poles, patients may be talkative and may exhibit bizarre postures. Their behavior may become agitated or violent, apparently in an unprovoked manner but usually in response to hallucinations. By contrast, in catatonic stupor, often referred to as catatonia, patients seem completely lifeless and may exhibit such signs as muteness, negativism, and automatic obedience. Waxy flexibility, once a common sign in catatonia, has become rare, as has manneristic behavior. A person with a less extreme subtype of catatonia may show marked social withdrawal and egocentricity, lack of spontaneous speech or movement, and an absence of goal-directed behavior. Patients with catatonia may sit immobile and speechless in their chairs, respond to questions with only short answers, and move only when directed to. Other obvious behavior may include odd clumsiness or stiffness in body movements, signs now seen as possibly indicating a disease process in the basal ganglia. Patients with schizophrenia often are poorly groomed, fail to bathe, and dress much too warmly for the prevailing temperatures. Other odd behaviors include tics, stereotypies, mannerisms, and, occasionally, echopraxia, in which patients imitate the posture or the behaviors of the examiner.

Precox Feeling.   Some experienced clinicians report a precox feeling, an intuitive experience of their inability to establish an emotional rapport with a patient. Although the experience is common, no data indicate that it is a valid or reliable criterion in the diagnosis of schizophrenia.

Mood, Feelings, and Affect

Two common affective symptoms in schizophrenia are reduced emotional responsiveness, sometimes severe enough to warrant the label of anhedonia, and overly active and inappropriate emotions such as extremes of rage, happiness, and anxiety. A flat or blunted affect can be a symptom of the illness itself, of the parkinsonian adverse effects of antipsychotic medications, or of depression, and differentiating these symptoms can be a clinical challenge. Overly emotional patients may describe exultant feelings of omnipotence, religious ecstasy, terror at the disintegration of their souls, or paralyzing anxiety about the destruction of the universe. Other feeling tones include perplexity, a sense of isolation, overwhelming ambivalence, and depression.

Perceptual Disturbances

Hallucinations.   Any of the five senses may be affected by hallucinatory experiences in patients with schizophrenia. The most common hallucinations, however, are auditory, with voices that are often threatening, obscene, accusatory, or insulting. Two or more voices may converse among themselves, or a voice may comment on the patient's life or behavior. Visual hallucinations are common, but tactile, olfactory, and gustatory hallucinations are unusual; their presence should prompt the clinician to consider the possibility of an underlying medical or neurological disorder that is causing the entire syndrome.

CENESTHETIC HALLUCINATIONS.   Cenesthetic hallucinations are unfounded sensations of altered states in bodily organs. Examples of cenesthetic hallucinations are a burning sensation in the brain, a pushing sensation in the blood vessels, and a cutting sensation in the bone marrow. Bodily distortions may also occur.

Illusions.   As differentiated from hallucinations, illusions are distortions of real images or sensations, whereas hallucinations are not based on real images or sensations. Illusions can occur in schizophrenia patients during active phases, but they can also occur during the prodromal phases and during periods of remission. Whenever illusions or hallucinations occur, clinicians should consider the possibility of a substance-related cause for the symptoms, even when patients have already received a diagnosis of schizophrenia.

Thought

Disorders of thought are the most difficult symptoms for many clinicians and students to understand, but they may be the core symptoms of schizophrenia. Dividing the disorders of thought into disorders of thought content, form of thought, and thought process is one way to clarify them.

Thought Content.   Disorders of thought content reflect the patient's ideas, beliefs, and interpretations of stimuli. Delusions, the most obvious example of a disorder of thought content, are varied in schizophrenia and may assume persecutory, grandiose, religious, or somatic forms.

Patients may believe that an outside entity controls their thoughts or behavior or, conversely, that they control outside events in an extraordinary fashion (such as causing the sun to rise and set or by preventing earthquakes). Patients may have an intense and consuming preoccupation with esoteric, abstract, symbolic, psychological, or philosophical ideas. Patients may also worry about allegedly life-threatening but bizarre and implausible somatic conditions, such as the presence of aliens inside the patient's testicles affecting his ability to father children.

The phrase *loss of ego boundaries* describes the lack of a clear sense of where the patient's body, mind, and influence end and where those of other animate and inanimate objects begin. For example, patients may think that other persons, the television, or the newspapers are referring to them (*ideas of reference*). Other symptoms of the loss of ego boundaries include the sense that the patient has physically fused with an outside object (e.g., a tree or another person) or that the patient has disintegrated and fused with the entire universe (*cosmic identity*). With such a state of mind, some patients with schizophrenia doubt their sex or their sexual orientation. These symptoms should not be confused with transvestism, transsexuality, or other gender identity problems.

Form of Thought.   Disorders of the form of thought are objectively observable in patients' spoken and written language. The disorders include looseness of associations, derailment, incoherence, tangentiality, circumstantiality, neologisms, echolalia, verbigeration, word salad, and mutism. Although looseness of associations was once described as pathognomonic for schizophrenia, the symptom is frequently seen in mania. Distinguishing between looseness of associations and tangentiality can be difficult for even the most experienced clinicians.

The following sample is taken from a memo typed by a schizophrenic secretary who was still able to work part time in an office. Note her preoccupation with the mind, the Trinity, and other esoteric matters. Also note that peculiar restructuring of concepts by hyphenating the words germ-any (the patient had a distinct fear of germs) and infer-no (inferring that there will be no salvation). The "chain reaction" is a reference to atomic piles:

> Mental health is the Blessed Trinity, and as man cannot be without God, it is futile to deny His Son. For the Creation understand germ-any in Voice New Order, not lie of chained reaction, spawning mark in temple Cain with Babel grave'n image to wanton V day "Israel."
>
> Lucifer fell Jew prostitute and lambeth walks by roam to sex ritual, in Bible six million of the Babylon woman, infer-no Salvation.

The one common factor in the foregoing thought process is a preoccupation with invisible forces, radiation, witchcraft, religion, philosophy, psychology and a leaning toward the esoteric, the abstract, and the symbolic. Consequently, a schizophrenic patient's thinking is characterized simultaneously by both an overly concrete and an overly symbolic nature.

Thought Process.   Disorders in thought process concern the way in which ideas and languages are formulated. The examiner infers a disorder from what and how the patient speaks, writes, or draws. The examiner may also assess the patient's thought process by observing his or her behavior, especially in carrying out discrete tasks (e.g., in occupational therapy). Disorders of thought process include flight of ideas, thought blocking, impaired attention, poverty of thought content, poor abstraction abilities, perseveration, idiosyncratic associations (e.g., identical predicates and clang associations), overinclusion, and circumstantiality. *Thought control*, in which outside forces are controlling what the patient thinks or feels, is common, as is *thought broadcasting*, in which patients think others can read their minds or that their thoughts are broadcast through television sets or radios.

Impulsiveness, Violence, Suicide, and Homicide

Patients with schizophrenia may be agitated and have little impulse control when ill. They may also have decreased social sensitivity and appear to be impulsive when, for example, they grab another patient's cigarettes, change television channels abruptly, or throw food on the floor. Some apparently impulsive behavior, including suicide and homicide attempts, may be in response to hallucinations commanding the patient to act.

Violence.   Violent behavior (excluding homicide) is common among untreated schizophrenia patients. Delusions of a persecutory nature, previous episodes of violence, and neurological deficits are risk factors for violent or impulsive behavior. Management includes appropriate antipsychotic medication. Emergency treatment consists of restraints and seclusion. Acute sedation with lorazepam (Ativan), 1 to 2 mg intramuscularly, repeated every hour as needed, may be necessary to prevent the patient from harming others. If a clinician feels fearful in the presence of a schizophrenia patient, it should be taken as an internal clue that the patient may be on the verge of acting out violently. In such cases, the interview should be terminated or be conducted with an attendant at the ready.

Suicide.   Suicide is the leading cause of premature death among people with schizophrenia. Suicide attempts are made by 20 to 50 percent of these patients, with long-term rates of suicide estimated to be 10 to 13 percent. These numbers reflect an approximately 20-fold increase over the suicide rate in the general population. Often, suicide in schizophrenia seems to occur "out of the blue," without prior warnings or expressions of verbal intent. The most important factor is the presence of a major depressive episode. Epidemiological studies indicate that up to 80 percent of schizophrenia patients may have a major depressive episode at some time in their lives. Some data suggest that those patients with the best prognosis (few negative symptoms, preservation of capacity to experience affects, better abstract thinking) can paradoxically also be at highest risk for suicide. The profile of the patient at greatest risk is a young man

who once had high expectations, declined from a higher level of functioning, realizes that his dreams are not likely to come true, and has lost faith in the effectiveness of treatment. Other possible contributors to the high rate of suicide include command hallucinations and drug abuse. Two thirds or more of schizophrenic patients who commit suicide have seen an apparently unsuspecting clinician within 72 hours of death. A large pharmacological study suggests that clozapine (Clozaril) may have particular efficacy in reducing suicidal ideation in schizophrenia patients with prior hospitalizations for suicidality. Adjunctive antidepressant medications have been shown to be effective in alleviating co-occurring major depression in schizophrenia.

The following is an example of an unpredictable suicide in a schizophrenic who had been responding to psychiatric treatment:

The patient had been an autistic child and did not speak until he was 7 years old. He had responded well to psychiatric treatment, and at age 13 his I.Q. was reported as 122. At age 17, he became violent toward his parents, shaved all his hair off, and made such statements as, "I like bank robbers knocking people unconscious" and "I think tough gangs are funny because they beat down people." While saying this, he laughed loudly. He was admitted to a mental hospital, where he responded with definite improvement to pharmacotherapy and psychotherapy, and he went home regularly for weekends.

He left various notes on his desk before committing suicide. Among these notes was an 8-page list giving 211 "inexcusable mistakes throughout my life." Each one was dated, for example, "1952, 2nd of November: throwing up in my friend's house on a shoe-box. 1953, 17th August: accidentally wearing a watch that wasn't water-proof in the bathtub. 1956, 23rd of September: slamming back-door of Meteor after getting in."

He then proceeded in his notes to give "the causes of the mistakes": "Montreal having a mountain; I have a receding hair-line; my height since I was nine years old; Canada having two languages..." He also wrote: "My feelings of tension since 1962 is getting worse most of the time. I planned the date of my death without the slightest trace of emotion..."

The boy hanged himself at age 18 in the family garage. An experienced psychiatrist who had repeatedly interviewed him noted no signs of depression only a week before. (Courtesy of Heinz E. Lehmann, M.D.)

Homicide.   In spite of the sensational attention that the news media provide when a patient with schizophrenia murders someone, the data indicate that these patients are no more likely to commit homicide than is a member of the general population. When a patient with schizophrenia does commit homicide, it may be for unpredictable or bizarre reasons based on hallucinations or delusions. Possible predictors of homicidal activity are a history of previous violence, dangerous behavior while hospitalized, and hallucinations or delusions involving such violence.

> A schizophrenic man who had been going home on weekends for many months was told by his sister that she would not ask for permission any more to take him out of the hospital if he would not do his part with the housework in the future, for instance, help with the dishes. On the next weekend visit, the patient killed his sister and mother. He had shown no signs of disturbance whatsoever during the preceding week, had been sleeping well, and had been attending occupational therapy classes as usual.
>
> A 19-year-old boy who had been discharged from a mental hospital in what appeared to be a residual state of chronic schizophrenia of the undifferentiated type stabbed his father to death when the latter, during a state of intoxication, told the patient that he was too much of a bother around the house and that he might as well return to the hospital.
>
> Another schizophrenic, whose condition had not yet been diagnosed, complained to a general practitioner about various physical ailments. When the physician finally told him that he should not come anymore because there was nothing else he could do for him, the patient quickly left the office but returned a few hours later and killed the doctor. (Courtesy of Heinz E. Lehmann, M.D.)

Sensorium and Cognition

Orientation. Patients with schizophrenia are usually oriented to person, time, and place. The lack of such orientation should prompt clinicians to investigate the possibility of a medical or neurological brain disorder. Some patients with schizophrenia may give incorrect or bizarre answers to questions about orientation, for example, "I am Christ; this is heaven; and it is AD 35."

> A schizophrenic patient asserted that he was in a prison elaborately disguised to look like a hospital with a staff of jailers disguised as doctors and nurses who were all engaged in a charade to elicit incriminating facts about the patient and his family. He made a severe suicidal attempt because he believed that only upon his death would the jailers spare the lives of his loved ones.

Memory. Memory, as tested in the mental status examination, is usually intact, but there can be minor cognitive deficiencies. It may be possible, however, to get the patient to attend closely enough to the memory tests for the ability to be assessed adequately.

Cognitive Impairment. An important development in the understanding of the psychopathology of schizophrenia is an appreciation of the importance of cognitive impairment in the disorder. In outpatients, cognitive impairment is a better predictor of level of function than is the severity of psychotic symptoms. Patients with schizophrenia typically exhibit subtle cognitive dysfunction in the domains of attention, executive function, working memory, and episodic memory. Although a substantial percentage of patients have normal intelligence quotients, it is possible that every person who has schizophrenia has cognitive dysfunction compared to what he or she would be able to do without the disorder. Although these impairments cannot function as diagnostic tools, they are strongly related to the functional outcome of the illness and, for that reason, have clinical value as prognostic variables, as well as for treatment planning.

The cognitive impairment seems already to be present when patients have their first episode and appears largely to remain stable over the course of early illness. (There may be a small subgroup of patients who have a true dementia in late life that is not due to other cognitive disorders, such as Alzheimer's disease.) Cognitive impairments are also present in attenuated forms in nonpsychotic relatives of schizophrenia patients.

The cognitive impairments of schizophrenia have become the target of pharmacological and psychosocial treatment trials. It is likely that effective treatments will become widely available within a few years, and these are likely to lead to an improvement in the quality of life and level of functioning of people with schizophrenia.

Judgment and Insight. Classically, patients with schizophrenia are described as having poor insight into the nature and the severity of their disorder. The so-called lack of insight is associated with poor compliance with treatment. When examining schizophrenia patients, clinicians should carefully define various aspects of insight, such as awareness of symptoms, trouble getting along with people, and the reasons for these problems. Such information can be clinically useful in tailoring a treatment strategy and theoretically useful in postulating what areas of the brain contribute to the observed lack of insight (e.g., the parietal lobes).

Reliability. A patient with schizophrenia is no less reliable than any other psychiatric patient. The nature of the disorder, however, requires the examiner to verify important information through additional sources.

Somatic Comorbidity

Neurological Findings. Localizing and nonlocalizing neurological signs (also known as hard and soft signs, respectively) have been reported to be more common in patients with schizophrenia than in other psychiatric patients. Nonlocalizing signs include dysdiadochokinesia, astereognosis, primitive reflexes, and diminished dexterity. The presence of neurological signs and symptoms correlates with increased severity of illness, affective blunting, and a poor prognosis. Other abnormal neurological signs include tics, stereotypies, grimacing, impaired fine motor skills, abnormal motor tone, and abnormal movements. One study has found that only about 25 percent of patients with schizophrenia are aware of their abnormal involuntary movements and that the lack of awareness is correlated with lack of insight about the primary psychiatric disorder and the duration of illness.

Eye Examination. In addition to the disorder of smooth ocular pursuit (saccadic movement), patients with schizophrenia have an elevated blink rate. The elevated blink rate is thought to reflect hyperdopaminergic activity. In primates, blinking can be increased by dopamine agonists and reduced by dopamine antagonists.

Speech.   Although the disorders of speech in schizophrenia (e.g., looseness of associations) are classically considered to indicate a thought disorder, they may also indicate a forme fruste of aphasia, perhaps implicating the dominant parietal lobe. The inability of schizophrenia patients to perceive the prosody of speech or to inflect their own speech can be seen as a neurological symptom of a disorder in the nondominant parietal lobe. Other parietal lobe–like symptoms in schizophrenia include the inability to carry out tasks (i.e., apraxia), right–left disorientation, and lack of concern about the disorder.

Other Comorbidity

Obesity.   Patients with schizophrenia appear to be more obese, with higher body mass indexes (BMIs) than age- and gender-matched cohorts in the general population. This is due, at least in part, to the effect of many antipsychotic medications, as well as poor nutritional balance and decreased motor activity. This weight gain, in turn, contributes to an increased risk of cardiovascular morbidity and mortality, an increased risk of diabetes, and other obesity-related conditions such as hyperlipidemia and obstructive sleep apnea.

Diabetes Mellitus.   Schizophrenia is associated with an increased risk of type II diabetes mellitus. This is probably due, in part, to the association with obesity noted previously, but there is also evidence that some antipsychotic medications cause diabetes through a direct mechanism.

Cardiovascular Disease.   Many antipsychotic medications have direct effects on cardiac electrophysiology. In addition, obesity, increased rates of smoking, diabetes, hyperlipidemia, and a sedentary lifestyle all independently increase the risk of cardiovascular morbidity and mortality.

Human Immunodeficiency Virus (HIV).   Patients with schizophrenia appear to have a risk of HIV infection that is 1.5 to 2 times that of the general population. This association is thought to be due to increased risk behaviors, such as unprotected sex, multiple partners, and increased drug use.

Chronic Obstructive Pulmonary Disease.   Rates of chronic obstructive pulmonary disease are reportedly increased in schizophrenia patients compared to the general population. The increased prevalence of smoking is an obvious contributor to this problem and may be the only cause.

Rheumatoid Arthritis.   Patients with schizophrenia have approximately one-third the risk of rheumatoid arthritis that is found in the general population. This inverse association has been replicated several times, the significance of which is unknown.

DIFFERENTIAL DIAGNOSIS

Secondary Psychotic Disorders

A wide range of nonpsychiatric medical conditions and a variety of substances can induce symptoms of psychosis and catatonia. The most appropriate diagnosis for such psychosis or catatonia is psychotic disorder due to a general medical condition, catatonic disorder due to a general medical condition, or substance-induced psychotic disorder.

When evaluating a patient with psychotic symptoms, clinicians should follow the general guidelines for assessing nonpsy-

chiatric conditions. First, clinicians should aggressively pursue an undiagnosed nonpsychiatric medical condition when a patient exhibits any unusual or rare symptoms or any variation in the level of consciousness. Second, clinicians should attempt to obtain a complete family history, including a history of medical, neurological, and psychiatric disorders. Third, clinicians should consider the possibility of a nonpsychiatric medical condition, even in patients with previous diagnoses of schizophrenia. A patient with schizophrenia is just as likely to have a brain tumor that produces psychotic symptoms as is a patient without schizophrenia.

Other Psychotic Disorders

The psychotic symptoms of schizophrenia can be identical with those of schizophreniform disorder, brief psychotic disorder, schizoaffective disorder, and delusional disorders. *Schizophreniform disorder* differs from schizophrenia in that the symptoms have a duration of at least 1 month but less than 6 months. *Brief psychotic disorder* is the appropriate diagnosis when the symptoms have lasted at least 1 day but less than 1 month and when the patient has not returned to the premorbid state of functioning within that time. There may also be a precipitating traumatic event. When a manic or depressive syndrome develops concurrently with the major symptoms of schizophrenia, *schizoaffective disorder* is the appropriate diagnosis. Nonbizarre delusions present for at least 1 month without other symptoms of schizophrenia or a mood disorder warrant the diagnosis of *delusional disorder*.

Mood Disorders

A patient with a major depressive episode may present with delusions and hallucinations, whether the patient has unipolar or bipolar mood disorder. Delusions seen with psychotic depression are typically mood congruent and involve themes such as guilt, self-depreciation, deserved punishment, and incurable illnesses. In mood disorders, psychotic symptoms resolve completely with the resolution of depression. A depressive episode that is this severe may also result in loss of functioning, decline in self-care, and social isolation, but these are secondary to the depressive symptoms and should not be confused with the negative symptoms of schizophrenia.

A full-blown manic episode often presents with delusions and sometimes hallucinations. Delusions in mania are most often mood congruent and typically involve grandiose themes. The flight of ideas seen in mania may, at times, be confused with the thought disorder of schizophrenia. Special attention during mental status examination of a patient with flight of ideas is required to note whether the associative links between topics are conserved, although the conservation is difficult for the observer to follow because of the patient's accelerated rate of thinking.

Personality Disorders

Various personality disorders may have some features of schizophrenia. Schizotypal, schizoid, and borderline personality disorders are the personality disorders with the most similar symptoms. Severe obsessive-compulsive personality disorder may mask an underlying schizophrenic process. Personality disorders, unlike schizophrenia, have mild symptoms and a history of occurring throughout a patient's life; they also lack an identifiable date of onset.

Malingering and Factitious Disorders

For a patient who imitates the symptoms of schizophrenia but does not actually have the disorder, either malingering or a factitious disorder may be an appropriate diagnosis. Persons have faked schizophrenic symptoms and have been admitted into, and treated at, psychiatric hospitals. The condition of patients who are completely in control of their symptom production may qualify for a diagnosis of malingering; such patients usually have some obvious financial or legal reason to be considered mentally ill. The condition of patients who are less in control of their falsification of psychotic symptoms may qualify for a diagnosis of a factitious disorder. Some patients with schizophrenia, however, may falsely complain of an exacerbation of psychotic symptoms to obtain increased assistance benefits or to gain admission to a hospital. (Factitious disorders are the subject of Chapter 15.)

COURSE AND PROGNOSIS

Course

A premorbid pattern of symptoms may be the first evidence of illness, although the import of the symptoms is usually recognized only retrospectively. Characteristically, the symptoms begin in adolescence and are followed by the development of prodromal symptoms in days to a few months. Social or environmental changes, such as going away to college, using a substance, or a relative's death, may precipitate the disturbing symptoms, and the prodromal syndrome may last a year or more before the onset of overt psychotic symptoms.

The classic course of schizophrenia is one of exacerbations and remissions. After the first psychotic episode, a patient gradually recovers and may then function relatively normally for a long time. Patients usually relapse, however, and the pattern of illness during the first 5 years after the diagnosis generally indicates the patient's course. Further deterioration in the patient's baseline functioning follows each relapse of the psychosis. This failure to return to baseline functioning after each relapse is the major distinction between schizophrenia and the mood disorders. Sometimes, a clinically observable postpsychotic depression follows a psychotic episode, and the schizophrenia patient's vulnerability to stress is usually life-long. Positive symptoms tend to become less severe with time, but the socially debilitating negative or deficit symptoms may increase in severity. Although about one third of all schizophrenia patients have some marginal or integrated social existence, most have lives characterized by aimlessness, inactivity, frequent hospitalizations, and, in urban settings, homelessness and poverty.

Prognosis

Several studies have shown that over the 5- to 10-year period after the first psychiatric hospitalization for schizophrenia, only about 10 to 20 percent of patients can be described as having a good outcome. More than 50 percent of patients can be described as having a poor outcome, with repeated hospital-izations, exacerbations of symptoms, episodes of major mood disorders, and suicide attempts. In spite of these glum figures, schizophrenia does not always run a deteriorating course, and several factors have been associated with a good prognosis (see Table 10–3).

Reported remission rates range from 10 to 60 percent, and a reasonable estimate is that 20 to 30 percent of all schizophrenia patients are able to lead somewhat normal lives. About 20 to 30 percent of patients continue to experience moderate symptoms, and 40 to 60 percent of patients remain significantly impaired by their disorder for their entire lives. Patients with schizophrenia do much less well than patients with mood disorders, although 20 to 25 percent of mood disorder patients are also severely disturbed at long-term follow-up.

TREATMENT

Although antipsychotic medications are the mainstay of the treatment for schizophrenia, research has found that psychosocial interventions, including psychotherapy, can augment the clinical improvement. Just as pharmacological agents are used to treat presumed chemical imbalances, nonpharmacological strategies must treat nonbiological issues. The complexity of schizophrenia usually renders any single therapeutic approach inadequate to deal with the multifaceted disorder. Psychosocial modalities should be integrated into the drug treatment regimen and should support it. Most patients with schizophrenia benefit more from the combined use of antipsychotic drugs and psychosocial treatment than from either treatment used alone.

Hospitalization

Hospitalization is indicated for diagnostic purposes, for stabilization of medications, for patients' safety because of suicidal or homicidal ideation, and for grossly disorganized or inappropriate behavior, including the inability to take care of basic needs such as food, clothing, and shelter. Establishing an effective association between patients and community support systems is also a primary goal of hospitalization.

Short stays of 4 to 6 weeks are just as effective as long-term hospitalizations, and those hospital settings with active behavioral approaches produce better results than do custodial institutions. Hospital treatment plans should be oriented toward practical issues of self-care, quality of life, employment, and social relationships. During hospitalization, patients should be coordinated with aftercare facilities including their family homes, foster families, board-and-care homes, and halfway houses. Day-care centers and home visits by therapists or nurses can help patients to remain out of the hospital for long periods and can improve the quality of their daily lives.

Pharmacotherapy

The introduction of chlorpromazine (Thorazine) in 1952 may be the most important single contribution to the treatment of a psychiatric illness. Henri Laborit, a surgeon in Paris, noticed that administering chlorpromazine to patients before surgery resulted in an unusual state in which they seemed less anxious regarding the procedure. Chlorpromazine was subsequently shown to be effective at reducing hallucinations and delusions, as well as excitement. It was also noted that it caused side effects that appeared similar to parkinsonism.

Antipsychotics diminish positive psychotic symptom expression and reduce relapse rates. Approximately 70 percent of patients treated with any antipsychotic achieve remission.

The drugs used to treat schizophrenia have a wide variety of pharmacological properties, but all share the capacity to antagonize postsynaptic dopamine receptors in the brain. Antipsychotics can be categorized into two main groups: the older conventional antipsychotics, which have also been called *first-generation antipsychotics*, or *dopamine receptor antagonists*, and the newer drugs, which have been called *second-generation antipsychotics*, or *SDAs*. Conventional antipsychotics are often referred to as DRAs or *neuroleptics* because of their parkinsonian-like side effects.

Clozapine (Clozaril), the first effective antipsychotic with negligible extrapyramidal side effects, was discovered in 1958 and first studied during the 1960s. However, in 1976, it was noted that clozapine was associated with a substantial risk of agranulocytosis. This property resulted in delays in the introduction of clozapine. In 1990, clozapine finally became available in the United States, but its use was restricted to patients who responded poorly to other agents.

PHASES OF TREATMENT IN SCHIZOPHRENIA

Treatment of Acute Psychosis

Acute psychotic symptoms require immediate attention. Treatment during the acute phase focuses on alleviating the most severe psychotic symptoms. This phase usually lasts from 4 to 8 weeks. Acute schizophrenia is typically associated with severe agitation, which can result from such symptoms as frightening delusions, hallucinations, or suspiciousness, or from other causes, including stimulant abuse. Patients with akathisia can appear agitated when they experience a subjective feeling of motor restlessness. Differentiating akathisia from psychotic agitation can be difficult, particularly when patients are incapable of describing their internal experience. If patients are receiving an agent associated with extrapyramidal side effects, usually a first-generation antipsychotic, a trial with an anticholinergic antiparkinson medication, benzodiazepine, or propranolol (Inderal) may be helpful in making the discrimination.

Clinicians have a number of options for managing agitation that results from psychosis. Antipsychotics and benzodiazepines can result in relatively rapid calming of patients. With highly agitated patients, intramuscular administration of antipsychotics produces a more rapid effect. An advantage of an antipsychotic is that a single intramuscular injection of haloperidol (Haldol), fluphenazine (Prolixin, Permitil), olanzapine (Zyprexa), or ziprasidone (Zeldox) will often result in calming without an excess of sedation. Low-potency antipsychotics are often associated with sedation and postural hypotension, particularly when they are administered intramuscularly. Intramuscular ziprasidone and olanzapine are similar to their oral counterparts in not causing substantial extrapyramidal side effects during acute treatment. This can be an important advantage over haloperidol or fluphenazine, which can cause frightening dystonias or akathisia in some patients. A rapidly dissolving oral formulation of olanzapine (Zydis) may also be helpful as an alternative to an intramuscular injection.

Benzodiazepines are also effective for agitation during acute psychosis. Lorazepam (Ativan) has the advantage of reliable absorption when it is administered either orally or intramuscularly. The use of benzodiazepines may also reduce the amount of antipsychotic that is needed to control psychotic patients.

Some studies suggest that a longer time between the first onset of psychosis and the initiation of treatment is related to a worse outcome. As a result, clinicians must consider the possibility that delayed treatment may worsen the patient's prognosis. However, these data do not mean that all patients need to be treated immediately. A brief delay may permit clinicians to develop a more thorough diagnostic evaluation and rule out causes of abnormal behavior, such as substance abuse, extreme stress, medical illnesses, and other psychiatric illnesses.

Treatment during Stabilization and Maintenance Phase

In the stable, or maintenance, phase the illness is in a relative stage of remission. The goals during this phase are to prevent psychotic relapse and to assist patients in improving their level of functioning. As newer medications have been introduced with a substantively reduced risk of tardive dyskinesia, one of the major concerns about long-term treatment has been diminished. During this phase, patients are usually in a relative state of remission with only minimal psychotic symptoms. Stable patients who are maintained on an antipsychotic have a much lower relapse rate than patients who have their medications discontinued. Data suggest that 16 to 23 percent of patients receiving treatment will experience a relapse within 1 year, and 53 to 72 percent will relapse without medications. Even patients who have had only one episode have a 4 in 5 chance of relapsing at least once over the following 5 years. Stopping medication increases this risk fivefold. Although published guidelines do not make definitive recommendations about the duration of maintenance treatment after the first episode, recent data suggest that 1 or 2 years might not be adequate. This is a particular concern when patients have achieved good employment status or are involved in educational programs, because they have an enormous amount to lose if they experience another psychotic decompensation.

It is generally recommended that multiepisode patients receive maintenance treatment for at least 5 years, and many experts recommend pharmacotherapy on an indefinite basis.

Noncompliance

Noncompliance with long-term antipsychotic treatment is very high. An estimated 40 to 50 percent of patients become noncompliant within 1 or 2 years. Compliance increases when long-acting medication is used instead of oral medication.

When beginning long-acting drugs, some oral supplementation is necessary while peak plasma levels are being achieved. Fluphenazine and haloperidol have been formulated as long-acting injectables. A long-acting form of risperidone is also available.

There are a number of advantages to using long-acting injectable medication. Clinicians know immediately when noncompliance occurs and have some time to initiate appropriate interventions before the medication effect dissipates; there is less day-to-day variability in blood levels, making it easier to establish a minimum effective dose; and, finally, many patients prefer it to having to remember dosage schedules of daily oral preparations.

STRATEGIES FOR POOR RESPONDERS

When patients with acute schizophrenia are administered an antipsychotic medication, approximately 60 percent will improve to the extent that they will achieve a complete remission or experience only mild symptoms; the remaining 40 percent of patients will improve but still demonstrate variable levels of positive symptoms that are resistant to the medications. Rather than categorize patients into responders and nonresponders, it is more accurate to consider the degree to which the illness is improved by medication. Some resistant patients are so severely ill that they require chronic institutionalization. Others will respond to an antipsychotic with substantial suppression of their psychotic symptoms but demonstrate persistent symptoms, such as hallucinations or delusions.

Before considering a patient a poor responder to a particular drug, it is important to assure that he or she received an adequate trial of the medication. A 4- to 6-week trial on an adequate dose of an antipsychotic represents a reasonable trial for most patients. Patients who demonstrate even a mild amount of improvement during this period may continue to improve at a steady rate for 3 to 6 months. It may be helpful to confirm that the patient is receiving an adequate amount of the drug by monitoring the plasma concentration. This information is available for a number of antipsychotics, including haloperidol, clozapine, fluphenazine, trifluoperazine (Stelazine), and perphenazine (Trilafon). A very low plasma concentration may indicate that the patient has been noncompliant or, more commonly, only partially compliant. It may also suggest that the patient is a rapid metabolizer of the antipsychotic or that the drug is not being adequately absorbed. Under these conditions, raising the dose may be helpful. If the level is relatively high, clinicians should consider whether side effects may be interfering with therapeutic response.

If the patient is responding poorly, one may increase the dose above the usual therapeutic level; however, higher doses are not usually associated with greater improvement than conventional doses. Changing to another drug is preferable to changing to a high dose.

If a patient has responded poorly to a conventional dopamine receptor antagonist, it is unlikely that this individual will do well on another dopamine receptor antagonist. Changing to an SDA is more likely to be helpful.

Clozapine is effective for patients who respond poorly to dopamine receptor antagonists. Double-blind studies comparing clozapine to other antipsychotics indicated that clozapine had the clearest advantage over conventional drugs in patients with the most severe psychotic symptoms, as well as in those who had previously responded poorly to other antipsychotics. When clozapine was compared with chlorpromazine in a severely psychotic group of individuals who had failed in trials with at least three antipsychotics, clozapine was significantly more effective in nearly every dimension of psychopathology, including both positive symptoms and negative symptoms.

MANAGING SIDE EFFECTS

Patients frequently experience side effects of an antipsychotic before they experience clinical improvement. Whereas a clinical response may be delayed for days or weeks after drugs are started, side effects may begin almost immediately. For low-potency drugs, these side effects are likely to include sedation, postural hypotension, and anticholinergic effects, whereas high-potency drugs are likely to cause extrapyramidal side effects.

Extrapyramidal Side Effects

Clinicians have a number of alternatives for treating extrapyramidal side effects. These include reducing the dose of the antipsychotic (which is most commonly a dopamine receptor antagonist), adding an antiparkinson medication, and changing the patient to an SDA that is less likely to cause extrapyramidal side effects. The most effective antiparkinson medications are the anticholinergic antiparkinson drugs. However, these medications have their own side effects, including dry mouth, constipation, blurred vision, and, often, memory loss. In addition, these medications are often only partially effective, leaving patients with substantial amounts of lingering extrapyramidal side effects. Centrally acting β-blockers, such as propranolol, also are often effective for treating akathisia. Most patients respond to doses between 30 and 90 mg per day.

If conventional antipsychotics are being prescribed, clinicians may consider prescribing prophylactic antiparkinson medications for patients who are likely to experience disturbing extrapyramidal side effects. These include patients who have a history of extrapyramidal side effect sensitivity and those who are being treated with relatively high doses of high-potency drugs. Prophylactic antiparkinson medications may also be indicated when high-potency drugs are prescribed for young men who tend to have an increased vulnerability for developing dystonias. Again, these patients should be candidates for newer drugs.

Some individuals are highly sensitive to extrapyramidal side effects at the dose that is necessary to control their psychosis. For many of these patients, medication side effects may seem worse than the illness itself. These patients should be treated routinely with an SDA because these agents result in substantially fewer extrapyramidal side effects than the dopamine receptor antagonists. However, these highly sensitive individuals may even experience extrapyramidal side effects on an SDA. Risperidone may cause extrapyramidal side effects even at low doses— for example, 0.5 mg—but the severity and risk are increased at higher doses—for example, more than 6 mg. Olanzapine and Ziprasidone are also associated with dose-related parkinsonism and akathisia.

Tardive Dyskinesia

About 20 to 30 percent of patients on long-term treatment with a conventional dopamine receptor antagonist exhibit symptoms of tardive dyskinesia. Three to five percent of young patients receiving a dopamine receptor antagonist develop tardive dyskinesia each year. The risk in elderly patients is much higher. Although seriously disabling dyskinesia is uncommon, when it occurs it can affect walking, breathing, eating, and talking. Individuals who are more sensitive to acute extrapyramidal side effects appear to be more vulnerable to developing tardive dyskinesia. Patients with organic mental illness and affective disorders may also be more vulnerable to tardive dyskinesia than those with schizophrenia.

The onset of the abnormal movements usually occurs either while the patient is receiving an antipsychotic, within 4 weeks of discontinuing an oral antipsychotic, or 8 weeks after the withdrawal of a depot antipsychotic. There is a slightly lower risk of tardive dyskinesia with new-generation drugs. However, the risk of tardive dyskinesia is not absent with SDAs.

Recommendations for preventing and managing tardive dyskinesia include (1) using the lowest effective dose of antipsychotic; (2) prescribing cautiously with children, elderly patients, and patients with mood disorders; (3) examining patients on a regular basis for evidence of tardive dyskinesia; (4) considering alternatives to the antipsychotic being used, obtaining informed consent, and considering dose reduction when tardive dyskinesia is diagnosed; and (5) considering a number of options if the tardive dyskinesia worsens, including discontinuing the antipsychotic or switching to a different drug. Clozapine has been shown to be effective in reducing severe tardive dyskinesia or tardive dystonia. The reader is referred to Section 32.2 for an extensive discussion of medication-induced movement disorders.

Other Side Effects

Sedation and postural hypotension can be important side effects for patients who are being treated with low-potency DRAs, such as perphenazine. These effects are often most severe during the initial dosing with these medications. As a result, patients treated with these medications may require weeks to reach a therapeutic dose. Although most patients develop tolerance to sedation and postural hypotension, sedation may continue to be a problem. In these patients, daytime drowsiness may interfere with a patient's attempts to return to community life.

All of the dopamine receptor antagonists, as well as risperidone, elevate prolactin levels, which can result in galactorrhea and irregular menses. Long-term elevations in prolactin and the resultant suppression in gonadotropin-releasing hormone can cause suppression in gonadal hormones. These, in turn, may have effects on libido and sexual functioning. There is also concern that elevated prolactin may cause decreases in bone density and lead to osteoporosis. The concerns about hyperprolactinemia and sexual functioning and bone density are based on experiences with prolactin elevations related to tumors and other causes. It is unclear if these risks are also associated with the lower elevations that occur with prolactin-elevating drugs.

Health Monitoring in Patients Receiving Antipsychotics

Because of the SDAs effects on insulin metabolism, psychiatrists should monitor a number of health indicators including BMI, fasting blood glucose, and lipid profiles. Patients should be weighed and their BMI calculated for every visit for 6 months after a medication change. See Section 19.3 on Obesity for a discussion of the metabolic syndrome.

Side Effects of Clozapine

Clozapine has a number of side effects that make it a difficult drug to administer. The most serious is a risk of agranulocytosis. This potentially fatal condition occurs in approximately 0.3 percent of patients treated with clozapine during the first year of exposure. Subsequently, the risk is substantially lower. As a result, patients who receive clozapine in the United States are required to be in a program of weekly blood monitoring for the first 6 months and biweekly monitoring for the next 6 months. After 1 year of treatment without hematological problems, monitoring can be done monthly.

Clozapine is also associated with a higher risk of seizures than other antipsychotics. The risk reaches nearly 5 percent at doses greater than 600 mg. Patients who develop seizures with clozapine can usually be managed by reducing the dose and adding an anticonvulsant, usually valproate (Depakene). Myocarditis has been reported to occur in approximately 5 patients per 100,000 patient-years. Other side effects with clozapine include hypersalivation, sedation, tachycardia, weight gain, diabetes, fever, and postural hypotension.

OTHER BIOLOGICAL THERAPIES

Electroconvulsive therapy (ECT) has been studied in both acute and chronic schizophrenia. Studies in recent-onset patients indicate that ECT is about as effective as antipsychotic medications and more effective than psychotherapy. Other studies suggest that supplementing antipsychotic medications with ECT is more effective than using antipsychotic medications alone. Antipsychotic medications should be administered during and after ECT treatment. Although psychosurgery is no longer considered an appropriate treatment, it is practiced on a limited experimental basis for severe, intractable cases.

PSYCHOSOCIAL THERAPIES

Psychosocial therapies include a variety of methods to increase social abilities, self-sufficiency, practical skills, and interpersonal communication in schizophrenia patients. The goal is to enable persons who are severely ill to develop social and vocational skills for independent living. Such treatment is carried out at many sites: hospitals, outpatient clinics, mental health centers, day hospitals, and home or social clubs.

Social Skills Training

Social skills training is sometimes referred to as behavioral skills therapy. The therapy can be directly supportive and useful to the patient along with pharmacological therapy. In addition to the psychotic symptoms seen in patients with schizophrenia, other noticeable symptoms involve the way the person relates to others, including poor eye contact, unusual delays in response, odd facial expressions, lack of spontaneity in social situations, and inaccurate perceptions or lack of perception of emotions in other people. Behavioral skills training addresses these behaviors through the use of videotapes of others and of the patient, role playing in therapy, and homework assignments for the specific skills being practiced. Social skills training has been shown to reduce relapse rates as measured by the need for hospitalization.

Family-Oriented Therapies

Because patients with schizophrenia are often discharged in an only partially remitted state, a family to which a patient returns can often benefit from a brief but intensive (as often as daily) course of family therapy. The therapy should focus on the immediate situation and should include identifying and avoiding potentially troublesome situations. When problems do emerge with the patient in the family, the aim of the therapy should be to resolve the problem quickly.

In wanting to help, family members too often encourage a relative with schizophrenia to resume regular activities too quickly, both from ignorance about the disorder and from denial of its severity. Without being overly discouraging, therapists must help the family and the patient understand and learn about schizophrenia and must encourage discussion of the psychotic episode and the events leading up to it. Ignoring the psychotic episode, a common occurrence, often increases the shame associated with the event and does not exploit the freshness of the episode to understand it better. Psychotic symptoms often frighten family members, and talking openly with the psychiatrist and with the relative with schizophrenia often eases all parties. Therapists can direct later family therapy toward long-range application of stress-reducing and coping strategies and toward the patient's gradual reintegration into everyday life.

Therapists must control the emotional intensity of family sessions with patients with schizophrenia. The excessive expression of emotion during a session can damage a patient's recovery process and can undermine potentially successful future family therapy. Several studies have shown that family therapy is especially effective in reducing relapses.

National Alliance for the Mentally Ill. NAMI and similar organizations are support groups for family members and friends of patients who are mentally ill and for patients themselves. These organizations offer emotional and practical advice about obtaining care in the sometimes-complex health care delivery system and are useful sources to which to refer family members. NAMI has also waged a campaign to destigmatize mental illness and to increase government awareness of the needs and rights of persons who are mentally ill and their families.

Case Management

Because a variety of professionals with specialized skills, such as psychiatrists, social workers, and occupational therapists, among others, are involved in a treatment program, it is helpful to have one person aware of all the forces acting on the patient. The case manager ensures that their efforts are coordinated and that the patient keeps appointments and complies with treatment plans; the case manager may make home visits and even accompany the patient to work. The success of the program depends on the educational background, training, and competence of the individual case manager, which vary. Case managers often have too many cases to manage effectively. The ultimate benefits of the program have yet to be demonstrated.

Assertive Community Treatment

The Assertive Community Treatment (ACT) program was originally developed by researchers in Madison, Wisconsin, in the 1970s, for the delivery of services for persons with chronic mental illness. Patients are assigned to one multidisciplinary team (case manager, psychiatrist, nurse, general physicians, etc.). The team has a fixed caseload of patients and delivers all services when and where needed by the patient, 24 hours a day, 7 days a week. This is mobile and intensive intervention that provides treatment, rehabilitation, and support activities. These include home delivery of medications, monitoring of mental and physical health, in vivo social skills, and frequent contact with family members. There is a high staff-to-patient ratio (1:12). ACT programs can effectively decrease the risk of rehospitalization for persons with schizophrenia, but they are labor-intensive and expensive programs to administer.

Group Therapy

Group therapy for persons with schizophrenia generally focuses on real-life plans, problems, and relationships. Groups may be behaviorally oriented, psychodynamically or insight oriented, or supportive. Some investigators doubt that dynamic interpretation and insight therapy are valuable for typical patients with schizophrenia. But group therapy is effective in reducing social isolation, increasing the sense of cohesiveness, and improving reality testing for patients with schizophrenia. Groups led in a supportive manner appear to be most helpful for schizophrenia patients.

Cognitive-Behavioral Therapy

Cognitive-behavioral therapy has been used in schizophrenia patients to improve cognitive distortions, reduce distractibility, and correct errors in judgment. There are reports of ameliorating delusions and hallucinations in some patients using this method. Patients who might benefit generally have some insight into their illness.

Individual Psychotherapy

Studies of the effects of individual psychotherapy in the treatment of schizophrenia have provided data that the therapy is helpful and that the effects are additive to those of pharmacological treatment. In psychotherapy with a schizophrenia patient, developing a therapeutic relationship that the patient experiences as safe is critical. The therapist's reliability, the emotional distance between the therapist and the patient, and the genuineness of the therapist as interpreted by the patient all affect the therapeutic experience. Psychotherapy for a schizophrenia patient should be thought of in terms of decades, rather than sessions, months, or even years.

Some clinicians and researchers have emphasized that the ability of a patient with schizophrenia to form a therapeutic alliance with a therapist is predictive of the outcome. Schizophrenia patients who are able to form a good therapeutic alliance are likely to remain in psychotherapy, remain compliant with their medications, and have good outcomes at 2-year follow-up evaluations.

The relationship between clinicians and patients differs from that encountered in the treatment of nonpsychotic patients. Establishing a relationship is often difficult. Persons with schizophrenia are desperately lonely yet defend against closeness and trust; they are likely to become suspicious, anxious, or hostile or to regress when someone attempts to draw close. Therapists should scrupulously respect a patient's distance and privacy and should demonstrate simple directness, patience, sincerity, and sensitivity to social conventions in preference to premature informality and the condescending use of first names. The patient is likely to perceive exaggerated warmth or professions of friendship as attempts at bribery, manipulation, or exploitation.

In the context of a professional relationship, however, flexibility is essential in establishing a working alliance with the patient. A therapist may have meals with the patient, sit on the floor, go for a walk, eat at a restaurant, accept and give gifts, play table tennis, remember the patient's birthday, or just sit silently with the patient. The major aim is to convey the idea that the therapist is trustworthy, wants to understand the patient and tries to do so, and has faith in the patient's potential as a human being, no matter how disturbed, hostile, or bizarre the patient may be at the moment.

Personal Therapy

A flexible type of psychotherapy called personal therapy is a recently developed form of individual treatment for schizophrenia patients. Its objective is to enhance personal and social adjustment and to forestall relapse. It is a select method using social skills and relaxation exercises, psychoeducation, self-reflection, self-awareness, and exploration of individual vulnerability to stress. The therapist provides a setting that stresses acceptance and empathy. Patients receiving personal therapy show improvement in social adjustment (a composite measure that includes work performance, leisure, and interpersonal relationships) and have a lower relapse rate after 3 years than patients not receiving personal therapy.

Dialectical Behavior Therapy

Dialectical behavior therapy (DBT) combines cognitive and behavioral theories in both individual and group settings and has proved useful in borderline states; it might have benefit in schizophrenia. Emphasis is placed on improving interpersonal skills in the presence of an active and empathic therapist.

Vocational Therapy

A variety of methods and settings are used to help patients regain old skills or develop new ones. These include sheltered workshops, job clubs, and part-time or transitional employment programs. Enabling patients to become gainfully employed is both a means toward, and a sign of, recovery. Many schizophrenia patients are capable of performing high-quality work in spite of their illness. Others may exhibit exceptional skill or even brilliance in a limited field as a result of some idiosyncratic aspect of their disorder.

Art Therapy

Many schizophrenic patients benefit from art therapy, which provides them with an outlet for their constant bombardment of imagery. It helps them to communicate with and share their inner, often-frightening world with others. In some circles, the art of the mentally ill is highly collectable; but whether purchased or not, the production of a work that is appreciated by others can do much to raise self-esteem.

Integrating Psychosocial and Medication Treatments

Antipsychotic medication has been established as the most effective treatment for schizophrenia; but it is not sufficient for many patients, who greatly benefit from the addition of psychosocial therapy. In fact, many studies show that combining both approaches produces the best results.

11 ▲

Other Psychotic Disorders

▲ 11.1 Schizophreniform Disorder

Gabriel Langfeldt (1895–1983) first used the term *schizophreniform* in 1939, at the University Psychiatric Clinic in Oslo, Norway, to describe a condition with sudden onset and benign course associated with mood symptoms and clouding of consciousness. The text revision of the fourth edition of the *Diagnostic and Statistical Manual of Mental Disorders* (DSM-IV-TR) describes schizophreniform disorder as similar to schizophrenia, except that its symptoms last at least 1 month but less than 6 months. Patients with schizophreniform disorder return to their baseline level of functioning once the disorder has resolved. In contrast, for a patient to meet the diagnostic criteria for schizophrenia, the symptoms must have been present for at least 6 months.

EPIDEMIOLOGY

Little is known about the incidence, prevalence, and sex ratio of schizophreniform disorder. The disorder is most common in adolescents and young adults and is less than half as common as schizophrenia. A lifetime prevalence rate of 0.2 percent and a 1-year prevalence rate of 0.1 percent have been reported.

Several studies have shown that the relatives of patients with schizophreniform disorder are at high risk of having other psychiatric disorders, but the distribution of the disorders differs from the distribution seen in the relatives of patients with schizophrenia and bipolar disorders. Specifically, the relatives of patients with schizophreniform disorders are more likely to have mood disorders than are the relatives of patients with schizophrenia. In addition, the relatives of patients with schizophreniform disorder are more likely to have a diagnosis of a psychotic mood disorder than are the relatives of patients with bipolar disorders.

ETIOLOGY

The cause of schizophreniform disorder is not known. As Langfeldt noted in 1939, patients with this diagnostic label are likely to be heterogeneous. In general, some patients have a disorder similar to schizophrenia, whereas others have a disorder similar to a mood disorder. Because of the generally good outcome, the disorder probably has similarities to the episodic nature of mood disorders. Some data, however, indicate a close relation to schizophrenia.

In support of the relation to mood disorders, several studies have shown that patients with schizophreniform disorder, as a group, have more affective symptoms (especially mania) and a better outcome than patients with schizophrenia. In addition, the increased occurrence of mood disorders in the relatives of patients with schizophreniform disorder indicates a relation to mood disorders. Thus, the biological and epidemiological data are most consistent with the hypothesis that the current diagnostic category defines a group of patients some of whom have a disorder similar to schizophrenia, whereas others have a disorder resembling a mood disorder.

Brain Imaging

A relative activation deficit in the inferior prefrontal region of the brain while the patient is performing a region-specific psychological task (the Wisconsin Card Sorting Test), as reported for patients with schizophrenia, has been reported in patients with schizophreniform disorder. One study showed the deficit to be limited to the left hemisphere and also found impaired striatal activity suppression limited to the left hemisphere during the activation procedure. The data can be interpreted to indicate a physiological similarity between the psychosis of schizophrenia and the psychosis of schizophreniform disorder. Additional central nervous system factors, as yet unidentified, may lead to either the long-term course of schizophrenia or the foreshortened course of schizophreniform disorder.

Although some data indicate that patients with schizophreniform disorder may have enlarged cerebral ventricles, as determined by computed tomography and magnetic resonance imaging, other data indicate that, unlike the enlargement seen in schizophrenia, the ventricular enlargement in schizophreniform disorder is not correlated with either outcome or other biological measures.

Other Biological Measures

Although brain imaging studies point to a similarity between schizophreniform disorder and schizophrenia, at least one study of electrodermal activity indicated a difference. Patients with schizophrenia who were born during the winter and spring months (a period of high risk for the birth of these patients) had hyporesponsive skin conductances, but this association was absent in patients with schizophreniform disorder. The significance and the meaning of this single study are difficult to interpret, but the results do suggest caution in assuming similarity between patients with schizophrenia and those with schizophreniform disorder. Data from at least one study of eye tracking in the two groups also indicate that they may differ in some biological measures.

DIAGNOSTIC AND CLINICAL FEATURES

The DSM-IV-TR criteria for schizophreniform disorder are listed in Table 11.1–1. Schizophreniform disorder is an acute psychotic

Table 11.1–1
DSM-IV-TR Diagnostic Criteria for Schizophreniform Disorder

A. Criteria A, D, and E of schizophrenia are met.
B. An episode of the disorder (including prodromal, active, and residual phases) lasts at least 1 month but less than 6 months. (When the diagnosis must be made without waiting for recovery, it should be qualified as "provisional.")

Specify if:

Without good prognostic features
With good prognostic features: as evidenced by two (or more) of the following:

(1) onset of prominent psychotic symptoms within 4 weeks of the first noticeable change in usual behavior or functioning
(2) confusion or perplexity at the height of the psychotic episode
(3) good premorbid social and occupational functioning
(4) absence of blunted or flat affect

From American Psychiatric Association. *Diagnostic and Statistical Manual of Mental Disorders.* 4th ed. Text rev. Washington, DC: American Psychiatric Association; copyright 2000, with permission.

disorder that has a rapid onset and lacks a long prodromal phase. Although many patients with schizophreniform disorder may experience functional impairment at the time of an episode, they are unlikely to report a progressive decline in social and occupational functioning. The initial symptom profile is the same as that of schizophrenia in that two or more psychotic symptoms (hallucinations, delusions, disorganized speech and behavior, or negative symptoms) must be present. Schneiderian first-rank symptoms are frequently observed. In addition, an increased likelihood is found of emotional turmoil and confusion, the presence of which may indicate a good prognosis. Although negative symptoms may be present, they are relatively uncommon in schizophreniform disorder and are considered poor prognostic features. In a small series of first-admission patients with schizophreniform disorder, one fourth had moderate to severe negative symptoms. Almost all were initially categorized as "schizophreniform disorder without good prognostic features," and 2 years later, 73 percent were rediagnosed with schizophrenia, compared with 38 percent of those with "good prognostic features."

By definition, patients with schizophreniform disorder return to their baseline state within 6 months. In some instances, the illness is episodic, with more than one episode occurring after long periods of full remission. If the combined duration of symptomatology exceeds 6 months, however, then schizophrenia should be considered.

Ms. V was a 30-year-old white woman from a working-class family. She was born prematurely and as a toddler had a seizure disorder that was treated with phenobarbital (Luminal, Solfoton) for 1 year. She did well in school, but dropped out in the 12th grade, obtained a General Educational Development (GED) diploma, and began working at 18 years of age. She described her adolescence as a time when she was happy, outgoing, and had several friends. She married at 21 years of age and had two children, but 9 months before her initial hospitalization, she and her husband separated. Ms. V began working in a local factory, and she and her children moved in with her mother. About 6 weeks before her initial admission, Ms. V started feeling that drug dealers and gangsters were out to hurt her and that people were poisoning her food. She also did not let her children eat, fearing they would die from food poisoning. She was admitted to the hospital for 2 weeks but did not receive any medications at that time. Three weeks after discharge, she was readmitted with the same symptoms and also experienced thought broadcasting, thought insertion, and olfactory hallucinations. She was treated with haloperidol (Haldol) and was discharged after 1 month. She later moved to Florida with her mother and children, worked full time, and remained free of symptoms without treatment for 9 years. At that time, she again became psychotic, but after treatment with olanzapine (Zyprexa) for 1 month, she recovered fully and resumed her usual social and occupational functioning. (Courtesy of Bushra Naz, M.D., Laura J. Fochtmann, M.D., and Evelyn J. Bromet, M.D.)

DIFFERENTIAL DIAGNOSIS

It is important to first differentiate schizophreniform disorder from psychoses that can arise from medical conditions. This is accomplished by taking a detailed history and physical examination and, when indicated, performing laboratory tests or imaging studies. A detailed history of medication use, including over-the-counter medications and herbal products, is essential because many therapeutic agents can also produce an acute psychosis. Although it is not always possible to distinguish substance-induced psychosis from other psychotic disorders cross-sectionally, a rapid onset of psychotic symptoms in a patient with a significant substance history should raise the suspicion of a substance-induced psychosis. A detailed substance use history and toxicological screen are also important for treatment planning in an individual with a new onset of psychosis.

The duration of psychotic symptoms is one of the factors that distinguish schizophreniform disorder from other syndromes. Schizophrenia is diagnosed if the duration of the prodromal, active, and residual phases lasts for more than 6 months, whereas symptoms that occur for less than 1 month indicate a brief psychotic disorder. In DSM-IV-TR, a diagnosis of brief psychotic disorder does not require that a major stressor be present.

It is sometimes difficult to distinguish mood disorders with psychotic features from schizophreniform disorder. Furthermore, schizophreniform disorder and schizophrenia can be highly comorbid with mood and anxiety disorders. Additional confounds are that mood symptoms, such as loss of interest and pleasure, may be difficult to distinguish from negative symptoms, avolition, and anhedonia. Some mood symptoms may also be present during the early course of schizophrenia. A thorough longitudinal history is important in elucidating the diagnosis because the presence of psychotic symptoms exclusively during periods of mood disturbance is an indication of a primary mood disorder.

COURSE AND PROGNOSIS

The course of schizophreniform disorder, for the most part, is defined in the criteria. It is a psychotic illness lasting more than

1 month and less than 6 months. The real issue is what happens to persons with this illness over time. Most estimates of progression to schizophrenia range between 60 and 80 percent. What happens to the other 20 to 40 percent is not known. Some will have a second or third episode during which they will deteriorate into a more chronic condition of schizophrenia. A few, however, may have only this single episode and then continue on with their lives, which is clearly the outcome desired by all clinicians and family members, although it is probably a rare occurrence and should not be held out as likely.

TREATMENT

Hospitalization, which is often necessary in treating patients with schizophreniform disorder, allows effective assessment, treatment, and supervision of a patient's behavior. The psychotic symptoms can usually be treated by a 3- to 6-month course of antipsychotic drugs (e.g., risperidone). Several studies have shown that patients with schizophreniform disorder respond to antipsychotic treatment much more rapidly than do patients with schizophrenia. In one study, about 75 percent of patients with schizophreniform disorder and only 20 percent of the patients with schizophrenia responded to antipsychotic medications within 8 days. A trial of lithium (Eskalith), carbamazepine (Tegretol), or valproate (Depakene) may be warranted for treatment and prophylaxis if a patient has a recurrent episode. Psychotherapy is usually necessary to help patients integrate the psychotic experience into their understanding of their minds and lives. Electroconvulsive therapy may be indicated for some patients, especially those with marked catatonic or depressed features.

Finally, most patients with schizophreniform disorder progress to full-blown schizophrenia despite treatment. In those cases, a course of management consistent with a chronic illness must be formulated.

▲ 11.2 Schizoaffective Disorder

As the term implies, *schizoaffective disorder* has features of both schizophrenia and affective disorders (now called *mood disorders*). In current diagnostic systems, patients can receive the diagnosis of schizoaffective disorder if they fit into one of the following six categories: (1) patients with schizophrenia who have mood symptoms; (2) patients with mood disorder who have symptoms of schizophrenia; (3) patients with both mood disorder and schizophrenia; (4) patients with a third psychosis unrelated to schizophrenia and mood disorder; (5) patients whose disorder is on a continuum between schizophrenia and mood disorder; and (6) patients with some combination of the foregoing. The text revision of the fourth edition of the *Diagnostic and Statistical Manual of Mental Disorders* (DSM-IV-TR) incorporated the stricter time frame of 1 month's duration of schizophrenia symptoms and required an "uninterrupted period of illness during which at some time, either there is a Major Depressive Episode, a Manic Episode, or a Mixed Episode concurrent with symptoms that meet Criterion A for Schizophrenia." DSM-IV-TR also elaborated more on the criterion of duration of the mood symp-

toms relative to the psychotic symptoms. In the tenth revision of *International Statistical Classification of Diseases and Related Health Problems* (ICD-10), schizoaffective disorder is a distinct entity and can be applied to patients who have co-occurring mood symptoms and schizophrenic-like mood-incongruent psychosis.

EPIDEMIOLOGY

The lifetime prevalence of schizoaffective disorder is less than 1 percent, possibly in the range of 0.5 to 0.8 percent. These figures, however, are estimates; various studies of schizoaffective disorder have used varying diagnostic criteria. In clinical practice, a preliminary diagnosis of schizoaffective disorder is frequently used when a clinician is uncertain of the diagnosis.

Gender and Age Differences

The literature describing gender and age differences among patients with schizoaffective disorder is limited. The depressive type of schizoaffective disorder may be more common in older persons than in younger persons, and the bipolar type may be more common in young adults than in older adults. The prevalence of the disorder has been reported to be lower in men than in women, particularly married women; the age of onset for women is later than that for men, as in schizophrenia. Men with schizoaffective disorder are likely to exhibit antisocial behavior and to have a markedly flat or inappropriate affect.

ETIOLOGY

The cause of schizoaffective disorder is unknown. The disorder may be a type of schizophrenia, a type of mood disorder, or the simultaneous expression of each. Schizoaffective disorder may also be a distinct third type of psychosis, one that is unrelated to either schizophrenia or a mood disorder. The most likely possibility is that schizoaffective disorder is a heterogeneous group of disorders encompassing all of these possibilities.

Studies designed to explore the etiology have examined family histories, biological markers, short-term treatment responses, and long-term outcomes. Most studies have considered patients with schizoaffective disorder to be a homogeneous group, but recent studies have examined the bipolar and depressive types of schizoaffective disorder separately, and DSM-IV-TR has a classification for each type.

Although much of the family and genetic research in schizoaffective disorder is based on the premise that schizophrenia and the mood disorders are completely separate entities, some data indicate that they may be genetically related. Studies of the relatives of patients with schizoaffective disorder have reported inconsistent results; however, according to DSM-IV-TR, an increased risk of schizophrenia exists among the relatives of probands with schizoaffective disorder.

As a group, patients with schizoaffective disorder have a better prognosis than patients with schizophrenia and a worse prognosis than patients with mood disorders. In addition, as a group, patients with schizoaffective disorder tend to have a nondeteriorating course and respond better to lithium than do patients with schizophrenia.

Consolidation of Data

A reasonable conclusion from the data is that patients with schizoaffective disorder are a heterogeneous group: Some have schizophrenia with prominent affective symptoms, others have a mood disorder with prominent schizophrenic symptoms, and still others have a distinct clinical syndrome. The hypothesis that patients with schizoaffective disorder have both schizophrenia and a mood disorder is untenable because the calculated co-occurrence of the two disorders is much lower than the incidence of schizoaffective disorder.

DIAGNOSIS AND CLINICAL FEATURES

The DSM-IV-TR diagnostic criteria are provided in Table 11.2–1. The diagnostic criteria, however, still leave much to interpretation. The clinician must accurately diagnose the affective illness, making sure it meets the criteria of either a manic or a depressive episode, but also determining the exact length of each episode (not always easy or even possible).

The length of each episode is critical for two reasons. First, to meet Criterion B (psychotic symptoms in the absence of the mood syndrome), it is important to know when the affective episode ends and the psychosis continues. Second, to meet Criterion C, the length of all mood episodes must be combined and compared with the total length of the illness. If the mood component is present for a substantial portion of the total illness, then that criterion is met. Calculating the total length of the episodes can be difficult, and the term "substantial portion" is not defined. In practice, most clinicians look for the mood component to be 15 to 20 percent of the total illness. Patients who have one full manic episode lasting 2 months but who have had symptoms of schizophrenia for 10 years do not meet the criteria for schizoaffective disorder. Instead, the diagnosis would be a mood episode superimposed on schizophrenia. Whether the bipolar

and depressive type specifiers are helpful is unclear, but they may direct treatment options. These subtypes are often confused with earlier subtypes (schizophrenic vs. affective type) thought to have implications in course and prognosis. As with most psychiatric diagnoses, schizoaffective disorder should not be used if the symptoms are caused by substance abuse or a secondary medical condition.

> Mrs. P was a 47-year-old, divorced, unemployed woman who lived alone and was chronically psychotic despite treatment with olanzapine, 20 mg per day, and citalopram (Celexa), 20 mg per day. She believed that she was getting messages from God and the police department to go on a mission to fight drug dealers. She also believed that the Mafia was trying to stop her in this pursuit. The onset of her illness began at 20 years of age, when she experienced the first of several depressive episodes. She also described periods when she felt more energetic, talkative, had decreased need for sleep, and was more active, sometimes cleaning her house the whole night. Approximately 4 years after the onset of her symptoms, she began to hear "voices" that became stronger when she got depressed but were still present and continued to disturb her even when her mood was euthymic. Approximately 10 years after her illness began, she developed the belief that policemen were everywhere and that the neighbors were spying on her. She was hospitalized voluntarily. Two years later, she had another depressive episode, and the voices told her she could not live in her apartment. She was tried on lithium, antidepressants, and antipsychotic medications but continued to be chronically symptomatic with mood symptoms as well as psychosis. (Courtesy of Shmuel Fennig, M.D., Laura J. Fochtmann, M.D., and Gabrielle A. Carlson, M.D.)

DIFFERENTIAL DIAGNOSIS

The psychiatric differential diagnosis includes all the possibilities usually considered for mood disorders and for schizophrenia. In any differential diagnosis of psychotic disorders, a complete medical workup should be performed to rule out organic causes for the symptoms. A history of substance use (with or without positive results on a toxicology screening test) may indicate a substance-induced disorder. Preexisting medical conditions, their treatment, or both can cause psychotic and mood disorders. Any suspicion of a neurological abnormality warrants consideration of a brain scan to rule out anatomical pathology and an electroencephalogram to determine any possible seizure disorders (e.g., temporal lobe epilepsy). Psychotic disorder caused by seizure disorder is more common than that seen in the general population. It tends to be characterized by paranoia, hallucinations, and ideas of reference. Patients with epilepsy with psychosis are believed to have a better level of function than patients with schizophrenic spectrum disorders. Better control of the seizures can reduce the psychosis.

Table 11.2–1
DSM-IV-TR Diagnostic Criteria for Schizoaffective Disorder

A. An uninterrupted period of illness during which, at some time, there is either a major depressive episode, a manic episode, or a mixed episode concurrent with symptoms that meet Criterion A for schizophrenia.
   Note: The major depressive episode must include Criterion A1: depressed mood.
B. During the same period of illness, there have been delusions or hallucinations for at least 2 weeks in the absence of prominent mood symptoms.
C. Symptoms that meet criteria for a mood episode are present for a substantial portion of the total duration of the active and residual periods of the illness.
D. The disturbance is not due to the direct physiological effects of a substance (e.g., a drug of abuse, a medication) or a general medical condition.

Specify type:
   Bipolar type: if the disturbance includes a manic or a mixed episode (or a manic or a mixed episode and major depressive episodes)
   Depressive type: if the disturbance only includes major depressive episodes

From American Psychiatric Association. *Diagnostic and Statistical Manual of Mental Disorders.* 4th ed. Text rev. Washington, DC: American Psychiatric Association; copyright 2000, with permission.

COURSE AND PROGNOSIS

Considering the uncertainty and evolving diagnosis of schizoaffective disorder, it is difficult to determine the long-term course and prognosis. Given the definition of the diagnosis, patients with schizoaffective disorder might be expected to have a course similar to an episodic mood disorder, a chronic schizophrenic course, or some intermediate outcome. It has been presumed that an increasing presence of schizophrenic symptoms predicted worse prognosis. After 1 year, patients with schizoaffective disorder had different outcomes depending on whether their predominant symptoms were affective (better prognosis) or schizophrenic (worse prognosis). One study that followed patients diagnosed with schizoaffective disorder for 8 years found that the outcomes of these patients more closely resembled outcomes of patients with schizophrenia than outcomes of patients with a mood disorder with psychotic features.

TREATMENT

Mood stabilizers are a mainstay of treatment for bipolar disorders and would be expected to be important in the treatment of patients with schizoaffective disorder. One study that compared lithium with carbamazepine (Tegretol) found that carbamazepine was superior for schizoaffective disorder, depressive type, but found no difference in the two agents for the bipolar type. In practice, however, these medications are used extensively alone, in combination with each other, or with an antipsychotic agent. In manic episodes, patients who are schizoaffective should be treated aggressively with doses of a mood stabilizer in the middle-to-high therapeutic blood concentration range. As the patient enters maintenance phase, the dose can be reduced to low to middle range to avoid adverse effects and potential effects on organ systems (e.g., thyroid and kidney) and to improve ease of use and compliance. Laboratory monitoring of plasma drug concentrations and periodic screening of thyroid, kidney, and hematological functioning should be performed.

By definition, many patients who are schizoaffective have major depressive episodes. Treatment with antidepressants mirrors treatment of bipolar depression. Care should be taken not to precipitate a cycle of rapid switches from depression to mania with the antidepressant. The choice of antidepressant should take into account previous antidepressant successes or failures. Selective serotonin reuptake inhibitors (e.g., fluoxetine [Prozac] and sertraline [Zoloft]) are often used as first-line agents because they have less effect on cardiac status and have a favorable overdose profile. Agitated or insomniac patients, however, may benefit from a tricyclic drug. As in all cases of intractable mania, the use of electroconvulsive therapy should be considered. As mentioned, antipsychotic agents are important in the treatment of the psychotic symptoms of schizoaffective disorder.

Psychosocial Treatment

Patients benefit from a combination of family therapy, social skills training, and cognitive rehabilitation. Because the psychiatric field has had difficulty deciding on the exact diagnosis and prognosis of schizoaffective disorder, this uncertainty must be explained to the patient. The range of symptoms can be vast as patients contend with both ongoing psychosis and varying mood states. It can be very difficult for family members to keep up with the changing nature and needs of these patients. Medication regimens can be complicated, with multiple medications from all classes of drugs.

▲ 11.3 Delusional Disorder and Shared Psychotic Disorder

Delusions are false fixed beliefs not in keeping with the culture. They are among the most interesting of psychiatric symptoms because of the great variety of false beliefs that can be held by so many people and because they are so difficult to treat. The diagnosis of delusional disorder is made when a person exhibits nonbizarre delusions of at least 1 month's duration that cannot be attributed to other psychiatric disorders. *Nonbizarre* means that the delusions must be about situations that can occur in real life, such as being followed, infected, loved at a distance, and so on; that is, they usually have to do with phenomena that, although not real, are nonetheless possible. Several types of delusions may be present, and the predominant type is specified when the diagnosis is made.

EPIDEMIOLOGY

An accurate assessment of the epidemiology of delusional disorder is hampered by the relative rareness of the disorder, as well as by its changing definitions in recent history. Moreover, delusional disorder may be underreported because delusional patients rarely seek psychiatric help unless forced to do so by their families or by the courts. Even with these limitations, however, the literature does support the contention that delusional disorder, although uncommon, has a relatively steady rate.

The prevalence of delusional disorder in the United States is estimated to be 0.025 to 0.03 percent. Thus, delusional disorder is much rarer than schizophrenia, which has a prevalence of about 1 percent, and the mood disorders, which have a prevalence of about 5 percent. The annual incidence of delusional disorder is 1 to 3 new cases per 100,000 persons. According to the text revision of the fourth edition of the *Diagnostic and Statistical Manual of Mental Disorders* (DSM-IV-TR), delusional disorders account for only 1 to 2 percent of all admissions to inpatient mental health facilities. The mean age of onset is about 40 years, but the range for age of onset runs from 18 years of age to the 90s. A slight preponderance of female patients exists. Men are more likely to develop paranoid delusions than women, who are more likely to develop delusions of erotomania. Many patients are married and employed, but some association is seen with recent immigration and low socioeconomic status.

ETIOLOGY

As with all major psychiatric disorders, the cause of delusional disorder is unknown. Moreover, patients currently classified as having delusional disorder probably have a heterogeneous group of conditions with delusions as the predominant symptom. The central concept about the cause of delusional disorder is its distinctness from schizophrenia and the mood disorders. Delusional disorder is much rarer than either schizophrenia or mood disorders, with a later onset than schizophrenia and a much less pronounced female predominance than the mood disorders. The most convincing data come from family studies that report an increased prevalence of delusional disorder and related personality traits (e.g., suspiciousness, jealousy, and secretiveness) in the relatives of delusional disorder probands. Family studies have reported neither an increased incidence of schizophrenia and mood disorders in the families of delusional disorder probands nor an increased incidence of delusional disorder in the families of probands with schizophrenia. Long-term follow-up of patients with delusional disorder indicates that the diagnosis of delusional disorder is relatively stable, with less than one fourth of the patients eventually being reclassified as having schizophrenia and less than 10 percent of patients eventually being reclassified as having a mood disorder. These data indicate that delusional disorder is not simply an early stage in the development of one or both of these two more common disorders.

Biological Factors

A wide range of nonpsychiatric medical conditions and substances, including clear-cut biological factors, can cause delusions, but not everyone with a brain tumor, for example, has delusions. Unique, and not yet understood, factors in a patient's brain and personality are likely to be relevant to the specific pathophysiology of delusional disorder.

The neurological conditions most commonly associated with delusions affect the limbic system and the basal ganglia. Patients whose delusions are caused by neurological diseases and who show no intellectual impairment tend to have complex delusions similar to those in patients with delusional disorder. Conversely, patients with neurological disorder with intellectual impairments often have simple delusions unlike those in patients with delusional disorder. Thus, delusional disorder may involve the limbic system or basal ganglia in patients who have intact cerebral cortical functioning.

Delusional disorder can arise as a normal response to abnormal experiences in the environment, the peripheral nervous system, or the central nervous system (CNS). Thus, if patients have erroneous sensory experiences of being followed (e.g., hearing footsteps), they may come to believe that they are actually being followed. This hypothesis hinges on the presence of hallucinatory-like experiences that need to be explained. The presence of such hallucinatory experiences in delusional disorder has not been proved.

Psychodynamic Factors

Practitioners have a strong clinical impression that many patients with delusional disorder are socially isolated and have attained less-than-expected levels of achievement. Specific psychodynamic theories about the cause and the evolution of delusional symptoms involve suppositions regarding hypersensitive persons and specific ego mechanisms: reaction formation, projection, and denial.

Freud's Contributions. Sigmund Freud believed that delusions, rather than being symptoms of the disorder, are part of a healing process. In 1896, he described projection as the main defense mechanism in paranoia. Later, Freud read *Memories of My Nervous Illness*, an autobiographical account by Daniel Paul Schreber. Although he never met Schreber, Freud theorized from his review of the autobiography that unconscious homosexual tendencies are defended against by denial and projection. According to classic psychodynamic theory, the dynamics underlying the formation of delusions for a female patient are the same as for a male patient. Careful studies of patients with delusions have been unable to corroborate Freud's theories, although they may be relevant in individual cases. Overall, no higher incidence of homosexual ideation or activity is found in patients with delusions than in other groups. Freud's major contribution, however, was to demonstrate the role of projection in the formation of delusional thought.

Paranoid Pseudocommunity. Norman Cameron described seven situations that favor the development of delusional disorders: an increased expectation of receiving sadistic treatment, situations that increase distrust and suspicion, social isolation, situations that increase envy and jealousy, situations that lower self-esteem, situations that cause persons to see their own defects in others, and situations that increase the potential for rumination over probable meanings and motivations. When frustration from any combination of these conditions exceeds the tolerable limit, persons become withdrawn and anxious; they realize that something is wrong, seek an explanation for the problem, and crystallize a delusional system as a solution. Elaboration of the delusion to include imagined persons and attribution of malevolent motivations to both real and imagined persons result in the organization of the *pseudocommunity*—a perceived community of plotters. This delusional entity hypothetically binds together projected fears and wishes to justify the patient's aggression and to provide a tangible target for the patient's hostilities.

Other Psychodynamic Factors. Clinical observations indicate that many, if not all, paranoid patients experience a lack of trust in relationships. A hypothesis relates this distrust to a consistently hostile family environment, often with an overcontrolling mother and a distant or sadistic father. Erik Erikson's concept of trust versus mistrust in early development is a useful model to explain the suspiciousness of the paranoid who never went through the healthy experience of having his or her needs satisfied by what Erikson termed the "outer-providers." Thus, they have a general distrust of their environment.

Defense Mechanisms. Patients with delusional disorder use primarily the defense mechanisms of reaction formation, denial, and projection. They use reaction formation as a defense against aggression, dependence needs, and feelings of affection and transform the need for dependence into staunch independence. Patients use denial to avoid awareness of painful reality. Consumed with anger and hostility and unable to face responsibility for the rage, they project their resentment and anger onto others and use projection to protect themselves from recognizing unacceptable impulses in themselves.

Other Relevant Factors. Delusions have been linked to a variety of additional factors such as social and sensory isolation, socioeconomic deprivation, and personality disturbance. The deaf, the visually impaired, and possibly immigrants with limited ability in a new language may be more vulnerable to delusion formation than the normal population. Vulnerability is heightened with advanced age. Delusional disturbance and other paranoid features are common in the elderly. In short, multiple factors are associated with the formation of delusions, and the source and pathogenesis of delusional disorders per se have yet to be specified.

DIAGNOSIS AND CLINICAL FEATURES

The DSM-IV-TR diagnostic criteria for delusional disorder are listed in Table 11.3–1.

Mental Status

General Description.   Patients are usually well groomed and well dressed, without evidence of gross disintegration of personality or of daily activities, yet they may seem eccentric, odd, suspicious, or hostile. They are sometimes litigious and may make this inclination clear to the examiner. The most remarkable feature of patients with delusional disorder is that the mental status examination shows them to be quite normal except for a markedly abnormal delusional system. Patients may attempt to engage clinicians as allies in their delusions, but a clinician should not pretend to accept the delusion; this collusion further confounds reality and sets the stage for eventual distrust between the patient and the therapist.

Table 11.3–1
DSM-IV-TR Diagnostic Criteria for Delusional Disorder

A. Nonbizarre delusions (i.e., involving situations that occur in real life, such as being followed, poisoned, infected, loved at a distance, or deceived by spouse or lover, or having a disease) of at least 1 month's duration.
B. Criterion A for schizophrenia has never been met.
   Note: Tactile and olfactory hallucinations may be present in delusional disorder if they are related to the delusional theme.
C. Apart from the impact of the delusion(s) or its ramifications, functioning is not markedly impaired, and behavior is not obviously odd or bizarre.
D. If mood episodes have occurred concurrently with delusions, their total duration has been brief relative to the duration of the delusional periods.
E. The disturbance is not due to the direct physiological effects of a substance (e.g., a drug of abuse, a medication) or a general medical condition.
Specify type (the following types are assigned based on the predominant delusional theme):
   Erotomanic type: delusions that another person, usually of higher status, is in love with the individual
   Grandiose type: delusions of inflated worth, power, knowledge, identity, or special relationship to a deity or famous person
   Jealous type: delusions that the individual's sexual partner is unfaithful
   Persecutory type: delusions that the person (or someone to whom the person is close) is being malevolently treated in some way
   Somatic type: delusions that the person has some physical defect or general medical condition
   Mixed type: delusions characteristic of more than one of the above types but no one theme predominates
   Unspecified type

From American Psychiatric Association. *Diagnostic and Statistical Manual of Mental Disorders.* 4th ed. Text rev. Washington, DC: American Psychiatric Association; copyright 2000, with permission.

Mood, Feelings, and Affect.   Patients' moods are consistent with the content of their delusions. A patient with grandiose delusions is euphoric; one with persecutory delusions is suspicious. Whatever the nature of the delusional system, the examiner may sense some mild depressive qualities.

Perceptual Disturbances.   By definition, patients with delusional disorder do not have prominent or sustained hallucinations. According to DSM-IV-TR, tactile or olfactory hallucinations may be present if they are consistent with the delusion (e.g., somatic delusion of body odor). A few delusional patients have other hallucinatory experiences—virtually always auditory rather than visual.

Thought.   Disorder of thought content, in the form of delusions, is the key symptom of the disorder. The delusions are usually systematized and are characterized as being possible; for example, delusions of being persecuted, having an unfaithful spouse, being infected with a virus, or being loved by a famous person. These examples of delusional content contrast with the bizarre and impossible delusional content in some patients with schizophrenia. The delusional system itself can be complex or simple. Patients lack other signs of thought disorder, although some may be verbose, circumstantial, or idiosyncratic in their speech when they talk about their delusions. Clinicians should not assume that all unlikely scenarios are delusional; the veracity of a patient's beliefs should be checked before deeming their content to be delusional.

Sensorium and Cognition

ORIENTATION.   Patients with delusional disorder usually have no abnormality in orientation unless they have a specific delusion about a person, place, or time.

MEMORY.   Memory and other cognitive processes are intact in patients with delusional disorder.

Impulse Control.   Clinicians must evaluate patients with delusional disorder for ideation or plans to act on their delusional material by suicide, homicide, or other violence. Although the incidence of these behaviors is not known, therapists should not hesitate to ask patients about their suicidal, homicidal, or other violent plans. Destructive aggression is most common in patients with a history of violence; if aggressive feelings existed in the past, therapists should ask patients how they managed those feelings. If patients cannot control their impulses, hospitalization is probably necessary. Therapists can sometimes help foster a therapeutic alliance by openly discussing how hospitalization can help patients gain additional control of their impulses.

Judgment and Insight.   Patients with delusional disorder have virtually no insight into their condition and are almost always brought to the hospital by the police, family members, or employers. Judgment can best be assessed by evaluating the patient's past, present, and planned behavior.

Reliability.   Patients with delusional disorder are usually reliable in their information, except when it impinges on their delusional system.

Types

Persecutory Type. The delusion of persecution is a classic symptom of delusional disorder; persecutory-type and jealousy-type delusions are probably the forms seen most frequently by psychiatrists. Patients with this subtype are convinced that they are being persecuted or harmed. The persecutory beliefs are often associated with querulousness, irritability, and anger, and the individual who acts out his or her anger may at times be assaultive or even homicidal. At other times, such individuals may become preoccupied with formal litigation against their perceived persecutors. In contrast to persecutory delusions in schizophrenia, the clarity, logic, and systematic elaboration of the persecutory theme in delusional disorder leave a remarkable stamp on this condition. The absence of other psychopathology, deterioration in personality, or deterioration in most areas of functioning also contrasts with the typical manifestations of schizophrenia.

Mrs. S, 62 years of age, was referred to a psychiatrist because of complaints of not being able to sleep. Before this episode, she worked full time taking care of children, played tennis almost every day, and managed her household chores. Her chief complaint was that her downstairs neighbor wanted to get her to move away and was doing a variety of things to harass her. At first, she based her belief on certain looks that he gave her and damage done to her mailbox, but later she believed he might be leaving empty bottles of cleaning solutions in the basement so she would be overcome by fumes. As a result, the patient was fearful of falling asleep, convinced that she might be asphyxiated and not awaken in time to get help. She felt somewhat depressed and believed her appetite might be diminished from the stress of being harassed. She had not lost weight and still enjoyed playing tennis and going out with friends. At one point, she considered moving to another apartment but then decided to fight back. The episode had gone on for 8 months when her daughter persuaded her to have a psychiatric assessment. She was pleasant and cooperative in the interview. Except for the specific delusion and mild depressive symptoms, her mental status was normal.

Her history revealed that she was depressed 30 years before, after the death of a close friend. She saw a counselor for several months, which she found helpful, but was not treated with medication. For the current episode, she agreed to take medications, although she believed her neighbor was more in need of treatment than she was. Her symptoms improved somewhat with oral risperidone (Risperdal), 2 mg every night, and oral clonazepam (Klonopin), 0.5 mg every morning and every night. (Courtesy of Shmuel Fennig, M.D., Laura J. Fochtmann, M.D., and Evelyn J. Bromet, PhD.)

Jealous Type. Delusional disorder with delusions of infidelity has been called *conjugal paranoia* when it is limited to the delusion that a spouse has been unfaithful. The eponym *Othello syndrome* has been used to describe morbid jealousy that can arise from multiple concerns. The delusion usually afflicts men, often those with no prior psychiatric illness. It may appear suddenly and serve to explain a host of present and past events involving the spouse's behavior. The condition is difficult to treat and may diminish only on separation, divorce, or death of the spouse.

Marked jealousy (usually termed *pathological* or *morbid jealousy*) is thus a symptom of many disorders—including schizophrenia (female patients more commonly display this feature), epilepsy, mood disorders, drug abuse, and alcoholism—for which treatment is directed at the primary disorder. Jealousy is a powerful emotion; when it occurs in delusional disorder or as part of another condition, it can be potentially dangerous and has been associated with violence, notably both suicide and homicide. The forensic aspects of the symptom have been noted repeatedly, especially its role as a motive for murder. Physical and verbal abuse occur more frequently, however, than do extreme actions among individuals with this symptom. Caution and care in deciding how to deal with such presentations are essential not only for diagnosis, but also from the point of view of safety.

F.M. was a 51-year-old married white man who lived with his wife in their own home and worked full time driving a sanitation truck. He was admitted to the hospital reporting that he was depressed because his wife was having an affair. He began to follow her, kept notes on his observations, and badgered her constantly about this, often waking her up in the middle of the night to make accusations. Shortly before admission, these arguments led to physical violence, and he was brought to the hospital by police. He was treated with oral thioridazine (Mellaril), 50 mg every night, and noted that he was less worried about his wife's behavior. He was seen by a psychiatrist monthly, but on follow-up 10 years later, he continued to believe that his wife was unfaithful. His wife noted that he sometimes became agitated about the delusion but that he generally controlled the impulse to act on it. (Courtesy of Shmuel Fennig, M.D., Laura J. Fochtmann, M.D., and Evelyn J. Bromet, PhD.)

Erotomanic Type. In erotomania, which has also been referred to as *de Clérambault syndrome* or *psychose passionelle*, the patient has the delusional conviction that another person, usually of higher status, is in love with him or her. Such patients also tend to be solitary, withdrawn, dependent, and sexually inhibited, and also have poor levels of social or occupational functioning. The following operational criteria for the diagnosis of erotomania have been suggested: (1) a delusional conviction of amorous communication; (2) object of much higher rank; (3) object being the first to fall in love; (4) object being the first to make advances; (5) sudden onset (within a 7-day period); (6) object remains unchanged; (7) patient rationalizes paradoxical behavior of the object; (8) chronic course; and (9) absence of hallucinations. Besides being the key symptom in some cases of delusional disorder, it is known to occur in schizophrenia, mood disorder, and other organic disorders.

Patients with erotomania frequently show certain characteristics: They are generally unattractive women in low-level jobs who lead withdrawn, lonely lives; they are single and have few sexual contacts. They select secret lovers who differ substantially from them. They exhibit what has been called *paradoxical conduct*, the delusional phenomenon of interpreting all denials of love, no matter how clear, as secret affirmations of love. The course may be chronic, recurrent, or brief. Separation from the love object may be the only satisfactory intervention. Although men are less commonly afflicted by this condition than women, they may be more aggressive and possibly violent in their pursuit of love. Hence, in forensic populations, men with this condition predominate. The object of aggression may not be the loved individual but companions or protectors of the love object who are viewed as trying to come between the lovers. The tendency toward violence among men with erotomania may lead initially to police, rather than psychiatric, contact. In certain cases, resentment and rage in response to an absence of reaction from all forms of love communication may sufficiently escalate to put the love object in danger. So-called stalkers, who continually follow their perceived lovers, frequently have delusions. Although most stalkers are men, women also stalk, and both groups have a high potential for violence.

Mrs. D was a 32-year-old nurse, married with two children, when she was referred to the clinic by her supervisor from a local hospital. She had assaulted one of the residents, claiming he was in love with her. She had worked in the hospital for 12 years and was considered a good nurse. She had previously fallen in love with another physician on the staff of the hospital. Her current delusion began when the young physician entered a room in which she was lying in bed after cosmetic surgery and pointed at her. She had not known him before, but at that moment, she became convinced that he was in love with her. She tried to approach him several times by letter and phone and, although he did not respond, she was sure he was trying to hide his love from her. She was convinced that he was trying to transmit his love through looks he gave her and through the tone of his voice. The resident met her and denied being in love with her, but she began stalking him. At that point, the head nurse forced her to go for a consultation. She was treated for several months during which she continued to work at the same unit and was able to avoid contact with the resident. She insisted that her husband did not know about this. She refused any medications. The therapist arranged a three-way meeting with himself, the patient, and the resident. As a result of this meeting, there was a small reduction in the intensity of her belief, but she continued to maintain it nonetheless. She subsequently agreed to take antipsychotic medications and was given perphenazine, 16 mg per day, but with no improvement. She continued to hold her belief, and the delusion subsided only after the resident moved to another hospital. (Reprinted with permission from *DSM-IV-TR Casebook.*)

Somatic Type.   Delusional disorder with somatic delusions has been called *monosymptomatic hypochondriacal psychosis*. The condition differs from other conditions with hypochondriacal symptoms in the degree of reality impairment. In delusional disorder, the delusion is fixed, unarguable, and presented intensely, because the patient is totally convinced of the physical nature of the disorder. In contrast, persons with hypochondriasis often admit that their fear of illness is largely groundless. The content of the somatic delusion can vary widely from case to case. The three main types are (1) delusions of infestation

(including parasitosis); (2) delusions of dysmorphophobia, such as of misshapenness, personal ugliness, or exaggerated size of body parts (this category seems closest to that of body dysmorphic disorder); and (3) delusions of foul body odors or halitosis. This third category, sometimes referred to as *olfactory reference syndrome*, appears somewhat different from the category of delusions of infestation in that patients with the former have an earlier age of onset (mean 25 years), male predominance, single status, and absence of past psychiatric treatment. Otherwise, the three groups, although individually low in prevalence, appear to overlap.

The onset of symptoms with the somatic type of delusional disorder may be gradual or sudden. In most patients, the illness is unremitting, although the delusion severity may fluctuate. Hyperalertness and high anxiety also characterize patients with this subtype. Some themes recur, such as concerns about infestation in delusional parasitosis, preoccupation with body features with the dysmorphic delusions, and delusional concerns about body odor, which are sometimes referred to as *bromosis*. In delusional parasitosis, tactile sensory phenomena are often linked to the delusional beliefs.

Patients with the somatic type of delusional disorder rarely present for psychiatric evaluation, and when they do, it is usually in the context of a psychiatric consultation or liaison service. Instead, patients generally present to a specific medical specialist for evaluation. Thus, these individuals are more often encountered by dermatologists, plastic surgeons, urologists, acquired immune deficiency syndrome specialists, and sometimes dentists or gastroenterologists.

Ms. G was a 56-year-old homemaker and mother of two who was hospitalized in the burn unit for wound care and skin grafting after sustaining chemical burns to her trunk and extremities. Six months before admission, Ms. G had become increasingly convinced that minute bugs had burrowed underneath her skin. She tried to rid herself of them by washing multiple times each day with medicated soap and lindane shampoo. She also visited several dermatologists and had shown them samples of "dead bugs" for them to examine under the microscope. All told her there was nothing wrong with her and suggested that her problems were psychiatric in nature. She became increasingly distressed by the infestation and worried that the bugs might invade her other organs if not eradicated. Consequently, she decided to asphyxiate the bugs by covering her body with gasoline and holding it against her skin with plastic wrap. She noted that her skin became red and felt as though it were burning, but she viewed this as a positive sign that the bugs were being killed and writhing around as they died. Several hours after she had applied the gasoline, her daughter came to the house, saw Ms. G's condition, and took her to the hospital. When evaluated in the burn unit, Ms. G spoke openly of her concerns about the bugs and was still unsure whether they were present or not. At the same time, she recognized that it had been a mistake to try to kill them with gasoline. She was oriented to person, place, and time and had no other delusional beliefs or auditory or visual hallucinations. She said her mood was "OK," although she was realistically concerned about the extensive treatment that she required and the difficult process of recovering from her injury. She reported no suicidal ideas or intent before admission and had no history of psychiatric treatment. She also did not report any use of substances except for drinking several beers socially approximately twice each month. During her stay in the hospital, she was treated with haloperidol in doses of up to 5 mg per day, with improvement in her concerns about the infestation. She continued to cooperate with treatment for her burns. (Courtesy of Shmuel Fennig, M.D., Laura J. Fochtmann, M.D., and Evelyn J. Bromet, Ph.D.)

Grandiose Type.   Delusions of grandeur (megalomania) have been noted for years. They were first described by Kraepelin.

A 51-year-old man was arrested for disturbing the peace. Police had been called to a local park to stop him from carving his initials and those of a recently formed religious cult into various trees surrounding a pond in the park. When confronted, he had scornfully argued that having been chosen to begin a new townwide religious revival, it was necessary for him to publicize his intent in a permanent fashion. The police were unsuccessful in preventing the man from cutting another tree and arrested him. Psychiatric examination was ordered at the state hospital, and the patient was observed there for several weeks. He denied any emotional difficulty and had never received psychiatric treatment. He had no history of euphoria or mood swings. The patient was angry about being hospitalized and only gradually permitted the doctor to interview him. In a few days, however, he was busy preaching to his fellow patients and letting them know that he had been given a special mandate from God to bring in new converts through his ability to heal. Eventually, his preoccupation with special powers diminished, and no other evidence of psychopathology was observed. The patient was discharged, having received no medication at all. Two months later he was arrested at a local theater, this time for disrupting the showing of a film that depicted subjects he believed to be satanic.

Mixed Type.   The category mixed type applies to patients with two or more delusional themes. This diagnosis should be reserved for cases in which no single delusional type predominates.

Unspecified Type.   The category unspecified type is reserved for cases in which the predominant delusion cannot be subtyped within the previous categories. A possible example is certain delusions of misidentification, for example, Capgras syndrome, named for the French psychiatrist who described the *illusion des sosies*, or the illusion of doubles. The delusion in Capgras syndrome is the belief that a familiar person has been replaced by an impostor. Others have described variants of the Capgras syndrome, namely, the delusion that persecutors or familiar persons can assume the guise of strangers (*Frégoli's phenomenon*) and the very rare delusion that familiar persons can

change themselves into other persons at will (*intermetamorphosis*). Each disorder is not only rare but may be associated with schizophrenia, dementia, epilepsy, and other organic disorders. Reported cases have been predominantly in women, have had associated paranoid features, and have included feelings of depersonalization or derealization. The delusion may be short lived, recurrent, or persistent. It is unclear whether delusional disorder can appear with such a delusion. Certainly, the Frégoli and intermetamorphosis delusions have bizarre content and are unlikely, but the delusion in Capgras syndrome is a possible candidate for delusional disorder. The role of hallucination or perceptual disturbance in this condition needs to be explicated. Cases have appeared after sudden brain damage.

In the 19th century, the French psychiatrist Jules Cotard described several patients who suffered from a syndrome called *délire de négation*, sometimes referred to as *nihilistic delusional disorder* or *Cotard syndrome*. Patients with the syndrome complain of having lost not only possessions, status, and strength, but also their heart, blood, and intestines. The world beyond them is reduced to nothingness. This relatively rare syndrome is usually considered a precursor to a schizophrenic or depressive episode. With the common use today of antipsychotic drugs, the syndrome is seen even less frequently than in the past.

Shared Psychotic Disorder

Shared psychotic disorder (also referred to over the years as *shared paranoid disorder, induced psychotic disorder, folie à deux, folie impose,* and *double insanity*) was first described by two French psychiatrists, Ernest-Charles Lasègue and Jean-Pierre Falret, in 1877. It is probably rare, but incidence and prevalence figures are lacking, and the literature consists almost entirely of case reports.

The disorder is characterized by the transfer of delusions from one person to another. Both persons are closely associated for a long time and typically live together in relative social isolation. In its most common form (which is covered by the DSM-IV-TR criteria in Table 11.3–2), the individual who first has the delusion (the primary case) is often chronically ill and typically is the influential member of a close relationship with a more suggestible person (the secondary case) who also develops the delusion. The person in the secondary case is frequently less intelligent, more gullible, more passive, or more lacking in self-esteem than the

Table 11.3–2
DSM-IV-TR Diagnostic Criteria for Shared Psychotic Disorder

A delusion develops in an individual in the context of a close relationship with another person(s), who has an already-established delusion.

The delusion is similar in content to that of the person who already has the established delusion.

The disturbance is not better accounted for by another psychotic disorder (e.g., schizophrenia) or a mood disorder with psychotic features and is not due to the direct physiological effects of a substance (e.g., a drug of abuse, a medication) or a general medical condition.

From American Psychiatric Association. *Diagnostic and Statistical Manual of Mental Disorders.* 4th ed. Text rev. Washington, DC: American Psychiatric Association; copyright 2000, with permission.

person in the primary case. If the pair separates, the secondary person may abandon the delusion, but this outcome is not seen uniformly. The occurrence of the delusion is attributed to the strong influence of the more dominant member. Old age, low intelligence, sensory impairment, cerebrovascular disease, and alcohol abuse are among the factors associated with this peculiar form of psychotic disorder. A genetic predisposition to idiopathic psychoses has also been suggested as a possible risk factor.

Other special forms have been reported, such as *folie simultanée*, in which two persons become psychotic simultaneously and share the same delusion. Occasionally, more than two individuals are involved (e.g., *folie à trois, quatre, cinq*; also *folie à famille*), but such cases are especially rare. The most common relationships in *folie à deux* are sister–sister, husband–wife, and mother–child, but other combinations have also been described. Almost all cases involve members of a single family.

DIFFERENTIAL DIAGNOSIS

Medical Conditions

In making a diagnosis of delusional disorder, the first step is to eliminate medical disorders as a potential cause of delusions. Many medical conditions can be associated with the development of delusions, at times accompanying a delirious state.

Toxic-metabolic conditions and disorders affecting the limbic system and basal ganglia are most often associated with the emergence of delusional beliefs. Complex delusions occur more frequently in patients with subcortical pathology. In Huntington's disease and in individuals with idiopathic basal ganglia calcifications, for example, more than 50 percent of patients demonstrated delusions at some point in their illness. After right cerebral infarction, types of delusions that are more prevalent include anosognosia and reduplicative paramnesia (i.e., individuals believing they are in different places at the same time). Capgras syndrome has been observed in a number of medical disorders, including CNS lesions, vitamin B_{12} deficiency, hepatic encephalopathy, diabetes, and hypothyroidism. Focal syndromes have more often involved the right rather than the left hemisphere. Delusions of infestation, lycanthropy (i.e., the false belief that the patient is an animal, often a wolf or "werewolf"), heutoscopy (i.e., the false belief that one has a double), and erotomania have been reported in small numbers of patients with epilepsy, CNS lesions, or toxic-metabolic disorders.

Delirium, Dementia, and Substance-Related Disorders

Delirium and dementia should be considered in the differential diagnosis of a patient with delusions. Delirium can be differentiated by the presence of a fluctuating level of consciousness or impaired cognitive abilities. Delusions early in the course of a dementing illness, as in dementia of the Alzheimer's type, can give the appearance of a delusional disorder; however, neuropsychological testing usually detects cognitive impairment. Although alcohol abuse is an associated feature for patients with delusional disorder, delusional disorder should be distinguished from alcohol-induced psychotic disorder with hallucinations. Intoxication with sympathomimetics (including amphetamine, marijuana, or L-dopa is likely to result in delusional symptoms.

Other Disorders

The psychiatric differential diagnosis for delusional disorder includes malingering and factitious disorder with predominantly psychological signs and symptoms. The nonfactitious disorders in the differential diagnosis are schizophrenia, mood disorders, obsessive-compulsive disorder, somatoform disorders, and paranoid personality disorder. Delusional disorder is distinguished from schizophrenia by the absence of other schizophrenic symptoms and by the nonbizarre quality of the delusions; patients with delusional disorder also lack the impaired functioning seen in schizophrenia. The somatic type of delusional disorder may resemble a depressive disorder or a somatoform disorder. The somatic type of delusional disorder is differentiated from depressive disorders by the absence of other signs of depression and the lack of a pervasive quality to the depression. Delusional disorder can be differentiated from somatoform disorders by the degree to which the somatic belief is held by the patient. Patients with somatoform disorders allow for the possibility that their disorder does not exist, whereas patients with delusional disorder do not doubt its reality. Separating paranoid personality disorder from delusional disorder requires the sometimes difficult clinical distinction between extreme suspiciousness and frank delusion. In general, if clinicians doubt that a symptom is a delusion, the diagnosis of delusional disorder should not be made.

COURSE AND PROGNOSIS

Some clinicians and some research data indicate that an identifiable psychosocial stressor often accompanies the onset of delusional disorder. The nature of the stressor, in fact, may warrant some suspicion or concern. Examples of such stressors are recent immigration, social conflict with family members or friends, and social isolation. A sudden onset is generally thought to be more common than an insidious onset. Some clinicians believe that a person with delusional disorder is likely to have below-average intelligence and that the premorbid personality of such a person is likely to be extroverted, dominant, and hypersensitive. The person's initial suspicions or concerns gradually become elaborate, consume much of the person's attention, and finally become delusional. Persons may begin quarreling with coworkers, may seek protection from the Federal Bureau of Investigation or the police, or may begin visiting many medical or surgical physicians to seek consultations, lawyers about suits, or police about delusional suspicions.

As mentioned, delusional disorder is considered a fairly stable diagnosis. About 50 percent of patients have recovered at long-term follow-up, 20 percent show decreased symptoms, and 30 percent exhibit no change. The following factors correlate with a good prognosis: high levels of occupational, social, and functional adjustments; female sex; onset before age 30 years; sudden onset; short duration of illness; and the presence of precipitating factors. Although reliable data are limited, patients with persecutory, somatic, and erotic delusions are thought to have a better prognosis than patients with grandiose and jealous delusions.

TREATMENT

Delusional disorder was generally regarded as resistant to treatment, and interventions often focused on managing the morbidity of the disorder by reducing the impact of the delusion on the patient's (and family's) life. In recent years, however, the outlook has become less pessimistic or restricted in planning effective treatment. The goals of treatment are to establish the diagnosis, decide on appropriate interventions, and manage complications. The success of these goals depends on an effective and therapeutic doctor–patient relationship, which is far from easy to establish. The patients do not complain about psychiatric symptoms and often enter treatment against their will; even the psychiatrist may be drawn into their delusional nets.

In shared psychiatric disorder, the patients must be separated. If hospitalization is indicated, they should be placed on different units and have no contact. In general, the healthier of the two will give up the delusional belief (sometimes without any other therapeutic intervention). The sicker of the two will maintain the false fixed belief.

Psychotherapy

The essential element in effective psychotherapy is to establish a relationship in which patients begin to trust a therapist. Individual therapy seems to be more effective than group therapy; insight-oriented, supportive, cognitive, and behavioral therapies are often effective. Initially, a therapist should neither agree with nor challenge a patient's delusions. Although therapists must ask about a delusion to establish its extent, persistent questioning about it should probably be avoided. Physicians may stimulate the motivation to receive help by emphasizing a willingness to help patients with their anxiety or irritability, without suggesting that the delusions be treated, but therapists should not actively support the notion that the delusions are real.

The unwavering reliability of therapists is essential in psychotherapy. Therapists should be on time and make appointments as regularly as possible, with the goal of developing a solid and trusting relationship with a patient. Overgratification may actually increase patients' hostility and suspiciousness because ultimately they must realize that not all demands can be met. Therapists can avoid overgratification by not extending the designated appointment period, by not giving extra appointments unless absolutely necessary, and by not being lenient about the fee.

Therapists should avoid making disparaging remarks about a patient's delusions or ideas but can sympathetically indicate to patients that their preoccupation with their delusions is both distressing to themselves and interferes with a constructive life. When patients begin to waver in their delusional beliefs, therapists may increase reality testing by asking the patients to clarify their concerns.

A useful approach in building a therapeutic alliance is to empathize with the patient's internal experience of being overwhelmed by persecution. It may be helpful to make such comments as, "You must be exhausted, considering what you have been through." Without agreeing with every delusional misperception, a therapist can acknowledge that from the patient's perspective, such perceptions create much distress. The ultimate goal is to help patients entertain the possibility of doubt about their perceptions. As they become less rigid, feelings of weakness and inferiority, associated with some depression, may surface. When a patient allows feelings of vulnerability to enter into the therapy, a positive therapeutic alliance has been established, and constructive therapy becomes possible.

When family members are available, clinicians may decide to involve them in the treatment plan. Without being delusionally seen as siding with the enemy, a clinician should attempt to enlist the family as allies in the treatment process. Consequently, both the patient and the family need to understand that the therapist maintains physician–patient confidentiality and that communications from relatives are discussed with the patient. The family may benefit from the therapist's support and, thus, may support the patient.

A good therapeutic outcome depends on a psychiatrist's ability to respond to the patient's mistrust of others and the resulting interpersonal conflicts, frustrations, and failures. The mark of successful treatment may be a satisfactory social adjustment rather than abatement of the patient's delusions.

Hospitalization

Patients with delusional disorder can generally be treated as outpatients, but clinicians should consider hospitalization for several reasons. First, patients may need a complete medical and neurological evaluation to determine whether a nonpsychiatric medical condition is causing the delusional symptoms. Second, patients need an assessment of their ability to control violent impulses (e.g., to commit suicide or homicide) that may be related to the delusional material. Third, patients' behavior about the delusions may have significantly affected their ability to function within their family or occupational settings; they may require professional intervention to stabilize social or occupational relationships.

If a physician is convinced that a patient would receive the best treatment in a hospital, then the physician should attempt to persuade the patient to accept hospitalization; failing that, legal commitment may be indicated. If a physician convinces a patient that hospitalization is inevitable, the patient often voluntarily enters a hospital to avoid legal commitment.

Pharmacotherapy

In an emergency, severely agitated patients should be given an antipsychotic drug intramuscularly. Although no adequately conducted clinical trials with large numbers of patients have been conducted, most clinicians consider antipsychotic drugs the treatment of choice for delusional disorder. Patients are likely to refuse medication because they can easily incorporate the administration of drugs into their delusional systems; physicians should not insist on medication immediately after hospitalization but, rather, should spend a few days establishing rapport with the patient. Physicians should explain potential adverse effects to patients, so that they do not later suspect that the physician lied.

A patient's history of medication response is the best guide to choosing a drug. A physician should often start with low doses (e.g., 2 mg of haloperidol [Haldol] or 2 mg of risperidone [Risperdal]) and increase the dose slowly. If a patient fails to respond to the drug at a reasonable dose in a 6-week trial, antipsychotic drugs from other classes should be tried. Some investigators have indicated that pimozide may be particularly effective in delusional disorder, especially in patients with somatic delusions. A common cause of drug failure is noncompliance, which should also be evaluated. Concurrent psychotherapy facilitates compliance with drug treatment.

If the patient receives no benefit from antipsychotic medication, discontinue use of the drug. In patients who do respond to antipsychotic drugs, some data indicate that maintenance doses can be low. Although essentially no studies evaluate the use of antidepressants, lithium (Eskalith), or anticonvulsants (e.g., carbamazepine [Tegretol] and valproate [Depakene]) in the treatment of delusional disorder, trials with these drugs may be warranted in patients who do not respond to antipsychotic drugs. Trials of these drugs should also be considered when a patient has either the features of a mood disorder or a family history of mood disorders.

▲ 11.4 Brief Psychotic Disorder, Psychotic Disorder Not Otherwise Specified, and Secondary Psychotic Disorders

BRIEF PSYCHOTIC DISORDER

Brief psychotic disorder is defined by the text revision of the fourth edition of *Diagnostic and Statistical Manual of Mental Disorders* (DSM-IV-TR) as a psychotic condition that involves the sudden onset of psychotic symptoms and lasts 1 day or more but less than 1 month. Remission is full, and the individual returns to the premorbid level of functioning. Brief psychotic disorder is an acute and transient psychotic syndrome, and, thus, most individuals diagnosed with brief psychotic disorder under DSM-IV-TR are classified as having acute and transient psychotic disorders under the tenth revision of the *International Statistical Classification of Diseases and Related Health Problems* (ICD-10).

History

Brief psychotic disorder has been poorly studied in psychiatry in the United States, partly because of the frequent changes in diagnostic criteria during the past 15 years. The diagnosis has been better appreciated and more completely studied in Scandinavia and other Western European countries than in the United States. Patients with disorders similar to brief psychotic disorder were previously classified as having reactive, hysterical, stress, and psychogenic psychoses.

Epidemiology

The exact incidence and prevalence of brief psychotic disorder is not known, but it is generally considered uncommon. The disorder occurs more often among younger patients (20s and 30s) than among older patients. Reliable data on sex and sociocultural determinants are limited, although some findings suggest a higher incidence in women and persons in developing countries. Such epidemiological patterns are sharply distinct from those of schizophrenia. Some clinicians indicate that the disorder may be seen most frequently in patients of low socioeconomic status and in those who have experienced disasters or major cultural changes (e.g., immigrants). The age of onset in industrialized settings may be higher than in developing countries. Persons who have gone through major psychosocial stressors may be at greater risk for subsequent brief psychotic disorder.

Comorbidity

The disorder is often seen in patients with personality disorders (most commonly, histrionic, narcissistic, paranoid, schizotypal, and borderline personality disorders).

Etiology

The cause of brief psychotic disorder is unknown. Patients who have a personality disorder may have a biological or psychological vulnerability for the development of psychotic symptoms, particularly those with borderline, schizoid, schizotypal, or paranoid qualities. Some patients with brief psychotic disorder have a history of schizophrenia or mood disorders in their families, but this finding is nonconclusive. Psychodynamic formulations have emphasized the presence of inadequate coping mechanisms and the possibility of secondary gain for patients with psychotic symptoms. Additional psychodynamic theories suggest that the psychotic symptoms are a defense against a prohibited fantasy, the fulfillment of an unattained wish, or an escape from a stressful psychosocial situation.

Diagnosis

The DSM-IV-TR describes a continuum of diagnoses for psychotic disorders, based primarily on the duration of the symptoms. For psychotic symptoms that last at least 1 day but less than 1 month and are not associated with a mood disorder, a substance-related disorder, or a psychotic disorder caused by a general medical condition, a diagnosis of brief psychotic disorder is likely to be appropriate (Table 11.4–1).

The DSM-IV-TR describes three subtypes: (1) the presence of stressors, (2) the absence of stressors, and (3) a postpartum onset, each of which is discussed here.

As with other acutely ill psychiatric patients, the history necessary to make the diagnosis may not be obtainable solely from the patient. Although psychotic symptoms may be obvious, information about prodromal symptoms, previous episodes of a mood disorder, and a recent history of ingestion of a psychotomimetic substance may not be available from the clinical interview alone. In addition, clinicians may not be able to obtain accurate information about the presence or absence of precipitating stressors. Such information is usually best and most accurately obtained from a relative or a friend.

Clinical Features

The symptoms of brief psychotic disorder always include at least one major symptom of psychosis, usually with an abrupt onset, but do not always include the entire symptom pattern seen in schizophrenia. Some clinicians have observed that labile mood, confusion, and impaired attention may be more common at the onset of brief psychotic disorder than at the onset of eventually chronic psychotic disorders. Characteristic symptoms in brief psychotic disorder include emotional volatility, strange or bizarre behavior, screaming or muteness, and impaired memory for recent events. Some of the symptoms suggest a diagnosis of delirium and warrant a medical workup, especially to rule out adverse reactions to drugs.

**Table 11.4–1
DSM-IV-TR Diagnostic Criteria for Brief
Psychotic Disorder**

A. Presence of one (or more) of the following symptoms:
   (1) delusions
   (2) hallucinations
   (3) disorganized speech (e.g., frequent derailment or
       incoherence)
   (4) grossly disorganized or catatonic behavior
   Note: Do not include a symptom if it is a culturally
   sanctioned response pattern.
B. Duration of an episode of the disturbance is at least 1 day
   but less than 1 month, with eventual full return to
   premorbid level of functioning.
C. The disturbance is not better accounted for by a mood
   disorder with psychotic features, schizoaffective disorder,
   or schizophrenia and is not due to the direct physiological
   effects of a substance (e.g., a drug of abuse, a medication)
   or a general medical condition.
Specify if:
   With marked stressor(s) (brief reactive psychosis): if
   symptoms occur shortly after and apparently in response
   to events that, singly or together, would be markedly
   stressful to almost anyone in similar circumstances in the
   person's culture
   Without marked stressor(s): if psychotic symptoms do not
   occur shortly after, or are not apparently in response to
   events that, singly or together, would be markedly stressful
   to almost anyone in similar circumstances in the person's
   culture
   With postpartum onset: if onset within 4 weeks postpartum

From American Psychiatric Association. *Diagnostic and Statistical
Manual of Mental Disorders.* 4th ed. Text rev. Washington, DC:
American Psychiatric Association; copyright 2000, with permission.

Scandinavian and other European literature describes several characteristic symptom patterns in brief psychotic disorder, although these may differ somewhat between Europe and America. The symptom patterns include acute paranoid reactions and reactive confusion, excitation, and depression. Some data suggest that, in the United States, paranoia is often the predominant symptom in the disorder. In French psychiatry, *bouffée délirante* is similar to brief psychotic disorder.

Precipitating Stressors.   The clearest examples of precipitating stressors are major life events that would cause any person significant emotional upset. Such events include the loss of a close family member or a severe automobile accident. Some clinicians argue that the severity of the event must be considered in relation to the patient's life. This view, although reasonable, may broaden the definition of precipitating stressor to include events unrelated to the psychotic episode. Others have argued that the stressor may be a series of modestly stressful events rather than a single markedly stressful event, but evaluating the amount of stress caused by a sequence of events calls for an almost impossibly high degree of clinical judgment.

A Norwegian lumberman was admitted to the psychiatric ward of a hospital shortly after starting his required military duty at 20 years of age. During the first week after his arrival at the military base, he believed the other recruits looked at him in a strange way. He watched the people around him to see

whether they were out "to get" him. He heard voices calling his name several times. He became increasingly suspicious and after another week had to be admitted to the psychiatric department at the University of Oslo. There he was guarded, scowling, skeptical, and depressed. He gave the impression of being very shy and inhibited. His psychotic symptoms disappeared rapidly when he was treated with an antipsychotic drug. However, he had difficulties in adjusting to hospital life. Transfer to a long-term mental hospital was considered; but after 3 months, a decision was made to discharge him to his home in the forest. He was subsequently judged unfit to return to military services and was struck from the military lists.

The patient, the eldest of five siblings, was the son of a farm laborer in one of the valleys of Norway. His father was an intemperate drinker who became angry and brutal when drunk. The family was very poor, and there were constant quarrels between the parents. As a child, the patient was inhibited and fearful and often ran into the woods when troubled. He had academic difficulties and barely passed elementary school.

When the patient became older, he preferred to spend most of his time in the woods, where he worked as a lumberman from 15 years of age. He had his own horse, lived in a log cabin, and disliked being with people. He sometimes took part in the youth dances in the village. Although never a heavy drinker, he often got into fights in the village when he had a drink or two. At the age of 16 years, he began to keep company with a girl 1 year his junior who sometimes kept house for him in the woods. They eventually became engaged. (Courtesy of Ramin Mojtabai, M.D., Ph.D., M.P.H.)

Differential Diagnosis

Clinicians must not assume that the correct diagnosis for a patient who is briefly psychotic is brief psychotic disorder, even when a clear precipitating psychosocial factor is identified. Such a factor may be merely coincidental. If psychotic symptoms are present longer than 1 month, the diagnoses of schizophreniform disorder, schizoaffective disorder, schizophrenia, mood disorders with psychotic features, delusional disorder, and psychotic disorder not otherwise specified must be entertained. If psychotic symptoms of sudden onset are present for less than 1 month in response to an obvious stressor, however, the diagnosis of brief psychotic disorder is strongly suggested. Other diagnoses to consider in the differential diagnosis include factitious disorder with predominantly psychological signs and symptoms, malingering, psychotic disorder caused by a general medical condition, and substance-induced psychotic disorder. In factitious disorder, symptoms are intentionally produced; in malingering, a specific goal is involved in appearing psychotic (e.g., to gain admission to the hospital); and when associated with a medical condition or drugs, the cause becomes apparent with proper medical or drug workups. If the patient admits to using illicit substances, the clinician can make the assessment of substance intoxication or substance withdrawal without the use of laboratory testing. Patients with epilepsy or delirium can also show psychotic symptoms that resemble those seen in brief psychotic disorder. Additional psychiatric disorders to be considered in the differential diagnosis include dissociative identity disorder and psychotic episodes associated with borderline and schizotypal personality disorders.

Course and Prognosis

By definition, the course of brief psychotic disorder is less than 1 month. Nonetheless, the development of such a significant psychiatric disorder may signify a patient's mental vulnerability. Approximately half of patients who are first classified as having brief psychotic disorder later display chronic psychiatric syndromes such as schizophrenia and mood disorders. Patients with brief psychotic disorder, however, generally have good prognoses, and European studies have indicated that 50 to 80 percent of all patients have no further major psychiatric problems.

The length of the acute and residual symptoms is often just a few days. Occasionally, depressive symptoms follow the resolution of the psychotic symptoms. Suicide is a concern during both the psychotic phase and the postpsychotic depressive phase. Several indicators have been associated with a good prognosis (Table 11.4–2). Patients with the features listed in Table 11.4–2 are unlikely to have subsequent episodes, and schizophrenia or a mood disorder is unlikely to develop later.

Treatment

Hospitalization.   A patient who is acutely psychotic may need brief hospitalization for both evaluation and protection. Evaluation requires close monitoring of symptoms and assessment of the patient's level of danger to self and others. In addition, the quiet, structured setting of a hospital may help patients regain their sense of reality. While clinicians wait for the setting or the drugs to have their effects, seclusion, physical restraints, or one-to-one monitoring of the patient may be necessary.

Pharmacotherapy.   The two major classes of drugs to be considered in the treatment of brief psychotic disorder are the antipsychotic drugs and the benzodiazepines. When an antipsychotic drug is chosen, a high-potency antipsychotic drug such as haloperidol or a serotonin-dopamine agonist such as ziprasidone may be used. In patients who are at high risk for the development of extrapyramidal adverse effects (e.g., young men), a serotonin-dopamine antagonist drug should be administered as prophylaxis against medication-induced movement disorder symptoms. Alternatively, benzodiazepines can be used in the short-term treatment of psychosis. Although benzodiazepines have limited or no usefulness in the long-term treatment of psychotic disorders,

Table 11.4–2
Good Prognostic Features for Brief Psychotic Disorder

Good premorbid adjustment
Few premorbid schizoid traits
Severe precipitating stressor
Sudden onset of symptoms
Affective symptoms
Confusion and perplexity during psychosis
Little affective blunting
Short duration of symptoms
Absence of schizophrenic relatives

they can be effective for a short time and are associated with fewer adverse effects than the antipsychotic drugs. In rare cases, the benzodiazepines are associated with increased agitation and, more rarely still, with withdrawal seizures, which usually occur only with the sustained use of high doses. The use of other drugs in the treatment of brief psychotic disorder, although reported in case studies, has not been supported in any large-scale studies. Anxiolytic medications, however, are often useful during the first 2 to 3 weeks after the resolution of the psychotic episode. Clinicians should avoid long-term use of any medication in the treatment of the disorder. If maintenance medication is necessary, a clinician may have to reconsider the diagnosis.

Psychotherapy.   Although hospitalization and pharmacotherapy are likely to control short-term situations, the difficult part of treatment is the psychological integration of the experience (and possibly the precipitating trauma, if one was present) into the lives of the patients and their families. Psychotherapy is of use in providing an opportunity to discuss the stressors and the psychotic episode. Exploration and development of coping strategies are the major topics in psychotherapy. Associated issues include helping patients to deal with the loss of self-esteem and to regain self-confidence. An individualized treatment strategy based on increasing problem-solving skills while strengthening the ego structure through psychotherapy appears to be the most efficacious. Family involvement in the treatment process may be crucial to a successful outcome.

PSYCHOTIC DISORDER NOT OTHERWISE SPECIFIED

Under the umbrella of psychosis not otherwise specified is a variety of clinical presentations that do not fit within current diagnostic rubrics. In DSM-IV-TR, it includes "psychotic symptomatology (i.e., delusions, hallucinations, disorganized speech, grossly disorganized or catatonic behavior) about which there is inadequate information to make a specific diagnosis or about which there is contradictory information, or disorders with psychotic symptoms that do not meet the criteria for any specific Psychotic Disorder." DSM-IV-TR lists some examples of the diagnosis to help guide clinicians (Table 11.4–3).

Autoscopic Psychosis

The characteristic symptom of autoscopic psychosis is a visual hallucination of all or part of the person's own body. The hallucinatory perception, which is called a *phantom*, is usually colorless and transparent, and because the phantom imitates the person's movements, it is perceived as though appearing in a mirror. The phantom tends to appear suddenly and without warning.

Epidemiology.   Autoscopy is a rare phenomenon. Some persons have an autoscopic experience only once or a few times; others have the experience more often. Although the data are limited, sex, age, heredity, and intelligence do not seem to be related to the occurrence of the syndrome.

Etiology.   The cause of the autoscopic phenomenon is unknown. A biological hypothesis is that abnormal, episodic activity in areas of the temporoparietal lobes is involved with the sense of self, perhaps combined with abnormal activity in parts of the visual cortex. Psychological

Table 11.4–3
DSM-IV-TR Diagnostic Criteria for Psychotic Disorder Not Otherwise Specified

This category includes psychotic symptomatology (i.e., delusions, hallucinations, disorganized speech, grossly disorganized or catatonic behavior) about which there is inadequate information to make a specific diagnosis or about which there is contradictory information, or disorders with psychotic symptoms that do not meet the criteria for any specific psychotic disorder.

Examples include

1. Postpartum psychosis that does not meet criteria for mood disorder with psychotic features, brief psychotic disorder, psychotic disorder due to a general medical condition, or substance-induced psychotic disorder
2. Psychotic symptoms that have lasted for less than 1 month but that have not yet remitted, so that the criteria for brief psychotic disorder are not met
3. Persistent auditory hallucinations in the absence of any other features
4. Persistent nonbizarre delusions with periods of overlapping mood episodes that have been present for a substantial portion of the delusional disturbance
5. Situations in which the clinician has concluded that a psychotic disorder is present, but is unable to determine whether it is primary, due to a general medical condition, or substance induced

From American Psychiatric Association. *Diagnostic and Statistical Manual of Mental Disorders.* 4th ed. Text rev. Washington, DC: American Psychiatric Association; copyright 2000, with permission.

theories have associated the syndrome with personalities characterized by imagination, visual sensitivity, and, possibly, narcissistic personality disorder traits. Such persons may likely experience autoscopic phenomena during periods of stress.

Course and Prognosis. The classic descriptions of the phenomenon indicate that, in most cases, the syndrome is neither progressive nor incapacitating. Affected persons usually maintain some emotional distance from the phenomenon, an observation that suggests a specific neuroanatomical lesion. Rarely do the symptoms reflect the onset of schizophrenia or other psychotic disorders.

Postpartum Psychosis

Postpartum psychosis (sometimes called *puerperal psychosis*) is an example of psychotic disorder not otherwise specified that occurs in women who have recently delivered a baby; the syndrome is most often characterized by the mother's depression, delusions, and thoughts of harming either her infant or herself. For a complete discussion on postpartum conditions and other disorders related to pregnancy see Chapter 26, Psychiatry and Reproductive Medicine.

PSYCHOTIC DISORDERS DUE TO A GENERAL MEDICAL CONDITION AND SUBSTANCE-INDUCED PSYCHOTIC DISORDER

The evaluation of a patient with psychotic disorders requires consideration of the possibility that the psychotic symptoms result from a general medical condition such as a brain tumor or the ingestion of a substance such as phencyclidine (PCP).

Epidemiology

Relevant epidemiological data about psychotic disorder caused by a general medical condition and substance-induced psychotic disorder are lacking. The disorders are most often encountered in patients who abuse alcohol or other substances on a long-term basis. The delusional syndrome that may accompany complex partial seizures is more common in women than in men.

Etiology

Physical conditions such as cerebral neoplasms, particularly of the occipital or temporal areas, can cause hallucinations. Sensory deprivation, as in people who are blind or deaf, can also result in hallucinatory or delusional experiences. Lesions involving the temporal lobe and other cerebral regions, especially the right hemisphere and the parietal lobe, are associated with delusions.

Psychoactive substances are common causes of psychotic syndromes. The most commonly involved substances are alcohol, indole hallucinogens, such as lysergic acid diethylamide, amphetamine, cocaine, mescaline, PCP, and ketamine. Many other substances, including steroids and thyroxine, can produce hallucinations.

Diagnosis

Psychotic Disorder Due to a General Medical Condition. The diagnosis of psychotic disorder due to a general medical condition (Table 11.4–4) is defined in DSM-IV-TR by specifying the predominant symptoms. When the diagnosis is used, the medical condition, along with the predominant symptoms pattern, should be included in the diagnosis; for example, psychotic disorder due to a brain tumor, with delusions. The DSM-IV-TR criteria further specify that the disorder does not occur exclusively while a patient is delirious or demented and

Table 11.4–4
DSM-IV-TR Diagnostic Criteria for Psychotic Disorder Due to a General Medical Condition

A. Prominent hallucinations or delusions
B. There is evidence from the history, physical examination, or laboratory findings that the disturbance is the direct physiological consequence of a general medical condition.
C. The disturbance is not better accounted for by another mental disorder.
D. The disturbance does not occur exclusively during the course of a delirium.

Code based on predominant symptom:
   With delusions: if delusions are the predominant symptom
   With hallucinations: if hallucinations are the predominant symptom
   Coding note: Include the name of the general medical condition on Axis I, e.g., psychotic disorder due to malignant lung neoplasm, with delusions; also code the general medical condition on Axis III.
   Coding note: If delusions are part of vascular dementia, indicate the delusions by coding the appropriate subtype, e.g., vascular dementia, with delusions.

From American Psychiatric Association. *Diagnostic and Statistical Manual of Mental Disorders.* 4th ed. Text rev. Washington, DC: American Psychiatric Association; copyright 2000, with permission.

that the symptoms are not better accounted for by another mental disorder.

Substance-Induced Psychotic Disorder

The diagnostic category of substance-induced psychotic disorder in DSM-IV-TR (Table 11.4–5) is reserved for those with substance-induced psychotic symptoms and impaired reality

Table 11.4–5
DSM-IV-TR Diagnostic Criteria for Substance-Induced Psychotic Disorder

A. Prominent hallucinations or delusions. **Note:** Do not include hallucinations if the person has insight that they are substance induced.
B. There is evidence from the history, physical examination, or laboratory findings of either (1) or (2):
  (1) the symptoms in Criterion A developed during, or within a month of, substance intoxication or withdrawal
  (2) medication use is etiologically related to the disturbance
C. The disturbance is not better accounted for by a psychotic disorder that is not substance induced. Evidence that the symptoms are better accounted for by a psychotic disorder that is not substance induced might include the following: the symptoms precede the onset of the substance use (or medication use); the symptoms persist for a substantial period of time (e.g., about a month) after the cessation of acute withdrawal or severe intoxication, or are substantially in excess of what would be expected given the type or amount of the substance used or the duration of use; or there is other evidence that suggests the existence of an independent non–substance-induced psychotic disorder (e.g., a history of recurrent non–substance-related episodes).
D. The disturbance does not occur exclusively during the course of a delirium.
Note: This diagnosis should be made instead of a diagnosis of substance intoxication or substance withdrawal only when the symptoms are in excess of those usually associated with the intoxication or withdrawal syndrome and when the symptoms are sufficiently severe to warrant independent clinical attention.

Code [Specific substance]-induced psychotic disorder: (Alcohol, with delusions; alcohol, with hallucinations; amphetamine [or amphetaminelike substance], with delusions; amphetamine [or amphetaminelike substance], with hallucinations; cannabis, with delusions; cannabis, with hallucinations; cocaine, with delusions; cocaine, with hallucinations; hallucinogen, with delusions; hallucinogen, with hallucinations; inhalant, with delusions; inhalant, with hallucinations; opioid, with delusions; opioid, with hallucinations; phencyclidine [or phencyclidinelike substance], with delusions; phencyclidine [or phencyclidinelike substance], with hallucinations; sedative, hypnotic, or anxiolytic, with delusions; sedative, hypnotic, or anxiolytic, with hallucinations; other [or unknown] substance, with delusions; other [or unknown] substance, with hallucinations)

Specify if:
  With onset during intoxication: if criteria are met for intoxication with the substance and the symptoms develop during the intoxication syndrome
  With onset during withdrawal: if criteria are met for withdrawal from the substance and the symptoms develop during, or shortly after, a withdrawal syndrome

testing. People with substance-induced psychotic symptoms (e.g., hallucinations) but with intact reality testing should be classified as having a substance-related disorder (e.g., PCP intoxication with perceptual disturbances). The diagnosis of substance-induced psychotic disorder is included with the other psychotic disorder diagnoses in DSM-IV-TR to prompt clinicians to consider the possibility that a substance is causally involved in the production of psychotic symptoms. The full diagnosis of substance-induced psychotic disorder should include the type of substance involved, the stage of substance use when the disorder began (e.g., during intoxication or withdrawal), and the clinical phenomena (e.g., hallucinations or delusions).

Clinical Features

Hallucinations.   Hallucinations can occur in one or more sensory modalities. Tactile hallucinations (e.g., a sensation of bugs crawling on the skin) are characteristic of cocaine use. Auditory hallucinations are usually associated with psychoactive substance abuse; auditory hallucinations can also occur in persons who are deaf. Olfactory hallucinations can result from temporal lobe epilepsy; visual hallucinations can occur in persons who are blind because of cataracts. Hallucinations are either recurrent or persistent and are experienced in a state of full wakefulness and alertness; a hallucinating patient shows no significant changes in cognitive functions. Visual hallucinations often take the form of scenes involving diminutive (lilliputian) human figures or small animals. Rare musical hallucinations typically feature religious songs. Patients with psychotic disorder caused by a general medical condition and substance-induced psychotic disorder may act on their hallucinations. In alcohol-related hallucinations, threatening, critical, or insulting third-person voices speak about the patients and may tell them to harm either themselves or others. Such patients are dangerous and are at significant risk for suicide or homicide. Patients may or may not believe that the hallucinations are real.

Delusions.   Secondary and substance-induced delusions are usually present in a state of full wakefulness. Patients experience no change in the level of consciousness, although mild cognitive impairment may be observed. Patients may appear confused, disheveled, or eccentric, with tangential or even incoherent speech. Hyperactivity and apathy may be present, and an associated dysphoric mood is thought to be common. The delusions can be systematized or fragmentary, with varying content, but persecutory delusions are the most common.

Differential Diagnosis

Psychotic disorder due to a general medical condition and substance-induced psychotic disorder must be distinguished from delirium (in which patients have a clouded sensorium), from dementia (in which patients have major intellectual deficits), and from schizophrenia (in which patients have other symptoms of thought disorder and impaired functioning). Psychotic disorder due to a general medical condition and substance-induced psychotic disorder must also be differentiated from psychotic mood disorders (in which other affective symptoms are pronounced).

Treatment

Treatment involves identifying the general medical condition or the particular substance involved. At this point, treatment is directed toward the underlying condition and the patient's immediate behavioral control. Hospitalization may be necessary to evaluate patients completely and to ensure their safety. Antipsychotic agents (e.g., olanzapine [Zyprexa] or haloperidol) may be necessary for immediate and short-term control of psychotic or aggressive behavior, although benzodiazepines may also be useful for controlling agitation and anxiety.

▲ 11.5 Culture-Bound Syndromes

The term *culture-bound syndrome* usually denotes specific arrays of behavioral and experiential phenomena that tend to present themselves preferentially in particular sociocultural contexts and that are readily recognized as illness behavior by most participants in that culture. The syndromes are commonly assigned culturally sanctioned explanations and interpretations that, in turn, generate a set of culturally congruent remedies, usually in the form of healing rituals performed by someone to whom the community assigns a therapeutic role.

Assessment of culture-bound syndromes must start with recognition that each human society has an indigenous body of beliefs and practices directed at explaining and treating disease and disorder and that patients internalize that worldview during the process of enculturation. They share their experiences and deal with distress through commonly understood symbols and meanings. In that light, the diagnostic encounter itself can be used as a point of entry into the patient's world. Although a person cannot become an anthropological expert about each and every possible cultural group, the clinician can try to learn by asking patients to share their cultural norms as they understand them.

EPIDEMIOLOGY

The last few decades have witnessed the production of significant research illuminating diverse aspects of cross-cultural practice. Of great interest for those responsible for the organization of psychiatric care are the ongoing findings of psychiatric epidemiology across cultures. Claims have repeatedly been made that African-Americans, Hispanics, Asians, and other minorities experience higher levels of psychological distress and disorder than the mainstream population. Lifetime rates for phobic disorder were significantly higher among African-American respondents, and young Hispanics showed a higher prevalence of alcohol abuse. Other studies conducted by the Institute for Health Statistics demonstrated that, despite similar demographic characteristics, the prevalence of major depressive disorder for mainland Puerto Ricans was significantly higher than for island Puerto Ricans. Mexican-Americans with low acculturation status are reported to display low prevalence for most psychiatric disorders.

REPRESENTATIVE SYNDROMES

Table 11.5–1 lists representative culture-bound syndromes from around the world with some of their clinical features. Two early descriptions of cases of cross-cultural syndromes are given as follows.

Amok

The patient, a healthy young adult man, originally came from the hinterlands of Abau, in Papua, New Guinea. At the time of the act, he was working with a building gang on Ferguson Island. He was a foreigner to his work mates, one of whom called him an "Abau bush pig"—a grave insult. One night, at approximately 6:30 PM, the others were in their dormitory reading or lying down, when the patient came in with a 12-inch bush knife and suddenly attacked them, going from bed to bed hacking at them with the knife, mostly in the vicinity of the head and neck. Six died, then or later, some with terrible wounds, their heads being almost chopped off. Finally, another man in the vicinity heard the noise and came in with a rifle and one cartridge. The patient who had run amok attempted to attack him, was fired at, and still did not cease attacking. He was then put out of action by the butt of the rifle and died. (Courtesy of Manuel Trujillo, M.D.)

Koro

A Chinese patrol officer asked the physician A. H. Vorstman to accompany him to a village in the Singtan district to provide medical aid to a member of the native elite. The patient was found in bed, surrounded by a retinue and with an old man sitting at the foot of the bed. Having no information about the patient's symptoms during the preceding days, Vorstman's examination and questioning failed to yield much insight into the man's problem. Vorstman concluded that alcohol abuse, a common native habit, was the background for this case. The Chinese official who accompanied Vorstman related to him that, for the last 8 days, the patient's penis had withdrawn into his abdomen, and, as a preventive measure, the old man at the foot of the bed had been gripping his master's "obstinate limb." Vorstman was the first person to publish cases of Koro. (Courtesy of Manuel Trujillo, M.D.)

COURSE AND PROGNOSIS

Limited data on the longitudinal course of patients with culture-bound syndromes suggest that some of them eventually develop clinical features compatible with a diagnosis of schizophrenia, bipolar disorder, cognitive disorder, or other psychotic disorders. Thus, gathering information from all possible sources is crucial. Because clinical pictures evolve over time, thorough reevaluations should be conducted periodically to refine the diagnosis and improve clinical care.

TREATMENT

Treatment of a culture-bound syndrome poses several diagnostic challenges, the first of which is determining whether the symptomatology represents a culturally appropriate adaptive response

Table 11.5–1
Examples of Culture-Bound Syndromes

amok A dissociative episode characterized by a period of brooding followed by an outburst of violent, aggressive, or homicidal behavior directed at persons and objects. The episode tends to be precipitated by a perceived slight or insult and seems to be prevalent only among men. The episode is often accompanied by persecutory ideation; automatism, amnesia, exhaustion, and a return to premorbid state follow the episode. Some instances of amok may occur during a brief psychotic episode or constitute the onset or an exacerbation of a chronic psychotic process. The original reports that used this term were from Malaysia. A similar behavior pattern is found in Laos, Philippines, Polynesia (*cafard* or *cathard*), Papua New Guinea, and Puerto Rico (*mal de pelea*) and among the Navajo (*iich'aa*).

ataque de nervios An idiom of distress principally reported among Latinos from the Caribbean but recognized among many Latin American and Latin Mediterranean groups. Commonly reported symptoms include uncontrollable shouting, attacks of crying, trembling, heat in the chest rising into the head, and verbal or physical aggression. Dissociative experiences, seizure-like or fainting episodes, and suicidal gestures are prominent in some attacks but absent in others. A general feature of an *ataque de nervios* is a sense of being out of control. *Ataques de nervios* frequently occur as a direct result of a stressful event relating to the family (e.g., death of a close relative, separation or divorce from a spouse, conflicts with a spouse or children, or witnessing an accident involving a family member). Persons may experience amnesia for what occurred during the *ataque de nervios*, but they otherwise return rapidly to their usual level of functioning. Although descriptions of some *ataques de nervios* most closely fit the *Diagnostic and Statistical Manual of Mental Disorders* (DSM) description of panic attacks, the association of most *ataques* with a precipitating event and the frequent absence of the hallmark symptoms of acute fear or apprehension distinguish them from panic disorder. *Ataques* span the range from normal expressions of distress not associated with a mental disorder to symptom presentations associated with anxiety, mood, dissociative, or somatoform disorders.

bilis and colera (also referred to as *muina*) The underlying cause is thought to be strongly experienced anger or rage. Anger is viewed among many Latino groups as a particularly powerful emotion that can have direct effects on the body and exacerbate existing symptoms. The major effect of anger is to disturb core body balances (which are understood as a balance between hot and cold valences in the body and between the material and spiritual aspects of the body). Symptoms can include acute nervous tension, headache, trembling, screaming, stomach disturbances, and, in more severe cases, loss of consciousness. Chronic fatigue may result from an acute episode.

bouffée délirante A syndrome observed in West Africa and Haiti. The French term refers to a sudden outburst of agitated and aggressive behavior, marked confusion, and psychomotor excitement. It may sometimes be accompanied by visual and auditory hallucinations or paranoid ideation. The episodes may resemble an episode of brief psychotic disorder.

brain fag A term initially used in West Africa to refer to a condition experienced by high school or university students in response to the challenges of schooling. Symptoms include difficulties in concentrating, remembering, and thinking. Students often state that their brains are "fatigued." Additional somatic symptoms are usually centered on the head and neck and include pain, pressure or tightness, blurring of vision, heat, or burning. "Brain tiredness" or fatigue from "too much thinking" is an idiom of distress in many cultures, and resulting syndromes can resemble certain anxiety, depressive, and somatoform disorders.

dhat A folk diagnostic term used in India to refer to severe anxiety and hypochondriacal concerns associated with the discharge of semen, whitish discoloration of the urine, and feelings of weakness and exhaustion. Similar to *jiryan* (India), *sukra prameha* (Sri Lanka), and *shen-k'uei* (China).

falling-out or blackout Episodes that occur primarily in southern U.S. and Caribbean groups. They are characterized by a sudden collapse, which sometimes occurs without warning but is sometimes preceded by feelings of dizziness or "swimming" in the head. The person's eyes are usually open, but the person claims an inability to see. Those affected usually hear and understand what is occurring around them but feel powerless to move. This may correspond to a diagnosis of conversion disorder or a dissociative disorder.

ghost sickness A preoccupation with death and the deceased (sometimes associated with witchcraft), frequently observed among members of many American Indian tribes. Various symptoms can be attributed to ghost sickness, including bad dreams, weakness, feeling of danger, loss of appetite, fainting, dizziness, fear, anxiety, hallucinations, loss of consciousness, confusion, feelings of futility, and a sense of suffocation.

hwa-byung (also known as *wool-hwa-byung*) A Korean folk syndrome literally translated into English as "anger syndrome" and attributed to the suppression of anger. The symptoms include insomnia, fatigue, panic, fear of impending death, dysphoric affect, indigestion, anorexia, dyspnea, palpitations, generalized aches and pains, and a feeling of a mass in the epigastrium.

koro A term, probably of Malaysian origin, that refers to an episode of sudden and intense anxiety that the penis (or, in women, the vulva and nipples) will recede into the body and possibly cause death. The syndrome is reported in South and East Asia, where it is known by a variety of local terms, such as *shuk yang*, *shook yong*, and *suo yang* (Chinese); *jinjinia bemar* (Assam); and *rok-joo* (Thailand). It is occasionally found in the West. *Koro* at times occurs in localized epidemic form in East Asian areas. The diagnosis is included in the second edition of *Chinese Classification of Mental Disorders* (CCMD-2).

latah Hypersensitivity to sudden fright, often with echopraxia, echolalia, command obedience, and dissociative or trance-like behavior. The term *latah* is of Malaysian or Indonesian origin, but the syndrome has been found in many parts of the world. Other terms for the condition are *amurakh, irkunil, ikota, olan, myriachit,* and *menkeiti* (Siberian groups); *bah tschi, bah-tsi,* and *baah-ji* (Thailand); *imu* (Ainu, Sakhalin, Japan); and *mali-mali* and *silok* (Philippines). In Malaysia it is more frequent in middle-aged women.

locura A term used by Latinos in the United States and Latin America to refer to a severe form of chronic psychosis. The condition is attributed to an inherited vulnerability, to the effect of multiple life difficulties, or to a combination of both factors. Symptoms exhibited by persons with *locura* include incoherence, agitation, auditory and visual hallucinations, inability to follow rules of social interaction, unpredictability, and possibly violence.

mal de ojo A concept widely found in Mediterranean cultures and elsewhere in the world. *Mal de ojo* is a Spanish phrase translated into English as "evil eye." Children are especially at risk. Symptoms include fitful sleep, crying without apparent cause, diarrhea, and vomiting and fever in a child or infant. Sometimes adults (especially women) have the condition.

nervios A common idiom of distress among Latinos in the United States and Latin America. A number of other ethnic groups have related, although often somewhat distinctive, ideas of "nerves" (such as *nerva* among Greeks in North America). *Nervios* refers both to a general state of vulnerability to stressful life experiences and to a syndrome brought on by difficult life circumstances. The term *nervios* includes a wide range of symptoms of emotional distress, somatic disturbance, and inability to function. Common symptoms include headaches and brain aches, irritability, stomach disturbances, sleep difficulties, nervousness, easy tearfulness, inability to concentrate, trembling, tingling sensations, and *mareos* (dizziness with occasional vertigo-like exacerbations). *Nervios* tends to be an ongoing problem, although variable in the degree

(continued)

**Table 11.5–1
(Continued)**

of disability that is manifest. *Nervios* is a very broad syndrome that spans the range from patients free of a mental disorder to presentations resembling adjustment, anxiety, depressive, dissociative, somatoform, or psychotic disorders. Differential diagnosis depends on the constellation of symptoms experienced, the kinds of social events that are associated with the onset and progress of *nervios*, and the level of disability experienced.

piblokto An abrupt dissociative episode accompanied by extreme excitement of up to 30 minutes' duration and frequently followed by convulsive seizures and coma lasting up to 12 hours. It is observed primarily in Arctic and subarctic Eskimo communities, although regional variations in name exist. The person may be withdrawn or mildly irritable for a period of hours or days before the attack and typically reports complete amnesia for the attack. During the attack persons may tear off their clothing, break furniture, shout obscenities, eat feces, flee from protective shelters, or perform other irrational or dangerous acts.

***qi-gong* psychotic reactions** Acute, time-limited episodes characterized by dissociative, paranoid, or other psychotic or nonpsychotic symptoms that may occur after participation in the Chinese folk health-enhancing practice of *qi-gong* (exercise of vital energy). Especially vulnerable are persons who become overly involved in the practice. This diagnosis is included in CCMD-2.

rootwork A set of cultural interpretations that ascribe illness to hexing, witchcraft, sorcery, or evil influence of another person. Symptoms may include generalized anxiety and gastrointestinal complaints (e.g., nausea, vomiting, diarrhea), weakness, dizziness, the fear of being poisoned, and sometimes fear of being killed (voodoo death). Roots, spells, or hexes can be put or placed on another person, causing a variety of emotional and psychological problems. The hexed person may even fear death until the root has been taken off (eliminated), usually through the work of a root doctor (a healer in this tradition), who can also be called on to bewitch an enemy. Rootwork is found in the southern United States among both African-American and European-American populations and in Caribbean societies. It is also known as *mal puesto* or *brujeria* in Latino societies.

sangue dormido ("sleeping blood") A syndrome found among Portuguese Cape Verde Islanders (and immigrants from there to the United States). It includes pain, numbness, tremor, paralysis, convulsions, stroke, blindness, heart attack, infection, and miscarriages.

Shenjing shuariuo ("neurasthenia") In China a condition characterized by physical and mental fatigue, dizziness, headaches, other pains, concentration difficulties, sleep disturbance, and memory loss. Other symptoms include gastrointestinal problems, sexual dysfunction, irritability, excitability, and various signs suggesting disturbance of the autonomic nervous system. In many cases the symptoms would meet the criteria for a DSM mood or anxiety disorder. The diagnosis is included in CCMD-2.

shen-k'uei (Taiwan), ***shenkui*** (China) A Chinese folk label describing marked anxiety or panic symptoms with accompanying somatic complaints for which no physical cause can be

demonstrated. Symptoms include dizziness, backache, fatigability, general weakness, insomnia, frequent dreams, and complaints of sexual dysfunction, such as premature ejaculation and impotence. Symptoms are attributed to excessive semen loss from frequent intercourse, masturbation, nocturnal emission, or passing of white turbid urine believed to contain semen. Excessive semen loss is feared because of the belief that it represents the loss of one's vital essence and can therefore be life threatening.

shin-byung A Korean folk label for a syndrome in which initial phases are characterized by anxiety and somatic complaints (general weakness, dizziness, fear, anorexia, insomnia, gastrointestinal problems), with subsequent dissociation and possession by ancestral spirits.

spell A trance state in which persons "communicate" with deceased relatives or spirits. At times the state is associated with brief periods of personality change. The culture-specific syndrome is seen among African-Americans and European-Americans from the southern United States. Spells are not considered to be medical events in the folk tradition but may be misconstrued as psychotic episodes in clinical settings.

susto (*frigh* or "soul loss") A folk illness prevalent among some Latinos in the United States and among people in Mexico, Central America, and South America. *Susto* is also referred to as *espanto, pasmo, tripa ida, perdida del alma,* or *chibih. Susto* is an illness attributed to a frightening event that causes the soul to leave the body and results in unhappiness and sickness. Persons with *susto* also experience significant strains in key social roles. Symptoms may appear any time from days to years after the fright is experienced. It is believed that in extreme cases, *susto* may result in death. Typical symptoms include appetite disturbances, inadequate or excessive sleep, troubled sleep or dreams, feelings of sadness, lack of motivation to do anything, and feelings of low self-worth or dirtiness. Somatic symptoms accompanying *susto* include muscle aches and pains, headache, stomachache, and diarrhea. Ritual healings are focused on calling the soul back to the body and cleansing the person to restore bodily and spiritual balance. Different experience of *susto* may be related to major depressive disorder, posttraumatic stress disorders, and somatoform disorders. Similar etiological beliefs and symptom configurations are found in many parts of the world.

taijin kyofu sho A culturally distinctive phobia in Japan, in some ways resembling social phobia in DSM. The syndrome refers to an intense fear that one's body, its parts or its functions, displease, embarrass, or are offensive to other people in appearance, odor, facial expressions, or movements. The syndrome is included in the official Japanese diagnostic system for mental disorders.

zar A general term applied in Ethiopia, Somalia, Egypt, Sudan, Iran, and other North African and Middle Eastern societies to the experience of spirits possessing a person. Persons possessed by a spirit may experience dissociative episodes that may include shouting, laughing, hitting the head against a wall, singing, or weeping. They may show apathy and withdrawal, refusing to eat or carry out daily tasks or may develop a long-term relationship with the possessing spirit. Such behavior is not considered pathological locally.

to a situation. Clinicians are well advised to (1) know or search out the demographics of the local population or catchment area being served; (2) recognize that a local pattern exists of conceptualization, naming, vocabulary, explanation, and treatment of patterns of distress that afflict a community, including mental disorders; and (3) talk with the family and learn about local customs or search out other modes of documentation. Persons within the culture will almost always recognize that one of their own is acting in a deviant manner, and their input can be extremely valuable in making an assessment of mental disorder.

When taking the history, ask the patients what they think could have caused the problem and how they explain it to themselves. Some useful questions: (1) What do you think has caused your problem? (2) Why do you think it started when it did?

(3) What do you think your sickness does to you? How does it work? (4) How severe is your sickness? Will it have a short or long course? (5) What kind of treatment do you think you should receive?

Insight into the dynamics of the patient's world facilitates the clinician's efforts to adapt his or her techniques (e.g., general activity level, mode of verbal intervention, content of remarks, tone of voice) to the patient's cultural background. It implies acceptance of, and respect for, the patient's cultural frame of reference and opens the possibility of direct intervention in the lives of patients, who may be willing to cooperate when they feel understood.

Therapies

Much knowledge has accrued about the applications of standard, psychoanalytically based psychotherapy to populations and ethnic backgrounds other than whites of Western origin. To the repeated observation that ethnic communities are accepted for psychotherapy treatment at lower rates and drop out earlier than their mainstream counterparts, researchers and clinicians have provided a bounty of adaptations ranging from preparations for psychotherapy to substantive framework modifications. The most daring step in this continuum is the development of culture-specific therapies empirically derived from culture-specific behavioral features. José Szapocznik, for example, has developed and proposed a model of family therapy for Miami's Cuban families guided by empirically derived values prevalent in that population, such as strong familial affiliation and a preference for hierarchical family structures.

While encouraging openness to such technologies, systems of care should establish standards and guidelines that aim to obtain clinical and functional outcomes equivalent to the mainstream state-of-the-art efficacy studies, equally avoiding, promoting, and discouraging particular approaches until unquestionable evidence of efficacy and effectiveness is developed.

Cognitive and cognitive behavior therapies may achieve some modicum of freedom from cultural bias to the degree that cognitive therapists work with the specific pathogenic beliefs of the patient, whatever the cultural origin of such beliefs. Its application to minority populations experiencing anxiety and depressive disorders may be an area of promising cross-cultural research.

Indigenous Healers

One promising avenue is collaboration with indigenous healers. Several researchers have reported on their success in the use of indigenous and traditional healers in the treatment of psychiatric patients, especially those whose psychotic conditions are substantially connected to culture-specific beliefs (e.g., fear of voodoo death). Decisions about involving indigenous healers should be individualized and planned thoughtfully, taking into consideration the setting, the thoughtfulness and flexibility of the available healers, the type of psychopathology, and the patient's characteristics. The World Health Organization has long advocated implementation at the local level of a policy of close collaboration between the conventional health system and traditional medicine, particularly between individual health professionals and traditional practitioners.

Pharmacogenetics

The field of pharmacogenetics grew out of observations of significant ethnic differences in response to drugs, in differential development, and in adverse-effect profiles, leading to the discovery of defects or deficiencies in the genetically controlled activity of enzyme systems responsible for the metabolism of psychotropic medications and toxins such as alcohol.

Acetylation Status.   Observations of ethnic differences in the adverse-effects profile of the antituberculosis drug isoniazid (Nydrazid, Rifamate) led to the classification of persons as slow or rapid acetylators, which, among other biological effects, determines their metabolism of psychotropic medications such as clonazepam (Klonopin) and phenelzine (Nardil).

Alcohol Metabolism.   P. H. Wolf, while studying racial differences in alcohol sensitivity, observed that about 80 percent of Asians and 50 percent of Native Americans exhibited the flushing response to alcohol (compared with 10 percent of whites) and concluded that these differences had a genetic basis. They have been proved to be related to genetic polymorphism of isozymes of alcohol dehydrogenase (ADH) and aldehyde dehydrogenase (ALDH), enzymes critical for complete metabolism of alcohol and other neurotransmitters and which play a role in development of alcoholism or its avoidance. For example, Asians who are either homozygous or heterozygous for the atypical Asian-type *ALDH2* gene are alcohol sensitive and have a low risk for alcoholism and alcoholic liver disease.

Native Americans have a high frequency of both alcohol flushing and alcohol-related problems, and Akira Yoshida's research team reported in 1993 that they had practically no detectable Asian-type *ADH2* and *ALDH2* genes, a major alcohol-rejecting genetic factor.

Cytochrome P450 Isozymes.   The cytochrome P450 enzyme system is key in the metabolism of psychotropic and nonpsychotropic drugs as well as a great variety of environmental toxins that find their way into the diets of animals and humans. The genetic defects that render these enzymes less effective and make humans poor metabolizers are unequally distributed among ethnic populations. This is particularly the case for two cytochrome P450 (CYP) isozymes: CYP 2D6 (debrisoquin hydroxylase), and CYP 2Cmp (mephenytoin hydroxylase). The percentage of CYP 2D6–poor metabolizers is lower for Asians (0.5 to 2.4 percent) and higher for whites (2.9 to 10 percent). Similar interethnic variance exists in the frequency of poor metabolizers of CYP 2Cmp: low among whites (3 percent), intermediate for African-Americans (18 percent), and higher (up to 20 percent) in Asian and Japanese populations.

These interethnic differences in the P450 isozymes are of great importance in psychiatry and psychopharmacology because of their role in the metabolism of antipsychotics, antidepressants, sedatives such as barbiturates and benzodiazepines, and β-adrenergic receptor antagonists (β-blockers) such as propranolol (Inderal).

Environmental Factors.   In addition to being genetically regulated, enzymes that participate in the metabolism of psychotropic medications respond to environmental variables such as diet, alcohol, smoking status, and caffeine intake. All of these factors can accelerate or slow the metabolism of drugs through enzyme induction or inhibition.

Herbal Medicines. In parallel with available Western medicine–oriented psychiatric services, immigrants often retain their loyalty to ethnically based folk-medicine systems. Mexican-Americans are willing to accept prescribed medications from psychiatrists and herbs from a community healer, just as other Americans use natural serotonin-enhancing herbs such as St. John's wort in addition to, or instead of, the more conventional psychotropics prescribed by their psychiatrists. Many of these herbs possess high levels of psychoactive activity, such as anticholinergics (*Swertia japonica* used by Japanese patients or *Datura candida* used by Cubans), stimulants (the caffeine-loaded *Ibexguazusa* of Latin America), and sedatives (*Schumanniophyton problematicans* of the Nigerians). Others, such as ginseng and glycyrrhiza, may stimulate or inhibit cytochrome P450.

12

Mood Disorders

▲ 12.1 Depression and Bipolar Disorder

Mood is a pervasive and sustained feeling tone that is experienced internally and that influences a person's behavior and perception of the world. Affect is the external expression of mood. Mood can be normal, elevated, or depressed. Healthy persons experience a wide range of moods and have an equally large repertoire of affective expressions; they feel in control of their moods and affects.

Mood disorders are a group of clinical conditions characterized by a loss of that sense of control and a subjective experience of great distress. Patients with elevated mood demonstrate expansiveness, flight of ideas, decreased sleep, and grandiose ideas. Patients with depressed mood experience a loss of energy and interest, feelings of guilt, difficulty in concentrating, loss of appetite, and thoughts of death or suicide. Other signs and symptoms of mood disorders include change in activity level, cognitive abilities, speech, and vegetative functions (e.g., sleep, appetite, sexual activity, and other biological rhythms). These disorders virtually always result in impaired interpersonal, social, and occupational functioning.

Patients afflicted with only major depressive episodes are said to have *major depressive disorder* or *unipolar depression*. Patients with both manic and depressive episodes or patients with manic episodes alone are said to have *bipolar disorder*. The terms "unipolar mania" and "pure mania" are sometimes used for patients who are bipolar but who do not have depressive episodes.

Three additional categories of mood disorders are hypomania, cyclothymia, and dysthymia. Hypomania is an episode of manic symptoms that does not meet the full criteria for manic episode of the text revision of the fourth edition of *Diagnostic and Statistical Manual of Mental Disorders* (DSM-IV-TR). Cyclothymia and dysthymia are defined by DSM-IV-TR as disorders that represent less severe forms of bipolar disorder and major depression, respectively.

The field of psychiatry has considered major depression and bipolar disorder to be two separate disorders, particularly in the last 20 years. The possibility that bipolar disorder is actually a more severe expression of major depression has been reconsidered recently, however. Many patients given a diagnosis of a major depressive disorder reveal, on careful examination, past episodes of manic or hypomanic behavior that have gone undetected. Many authorities see considerable continuity between recurrent depressive and bipolar disorders. This has led to widespread discussion and debate about the bipolar spectrum, which incorporates classic bipolar disorder, bipolar II, and recurrent depressions.

DSM-IV-TR CLASSIFICATION OF MOOD DISORDERS

Depression

According to DSM-IV-TR, a major depressive disorder occurs without a history of a manic, mixed, or hypomanic episode. A major depressive episode must last at least 2 weeks, and typically a person with a diagnosis of a major depressive episode also experiences at least four symptoms from a list that includes changes in appetite and weight, changes in sleep and activity, lack of energy, feelings of guilt, problems with thinking and making decisions, and recurring thoughts of death or suicide.

Mania

A manic episode is a distinct period of an abnormally and persistently elevated, expansive, or irritable mood lasting for at least 1 week, or less if a patient must be hospitalized. A hypomanic episode lasts at least 4 days and is similar to a manic episode except that it is not sufficiently severe to cause impairment in social or occupational functioning and no psychotic features are present. Both mania and hypomania are associated with inflated self-esteem, decreased need for sleep, distractibility, great physical and mental activity, and overinvolvement in pleasurable behavior. According to DSM-IV-TR, bipolar I disorder is defined as having a clinical course of one or more manic episodes and, sometimes, major depressive episodes. A mixed episode is a period of at least 1 week in which both a manic episode and a major depressive episode occur almost daily. A variant of bipolar disorder characterized by episodes of major depression and hypomania rather than mania is known as *bipolar II disorder*.

Dysthymia and Cyclothymia

Two additional mood disorders, dysthymic disorder and cyclothymic disorder (discussed fully in Section 12.2), have also been appreciated clinically for some time. Dysthymic disorder and cyclothymic disorder are characterized by the presence of symptoms that are less severe than those of major depressive disorder and bipolar I disorder, respectively. DSM-IV-TR defines dysthymic disorder as characterized by at least 2 years of depressed mood that is not sufficiently severe to fit the diagnosis of major depressive episode. Cyclothymic disorder is characterized by at least 2 years of frequently occurring hypomanic symptoms that cannot fit the diagnosis of manic episode and of depressive symptoms that cannot fit the diagnosis of major depressive episode.

Other Categories

The DSM-IV-TR includes three mood disorder research categories (minor depressive disorder, recurrent brief depressive disorder, and premenstrual dysphoric disorder). Other DSM-IV-TR diagnoses are mood disorder due to a general medical condition and substance-induced mood disorder. These categories are designed to broaden the recognition of mood disorder diagnoses, to describe mood disorder symptoms more specifically than in the past, and to facilitate the differential diagnosis of mood disorders. Finally, DSM-IV-TR includes three residual disorders: bipolar disorder not otherwise specified, depressive disorder not otherwise specified, and mood disorder not otherwise specified (see Section 12.3).

EPIDEMIOLOGY

Incidence and Prevalence

Mood disorders are common. In the most recent surveys, major depressive disorder has the highest lifetime prevalence (almost 17 percent) of any psychiatric disorder. The annual incidence (number of new cases) of a major depressive episode is 1.59 percent (women, 1.89 percent; men, 1.10 percent). The annual incidence of bipolar illness is less than 1 percent, but it is difficult to estimate because milder forms of bipolar disorder are often missed.

Sex

An almost universal observation, independent of country or culture, is the twofold greater prevalence of major depressive disorder in women than in men. The reasons for the difference are hypothesized to involve hormonal differences, the effects of childbirth, differing psychosocial stressors for women and for men, and behavioral models of learned helplessness. In contrast to major depressive disorder, bipolar I disorder has an equal prevalence among men and women. Manic episodes are more common in men, and depressive episodes are more common in women. When manic episodes occur in women, they are more likely than men to present a mixed picture (e.g., mania and depression). Women also have a higher rate of being rapid cyclers, defined as having four or more manic episodes in a 1-year period.

Age

The onset of bipolar I disorder is earlier than that of major depressive disorder. The age of onset for bipolar I disorder ranges from childhood (as early as age 5 or 6 years) to 50 years or even older in rare cases, with a mean age of 30 years. The mean age of onset for major depressive disorder is about 40 years, with 50 percent of all patients having an onset between the ages of 20 and 50 years. Major depressive disorder can also begin in childhood or in old age. Recent epidemiological data suggest that the incidence of major depressive disorder may be increasing among people younger than 20 years of age. This may be related to the increased use of alcohol and drugs of abuse in this age group.

Marital Status

Major depressive disorder occurs most often in persons without close interpersonal relationships or in those who are divorced or separated. Bipolar I disorder is more common in divorced and single persons than among married persons, but this difference may reflect the early onset and the resulting marital discord characteristic of the disorder.

Socioeconomic and Cultural Factors

No correlation has been found between socioeconomic status and major depressive disorder. A higher-than-average incidence of bipolar I disorder is found among the upper socioeconomic groups. Bipolar I disorder is more common in persons who did not graduate from college than in college graduates, however, which may also reflect the relatively early age of onset for the disorder. Depression is more common in rural areas than in urban areas. The prevalence of mood disorder does not differ among races. A tendency exists, however, for examiners to underdiagnose mood disorder and overdiagnose schizophrenia in patients whose racial or cultural background differs from theirs.

COMORBIDITY

Individuals with major mood disorders are at an increased risk of having one or more additional comorbid Axis I disorders. The most frequent disorders are alcohol abuse or dependence, panic disorder, obsessive-compulsive disorder (OCD), and social anxiety disorder. Conversely, individuals with substance use disorders and anxiety disorders also have an elevated risk of lifetime or current comorbid mood disorder. In both unipolar and bipolar disorder, men more frequently present with substance use disorders, whereas women more frequently present with comorbid anxiety and eating disorders. In general, patients who are bipolar more frequently show comorbidity of substance use and anxiety disorders than do patients with unipolar major depression. In the Epidemiological Catchment Area study, the lifetime history of substance use disorders, panic disorder, and OCD was approximately twice as high among patients with bipolar I disorder (61 percent, 21 percent, and 21 percent, respectively) than in patients with unipolar major depression (27 percent, 10 percent, and 12 percent, respectively). Comorbid substance use disorders and anxiety disorders worsen the prognosis of the illness and markedly increase the risk of suicide among patients who are unipolar major depressive and bipolar.

ETIOLOGY

Biological Factors

Many studies have reported biological abnormalities in patients with mood disorders. Until recently, the monoamine neurotransmitters—norepinephrine, dopamine, serotonin, and histamine—were the main focus of theories and research about the etiology of these disorders. A progressive shift has occurred from focusing on disturbances of single neurotransmitter systems in favor of studying neurobehavioral systems, neural circuits, and more intricate neuroregulatory mechanisms. The monoaminergic systems, thus, are now viewed as broader, neuromodulatory systems, and disturbances are as likely to be secondary or epiphenomenal effects as they are directly or causally related to etiology and pathogenesis.

Biogenic Amines.   Of the biogenic amines, norepinephrine and serotonin are the two neurotransmitters most implicated in the pathophysiology of mood disorders.

NOREPINEPHRINE.   The correlation suggested by basic science studies between the downregulation or decreased sensitivity of β-adrenergic receptors and clinical antidepressant responses is probably the most compelling piece of evidence indicating a direct role for the noradrenergic system in depression. Other evidence has also implicated the presynaptic β_2 receptors in depression because activation of these receptors results in a decrease of the amount of norepinephrine released. Presynaptic β_2 receptors are also located on serotonergic neurons and regulate the amount of serotonin released. The clinical effectiveness of antidepressant drugs with noradrenergic effects—for example, venlafaxine (Effexor)—further supports a role for norepinephrine in the pathophysiology of at least some of the symptoms of depression.

SEROTONIN.   With the huge effect that the selective serotonin reuptake inhibitors (SSRIs)—for example, fluoxetine (Prozac)—have made on the treatment of depression, serotonin has become the biogenic amine neurotransmitter most commonly associated with depression. The identification of multiple serotonin receptor subtypes has also increased the excitement within the research community about the development of even more specific treatments for depression. In addition to the fact that SSRIs and other serotonergic antidepressants are effective in the treatment of depression, other data indicate that serotonin is involved in the pathophysiology of depression. Depletion of serotonin may precipitate depression, and some patients with suicidal impulses have low cerebrospinal fluid (CSF) concentrations of serotonin metabolites and low concentrations of serotonin uptake sites on platelets.

DOPAMINE.   Although norepinephrine and serotonin are the biogenic amines most often associated with the pathophysiology of depression, dopamine has also been theorized to play a role. The data suggest that dopamine activity may be reduced in depression and increased in mania. The discovery of new subtypes of the dopamine receptors and an increased understanding of the presynaptic and postsynaptic regulation of dopamine function have further enriched research into the relation between dopamine and mood disorders. Drugs that reduce dopamine concentrations (e.g., reserpine [Serpasil]) and diseases that reduce dopamine concentrations (e.g., Parkinson's disease) are associated with depressive symptoms. In contrast, drugs that increase dopamine concentrations, such as tyrosine, amphetamine, and bupropion (Wellbutrin), reduce the symptoms of depression. Two recent theories about dopamine and depression are that the mesolimbic dopamine pathway may be dysfunctional in depression and that the dopamine D_1 receptor may be hypoactive in depression.

Other Neurotransmitter Disturbances.   Acetylcholine (ACh) is found in neurons that are distributed diffusely throughout the cerebral cortex. Cholinergic neurons have reciprocal or interactive relationships with all three monoamine systems. Abnormal levels of choline, which is a precursor to ACh, have been found at autopsy in the brains of some depressed patients, perhaps reflecting abnormalities in cell phospholipid composition. Cholinergic agonist and antagonist drugs have differential clinical effects on depression and mania. Agonists can produce lethargy, anergia, and psychomotor retardation in healthy subjects, can exacerbate symptoms in depression, and can reduce symptoms in mania. These effects generally are not sufficiently robust to have clinical applications, and adverse effects are problematic. In an animal model of depression, strains of mice that are super- or subsensitive to cholinergic agonists have been found to

be susceptible or more resistant to developing learned helplessness (discussed later). Cholinergic agonists can induce changes in hypothalamic-pituitary-adrenal (HPA) activity and sleep that mimic those associated with severe depression. Some patients with mood disorders in remission, as well as their never-ill first-degree relatives, have a trait-like increase in sensitivity to cholinergic agonists.

γ-Aminobutyric acid (GABA) has an inhibitory effect on ascending monoamine pathways, particularly the mesocortical and mesolimbic systems. Reductions have been observed in plasma, CSF, and brain GABA levels in depression. Animal studies have also found that chronic stress can reduce and eventually deplete GABA levels. By contrast, GABA receptors are upregulated by antidepressants, and some GABAergic medications have weak antidepressant effects.

The amino acids glutamate and glycine are the major excitatory and inhibitory neurotransmitters in the CNS. Glutamate and glycine bind to sites associated with the N-methyl-D-aspartate (NMDA) receptor, and an excess of glutamatergic stimulation can cause neurotoxic effects. Of importance, a high concentration of NMDA receptors exists in the hippocampus. Glutamate, thus, may work in conjunction with hypercortisolemia to mediate the deleterious neurocognitive effects of severe recurrent depression. Emerging evidence suggests that drugs that antagonize NMDA receptors have antidepressant effects.

Second Messengers and Intracellular Cascades.   The binding of a neurotransmitter and a postsynaptic receptor triggers a cascade of membrane-bound and intracellular processes mediated by second messenger systems. Receptors on cell membranes interact with the intracellular environment via guanine nucleotide-binding proteins (G proteins). The G proteins, in turn, connect to various intracellular enzymes (e.g., adenylate cyclase, phospholipase C, and phosphodiesterase) that regulate utilization of energy and formation of second messengers, such as cyclic nucleotide (e.g., cyclic adenosine monophosphate [cAMP] and cyclic guanosine monophosphate), as well as phosphatidylinositols (e.g., inositol triphosphate and diacylglycerol) and calcium-calmodulin. Second messengers regulate the function of neuronal membrane ion channels. Increasing evidence also indicates that mood-stabilizing drugs act on G proteins or other second messengers.

Alterations of Hormonal Regulation.   Lasting alterations in neuroendocrine and behavioral responses can result from severe early stress. Animal studies indicate that even transient periods of maternal deprivation can alter subsequent responses to stress. Activity of the gene coding for the neurokinin brain-derived neurotrophic growth factor is decreased after chronic stress, as is the process of neurogenesis. Protracted stress thus can induce changes in the functional status of neurons and, eventually, cell death. Recent studies in depressed humans indicate that a history of early trauma is associated with increased HPA activity accompanied by structural changes (i.e., atrophy or decreased volume) in the cerebral cortex.

THYROID AXIS ACTIVITY.   Approximately 5 to 10 percent of people evaluated for depression have previously undetected thyroid dysfunction, as reflected by an elevated basal thyroid-stimulating hormone (TSH) level or an increased TSH response to a 500-mg infusion of the hypothalamic neuropeptide thyroid-releasing hormone (TRH). Such abnormalities are often associated with elevated antithyroid antibody levels and, unless corrected with hormone replacement therapy, can compromise response to treatment. An even larger subgroup of depressed patients (e.g., 20 to 30 percent) shows a blunted TSH response to TRH challenge. The major therapeutic implication of a blunted TSH response is evidence of an increased risk of relapse despite preventive antidepressant therapy. Of note, unlike the dexamethasone-suppression test (DST), blunted TSH response to TRH does not usually normalize with effective treatment.

GROWTH HORMONE.   Growth hormone (GH) is secreted from the anterior pituitary after stimulation by norepinephrine and dopamine (DA). Secretion is inhibited by somatostatin, a hypothalamic neuropeptide, and corticotropin-releasing hormone. Decreased CSF somatostatin levels have been reported in depression, and increased levels have been observed in mania.

PROLACTIN.   Prolactin is released from the pituitary by serotonin stimulation and inhibited by DA. Most studies have not found significant abnormalities of basal or circadian prolactin secretion in depression, although a blunted prolactin response to various serotonin agonists has been described. This response is uncommon among premenopausal women, suggesting that estrogen has a moderating effect.

Alterations of Sleep Neurophysiology.   Depression is associated with a premature loss of deep (slow wave) sleep and an increase in nocturnal arousal. The latter is reflected by four types of disturbance: (1) an increase in nocturnal awakenings, (2) a reduction in total sleep time, (3) increased phasic rapid eye movement (REM) sleep, and (4) increased core body temperature. The combination of increased REM drive and decreased slow wave sleep results in a significant reduction in the first period of non-REM (NREM) sleep, a phenomenon referred to as *reduced REM latency*. Reduced REM latency and deficits of slow wave sleep typically persist after recovery of a depressive episode. Blunted secretion of GH after sleep onset is associated with decreased slow wave sleep and shows similar state-independent or trait-like behavior. The combination of reduced REM latency, increased REM density, and decreased sleep maintenance identifies approximately 40 percent of depressed outpatients and 80 percent of depressed inpatients. False-negative findings are commonly seen in younger, hypersomnolent patients, who may actually experience an increase in slow wave sleep during episodes of depression. Approximately 10 percent of otherwise healthy individuals have abnormal sleep profiles, and, as with dexamethasone nonsuppression, false-positive cases are not uncommonly seen in other psychiatric disorders.

Patients manifesting a characteristically abnormal sleep profile have been found to be less responsive to psychotherapy and to have a greater risk of relapse or recurrence and may benefit preferentially from pharmacotherapy.

Immunological Disturbance.   Depressive disorders are associated with several immunological abnormalities, including decreased lymphocyte proliferation in response to mitogens and other forms of impaired cellular immunity. These lymphocytes produce neuromodulators, such as corticotropin-releasing factor, and cytokines, peptides known as *interleukins*. There appears to be an association with clinical severity, hypercortisolism, and immune dysfunction, and the cytokine interleukin-1 may induce gene activity for glucocorticoid synthesis.

Structural and Functional Brain Imaging.   Computed axial tomography and magnetic resonance imaging scans have permitted the use of sensitive, noninvasive methods to assess the living brain, including cortical and subcortical tracts, as well as white matter lesions. The most consistent abnormality observed in the depressive disorders is increased frequency of abnormal hyperintensities in subcortical regions, such as periventricular regions, the basal ganglia, and the thalamus. More common in bipolar I disorder and among the elderly, these hyperintensities appear to reflect the deleterious neurodegenerative effects of recurrent affective episodes. Ventricular enlargement, cortical atrophy, and sulcal widening also have been reported in some studies. Some depressed patients also may have reduced hippocampal or caudate nucleus volumes, or both, suggesting more focal defects in relevant neurobehavioral systems. Diffuse and focal areas of atrophy have been associated with increased illness severity, bipolarity, and increased cortisol levels.

The most widely replicated positron emission tomography finding in depression is decreased anterior brain metabolism, which is generally more pronounced on the left side. From a different vantage point, depression may be associated with a relative increase in nondominant hemispheric activity. Furthermore, a reversal of hypofrontality occurs after shifts from depression into hypomania, such that greater left hemisphere reductions are seen in depression compared with greater right hemisphere reductions in mania. Other studies have observed more specific reductions of reduced cerebral blood flow or metabolism, or both, in the dopaminergically innervated tracts of the mesocortical and mesolimbic systems in depression. Again, evidence suggests that antidepressants at least partially normalize these changes.

In addition to a global reduction of anterior cerebral metabolism, increased glucose metabolism has been observed in several limbic regions, particularly among patients with relatively severe recurrent depression and a family history of mood disorder. During episodes of depression, increased glucose metabolism is correlated with intrusive ruminations.

Neuroanatomical Considerations.   Both the symptoms of mood disorders and biological research findings support the hypothesis that mood disorders involve pathology of the brain. Modern affective neuroscience focuses on the importance of four brain regions in the regulation of normal emotions: the prefrontal cortex (PFC), the anterior cingulate, the hippocampus, and the amygdala. The PFC is viewed as the structure that holds representations of goals and appropriate responses to obtain these goals. Such activities are particularly important when multiple, conflicting behavioral responses are possible or when it is necessary to override affective arousal. Evidence indicates some hemispherical specialization in PFC function. For example, left-sided activation of regions of the PFC is more involved in goal-directed or appetitive behaviors, whereas regions of the right PFC are implicated in avoidance behaviors and inhibition of appetitive pursuits. Subregions in the PFC appear to localize representations of behaviors related to reward and punishment.

The anterior cingulate cortex (ACC) is thought to serve as the point of integration of attentional and emotional inputs. Two subdivisions have been identified: an affective subdivision in the rostral and ventral regions of the ACC and a cognitive subdivision involving the dorsal ACC. The former subdivision shares extensive connections with other limbic regions, and the latter interacts more with the PFC and other cortical regions. It is proposed that activation of the ACC facilitates control of emotional arousal, particularly when goal attainment has been thwarted or when novel problems have been encountered.

The hippocampus is most clearly involved in various forms of learning and memory, including fear conditioning, as well as inhibitory regulation of HPA-axis activity. Emotional or contextual learning appears to involve a direct connection between the hippocampus and the amygdala.

The amygdala appears to be a crucial way station for processing novel stimuli of emotional significance and coordinating or organizing cortical responses. Located just above the hippocampi bilaterally, the amygdala has long been viewed as the heart of the limbic system. Although most research has focused on the role of the amygdala in responding to fearful or painful stimuli, it may be ambiguity or novelty, rather than the aversive nature of the stimulus per se, that brings the amygdala on line.

Genetic Factors

Numerous family, adoption, and twin studies have long documented the heritability of mood disorders. Recently, however, the primary focus of genetic studies has been to identify specific susceptibility genes by using molecular genetic methods.

Family Studies.   Family studies address the question of whether a disorder is familial. More specifically, is the rate of illness in the family members of someone with the disorder greater than that of the general population? Family data indicate that if one parent has a mood disorder, a child will have a risk of between 10 and 25 percent for mood disorder. If both parents are affected, this risk roughly doubles. The more members of the family who are affected, the greater the risk is to a child. The risk is greater if the affected family members are first-degree relatives rather than more distant relatives. A family history of bipolar disorder conveys a greater risk for mood disorders in general and, specifically, a much greater risk for bipolar disorder. Unipolar disorder is typically the most common form of mood disorder in families of bipolar probands. This familial overlap suggests some degree of common genetic underpinning between these two forms of mood disorder. The presence of more-severe illness in the family also conveys a greater risk.

Adoption Studies.   Adoption studies provide an alternative approach to separating genetic and environmental factors in familial transmission. Only a limited number of such studies have been reported, and their results have been mixed. One large study found a threefold increase in the rate of bipolar disorder and a twofold increase in unipolar disorder in the biological relatives of bipolar probands. Similarly, in a Danish sample, a threefold increase in the rate of unipolar disorder and a sixfold increase in the rate of completed suicide in the biological relatives of affectively ill probands were reported. Other studies, however, have been less convincing and have found no difference in the rates of mood disorders.

Twin Studies.   Twin studies provide the most powerful approach to separating genetic from environmental factors, or "nature" from "nurture." The twin data provide compelling evidence that genes explain only 50 to 70 percent of the etiology of mood disorders. Environment or other nonheritable factors must explain the remainder. Therefore, it is a predisposition or susceptibility to disease that is inherited. Considering unipolar and bipolar disorders together, these studies find a concordance rate for mood disorder in monozygotic twins of 70 to 90 percent compared with a rate in same-sex dizygotic twins of 16 to 35 percent. This is the most compelling data for the role of genetic factors in mood disorders.

Linkage Studies.   **Deoxyribonucleic acid** (DNA) markers are segments of DNA of known chromosomal location, which are highly variable among individuals. They are used to track the segregation of specific chromosomal regions within families affected with a disorder. When a marker is identified with disease in families, the disease is said to be *genetically linked*. Chromosomes 18q and 22q are the two regions

with strongest evidence for linkage to bipolar disorder. Several linkage studies have found evidence for the involvement of specific genes in clinical subtypes. For example, the linkage evidence on 18q has been shown to be derived largely from bipolar II–bipolar II sibling pairs and from families in which the probands had panic symptoms.

Gene-mapping studies of unipolar depression have found very strong evidence of linkage to the locus for cAMP response element-binding protein (CREB1) on chromosome 2. Eighteen other genomic regions were found to be linked; some of these displayed interactions with the CREB1 locus. Another study has reported evidence for a gene–environment interaction in the development of major depression. Subjects who underwent adverse life events were shown, in general, to be at an increased risk for depression. Of such subjects, however, those with a variant in the serotonin transporter gene showed the greatest increase in risk. This is one of the first reports of a specific gene–environment interaction in a psychiatric disorder.

Psychosocial Factors

Life Events and Environmental Stress.   A long-standing clinical observation is that stressful life events more often precede first, rather than subsequent, episodes of mood disorders. This association has been reported for both patients with major depressive disorder and patients with bipolar I disorder. One theory proposed to explain this observation is that the stress accompanying the first episode results in long-lasting changes in the brain's biology. These long-lasting changes may alter the functional states of various neurotransmitter and intraneuronal signaling systems, changes that may even include the loss of neurons and an excessive reduction in synaptic contacts. As a result, a person has a high risk of undergoing subsequent episodes of a mood disorder, even without an external stressor.

Some clinicians believe that life events play the primary or principal role in depression; others suggest that life events have only a limited role in the onset and timing of depression. The most compelling data indicate that the life event most often associated with development of depression is losing a parent before age 11 years. The environmental stressor most often associated with the onset of an episode of depression is the loss of a spouse. Another risk factor is unemployment; persons out of work are three times more likely to report symptoms of an episode of major depression than those who are employed.

Personality Factors.   No single personality trait or type uniquely predisposes a person to depression; all humans, of whatever personality pattern, can and do become depressed under appropriate circumstances. Persons with certain personality disorders—obsessive-compulsive, histrionic, and borderline—may be at greater risk for depression than persons with antisocial or paranoid personality disorder. The latter can use projection and other externalizing defense mechanisms to protect themselves from their inner rage. No evidence indicates that any particular personality disorder is associated with later development of bipolar I disorder; however, patients with dysthymic disorder and cyclothymic disorder are at risk of later developing major depression or bipolar I disorder.

Recent stressful events are the most powerful predictors of the onset of a depressive episode. From a psychodynamic perspective, the clinician is always interested in the meaning of the stressor. Research has demonstrated that stressors that the patient experiences as reflecting negatively on his or her self-esteem are more likely to produce depression. Moreover, what may seem to be a relatively mild stressor to outsiders may be devastating to the patient because of particular idiosyncratic meanings attached to the event.

Psychodynamic Factors in Depression.

The psychodynamic understanding of depression defined by Sigmund Freud and expanded by Karl Abraham is known as the classic view of depression. That theory involves four key points: (1) disturbances in the infant–mother relationship during the oral phase (the first 10 to 18 months of life) predispose to subsequent vulnerability to depression; (2) depression can be linked to real or imagined object loss; (3) introjection of the departed objects is a defense mechanism invoked to deal with the distress connected with the object's loss; and (4) because the lost object is regarded with a mixture of love and hate, feelings of anger are directed inward at the self.

Melanie Klein understood depression as involving the expression of aggression toward loved ones, much as Freud did. Edward Bibring regarded depression as a phenomenon that sets in when a person becomes aware of the discrepancy between extraordinarily high ideals and the inability to meet those goals. Edith Jacobson saw the state of depression as similar to the situation of a powerless, helpless child victimized by a tormenting parent. Silvano Arieti observed that many depressed people have lived their lives for someone else rather than for themselves. He referred to the person for whom depressed patients live as the dominant other, which may be a principle, an ideal, or an institution, as well as an individual. Depression sets in when patients realize that the person or ideal for which they have been living is never going to respond in a manner that will meet their expectations. Heinz Kohut's conceptualization of depression, derived from his self-psychological theory, rests on the assumption that the developing self has specific needs that must be met by parents to give the child a positive sense of self-esteem and self-cohesion. When others do not meet these needs, there is a massive loss of self-esteem that presents as depression. John Bowlby believed that damaged early attachments and traumatic separation in childhood predispose to depression. Adult losses are said to revive the traumatic childhood loss and so precipitate adult depressive episodes.

Psychodynamic Factors in Mania.

Most theories of mania view manic episodes as a defense against underlying depression. Abraham, for example, believed that the manic episodes may reflect an inability to tolerate a developmental tragedy, such as the loss of a parent. The manic state may also result from a tyrannical superego, which produces intolerable self-criticism that is then replaced by euphoric self-satisfaction. Bertram Lewin regarded the manic patient's ego as overwhelmed by pleasurable impulses, such as sex, or by feared impulses, such as aggression. Klein also viewed mania as a defensive reaction to depression, using manic defenses such as omnipotence, in which the person develops delusions of grandeur.

Other Formulations of Depression

Cognitive Theory.

According to cognitive theory, depression results from specific cognitive distortions present in persons susceptible to depression. Those distortions, referred to as *depressogenic schemata*, are cognitive templates that perceive both internal and external data in ways that are altered by early experiences. Aaron Beck postulated a cognitive triad of depression that consists of views about (1) the self—a negative self-precept; (2) the environment—a tendency to experience the world as hostile and demanding; and (3) the future—the expectation of suffering and failure. Therapy consists in modifying these distortions.

Learned Helplessness.

The learned helplessness theory of depression connects depressive phenomena to the experience of uncontrollable events. For example, when dogs in a laboratory were exposed to electrical shocks from which they could not escape, they showed behaviors that differentiated them from dogs that had not been exposed to such uncontrollable events. The dogs exposed to the shocks would not cross a barrier to stop the flow of electric shock when put in a new learning situation. They remained passive and did not move. According to the learned helplessness theory, the shocked dogs learned that outcomes were independent of responses, so they had both cognitive motivational deficit (i.e., they would not attempt to escape the shock) and emotional deficit (indicating decreased reactivity to the shock). In the reformulated view of learned helplessness as applied to human depression, internal causal explanations are thought to produce a loss of self-esteem after adverse external events. Behaviorists who subscribe to the theory stress that improvement of depression is contingent on the patient's learning a sense of control and mastery of the environment.

DIAGNOSIS

In addition to the diagnostic criteria for major depressive disorder and bipolar disorders, DSM-IV-TR includes specific criteria for mood episodes (Tables 12.1–1 through 12.1–4) and criteria, such as severity (Tables 12.1–5 through 12.1–7), to qualify the most recent episode.

Major Depressive Disorder

The DSM-IV-TR lists the criteria for a major depressive episode separately from the diagnostic criteria for depression-related diagnoses (Table 12.1–1) and also lists severity descriptors for a major depressive episode (Table 12.1–5).

Major Depressive Disorder, Single Episode.

DSM-IV-TR specifies the diagnostic criteria for the first episode of major depressive disorder (Table 12.1–8). Differentiation between these patients and those who have two or more episodes of major depressive disorder is justified because of the uncertain course of the former patients' disorder. Several studies have reported data consistent with the notion that major depression covers a heterogeneous population of disorders. One type of study assessed the stability of a diagnosis of major depression in a patient over time. The study found that 25 to 50 percent of the patients were later reclassified as having a different psychiatric condition or a nonpsychiatric medical condition with psychiatric symptoms. A second type of study evaluated first-degree relatives of affectively ill patients to determine the presence and types of psychiatric diagnoses for these relatives over time. Both types of studies found that depressed patients with more depressive symptoms are more likely to have stable diagnoses over time and are more likely to have affectively ill relatives than are depressed patients with fewer depressive symptoms. In addition, patients with bipolar I disorder and those with bipolar II disorder (recurrent major depressive episodes with hypomania) are likely to have stable diagnoses over time.

Major Depressive Disorder, Recurrent.

Patients who are experiencing at least a second episode of depression are

Table 12.1–1
DSM-IV-TR Criteria for Major Depressive Episode

A. Five (or more) of the following symptoms have been present during the same 2-week period and represent a change from previous functioning; at least one of the symptoms is either (1) depressed mood or (2) loss of interest or pleasure. **Note:** Do not include symptoms that are clearly due to a general medical condition, or mood-incongruent delusions or hallucinations.

   (1) depressed mood most of the day, nearly every day, as indicated by either subjective report (e.g., feels sad or empty) or observation made by others (e.g., appears tearful). **Note:** In children and adolescents, can be irritable mood

   (2) markedly diminished interest or pleasure in all, or almost all, activities most of the day, nearly every day (as indicated by either subjective account or observation made by others)

   (3) significant weight loss when not dieting or weight gain (e.g., a change of more than 5% of body weight in a month), or decrease or increase in appetite nearly every day. **Note:** In children, consider failure to make expected weight gains.

   (4) insomnia or hypersomnia nearly every day

   (5) psychomotor agitation or retardation nearly every day (observable by others, not merely subjective feelings of restlessness or being slowed down)

   (6) fatigue or loss of energy nearly every day

   (7) feelings of worthlessness or excessive or inappropriate guilt (which may be delusional) nearly every day (not merely self-reproach or guilt about being sick)

   (8) diminished ability to think or concentrate, or indecisiveness, nearly every day (either by subjective account or as observed by others)

   (9) recurrent thoughts of death (not just fear of dying), recurrent suicidal ideation without a specific plan, or a suicide attempt or a specific plan for committing suicide

B. The symptoms do not meet criteria for a mixed episode.

C. The symptoms cause clinically significant distress or impairment in social, occupational, or other important areas of functioning.

D. The symptoms are not due to the direct physiological effects of a substance (e.g., a drug of abuse, a medication) or a general medical condition (e.g., hypothyroidism).

E. The symptoms are not better accounted for by bereavement, i.e., after the loss of a loved one, the symptoms persist for longer than 2 months or are characterized by marked functional impairment, morbid preoccupation with worthlessness, suicidal ideation, psychotic symptoms, or psychomotor retardation.

From American Psychiatric Association. *Diagnostic and Statistical Manual of Mental Disorders.* 4th ed. Text rev. Washington, DC: American Psychiatric Association; copyright 2000, with permission.

Table 12.1–2
DSM-IV-TR Criteria for Manic Episode

A. A distinct period of abnormally and persistently elevated, expansive, or irritable mood, lasting at least 1 week (or any duration if hospitalization is necessary).

B. During the period of mood disturbance, three (or more) of the following symptoms have persisted (four if the mood is only irritable) and have been present to a significant degree:

   (1) inflated self-esteem or grandiosity

   (2) decreased need for sleep (e.g., feels rested after only 3 hours of sleep)

   (3) more talkative than usual or pressure to keep talking

   (4) flight of ideas or subjective experience that thoughts are racing

   (5) distractibility (i.e., attention too easily drawn to unimportant or irrelevant external stimuli)

   (6) increase in goal-directed activity (either socially, at work or school, or sexually) or psychomotor agitation

   (7) excessive involvement in pleasurable activities that have a high potential for painful consequences (e.g., engaging in unrestrained buying sprees, sexual indiscretions, or foolish business investments)

C. The symptoms do not meet criteria for a mixed episode.

D. The mood disturbance is sufficiently severe to cause marked impairment in occupational functioning or in usual social activities or relationships with others, or to necessitate hospitalization to prevent harm to self or others, or there are psychotic features.

E. The symptoms are not due to the direct physiological effects of a substance (e.g., a drug of abuse, a medication, or other treatment) or a general medical condition (e.g., hyperthyroidism).

Note: Manic-like episodes that are clearly caused by somatic antidepressant treatment (e.g., medication, electroconvulsive therapy, light therapy) should not count toward a diagnosis of bipolar I disorder.

From American Psychiatric Association. *Diagnostic and Statistical Manual of Mental Disorders.* 4th ed. Text rev. Washington, DC: American Psychiatric Association; copyright 2000, with permission.

---

classified in DSM-IV-TR as having major depressive disorder, recurrent (Table 12.1–9). The essential problem with diagnosing recurrent episodes of major depressive disorder is choosing the criteria with which to designate the resolution of each period. Two variables are the degree of resolution of the symptoms and the length of the resolution. DSM-IV-TR requires that distinct episodes of depression be separated by at least 2 months during which a patient has no significant symptoms of depression.

Bipolar I Disorder

The DSM-IV-TR criteria for a manic episode (Table 12.1–2) requires the presence of a distinct period of abnormal mood

lasting at least 1 week and includes separate bipolar I disorder diagnoses for a single manic episode and a recurrent episode, based on the symptoms of the most recent episode as described later.

The designation bipolar I disorder is synonymous with what was formerly known as bipolar disorder—a syndrome in which a complete set of mania symptoms occurs during the course of the disorder. The diagnostic criteria for bipolar II disorder are depressive episodes and hypomanic episodes (Table 12.1–3) during the course of the disorder, but with the episodes of manic-like symptoms not quite meeting the diagnostic criteria for a full manic syndrome.

Manic episodes clearly precipitated by antidepressant treatment (e.g., pharmacotherapy, electroconvulsive therapy [ECT]) do not indicate bipolar I disorder.

Bipolar I Disorder, Single Manic Episode.   According to DSM-IV-TR, patients must be experiencing their first manic episode to meet the diagnostic criteria for bipolar I disorder, single manic episode (Table 12.1–10). This requirement rests on the fact that patients who are having their first episode of bipolar I disorder depression cannot be distinguished from patients with major depressive disorder.

Table 12.1–3
DSM-IV-TR Criteria for Hypomanic Episode

A. A distinct period of persistently elevated, expansive, or irritable mood, lasting throughout at least 4 days, that is clearly different from the usual nondepressed mood.

B. During the period of mood disturbance, three (or more) of the following symptoms have persisted (four if the mood is only irritable) and have been present to a significant degree:

(1) inflated self-esteem or grandiosity

(2) decreased need for sleep (e.g., feels rested after only 3 hours of sleep)

(3) more talkative than usual or pressure to keep talking

(4) flight of ideas or subjective experience that thoughts are racing

(5) distractibility (i.e., attention too easily drawn to unimportant or irrelevant external stimuli)

(6) increase in goal-directed activity (either socially, at work or school, or sexually) or psychomotor agitation

(7) excessive involvement in pleasurable activities that have a high potential for painful consequences (e.g., the person engages in unrestrained buying sprees, sexual indiscretions, or foolish business investments)

C. The episode is associated with an unequivocal change in functioning that is uncharacteristic of the person when not symptomatic.

D. The disturbance in mood and the change in functioning are observable by others.

E. The episode is not severe enough to cause marked impairment in social or occupational functioning, or to necessitate hospitalization, and there are no psychotic features.

F. The symptoms are not due to the direct physiological effects of a substance (e.g., a drug of abuse, a medication, or other treatment) or a general medical condition (e.g., hyperthyroidism).

Note: Hypomanic-like episodes that are clearly caused by somatic antidepressant treatment (e.g., medication, electroconvulsive therapy, light therapy) should not count toward a diagnosis of bipolar II disorder.

From American Psychiatric Association. *Diagnostic and Statistical Manual of Mental Disorders.* 4th ed. Text rev. Washington, DC: American Psychiatric Association; copyright 2000, with permission.

Table 12.1–4
DSM-IV-TR Criteria for Mixed Episode

A. The criteria are met both for a manic episode and for a major depressive episode (except for duration) nearly every day during at least a 1-week period.

B. The mood disturbance is sufficiently severe to cause marked impairment in occupational functioning or in usual social activities or relationships with others, or to necessitate hospitalization to prevent harm to self or others, or there are psychotic features.

C. The symptoms are not due to the direct physiological effects of a substance (e.g., a drug of abuse, a medication, or other treatment) or a general medical condition (e.g., hyperthyroidism).

Note: Mixed-like episodes that are clearly caused by somatic antidepressant treatment (e.g., medication, electroconvulsive therapy, light therapy) should not count toward a diagnosis of bipolar I disorder.

From American Psychiatric Association. *Diagnostic and Statistical Manual of Mental Disorders.* 4th ed. Text rev. Washington, DC: American Psychiatric Association; copyright 2000, with permission.

Table 12.1–5
DSM-IV-TR Criteria for Severity/Psychotic/Remission Specifiers for Current (or Most Recent) Major Depressive Episode

Note: Code in fifth digit. Mild, moderate, severe without psychotic features, and severe with psychotic features can be applied only if the criteria are currently met for a major depressive episode. In partial remission and in full remission can be applied to the most recent major depressive episode in major depressive disorder and to a major depressive episode in bipolar I or II disorder only if it is the most recent type of mood episode.

Mild: Few, if any, symptoms in excess of those required to make the diagnosis and symptoms result in only minor impairment in occupational functioning or in usual social activities or relationships with others.

Moderate: Symptoms or functional impairment between "mild" and "severe."

Severe without psychotic features: Several symptoms in excess of those required to make the diagnosis, and symptoms markedly interfere with occupational functioning or with usual social activities or relationships with others.

Severe with psychotic features: Delusions or hallucinations. If possible, specify whether the psychotic features are mood-congruent or mood-incongruent:

Mood-congruent psychotic features: Delusions or hallucinations whose content is entirely consistent with the typical depressive themes of personal inadequacy, guilt, disease, death, nihilism, or deserved punishment.

Mood-incongruent psychotic features: Delusions or hallucinations whose content does not involve typical depressive themes of personal inadequacy, guilt, disease, death, nihilism, or deserved punishment. Included are such symptoms as persecutory delusions (not directly related to depressive themes), thought insertion, thought broadcasting, and delusions of control.

In partial remission: Symptoms of a major depressive episode are present but full criteria are not met, or there is a period without any significant symptoms of a major depressive episode lasting less than 2 months following the end of the major depressive episode. (If the major depressive episode was superimposed on dysthymic disorder, the diagnosis of dysthymic disorder alone is given once the full criteria for a major depressive episode are no longer met.)

In full remission: During the past 2 months, no significant signs or symptoms of the disturbance were present.

Unspecified

From American Psychiatric Association. *Diagnostic and Statistical Manual of Mental Disorders.* 4th ed. Text rev. Washington, DC: American Psychiatric Association; copyright 2000, with permission.

Bipolar I Disorder, Recurrent. The issues about defining the end of an episode of depression also apply to defining the end of an episode of mania. Manic episodes are considered distinct when they are separated by at least 2 months without significant symptoms of mania or hypomania. DSM-IV-TR specifies diagnostic criteria for recurrent bipolar I disorder on the basis of the symptoms of the most recent episode: bipolar I disorder, most recent episode manic (Table 12.1–11); bipolar I disorder, most recent episode hypomanic (Table 12.1–12); bipolar I disorder, most recent episode depressed (Table 12.1–13); bipolar I disorder, most recent episode mixed (Table 12.1–14); and bipolar I disorder, most recent episode unspecified (Table 12.1–15).

Table 12.1–6
DSM-IV-TR Criteria for Severity/Psychotic/
Remission Specifiers for Current (or Most Recent)
Manic Episode

Note: Code in fifth digit. Mild, moderate, severe without psychotic features, and severe with psychotic features can be applied only if the criteria are currently met for a manic episode. In partial remission and in full remission can be applied to a manic episode in bipolar I disorder only if it is the most recent type of mood episode.

Mild: Minimum symptom criteria are met for a manic episode.

Moderate: Extreme increase in activity or impairment in judgment.

Severe without psychotic features: Almost continual supervision required to prevent physical harm to self or others.

Severe with psychotic features: Delusions or hallucinations. If possible, specify whether the psychotic features are mood-congruent or mood-incongruent:

  Mood-congruent psychotic features: Delusions or hallucinations whose content is entirely consistent with the typical manic themes of inflated worth, power, knowledge, identity, or special relationship to a deity or famous person.

  Mood-incongruent psychotic features: Delusions or hallucinations whose content does not involve typical manic themes of inflated worth, power, knowledge, identity, or special relationship to a deity or famous person. Included are such symptoms as persecutory delusions (not directly related to grandiose ideas or themes), thought insertion, and delusions of being controlled.

In partial remission: Symptoms of a manic episode are present but full criteria are not met, or there is a period without any significant symptoms of a manic episode lasting less than 2 months following the end of the manic episode.

In full remission: During the past 2 months no significant signs or symptoms of the disturbance were present.

Unspecified

From American Psychiatric Association. *Diagnostic and Statistical Manual of Mental Disorders.* 4th ed. Text rev. Washington, DC: American Psychiatric Association; copyright 2000, with permission.

Table 12.1–7
DSM-IV-TR Criteria for Severity/Psychotic/
Remission Specifiers for Current (or Most Recent)
Mixed Episode

Note: Code in fifth digit. Mild, moderate, severe without psychotic features, and severe with psychotic features can be applied only if the criteria are currently met for a mixed episode. In partial remission and in full remission can be applied to a mixed episode in bipolar I disorder only if it is the most recent type of mood episode.

Mild: No more than minimum symptom criteria are met for both a manic episode and a major depressive episode.

Moderate: Symptoms or functional impairment between "mild" and "severe."

Severe without psychotic features: Almost continual supervision required to prevent physical harm to self or others.

Severe with psychotic features: Delusions or hallucinations. If possible, specify whether the psychotic features are mood-congruent or mood-incongruent:

  Mood-congruent psychotic features: Delusions or hallucinations whose content is entirely consistent with the typical manic or depressive themes.

  Mood-incongruent psychotic features: Delusions or hallucinations whose content does not involve typical manic or depressive themes. Included are such symptoms as persecutory delusions (not directly related to grandiose or depressive themes), thought insertion, and delusions of being controlled.

In partial remission: Symptoms of a mixed episode are present but full criteria are not met, or there is a period without any significant symptoms of a mixed episode lasting less than 2 months following the end of the mixed episode.

In full remission: During the past 2 months, no significant signs or symptoms of the disturbance were present.

Unspecified

From American Psychiatric Association. *Diagnostic and Statistical Manual of Mental Disorders.* 4th ed. Text rev. Washington, DC: American Psychiatric Association; copyright 2000, with permission.

Bipolar II Disorder

The diagnostic criteria for bipolar II disorder specify the particular severity, frequency, and duration of the hypomanic symptoms. The diagnostic criteria for a hypomanic episode (Table 12.1–3) are listed separately from the criteria for bipolar II disorder (Table 12.1–16). The criteria have been established to decrease overdiagnosis of hypomanic episodes and the incorrect classification of patients with major depressive disorder as patients with bipolar II disorder. Clinically, psychiatrists may find it difficult to distinguish euthymia from hypomania in a patient who has been chronically depressed for many months or years. As with bipolar I disorder, antidepressant-induced hypomanic episodes are not diagnostic of bipolar II disorder.

Specifiers Describing Most Recent Episode

In addition to the severity, psychotic, and remission specifiers (Tables 12.1–3 through 12.1–7), DSM-IV-TR defines additional symptom features that can be used to describe patients with various mood disorders. Two of the features (melancholic and atypical) are limited to describing depressive episodes. Two others

(catatonic features and with postpartum onset) can be applied to depressive and manic episodes. These are described in what follows.

With Psychotic Features.   The presence of psychotic features (Table 12.1–3) in major depressive disorder reflects severe disease and is a poor prognostic indicator. A review of the literature comparing psychotic with nonpsychotic major depressive disorder indicates that the two conditions may be distinct in their pathogenesis. One difference is that bipolar I disorder is more common in the families of probands with psychotic depression than in the families of probands with nonpsychotic depression.

The psychotic symptoms themselves are often categorized as either mood congruent, that is, in harmony with the mood disorder ("I deserve to be punished because I am so bad"), or mood incongruent, not in harmony with the mood disorder. Patients with mood disorder with mood-congruent psychoses have a psychotic type of mood disorder; however, patients with mood disorder with mood-incongruent psychotic symptoms may have schizoaffective disorder or schizophrenia.

The following factors have been associated with a poor prognosis for patients with mood disorders: long duration of episodes,

Table 12.1–8
DSM-IV-TR Diagnostic Criteria for Major Depressive Disorder, Single Episode

A. Presence of a single major depressive episode.
B. The major depressive episode is not better accounted for by schizoaffective disorder and is not superimposed on schizophrenia, schizophreniform disorder, delusional disorder, or psychotic disorder not otherwise specified.
C. There has never been a manic episode, a mixed episode, or a hypomanic episode. **Note:** This exclusion does not apply if all of the manic-like, mixed-like, or hypomanic-like episodes are substance or treatment induced or are due to the direct physiological effects of a general medical condition.

If the full criteria are currently met for a major depressive episode, specify its current clinical status and/or features:

Mild, moderate, severe without psychotic features/severe with psychotic features
Chronic
With catatonic features
With melancholic features
With atypical features
With postpartum onset

If the full criteria are not currently met for a major depressive episode, specify the current clinical status of the major depressive disorder or features of the most recent episode:

In partial remission, in full remission
Chronic
With catatonic features
With melancholic features
With atypical features
With postpartum onset

Table 12.1–9
DSM-IV-TR Diagnostic Criteria for Major Depressive Disorder, Recurrent

A. Presence of two or more major depressive episodes. **Note:** To be considered separate episodes, there must be an interval of at least 2 consecutive months in which criteria are not met for a major depressive episode.
B. The major depressive episodes are not better accounted for by schizoaffective disorder and are not superimposed on schizophrenia, schizophreniform disorder, delusional disorder, or psychotic disorder not otherwise specified.
C. There has never been a manic episode, a mixed episode, or a hypomanic episode. **Note:** This exclusion does not apply if all of the manic-like, mixed-like, or hypomanic-like episodes are substance or treatment induced or are due to the direct physiological effects of a general medical condition.

If the full criteria are currently met for a major depressive episode, specify its current clinical status and/or features:

Mild, moderate, severe without psychotic features/severe with psychotic features
Chronic
With catatonic features
With melancholic features
With atypical features
With postpartum onset

If the full criteria are not currently met for a major depressive episode, specify the current clinical status of the major depressive disorder or features of the most recent episode:

In partial remission, in full remission
Chronic
With catatonic features
With melancholic features
With atypical features
With postpartum onset
Specify if:
   Longitudinal course specifiers (with and without interepisode recovery)
   With seasonal pattern

temporal dissociation between the mood disorder and the psychotic symptoms, and a poor premorbid history of social adjustment. The presence of psychotic features also has significant treatment implications. These patients typically require antipsychotic drugs in addition to antidepressants or mood stabilizers and may need ECT to obtain clinical improvement.

With Melancholic Features. Melancholia is one of the oldest terms used in psychiatry, dating back to its use by Hippocrates in the 4th century to describe the dark mood of depression. It is still used to refer to a depression characterized by severe anhedonia, early-morning awakening, weight loss, and profound feelings of guilt (often over trivial events). It is not uncommon for patients who are melancholic to have suicidal ideation. Melancholia is associated with changes in the autonomic nervous system and in endocrine functions. For that reason, melancholia is sometimes referred to as "endogenous depression" or depression that arises in the absence of external life stressors or precipitants. The DSM-IV-TR melancholic features can be applied to major depressive episodes in major depressive disorder, bipolar I disorder, or bipolar II disorder (Table 12.1–17).

With Atypical Features. The introduction of a formally defined depression with atypical features is a response to research and clinical data indicating that patients with atypical features have specific, predictable characteristics: overeating and

oversleeping. These symptoms have sometimes been referred to as *reversed vegetative symptoms*, and the symptom pattern has sometimes been called *hysteroid dysphoria*. When patients with major depressive disorder with atypical features are compared with patients with typical depression features, the patients with atypical features are found to have a younger age of onset, more severe psychomotor slowing, and more frequent coexisting diagnoses of panic disorder, substance abuse or dependence, and somatization disorder. The high incidence and severity of anxiety symptoms in patients with atypical features have sometimes been correlated with the likelihood of their being misclassified as having an anxiety disorder rather than a mood disorder. Patients with atypical features may also have a long-term course, a diagnosis of bipolar I disorder, or a seasonal pattern to their disorder.

The DSM-IV-TR atypical features can be applied to the most recent major depressive episode in major depressive disorder, bipolar I disorder, bipolar II disorder, or dysthymic disorder (Table 12.1–18).

Table 12.1–10
DSM-IV-TR Diagnostic Criteria for Bipolar I Disorder, Single Manic Episode

A. Presence of only one manic episode and no past major depressive episodes. **Note:** Recurrence is defined as either a change in polarity from depression or an interval of at least 2 months without manic symptoms.
B. The manic episode is not better accounted for by schizoaffective disorder and is not superimposed on schizophrenia, schizophreniform disorder, delusional disorder, or psychotic disorder not otherwise specified.

Specify if:
   Mixed: if symptoms meet criteria for a mixed episode
If the full criteria are currently met for a manic, mixed, or major depressive episode, specify its current clinical status and/or features:
   Mild, moderate, severe without psychotic features/severe with psychotic features
   With catatonic features
   With postpartum onset
If the full criteria are not currently met for a manic, mixed, or major depressive episode, specify the current clinical status of the bipolar I disorder or features of the most recent episode:
   In partial remission, in full remission
   With catatonic features
   With postpartum onset

From American Psychiatric Association. *Diagnostic and Statistical Manual of Mental Disorders.* 4th ed. Text rev. Washington, DC: American Psychiatric Association; copyright 2000, with permission.

Table 12.1–11
DSM-IV-TR Diagnostic Criteria for Bipolar I Disorder, Most Recent Episode Manic

A. Currently (or most recently) in a manic episode.
B. There has previously been at least one major depressive episode, manic episode, or mixed episode.
C. The mood episodes in Criteria A and B are not better accounted for by schizoaffective disorder and are not superimposed on schizophrenia, schizophreniform disorder, delusional disorder, or psychotic disorder not otherwise specified.

If the full criteria are currently met for a manic episode, specify its current clinical status and/or features:
   Mild, moderate, severe without psychotic features/severe with psychotic features
   With catatonic features
   With postpartum onset
If the full criteria are not currently met for a manic episode, specify the current clinical status of the bipolar I disorder and/or features of the most recent manic episode:
   In partial remission, in full remission
   With catatonic features
   With postpartum onset
Specify if:
   Longitudinal course specifiers (with and without interepisode recovery)
   With seasonal pattern (applies only to the pattern of major depressive episodes)
   With rapid cycling

From American Psychiatric Association. *Diagnostic and Statistical Manual of Mental Disorders.* 4th ed. Text rev. Washington, DC: American Psychiatric Association; copyright 2000, with permission.

Table 12.1–12
DSM-IV-TR Diagnostic Criteria for Bipolar I Disorder, Most Recent Episode Hypomanic

A. Currently (or most recently) in a hypomanic episode.
B. There has previously been at least one manic episode or mixed episode.
C. The mood symptoms cause clinically significant distress or impairment in social, occupational, or other important areas of functioning.
D. The mood episodes in Criteria A and B are not better accounted for by schizoaffective disorder and are not superimposed on schizophrenia, schizophreniform disorder, delusional disorder, or psychotic disorder not otherwise specified.

Specify if:
   Longitudinal course specifiers (with and without interepisode recovery)
   With seasonal pattern (applies only to the pattern of major depressive episodes)
   With rapid cycling

From American Psychiatric Association. *Diagnostic and Statistical Manual of Mental Disorders.* 4th ed. Text rev. Washington, DC: American Psychiatric Association; copyright 2000, with permission.

Table 12.1–13
DSM-IV-TR Diagnostic Criteria for Bipolar I Disorder, Most Recent Episode Depressed

A. Currently (or most recently) in a major depressive episode.
B. There has previously been at least one manic episode or mixed episode.
C. The mood episodes in Criteria A and B are not better accounted for by schizoaffective disorder and are not superimposed on schizophrenia, schizophreniform disorder, delusional disorder, or psychotic disorder not otherwise specified.

If the full criteria are currently met for a major depressive episode, specify its current clinical status and/or features:
   Mild, moderate, severe without psychotic features/severe with psychotic features
   Chronic
   With catatonic features
   With melancholic features
   With atypical features
   With postpartum onset
If the full criteria are not currently met for a major depressive episode, specify the current clinical status of the bipolar I disorder and/or features of the most recent major depressive episode:
   In partial remission, in full remission
   Chronic
   With catatonic features
   With melancholic features
   With atypical features
   With postpartum onset
Specify if:
   Longitudinal course specifiers (with and without interepisode recovery)
   With seasonal pattern (applies only to the pattern of major depressive episodes)
   With rapid cycling

From American Psychiatric Association. *Diagnostic and Statistical Manual of Mental Disorders.* 4th ed. Text rev. Washington, DC: American Psychiatric Association; copyright 2000, with permission.

Table 12.1–14
DSM-IV-TR Diagnostic Criteria for Bipolar I Disorder, Most Recent Episode Mixed

A. Currently (or most recently) in a mixed episode.
B. There has previously been at least one major depressive episode, manic episode, or mixed episode.
C. The mood episodes in Criteria A and B are not better accounted for by schizoaffective disorder and are not superimposed on schizophrenia, schizophreniform disorder, delusional disorder, or psychotic disorder not otherwise specified.

If the full criteria are currently met for a mixed episode, specify its current clinical status and/or features:

Mild, moderate, severe without psychotic features/severe with psychotic features
With catatonic features
With postpartum onset

If the full criteria are not currently met for a mixed episode, specify the current clinical status of the bipolar I disorder and/or features of the most recent mixed episode:

In partial remission, in full remission
With catatonic features
With postpartum onset

Specify if:
Longitudinal course specifiers (with and without interepisode recovery)
With seasonal pattern (applies only to the pattern of major depressive episodes)
With rapid cycling

From American Psychiatric Association. *Diagnostic and Statistical Manual of Mental Disorders.* 4th ed. Text rev. Washington, DC: American Psychiatric Association; copyright 2000, with permission.

Table 12.1–15
DSM-IV-TR Diagnostic Criteria for Bipolar I Disorder, Most Recent Episode Unspecified

A. Criteria, except for duration, are currently (or most recently) met for a manic, a hypomanic, a mixed, or a major depressive episode.
B. There has previously been at least one manic episode or mixed episode.
C. The mood symptoms cause clinically significant distress or impairment in social, occupational, or other important areas of functioning.
D. The mood symptoms in Criteria A and B are not better accounted for by schizoaffective disorder and are not superimposed on schizophrenia, schizophreniform disorder, delusional disorder, or psychotic disorder not otherwise specified.
E. The mood symptoms in Criteria A and B are not due to the direct physiological effects of a substance (e.g., a drug of abuse, a medication, or other treatment) or a general medical condition (e.g., hyperthyroidism).

Specify if:
Longitudinal course specifiers (with and without interepisode recovery)
With seasonal pattern (applies only to the pattern of major depressive episodes)
With rapid cycling

From American Psychiatric Association. *Diagnostic and Statistical Manual of Mental Disorders.* 4th ed. Text rev. Washington, DC: American Psychiatric Association; copyright 2000, with permission.

Table 12.1–16
DSM-IV-TR Diagnostic Criteria for Bipolar II Disorder

A. Presence (or history) of one or more major depressive episodes.
B. Presence (or history) of at least one hypomanic episode.
C. There has never been a manic episode or a mixed episode.
D. The mood symptoms in Criteria A and B are not better accounted for by schizoaffective disorder and are not superimposed on schizophrenia, schizophreniform disorder, delusional disorder, or psychotic disorder not otherwise specified.
E. The symptoms cause clinically significant distress or impairment in social, occupational, or other important areas of functioning.

Specify current or most recent episode:
Hypomanic: if currently (or most recently) in a hypomanic episode
Depressed: if currently (or most recently) in a major depressive episode

If the full criteria are currently met for a major depressive episode, specify its current clinical status and/or features:

Mild, moderate, severe without psychotic features/severe with psychotic features. Note: Fifth-digit codes cannot be used here because the code for bipolar II disorder already uses the fifth digit.
Chronic
With catatonic features
With melancholic features
With atypical features
With postpartum onset

If the full criteria are not currently met for a hypomanic or major depressive episode, specify the clinical status of the bipolar II disorder and/or features of the most recent major depressive episode (only if it is the most recent type of mood episode):

In partial remission, in full remission. Note: Fifth-digit codes cannot be used here because the code for bipolar II disorder already uses the fifth digit.
Chronic
With catatonic features
With melancholic features
With atypical features
With postpartum onset

Specify if:
Longitudinal course specifiers (with and without interepisode recovery)
With seasonal pattern (applies only to the pattern of major depressive episodes)
With rapid cycling

From American Psychiatric Association. *Diagnostic and Statistical Manual of Mental Disorders.* 4th ed. Text rev. Washington, DC: American Psychiatric Association; copyright 2000, with permission.

Ms. G is a 17-year-old high school senior, referred for evaluation after she attempted suicide with an overdose of pills. Earlier on the night of the suicide attempt, she had a fight with her mother over a request to order pizza. Ms. G remembers her mother saying that she was a "spoiled brat" and asking whether she would be happier living elsewhere. Ms. G, feeling rejected and despondent, went to her room and wrote a note saying that she was having a mental breakdown and that she loved her parents but could not communicate with them. She added a request that her favorite glass animals be given to a particular friend. The parents, who had gone out to a movie, returned home later that evening to find their daughter comatose and immediately rushed her to the hospital emergency room.

During the last couple of months, Ms. G had been crying frequently and had lost interest in her friends, school, and social activities. She had been eating more and more and had recently begun to gain weight, which her mother is very unhappy about. Ms. G says that her mother is always harping about "taking care of herself," and in fact, the argument on the night of her suicide attempt was about Ms. G's desire to order a pizza that her mother did not think she needed. Ms. G's mother reports that all her daughter seems to want to do is sleep and that she never wants to go out with her friends or help around the house. When questioned about changes in her sleep habits, Ms. G admits that she has been feeling very tired lately and that she often feels as if there is nothing to make it worth getting out of bed. She does mention that she is excited about an upcoming visit from her boyfriend, who attends a college a considerable distance away and has not been home for several months.

Upon evaluation, it is apparent that Ms. G, the third of three children of upper-middle-class and very intelligent parents, is struggling with a view of herself as less bright, clever, and attractive than her two siblings. She feels ignored and essentially rejected by her seemingly omnipresent mother. Ms. G is having difficulty developing a sense of separation from her mother and an individual sense of identity. She experiences her mother's directives as interference with her efforts to express autonomy and independence. (Reprinted with permission from *DSM-IV Case Studies*.)

Table 12.1–17
DSM-IV-TR Criteria for Melancholic Features Specifier

Specify if:
With melancholic features (can be applied to the current or most recent major depressive episode in major depressive disorder and to a major depressive episode in bipolar I or bipolar II disorder only if it is the most recent type of mood episode)
A. Either of the following, occurring during the most severe period of the current episode:
　(1) loss of pleasure in all, or almost all, activities
　(2) lack of reactivity to usually pleasurable stimuli (does not feel much better, even temporarily, when something good happens)
B. Three (or more) of the following:
　(1) distinct quality of depressed mood (i.e., the depressed mood is experienced as distinctly different from the kind of feeling experienced after the death of a loved one)
　(2) depression regularly worse in the morning
　(3) early morning awakening (at least 2 hours before usual time of awakening)
　(4) marked psychomotor retardation or agitation
　(5) significant anorexia or weight loss
　(6) excessive or inappropriate guilt

From American Psychiatric Association. *Diagnostic and Statistical Manual of Mental Disorders*. 4th ed. Text rev. Washington, DC: American Psychiatric Association; copyright 2000, with permission.

Table 12.1–18
DSM-IV-TR Criteria for Atypical Features Specifier

Specify if:
With atypical features (can be applied when these features predominate during the most recent 2 weeks of a current major depressive episode in major depressive disorder or in bipolar I or bipolar II disorder when a current major depressive episode is the most recent type of mood episode, or when these features predominate during the most recent 2 years of dysthymic disorder; if the major depressive episode is not current, it applies if the feature predominates during any 2-week period)
A. Mood reactivity (i.e., mood brightens in response to actual or potential positive events)
B. Two (or more) of the following features:
　(1) significant weight gain or increase in appetite
　(2) hypersomnia
　(3) leaden paralysis (i.e., heavy, leaden feelings in arms or legs)
　(4) long-standing pattern of interpersonal rejection sensitivity (not limited to episodes of mood disturbance) that results in significant social or occupational impairment
C. Criteria are not met for with melancholic features or with catatonic features during the same episode.

From American Psychiatric Association. *Diagnostic and Statistical Manual of Mental Disorders*. 4th ed. Text rev. Washington, DC: American Psychiatric Association; copyright 2000, with permission.

With Catatonic Features.   As a symptom, catatonia (Table 12.1–19) can be present in several mental disorders, most commonly, schizophrenia and the mood disorders. The presence of catatonic features in patients with mood disorders may have prognostic and treatment significance.

The hallmark symptoms of catatonia—stuporousness, blunted affect, extreme withdrawal, negativism, and marked psychomotor retardation—can be seen in both catatonic and noncatatonic schizophrenia, major depressive disorder (often

Table 12.1–19
DSM-IV-TR Criteria for Catatonic Features Specifier

Specify if:
With catatonic features (can be applied to the current or most recent major depressive episode, manic episode, or mixed episode in major depressive disorder, bipolar I disorder, or bipolar II disorder)
　The clinical picture is dominated by at least two of the following:
　(1) motoric immobility as evidenced by catalepsy (including waxy flexibility) or stupor
　(2) excessive motor activity (that is apparently purposeless and not influenced by external stimuli)
　(3) extreme negativism (an apparently motiveless resistance to all instructions or maintenance of a rigid posture against attempts to be moved) or mutism
　(4) peculiarities of voluntary movement as evidenced by posturing (voluntary assumption of inappropriate or bizarre postures), stereotyped movements, prominent mannerisms, or prominent grimacing
　(5) echolalia or echopraxia

From American Psychiatric Association. *Diagnostic and Statistical Manual of Mental Disorders*. 4th ed. Text rev. Washington, DC: American Psychiatric Association; copyright 2000, with permission.

Table 12.1–20
DSM-IV-TR Criteria for Postpartum Onset Specifier

Specify if:
   With postpartum onset (can be applied to the current or most recent major depressive, manic, or mixed episode in major depressive disorder, bipolar I disorder, or bipolar II disorder; or to brief psychotic disorder)
      Onset of episode within 4 weeks postpartum

From American Psychiatric Association. *Diagnostic and Statistical Manual of Mental Disorders.* 4th ed. Text rev. Washington, DC: American Psychiatric Association; copyright 2000, with permission.

with psychotic features), and medical and neurological disorders. Clinicians often do not associate catatonic symptoms with bipolar I disorder because of the marked contrast between the symptoms of stuporous catatonia and the classic symptoms of mania. Because catatonic symptoms are a behavioral syndrome appearing in several medical and psychiatric conditions, catatonic symptoms do not imply a single diagnosis.

Postpartum Onset.   DSM-IV-TR allows the specification of a postpartum mood disturbance if the onset of symptoms is within 4 weeks postpartum (Table 12.1–20). Postpartum mental disorders commonly include psychotic symptoms. (Postpartum psychosis is discussed in Section 11.4 and in Chapter 26 on reproductive psychiatry.)

Chronic.   DSM-IV-TR allows the specification of chronic to describe major depressive episodes that occur as a part of major depressive disorder, bipolar I disorder, and bipolar II disorder (Table 12.1–21).

Describing Course of Recurrent Episodes

The DSM-IV-TR includes criteria for three distinct course specifiers for mood disorders. One of the course specifiers, with rapid cycling (Table 12.1–22), is restricted to bipolar I disorder and bipolar II disorder. Two other course specifiers, with seasonal pattern (Table 12.1–23) and with or without full interepisode recovery (Table 12.1–24), can be applied to bipolar I disorder, bipolar II disorder, and major depressive disorder, recurrent. The course specifier with postpartum onset can be applied to major depressive or manic episodes in bipolar I disorder, bipolar II disorder, major depressive disorder, and brief psychotic disorder.

Table 12.1–21
DSM-IV-TR Criteria for Chronic Specifier

Specify if:
   Chronic (can be applied to the current or most recent major depressive episode in major depressive disorder and to a major depressive episode in bipolar I or II disorder only if it is the most recent type of mood episode)
      Full criteria for a major depressive episode have been met continuously for at least the past 2 years.

From American Psychiatric Association. *Diagnostic and Statistical Manual of Mental Disorders.* 4th ed. Text rev. Washington, DC: American Psychiatric Association; copyright 2000, with permission.

Table 12.1–22
DSM-IV-TR Criteria for Rapid-Cycling Specifier

Specify if:
   With rapid cycling (can be applied to bipolar I disorder or bipolar II disorder)   At least four episodes of a mood disturbance in the previous 12 months that meet criteria for a major depressive, manic, mixed, or hypomanic episode.
   Note: Episodes are demarcated either by partial or full remission for at least 2 months or a switch to an episode of opposite polarity (e.g., major depressive episode to manic episode).

From American Psychiatric Association. *Diagnostic and Statistical Manual of Mental Disorders.* 4th ed. Text rev. Washington, DC: American Psychiatric Association; copyright 2000, with permission.

Rapid Cycling.   Patients with rapid cycling bipolar I disorder are likely to be female and to have had depressive and hypomanic episodes. No data indicate that rapid cycling has a familial pattern of inheritance, and, thus, an external factor such as stress or drug treatment may be involved in the pathogenesis of rapid cycling. The DSM-IV-TR criteria specify that the patient must have at least four episodes within a 12-month period (Table 12.1–22).

Seasonal Pattern.   Patients with a seasonal pattern to their mood disorders tend to experience depressive episodes during a particular season, most commonly winter. The pattern has become known as seasonal affective disorder (SAD), although this term is not used in DSM-IV-TR (Table 12.1–23). Two types of evidence indicate that the seasonal pattern may represent a separate diagnostic entity. First, the patients are likely to respond to treatment with light therapy, although no studies with controls to evaluate light therapy in nonseasonally depressed patients have

Table 12.1–23
DSM-IV-TR Criteria for Seasonal Pattern Specifier

Specify if:
   With seasonal pattern (can be applied to the pattern of major depressive episodes in bipolar I disorder, bipolar II disorder, or major depressive disorder, recurrent).
   A. There has been a regular temporal relationship between the onset of major depressive episodes in bipolar I or bipolar II disorder or major depressive disorder, recurrent, and a particular time of the year (e.g., regular appearance of the major depressive episode in the fall or winter).
      Note: Do not include cases in which there is an obvious effect of seasonal-related psychosocial stressors (e.g., regularly being unemployed every winter).
   B. Full remissions (or a change from depression to mania or hypomania) also occur at a characteristic time of the year (e.g., depression disappears in the spring).
   C. In the last 2 years, two major depressive episodes have occurred that demonstrate the temporal seasonal relationships defined in Criteria A and B, and no nonseasonal major depressive episodes have occurred during that same period.
   D. Seasonal major depressive episodes (as described above) substantially outnumber the nonseasonal major depressive episodes that may have occurred over the individual's lifetime.

From American Psychiatric Association. *Diagnostic and Statistical Manual of Mental Disorders.* 4th ed. Text rev. Washington, DC: American Psychiatric Association; copyright 2000, with permission.

Table 12.1–24
DSM-IV-TR Criteria for Longitudinal Course Specifiers

Specify if (can be applied to recurrent major depressive disorder or bipolar I or II disorder):

With full interepisode recovery: if full remission is attained between the two most recent mood episodes

Without full interepisode recovery: if full remission is not attained between the two most recent mood episodes

From American Psychiatric Association. *Diagnostic and Statistical Manual of Mental Disorders.* 4th ed. Text rev. Washington, DC: American Psychiatric Association; copyright 2000, with permission.

been conducted. Second, research has shown that patients evince decreased metabolic activity in the orbital frontal cortex and in the left inferior parietal lobe. Further studies are necessary to differentiate depressed persons with seasonal pattern from other depressed persons.

Longitudinal Course Specifiers.   DSM-IV-TR includes specific descriptions of longitudinal courses for major depressive disorder, bipolar I disorder, and bipolar II disorder (Table 12.1–24). These longitudinal course specifiers help clinicians and researchers to identify appropriate treatment and prognosticate based on various longitudinal courses.

Non–DSM-IV-TR Types.   Other systems that identify types of patients with mood disorders usually separate patients with good and poor prognoses or patients who may respond to one treatment or another. They also differentiate endogenous–reactive and primary–secondary schemes.

The endogenous–reactive continuum is a controversial division. It implies that endogenous depressions are biological and that reactive depressions are psychological, primarily on the basis of the presence or absence of an identifiable precipitating stress. Other symptoms of endogenous depression have been described as diurnal variation, delusions, psychomotor retardation, early-morning awakening, and feelings of guilt; thus, endogenous depression is similar to the DSM-IV-TR diagnosis of major depressive disorder with psychotic features or melancholic features or both. Symptoms of reactive depression have included initial insomnia, anxiety, emotional lability, and multiple somatic complaints.

Primary depressions are what DSM-IV-TR refers to as mood disorders, except for the diagnoses of mood disorder caused by a general medical condition and substance-induced mood disorder, which are considered secondary depressions. Double depression is the condition in which major depressive disorder is superimposed on dysthymic disorder. A depressive equivalent is a symptom or syndrome that may be a *forme fruste* of a depressive episode. For example, a triad of truancy, alcohol abuse, and sexual promiscuity in a formerly well-behaved adolescent may constitute a depressive equivalent.

CLINICAL FEATURES

The two basic symptom patterns in mood disorders are depression and mania. Depressive episodes can occur in both major

depressive disorder and bipolar I disorder. Researchers have attempted to find reliable differences between bipolar I disorder depressive episodes and episodes of major depressive disorder, but the differences are elusive. In a clinical situation, only the patient's history, family history, and future course can help differentiate the two conditions. Some patients with bipolar I disorder have mixed states with both manic and depressive features, and some seem to experience brief—minutes to a few hours—episodes of depression during manic episodes.

Depressive Episodes

A depressed mood and a loss of interest or pleasure are the key symptoms of depression. Patients may say that they feel blue, hopeless, in the dumps, or worthless. For a patient, the depressed mood often has a distinct quality that differentiates it from the normal emotion of sadness or grief. Patients often describe the symptom of depression as one of agonizing emotional pain and sometimes complain about being unable to cry, a symptom that resolves as they improve.

About two thirds of all depressed patients contemplate suicide, and 10 to 15 percent commit suicide. Those recently hospitalized with a suicide attempt or suicidal ideation have a higher lifetime risk of successful suicide than those never hospitalized for suicidal ideation. Some depressed patients sometimes seem unaware of their depression and do not complain of a mood disturbance, even though they exhibit withdrawal from family, friends, and activities that previously interested them. Almost all depressed patients (97 percent) complain about reduced energy; they have difficulty finishing tasks, are impaired at school and work, and have less motivation to undertake new projects. About 80 percent of patients complain of trouble sleeping, especially early-morning awakening (i.e., terminal insomnia) and multiple awakenings at night, during which they ruminate about their problems. Many patients have decreased appetite and weight loss, but others experience increased appetite and weight gain and sleep longer than usual. These patients are classified in DSM-IV-TR as having atypical features.

Anxiety, a common symptom of depression, affects as many as 90 percent of all depressed patients. The various changes in food intake and rest can aggravate coexisting medical illnesses such as diabetes, hypertension, chronic obstructive lung disease, and heart disease. Other vegetative symptoms include abnormal menses and decreased interest and performance in sexual activities. Sexual problems can sometimes lead to inappropriate referrals, such as to marital counseling and sex therapy, when clinicians fail to recognize the underlying depressive disorder. Anxiety (including panic attacks), alcohol abuse, and somatic complaints (e.g., constipation and headaches) often complicate the treatment of depression. About 50 percent of all patients describe a diurnal variation in their symptoms, with increased severity in the morning and lessening of symptoms by evening. Cognitive symptoms include subjective reports of an inability to concentrate (84 percent of patients in one study) and impairments in thinking (67 percent of patients in another study).

Depression in Children and Adolescents.   School phobia and excessive clinging to parents may be symptoms of depression in children. Poor academic performance, substance abuse, antisocial behavior, sexual promiscuity, truancy, and running away may be symptoms of depression in adolescents. (This subject is further discussed in Section 45.1.)

Depression in Older People. Depression is more common in older persons than it is in the general population. Various studies have reported prevalence rates ranging from 25 to almost 50 percent, although the percentage of these cases that are caused by major depressive disorder is uncertain. Several studies indicate that depression in older persons may be correlated with low socioeconomic status, the loss of a spouse, a concurrent physical illness, and social isolation. Other studies have indicated that depression in older persons is underdiagnosed and undertreated, perhaps particularly by general practitioners. The underrecognition of depression in older persons may occur because the disorder appears more often with somatic complaints in older, than in younger, age groups. Furthermore, ageism may influence and cause clinicians to accept depressive symptoms as normal in older patients.

Manic Episodes

An elevated, expansive, or irritable mood is the hallmark of a manic episode. The elevated mood is euphoric and often infectious and can even cause a countertransferential denial of illness by an inexperienced clinician. Although uninvolved persons may not recognize the unusual nature of a patient's mood, those who know the patient recognize it as abnormal. Alternatively, the mood may be irritable, especially when a patient's overtly ambitious plans are thwarted. Patients often exhibit a change of predominant mood from euphoria early in the course of the illness to later irritability.

The treatment of manic patients in an inpatient ward can be complicated by their testing of the limits of ward rules, their tendency to shift responsibility for their acts onto others, their exploitation of the weaknesses of others, and their propensity to create conflicts among staff members. Outside the hospital, manic patients often drink alcohol excessively, perhaps in an attempt to self-medicate. Their disinhibited nature is reflected in excessive use of the telephone, especially in making long-distance calls during the early-morning hours.

Pathological gambling, a tendency to disrobe in public places, wearing clothing and jewelry of bright colors in unusual or outlandish combinations, and inattention to small details (e.g., forgetting to hang up the telephone) are also symptomatic of the disorder. Patients act impulsively and at the same time with a sense of conviction and purpose. They are often preoccupied by religious, political, financial, sexual, or persecutory ideas that can evolve into complex delusional systems. Occasionally, manic patients become regressed and play with their urine and feces.

Mania in Adolescents. Mania in adolescents is often misdiagnosed as antisocial personality disorder or schizophrenia. Symptoms of mania in adolescents may include psychosis, alcohol or other substance abuse, suicide attempts, academic problems, philosophical brooding, OCD symptoms, multiple somatic complaints, marked irritability resulting in fights, and other antisocial behaviors. Although many of these symptoms are seen in normal adolescents, severe or persistent symptoms should cause clinicians to consider bipolar I disorder in the differential diagnosis.

Bipolar II Disorder

The clinical features of bipolar II disorder are those of major depressive disorder combined with those of a hypomanic episode. Although the data are limited, a few studies indicate that bipolar II disorder is associated with more marital disruption and with onset at an earlier age than bipolar I disorder. Evidence also indicates that patients with bipolar II disorder are at greater risk of both attempting and completing suicide than patients with bipolar I disorder and major depressive disorder.

Coexisting Disorders

Anxiety. In the anxiety disorders, DSM-IV-TR notes the existence of mixed anxiety–depressive disorder. Significant symptoms of anxiety can and often do coexist with significant symptoms of depression. Whether patients who exhibit significant symptoms of both anxiety and depression are affected by two distinct disease processes or by a single disease process that produces both sets of symptoms is not yet resolved. Patients of both types may constitute the group of patients with mixed anxiety–depressive disorder.

Alcohol Dependence. Alcohol dependence frequently coexists with mood disorders. Both patients with major depressive disorder and those with bipolar I disorder are likely to meet the diagnostic criteria for an alcohol use disorder. The data indicate that alcohol dependence is more strongly associated with a coexisting diagnosis of depression in women than in men. In contrast, the genetic and family data about men who have both a mood disorder and alcohol dependence indicate that they are likely to have two genetically distinct disease processes.

Other Substance-Related Disorders. Substance-related disorders other than alcohol dependence are also commonly associated with mood disorders. The abuse of substances may be involved in precipitating an episode of illness or, conversely, may represent patients' attempts to treat their own illnesses. Although manic patients seldom use sedatives to dampen their euphoria, depressed patients often use stimulants, such as cocaine and amphetamines, to relieve their depression.

Medical Conditions. Depression commonly coexists with medical conditions, especially in older persons. When depression and medical conditions coexist, clinicians must try to determine whether the underlying medical condition is pathophysiologically related to the depression or whether any drugs that the patient is taking for the medical condition are causing the depression. Many studies indicate that treatment of a coexisting major depressive disorder can improve the course of the underlying medical disorder, including cancer.

MENTAL STATUS EXAMINATION

Depressive Episodes

General Description.   Generalized psychomotor retardation is the most common symptom of depression, although psychomotor agitation is also seen, especially in older patients. Hand-wringing and hair-pulling are the most common symptoms of agitation. Classically, a depressed patient has a stooped posture, no spontaneous movements, and a downcast, averted gaze. On clinical examination, depressed patients exhibiting gross symptoms of psychomotor retardation may appear identical to patients with catatonic schizophrenia. This fact is recognized in DSM-IV-TR by the inclusion of the symptom qualifier "with catatonic features" for some mood disorders.

Mood, Affect, and Feelings.   Depression is the key symptom, although about 50 percent of patients deny depressive feelings and do not appear to be particularly depressed. Family members or employers often bring or send these patients for treatment because of social withdrawal and generally decreased activity.

Speech.   Many depressed patients have decreased rate and volume of speech; they respond to questions with single words and exhibit delayed responses to questions. The examiner may literally have to wait 2 or 3 minutes for a response to a question.

Perceptual Disturbances.   Depressed patients with delusions or hallucinations are said to have a major depressive episode with psychotic features. Even in the absence of delusions or hallucinations, some clinicians use the term *psychotic depression* for grossly regressed depressed patients—mute, not bathing, soiling. Such patients are probably better described as having catatonic features.

Delusions and hallucinations that are consistent with a depressed mood are said to be mood congruent. Mood-congruent delusions in a depressed person include those of guilt, sinfulness, worthlessness, poverty, failure, persecution, and terminal somatic illnesses (such as cancer and "rotting" brain). The content of mood-incongruent delusions or hallucinations is not consistent with a depressed mood. For example, a mood-incongruent delusion in a depressed person might involve grandiose themes of exaggerated power, knowledge, and worth. When that occurs, a schizophrenic disorder should be considered.

Thought.   Depressed patients customarily have negative views of the world and of themselves. Their thought content often includes nondelusional ruminations about loss, guilt, suicide, and death. About 10 percent of all depressed patients have marked symptoms of a thought disorder, usually thought blocking and profound poverty of content.

Sensorium and Cognition

ORIENTATION.   Most depressed patients are oriented to person, place, and time, although some may not have sufficient energy or interest to answer questions about these subjects during an interview.

MEMORY.   About 50 to 75 percent of all depressed patients have a cognitive impairment, sometimes referred to as *depressive pseudodementia*. Such patients commonly complain of impaired concentration and forgetfulness.

Impulse Control.   About 10 to 15 percent of all depressed patients commit suicide, and about two thirds have suicidal ideation. Depressed patients with psychotic features occasionally consider killing a person as a result of their delusional systems, but the most severely depressed patients often lack the motivation or the energy to act in an impulsive or violent way. Patients with depressive disorders are at increased risk of suicide as they begin to improve and regain the energy needed to plan and carry out a suicide (paradoxical suicide). It is usually clinically unwise to give a depressed patient a large prescription for a large number of antidepressants, especially tricyclic drugs, at the time of their discharge from the hospital. Similarly, drugs that may be activating, such as fluoxetine, may be prescribed in such a way that the energizing qualities are minimized (e.g., be given a benzodiazepine at the same time).

Judgment and Insight.   Judgment is best assessed by reviewing patients' actions in the recent past and their behavior during the interview. Depressed patients' description of their disorder is often hyperbolic; they overemphasize their symptoms, their disorder, and their life problems. It is difficult to convince such patients that improvement is possible.

Reliability.   In interviews and conversations, depressed patients overemphasize the bad and minimize the good. A common clinical mistake is unquestioningly to believe a depressed patient who states that a previous trial of antidepressant medications did not work. Such statements may be false, and they require confirmation from another source. Psychiatrists should not view patients' misinformation as an intentional fabrication; the admission of any hopeful information may be impossible for a person in a depressed state of mind.

Objective Rating Scales for Depression.   Objective rating scales for depression can be useful in clinical practice for documenting the depressed patient's clinical state.

ZUNG.   The Zung Self-Rating Depression Scale is a 20-item report scale. A normal score is 34 or less; a depressed score is 50 or more. The scale provides a global index of the intensity of a patient's depressive symptoms, including the affective expression of depression.

RASKIN.   The Raskin Depression Scale is a clinician-rated scale that measures the severity of a patient's depression, as reported by the patient and as observed by the physician, on a 5-point scale of three dimensions: verbal report, displayed behavior, and secondary symptoms. The scale has a range of 3 to 13; a normal score is 3, and a depressed score is 7 or more.

HAMILTON.   The Hamilton Rating Scale for Depression is a widely used depression scale with up to 24 items, each of which is rated 0 to 4 or 0 to 2, with a total score of 0 to 76. The clinician evaluates the patient's answers to questions about feelings of guilt, thoughts of suicide, sleep habits, and other symptoms of depression, and the ratings are derived from the clinical interview.

Manic Episodes

General Description.
Manic patients are excited, talkative, sometimes amusing, and frequently hyperactive. At times, they are grossly psychotic and disorganized and require physical restraints and the intramuscular injection of sedating drugs.

Mood, Affect, and Feelings.
Manic patients classically are euphoric, but they can also be irritable, especially when mania has been present for some time. They also have a low frustration tolerance, which can lead to feelings of anger and hostility. Manic patients may be emotionally labile, switching from laughter to irritability to depression in minutes or hours.

Speech.
Manic patients often cannot be interrupted while they are speaking, and they are often intrusive nuisances to those around them. Their speech is often disturbed. As the mania gets more intense, speech becomes louder, more rapid, and difficult to interpret. As the activated state increases, their speech is filled with puns, jokes, rhymes, plays on words, and irrelevancies. At a still greater activity level, associations become loosened, the ability to concentrate fades, and flight of ideas, clanging, and neologisms appear. In acute manic excitement, speech can be totally incoherent and indistinguishable from that of a person with schizophrenia.

Perceptual Disturbances.
Delusions occur in 75 percent of all manic patients. Mood-congruent manic delusions are often concerned with great wealth, extraordinary abilities, or power. Bizarre and mood-incongruent delusions and hallucinations may also appear in mania.

Thought.
The manic patient's thought content includes themes of self-confidence and self-aggrandizement. Manic patients are often easily distracted, and their cognitive functioning in the manic state is characterized by an unrestrained and accelerated flow of ideas.

Sensorium and Cognition.
Although the cognitive deficits of patients with schizophrenia have been much discussed, less has been written about similar deficits in patients with bipolar I disorder. These deficits can be interpreted as reflecting diffuse cortical dysfunction; subsequent work may localize the abnormal areas. Grossly, orientation and memory are intact, although some manic patients may be so euphoric that they answer questions testing orientation incorrectly. Emil Kraepelin called the symptom "delirious mania."

Impulse Control.
About 75 percent of all manic patients are assaultive or threatening. Manic patients do attempt suicide and homicide, but the incidence of these behaviors is unknown, but probably low.

Judgment and Insight.
Impaired judgment is a hallmark of manic patients. They may break laws about credit cards, sexual activities, and finances and sometimes involve their families in financial ruin. Manic patients also have little insight into their disorder.

Reliability.
Manic patients are notoriously unreliable in their information. Because lying and deceit are common in mania, inexperienced clinicians may treat manic patients with inappropriate disdain.

DIFFERENTIAL DIAGNOSIS

Major Depressive Disorder

Medical Disorders.
The DSM-IV-TR diagnosis of mood disorder due to a general medical condition describes a mood disorder caused by a nonpsychiatric medical condition. The DSM-IV-TR diagnosis of substance-induced mood disorder describes a mood disorder caused by a substance. Both these diagnostic categories are discussed in Section 12.3.

Failure to obtain a good clinical history or to consider the context of a patient's current life situation can lead to diagnostic errors. Clinicians should have depressed adolescents tested for mononucleosis, and patients who are markedly overweight or underweight should be tested for adrenal and thyroid dysfunctions. Homosexuals, bisexual men, prostitutes, and persons who abuse a substance intravenously should be tested for acquired immune deficiency syndrome. Older patients should be evaluated for viral pneumonia and other medical conditions.

Many neurological and medical disorders and pharmacological agents can produce symptoms of depression. Patients with depressive disorders often first visit their general practitioners with somatic complaints. Most medical causes of depressive disorders can be detected with a comprehensive medical history, a complete physical and neurological examination, and routine blood and urine tests. The workup should include tests for thyroid and adrenal functions because disorders of both of these endocrine systems can appear as depressive disorders. In substance-induced mood disorder, a reasonable rule of thumb is that any drug a depressed patient is taking should be considered a potential factor in the mood disorder. Cardiac drugs, antihypertensives, sedatives, hypnotics, antipsychotics, antiepileptics, antiparkinsonian drugs, analgesics, antibacterials, and antineoplastics are all commonly associated with depressive symptoms.

NEUROLOGICAL CONDITIONS. The most common neurological problems that manifest depressive symptoms are Parkinson's disease, dementing illnesses (including dementia of the Alzheimer's type), epilepsy, cerebrovascular diseases, and tumors. About 50 to 75 percent of all patients with Parkinson's disease have marked symptoms of depressive disorder that do not correlate with the patient's physical disability, age, or duration of illness but do correlate with the presence of abnormalities found on neuropsychological tests. The symptoms of depressive disorder can be masked by the almost identical motor symptoms of Parkinson's disease. Depressive symptoms often respond to antidepressant drugs or ECT. The interictal changes associated with temporal lobe epilepsy can mimic a depressive disorder, especially if the epileptic focus is on the right side. Depression is a common complicating feature of cerebrovascular diseases, particularly in the 2 years after the episode. Depression is more common in anterior brain lesions than in posterior brain lesions and, in both cases, often responds to antidepressant medications. Tumors of the diencephalic and temporal regions are particularly likely to be associated with depressive disorder symptoms.

PSEUDODEMENTIA.   Clinicians can usually differentiate the pseudodementia of major depressive disorder from the dementia of a disease, such as dementia of the Alzheimer's type, on clinical grounds. The cognitive symptoms in major depressive disorder have a sudden onset, and other symptoms of the disorder, such as self-reproach, are also present. A diurnal variation in the cognitive problems, which is not seen in primary dementias, may occur. Depressed patients with cognitive difficulties often do not try to answer questions ("I don't know"), whereas patients with dementia may confabulate. During an interview, depressed patients can sometimes be coached and encouraged into remembering, an ability that demented patients lack.

Mental Disorders.   Depression can be a feature of virtually any mental disorder listed in DSM-IV-TR, but the mental disorders such as anxiety and schizophrenia deserve particular consideration in the differential diagnosis.

OTHER MOOD DISORDERS.   Clinicians must consider a range of DSM-IV-TR diagnostic categories before arriving at a final diagnosis. Mood disorder caused by a general medical condition and substance-induced mood disorder must be ruled out. Clinicians must also determine whether a patient has had episodes of mania-like symptoms, indicating bipolar I disorder (complete manic and depressive syndromes), bipolar II disorder (recurrent major depressive episodes with hypomania), or cyclothymic disorder (incomplete depressive and manic syndromes). If a patient's symptoms are limited to those of depression, clinicians must assess the severity and duration of the symptoms to differentiate among major depressive disorder (complete depressive syndrome for 2 weeks), minor depressive disorder (incomplete but episodic depressive syndrome), recurrent brief depressive disorder (complete depressive syndrome but for less than 2 weeks per episode), and dysthymic disorder (incomplete depressive syndrome without clear episodes).

OTHER MENTAL DISORDERS.   Substance-related disorders, psychotic disorders, eating disorders, adjustment disorders, somatoform disorders, and anxiety disorders are all commonly associated with depressive symptoms and should be considered in the differential diagnosis of a patient with depressive symptoms. Perhaps the most difficult differential is that between anxiety disorders with depression and depressive disorders with marked anxiety. The difficulty of distinguishing these is reflected in the inclusion of the diagnosis of mixed anxiety-depressive disorder in DSM-IV-TR. An abnormal result on the dexamethasone-suppression test, the presence of shortened REM latency on a sleep electroencephalogram, and a negative lactate infusion test result support a diagnosis of major depressive disorder in particularly ambiguous cases.

UNCOMPLICATED BEREAVEMENT.   Uncomplicated bereavement is not considered a mental disorder, even though about one third of all bereaved spouses for a time meet the diagnostic criteria for major depressive disorder. Some patients with uncomplicated bereavement do develop major depressive disorder, but the diagnosis is not made unless no resolution of the grief occurs. The differentiation is based on the symptoms' severity and length. In major depressive disorder, common symptoms that evolve from unresolved bereavement are a morbid preoccupation with worthlessness, suicidal ideation, feelings that the person has committed an act (not just an omission) that caused the spouse's death, mummification (keeping the deceased's belongings exactly as they were), and a particularly severe anniversary reaction, which sometimes includes a suicide attempt.

In severe forms of bereavement depression, the patient simply pines away, unable to live without the departed person, usually a spouse. Such persons do have a serious medical condition. Their immune function is often depressed, and their cardiovascular status is precarious. Death can ensue within a few months of that of a spouse, especially among elderly men. Such considerations suggest that it would be clinically unwise to withhold antidepressants from many persons experiencing such an intense mourning.

A 75-year-old widow was brought to treatment by her daughter because of severe insomnia and total loss of interest in daily routines after her husband's death 1 year before. She had been agitated for the first 2 to 3 months and thereafter "sank into total inactivity—not wanting to get out of bed, not wanting to do anything, not wanting to go out." According to her daughter, she was married at 21 years of age, had four children, and had been a housewife until her husband's death from a heart attack. Past psychiatric history was negative; premorbid adjustment had been characterized by compulsive traits. During the interview, she was dressed in black, appeared moderately slowed, and sobbed intermittently, saying "I search everywhere for him ... I don't find him." When asked about life, she said "everything I see is black." Although she expressed no interest in food, she did not seem to have lost an appreciable amount of weight. Her DST [dexamethasone suppression test] result was 18 mg/dL. The patient declined psychiatric care, stating that she "preferred to join her husband rather than get well." She was too religious to commit suicide, but, by refusing treatment, she felt that she would "pine away ... find relief in death and reunion." (Courtesy of Hagop Akiskal, M.D.)

Schizophrenia.   Much has been published about the clinical difficulty of distinguishing a manic episode from schizophrenia. Although difficult, a differential diagnosis is possible. Merriment, elation, and infectiousness of mood are much more common in manic episodes than in schizophrenia. The combination of a manic mood, rapid or pressured speech, and hyperactivity weighs heavily toward a diagnosis of a manic episode. The onset in a manic episode is often rapid and is perceived as a marked change from a patient's previous behavior. Half of all patients with bipolar I disorder have a family history of mood disorder. Catatonic features may be part of a depressive phase of bipolar I disorder. When evaluating patients with catatonia, clinicians should look carefully for a past history of manic or depressive episodes and for a family history of mood disorders. Manic symptoms in persons from minority groups (particularly blacks and Hispanics) are often misdiagnosed as schizophrenic symptoms.

Medical Conditions.   In contrast to depressive symptoms, which are present in almost all psychiatric disorders, manic symptoms are more distinctive, although they can be caused by a wide range of medical and neurological conditions and substances. Antidepressant treatment can also be associated with the precipitation of mania in some patients.

Bipolar I Disorder

When a patient with bipolar I disorder has a depressive episode, the differential diagnosis is the same as that for a patient being considered for a diagnosis of major depressive disorder. When a patient is manic, however, the differential diagnosis includes bipolar I disorder, bipolar II disorder, cyclothymic disorder, mood disorder caused by a general medical condition, and substance-induced mood disorder. For manic symptoms, borderline, narcissistic, histrionic, and antisocial personality disorders need special consideration.

Bipolar II Disorder

The differential diagnosis of patients being evaluated for a mood disorder should include the other mood disorders, psychotic disorders, and borderline disorder. The differentiation between major depressive disorder and bipolar I disorder, on one hand, and bipolar II disorder, on the other hand, rests on the clinical evaluation of the mania-like episodes. Clinicians should not mistake euthymia in a chronically depressed patient for a hypomanic or manic episode. Patients with borderline personality disorder often have a severely disrupted life, similar to that of patients with bipolar II disorder, because of the multiple episodes of significant mood disorder symptoms.

Major Depressive Disorder versus Bipolar Disorder

The question of whether a patient has major depressive disorder or bipolar disorder has emerged as a major challenge in clinical practice. Numerous studies have shown that bipolar disorder is not only confused with personality, substance use, and schizophrenic disorders, but also with depressive and anxiety disorders. Certain features—especially in combination—are predictive of bipolar disorder.

Broader indicators of bipolarity include the following conditions, none of which, by itself, confirms a bipolar diagnosis, but should raise clinical suspicion in that direction: agitated depression, cyclical depression, episodic sleep dysregulation, or a combination of these; refractory depression (failed antidepressants from three different classes); depression in someone with an extroverted profession, periodic impulsivity, such as gambling, sexual misconduct, and wanderlust, or periodic irritability, suicidal crises, or both; and depression with erratic personality disorders.

COURSE AND PROGNOSIS

Studies of the course and prognosis of mood disorders have generally concluded that mood disorders tend to have long courses and that patients tend to have relapses. Although mood disorders are often considered benign in contrast to schizophrenia, they exact a profound toll on affected patients.

Major Depressive Disorder
Course

ONSET.   About 50 percent of patients having their first episode of major depressive disorder exhibited significant depressive symptoms before the first identified episode. Therefore, early identification and treatment of early symptoms may prevent the development of a full depressive episode. Although symptoms may have been present, patients with major depressive disorder usually have not had a premorbid personality disorder. The first depressive episode occurs before age 40 years in about 50 percent of patients. A later onset is associated with the absence of a family history of mood disorders, antisocial personality disorder, and alcohol abuse.

DURATION.   An untreated depressive episode lasts 6 to 13 months; most treated episodes last about 3 months. The withdrawal of antidepressants before 3 months has elapsed almost always results in the return of the symptoms. As the course of the disorder progresses, patients tend to have more frequent episodes that last longer. Over a 20-year period, the mean number of episodes is five or six.

DEVELOPMENT OF MANIC EPISODES.   About 5 to 10 percent of patients with an initial diagnosis of major depressive disorder have a manic episode 6 to 10 years after the first depressive episode. The mean age for this switch is 32 years, and it often occurs after two to four depressive episodes. Although the data are inconsistent and controversial, some clinicians report that the depression of patients who are later classified as having bipolar I disorder is often characterized by hypersomnia, psychomotor retardation, psychotic symptoms, a history of postpartum episodes, a family history of bipolar I disorder, and a history of antidepressant-induced hypomania.

Prognosis.   Major depressive disorder is not a benign disorder. It tends to be chronic, and patients tend to relapse. Patients who have been hospitalized for a first episode of major depressive disorder have about a 50 percent chance of recovering in the first year. The percentage of patients recovering after repeated hospitalization decreases with passing time. Many unrecovered patients remain affected with dysthymic disorder. About 25 percent of patients experience a recurrence of major depressive disorder in the first 6 months after release from a hospital, about 30 to 50 percent in the following 2 years, and about 50 to 75 percent in 5 years. The incidence of relapse is lower than these figures in patients who continue prophylactic psychopharmacological treatment and in patients who have had only one or two depressive episodes. Generally, as a patient experiences more and more depressive episodes, the time between the episodes decreases, and the severity of each episode increases.

PROGNOSTIC INDICATORS.   Many studies have focused on identifying both good and bad prognostic indicators in the course of major depressive disorder. Mild episodes, the absence of psychotic symptoms, and a short hospital stay are good prognostic indicators. Psychosocial indicators of a good course include a history of solid friendships during adolescence, stable family functioning, and generally sound social functioning for the 5 years preceding the illness. Additional good prognostic signs are the absence of a comorbid psychiatric disorder and of a personality disorder, no more than one previous hospitalization for major depressive disorder, and an advanced age of onset. The possibility of a poor prognosis is increased by coexisting dysthymic disorder, abuse of alcohol and other substances, anxiety disorder symptoms, and a history of more than one previous depressive episode. Men are more likely than women to experience a chronically impaired course.

Bipolar I Disorder

Course.   The natural history of bipolar I disorder is such that it is often useful to make a graph of a patient's disorder and to keep it up to date as treatment progresses. Although cyclothymic disorder is sometimes diagnosed retrospectively in patients with bipolar I disorder, no identified personality traits are specifically associated with bipolar I disorder.

Bipolar I disorder most often starts with depression (75 percent of the time in women, 67 percent in men) and is a recurring disorder. Most patients experience both depressive and manic episodes, although 10 to 20 percent experience only manic episodes. The manic episodes typically have a rapid onset (hours or days), but may evolve over a few weeks. An untreated manic episode lasts about 3 months; therefore, clinicians should not discontinue giving drugs before that time. Of persons who have a single manic episode, 90 percent are likely to have another. As the disorder progresses, the time between episodes often decreases. After about five episodes, however, the interepisode interval often stabilizes at 6 to 9 months. Of persons with bipolar disorder, 5 to 15 percent have four or more episodes per year and can be classified as rapid cyclers.

BIPOLAR I DISORDER IN CHILDREN AND OLDER PERSONS. Bipolar I disorder can affect both the very young and older persons. The incidence of bipolar I disorder in children and adolescents is about 1 percent, and the onset can be as early as age 8 years. Common misdiagnoses are schizophrenia and oppositional defiant disorder.

Bipolar I disorder with such an early onset is associated with a poor prognosis. Manic symptoms are common in older persons, although the range of causes is broad and includes nonpsychiatric medical conditions, dementia, and delirium, as well as bipolar I disorder. The onset of true bipolar I disorder in older persons is relatively uncommon.

Prognosis.   Patients with bipolar I disorder have a poorer prognosis than do patients with major depressive disorder. About 40 to 50 percent of patients with bipolar I disorder may have a second manic episode within 2 years of the first episode. Although lithium prophylaxis improves the course and prognosis of bipolar I disorder, probably only 50 to 60 percent of patients achieve significant control of their symptoms with lithium. One 4-year follow-up study of patients with bipolar I disorder found that a premorbid poor occupational status, alcohol dependence, psychotic features, depressive features, interepisode depressive features, and male gender were all factors that contributed to a poor prognosis. Short duration of manic episodes, advanced age of onset, few suicidal thoughts, and few coexisting psychiatric or medical problems predict a better outcome.

About 7 percent of patients with bipolar I disorder do not have a recurrence of symptoms, 45 percent have more than one episode, and 40 percent have a chronic disorder. Patients may have from 2 to 30 manic episodes, although the mean number is about 9. About 40 percent of all patients have more than 10 episodes. On long-term follow-up, 15 percent of all patients with bipolar I disorder are well, 45 percent are well but have multiple relapses, 30 percent are in partial remission, and 10 percent are chronically ill. One third of all patients with bipolar I disorder have chronic symptoms and evidence of significant social decline.

Bipolar II Disorder

The course and prognosis of bipolar II disorder have just begun to be studied. Preliminary data indicate, however, that the diagnosis is stable, as shown by the high likelihood that patients with bipolar II disorder will have the same diagnosis up to 5 years later. Bipolar II disorder is a chronic disease that warrants long-term treatment strategies.

TREATMENT

Treatment of patients with mood disorders should be directed toward several goals. First, the patient's safety must be guaranteed. Second, a complete diagnostic evaluation of the patient is necessary. Third, a treatment plan that addresses not only the immediate symptoms but also the patient's prospective well-being should be initiated. Although current treatment emphasizes pharmacotherapy and psychotherapy addressed to the individual patient, stressful life events are also associated with increases in relapse rates. Thus, treatment should address the number and severity of stressors in patients' lives.

Overall, the treatment of mood disorders is rewarding for psychiatrists. Specific treatments are now available for both manic and depressive episodes, and data indicate that prophylactic treatment is also effective. Because the prognosis for each episode is good, optimism is always warranted and is welcomed by both the patient and the patient's family. Mood disorders are chronic, however, and the psychiatrist must educate the patient and the family about future treatment strategies.

Hospitalization

The first and most critical decision a physician must make is whether to hospitalize a patient or attempt outpatient treatment. Clear indications for hospitalization are the risk of suicide or homicide, a patient's grossly reduced ability to get food and shelter, and the need for diagnostic procedures. A history of rapidly progressing symptoms and the rupture of a patient's usual support systems are also indications for hospitalization.

A physician may safely treat mild depression or hypomania in the office if he or she evaluates the patient frequently. Clinical signs of impaired judgment, weight loss, or insomnia should be minimal. The patient's support system should be strong, neither overinvolved nor withdrawing from the patient. Any adverse changes in the patient's symptoms or behavior or the attitude of the patient's support system may suffice to warrant hospitalization.

Patients with mood disorders are often unwilling to enter a hospital voluntarily, and may have to be involuntarily committed. These patients often cannot make decisions because of their slowed thinking, negative *Weltanschauung* (world view), and hopelessness. Patients who are manic often have such a complete lack of insight into their disorder that hospitalization seems absolutely absurd to them.

Psychosocial Therapy

Although most studies indicate—and most clinicians and researchers believe—that a combination of psychotherapy and pharmacotherapy is the most effective treatment for major depressive disorder, some data suggest another view: Either pharmacotherapy or psychotherapy alone is effective, at least in patients with mild major depressive episodes, and the use of combined therapy adds to the cost of treatment.

Three types of short-term psychotherapies—cognitive therapy, interpersonal therapy, and behavior therapy—have been studied to determine their efficacy in the treatment of major depressive disorder. Although its efficacy in treating major depressive disorder is not as well researched as these three therapies, psychoanalytically oriented psychotherapy has long been used for depressive disorders, and many clinicians use the technique as their primary method. What differentiates the three short-term psychotherapy methods from the psychoanalytically oriented approach are the active and directive roles of the therapist, the directly recognizable goals, and the end points for short-term therapy.

Accumulating evidence is encouraging about the efficacy of dynamic therapy. In a randomized, controlled trial comparing psychodynamic therapy with cognitive-behavior therapy, the outcome of the depressed patients was the same in the two treatments.

The National Institute of Mental Health (NIMH) Treatment of Depression Collaborative Research Program found the following predictors of response to various treatments: low social dysfunction suggested a good response to interpersonal therapy; low cognitive dysfunction suggested a good response to cognitive-behavioral therapy and pharmacotherapy; high work dysfunction suggested a good response to pharmacotherapy; and high depression severity suggested a good response to interpersonal therapy and pharmacotherapy.

Cognitive Therapy.
Cognitive therapy, originally developed by Aaron Beck, focuses on the cognitive distortions postulated to be present in major depressive disorder. Such distortions include selective attention to the negative aspects of circumstances and unrealistically morbid inferences about consequences. For example, apathy and low energy result from a patient's expectation of failure in all areas. The goal of cognitive therapy is to alleviate depressive episodes and prevent their recurrence by helping patients identify and test negative cognitions; develop alternative, flexible, and positive ways of thinking; and rehearse new cognitive and behavioral responses.

Studies have shown that cognitive therapy is effective in the treatment of major depressive disorder. Most studies have found that cognitive therapy is equal in efficacy to pharmacotherapy and is associated with fewer adverse effects and better follow-up than pharmacotherapy. Some of the best-controlled studies have indicated that the combination of cognitive therapy and pharmacotherapy is more efficacious than either therapy alone, although other studies have not found that additive effect. At least

one study, the NIMH Treatment of Depression Collaborative Research Program, found that pharmacotherapy, either alone or with psychotherapy, may be the treatment of choice for patients with severe major depressive episodes.

Interpersonal Therapy.
Interpersonal therapy, developed by Gerald Klerman, focuses on one or two of a patient's current interpersonal problems. This therapy is based on two assumptions. First, current interpersonal problems are likely to have their roots in early dysfunctional relationships. Second, current interpersonal problems are likely to be involved in precipitating or perpetuating the current depressive symptoms. Controlled trials have indicated that interpersonal therapy is effective in the treatment of major depressive disorder and, not surprisingly, may be specifically helpful in addressing interpersonal problems. Some studies indicate that interpersonal therapy may be the most effective method for severe major depressive episodes when the treatment choice is psychotherapy alone.

The interpersonal therapy program usually consists of 12 to 16 weekly sessions and is characterized by an active therapeutic approach. Intrapsychic phenomena, such as defense mechanisms and internal conflicts, are not addressed. Discrete behaviors—such as lack of assertiveness, impaired social skills, and distorted thinking—may be addressed but only in the context of their meaning in, or their effect on, interpersonal relationships.

Behavior Therapy.
Behavior therapy is based on the hypothesis that maladaptive behavioral patterns result in a person's receiving little positive feedback and perhaps outright rejection from society. By addressing maladaptive behaviors in therapy, patients learn to function in the world in such a way that they receive positive reinforcement. Behavior therapy for major depressive disorder has not yet been the subject of many controlled studies. The limited data indicate that it is an effective treatment for major depressive disorder.

Psychoanalytically Oriented Therapy.
The psychoanalytic approach to mood disorders is based on psychoanalytic theories about depression and mania. The goal of psychoanalytic psychotherapy is to effect a change in a patient's personality structure or character, not simply to alleviate symptoms. Improvements in interpersonal trust, capacity for intimacy, coping mechanisms, the capacity to grieve, and the ability to experience a wide range of emotions are some of the aims of psychoanalytic therapy. Treatment often requires the patient to experience periods of heightened anxiety and distress during the course of therapy, which may continue for several years.

Family Therapy.
Family therapy is not generally viewed as a primary therapy for the treatment of major depressive disorder, but increasing evidence indicates that helping a patient with a mood disorder to reduce and cope with stress can lessen the chance of a relapse. Family therapy is indicated if the disorder jeopardizes a patient's marriage or family functioning or if the mood disorder is promoted or maintained by the family situation. Family therapy examines the role of the mood-disordered member in the overall psychological well-being of the whole family; it also examines the role of the entire family in the maintenance of the patient's symptoms. Patients with mood disorders have a high rate of divorce, and about 50 percent of all

spouses report that they would not have married or had children if they had known that the patient was going to develop a mood disorder.

Vagal Nerve Stimulation

Experimental stimulation of the vagus nerve in several studies designed for the treatment of epilepsy found that patients showed improved mood. This observation led to the use of left vagal nerve stimulation (VNS) using an electronic device implanted in the skin, similar to a cardiac pacemaker. Preliminary studies have shown that a number of patients with chronic, recurrent major depressive disorder went into remission when treated with VNS. The mechanism of action of VNS to account for improvement is unknown. The vagus nerve connects to the enteric nervous system and, when stimulated, may cause release of peptides that act as neurotransmitters. Extensive clinical trials are being conducted to determine the efficacy of VNS. Section 32.38 covers this and other brain stimulation methods.

Sleep Deprivation

Mood disorders are characterized by sleep disturbance. Mania tends to be characterized by a decreased need for sleep, whereas depression can be associated with either hypersomnia or insomnia. Sleep deprivation may precipitate mania in patients who are bipolar I and temporarily relieve depression in those who are unipolar. Approximately 60 percent of depressive disorder patients exhibit significant but transient benefit from total sleep deprivation. The positive results are typically reversed by the next night of sleep. Several strategies have been used in an attempt to achieve a more sustained response to sleep deprivation. One method used serial total sleep deprivation with a day or two of normal sleep in between. This method does not achieve a sustained antidepressant response because the depression tends to return with normal sleep cycles. Another approach used phase delay in the time patients go to sleep each night, or partial sleep deprivation. In this method, patients may stay awake from 2 AM to 10 PM daily. Up to 50 percent of patients get same-day antidepressant effects from partial sleep deprivation, but this benefit also tends to wear off in time. In some reports, however, serial partial sleep deprivation has been used successfully to treat insomnia associated with depression. The third, and probably most effective, strategy combines sleep deprivation with pharmacological treatment of depression. A number of studies have suggested that total and partial sleep deprivation followed by immediate treatment with an antidepressant or lithium (Eskalith) sustains the antidepressant effects of sleep deprivation. Likewise, several reports have suggested that sleep deprivation accelerates the response to antidepressants, including fluoxetine (Prozac) and nortriptyline (Aventyl, Pamelor). Sleep deprivation has also been noted to improve premenstrual dysphoria.

Phototherapy

Phototherapy (light therapy) was introduced in 1984 as a treatment for SAD (mood disorder with seasonal pattern). In this disorder, patients typically experience depression as the photoperiod of the day decreases with advancing winter. Women represent at least 75 percent of all patients with seasonal depression, and the mean age of presentation is 40 years. Patients rarely present older than the age of 55 years with seasonal affective disorder.

Phototherapy typically involves exposing the afflicted patient to bright light in the range of 1,500 to 10,000 lux or more, typically with a light box that sits on a table or desk. Patients sit in front of the box for approximately 1 to 2 hours before dawn each day, although some patients may also benefit from exposure after dusk. Alternatively, some manufacturers have developed light visors, with a light source built into the brim of the hat. These light visors allow mobility, but recent controlled studies have questioned the use of this type of light exposure. Trials have typically lasted 1 week, but longer treatment durations may be associated with greater response.

Phototherapy tends to be well tolerated. Newer light sources tend to use lower light intensities and come equipped with filters; patients are instructed not to look directly at the light source. As with any effective antidepressant, phototherapy, on rare occasions, has been implicated in switching some depressed patients into mania or hypomania.

In addition to seasonal depression, the other major indication for phototherapy may be in sleep disorders. Phototherapy has been used to decrease the irritability and diminished functioning associated with shift work. Sleep disorders in geriatric patients have reportedly improved with exposure to bright light during the day. Likewise, some evidence suggests that jet lag might respond to light therapy. Preliminary data indicate that phototherapy may benefit some patients with OCD that has a seasonal variation.

Pharmacotherapy

Once a diagnosis has been established, a pharmacological treatment strategy can be formulated. Accurate diagnosis is crucial because unipolar and bipolar spectrum disorders require different treatment regimens.

The objective of pharmacologic treatment is symptom remission, not just symptom reduction. Patients with residual symptoms, as opposed to full remission, are more likely to experience a relapse or recurrence of mood episodes and to experience ongoing impairment of daily functioning.

Major Depressive Disorder.   The use of specific pharmacotherapy approximately doubles the chances that a depressed patient will recover in 1 month. All available antidepressants may take up to 3 to 4 weeks to exert significant therapeutic effects, although they may begin to show their effects earlier. Choice of antidepressants is determined by the side effect profile least objectionable to a given patient's physical status, temperament, and lifestyle. That numerous classes of antidepressants are available, many with different mechanisms of action, represents indirect evidence for heterogeneity of putative biochemical lesions. Although the first antidepressant drugs, the monoamine oxidase inhibitors (MAOIs) and tricyclic antidepressants, are still in use, newer compounds have made the treatment of depression more "clinician and patient friendly."

GENERAL CLINICAL GUIDELINES.   The most common clinical mistake leading to an unsuccessful trial of an antidepressant drug is the use of too low a dose for too short a time. Unless adverse events prevent it, the dose of an antidepressant should be raised to the maximum recommended level and maintained at that level for at least 4 or 5 weeks before a drug trial is considered unsuccessful. Alternatively, if a patient is improving clinically on a low dose of the drug, this dose should not be raised unless clinical improvement stops before maximal benefit is obtained. When a patient does not begin to respond to appropriate doses of a drug after 2 or 3 weeks, clinicians may decide to obtain a plasma concentration of the drug if the test is available for the particular drug being used. The test may indicate either noncompliance or particularly unusual pharmacokinetic disposition of the drug and may thereby suggest an alternative dose.

DURATION AND PROPHYLAXIS. Antidepressant treatment should be maintained for at least 6 months or the length of a previous episode, whichever is greater. Prophylactic treatment with antidepressants is effective in reducing the number and severity of recurrences. One study concluded that when episodes are less than $2^1/_2$ years apart, prophylactic treatment for 5 years is probably indicated. Another factor suggesting prophylactic treatment is the seriousness of previous depressive episodes. Episodes that have involved significant suicidal ideation or impairment of psychosocial functioning may indicate that clinicians should consider prophylactic treatment. When antidepressant treatment is stopped, the drug dose should be tapered gradually over 1 to 2 weeks, depending on the half-life of the particular compound. Several studies indicate that maintenance antidepressant medication appears to be safe and effective for the treatment of chronic depression.

Prevention of new mood episodes (i.e., recurrences) is the aim of the maintenance phase of treatment. Only those patients with recurrent or chronic depressions are candidates for maintenance treatment.

INITIAL MEDICATION SELECTION. The available antidepressants do not differ in overall efficacy, speed of response, or long-term effectiveness. Antidepressants, however, do differ in their pharmacology, drug–drug interactions, short- and long-term side effects, likelihood of discontinuation symptoms, and ease of dose adjustment. Failure to tolerate or to respond to one medication does not imply that other medications will also fail. Selection of the initial treatment depends on the chronicity of the condition, course of illness (a recurrent or chronic course is associated with increased likelihood of subsequent depressive symptoms without treatment), family history of illness and treatment response, symptom severity, concurrent general medical or other psychiatric conditions, prior treatment responses to other acute phase treatments, potential drug–drug interactions, and patient preference. In general, approximately 45 to 60 percent of all outpatients with uncomplicated (i.e., minimal psychiatric and general medical comorbidity), nonchronic, nonpsychotic major depressive disorder who begin treatment with medication respond (i.e., achieve at least a 50 percent reduction in baseline symptoms); however, only 35 to 50 percent achieve remission (i.e., the virtual absence of depressive symptoms).

TREATMENT OF DEPRESSIVE SUBTYPES. Clinical types of major depressive episodes may have varying responses to particular antidepressants or to drugs other than antidepressants. Patients with major depressive disorder with atypical features may preferentially respond to treatment with MAOIs or SSRIs. Antidepressants with dual action on both serotonergic and noradrenergic re-

ceptors demonstrate greater efficacy in melancholic depressions. Patients with seasonal winter depression can be treated with light therapy. Treatment of major depressive episodes with psychotic features may require a combination of an antidepressant and an atypical antipsychotic. Several studies have also shown that ECT is effective for this indication—perhaps more effective than pharmacotherapy. For those with atypical symptom features, strong evidence exists for the effectiveness of MAOIs. SSRIs and bupropion (Wellbutrin) are also of use in atypical depression.

COMORBID DISORDERS. The concurrent presence of another disorder can affect initial treatment selection. For example, the successful treatment of OCD associated with depressive symptoms usually results in remission of the depression. Similarly, when panic disorder occurs with major depression, medications with demonstrated efficacy in both conditions are preferred (e.g., tricyclics and SSRIs). In general, the nonmood disorder dictates the choice of treatment in comorbid states.

Concurrent substance abuse raises the possibility of a substance-induced mood disorder, which must be evaluated by history or by requiring abstinence for several weeks. Abstinence often results in remission of depressive symptoms in substance-induced mood disorders. For those with continuing significant depressive symptoms, even with abstinence, an independent mood disorder is diagnosed and treated.

General medical conditions are established risk factors in the development of depression. The presence of a major depressive episode is associated with increased morbidity or mortality of many general medical conditions (e.g., cardiovascular disease, diabetes, cerebrovascular disease, and cancer).

THERAPEUTIC USE OF SIDE EFFECTS. Choosing more-sedating antidepressants (e.g., amitriptyline [Elavil, Endep]) for more-anxious, depressed patients or more-activating agents (e.g., desipramine) for more-psychomotor–retarded patients is not generally helpful. For example, any short-term benefits with paroxetine, mirtazapine, or amitriptyline (more-sedating drugs) on symptoms of anxiety or insomnia may become liabilities over time. These drugs often continue to be sedating in the longer run, which can lead to patients prematurely discontinuing medication and increase the risk of relapse or recurrence. Some practitioners use adjunctive medications (e.g., sleeping pills or anxiolytics) combined with antidepressants to provide more immediate symptom relief or to cover those side effects to which most patients ultimately adapt.

A patient's prior treatment history is important because an earlier response typically predicts current response. A documented failure on a properly conducted trial of a particular antidepressant class (e.g., SSRIs, tricyclics, or MAOIs) suggests choosing an agent from an alternative class. The history of a first-degree relative responding to a particular drug is associated with a good response to the same class of agents in the patient.

ACUTE TREATMENT FAILURES. Patients may not respond to a medication because (1) they cannot tolerate the side effects, even in the face of a good clinical response; (2) an idiosyncratic adverse event may occur; (3) the clinical response is not adequate; or (4) the wrong diagnosis has been made. Acute-phase medication trials should last 4 to 6 weeks to determine if meaningful symptom reduction is attained. Most (but not all) patients who ultimately respond fully show at least a partial response (i.e., at least a 30 percent reduction in pretreatment depressive symptom severity) by week 4 if the dose is adequate during the initial weeks of treatment. Lack of a partial response by 4 to 6 weeks indicates that a treatment change is needed. Longer time periods—8 to 12 weeks or longer—are needed to define the ultimate degree of symptom reduction achievable with a medication. Approximately one half of patients require a second medication treatment trial because the initial treatment is poorly tolerated or ineffective.

SELECTING SECOND TREATMENT OPTIONS.   When the initial treatment is unsuccessful, switching to an alternative treatment or augmenting the current treatment is a common option. The choice between switching from the initial single treatment to a new single treatment (as opposed to adding a second treatment to the first one) rests on the patient's prior treatment history, the degree of benefit achieved with the initial treatment, and patient preference. As a rule, switching rather than augmenting is preferred after an initial medication failure. On the other hand, augmentation strategies are helpful with patients who have gained some benefit from the initial treatment but who have not achieved remission. The best-documented augmentation strategies involve lithium (Eskalith) or thyroid hormone. A combination of an SSRI and bupropion is also widely employed. In fact, no combination strategy has been conclusively shown to be more effective than another. ECT is effective in psychotic and nonpsychotic forms of depression but is recommended generally only for repeatedly nonresponsive cases or in patients with very severe disorders.

STAR*D (SEQUENCED TREATMENT ALTERNATIVE TO RELIEVE DEPRESSION STUDY).   An important evidence-based study evaluating treatment methods for depressed patients was conducted and published in the *American Journal of Psychiatry* in 2006. Each of four levels of the study tested a different medication or medication combination. The primary goal of each level was to determine if the treatment used during that level could adequately treat participants' major depressive disorder. Those who did not become symptom-free could proceed to the next level of treatment.

The study found that patients who did not respond to 6 weeks of treatment with a given SSRI (the study used citalopram) might respond when switched to another SSRI. If patients did not respond to the new SSRI, another medication to augment the SSRI such as bupropion was added and would produce a response in some patients. If there were still no response, further augmentation with nortyptaline, mirtazapine, lithium, or thyroid hormone would help some additional patients. Continued nonresponse required a third step—switching treatments or adding to existing medication using tranylcypromine or a combination of venlafaxine plus mirtazapine. About 50 percent of patients became symptom-free after two treatment levels. Overall, the study found that 70 percent of patients could go into remission with treatment.

The study found that in some cases the addition of psychotherapy (in the study, cognitive therapy was used) appeared to improve response outcomes. Some patients responded to cognitive therapy without medication.

COMBINED TREATMENT.   Medication and formal psychotherapy are often combined in practice. If physicians view mood disorders as fundamentally evolving from psychodynamic issues, their ambivalence about the use of drugs may result in a poor response, noncompliance, and probably inadequate doses for too short a treatment period. Alternatively, if physicians ignore the psychosocial needs of a patient, the outcome of pharmacotherapy may be compromised. Several trials of a combination of pharmacotherapy and psychotherapy for chronically depressed outpatients have shown a higher response and higher remission rates for the combination than for either treatment used alone.

Bipolar Disorders.   The pharmacological treatment of bipolar disorders is divided into acute and maintenance phases. Bipolar treatment, however, also involves the formulation of different strategies for the patient who is experiencing mania or hypomania or depression. No one drug is predictably effective for all patients. Often, it is necessary to try several so-called "mood stabilizers" before an optimal treatment is found.

TREATMENT OF ACUTE MANIA.   Acute mania, or hypomania, usually is the easiest phase of bipolar disorder to treat. Agents can be used alone or in combination to bring the patient down from a high. Patients with severe mania are best treated in the hospital, where aggressive dosing is possible and an adequate response can be achieved within days or weeks. Adherence to treatment, however, is often a problem because patients with mania frequently lack insight into their illness and refuse to take medication. Because impaired judgment, impulsivity, and aggressiveness combine to put the patient or others at risk, many patients in the manic phase are medicated to protect themselves and others from harm.

Lithium Carbonate.   Lithium carbonate is considered the prototypical "mood stabilizer." Yet, because the onset of antimanic action with lithium can be slow, it usually is supplemented in the early phases of treatment by atypical antipsychotics, mood-stabilizing anticonvulsants, or high-potency benzodiazepines. Therapeutic lithium levels are between 0.6 and 1.2 mEq/L. The acute use of lithium has been limited in recent years by its unpredictable efficacy, problematic side effects, and the need for frequent laboratory tests. The introduction of newer drugs with more favorable side effects, lower toxicity, and less need for frequent laboratory testing has resulted in a decline in lithium use. For many patients, however, its clinical benefits can be remarkable.

Valproate.   Valproate (valproic acid [Depakene] or divalproex sodium [Depakote]) has surpassed lithium in use for acute mania. Unlike lithium, Valproate is only indicated for acute mania, although most experts agree it also has prophylactic effects. Typical dose levels of valproic acid are 750 to 2,500 mg per day, achieving blood levels between 50 and 120 μg/mL. Rapid oral loading with 15 to 20 mg/kg of divalproex sodium from day 1 of treatment has been well tolerated and associated with a rapid onset of response. A number of laboratory tests are required during valproate treatment.

Carbamazepine and Oxcarbazepine.   Carbamazepine has been used worldwide for decades as a first-line treatment for acute mania but has only gained approval in the United States in 2004. Typical doses of carbamazepine to treat acute mania range between 600 and 1,800 mg per day, associated with blood levels of between 4 and 12 μg/mL. The keto congener of carbamazepine, oxcarbazepine, may possess similar antimanic properties. Higher doses than those of carbamazepine are required because 1,500 mg of oxcarbazepine approximates 1,000 mg of carbamazepine.

Clonazepam and Lorazepam.   The high-potency benzodiazepine anticonvulsants used in acute mania include clonazepam (Klonopin) and lorazepam (Ativan). Both may be effective and are widely used for adjunctive treatment of acute manic agitation, insomnia, aggression, and dysphoria, as well as panic. The safety and the benign side effect profile of these agents render them ideal adjuncts to lithium, carbamazepine, or valproate.

Atypical and Typical Antipsychotics.   All of the atypical antipsychotics—olanzapine, risperidone, quetiapine, ziprasidone, and aripiprazole—have demonstrated antimanic efficacy and are approved by the U.S. Food and Drug Administration for this indication. Compared with older agents, such as haloperidol (Haldol) and chlorpromazine (Thorazine), atypical antipsychotics have a lesser liability for excitatory postsynaptic potential and tardive dyskinesia; many do not increase prolactin. However, they have a wide range of substantial to no risk for weight gain with its associated problems of insulin resistance, diabetes, hyperlipidemia, hypercholesteremia, and cardiovascular impairment. Some patients, however, require maintenance treatment with an antipsychotic medication.

TREATMENT OF ACUTE BIPOLAR DEPRESSION.   The relative usefulness of standard antidepressants in bipolar illness, in general, and in rapid cycling and mixed states, in particular, remains controversial because of their propensity to induce cycling, mania, or hypomania. Accordingly, antidepressant drugs are often enhanced by a mood stabilizer in the first-line treatment for a first or isolated episode of bipolar depression. A fixed combination of olanzapine and fluoxetine (Symbyax) has been shown to be effective in treating acute bipolar depression for an 8-week period without inducing a switch to mania or hypomania.

Paradoxically, many patients who are bipolar in the depressed phase do not respond to treatment with standard antidepressants. In these instances, lamotrigine or low-dose ziprasidone (20 to 80 mg per day) may prove effective.

Electroconvulsive therapy may also be useful for bipolar depressed patients who do not respond to lithium or other mood stabilizers and their adjuncts, particularly in cases in which intense suicidal tendency presents as a medical emergency.

Other Agents.   When standard treatments fail, other types of compounds may prove effective. The calcium channel antagonist verapamil (Calan, Isoptin) has acute antimanic efficacy. Gabapentin, topiramate, zonisamide, levetiracetam, and tiagabine have not been shown to have acute antimania effects, although some patients may benefit from a trial of these agents when standard therapies have failed. Lamotrigine does not possess acute antimanic properties but does help prevent recurrence of manic episodes. Small studies suggest the potential acute antimanic and prophylactic efficacy of phenytoin. ECT is effective in acute mania. Bilateral treatments are required because unilateral, nondominant treatments have been reported to be ineffective or even to exacerbate manic symptoms. ECT is reserved for the patient with rare refractory mania or for the patient with medical complications, as well as extreme exhaustion (malignant hyperthermia or lethal catatonia).

MAINTENANCE TREATMENT OF BIPOLAR DISORDER.   Preventing recurrences of mood episodes is the greatest challenge facing the clinician. Not only must the chosen regimen achieve its primary goal—sustained euthymia—but in addition the medications should not produce unwanted side effects that affect functioning. Sedation, cognitive impairment, tremor, weight gain, and rash are some side effects that lead to treatment discontinuation.

Lithium, carbamazepine, and valproic acid, alone or in combination, are the most widely used agents in the long-term treatment of patients who are bipolar. Lamotrigine has prophylactic antidepressant and, potentially, mood-stabilizing properties. Patients on lamotrigine with bipolar I disorder depression exhibit a rate of switch into mania that is the same as the rate with placebo. Lamotrigine appears to have superior acute and prophylactic antidepressant properties compared with antimanic properties. Given that breakthrough depressions are a difficult problem during prophylaxis, lamotrigine has a unique therapeutic role. Very slow increases of lamotrigine help to avoid the rare side effect of lethal rash. A dose of 200 mg per day appears to be the average in many studies. The incidence of severe rash (i.e., Stevens-Johnson syndrome, a toxic epidermal necrolysis) is now thought to be approximately 2 in 10,000 adults and 4 in 10,000 children.

Thyroid supplementation is frequently necessary during long-term treatment. Many patients treated with lithium develop hypothyroidism, and many patients with bipolar disorder have idiopathic thyroid dysfunction. Triiodothyronine (25 to 50 μg per day), because of its short half-life, is often recommended for acute augmentation strategies, whereas thyroxine (T_4) is frequently used for long-term maintenance. In some centers, hypermetabolic doses of thyroid hormone are used. Data indicate improvement in both manic and depressive phases with hypermetabolic T_4 augmenting strategies.

Depression Awareness, Recognition and Treatment Program

The Depression Awareness, Recognition and Treatment program (D/ART) is a multiphase information and education program designed to alert health professionals and the general public to the fact that depressive disorders are common, serious, and treatable. It was launched by the NIMH in 1988 to enhance the availability and quality of treatment for depression.

▲ 12.2 Dysthymia and Cyclothymia

DYSTHYMIC DISORDER

According to the text revision of the fourth edition of *Diagnostic and Statistical Manual of Mental Disorders* (DSM-IV-TR), the most typical features of dysthymic disorder is the presence of a depressed mood that lasts most of the day and is present almost continuously. There are associated feelings of inadequacy, guilt, irritability, and anger; withdrawal from society; loss of interest; and inactivity and lack of productivity. The term *dysthymia*, which means "ill humored," was introduced in 1980. Before that time, most patients now classified as having dysthymic disorder were classified as having depressive neurosis (also called neurotic depression).

Dysthymic disorder is distinguished from major depressive disorder by the fact that patients complain that they have always been depressed. Thus, most cases are of early onset, beginning in childhood or adolescence and certainly occurring by the time patients reach their 20s. A late-onset subtype, much less prevalent and not well characterized clinically, has been identified among middle-aged and geriatric populations, largely through epidemiological studies in the community.

Although dysthymia can occur as a secondary complication of other psychiatric disorders, the core concept of dysthymic disorder refers to a subaffective or subclinical depressive disorder with (1) low-grade chronicity for at least 2 years; (2) insidious onset, with origin often in childhood or adolescence; and (3) persistent or intermittent course. The family history of patients with dysthymia is typically replete with both depressive and bipolar disorders, which is one of the more robust findings supporting its link to primary mood disorder.

Epidemiology

Dysthymic disorder is common among the general population and affects 5 to 6 percent of all persons. It is seen among patients in general psychiatric clinics, where it affects between one half and one third of all patients. No gender differences are seen for incidence rates. The disorder is more common in women younger than 64 years of age than in men of any age and is more common among unmarried and young persons and in those with low incomes. Dysthymic disorder frequently coexists with other mental disorders, particularly major depressive disorder, and in persons with major depressive disorder there is less likelihood of full remission between episodes. The patients may also have co-existing anxiety disorders (especially panic disorder), substance abuse, and borderline personality disorder. The disorder is more common among those with first-degree relatives with major depressive disorder. Patients with dysthymic disorder are likely to be taking a wide range of psychiatric medications, including antidepressants, antimania agents such as lithium (Eskalith) and carbamazepine (Tegretol), and sedative-hypnotics.

Etiology

Biological Factors.   The biological basis for the symptoms of dysthymic disorder and major depressive disorder are similar, but the biological bases for the underlying pathophysiology in the two disorders differ.

SLEEP STUDIES.   Decreased rapid eye movement (REM) latency and increased REM density are two state markers of depression in major depressive disorder that also occur in a significant proportion of patients with dysthymic disorder.

NEUROENDOCRINE STUDIES.   The two most studied neuroendocrine axes in major depressive disorder and dysthymic disorder are the adrenal axis and the thyroid axis, which have been tested by using the dexamethasone-suppression test (DST) and the thyrotropin-releasing hormone–stimulation test, respectively. Although the results of studies are not absolutely consistent, most indicate that patients with dysthymic disorder are less likely to have abnormal results on a DST than are patients with major depressive disorder.

Psychosocial Factors.   Psychodynamic theories about the development of dysthymic disorder posit that the disorder results from personality and ego development and culminates in difficulty adapting to adolescence and young adulthood. Karl Abraham, for example, thought that the conflicts of depression center on oral- and anal-sadistic traits. Anal traits include excessive orderliness, guilt, and concern for others; they are postulated to be a defense against preoccupation with anal matter and with disorganization, hostility, and self-preoccupation. A major defense mechanism used is reaction formation. Low self-esteem,

anhedonia, and introversion are often associated with the depressive character.

FREUD.   In *Mourning and Melancholia*, Sigmund Freud asserted that an interpersonal disappointment early in life can cause a vulnerability to depression that leads to ambivalent love relationships as an adult; real or threatened losses in adult life then trigger depression. Persons susceptible to depression are orally dependent and require constant narcissistic gratification. When deprived of love, affection, and care, they become clinically depressed; when they experience a real loss, they internalize or introject the lost object and turn their anger on it and, thus, on themselves.

COGNITIVE THEORY.   The cognitive theory of depression also applies to dysthymic disorder. It holds that a disparity between actual and fantasized situations leads to diminished self-esteem and a sense of helplessness. The success of cognitive therapy in the treatment of some patients with dysthymic disorder may provide some support for the theoretical model.

Diagnosis and Clinical Features

The DSM-IV-TR diagnosis criteria for dysthymic disorder (Table 12.2–1) stipulate the presence of a depressed mood most of the time for at least 2 years (or 1 year for children and adolescents). To meet the diagnostic criteria, a patient should not have symptoms that are better accounted for as major depressive disorder and should never have had a manic or hypomanic episode. DSM-IV-TR allows clinicians to specify whether the onset was early (before age 21 years) or late (age 21 years or older). DSM-IV-TR also allows specification of atypical features in dysthymic disorder.

The profile of dysthymic disorder overlaps with that of major depressive disorder but differs from it in that symptoms tend to outnumber signs (more subjective than objective depression). This means that disturbances in appetite and libido are uncharacteristic, and psychomotor agitation or retardation is not observed. This all translates into a depression with attenuated symptomatology. Subtle endogenous features are observed, however: inertia, lethargy, and anhedonia that are characteristically worse in the morning. Because patients presenting clinically often fluctuate in and out of a major depression, the core DSM-IV-TR criteria for dysthymic disorder tend to emphasize vegetative dysfunction, whereas the alternative Criterion B for dysthymic disorder (Table 12.2–2) in a DSM-IV-TR appendix lists cognitive symptoms.

Dysthymic disorder is quite heterogeneous. Anxiety is not a necessary part of its clinical picture, yet dysthymic disorder is often diagnosed in patients with anxiety and phobic disorders. That clinical situation is sometimes diagnosed as mixed anxiety-depressive disorder. For greater operational clarity, it is best to restrict dysthymic disorder to a primary disorder, one that cannot be explained by another psychiatric disorder. The essential features of such primary dysthymic disorder include habitual gloom, brooding, lack of joy in life, and preoccupation with inadequacy. Dysthymic disorder then is best characterized as long-standing, fluctuating, low-grade depression experienced as part of the habitual self and representing an accentuation of traits observed in the depressive temperament. The clinical picture of dysthymic

Table 12.2–1
DSM-IV-TR Diagnostic Criteria for Dysthymic Disorder

A. Depressed mood for most of the day, for more days than not, as indicated either by subjective account or observation by others, for at least 2 years. **Note:** In children and adolescents, mood can be irritable and duration must be at least 1 year.

B. Presence, while depressed, of two (or more) of the following:

(1) poor appetite or overeating
(2) insomnia or hypersomnia
(3) low energy or fatigue
(4) low self-esteem
(5) poor concentration or difficulty making decisions
(6) feelings of hopelessness

C. During the 2-year period (1 year for children or adolescents) of the disturbance, the person has never been without the symptoms in Criteria A and B for more than 2 months at a time.

D. No major depressive episode has been present during the first 2 years of the disturbance (1 year for children and adolescents); i.e., the disturbance is not better accounted for by chronic major depressive disorder, or major depressive disorder, in partial remission.
Note: There may have been a previous major depressive episode provided there was a full remission (no significant signs or symptoms for 2 months) before development of the dysthymic disorder. In addition, after the initial 2 years (1 year in children or adolescents) of dysthymic disorder, there may be superimposed episodes of major depressive disorder, in which case both diagnoses may be given when the criteria are met for a major depressive episode.

E. There has never been a manic episode, a mixed episode, or a hypomanic episode, and criteria have never been met for cyclothymic disorder.

F. The disturbance does not occur exclusively during the course of a chronic psychotic disorder, such as schizophrenia or delusional disorder.

G. The symptoms are not due to the direct physiological effects of a substance (e.g., a drug of abuse, a medication) or a general medical condition (e.g., hypothyroidism).

H. The symptoms cause clinically significant distress or impairment in social, occupational, or other important areas of functioning.

Specify if:
Early onset: if onset is before age 21 years
Late onset: if onset is age 21 years or older
Specify (for most recent 2 years of dysthymic disorder) if
With atypical features

From American Psychiatric Association. *Diagnostic and Statistical Manual of Mental Disorders.* 4th ed. Text rev. Washington, DC: American Psychiatric Association; copyright 2000, with permission.

Table 12.2–2
DSM-IV-TR Alternative Research Criterion B for Dysthymic Disorder

A. Presence, while depressed, of three (or more) of the following:

(1) low self-esteem or self-confidence, or feelings of inadequacy
(2) feelings of pessimism, despair, or hopelessness
(3) generalized loss of interest or pleasure
(4) social withdrawal
(5) chronic fatigue or tiredness
(6) feelings of guilt, brooding about the past
(7) subjective feelings of irritability or excessive anger
(8) decreased activity, effectiveness, or productivity
(9) difficulty in thinking, reflected by poor concentration, poor memory, or indecisiveness

From American Psychiatric Association. *Diagnostic and Statistical Manual of Mental Disorders.* 4th ed. Text rev. Washington, DC: American Psychiatric Association; copyright 2000, with permission.

Minor Depressive Disorder. Minor depressive disorder (discussed in Section 12.3) is characterized by episodes of depressive symptoms that are less severe than those seen in major depressive disorder. The difference between dysthymic disorder and minor depressive disorder is primarily the episodic nature of the symptoms in the latter. Between episodes, patients with minor depressive disorder have a euthymic mood, whereas patients with dysthymic disorder have virtually no euthymic periods.

Recurrent Brief Depressive Disorder. Recurrent brief depressive disorder (discussed in Section 12.3) is characterized by brief periods (less than 2 weeks) during which depressive episodes are present. Patients with the disorder would meet the diagnostic criteria for major depressive disorder if their episodes lasted longer. Patients with recurrent brief depressive disorder differ from patients with dysthymic disorder on two counts: They have an episodic disorder, and their symptoms are more severe.

Double Depression. An estimated 40 percent of patients with major depressive disorder also meet the criteria for dysthymic disorder, a combination often referred to as *double depression*. Data support the conclusion that patients with double depression have a poorer prognosis than patients with only major depressive disorder. The treatment of patients with double depression should be directed toward both disorders because the resolution of the symptoms of major depressive episode still leaves these patients with significant psychiatric impairment.

Alcohol and Substance Abuse. Patients with dysthymic disorder commonly meet the diagnostic criteria for a substance-related disorder. This comorbidity can be logical; patients with dysthymic disorder tend to develop coping methods for their chronically depressed state that involve substance abuse. Therefore, they are likely to use alcohol, stimulants such as cocaine, or marijuana, the choice perhaps depending primarily on a patient's social context. The presence of a comorbid diagnosis of substance abuse presents a diagnostic dilemma for clinicians; the long-term use of many substances can result in a symptom picture indistinguishable from that of dysthymic disorder.

disorder is varied, with some patients proceeding to major depression, whereas others manifest the pathology largely at the personality level.

Differential Diagnosis

The differential diagnosis for dysthymic disorder is essentially identical to that for major depressive disorder. Many substances and medical illnesses can cause chronic depressive symptoms. Two disorders are particularly important to consider in the differential diagnosis of dysthymic disorder—minor depressive disorder and recurrent brief depressive disorder.

Course and Prognosis

About 50 percent of patients with dysthymic disorder experience an insidious onset of symptoms before age 25 years. Despite the early onset, patients often suffer with the symptoms for a decade before seeking psychiatric help and may consider early-onset dysthymic disorder simply part of life. Patients with an early onset of symptoms are at risk for either major depressive disorder or bipolar I disorder in the course of their disorder. Studies of patients with the diagnosis of dysthymic disorder indicate that about 20 percent progressed to major depressive disorder, 15 percent to bipolar II disorder, and less than 5 percent to bipolar I disorder.

The prognosis for patients with dysthymic disorder varies. Antidepressive agents and specific types of psychotherapies (e.g., cognitive and behavior therapies) have positive effects on the course and prognosis of dysthymic disorder. The data on previously available treatments indicate that only 10 to 15 percent of patients are in remission 1 year after the initial diagnosis. About 25 percent of all patients with dysthymic disorder never attain a complete recovery. Overall, however, the prognosis is good with treatment.

Treatment

Historically, patients with dysthymic disorder either received no treatment or were seen as candidates for long-term, insight-oriented psychotherapy. Contemporary data offer the most objective support for cognitive therapy, behavior therapy, and pharmacotherapy. The combination of pharmacotherapy and some form of psychotherapy may be the most effective treatment for the disorder.

Cognitive Therapy.   Cognitive therapy is a technique in which patients are taught new ways of thinking and behaving to replace faulty negative attitudes about themselves, the world, and the future. It is a short-term therapy program oriented toward current problems and their resolution.

Behavior Therapy.   Behavior therapy for depressive disorders is based on the theory that depression is caused by a loss of positive reinforcement as a result of separation, death, or sudden environmental change. The various treatment methods focus on specific goals to increase activity, to provide pleasant experiences, and to teach patients how to relax. Altering personal behavior in depressed patients is believed to be the most effective way to change the associated depressed thoughts and feelings. Behavior therapy is often used to treat the learned helplessness of some patients who seem to meet every life challenge with a sense of impotence.

Insight-Oriented (Psychoanalytic) Psychotherapy. Individual insight-oriented psychotherapy is the most common treatment method for dysthymic disorder, and many clinicians consider it the treatment of choice. The psychotherapeutic approach attempts to relate the development and maintenance of depressive symptoms and maladaptive personality features to unresolved conflicts from early childhood. Insight into depressive equivalents (e.g., substance abuse) or into childhood disappointments as antecedents to adult depression can be gained

through treatment. Ambivalent current relationships with parents, friends, and others in the patient's current life are examined. Patients' understanding of how they try to gratify an excessive need for outside approval to counter low self-esteem and a harsh superego is an important goal in this therapy.

Interpersonal Therapy.   In interpersonal therapy for depressive disorders, a patient's current interpersonal experiences and ways of coping with stress are examined to reduce depressive symptoms and to improve self-esteem. Interpersonal therapy lasts for about 12 to 16 weekly sessions and can be combined with antidepressant medication.

Family and Group Therapies.   Family therapy may help both the patient and the patient's family deal with the symptoms of the disorder, especially when a biologically based subaffective syndrome seems to be present. Group therapy may help withdrawn patients learn new ways to overcome their interpersonal problems in social situations.

Pharmacotherapy.   Because of long-standing and commonly held theoretical beliefs that dysthymic disorder is primarily a psychologically determined disorder, many clinicians avoid prescribing antidepressants for patients; however, many studies have shown therapeutic success with antidepressants. The data generally indicate that selective serotonin reuptake inhibitors venlafaxine and bupropion are an effective treatment for patients with dysthymic disorder. Monoamine oxidase inhibitors are effective in a subgroup of patients with dysthymic disorder, a group who may also respond to the judicious use of amphetamines.

Hospitalization.   Hospitalization is usually not indicated for patients with dysthymic disorder, but particularly severe symptoms, marked social or professional incapacitation, the need for extensive diagnostic procedures, and suicidal ideation are all indications for hospitalization.

CYCLOTHYMIC DISORDER

Cyclothymic disorder is symptomatically a mild form of bipolar II disorder, characterized by episodes of hypomania and mild depression. In DSM-IV-TR, cyclothymic disorder is defined as a "chronic, fluctuating disturbance" with many periods of hypomania and of depression. The disorder is differentiated from bipolar II disorder, which is characterized by the presence of major (not minor) depressive and hypomanic episodes. As with dysthymic disorder, the inclusion of cyclothymic disorder with the mood disorders implies a relation, probably biological, to bipolar I disorder. Some psychiatrists, however, consider cyclothymic disorder to have no biological component and to result from chaotic object relations early in life.

Epidemiology

Patients with cyclothymic disorder may constitute from 3 to 5 percent of all psychiatric outpatients, perhaps particularly those with significant complaints about marital and interpersonal difficulties. In the general population, the lifetime prevalence of cyclothymic disorder is estimated to be about 1 percent. This figure is probably lower than the actual prevalence because, as with patients with bipolar I disorder, the patients may not be aware that they have a psychiatric problem. Cyclothymic disorder, as with dysthymic disorder, frequently coexists with borderline personality disorder. An estimated 10 percent of outpatients and 20 percent of inpatients with borderline personality disorder have a coexisting diagnosis of cyclothymic disorder. The female-to-male ratio in cyclothymic disorder is about 3 to 2, and 50 to 75 percent of all patients have an onset between ages 15 and 25 years. Families of persons with cyclothymic disorder often contain members with substance-related disorder.

Etiology

As with dysthymic disorder, controversy exists about whether cyclothymic disorder is related to the mood disorders, either biologically or psychologically. Some researchers have postulated that cyclothymic disorder has a closer relation to borderline personality disorder than to the mood disorders. Despite these controversies, the preponderance of biological and genetic data favors the idea of cyclothymic disorder as a bona fide mood disorder.

Biological Factors.   About 30 percent of all patients with cyclothymic disorder have positive family histories for bipolar I disorder; this rate is similar to the rate for patients with bipolar I disorder. Moreover, the pedigrees of families with bipolar I disorder often contain generations of patients with bipolar I disorder linked by a generation with cyclothymic disorder. Conversely, the prevalence of cyclothymic disorder in the relatives of patients with bipolar I disorder is much higher than the prevalence of cyclothymic disorder either in the relatives of patients with other mental disorders or in persons who are mentally healthy. The observations that about one third of patients with cyclothymic disorder subsequently have major mood disorders, that they are particularly sensitive to antidepressant-induced hypomania, and that about 60 percent respond to lithium add further support to the idea of cyclothymic disorder as a mild or attenuated form of bipolar II disorder.

Psychosocial Factors.   Most psychodynamic theories postulate that the development of cyclothymic disorder lies in traumas and fixations during the oral stage of infant development. Freud hypothesized that the cyclothymic state is the ego's attempt to overcome a harsh and punitive superego. Hypomania is explained psychodynamically as the lack of self-criticism and an absence of inhibitions occurring when a depressed person throws off the burden of an overly harsh superego. The major defense mechanism in hypomania is denial, by which the patient avoids external problems and internal feelings of depression.

Patients with cyclothymic disorder are characterized by periods of depression alternating with periods of hypomania. Psychoanalytic exploration reveals that such patients defend themselves against underlying depressive themes with their euphoric or hypomanic periods. Hypomania is frequently triggered by a profound interpersonal loss. The false euphoria generated in such instances is a patient's way to deny dependence on love objects and simultaneously disavow any aggression or destructiveness that may be associated with the loss of the loved person.

Diagnosis and Clinical Features

Although many patients seek psychiatric help for depression, their problems are often related to the chaos that their manic episodes have caused. Clinicians must consider a diagnosis of cyclothymic disorder when a patient appears with what may seem to be sociopathic behavioral problems. Marital difficulties and instability in relationships are common complaints because patients with cyclothymic disorder are often promiscuous and irritable while in manic and mixed states. Although there are anecdotal reports of increased productivity and creativity when patients are hypomanic, most clinicians report that their patients become disorganized and ineffective in work and school during these periods.

The DSM-IV-TR diagnostic criteria for cyclothymic disorder (Table 12.2–3) stipulate that a patient has never met the criteria for a major depressive episode and did not meet the criteria for a manic episode during the first 2 years of the disturbance. The criteria also require the more or less constant presence of symptoms for 2 years (or 1 year for children and adolescents).

Signs and Symptoms.   The symptoms of cyclothymic disorder are identical to the symptoms of bipolar II disorder, except that they are generally less severe. On occasion, however, the symptoms may be equally severe but of shorter duration than those seen in bipolar II disorder. About half of all patients with cyclothymic disorder have depression as their major symptom, and these patients are most likely to seek psychiatric help while

Table 12.2–3
DSM-IV-TR Diagnostic Criteria for Cyclothymic Disorder

A. For at least 2 years, the presence of numerous periods with hypomanic symptoms and numerous periods with depressive symptoms that do not meet criteria for a major depressive episode. **Note:** In children and adolescents, the duration must be at least 1 year.

B. During the above 2-year period (1 year in children and adolescents), the person has not been without the symptoms in Criterion A for more than 2 months at a time.

C. No major depressive episode, manic episode, or mixed episode has been present during the first 2 years of the disturbance.
Note: After the initial 2 years (1 year in children and adolescents) of cyclothymic disorder, there may be superimposed manic or mixed episodes (in which case both bipolar I disorder and cyclothymic disorder may be diagnosed) or major depressive episodes (in which case both bipolar II disorder and cyclothymic disorder may be diagnosed).

D. The symptoms in Criterion A are not better accounted for by schizoaffective disorder and are not superimposed on schizophrenia, schizophreniform disorder, delusional disorder, or psychotic disorder not otherwise specified.

E. The symptoms are not due to the direct physiological effects of a substance (e.g., a drug of abuse, a medication) or a general medical condition (e.g., hyperthyroidism).

F. The symptoms cause clinically significant distress or impairment in social, occupational, or other important areas of functioning.

From American Psychiatric Association. *Diagnostic and Statistical Manual of Mental Disorders.* 4th ed. Text rev. Washington, DC: American Psychiatric Association; copyright 2000, with permission.

depressed. Some patients with cyclothymic disorder have primarily hypomanic symptoms and are less likely to consult a psychiatrist than are primarily depressed patients. Almost all patients with cyclothymic disorder have periods of mixed symptoms with marked irritability.

Most patients with cyclothymic disorder seen by psychiatrists have not succeeded in their professional and social lives as a result of their disorder, but a few have become high achievers who have worked especially long hours and have required little sleep. Some persons' ability to control the symptoms of the disorder successfully depends on multiple individual, social, and cultural attributes.

The lives of most patients with cyclothymic disorder are difficult. The cycles of the disorder tend to be much shorter than those in bipolar I disorder. In cyclothymic disorder, the changes in mood are irregular and abrupt and sometimes occur within hours. The unpredictable nature of the mood changes produces great stress. Patients often feel that their moods are out of control. In irritable, mixed periods, they may become involved in unprovoked disagreements with friends, family, and coworkers.

Substance Abuse.   Alcohol abuse and other substance abuse are common in patients with cyclothymic disorder, who use substances either to self-medicate (with alcohol, benzodiazepines, and marijuana) or to achieve even further stimulation (with cocaine, amphetamines, and hallucinogens) when they are manic. About 5 to 10 percent of all patients with cyclothymic disorder have substance dependence. Persons with this disorder often have a history of multiple geographical moves, involvements in religious cults, and dilettantism.

Differential Diagnosis

When a diagnosis of cyclothymic disorder is under consideration, all the possible medical and substance-related causes of depression and mania, such as seizures and particular substances (cocaine, amphetamines, and steroids), must be considered. Borderline, antisocial, histrionic, and narcissistic personality disorders should also be considered in the differential diagnosis. Attention-deficit/hyperactivity disorder (ADHD) can be difficult to differentiate from cyclothymic disorder in children and adolescents. A trial of stimulants helps most patients with ADHD and exacerbates the symptoms of most patients with cyclothymic disorder. The diagnostic category of bipolar II disorder (discussed in Section 12.1) is characterized by the combination of major depressive and hypomanic episodes.

Course and Prognosis

Some patients with cyclothymic disorder are characterized as having been sensitive, hyperactive, or moody as young children. The onset of frank symptoms of cyclothymic disorder often occurs insidiously in the teens or early 20s. The emergence of symptoms at that time hinders a person's performance in school and the ability to establish friendships with peers. The reactions of patients to such a disorder vary; patients with adaptive coping strategies or ego defenses have better outcomes than patients with poor coping strategies. About one third of all patients with cyclothymic disorder develop a major mood disorder, most often bipolar II disorder.

Treatment

Biological Therapy.   The mood stabilizers and antimania drugs are the first line of treatment for patients with cyclothymic disorder. Although the experimental data are limited to studies with lithium, other antimania agents—for example, carbamazepine and valproate (Depakene)—are reported to be effective. Doses and plasma concentrations of these agents should be the same as those in bipolar I disorder. Antidepressant treatment of depressed patients with cyclothymic disorder should be done with caution because these patients have increased susceptibility to antidepressant-induced hypomanic or manic episodes. About 40 to 50 percent of all patients with cyclothymic disorder who are treated with antidepressants experience such episodes.

Psychosocial Therapy.   Psychotherapy for patients with cyclothymic disorder is best directed toward increasing patients' awareness of their condition and helping them develop coping mechanisms for their mood swings. Therapists usually need to help patients repair any damage, both work and family related, done during episodes of hypomania. Because of the long-term nature of cyclothymic disorder, patients often require lifelong treatment. Family and group therapies may be supportive, educational, and therapeutic for patients and for those involved in their lives. The psychiatrist conducting psychotherapy is able to evaluate the degree of cyclothymia and so provide an early-warning system to prevent full-blown manic attacks before they occur.

▲ 12.3 Other Mood Disorders

DEPRESSIVE DISORDER NOT OTHERWISE SPECIFIED

The diagnostic category depressive disorder not otherwise specified is used for patients who exhibit depressive symptoms as the major feature but who do not meet the diagnostic criteria for any other mood disorder (Table 12.3–1). Three disorders meet this criterion: (1) minor depressive disorder, (2) recurrent brief depressive disorder, and (3) premenstrual dysphoric disorder.

Minor Depressive Disorder

The literature in the United States on minor depressive disorder is limited, in part, because the term is used to describe a wide range of disorders, including dysthymic disorder, which is listed as a diagnosis in the text revision of the fourth edition of the *Diagnostic and Statistical Manual of Mental Disorders* (DSM-IV-TR).

Epidemiology.   Minor depressive disorder may be as common as major depressive disorder—that is, about 5 percent prevalence in the general population. The disorder is more common in women than in men and affects people of virtually any age, from childhood onward.

Etiology.   The cause of minor depressive disorder is unknown. Both biological and psychological factors are implicated.

Table 12.3–1
DSM-IV-TR Diagnostic Criteria for Depressive Disorder Not Otherwise Specified

The depressive disorder not otherwise specified category includes disorders with depressive features that do not meet the criteria for major depressive disorder, dysthymic disorder, adjustment disorder with depressed mood, or adjustment disorder with mixed anxiety and depressed mood. Sometimes depressive symptoms can present as part of an anxiety disorder not otherwise specified. Examples of depressive disorder not otherwise specified include

1. Premenstrual dysphoric disorder: in most menstrual cycles during the past year, symptoms (e.g., markedly depressed mood, marked anxiety, marked affective lability, decreased interest in activities) regularly occurred during the last week of the luteal phase (and remitted within a few days of the onset of menses). These symptoms must be severe enough to markedly interfere with work, school, or usual activities and be entirely absent for at least 1 week postmenses.
2. Minor depressive disorder: episodes of at least 2 weeks of depressive symptoms but with fewer than the five items required for major depressive disorder.
3. Recurrent brief depressive disorder: depressive episodes lasting from 2 days up to 2 weeks, occurring at least once a month for 12 months (not associated with the menstrual cycle).
4. Postpsychotic depressive disorder of schizophrenia: a major depressive episode that occurs during the residual phase of schizophrenia.
5. A major depressive episode superimposed on delusional disorder, psychotic disorder not otherwise specified, or the active phase of schizophrenia.
6. Situations in which the clinician has concluded that a depressive disorder is present but is unable to determine whether it is primary, due to a general medical condition, or substance induced.

From American Psychiatric Association. *Diagnostic and Statistical Manual of Mental Disorders.* 4th ed. Text rev. Washington, DC: American Psychiatric Association; copyright 2000, with permission.

Diagnosis and Clinical Features. The criteria for minor depressive disorder include symptoms equal in duration to those of major depressive disorder but less severe (Table 12.3–2). The central symptom of both disorders is the same—a depressed mood.

Differential Diagnosis. The differential diagnosis of minor depressive disorder includes dysthymic disorder and recurrent brief depressive disorder. Dysthymic disorder is characterized by the presence of chronic depressive symptoms, whereas recurrent brief depressive disorder is characterized by multiple brief episodes of severe depressive symptoms.

Course and Prognosis. No definitive data on the course and the prognosis of minor depressive disorder are available, but minor depressive disorder, as with major depressive disorder, has a long-term course that requires long-term treatment. Some cases remit spontaneously, however.

Treatment. The treatment of minor depressive disorder can include psychotherapy, pharmacotherapy, or both. Insight-oriented psychotherapy, cognitive therapy, interpersonal therapy, and behavior therapy are the psychotherapeutic treatments for major depressive disorder and, by implication, for minor depressive disorder. Patients with minor depressive disorder are prob-

Table 12.3–2
DSM-IV-TR Research Criteria for Minor Depressive Disorder

A. A mood disturbance, defined as follows:
  (1) at least two (but less than five) of the following symptoms have been present during the same 2-week period and represent a change from previous functioning; at least one of the symptoms is either (a) or (b):
    (a) depressed mood most of the day, nearly every day, as indicated by either subjective report (e.g., feels sad or empty) or observation made by others (e.g., appears tearful). **Note:** In children and adolescents, can be irritable mood.
    (b) markedly diminished interest or pleasure in all, or almost all, activities most of the day, nearly every day (as indicated by either subjective account or observation made by others)
    (c) significant weight loss when not dieting or weight gain (e.g., a change of more than 5% of body weight in a month), or decrease or increase in appetite nearly every day. **Note:** In children, consider failure to make expected weight gains.
    (d) insomnia or hypersomnia nearly every day
    (e) psychomotor agitation or retardation nearly every day (observable by others, not merely subjective feelings of restlessness or being slowed down)
    (f) fatigue or loss of energy nearly every day
    (g) feelings of worthlessness or excessive or inappropriate guilt (which may be delusional) nearly every day (not merely self-reproach or guilt about being sick)
    (h) diminished ability to think or concentrate, or indecisiveness, nearly every day (either by subjective account or as observed by others)
    (i) recurrent thoughts of death (not just fear of dying), recurrent suicidal ideation without a specific plan, or a suicide attempt or a specific plan for committing suicide
  (2) the symptoms cause clinically significant distress or impairment in social, occupational, or other important areas of functioning
  (3) the symptoms are not due to the direct physiological effects of a substance (e.g., a drug of abuse, a medication) or a general medical condition (e.g., hypothyroidism)
  (4) the symptoms are not better accounted for by bereavement (i.e., a normal reaction to the death of a loved one)
B. There has never been a major depressive episode, and criteria are not met for dysthymic disorder.
C. There has never been a manic episode, a mixed episode, or a hypomanic episode, and criteria are not met for cyclothymic disorder. **Note:** This exclusion does not apply if all of the manic-, mixed-, or hypomanic-like episodes are substance or treatment induced.
D. The mood disturbance does not occur exclusively during schizophrenia, schizophreniform disorder, schizoaffective disorder, delusional disorder, or psychotic disorder not otherwise specified.

From American Psychiatric Association. *Diagnostic and Statistical Manual of Mental Disorders.* 4th ed. Text rev. Washington, DC: American Psychiatric Association; copyright 2000, with permission.

ably responsive to pharmacotherapy, particularly selective serotonin reuptake inhibitors (SSRIs) and bupropion (Wellbutrin).

Recurrent Brief Depressive Disorder

Recurrent brief depressive disorder is characterized by multiple, relatively brief episodes (less than 2 weeks) of depressive

symptoms that, except for their brief duration, meet the diagnostic criteria for major depressive disorder.

Epidemiology.   The 10-year prevalence rate for the disorder is estimated to be 10 percent for people in their 20s; the 1-year prevalence rate for the general population is estimated to be 5 percent. These numbers indicate that recurrent brief depressive disorder is most common among young adults.

Etiology.   Patients with recurrent brief depressive disorder may share several biological abnormalities with patients with major depressive disorder. The variables include nonsuppression on the dexamethasone-suppression test, a blunt response to thyrotropin-releasing hormone, and a shortening of rapid eye movement sleep latency. The data are consistent with the idea that recurrent brief depressive disorder is closely related to major depressive disorder in its cause and pathophysiology.

Diagnosis and Clinical Features.   The criteria for recurrent brief depressive disorder specify that the symptom duration for each episode is less than 2 weeks (Table 12.3–3). Otherwise, the diagnostic criteria for recurrent brief depressive disorder and major depressive disorder are essentially identical. One subtle difference is that the frequent changes in their moods may make the lives of patients with recurrent brief depressive disorder seem more disrupted or chaotic than those of patients with major depressive disorder, whose depressive episodes occur at a measured pace.

Differential Diagnosis.   Clinicians should consider bipolar disorder and major depressive disorder with seasonal pattern in the differential diagnosis. Recurrent brief depressive disorder

Table 12.3–3
DSM-IV-TR Research Criteria for Recurrent Brief Depressive Disorder

A. Criteria, except for duration, are met for a major depressive episode.
B. The depressive periods in Criterion A last at least 2 days but less than 2 weeks.
C. The depressive periods occur at least once a month for 12 consecutive months and are not associated with the menstrual cycle.
D. The periods of depressed mood cause clinically significant distress or impairment in social, occupational, or other important areas of functioning.
E. The symptoms are not due to the direct physiological effects of a substance (e.g., a drug of abuse, a medication) or a general medical condition (e.g., hypothyroidism).
F. There has never been a major depressive episode, and criteria are not met for dysthymic disorder.
G. There has never been a manic episode, a mixed episode, or a hypomanic episode, and criteria are not met for cyclothymic disorder. **Note:** This exclusion does not apply if all of the manic-, mixed-, or hypomanic-like episodes are substance or treatment induced.
H. The mood disturbance does not occur exclusively during schizophrenia, schizophreniform disorder, schizoaffective disorder, delusional disorder, or psychotic disorder not otherwise specified.

From American Psychiatric Association. *Diagnostic and Statistical Manual of Mental Disorders.* 4th ed. Text rev. Washington, DC: American Psychiatric Association; copyright 2000, with permission.

can be associated with the rapid cycling type of bipolar disorder. Clinicians should also determine whether a seasonal pattern exists to the recurrence of depressive episodes.

Course and Prognosis.   The course, including age of onset, and prognosis are similar to those of major depressive disorder.

Treatment.   The treatment of patients with recurrent brief depressive disorder should be similar to the treatment of patients with major depressive disorder. Some of the treatments for bipolar I disorder—lithium (Eskalith) and anticonvulsants—may be of therapeutic value.

Premenstrual Dysphoric Disorder

Premenstrual dysphoric disorder is also called *late luteal-phase dysphoric disorder*. The syndrome involves mood symptoms (e.g., lability), behavior symptoms (e.g., changes in eating patterns), and physical symptoms (e.g., breast tenderness, edema, and headaches). This pattern of symptoms occurs at a specific time during the menstrual cycle, and the symptoms resolve for some period of time between menstrual cycles. (Chapter 26 provides an extensive overview of this and other disorders related to the reproductive cycle.)

Postpsychotic Depressive Disorder of Schizophrenia

Postpsychotic depressive disorder in patients with schizophrenia is categorized in an appendix in DSM-IV-TR.

Epidemiology.   The reported incidence of postpsychotic depression of schizophrenia varies widely, from less than 10 percent to more than 70 percent.

Etiology.   The etiology is unknown. Psychologically, some patients became depressed after realizing their vulnerability to mental illness, which lowers their self-esteem.

Prognostic Significance.   Patients with postpsychotic depressive disorder of schizophrenia are likely to have had poor premorbid adjustment, marked schizoid personality disorder traits, and an insidious onset of their psychotic symptoms. They are also likely to have first-degree relatives with mood disorders. Although the findings have not been consistent, postpsychotic depressive disorder of schizophrenia has been associated with a less-favorable prognosis, a higher likelihood of relapse, and a higher incidence of suicide than is seen in patients with schizophrenia without postpsychotic depressive disorder.

Diagnosis and Differential Diagnosis.   The symptoms of postpsychotic depressive disorder of schizophrenia can closely resemble the symptoms of the residual phase of schizophrenia as well as the adverse effects of commonly used antipsychotic medications. Clinicians should not confuse the antipsychotic-induced adverse effects of akathisia and akinesia with symptoms of postpsychotic depressive disorder. Distinguishing the diagnosis from schizoaffective disorder, depressive type, is also difficult (Table 12.3–4).

Table 12.3–4
DSM-IV-TR Research Criteria for Postpsychotic Depressive Disorder of Schizophrenia

A. Criteria are met for a major depressive episode.
 Note: The major depressive episode must include Criterion A1: depressed mood. Do not include symptoms that are better accounted for as medication side effects or negative symptoms of schizophrenia.
B. The major depressive episode is superimposed on and occurs only during the residual phase of schizophrenia.
C. The major depressive episode is not due to the direct physiological effects of a substance or a general medical condition.

From American Psychiatric Association. *Diagnostic and Statistical Manual of Mental Disorders.* 4th ed. Text rev. Washington, DC: American Psychiatric Association; copyright 2000, with permission.

Treatment.   The use of antidepressants is indicated in the treatment of postpsychotic depressive disorder of schizophrenia, but response rates vary and are unpredictable.

BIPOLAR DISORDER NOT OTHERWISE SPECIFIED

If patients exhibit depressive and manic symptoms as the major features of their disorder and do not meet the diagnostic criteria for any other mood disorder or other DSM-IV-TR mental disorder, the most appropriate diagnosis is bipolar disorder not otherwise specified (Table 12.3–5). This category should be used rarely.

Mixed Anxiety-Depressive Disorder

Mixed anxiety-depressive disorder is characterized by a persistent or recurrent depressed mood lasting at least 1 month and

Table 12.3–5
DSM-IV-TR Diagnostic Criteria for Bipolar Disorder Not Otherwise Specified

The bipolar disorder not otherwise specified category includes disorders with bipolar features that do not meet criteria for any specific bipolar disorder. Examples include
1. Very rapid alternation (over days) between manic symptoms and depressive symptoms that meet symptom threshold criteria but not minimal duration criteria for manic, hypomanic, or major depressive episodes
2. Recurrent hypomanic episodes without intercurrent depressive symptoms
3. A manic or mixed episode superimposed on delusional disorder, residual schizophrenia, or psychotic disorder not otherwise specified
4. Hypomanic episodes, along with chronic depressive symptoms, that are too infrequent to qualify for a diagnosis of cyclothymic disorder
5. Situations in which the clinician has concluded that a bipolar disorder is present but is unable to determine whether it is primary, due to a general medical condition, or substance induced

From American Psychiatric Association. *Diagnostic and Statistical Manual of Mental Disorders.* 4th ed. Text rev. Washington, DC: American Psychiatric Association; copyright 2000, with permission.

Table 12.3–6
Research Criteria for Mixed Anxiety-Depressive Disorder

A. Persistent or recurrent dysphoric mood lasting at least 1 month.
B. The dysphoric mood is accompanied by at least 1 month of four (or more) of the following symptoms:
 (1) difficulty concentrating or mind going blank
 (2) sleep disturbance (difficulty falling or staying asleep, or restless, unsatisfying sleep)
 (3) fatigue or low energy
 (4) irritability
 (5) worry
 (6) being easily moved to tears
 (7) hypervigilance
 (8) anticipating the worst
 (9) hopelessness (pervasive pessimism about the future)
 (10) low self-esteem or feelings of worthlessness
C. The symptoms cause clinically significant distress or impairment in social, occupational, or other important areas of functioning.
D. The symptoms are not due to the direct physiological effects of a substance (e.g., a drug of abuse, a medication) or a general medical condition.
E. All of the following:
 (1) criteria have never been met for Major Depressive Disorder, Dysthymic Disorder, Panic Disorder, or Generalized Anxiety Disorder
 (2) criteria are not currently met for any other Anxiety or Mood Disorder (including an Anxiety or Mood Disorder, In Partial Remission)
 (3) the symptoms are not better accounted for by any other mental disorder

From American Psychiatric Association. *Diagnostic and Statistical Manual of Mental Disorders.* 4th ed. Text rev. Washington DC: American Psychiatric Association; copyright 2000, with permission.

by symptoms of anxiety, such as sleep disturbance, fatigue or low energy, irritability, and worry (Table 12.3–6). The symptoms must cause clinically significant distress or impairment in social, occupational, or other important areas of functioning.

Patients with mixed pictures are reportedly most prevalent in general medical settings because they have many somatic complaints about which they are anxious, one of the most prominent being chronic fatigue. In the tenth revision of *International Statistical Classification of Diseases and Related Health Problems* (ICD-10), these patients are diagnosed with neurasthenia. Some patients with chronic fatigue syndrome also have mixed anxiety and depressive symptomatology.

Atypical Depression

Atypical depression refers to fatigue superimposed on a history of somatic anxiety and phobias, together with reverse vegetative signs (mood worse in the evening, insomnia, tendency to oversleep and overeat), so that weight gain occurs rather than weight loss. Sleep is disturbed in the first half of the night in many persons with atypical depressive disorder, so irritability, hypersomnolence, and daytime fatigue would be expected. The temperaments of these patients are characterized by extreme sensitivity, especially to rejection. SSRIs and monoamine oxidase inhibitors seem to show some specificity for such patients. Others are helped by psychostimulants, such as amphetamine.

SECONDARY MOOD DISORDERS

Secondary mood disorders consist of two broad categories that must be considered in the differential diagnosis of any patient with mood disorder symptoms. They are (1) mood disorder caused by a general medical condition and (2) substance-induced mood disorder.

Mood Disorders Due to a General Medical Condition

When depressive or manic symptoms are present in a patient with a general medical condition, attributing the depressive symptoms either to the general medical condition or to a mood disorder can be difficult. Many general medical conditions present depressive symptoms, such as poor sleep, agitation, decreased appetite, increased appetite, and fatigue. Table 12.3–7 lists the DSM-IV-TR criteria for the disorder. This category is discussed extensively in Section 7.5.

Table 12.3–7
DSM-IV-TR Diagnostic Criteria for Mood Disorder Due to a General Medical Condition

A. A prominent and persistent disturbance in mood predominates in the clinical picture and is characterized by either (or both) of the following:
   (1) depressed mood or markedly diminished interest or pleasure in all, or almost all, activities
   (2) elevated, expansive, or irritable mood
B. There is evidence from the history, physical examination, or laboratory findings that the disturbance is the direct physiological consequence of a general medical condition.
C. The disturbance is not better accounted for by another mental disorder (e.g., adjustment disorder with depressed mood in response to the stress of having a general medical condition).
D. The disturbance does not occur exclusively during the course of a delirium.
E. The symptoms cause clinically significant distress or impairment in social, occupational, or other important areas of functioning.
Specify type:
   With depressive features: if the predominant mood is depressed but the full criteria are not met for a major depressive episode
   With major depressive-like episode: if the full criteria are met (except Criterion D) for a major depressive episode
   With manic features: if the predominant mood is elevated, euphoric, or irritable
   With mixed features: if the symptoms of both mania and depression are present but neither predominates
   Coding note: Include the name of the general medical condition on Axis I, e.g., mood disorder due to hypothyroidism, with depressive features; also code the general medical condition on Axis III.
   Coding note: If depressive symptoms occur as part of a preexisting vascular dementia, indicate the depressive symptoms by coding the appropriate subtype, i.e., vascular dementia, with depressed mood.

From American Psychiatric Association. *Diagnostic and Statistical Manual of Mental Disorders.* 4th ed. Text rev. Washington, DC: American Psychiatric Association; copyright 2000, with permission.

Table 12.3–8
DSM-IV-TR Diagnostic Criteria for Substance-Induced Mood Disorder

A. A prominent and persistent disturbance in mood predominates in the clinical picture and is characterized by either (or both) of the following:
   (1) depressed mood or markedly diminished interest or pleasure in all, or almost all, activities
   (2) elevated, expansive, or irritable mood
B. There is evidence from the history, physical examination, or laboratory findings of either (1) or (2):
   (1) the symptoms in Criterion A developed during, or within a month of, substance intoxication or withdrawal
   (2) medication use is etiologically related to the disturbance
C. The disturbance is not better accounted for by a mood disorder that is not substance induced. Evidence that the symptoms are better accounted for by a mood disorder that is not substance induced might include the following: the symptoms precede the onset of the substance use (or medication use); the symptoms persist for a substantial period of time (e.g., about a month) after the cessation of acute withdrawal or severe intoxication or are substantially in excess of what would be expected given the type or amount of the substance used or the duration of use; or there is other evidence that suggests the existence of an independent non–substance-induced mood disorder (e.g., a history of recurrent major depressive episodes).
D. The disturbance does not occur exclusively during the course of a delirium.
E. The symptoms cause clinically significant distress or impairment in social, occupational, or other important areas of functioning.
Note: This diagnosis should be made instead of a diagnosis of substance intoxication or substance withdrawal only when the mood symptoms are in excess of those usually associated with the intoxication or withdrawal syndrome and when the symptoms are sufficiently severe to warrant independent clinical attention.
Code [Specific substance]-induced mood disorder:
Alcohol; amphetamine [or amphetamine-like substance]; cocaine; hallucinogen; inhalant; opioid; phencyclidine [or phencyclidine-like substance]; sedative, hypnotic, or anxiolytic; other [or unknown] substance
Specify type:
   With depressive features: if the predominant mood is depressed
   With manic features: if the predominant mood is elevated, euphoric, or irritable
   With mixed features: if symptoms of both mania and depression are present and neither predominates
Specify if:
   With onset during intoxication: if the criteria are met for intoxication with the substance and the symptoms develop during the intoxication syndrome
   With onset during withdrawal: if criteria are met for withdrawal from the substance and the symptoms develop during, or shortly after, a withdrawal syndrome

From American Psychiatric Association. *Diagnostic and Statistical Manual of Mental Disorders.* 4th ed. Text rev. Washington, DC: American Psychiatric Association; copyright 2000, with permission.

Substance-Induced Mood Disorder

Substance-induced mood disorder must always be considered in the differential diagnosis of mood disorder symptoms. Clinicians should consider three possibilities: (1) a patient may be taking drugs for the treatment of nonpsychiatric medical problems;

(2) a patient may have been accidentally, and perhaps unknowingly, exposed to neurotoxic chemicals; and (3) the patient may have taken a substance for recreational purposes or may be dependent on such a substance.

Epidemiology. The epidemiology of substance-induced mood disorder is unknown. The prevalence is probably high, given the widespread use of so-called recreational drugs, the many prescription drugs that can cause depression and mania, and the toxic chemicals that abound in the environment and the workplace.

Etiology. A wide range of drugs can produce depression and mania (e.g., antihypertensives, steroids).

Diagnosis and Clinical Features. When making the diagnosis of substance-induced mood disorder, the clinician should specify the substance involved, the time of onset (during intoxication or withdrawal), and the nature of the symptoms (e.g., manic or depressed) (Table 12.3–8). A maximum of 1 month between the use of the substance and the appearance of the symptoms is allowed in DSM-IV-TR, but the time frame is usually much shorter.

Substance-induced manic and depressive features can be identical to those of bipolar I disorder and major depressive disorder. Substance-induced mood disorder, however, may show more waxing and waning of symptoms and a fluctuation in a patient's level of consciousness.

Differential Diagnosis. A history of mood disorders in the patient or the patient's family weighs toward the diagnosis of a primary mood disorder, although such a history does not rule out the possibility of substance-induced mood disorder. Substances can also trigger an underlying mood disorder in a patient who is biologically vulnerable to mood disorders.

Table 12.3–9
DSM-IV-TR Diagnostic Criteria for Mood Disorder Not Otherwise Specified

This category includes disorders with mood symptoms that do not meet the criteria for any specific mood disorder and in which it is difficult to choose between depressive disorder not otherwise specified and bipolar disorder not otherwise specified (e.g., acute agitation).

From American Psychiatric Association. *Diagnostic and Statistical Manual of Mental Disorders.* 4th ed. Text rev. Washington, DC: American Psychiatric Association; copyright 2000, with permission.

Course and Prognosis. The course and prognosis of substance-induced mood disorder vary. Shortly after the substance has been cleared from the body, a normal mood usually returns. Sometimes, however, the substance exposure seems to precipitate a long-lasting mood disorder that may take weeks or months to resolve completely.

Treatment. The primary treatment of substance-induced mood disorder is the identification of the causally involved substance. Stopping the intake of the substance usually suffices to cause the mood disorder symptoms to abate. If the symptoms linger, treatment with appropriate psychiatric drugs may be necessary.

Mood Disorder Not Otherwise Specified

If patients exhibit mood symptoms that are difficult to distinguish between depression and mania and do not meet the diagnostic criteria for any other mood disorder or other DSM-IV-TR mental disorder, the most appropriate diagnosis is mood disorder not otherwise specified (Table 12.3–9). Clinicians are encouraged to try to make a more specific diagnosis, however.

13 ▲

Anxiety Disorders

▲ 13.1 Overview

Anxiety disorders are among the most prevalent mental disorders in the general population. Nearly 30 million persons are affected in the United States, with women affected nearly twice as frequently as men. Anxiety disorders are associated with significant morbidity and often are chronic and resistant to treatment. Anxiety disorders can be viewed as a family of related but distinct mental disorders, which include the following, as classified in the text revision of the fourth edition of *Diagnostic and Statistical Manual of Mental Disorders* (DSM-IV-TR): (1) panic disorder with or without agoraphobia; (2) agoraphobia with or without panic disorder; (3) specific phobia; (4) social phobia; (5) obsessive-compulsive disorder (OCD); (5) posttraumatic stress disorder (PTSD); (6) acute stress disorder; and (7) generalized anxiety disorder. Each of these disorders is discussed in detail in the sections that follow.

A fascinating aspect of anxiety disorders is the exquisite interplay of genetic and experiential factors. Little doubt exists that abnormal genes predispose to pathological anxiety states; however, evidence clearly indicates that traumatic life events and stress are also etiologically important. Thus, the study of anxiety disorders presents a unique opportunity to understand the relation between nature and nurture in the etiology of mental disorders.

NORMAL ANXIETY

Everyone experiences anxiety. It is characterized most commonly as a diffuse, unpleasant, vague sense of apprehension, often accompanied by autonomic symptoms such as headache, perspiration, palpitations, tightness in the chest, mild stomach discomfort, and restlessness, indicated by an inability to sit or stand still for long. The particular constellation of symptoms present during anxiety tends to vary among persons.

Fear versus Anxiety

Anxiety is an alerting signal; it warns of impending danger and enables a person to take measures to deal with a threat. Fear is a similar alerting signal, but it should be differentiated from anxiety. Fear is a response to a known, external, definite, or nonconflictual threat; anxiety is a response to a threat that is unknown, internal, vague, or conflictual.

This distinction between fear and anxiety arose accidentally. When Sigmund Freud's early translator mistranslated *angst*, the

German word for "fear," as anxiety, Freud generally ignored the distinction that associates anxiety with a repressed, unconscious object and fear with a known, external object. The distinction may be difficult to make because fear can also be caused by an unconscious, repressed, internal object displaced to another object in the external world. For example, a boy may fear barking dogs because he actually fears his father and unconsciously associates his father with barking dogs.

Nevertheless, according to postfreudian psychoanalytic formulations, the separation of fear and anxiety is psychologically justifiable. The emotion caused by a rapidly approaching car as a person crosses the street differs from the vague discomfort a person may experience when meeting new persons in a strange setting. The main psychological difference between the two emotional responses is the suddenness of fear and the insidiousness of anxiety.

Stress and Anxiety

Whether an event is perceived as stressful depends on the nature of the event and on the person's resources, psychological defenses, and coping mechanisms. All involve the ego, a collective abstraction for the process by which a person perceives, thinks, and acts on external events or internal drives. A person whose ego is functioning properly is in adaptive balance with both external and internal worlds; if the ego is not functioning properly and the resulting imbalance continues sufficiently long, the person experiences chronic anxiety.

Whether the imbalance is external, between the pressures of the outside world and the person's ego, or internal, between the person's impulses (e.g., aggressive, sexual, and dependent impulses) and conscience, the imbalance produces a conflict. Externally caused conflicts are usually interpersonal, whereas those that are internally caused are intrapsychic or intrapersonal. A combination of the two is possible, as in the case of employees whose excessively demanding and critical boss provokes impulses that they must control for fear of losing their jobs. Interpersonal and intrapsychic conflicts, in fact, are usually intertwined. Because human beings are social, their main conflicts are usually with other persons.

Symptoms of Anxiety

The experience of anxiety has two components: the awareness of the physiological sensations (e.g., palpitations and sweating) and the awareness of being nervous or frightened. A feeling of shame may increase anxiety—"Others will recognize that I am frightened." Many persons are astonished to find out that others are not aware of their anxiety or, if they are, do not appreciate its intensity.

In addition to motor and visceral effects, anxiety affects thinking, perception, and learning. It tends to produce confusion and distortions of perception, not only of time and space, but also of persons and the meanings of events. These distortions can interfere with learning by lowering concentration, reducing recall, and impairing the ability to relate one item to another—that is, to make associations.

An important aspect of emotions is their effect on the selectivity of attention. Anxious persons likely select certain things in their environment and overlook others in their effort to prove that they are justified in considering the situation frightening. If they falsely justify their fear, they augment their anxieties by the selective response and set up a vicious circle of anxiety, distorted perception, and increased anxiety. If, alternatively, they falsely reassure themselves by selective thinking, appropriate anxiety may be reduced, and they may fail to take necessary precautions.

PATHOLOGICAL ANXIETY

Epidemiology

The anxiety disorders make up one of the most common groups of psychiatric disorders. The National Comorbidity Study reported that one of four persons met the diagnostic criteria for at least one anxiety disorder and that there is a 12-month prevalence rate of 17.7 percent. Women (30.5 percent lifetime prevalence) are more likely to have an anxiety disorder than are men (19.2 percent lifetime prevalence). The prevalence of anxiety disorders decreases with higher socioeconomic status.

Contributions of Psychological Sciences

Three major schools of psychological theory—psychoanalytic, behavioral, and existential —have contributed theories about the causes of anxiety. Each theory has both conceptual and practical usefulness in treating anxiety disorders.

Psychoanalytic Theories.   Although Freud originally believed that anxiety stemmed from a physiological buildup of libido, he ultimately redefined anxiety as a signal of the presence of danger in the unconscious. Anxiety was viewed as the result of psychic conflict between unconscious sexual or aggressive wishes and corresponding threats from the superego or external reality. In response to this signal, the ego mobilized defense mechanisms to prevent unacceptable thoughts and feelings from emerging into conscious awareness. In his classic paper "Inhibitions, Symptoms, and Anxiety," Freud states that "it was anxiety which produced repression and not, as I formerly believed, repression which produced anxiety." Today, many neurobiologists continue to substantiate many of Freud's original ideas and theories. One example is the role of the amygdala, which subserves the fear response without any reference to conscious memory and substantiates Freud's concept of an unconscious memory system for anxiety responses. One of the unfortunate consequences of regarding the symptom of anxiety as a disorder rather than a signal is that the underlying sources of the anxiety may be ignored. From a psychodynamic perspective, the goal of therapy is not necessarily to eliminate all anxiety, but rather to increase anxiety tolerance, that is, the capacity to experience anxiety and use it as a signal to investigate the underlying conflict that has created it. Anxiety appears in response to various situations during the life cycle and, although psychopharmacological agents may ameliorate symptoms, they may do nothing to address the life situation or its internal correlates that have induced the state of anxiety. In the following case a disturbing fantasy precipitated an anxiety attack.

A married man 32 years of age was referred for therapy for severe and incapacitating anxiety, which was clinically manifested as repeated outbreaks of acute attacks of panic. Initially, he had absolutely no idea what had precipitated his attacks, nor were they associated with any conscious mental content. In the early weeks of treatment, he spent most of his time trying to impress the doctor with how hard he had worked and how effectively he had functioned before he was taken ill. At the same time, he described how fearful he was that he would fail at a new business venture he had embarked on. One day, with obvious acute anxiety that practically prevented him from talking, he revealed a fantasy that had suddenly popped into his mind a day or two before and had led to the outbreak of a severe anxiety attack. He had had the image of a large spike being driven through his penis. He also recalled that, as a child of 7, he was fascinated by his mother's clothing and that, on occasion, when she was out of the house, he dressed himself up in them. As an adult, he was fascinated by female lingerie and would sometimes find himself impelled by a desire to wear women's clothing. He had never yielded to the impulse, but on those occasions when the idea entered his consciousness, he became overwhelmed by acute anxiety and panic.

Behavioral Theories.   The behavioral or learning theories of anxiety postulate that anxiety is a conditioned response to a specific environmental stimulus. In a model of classic conditioning, a girl raised by an abusive father, for example, may become anxious as soon as she sees him. Through generalization, she may come to distrust all men. In the social learning model, a child may develop an anxiety response by imitating the anxiety in the environment, such as in anxious parents.

Existential Theories.   Existential theories of anxiety provide models for generalized anxiety, in which no specifically identifiable stimulus exists for a chronically anxious feeling. The central concept of existential theory is that persons experience feelings of living in a purposeless universe. Anxiety is their response to the perceived void in existence and meaning. Such existential concerns may have increased since the development of nuclear weapons and bioterrorism.

Contributions of Biological Sciences

Autonomic Nervous System.   Stimulation of the autonomic nervous system causes certain symptoms—cardiovascular (e.g., tachycardia), muscular (e.g., headache), gastrointestinal (e.g., diarrhea), and respiratory (e.g., tachypnea). The autonomic nervous systems of some patients with anxiety disorder, especially those with panic disorder, exhibit increased sympathetic tone, adapt slowly to repeated stimuli, and respond excessively to moderate stimuli.

Neurotransmitters.   The three major neurotransmitters associated with anxiety on the bases of animal studies and responses to drug treatment are norepinephrine, serotonin, and γ-aminobutyric acid (GABA). Much of the basic neuroscience information about anxiety comes from animal experiments involving behavioral paradigms and psychoactive agents. One such experiment used to study anxiety is the conflict test, in which an animal is simultaneously presented with stimuli that are positive (e.g., food) and negative (e.g., electric shock). Anxiolytic drugs (e.g., benzodiazepines) tend to facilitate the adaptation of the animal to this situation, whereas other drugs (e.g., amphetamines) further disrupt the animal's behavioral responses.

NOREPINEPHRINE.   Chronic symptoms experienced by patients with anxiety disorder, such as panic attacks, insomnia, startle, and autonomic hyperarousal, are characteristic of increased noradrenergic function. The general theory about the role of norepinephrine in anxiety disorders is that affected patients may have a poorly regulated noradrenergic system with occasional bursts of activity. The cell bodies of the noradrenergic system are primarily localized to the locus ceruleus in the rostral pons, and they project their axons to the cerebral cortex, the limbic system, the brainstem, and the spinal cord. Experiments in primates have demonstrated that stimulation of the locus ceruleus produces a fear response in the animals and that ablation of the same area inhibits or completely blocks the ability of the animals to form a fear response.

Human studies have found that in patients with panic disorder, β-adrenergic receptor agonists (e.g., isoproterenol [Isuprel]) and α_2-adrenergic receptor antagonists (e.g., yohimbine [Yocon]) can provoke frequent and severe panic attacks. Conversely, clonidine (Catapres), an α_2-receptor agonist, reduces anxiety symptoms in some experimental and therapeutic situations. A less-consistent finding is that patients with anxiety disorders, particularly panic disorder, have elevated cerebrospinal fluid or urinary levels of the noradrenergic metabolite 3-methoxy-4-hydroxyphenylglycol.

HYPOTHALAMIC-PITUITARY-ADRENAL AXIS.   Consistent evidence indicates that many forms of psychological stress increase the synthesis and release of cortisol. Cortisol serves to mobilize and to replenish energy stores and contributes to increased arousal, vigilance, focused attention, and memory formation; inhibition of the growth and reproductive system; and containment of the immune response. Excessive and sustained cortisol secretion can have serious adverse effects, including hypertension, osteoporosis, immunosuppression, insulin resistance, dyslipidemia, dyscoagulation, and, ultimately, atherosclerosis and cardiovascular disease. Alterations in hypothalamic-pituitary-adrenal (HPA) axis function have been demonstrated in PTSD. In patients with panic disorder, blunted adrenocorticoid hormone responses to corticotropin-releasing factor (CRF) have been reported in some studies and not in others.

CORTICOTROPIN-RELEASING HORMONE.   One of the most important mediators of the stress response, **corticotropin-releasing hormone** (CRH) coordinates the adaptive behavioral and physiological changes that occur during stress. Hypothalamic levels of CRH are increased by stress, resulting in activation of the HPA axis and increased release of cortisol and dehydroepiandrosterone. CRH also inhibits a variety of neurovegetative functions, such as food intake, sexual activity, and endocrine programs for growth and reproduction.

SEROTONIN.   The identification of many serotonin receptor types has stimulated the search for the role of serotonin in the pathogenesis of anxiety disorders. Different types of acute stress result in increased 5-hydroxytryptamine (5-HT) turnover in the prefrontal cortex, nucleus accumbens, amygdala, and lateral hypothalamus. The interest in this relation was initially motivated by the observation that serotonergic antidepressants have therapeutic effects in some anxiety disorders—for example, clomipramine (Anafranil) in OCD. The effectiveness of buspirone (BuSpar), a serotonin 5-HT$_{1A}$ receptor agonist, in the treatment of anxiety disorders also suggests the possibility of an association between

serotonin and anxiety. The cell bodies of most serotonergic neurons are located in the raphe nuclei in the rostral brainstem and project to the cerebral cortex, the limbic system (especially the amygdala and the hippocampus), and the hypothalamus. Several reports indicate that *meta*-chlorophenylpiperazine, a drug with multiple serotonergic and nonserotonergic effects, and fenfluramine (Pondimin), which causes the release of serotonin, do cause increased anxiety in patients with anxiety disorders; in addition, many anecdotal reports indicate that serotonergic hallucinogens and stimulants—for example, lysergic acid diethylamide and 3,4-methylenedioxymethamphetamine—are associated with the development of both acute and chronic anxiety disorders in persons who use these drugs. Clinical studies of 5-HT function in anxiety disorders have had mixed results. One study found that patients with panic disorder had lower levels of circulating 5-HT compared with controls. Thus, no clear pattern of abnormality in 5-HT function in panic disorder has emerged from analysis of peripheral blood elements.

GABA.   A role of GABA in anxiety disorders is most strongly supported by the undisputed efficacy of benzodiazepines, which enhance the activity of GABA at the GABA type A (GABA$_A$) receptor, in the treatment of some types of anxiety disorders. Although low-potency benzodiazepines are most effective for the symptoms of generalized anxiety disorder, high-potency benzodiazepines, such as alprazolam (Xanax), and clonazepam are effective in the treatment of panic disorder. Studies in primates have found that autonomic nervous system symptoms of anxiety disorders are induced when a benzodiazepine inverse agonist, β-carboline-3-carboxylic acid (BCCE), is administered. BCCE also causes anxiety in normal control volunteers. A benzodiazepine antagonist, flumazenil (Romazicon), causes frequent severe panic attacks in patients with panic disorder. These data have led researchers to hypothesize that some patients with anxiety disorders have abnormal functioning of their GABA$_A$ receptors, although this connection has not been shown directly.

APLYSIA.   A neurotransmitter model for anxiety disorders is based on the study of *Aplysia californica* by Nobel Prize winner Eric Kandel, M.D. *Aplysia* is a sea snail that reacts to danger by moving away, withdrawing into its shell, and decreasing its feeding behavior. These behaviors can be classically conditioned, so that the snail responds to a neutral stimulus as if it were a dangerous stimulus. The snail can also be sensitized by random shocks, so that it exhibits a flight response in the absence of real danger. Parallels have been drawn between classic conditioning and human phobic anxiety. The classically conditioned *Aplysia* shows measurable changes in presynaptic facilitation, resulting in the release of increased amounts of neurotransmitter. Although the sea snail is a simple animal, this work shows an experimental approach to complex neurochemical processes potentially involved in anxiety disorders in humans.

NEUROPEPTIDE Y.   Neuropeptide Y (NPY) is a highly conserved 36-amino acid peptide, which is among the most abundant peptides found in mammalian brain. Evidence suggesting the involvement of the amygdala in the anxiolytic effects of NPY is robust, and it probably occurs via the NPY-Y1 receptor. NPY has counterregulatory effects on CRH and locus ceruleus-norepinephrine systems at brain sites that are important in the expression of anxiety, fear, and depression. Preliminary studies in special operations soldiers under extreme training stress indicate that high NPY levels are associated with better performance.

GALANIN.   Galanin is a peptide that, in humans, contains 30 amino acids. It has been demonstrated to be involved in a number of physiological and behavioral functions, including learning and memory, pain control, food intake, neuroendocrine control, cardiovascular regulation, and, most recently, anxiety. A dense galanin immunoreactive fiber system originating in the LC innervates forebrain and midbrain structures, including the hippocampus, hypothalamus, amygdala, and prefrontal cortex. Studies in rats have shown that galanin administered centrally modulates anxiety-related behaviors. Galanin and NPY receptor agonists may be novel targets for antianxiety drug development.

Brain-Imaging Studies.

A range of brain-imaging studies, almost always conducted with a specific anxiety disorder, has produced several possible leads in the understanding of anxiety disorders. Structural studies—for example, computed tomography and magnetic resonance imaging (MRI)—occasionally show some increase in the size of cerebral ventricles. In one study, the increase was correlated with the length of time patients had been taking benzodiazepines. In one MRI study, a specific defect in the right temporal lobe was noted in patients with panic disorder. Several other brain-imaging studies have reported abnormal findings in the right hemisphere but not the left hemisphere; this finding suggests that some types of cerebral asymmetries may be important in the development of anxiety disorder symptoms in specific patients. Functional brain-imaging (fMRI) studies—for example, positron emission tomography, single photon emission computed tomography, and electroencephalography—of patients with anxiety disorder have variously reported abnormalities in the frontal cortex, the occipital and temporal areas, and, in a study of panic disorder, the parahippocampal gyrus.

Several functional neuroimaging studies have implicated the caudate nucleus in the pathophysiology of OCD. In posttraumatic stress disorder, fMRI studies have found increased activity in the amygdala, a brain region associated with fear. A conservative interpretation of these data is that some patients with anxiety disorders have a demonstrable functional cerebral pathological condition and that the condition may be causally relevant to their anxiety disorder symptoms.

Genetic Studies.

Genetic studies have produced solid evidence that at least some genetic component contributes to the development of anxiety disorders. Heredity has been recognized as a predisposing factor in the development of anxiety disorders. Almost half of all patients with panic disorder have at least one affected relative. The figures for other anxiety disorders, although not as high, also indicate a higher frequency of the illness in first-degree relatives of affected patients than in the relatives of nonaffected persons. Although adoption studies on anxiety disorders have not been reported, data from twin registers also support the hypothesis that anxiety disorders are at least partially genetically determined. Clearly, a linkage exists between genetics and anxiety disorders, but no anxiety disorder is likely to result from a simple mendelian abnormality. One report attributed about 4 percent of the intrinsic variability of anxiety within the general population to a polymorphic variant of the gene for the serotonin transporter, which is the site of action of many serotonergic drugs. Persons with the variant produce less transporter and have higher levels of anxiety.

In 2005, a scientific team led by National Institute of Mental Health grantee Eric Kandel demonstrated that knocking out a gene in the brain's fear hub creates mice unperturbed by situations that would normally trigger instinctive or learned fear responses. The gene codes for stathmin, a protein that is critical for the amygdala to form fear memories. Stathmin-knockout mice showed less anxiety when they heard a tone that had previously been associated with a shock, indicating less learned fear. The knockout mice also were more susceptible to exploring novel open space and maze environments, a reflection of less innate fear. Kandel suggests that stathmin-knockout mice can be used as a model of anxiety states of mental disorders with innate and learned fear components: These animals could be used to develop new antianxiety agents. Whether stathmin is similarly expressed and pivotal for anxiety in the human amygdala remains to be confirmed.

Neuroanatomical Considerations.

The locus ceruleus and the raphe nuclei project primarily to the limbic system and the cerebral cortex. In combination with the data from brain-imaging studies, these areas have become the focus of much hypothesis forming about the neuroanatomical substrates of anxiety disorders.

LIMBIC SYSTEM. In addition to receiving noradrenergic and serotonergic innervation, the limbic system also contains a high concentration of $GABA_A$ receptors. Ablation and stimulation studies in nonhuman primates have also implicated the limbic system in the generation of anxiety and fear responses. Increased activity in two areas of the limbic system has received special attention in the literature: the septohippocampal pathway, which may lead to anxiety, and the cingulate gyrus, which has been implicated particularly in the pathophysiology of OCD.

CEREBRAL CORTEX. The frontal cerebral cortex is connected with the parahippocampal region, the cingulate gyrus, and the hypothalamus and, thus, may be involved in the production of anxiety disorders. The temporal cortex has also been implicated as a pathophysiological site in anxiety disorders. This association is based in part on the similarity in clinical presentation and electrophysiology between some patients with temporal lobe epilepsy and patients with OCD.

▲ 13.2 Panic Disorder and Agoraphobia

An acute intense attack of anxiety accompanied by feelings of impending doom is known as *panic disorder*. The anxiety is characterized by discrete periods of intense fear that can vary from several attacks during one day to only a few attacks during a year. Patients with panic disorder present with a number of comorbid conditions, most commonly agoraphobia, which refers to a fear of or anxiety regarding places from which escape might be difficult.

Agoraphobia can be the most disabling of the phobias because it can significantly interfere with a person's ability to function in work and social situations outside the home. In the United States, most researchers of panic disorder believe that agoraphobia almost always develops as a complication in patients with panic disorder. That is, the fear of having a panic attack in a public place from which escape would be formidable is thought to cause the agoraphobia. Researchers in other countries as well as some researchers and clinicians in the United States disagree with this theory, but the text revision of the fourth edition of the *Diagnostic and Statistical Manual of Mental Disorders* (DSM-IV-TR) establishes panic disorder as the predominant disorder in the dyad. DSM-IV-TR includes diagnoses for panic disorder with and without agoraphobia and also for agoraphobia without a history of panic disorder. Panic attacks can also occur in many mental disorders (e.g., depressive disorders) and medical conditions (e.g., substance withdrawal or intoxication), and the presence of a panic attack does not in itself necessitate a diagnosis of panic disorder.

HISTORY

The idea of panic disorder may have its roots in the concept of irritable heart syndrome, which the physician Jacob Mendes DaCosta (1833–1900) noted in soldiers in the U.S. Civil War. DaCosta's syndrome included many psychological and somatic symptoms that have since been included among the diagnostic criteria for panic disorder. In 1895, Sigmund Freud introduced the concept of anxiety neurosis, consisting of acute and chronic psychological and somatic symptoms. Freud's acute anxiety neurosis was similar to panic disorder as defined in DSM-IV-TR, and Freud first noted the relation between panic attacks and agoraphobia. The term agoraphobia was coined in 1871 to describe the condition of patients who were afraid to venture alone into public places. The term is derived from the Greek words *agora* and *phobos*, meaning "fear of the marketplace."

EPIDEMIOLOGY

The lifetime prevalence of panic disorder is in the 1 to 4 percent range; the 6-month prevalence is approximately 0.5 to 1.0 percent, and that for panic attacks is 3 to 5.6 percent. Women are two to three times more likely to be affected than men, although underdiagnosis of panic disorder in men may contribute to the skewed distribution. The differences among Hispanics, whites, and blacks are few. The only social factor identified as contributing to the development of panic disorder is a recent history of divorce or separation. Panic disorder most commonly develops in young adulthood—the mean age of presentation is about 25 years—but both panic disorder and agoraphobia can develop at any age. Panic disorder has been reported in children and adolescents, and it is probably underdiagnosed in these age groups.

The lifetime prevalence of agoraphobia is somewhat more controversial, varying between 2 and 6 percent across studies. The major factor leading to this wide range of estimates relates to disagreement about the conceptualization of agoraphobia's relationship to panic disorder. Although studies of agoraphobia in psychiatric settings have reported that at least three fourths of the affected patients have panic disorder as well, studies of agoraphobia in community samples have found that as many as half of the patients have agoraphobia without panic disorder. The reasons for these divergent findings are unknown, but they probably involve differences in ascertainment techniques. In many cases, the onset of agoraphobia follows a traumatic event.

COMORBIDITY

Of patients with panic disorder, 91 percent have at least one other psychiatric disorder, as do 84 percent of those with agoraphobia. According to DSM-IV-TR, 10 to 15 percent of persons with panic disorder have comorbid major depressive disorder. About one third of persons with both disorders have major depressive disorder before the onset of panic disorder; about two thirds first experience panic disorder during or after the onset of major depression.

Anxiety disorders also commonly occur in persons with panic disorder and agoraphobia. Of persons with panic disorder, 15 to 30 percent also have social phobia, 2 to 20 percent have specific phobia, 15 to 30 percent have generalized anxiety disorder, 2 to 10 percent have posttraumatic stress disorder (PTSD), and up to 30 percent have obsessive-compulsive disorder (OCD). Other common comorbid conditions are hypochondriasis, personality disorders, and substance-related disorders.

ETIOLOGY
Biological Factors

Research on the biological basis of panic disorder has produced a range of findings; one interpretation is that the symptoms of panic disorder are related to a range of biological abnormalities in brain structure and function. Most work has used biological stimulants to induce panic attacks in patients with panic disorder. Considerable evidence indicates that abnormal regulation of brain noradrenergic systems is also involved in the pathophysiology of panic disorder. These and other studies have produced hypotheses implicating both peripheral and central nervous system (CNS) dysregulation in the pathophysiology of panic disorder. The autonomic nervous systems of some patients with panic disorder have been reported to exhibit increased sympathetic tone, to adapt slowly to repeated stimuli, and to respond excessively to moderate stimuli. Studies of the neuroendocrine status of these patients have shown several abnormalities, although the studies have been inconsistent in their findings.

The major neurotransmitter systems that have been implicated are those for norepinephrine, serotonin, and γ-aminobutyric acid (GABA). Serotonergic dysfunction is quite evident in panic disorder, and various studies with mixed serotonin agonist-antagonist drugs have demonstrated increased rates of anxiety. Such responses may be caused by postsynaptic serotonin hypersensitivity in panic disorder. Preclinical evidence suggests that attenuation of local inhibitory GABAergic transmission in the basolateral amygdala, midbrain, and hypothalamus can elicit anxiety-like physiological responses. The biological data have led to a focus on the brainstem (particularly the noradrenergic neurons of the locus ceruleus and the serotonergic neurons of the median raphe nucleus), the limbic system (possibly responsible for the generation of anticipatory anxiety), and the prefrontal cortex (possibly responsible for the generation of phobic avoidance). Among the various neurotransmitters involved, the noradrenergic system has also attracted much attention, with the presynaptic α_2-adrenergic receptors, in particular, playing a significant role. Patients with panic disorder are sensitive to the anxiogenic effects of yohimbine in addition to having exaggerated plasma 3-methoxy-4-hydroxyphenylglycol, cortisol, and cardiovascular responses. They have been identified by pharmacological challenges with the α_2-receptor agonist clonidine (Catapres) and the α_2-receptor antagonist yohimbine (Yocon), which stimulates firing of the locus ceruleus and elicits high rates of panic-like activity in those with panic disorder.

Panic-Inducing Substances. Panic-inducing substances (sometimes called *panicogens*) induce panic attacks in most patients with panic disorder and in a much smaller proportion of persons without panic disorder or a history of panic attacks. (The use of panic-inducing substances is strictly limited to research settings; no clinically indicated reasons exist to stimulate panic attacks in patients.) So-called respiratory panic-inducing substances cause respiratory stimulation and a shift in the acid-base balance. These substances include carbon dioxide (5 to 35 percent mixtures), sodium lactate, and bicarbonate. Neurochemical panic-inducing substances that act through specific neurotransmitter systems include yohimbine, an α_2-adrenergic receptor antagonist; *meta*-chlorophenylpiperazine, an agent with multiple serotonergic effects; GABA$_B$ receptor inverse agonists; flumazenil (Romazicon), a GABA$_B$ receptor antagonist; cholecystokinin; and caffeine. Isoproterenol (Isuprel) is also a panic-inducing substance, although its mechanism of action in inducing panic attacks is poorly understood. The respiratory panic-inducing substances may act initially at the peripheral cardiovascular baroreceptors and relay their signal by vagal afferents to the nucleus tractus solitarii and then on to the nucleus paragigantocellularis of the medulla. The hyperventilation in panic disorder patients may be caused by a hypersensitive suffocation alarm system whereby increasing partial pressure of carbon dioxide and brain lactate concentrations prematurely activates a physiological asphyxia monitor. The neurochemical panic-inducing substances are presumed primarily to affect the noradrenergic, serotonergic, and GABA receptors of the CNS directly.

Brain Imaging.   Structural brain-imaging studies, for example, magnetic resonance imaging (MRI), in patients with panic disorder have implicated pathological involvement in the temporal lobes, particularly the hippocampus and the amygdala. One MRI study reported abnormalities, especially cortical atrophy, in the right temporal lobe of these patients. Functional brain-imaging studies, for example, positron emission tomography (PET), have implicated dysregulation of cerebral blood flow (smaller increase or an actual decrease in cerebral blood flow). Specifically, anxiety disorders and panic attacks are associated with cerebral vasoconstriction, which may result in CNS symptoms, such as dizziness, and in peripheral nervous system symptoms that may be induced by hyperventilation and hypocapnia. Most functional brain-imaging studies have used a specific panic-inducing substance (e.g., lactate, caffeine, or yohimbine) in combination with PET or single photon emission computed tomography to assess the effects of the panic-inducing substance and the induced panic attack on cerebral blood flow.

Mitral Valve Prolapse.   Although great interest was formerly expressed in an association between mitral valve prolapse and panic disorder, research has almost completely erased any clinical significance or relevance to the association. Mitral valve prolapse is a heterogeneous syndrome consisting of the prolapse of one of the mitral valve leaflets, resulting in a midsystolic click on cardiac auscultation. Studies have found that the prevalence of panic disorder in patients with mitral valve prolapse is the same as the prevalence of panic disorder in patients without mitral valve prolapse.

Genetic Factors

Although few well-controlled studies of the genetic basis of panic disorder and agoraphobia have been conducted, the data support the conclusion that the disorders have a distinct genetic component. In addition, some data indicate that panic disorder with agoraphobia is a severe form of panic disorder and, thus, is more likely to be inherited. Various studies have found that the first-degree relatives of patients with panic disorder have a four- to eightfold higher risk for panic disorder than do first-degree relatives of other psychiatric patients. Twin studies have generally reported that monozygotic twins are more likely to be concordant for panic disorder than are dizygotic twins. No data exist indicating an association between a specific chromosomal location or mode of transmission and this disorder.

Psychosocial Factors

Both cognitive-behavioral and psychoanalytic theories have been developed to explain the pathogenesis of panic disorder and agoraphobia. The success of cognitive-behavioral approaches in the treatment of these disorders may add credence to the cognitive-behavioral theories.

Cognitive-Behavioral Theories.   Behavioral theories posit that anxiety is a response learned either from parental behavior or through the process of classic conditioning. In a classic conditioning approach to panic disorder and agoraphobia, a noxious stimulus (e.g., a panic attack) that occurs with a neutral stimulus (e.g., a bus ride) can result in the avoidance of the neutral stimulus. Other behavioral theories posit a linkage between the sensation of minor somatic symptoms (e.g., palpitations) and generation of a panic attack. Although cognitive-behavioral theories can help explain the development of agoraphobia or an increase in the number or severity of panic attacks, they do not explain the occurrence of the first unprovoked and unexpected panic attack that an affected patient experiences.

Psychoanalytic Theories.   Psychoanalytic theories conceptualize panic attacks as arising from an unsuccessful defense against anxiety-provoking impulses. What was previously a mild signal anxiety becomes an overwhelming feeling of apprehension, complete with somatic symptoms. To explain agoraphobia, psychoanalytic theories emphasize the loss of a parent in childhood and a history of separation anxiety. Being alone in public places revives the childhood anxiety about being abandoned. The defense mechanisms used include repression, displacement, avoidance, and symbolization. Traumatic separations during childhood can affect children's developing nervous systems in such a manner that they become susceptible to anxieties in adulthood. A predisposing neurophysiological vulnerability may interact with certain kinds of environmental stressors to produce the resulting panic attack.

DIAGNOSIS

Panic Attacks

The criteria for a panic attack are listed separately in the DSM-IV-TR (Table 13.2–1). Panic attacks can occur in mental disorders other than panic disorder, particularly in specific phobia, social phobia, and PTSD. Unexpected panic attacks occur at any time and are not associated with any identifiable situational stimulus, but panic attacks need not be unexpected. Attacks in patients with social and specific phobias are usually expected or cued to a recognized or specific stimulus. Some panic attacks do not fit easily into the distinction between unexpected and expected, and these attacks are referred to as *situationally predisposed panic attacks*. They may or may not occur when a patient is exposed to a specific trigger, or they may occur either immediately after exposure or after a considerable delay.

Table 13.2–1
DSM-IV-TR Criteria for Panic Attack

Note: A panic attack is not a codable disorder. Code the specific diagnosis in which the panic attack occurs (e.g., panic disorder with agoraphobia).

A discrete period of intense fear or discomfort, in which four (or more) of the following symptoms developed abruptly and reached a peak within 10 minutes:

(1) palpitations, pounding heart, or accelerated heart rate
(2) sweating
(3) trembling or shaking
(4) sensations of shortness of breath or smothering
(5) feeling of choking
(6) chest pain or discomfort
(7) nausea or abdominal distress
(8) feeling dizzy, unsteady, lightheaded, or faint
(9) derealization (feelings of unreality) or depersonalization (being detached from oneself)
(10) fear of losing control or going crazy
(11) fear of dying
(12) paresthesias (numbness or tingling sensations)
(13) chills or hot flushes

From American Psychiatric Association. *Diagnostic and Statistical Manual of Mental Disorders.* 4th ed. Text rev. Washington, DC: American Psychiatric Association; copyright 2000, with permission.

Panic Disorder

The DSM-IV-TR contains two diagnostic criteria for panic disorder, one without agoraphobia (Table 13.2–2) and the other with agoraphobia (Table 13.2–3), but both require the presence of panic attacks. Some community surveys have indicated that panic attacks are common, and a major issue in developing diagnostic criteria for panic disorder was determining a threshold

Table 13.2–2
DSM-IV-TR Diagnostic Criteria for Panic Disorder without Agoraphobia

A. Both (1) and (2):
  (1) recurrent unexpected panic attacks
  (2) at least one of the attacks has been followed by 1 month (or more) of one (or more) of the following:
    (a) persistent concern about having additional attacks
    (b) worry about the implications of the attack or its consequences (e.g., losing control, having a heart attack, "going crazy")
    (c) a significant change in behavior related to the attacks
B. Absence of agoraphobia
C. The panic attacks are not due to the direct physiological effects of a substance (e.g., a drug of abuse, a medication) or a general medical condition (e.g., hyperthyroidism).
D. The panic attacks are not better accounted for by another mental disorder, such as social phobia (e.g., occurring on exposure to feared social situations), specific phobia (e.g., on exposure to a specific phobic situation), obsessive-compulsive disorder (e.g., on exposure to dirt in someone with an obsession about contamination), posttraumatic stress disorder (e.g., in response to stimuli associated with a severe stressor), or separation anxiety disorder (e.g., in response to being away from home or close relatives).

From American Psychiatric Association. *Diagnostic and Statistical Manual of Mental Disorders.* 4th ed. Text rev. Washington, DC: American Psychiatric Association; copyright 2000, with permission.

Table 13.2–3
DSM-IV-TR Diagnostic Criteria for Panic Disorder with Agoraphobia

A. Both (1) and (2):
  (1) recurrent unexpected panic attacks
  (2) at least one of the attacks has been followed by 1 month (or more) of one (or more) of the following:
    (a) persistent concern about having additional attacks
    (b) worry about the implications of the attack or its consequences (e.g., losing control, having a heart attack, "going crazy")
    (c) a significant change in behavior related to the attacks
B. The presence of agoraphobia
C. The panic attacks are not due to the direct physiological effects of a substance (e.g., a drug of abuse, a medication) or a general medical condition (e.g., hyperthyroidism).
D. The panic attacks are not better accounted for by another mental disorder, such as social phobia (e.g., occurring on exposure to feared social situations), specific phobia (e.g., on exposure to a specific phobic situation), obsessive-compulsive disorder (e.g., on exposure to dirt in someone with an obsession about contamination), posttraumatic stress disorder (e.g., in response to stimuli associated with a severe stressor), or separation anxiety disorder (e.g., in response to being away from home or close relatives).

From American Psychiatric Association. *Diagnostic and Statistical Manual of Mental Disorders.* 4th ed. Text rev. Washington, DC: American Psychiatric Association; copyright 2000, with permission.

number or frequency of panic attacks required to meet the diagnosis. Setting the threshold too low results in the diagnosis of panic disorder in patients who do not have an impairment from an occasional panic attack; setting the threshold too high results in a situation in which patients who are impaired by their panic attacks do not meet the diagnostic criteria. The vagaries of setting a threshold are evidenced by the range of thresholds set in various diagnostic criteria. The Research Diagnostic Criteria require six panic attacks during a 6-week period. The 10th revision of the *International Statistical Classification of Diseases and Related Health Problems* (ICD-10) requires three attacks in 3 weeks (for moderate disease) or four attacks in 4 weeks (for severe disease). DSM-IV-TR does not specify a minimal number of panic attacks or a time frame but does require that at least one attack be followed by at least a month-long period of concern about having another panic attack or about the implications of the attack or a significant change in behavior. DSM-IV-TR also requires that the panic attacks generally be unexpected but allows for expected or situationally predisposed attacks.

Agoraphobia without History of Panic Disorder

Table 13.2–4 lists criteria for agoraphobia. The DSM-IV-TR diagnostic criteria for agoraphobia without history of panic disorder (Table 13.2–5) are based on the fear of a sudden incapacitating or embarrassing symptom. In contrast, the ICD-10 criteria require the presence of interrelated or overlapping phobias but do not require fear of incapacitating or embarrassing symptoms.

The DSM-IV-TR criteria also address the avoidance of situations that are based on a concern related to a medical disorder (e.g., fear of a myocardial infarction in a patient with severe heart disease).

**Table 13.2–4
DSM-IV-TR Criteria for Agoraphobia**

Note: Agoraphobia is not a codable disorder. Code the specific disorder in which the agoraphobia occurs (e.g., panic disorder with agoraphobia or agoraphobia without history of panic disorder).

A. Anxiety about being in places or situations from which escape might be difficult (or embarrassing) or in which help may not be available in the event of having an unexpected or situationally predisposed panic attack or panic-like symptoms. Agoraphobic fears typically involve characteristic clusters of situations that include being outside the home alone; being in a crowd or standing in a line; being on a bridge; and traveling in a bus, train, or automobile.
   Note: Consider the diagnosis of specific phobia if the avoidance is limited to one or only a few specific situations, or social phobia if the avoidance is limited to social situations.

B. The situations are avoided (e.g., travel is restricted) or else are endured with marked distress or with anxiety about having a panic attack or panic-like symptoms, or require the presence of a companion.

C. The anxiety or phobic avoidance is not better accounted for by another mental disorder, such as social phobia (e.g., avoidance limited to social situations because of fear of embarrassment), specific phobia (e.g., avoidance limited to a single situation like elevators), obsessive-compulsive disorder (e.g., avoidance of dirt in someone with an obsession about contamination), posttraumatic stress disorder (e.g., avoidance of stimuli associated with a severe stressor), or separation anxiety disorder (e.g., avoidance of leaving home or relatives).

From American Psychiatric Association. *Diagnostic and Statistical Manual of Mental Disorders*. 4th ed. Text rev. Washington, DC: American Psychiatric Association; copyright 2000, with permission.

CLINICAL FEATURES

Panic Disorder

The first panic attack is often completely spontaneous, although panic attacks occasionally follow excitement, physical exertion, sexual activity, or moderate emotional trauma. DSM-IV-TR emphasizes that at least the first attacks must be unexpected (uncued) to meet the diagnostic criteria for panic disorder. Clinicians should attempt to ascertain any habit or situation that commonly precedes a patient's panic attacks. Such activities may include

**Table 13.2–5
DSM-IV-TR Diagnostic Criteria for Agoraphobia without History of Panic Disorder**

A. The presence of agoraphobia related to fear of developing panic-like symptoms (e.g., dizziness or diarrhea).
B. Criteria have never been met for panic disorder.
C. The disturbance is not due to the direct physiological effects of a substance (e.g., a drug of abuse, a medication) or a general medical condition.
D. If an associated general medical condition is present, the fear described in Criterion A is clearly in excess of that usually associated with the condition.

From American Psychiatric Association. *Diagnostic and Statistical Manual of Mental Disorders*. 4th ed. Text rev. Washington, DC: American Psychiatric Association; copyright 2000, with permission.

the use of caffeine, alcohol, nicotine, or other substances; unusual patterns of sleeping or eating; and specific environmental settings, such as harsh lighting at work.

The attack often begins with a 10-minute period of rapidly increasing symptoms. The major mental symptoms are extreme fear and a sense of impending death and doom. Patients usually cannot name the source of their fear; they may feel confused and have trouble concentrating. The physical signs often include tachycardia, palpitations, dyspnea, and sweating. Patients often try to leave whatever situation they are in to seek help. The attack generally lasts 20 to 30 minutes and rarely more than 1 hour. A formal mental status examination during a panic attack may reveal rumination, difficulty speaking (e.g., stammering), and impaired memory. Patients may experience depression or depersonalization during an attack. The symptoms can disappear quickly or gradually. Between attacks, patients may have anticipatory anxiety about having another attack. The differentiation between anticipatory anxiety and generalized anxiety disorder can be difficult, although patients with pain disorder with anticipatory anxiety can name the focus of their anxiety.

Somatic concerns of death from a cardiac or respiratory problem may be the major focus of patients' attention during panic attacks. Patients may believe that the palpitations and chest pain indicate that they are about to die. As many as 20 percent of such patients actually have syncopal episodes during a panic attack. The patients may be seen in emergency rooms as young (20s), physically healthy persons who nevertheless insist that they are about to die from a heart attack. Rather than immediately diagnosing hypochondriasis, the emergency room physician should consider a diagnosis of panic disorder. Hyperventilation can produce respiratory alkalosis and other symptoms. The age-old treatment of breathing into a paper bag sometimes helps because it decreases alkalosis.

Agoraphobia

Patients with agoraphobia rigidly avoid situations in which it would be difficult to obtain help. They prefer to be accompanied by a friend or a family member in busy streets, crowded stores, closed-in spaces (e.g., tunnels, bridges, and elevators), and closed-in vehicles (e.g., subways, buses, and airplanes). Patients may insist that they be accompanied every time they leave the house. The behavior can result in marital discord, which may be misdiagnosed as the primary problem. Severely affected patients may simply refuse to leave the house. Particularly before a correct diagnosis is made, patients may be terrified that they are going crazy.

Associated Symptoms

Depressive symptoms are often present in panic disorder and agoraphobia, and in some patients, a depressive disorder coexists with the panic disorder. Some studies have found that the lifetime risk of suicide in persons with panic disorder is higher than it is in persons with no mental disorder. Clinicians should be alert to the risk of suicide. In addition to agoraphobia, other phobias and OCD can coexist with panic disorder. The psychosocial consequences of panic disorder and agoraphobia, in addition to marital discord, can include time lost from work, financial difficulties related to the loss of work, and alcohol and other substance abuse.

DIFFERENTIAL DIAGNOSIS
Panic Disorder

The differential diagnosis for a patient with panic disorder includes many medical disorders, as well as many mental disorders.

Medical Disorders

Panic disorder, with or without agoraphobia, must be differentiated from a number of medical conditions that produce similar symptomatology. Panic attacks are associated with a variety of endocrinological disorders, including both hypo- and hyperthyroid states, hyperparathyroidism, and pheochromocytomas. Episodic hypoglycemia associated with insulinomas can also produce panic-like states, as can primary neuropathological processes. These include seizure disorders, vestibular dysfunction, neoplasms, or the effects of both prescribed and illicit substances on the CNS. Finally, disorders of the cardiac and pulmonary systems, including arrhythmias, chronic obstructive pulmonary disease, and asthma, can produce autonomic symptoms and accompanying crescendo anxiety that can be difficult to distinguish from panic disorder. Clues of an underlying medical etiology to panic-like symptoms include the presence of atypical features during panic attacks, such as ataxia, alterations in consciousness, or bladder dyscontrol; onset of panic disorder relatively late in life; and physical signs or symptoms indicative of a medical disorder.

Mental Disorders

Panic disorder also must be differentiated from a number of psychiatric disorders, particularly other anxiety disorders. Panic attacks occur in many anxiety disorders, including social and specific phobia, PTSD, and even OCD. The key to correctly diagnosing panic disorder and differentiating the condition from other anxiety disorders involves the documentation of recurrent spontaneous panic attacks at some point in the illness. Differentiation from generalized anxiety disorder can also be difficult. Classically, panic attacks are characterized by their rapid onset (within minutes) and short duration (usually less than 10 to 15 minutes), in contrast to the anxiety associated with generalized anxiety disorder, which emerges and dissipates more slowly. Making this distinction can be difficult, however, because the anxiety surrounding panic attacks can be more diffuse and slower to dissipate than is typical. Because anxiety is a frequent concomitant of many other psychiatric disorders, including the psychoses and affective disorders, discrimination between panic disorder and a multitude of disorders can also be difficult.

Specific and Social Phobias

DSM-IV-TR addresses the sometimes difficult diagnostic task of distinguishing between panic disorder with agoraphobia, on the one hand, and specific and social phobias, on the other hand. Some patients who experience a single panic attack in a specific setting (e.g., an elevator) may go on to have long-lasting avoidance of the specific setting, regardless of whether they ever have another panic attack. These patients meet the diagnostic criteria for a specific phobia, and clinicians must use their judgment about what is the most appropriate diagnosis. In another example, a person who experiences one or more panic attacks may then fear speaking in public. Although the clinical picture is almost identical to the clinical picture in social phobia, a diagnosis of social phobia is excluded because the avoidance of the public situation is based on fear of having a panic attack rather than on fear of the public speaking itself. Because empirical data on the distinctions are limited, DSM-IV-TR advises clinicians to use their clinical judgment to diagnose difficult cases.

Agoraphobia without History of Panic Disorder

The differential diagnosis for agoraphobia without a history of panic disorder includes all of the medical disorders that can cause anxiety or depression. The psychiatric differential diagnosis includes major depressive disorder, schizophrenia, paranoid personality disorder, avoidance personality disorder, and dependent personality disorder.

COURSE AND PROGNOSIS
Panic Disorder

Panic disorder usually has its onset in late adolescence or early adulthood, although onset during childhood, early adolescence, and midlife does occur. Some data implicate increased psychosocial stressors with the onset of panic disorder, although no psychosocial stressor can be definitely identified in most cases.

Panic disorder, in general, is a chronic disorder, although its course is variable, both among patients and within a single patient. Long-term follow-up studies of panic disorder are difficult to interpret because they have not controlled for the effects of treatment. Nevertheless, about 30 to 40 percent of patients seem to be symptom free at long-term follow-up; about 50 percent have symptoms that are sufficiently mild not to affect their lives significantly; and about 10 to 20 percent continue to have significant symptoms.

After the first one or two panic attacks, patients may be relatively unconcerned about their condition; with repeated attacks, however, the symptoms may become a major concern. Patients may attempt to keep the panic attacks secret and thereby cause their families and friends concern about unexplained changes in behavior. The frequency and severity of the attacks can fluctuate. Panic attacks can occur several times in a day or less than once a month. Excessive intake of caffeine or nicotine can exacerbate the symptoms.

Depression can complicate the symptom picture in 40 to 80 percent of all patients, as estimated by various studies. Although the patients do not tend to talk about suicidal ideation, they are at increased risk for committing suicide. Alcohol and other substance dependence occurs in about 20 to 40 percent of all patients, and OCD may also develop. Family interactions and performance in school and at work commonly suffer. Patients with good premorbid functioning and symptoms of brief duration tend to have good prognoses.

Agoraphobia

Most cases of agoraphobia are thought to be caused by panic disorder. When the panic disorder is treated, the agoraphobia often improves with time. For rapid and complete reduction of agoraphobia, behavior therapy is sometimes indicated. Agoraphobia without a history of panic disorder is often incapacitating and chronic, and depressive disorders and alcohol dependence often complicate its course.

TREATMENT

With treatment, most patients exhibit dramatic improvement in the symptoms of panic disorder and agoraphobia. The two most effective treatments are pharmacotherapy and cognitive-behavioral therapy. Family and group therapy may help affected patients and their families adjust to the patient's disorder and to the psychosocial difficulties that the disorder may have precipitated.

Pharmacotherapy

Overview.   Alprazolam (Xanax) and paroxetine (Paxil) are the two drugs approved by the U.S. Food and Drug Administration (FDA) for the treatment of panic disorder. In general, experience is showing superiority of the selective serotonin reuptake inhibitors (SSRIs) and clomipramine (Anafranil) over the benzodiazepines, monoamine oxidase inhibitors (MAOIs), and tricyclic and tetracyclic drugs in terms of effectiveness and tolerance of adverse effects. A few reports have suggested a role for venlafaxine (Effexor), and buspirone (BuSpar) has been suggested as an additive medication in some cases. Venlafaxine is approved by the FDA for treatment of generalized anxiety disorder, and it may be useful in panic disorder combined with depression. β-Adrenergic receptor antagonists have not been found to be particularly useful for panic disorder. A conservative approach is to begin treatment with paroxetine, sertraline (Zoloft), citalopram (Celexa), or fluvoxamine (Luvox) in isolated panic disorder. If rapid control of severe symptoms is desired, a brief course of alprazolam should be initiated concurrently with the SSRI, followed by slowly tapering use of the benzodiazepine. In long-term use, fluoxetine (Prozac) is an effective drug for panic with comorbid depression, although its initial activating properties may mimic panic symptoms for the first several weeks, and it may be poorly tolerated on this basis. Clonazepam (Klonopin) can be prescribed for patients who anticipate a situation in which panic may occur (0.5 to 1 mg as required).

Selective Serotonin Reuptake Inhibitors.   All SSRIs are effective for panic disorder. Paroxetine and paroxetine CR have sedative effects and tend to calm patients immediately, which leads to greater compliance and less discontinuation. Citalopram, escitalopram (Lexapro), fluvoxamine, and sertraline are the next best tolerated. Anecdotal reports suggest that patients with panic disorder are particularly sensitive to the activating effects of SSRIs, particularly fluoxetine, so they should be given initially at small doses and titrated up slowly. Once at therapeutic doses—for example, 20 mg a day of paroxetine— some patients may experience increased sedation. One approach for patients with panic disorder is to give 5 or 10 mg a day of

paroxetine or 12.5 to 25 mg of paroxetine CR for 1 to 2 weeks, then increase the dose by 10 mg of paroxetine or 12.5 mg of paroxetine CR a day every 1 to 2 weeks to a maximum of 60 mg of paroxetine or 62.5 mg of paroxetine CR. If sedation becomes intolerable, then taper the paroxetine dose down to 10 mg a day of paroxetine or 12.5 mg of paroxetine CR and switch to fluoxetine at 10 mg a day and titrate upward slowly. Other strategies can be used, based on the experience of the clinician.

Benzodiazepines.   Benzodiazepines have the most rapid onset of action against panic, often within the first week, and they can be used for long periods without the development of tolerance to the antipanic effects. Alprazolam has been the most widely used benzodiazepine for panic disorder, but controlled studies have demonstrated equal efficacy for lorazepam (Ativan), and case reports have also indicated that clonazepam may be effective. Some patients use benzodiazepines as needed when faced with a phobic stimulus. Benzodiazepines can reasonably be used as the first agent for treatment of panic disorder while a serotonergic drug is being slowly titrated to a therapeutic dose. After 4 to 12 weeks, benzodiazepine use can be slowly tapered (over 4 to 10 weeks) while the serotonergic drug is continued. The major reservation among clinicians regarding the use of benzodiazepines for panic disorder is the potential for dependence, cognitive impairment, and abuse, especially after long-term use. Patients should be instructed not to drive, to abstain from alcohol or other CNS-depressant medications, and not to operate dangerous equipment while taking benzodiazepines. Benzodiazepines elicit a sense of well-being, whereas discontinuation of benzodiazepines produces a well-documented and unpleasant withdrawal syndrome. Anecdotal reports and small case series have indicated that addiction to alprazolam is one of the most difficult to overcome, and it may require a comprehensive program of detoxification. Benzodiazepine dosage should be tapered slowly, and all anticipated withdrawal effects should be thoroughly explained to the patient.

Tricyclic and Tetracyclic Drugs.   SSRIs are considered the first-line agents for the treatment of panic disorder. Data, however, show that among tricyclic drugs, clomipramine and imipramine (Tofranil) are the most effective in the treatment of panic disorder. Clinical experience indicates that the doses must be titrated slowly upward to avoid overstimulation and that the full clinical benefit requires full doses and may not be achieved for 8 to 12 weeks. Some data support the efficacy of desipramine (Norpramin), and less evidence suggests a role for maprotiline (Ludiomil), trazodone (Desyrel), nortriptyline (Pamelor), amitriptyline (Elavil), and doxepin (Adapin). Tricyclic drugs are less widely used than SSRIs because the tricyclic drugs generally have more severe adverse effects at the higher doses required for effective treatment of panic disorder.

Monoamine Oxidase Inhibitors.   The most robust data support the effectiveness of phenelzine (Nardil), and some data also support the use of tranylcypromine (Parnate). MAOIs appear less likely to cause overstimulation than either SSRIs or tricyclic drugs, but they may require full doses for at least 8 to 12 weeks to be effective. The need for dietary restrictions has limited the use of MAOIs, particularly since the appearance of the SSRIs.

Treatment Nonresponse.   If patients fail to respond to one class of drugs, another should be tried. Recent data support the effectiveness of venlafaxine. The combination of an SSRI or a tricyclic drug and a benzodiazepine or of an SSRI and lithium or a tricyclic drug can be tried. Case reports have suggested the effectiveness of carbamazepine (Tegretol), valproate (Depakene), and calcium channel inhibitors. Buspirone may have a role in the augmentation of other medications but has little effectiveness by itself. Clinicians should reassess the patient, particularly to establish the presence of comorbid conditions such as depression, alcohol use, or other substance use.

Duration of Pharmacotherapy.   Once it becomes effective, pharmacological treatment should generally continue for 8 to 12 months. Data indicate that panic disorder is a chronic, perhaps lifelong condition that recurs when treatment is discontinued. Studies have reported that 30 to 90 percent of patients with panic disorder who have had successful treatment have a relapse when their medication is discontinued. Patients may be likely to relapse if they have been given benzodiazepines and the benzodiazepine therapy is terminated in a way that causes withdrawal symptoms.

Cognitive and Behavior Therapies

Cognitive and behavior therapies are effective treatments for panic disorder. Various reports have concluded that cognitive and behavior therapies are superior to pharmacotherapy alone; other reports have concluded the opposite. Several studies and reports have found that the combination of cognitive or behavior therapy with pharmacotherapy is more effective than either approach alone. Several studies that included long-term follow-up of patients who received cognitive or behavior therapy indicate that the therapies are effective in producing long-lasting remission of symptoms.

Cognitive Therapy.   The two major foci of cognitive therapy for panic disorder are instruction about a patient's false beliefs and information about panic attacks. The instruction about false beliefs centers on the patient's tendency to misinterpret mild bodily sensations as indicating impending panic attacks, doom, or death. The information about panic attacks includes explanations that when panic attacks occur, they are time limited and not life threatening.

Mr. J was a 27-year-old laboratory technician who began having full-blown panic attacks 8 months before seeking help. Although he was unable to identify specific situations that elicited attacks, he was particularly concerned about the possibility of their occurring while he was engaged in laboratory procedures with patients. His attacks typically involved a sudden explosion of autonomic arousal and included palpitations, sweating, dizziness, feelings of unreality, and tingling in his arms and legs. He dreaded the idea that the attacks might recur. In the beginning of his cognitive-behavioral program, he found an educational handout that described the myths of panic attacks (e.g., that they will lead to heart attacks, losing control, or going crazy) particularly reassuring.

He began practicing diaphragmatic breathing each evening and, after several weeks, became effective in challenging his negative way of thinking about the consequences of panic attacks. In the latter few weeks of his 12-week program, he practiced exposing himself to physical sensations of panic by doing a variety of interoceptive exercises at home, including hyperventilating for 1 or 2 minutes at a time (designed to help Mr. J acclimate to the physical sensations associated with overbreathing), and spinning in a chair repeatedly (designed to help acclimate him to symptoms of dizziness and feelings of unreality). At the conclusion of the treatment program Mr. J's panic attacks had disappeared, and at 6-month follow-up he had maintained his treatment gains by attending "booster sessions" with his therapist once every 2 months.

Applied Relaxation.   The goal of applied relaxation (e.g., Herbert Benson's relaxation training) is to instill in patients a sense of control over their levels of anxiety and relaxation. Through the use of standardized techniques for muscle relaxation and the imagining of relaxing situations, patients learn techniques that may help them through a panic attack.

Respiratory Training.   Because the hyperventilation associated with panic attacks is probably related to some symptoms, such as dizziness and faintness, one direct approach to control panic attacks is to train patients to control the urge to hyperventilate. After such training, patients can use the technique to help control hyperventilation during a panic attack.

In Vivo Exposure.   In vivo exposure used to be the primary behavior treatment for panic disorder. The technique involves sequentially greater exposure of a patient to the feared stimulus; over time, the patient becomes desensitized to the experience. Previously, the focus was on external stimuli; recently, the technique has included exposure of the patient to internal feared sensations (e.g., tachypnea and fear of having a panic attack).

Other Psychosocial Therapies

Family Therapy.   Families of patients with panic disorder and agoraphobia may also have been affected by the family member's disorder. Family therapy directed toward education and support is often beneficial.

Insight-Oriented Psychotherapy.   Insight-oriented psychotherapy can be of benefit in the treatment of panic disorder and agoraphobia. Treatment focuses on helping patients understand the hypothesized unconscious meaning of the anxiety, the symbolism of the avoided situation, the need to repress impulses, and the secondary gains of the symptoms. A resolution of early infantile and oedipal conflicts is hypothesized to correlate with the resolution of current stresses.

Combined Psychotherapy and Pharmacotherapy

Even when pharmacotherapy is effective in eliminating the primary symptoms of panic disorder, psychotherapy may be needed to treat secondary symptoms. Glen O. Gabbard wrote

Panic-disordered patients frequently require a combination of drug therapy and psychotherapy. . . . Even when patients with panic attacks and agoraphobia have their symptoms pharmacologically controlled, they are often reluctant to venture out into the world again and may require psychotherapeutic interventions to help them overcome this fear. . . . Some patients will adamantly refuse any medication because they believe that it stigmatizes them as being mentally ill, so psychotherapeutic intervention is required to help them understand and eliminate their resistance to pharmacotherapy. For a comprehensive and effective treatment plan, these patients require psychotherapeutic approaches in addition to appropriate medications. In all patients with symptoms of panic disorder or agoraphobia, a careful psychodynamic evaluation will help weigh the contributions of biological and dynamic factors.

▲ 13.3 Specific Phobia and Social Phobia

The term *phobia* refers to an excessive fear of a specific object, circumstance, or situation. A specific phobia is a strong, persisting fear of an object or situation, whereas a social phobia is a strong, persisting fear of situations in which embarrassment can occur. The diagnosis of both specific and social phobias requires the development of intense anxiety, even to the point of panic, when exposed to the feared object or situation. Persons with specific phobias may anticipate harm, such as being bitten by a dog, or may panic at the thought of losing control; for instance, if they fear being in an elevator, they may also worry about fainting after the door closes. Persons with social phobias (also called *social anxiety disorder*) have excessive fears of humiliation or embarrassment in various social settings, such as in speaking in public, urinating in a public restroom (also called shy bladder), and speaking to a date. A generalized social phobia, which is often a chronic and disabling condition characterized by a phobic avoidance of most social situations, can be difficult to distinguish from avoidant personality disorder.

EPIDEMIOLOGY

Phobias are among the most common mental disorders in the United States; approximately 5 to 10 percent of the population is estimated to be afflicted with these troubling and sometimes disabling disorders. Less-conservative estimates have ranged as high as 25 percent of the population. The distress associated with phobias, especially when they are not recognized or acknowledged as mental disorders, can lead to further psychiatric complications, including other anxiety disorders, major depressive disorder, and substance-related disorders, especially alcohol use disorders.

Although phobias are common mental disorders, many persons with phobias either do not seek help to overcome their phobias or have their condition misdiagnosed when they do seek psychiatric or medical attention. The lifetime prevalence of specific phobia is about 11 percent, and the lifetime prevalence of social phobia has been reported to be 3 to 13 percent.

Specific Phobia

Specific phobia is more common than social phobia. Specific phobia is the most common mental disorder among women and the second most common among men, second only to substance-related disorders. The 6-month prevalence of specific phobia is about 5 to 10 per 100 persons. The rates of specific phobias in women (13.6 to 16.1 percent) are double those of men (5.2 to 6.7 percent), although the ratio is closer to 1 to 1 for the fear of blood, injection, or injury type. (Types of phobias are discussed later in this section.) The peak age of onset for the natural environment type and the blood-injection-injury type is in the range of 5 to 9 years, although onset also occurs at older ages. In contrast, the peak age of onset for the situational type (except fear of heights) is higher, in the mid-20s, which is closer to the age of onset for agoraphobia. The feared objects and situations in specific phobias (listed in descending frequency of appearance) are animals, storms, heights, illness, injury, and death.

Social Phobia

Various studies have reported a lifetime prevalence ranging from 3 to 13 percent for social phobia. The 6-month prevalence is about 2 to 3 per 100 persons. In epidemiological studies, females are affected more often than males, but in clinical samples, the reverse is often true. The reasons for these varying observations are unknown. The peak age of onset for social phobia is in the teens, although onset is common as young as 5 years of age and as old as 35 years of age.

COMORBIDITY

Persons with social phobia may have a history of other anxiety disorders, mood disorders, substance-related disorders, and bulimia nervosa. In addition, avoidant personality disorder frequently occurs in persons with generalized social phobia.

Reports of comorbidity in specific phobia range from 50 to 80 percent. Common comorbid disorders with specific phobia include anxiety, mood, and substance-related disorders.

ETIOLOGY

Both specific phobia and social phobia have types, and the precise causes of these types are likely to differ. Even within the types, as in all mental disorders, causative heterogeneity is found. The pathogenesis of the phobias, once it is understood, may prove to be a clear model for interactions between biological and genetic factors, on the one hand, and environmental events, on the other hand. In the blood-injection-injury type of specific phobia, affected persons may have inherited a particularly strong vasovagal reflex, which becomes associated with phobic emotions.

General Principles

Behavioral Factors. In 1920, John B. Watson wrote an article entitled "Conditioned Emotional Reactions" in which he recounted his experiences with Little Albert, an infant with a fear of rats and rabbits. Unlike Sigmund Freud's case of Little Hans, who had phobic symptoms (of horses) in the natural course of his maturation, Little Albert's difficulties were the direct result of the scientific experiments of two psychologists who used techniques that had successfully induced conditioned responses in laboratory animals.

Watson's hypothesis invoked the traditional pavlovian stimulus-response model of the conditioned reflex to account for the creation of the phobia: Anxiety is aroused by a naturally frightening stimulus that occurs in contiguity with a second, inherently neutral stimulus. As a result of the contiguity, especially when the two stimuli are paired on several successive occasions, the originally neutral stimulus becomes capable of arousing anxiety by itself. The neutral stimulus, therefore, becomes a conditioned stimulus for anxiety production.

In the classic stimulus-response theory, the conditioned stimulus gradually loses its potency to arouse a response if it is not reinforced by periodic repetition of the unconditioned stimulus. In phobias, attenuation of the response to the stimulus does not occur; the symptom may last for years without any apparent external reinforcement. Operant conditioning theory provides a model to explain this phenomenon: Anxiety is a drive that motivates the organism to do whatever it can to obviate a painful affect. In the course of its random behavior, the organism learns that certain actions enable it to avoid the anxiety-provoking stimulus. These avoidance patterns remain stable for long periods as a result of the reinforcement they receive from their capacity to diminish anxiety. This model is readily applicable to phobias, in that avoidance of the anxiety-provoking object or situation plays a central part. Such avoidance behavior becomes fixed as a stable symptom because of its effectiveness in protecting the person from the phobic anxiety.

Learning theory, which is particularly relevant to phobias, provides simple and intelligible explanations for many aspects of phobic symptoms. Critics contend, however, that learning theory deals mostly with surface mechanisms of symptom formation and is less useful than psychoanalytic theories in clarifying some of the complex underlying psychic processes involved.

Psychoanalytic Factors.   Freud's formulation of phobic neurosis is still the analytic explanation of specific phobia and social phobia. Freud hypothesized that the major function of anxiety is to signal the ego that a forbidden unconscious drive is pushing for conscious expression and to alert the ego to strengthen and marshal its defenses against the threatening instinctual force. Freud viewed the phobia—anxiety hysteria, as he continued to call it—as a result of conflicts centered on an unresolved childhood oedipal situation. Because sex drives continue to have a strong incestuous coloring in adults, sexual arousal can kindle an anxiety that is characteristically a fear of castration. When repression fails to be entirely successful, the ego must call on auxiliary defenses. In patients with phobias, the primary defense involved is displacement; that is, the sexual conflict is displaced from the person who evokes the conflict to a seemingly unimportant, irrelevant object or situation, which then has the power to arouse a constellation of affects, one of which is called *signal anxiety*. The phobic object or situation may have a direct associative connection with the primary source of the conflict and thus symbolizes it (the defense mechanism of symbolization).

Furthermore, the situation or the object is usually one that the person can avoid; with the additional defense mechanism of avoidance, the person can escape suffering serious anxiety. The end result is that the three combined defenses (repression, displacement, and symbolization) may eliminate the anxiety. The anxiety is controlled at the cost of creating a phobic neurosis, however. Freud first discussed the theoretical formulation of phobia formation in his famous case history of Little Hans, a 5-year-old boy who feared horses.

Although psychiatrists followed Freud's thought that phobias resulted from castration anxiety, recent psychoanalytic theorists have suggested that other types of anxiety may be involved. In agoraphobia, for example, separation anxiety clearly plays a leading role, and in erythrophobia (a fear of red that can be manifested as a fear of blushing), the element of shame implies the involvement of superego anxiety. Clinical observations have led to the view that anxiety associated with phobias has a variety of sources and colorings.

Phobias illustrate the interaction between a genetic constitutional diathesis and environmental stressors. Longitudinal studies suggest that certain children are constitutionally predisposed to phobias because they are born with a specific temperament known as *behavioral inhibition to the unfamiliar*, but a chronic environmental stress must act on a child's temperamental disposition to create a full-blown phobia. Stressors, such as the death of a parent, separation from a parent, criticism or humiliation by an older sibling, and violence in the household, may activate the latent diathesis within the child, who then becomes symptomatic.

Specific Phobia

The development of specific phobia may result from the pairing of a specific object or situation with the emotions of fear and panic. Various mechanisms for the pairing have been postulated. In general, a nonspecific tendency to experience fear or anxiety forms the backdrop; when a specific event (e.g., driving) is paired with an emotional experience (e.g., an accident), the person is susceptible to a permanent emotional association between driving or cars and fear or anxiety. The emotional experience itself can be in response to an external incident, as a traffic accident, or to an internal incident, most commonly a panic attack. Although a person may never again experience a panic attack and may not meet the diagnostic criteria for panic disorder, he or she may have a generalized fear of driving, not an expressed fear of having a panic attack while driving. Other mechanisms of association between the phobic object and the phobic emotions include modeling, in which a person observes the reaction in another (e.g., a parent), and information transfer, in which a person is taught or warned about the dangers of specific objects (e.g., venomous snakes).

Genetic Factors

Specific phobia tends to run in families. The blood-injection-injury type has a particularly high familial tendency. Studies have reported that two thirds to three fourths of affected probands have at least one first-degree relative with specific phobia of the same type, but the necessary twin and adoption studies have not been conducted to rule out a significant contribution by nongenetic transmission of specific phobia.

Social Phobia

Several studies have reported that some children possibly have a trait characterized by a consistent pattern of behavioral inhibition. This trait may be particularly common in the children of parents who are affected with panic disorder, and it may develop into severe shyness as the children grow older. At least some persons with social phobia may have exhibited behavioral inhibition during childhood. Perhaps associated with this trait, which is thought to be biologically based, are the psychologically based data indicating that the parents of persons with social phobia, as a group, were less caring, more rejecting, and more overprotective of their children than were other parents. Some social phobia research has referred to the spectrum from dominance to submission observed in the animal kingdom. For example, dominant humans may tend to walk with their chins in the air and to make eye contact, whereas submissive humans may tend to walk with their chins down and to avoid eye contact.

Neurochemical Factors. The success of pharmacotherapies in treating social phobia has generated two specific neurochemical hypotheses about two types of social phobia. Specifically, the use of β-adrenergic receptor antagonists—for example, propranolol (Inderal)—for performance phobias (e.g., public speaking) has led to the development of an adrenergic theory for these phobias. Patients with performance phobias may release more norepinephrine or epinephrine, both centrally and peripherally, than do nonphobic persons, or such patients may be sensitive to a normal level of adrenergic stimulation. The observation that monoamine oxidase inhibitors (MAOIs) may be more effective than tricyclic drugs in the treatment of generalized social phobia, in combination with preclinical data, has led some investigators to hypothesize that dopaminergic activity is related to the pathogenesis of the disorder. One study has shown significantly lower homovanillic acid concentrations. Another study, using single photon emission computed tomography, demonstrated decreased striatal dopamine reuptake site density. Thus, some evidence suggests dopaminergic dysfunction in social phobia.

Genetic Factors. First-degree relatives of persons with social phobia are about three times more likely to be affected with social phobia than are first-degree relatives of those without mental disorders. In addition, some preliminary data indicate that monozygotic twins are more often concordant than are dizygotic twins, although in social phobia it is particularly important to study twins reared apart to help control for environmental factors.

DIAGNOSIS

Specific Phobia

The text revision of the fourth edition of the *Diagnostic and Statistical Manual of Mental Disorders* (DSM-IV-TR) uses the term specific phobia to match the nomenclature in the 10th revision of the *International Statistical Classification of Diseases and Related Health Problems* (ICD-10). Table 13.3–1 lists the diagnostic criteria. Criteria A (excessive fear) and B (stimulus exposure) have been carefully worded in DSM-IV-TR to allow for the possibility that exposure to a phobic stimulus may result in a panic attack. In contrast to panic disorder, however, in specific phobia, the panic attack is situationally bound to the specific phobic stimulus. Criterion G (the anxiety attack) in DSM-IV-TR includes the words "not better accounted for" to emphasize the need for clinicians' judgment about diagnosing the symptoms. The specific content of the phobia and the strength of the relation (e.g., cued or noncued) between the stimulus and a panic attack also need to be considered.

The DSM-IV-TR includes distinctive types of specific phobia: animal type, natural environment type (e.g., storms), blood-injection-injury type, situational type (e.g., cars), and other type (for specific phobias that do not fit into the previous four types). Preliminary data indicate that the natural environment type is most common in children younger than 10 years of age and the situational type most often occurs in persons in their early 20s. The blood-injection-injury type is differentiated from the others in that bradycardia and hypotension often follow the initial tachycardia that is common to all phobias. The blood-injection-injury

Table 13.3–1
DSM-IV-TR Diagnostic Criteria for Specific Phobia

A. Marked and persistent fear that is excessive or unreasonable, cued by the presence or anticipation of a specific object or situation (e.g., flying, heights, animals, receiving an injection, seeing blood).
B. Exposure to the phobic stimulus almost invariably provokes an immediate anxiety response, which may take the form of a situationally bound or situationally predisposed panic attack.
Note: In children, the anxiety may be expressed by crying, tantrums, freezing, or clinging.
C. The person recognizes that the fear is excessive or unreasonable.
Note: In children, this feature may be absent.
D. The phobic situation(s) is avoided or else is endured with intense anxiety or distress.
E. The avoidance, anxious anticipation, or distress in the feared situation(s) interferes significantly with the person's normal routine, occupational (or academic) functioning, or social activities or relationships, or there is marked distress about having the phobia.
F. In individuals under age 18 years, the duration is at least 6 months.
G. The anxiety, panic attacks, or phobic avoidance associated with the specific object or situation are not better accounted for by another mental disorder, such as obsessive-compulsive disorder (e.g., fear of dirt in someone with an obsession about contamination), posttraumatic stress disorder (e.g., avoidance of stimuli associated with a severe stressor), separation anxiety disorder (e.g., avoidance of school), social phobia (e.g., avoidance of social situations because of fear of embarrassment), panic disorder with agoraphobia, or agoraphobia without history of panic disorder.
Specify type:
  Animal type
  Natural environment type (e.g., heights, storms, water)
  Blood-injection-injury type
  Situational type (e.g., airplanes, elevators, enclosed places)
  Other type (e.g., fear of choking, vomiting, or contracting an illness; in children, fear of loud sounds or costumed characters)

From American Psychiatric Association. *Diagnostic and Statistical Manual of Mental Disorders.* 4th ed. Text rev. Washington, DC: American Psychiatric Association; copyright 2000, with permission.

type of specific phobia is particularly likely to affect many members and generations of a family. One type of recently reported specific phobia is space phobia, in which persons are afraid of falling when there is no nearby support like a wall or a chair. Some data indicate that affected persons may have abnormal right hemisphere function, possibly resulting in visual-spatial impairment. Balance disorders should also be ruled out in such patients.

Focus. Phobias have traditionally been classified according to the specific fear by means of Greek or Latin prefixes, as indicated in Table 13.3–2: Other phobias that are related to changes in the society are fear of electromagnetic fields, fear of microwaves, and fear of society as a whole (amaxophobia).

Social Phobia. The DSM-IV-TR diagnostic criteria for social phobia (Table 13.3–3) acknowledge that the disorder can be associated with panic attacks. DSM-IV-TR also includes a

Table 13.3–2
Phobias

Acrophobia	Fear of heights
Agoraphobia	Fear of open places
Ailurophobia	Fear of cats
Hydrophobia	Fear of water
Claustrophobia	Fear of closed spaces
Cynophobia	Fear of dogs
Mysophobia	Fear of dirt and germs
Pyrophobia	Fear of fire
Xenophobia	Fear of strangers
Zoophobia	Fear of animals

specifier for generalized type, which may be useful in predicting course, prognosis, and treatment response. DSM-IV-TR excludes a diagnosis of social phobia when the symptoms are a result of social avoidance stemming from embarrassment about another psychiatric or nonpsychiatric medical condition.

Table 13.3–3
DSM-IV-TR Diagnostic Criteria for Social Phobia

A. A marked and persistent fear of one or more social or performance situations in which the person is exposed to unfamiliar people or to possible scrutiny by others. The individual fears that he or she will act in a way (or show anxiety symptoms) that will be humiliating or embarrassing. **Note:** In children, there must be evidence of the capacity for age-appropriate social relationships with familiar people and the anxiety must occur in peer settings, not just in interactions with adults.

B. Exposure to the feared social situation almost invariably provokes anxiety, which may take the form of a situationally bound or situationally predisposed panic attack. **Note:** In children, the anxiety may be expressed by crying, tantrums, freezing, or shrinking from social situations with unfamiliar people.

C. The person recognizes that the fear is excessive or unreasonable. **Note:** In children, this feature may be absent.

D. The feared social or performance situations are avoided or else are endured with intense anxiety or distress.

E. The avoidance, anxious anticipation, or distress in the feared social or performance situation(s) interferes significantly with the person's normal routine, occupational (academic) functioning, or social activities or relationships, or there is marked distress about having the phobia.

F. In individuals under age 18 years, the duration is at least 6 months.

G. The fear or avoidance is not due to the direct physiological effects of a substance (e.g., a drug of abuse, a medication) or a general medical condition and is not better accounted for by another mental disorder (e.g., panic disorder with or without agoraphobia, separation anxiety disorder, body dysmorphic disorder, a pervasive developmental disorder, or schizoid personality disorder).

H. If a general medical condition or another mental disorder is present, the fear in Criterion A is unrelated to it (e.g., the fear is not of stuttering, trembling in Parkinson's disease, or exhibiting abnormal eating behavior in anorexia nervosa or bulimia nervosa).

Specify if:
  Generalized: if the fears include most social situations (also consider the additional diagnosis of avoidant personality disorder)

From American Psychiatric Association. *Diagnostic and Statistical Manual of Mental Disorders.* 4th ed. Text rev. Washington, DC: American Psychiatric Association; copyright 2000, with permission.

Andy, a 25-year-old single man, lives with his mother and brother. He works as a mail sorter at the post office, a job he has had since he dropped out of college after 2 years. He came to an anxiety disorders clinic after reading a newspaper advertisement of the availability of free treatment if he participated in a research study of anxiety disorders. His chief complaint is of "nervousness." He says that right now he is "just going through the motions" and wants "to lead a normal life and go back to college."

During his adolescence and young adulthood, Andy had no close friends and usually preferred to be by himself. When he entered college, he formed several close friendships but became "super self-conscious" when speaking to strangers, classmates, and sometimes even friends. He would feel nervous, and his face would become so "stiff" that he had difficulty speaking. He had a "buzzing" in his head, felt as if he were "outside [his] body," had hot flashes, and perspired. These "panic attacks" (his term) came on suddenly, within seconds, and only when he was with people. When a classmate spoke to him, he sometimes "couldn't hear" what the classmate was saying because of his nervousness.

Outside of class, Andy began to feel increasingly uncomfortable in social situations. "I think that I was afraid of saying or doing something stupid." He began to turn down invitations to parties and to withdraw from other social activities (e.g., a bowling league). Eventually, he dropped out of college entirely.

Andy explains that the reason he chose to work at the post office is that the job does not require him to deal with people. When asked about other things that make him nervous, he says he tries to avoid using public lavatories and feels more comfortable in a public bathroom when the lights are dim, when there are few people present, and when he can use a stall rather than a urinal.

Andy has two long-standing "best" friends with whom he socializes regularly and feels completely comfortable. However, he hasn't dated since college, and he totally avoids group settings, such as weddings and dances. He has no problem with authority figures, and even welcomes constructive criticism from his supervisor at the post office. "My problem is nervousness, not obstinacy." (Reprinted with permission from *DSM-IV-TR Casebook.*)

CLINICAL FEATURES

Phobias are characterized by the arousal of severe anxiety, which is caused by exposure, or anticipated exposure, to specific objects or situations. DSM-IV-TR emphasizes the possibility that panic attacks can, and frequently do, occur in patients with specific and social phobias. The panic attacks, except perhaps for the first few, are to be expected. Exposure to the phobic stimulus or anticipation of it almost invariably results in a panic attack in a person who is susceptible to it.

Persons with phobias, by definition, try to avoid the phobic stimulus; some go to great trouble to avoid anxiety-provoking situations. For example, a patient with a phobia may take a bus across the United States rather than fly, to avoid contact with the object of the patient's phobia, an airplane. Perhaps as another way to avoid the stress of the phobic stimulus, many patients have substance-related disorders, particularly alcohol use disorders. Moreover, an estimated one third of patients with social phobia have major depressive disorder.

The major finding on the mental status examination is the presence of an irrational and ego-dystonic fear of a specific situation, activity, or object; patients are able to describe how they avoid contact with the phobia. Depression is commonly found on the mental status examination and may be present in as many as one third of all patients with phobia.

DIFFERENTIAL DIAGNOSIS

Specific phobia and social phobia need to be differentiated from appropriate fear and normal shyness, respectively. DSM-IV-TR aids in the differentiation by requiring that the symptoms impair the patient's ability to function appropriately. Nonpsychiatric medical conditions that can result in the development of a phobia include the use of substances (particularly hallucinogens and sympathomimetics), central nervous system tumors, and cerebrovascular diseases. Phobic symptoms in these instances are unlikely in the absence of additional suggestive findings on physical, neurological, and mental status examinations. Schizophrenia is also in the differential diagnosis of both specific phobia and social phobia because patients with schizophrenia can have phobic symptoms as part of their psychoses. Unlike patients with schizophrenia, however, patients with phobia have insight into the irrationality of their fears and lack the bizarre quality and other psychotic symptoms that accompany schizophrenia.

In the differential diagnosis of both specific phobia and social phobia, clinicians must consider panic disorder, agoraphobia, and avoidant personality disorder. Differentiation among panic disorder, agoraphobia, social phobia, and specific phobia can be difficult in individual cases. In general, however, patients with specific phobia or nongeneralized social phobia tend to experience anxiety immediately when presented with the phobic stimulus. Furthermore, the anxiety or panic is limited to the identified situation; patients are not abnormally anxious when they are neither confronted with the phobic stimulus nor caused to anticipate the stimulus.

A patient with agoraphobia is often comforted by the presence of another person in an anxiety-provoking situation, whereas a patient with social phobia is made more anxious than before by the presence of other persons. Whereas breathlessness, dizziness, a sense of suffocation, and a fear of dying are common in panic disorder and agoraphobia, the symptoms associated with social phobia usually involve blushing, muscle twitching, and anxiety about scrutiny. Differentiation between social phobia and avoidant personality disorder can be difficult and can require extensive interviews and psychiatric histories.

Specific Phobia

Other diagnoses to consider in the differential diagnosis of specific phobia are hypochondriasis, obsessive-compulsive disorder (OCD), and paranoid personality disorder. Hypochondriasis is the fear of having a disease, whereas specific phobia of the illness type is the fear of contracting the disease. Some patients with OCD manifest behavior indistinguishable from that of a patient with specific phobia. For example, patients with OCD may avoid knives because they have compulsive thoughts about killing their children, whereas patients with specific phobia about knives may avoid them for fear of cutting themselves. Patients with paranoid personality disorder have generalized fear that distinguishes them from those with specific phobia.

Social Phobia

Two additional differential diagnostic considerations for social phobia are major depressive disorder and schizoid personality disorder. The avoidance of social situations can often be a symptom in depression, but a psychiatric interview with the patient is likely to elicit a broad constellation of depressive symptoms. In patients with schizoid personality disorder, the lack of interest in socializing, not the fear of socializing, leads to the avoidant social behavior.

COURSE AND PROGNOSIS

Specific phobia exhibits a bimodal age of onset, with a childhood peak for animal phobia, natural environment phobia, and blood-injection-injury phobia and an early-adulthood peak for other phobias, such as situational phobia. As with other anxiety disorders, limited prospective epidemiological data exist on the natural course of specific phobia. Because patients with isolated specific phobias rarely present for treatment, research on the course of the disorder in the clinic is limited. The available information suggests that most specific phobias that begin in childhood and persist into adulthood continue to persist for many years. The severity of the condition is thought to remain relatively constant, without the waxing and waning course seen with other anxiety disorders.

Mr. A was a successful businessman who presented for treatment following a change in his business schedule. While he had formerly worked largely from an office near his home, a promotion led to a schedule of frequent out-of-town meetings, requiring weekly flights. Mr. A reported being "deathly afraid" of flying. Even the thought of getting on an airplane led to thoughts of impending doom as he envisioned his airplane crashing to the ground. These thoughts were associated with intense fear, palpitations, sweating, clammy palms, and stomach upset. While the thought of flying was terrifying enough, Mr. A became nearly incapacitated when he went to the airport. Immediately before boarding, Mr. A often had to turn back from the plane and run to the bathroom to vomit. (Courtesy of Daniel S. Pine, M.D.)

Social phobia tends to have its onset in late childhood or early adolescence. Social phobia tends to be a chronic disorder, although, as with the other anxiety disorders, prospective epidemiological data are limited. Both retrospective epidemiological studies and prospective clinical studies suggest that the disorder can profoundly disrupt the life of an individual over many years. This can include disruption in school or academic achievement and interference with job performance and social development.

TREATMENT

Behavior Therapy

The most studied and most effective treatment for phobias is probably behavior therapy. The key aspects of successful treatment are (1) the patient's commitment to treatment, (2) clearly identified problems and objectives, and (3) alternative strategies for coping with the feelings. A variety of behavioral treatment techniques have been used, the most common being systematic desensitization, a method pioneered by Joseph Wolpe. In this method, the patient is exposed serially to a predetermined list of anxiety-provoking stimuli graded in a hierarchy from the least to the most frightening. Through the use of antianxiety drugs, hypnosis, and instruction in muscle relaxation, patients are taught how to induce in themselves both mental and physical repose. Once they have mastered the techniques, patients are taught to use them to induce relaxation in the face of each anxiety-provoking stimulus. As they become desensitized to each stimulus in the scale, the patients move up to the next stimulus until, ultimately, what previously produced the most anxiety no longer elicits the painful affect.

Other behavioral techniques that have been used more recently involve intensive exposure to the phobic stimulus through either imagery or desensitization in vivo. In imaginal flooding, patients are exposed to the phobic stimulus for as long as they can tolerate the fear until they reach a point at which they can no longer feel it. Flooding (also known as implosion) in vivo requires patients to experience similar anxiety through exposure to the actual phobic stimulus.

Insight-Oriented Psychotherapy

Early in the development of psychoanalysis and the dynamically oriented psychotherapies, theorists believed that these methods were the treatments of choice for phobic neurosis, which at that time was thought to stem from oedipal-genital conflicts. Soon, however, therapists recognized that, despite progress in uncovering and analyzing unconscious conflicts, patients frequently failed to lose their phobic symptoms. Moreover, by continuing to avoid phobic situations, patients excluded a significant degree of anxiety and its related associations from the analytic process. Both Sigmund Freud and his pupil Sandor Ferenczi recognized that if progress in analyzing these symptoms was to be made, therapists had to go beyond their analytic roles and actively urge patients with phobia to seek the phobic situation and experience the anxiety and resultant insight. Since then, psychiatrists have generally agreed that a measure of activity on the therapist's part is often required to treat phobic anxiety successfully. The decision to apply the techniques of psychodynamic insight-oriented therapy should be based not on the presence of phobic symptoms alone, but also on positive indications from the patient's ego structure and life patterns for the use of this method of treatment. Insight-oriented therapy enables patients to understand the origin of the phobia, the phenomenon of secondary gain, and the role of resistance and enables them to seek healthy ways of dealing with anxiety-provoking stimuli.

Other Therapeutic Modalities

Hypnosis, supportive therapy, and family therapy may be useful in the treatment of phobic disorders. Hypnosis is used to enhance the therapist's suggestion that the phobic object is not dangerous, and self-hypnosis can be taught to the patient as a method of relaxation when confronted with the phobic object. Supportive psychotherapy and family therapy are often useful in helping the patient to actively confront the phobic object during treatment. Not only can family therapy enlist the aid of the family in treating the patient, but also it may help the family to understand the nature of the patient's problem.

Specific Phobia

A common treatment for specific phobia is exposure therapy. In this method, therapists desensitize patients by using a series of gradual, self-paced exposures to the phobic stimuli, and they teach patients various techniques to deal with anxiety, including relaxation, breathing control, and cognitive approaches. The cognitive-behavioral approaches include reinforcing the realization that the phobic situation is, in fact, safe. The key aspects of successful behavior therapy are the patient's commitment to treatment, clearly identified problems and objectives, and alternative strategies for coping with the patient's feelings. In the special situation of blood-injection-injury phobia, some therapists recommend that patients tense their bodies and remain seated during the exposure to help avoid the possibility of fainting from a vasovagal reaction to the phobic stimulation. β-Adrenergic receptor antagonists may be useful in the treatment of specific phobia, especially when the phobia is associated with panic attacks. Pharmacotherapy (e.g., benzodiazepines), psychotherapy, or combined therapy directed to the attacks may also be of benefit.

Social Phobia

Both psychotherapy and pharmacotherapy are useful in treating social phobias, and varying approaches are indicated for the generalized type and for performance situations. Some studies indicate that the use of both pharmacotherapy and psychotherapy produces better results than either therapy alone, although the finding may not be applicable to all situations and patients.

Effective drugs for the treatment of social phobia include (1) selective serotonin reuptake inhibitors (SSRIs), (2) the benzodiazepines, (3) venlafaxine (Effexor), and (4) buspirone (BuSpar). Most clinicians consider SSRIs the first-line treatment choice for patients with generalized social phobia. The benzodiazepines alprazolam (Xanax) and clonazepam (Klonopin) are also efficacious in both generalized and specific social phobia. Buspirone has shown additive effects when used to augment treatment with SSRIs.

In severe cases, successful treatment of social phobia with both irreversible MAOIs such as phenelzine (Nardil) and reversible inhibitors of monoamine oxidase such as moclobemide (Aurorix) and brofaromine (Consonar) (which are not available in the United States) has been reported. Therapeutic doses of phenelzine range from 45 to 90 mg a day, with response rates ranging from 50 to 70 percent, and approximately 5 to 6 weeks are needed to assess the efficacy.

The treatment of social phobia associated with performance situations frequently involves the use of β-adrenergic receptor antagonists shortly before exposure to a phobic stimulus. The two compounds most widely used are atenolol (Tenormin), 50 to 100 mg every morning or 1 hour before the performance, and propranolol (20 to 40 mg). Another option to help with performance anxiety is a relatively short- or intermediate-acting benzodiazepine, such as lorazepam or alprazolam. Cognitive, behavioral, and exposure techniques are also useful in performance situations.

Psychotherapy for the generalized type of social phobia usually involves a combination of behavioral and cognitive methods, including cognitive retraining, desensitization, rehearsal during sessions, and a range of homework assignments.

▲ 13.4 Obsessive-Compulsive Disorder

Obsessive-compulsive disorder (OCD) is represented by a diverse group of symptoms that include intrusive thoughts, rituals, preoccupations, and compulsions. These recurrent obsessions or compulsions cause severe distress to the person. The obsessions or compulsions are time-consuming and interfere significantly with the person's normal routine, occupational functioning, usual social activities, or relationships. A patient with OCD may have an obsession, a compulsion, or both.

An obsession is a recurrent and intrusive thought, feeling, idea, or sensation. In contrast to an obsession, which is a mental event, a compulsion is a behavior. Specifically, a compulsion is a conscious, standardized, recurrent behavior, such as counting, checking, or avoiding. A patient with OCD realizes the irrationality of the obsession and experiences both the obsession and the compulsion as ego-dystonic (i.e., unwanted behavior).

Although the compulsive act may be carried out in an attempt to reduce the anxiety associated with the obsession, it does not always succeed in doing so. The completion of the compulsive act may not affect the anxiety, and it may even increase the anxiety. Anxiety is also increased when a person resists carrying out a compulsion.

EPIDEMIOLOGY

The rates of OCD are fairly consistent, with a lifetime prevalence in the general population estimated at 2 to 3 percent. Some researchers have estimated that the disorder is found in as many as 10 percent of outpatients in psychiatric clinics. These figures make OCD the fourth-most-common psychiatric diagnosis after phobias, substance-related disorders, and major depressive disorder. Epidemiological studies in Europe, Asia, and Africa have confirmed these rates across cultural boundaries.

Among adults, men and women are equally likely to be affected, but among adolescents, boys are more commonly affected than girls. The mean age of onset is about 20 years, although men have a slightly earlier age of onset (mean about 19 years) than women (mean about 22 years). Overall, the symptoms of about two thirds of affected persons have an onset before age 25 years, and the symptoms of fewer than 15 percent have an onset after age 35 years. The onset of the disorder can occur in adolescence or childhood, in some cases as early as 2 years of age. Single persons are more frequently affected with OCD than are married persons, although this finding probably reflects the difficulty that persons with the disorder have in maintaining a relationship. OCD occurs less often among blacks than among whites, although access to health care rather than differences in prevalence may explain the variation.

COMORBIDITY

Persons with OCD are commonly affected by other mental disorders. The lifetime prevalence for major depressive disorder in persons with OCD is about 67 percent, and for social phobia it is about 25 percent. Other common comorbid psychiatric diagnoses in patients with OCD include alcohol use disorders, generalized anxiety disorder, specific phobia, panic disorder, eating disorders, and personality disorders. OCD exhibits a superficial resemblance to obsessive-compulsive personality disorder, which is associated with an obsessive concern for details, perfectionism, and other similar personality traits. The incidence of Tourette's disorder in patients with OCD is 5 to 7 percent, and 20 to 30 percent of patients with OCD have a history of tics.

ETIOLOGY

Biological Factors

Neurotransmitters

SEROTONERGIC SYSTEM.   The many clinical drug trials that have been conducted support the hypothesis that dysregulation of serotonin is involved in the symptom formation of obsessions and compulsions in the disorder. Data show that serotonergic drugs are more effective than drugs that affect other neurotransmitter systems, but whether serotonin is involved in the cause of OCD is not clear. Clinical studies have assayed cerebrospinal fluid (CSF) concentrations of serotonin metabolites (e.g., 5-hydroxyindoleacetic acid [5-HIAA]) and affinities and numbers of platelet-binding sites of tritiated imipramine (Tofranil), which binds to serotonin reuptake sites, and have reported variable findings of these measures in patients with OCD. In one study, the CSF concentration of 5-HIAA decreased after treatment with clomipramine (Anafranil), which has focused research attention on the serotonergic system.

NORADRENERGIC SYSTEM.   Less evidence exists for dysfunction in the noradrenergic system in OCD. Anecdotal reports show some improvement in OCD symptoms with use of oral clonidine (Catapres), a drug that lowers the amount of norepinephrine released from the presynaptic nerve terminals.

NEUROIMMUNOLOGY.   Some interest exists in a positive link between streptococcal infection and OCD. Group A β-hemolytic streptococcal infection can cause rheumatic fever, and approximately 10 to 30 percent of the patients develop Sydenham's chorea and show obsessive-compulsive symptoms.

Brain-Imaging Studies.   Neuroimaging in patients with OCD has produced converging data implicating altered function in the neurocircuitry between orbitofrontal cortex, caudate, and thalamus. Various functional brain-imaging studies—for example, positron emission tomography (PET)—have shown increased activity (e.g., metabolism and blood flow) in the frontal lobes, the basal ganglia (especially the caudate), and the cingulum of patients with OCD. The involvement of these areas in the pathology of OCD appears to be more associated with corticostriatal pathways than with the amygdala pathways that are the current focus of much anxiety disorder research. Pharmacological and behavioral treatments reportedly reverse these abnormalities. Data from functional brain-imaging studies are

consistent with data from structural brain-imaging studies. Both computed tomographic and magnetic resonance imaging (MRI) studies have found bilaterally smaller caudates in patients with OCD. Both functional and structural brain-imaging study results are also compatible with the observation that neurological procedures involving the cingulum are sometimes effective in the treatment of OCD. One recent MRI study reported increased T1 relaxation times in the frontal cortex, a finding consistent with the location of abnormalities discovered in PET studies.

Genetics. Genetic data on OCD support the hypothesis that the disorder has a significant genetic component. Relatives of probands with OCD consistently have a three- to fivefold higher probability of having OCD or obsessive-compulsive features than families of control probands. The data, however, do not yet distinguish the heritable factors from the influence of cultural and behavioral effects on the transmission of the disorder. Studies of concordance for the disorder in twins have consistently found a significantly higher concordance rate for monozygotic twins than for dizygotic twins. Some studies also demonstrate increased rates of a variety of conditions among relatives of OCD probands, including generalized anxiety disorder, tic disorders, body dysmorphic disorder, hypochondriasis, eating disorders, and habits such as nail-biting.

Other Biological Data. Electrophysiological studies, sleep electroencephalogram (EEG) studies, and neuroendocrine studies have contributed data that indicate some commonalities between depressive disorders and OCD. A higher-than-usual incidence of nonspecific EEG abnormalities occurs in patients with OCD. Sleep EEG studies have found abnormalities similar to those in depressive disorders, such as decreased rapid eye movement latency. Neuroendocrine studies have also produced some analogies to depressive disorders, such as nonsuppression on the dexamethasone-suppression test in about one third of patients and decreased growth hormone secretion with clonidine infusions.

As mentioned, studies have suggested a possible link between a subset of OCD cases and certain types of motor tic syndromes (i.e., Tourette's disorder and chronic motor tics). Higher rates of OCD, Tourette's disorder, and chronic motor tics are found in relatives of patients with Tourette's disorder than in relatives of controls, whether or not they had OCD. Most family studies of probands with OCD have found increased rates of Tourette's disorder and chronic motor tics only among the relatives of probands with OCD who also have some form of tic disorder. Evidence also suggests cotransmission of Tourette's syndrome, OCD, and chronic motor tics within families.

Behavioral Factors

According to learning theorists, obsessions are conditioned stimuli. A relatively neutral stimulus becomes associated with fear or anxiety through a process of respondent conditioning by being paired with events that are noxious or anxiety producing. Thus, previously neutral objects and thoughts become conditioned stimuli capable of provoking anxiety or discomfort.

Compulsions are established in a different way. When a person discovers that a certain action reduces anxiety attached to an obsessional thought, he or she develops active avoidance strategies in the form of compulsions or ritualistic behaviors to control the anxiety. Gradually, because of their efficacy in reducing a painful secondary drive (anxiety), the avoidance strategies become fixed as learned patterns of compulsive behaviors. Learning theory provides useful concepts for explaining certain aspects of obsessive-compulsive phenomena—for example, the anxiety-provoking capacity of ideas not necessarily frightening in themselves and the establishment of compulsive patterns of behavior.

Psychosocial Factors

Personality Factors. OCD differs from obsessive-compulsive personality disorder, which is associated with an obsessive concern for details, perfectionism, and similar personality traits. Most persons with OCD do not have premorbid compulsive symptoms, and such personality traits are neither necessary nor sufficient for the development of OCD. Only about 15 to 35 percent of patients with OCD have had premorbid obsessional traits.

Psychodynamic Factors. Psychodynamic insight may be of great help in understanding problems with treatment compliance, interpersonal difficulties, and personality problems accompanying the Axis I disorder. Many patients with OCD may refuse to cooperate with effective treatments such as selective serotonin reuptake inhibitors (SSRIs) and behavior therapy. Even though the symptoms of OCD may be biologically driven, psychodynamic meanings may be attached to them. Patients may become invested in maintaining the symptomatology because of secondary gains. For example, a male patient whose mother stays home to take care of him may unconsciously wish to hang on to his OCD symptoms because they keep the attention of his mother.

Another contribution of psychodynamic understanding involves the interpersonal dimensions. Studies have shown that relatives will accommodate the patient through active participation in rituals or significant modifications of their daily routines. This form of family accommodation is correlated with stress in the family, rejecting attitudes toward the patient, and poor family functioning. Often, the family members are involved in an effort to reduce the patient's anxiety or to control the patient's expressions of anger. This pattern of relatedness may become internalized and be recreated when the patient enters a treatment setting. By looking at recurring patterns of interpersonal relationships from a psychodynamic perspective, patients may learn how their illness affects others.

SIGMUND FREUD. In classic psychoanalytic theory, OCD was termed *obsessive-compulsive neurosis* and was considered a regression from the oedipal phase to the anal psychosexual phase of development. When patients with OCD feel threatened by anxiety about retaliation for unconscious impulses or by the loss of a significant object's love, they retreat from the oedipal position and regress to an intensely ambivalent emotional stage associated with the anal phase. The ambivalence is connected to the unraveling of the smooth fusion between sexual and aggressive drives characteristic of the oedipal phase. The coexistence of hatred and love toward the same person leaves patients paralyzed with doubt and indecision.

An example of how Freud viewed OCD symptoms is described by Otto Fenichel in the following case.

A patient, who was not analyzed, complained in the first interview that he suffered from the compulsion to look backward constantly, from fear that he might have overlooked something important behind him. These ideas were predominant; he might overlook a coin lying on the ground; he might have injured an insect by stepping on it; or an insect might have fallen on its back and need his help. The patient was also afraid of touching anything, and whenever he had touched an object he had to convince himself that he had not destroyed it. He had no vocation because the severe compulsions disturbed all his working activity; however, he had one passion: housecleaning. He liked to visit his neighbors and clean their houses, just for fun. Another symptom was described by the patient as his "clothes consciousness;" he was constantly preoccupied with the question whether or not his suit fitted. He, too, stated that sexuality did not play an important part in his life. He had sexual intercourse two or three times a year only, and exclusively with girls in whom he had no personal interest. Later on, he mentioned another symptom. As a child, he had felt his mother to be disgusting and had been terribly afraid of touching her. There was no real reason whatsoever for such a disgust, for the mother had been a nice person. (From Fenichel O. *The Psychoanalytic Theory of Neurosis.* New York: Norton; 1945:274, with permission.)

In this clinical picture, Freud believed the need to be clean and not to touch is related to anal sexuality, and the disgust for the mother is a reaction against incestuous fears.

One of the striking features of patients with OCD is the degree to which they are preoccupied with aggression or cleanliness, either overtly in the content of their symptoms or in the associations that lie behind them. The psychogenesis of OCD, therefore, may lie in disturbances in normal growth and development related to the anal-sadistic phase of development.

Ambivalence. Ambivalence is an important feature of normal children during the anal-sadistic developmental phase; children feel both love and murderous hate toward the same object, sometimes simultaneously. Patients with OCD often consciously experience both love and hate toward an object. This conflict of opposing emotions is evident in a patient's doing and undoing patterns of behavior and in paralyzing doubt in the face of choices.

Magical Thinking. In magical thinking, regression uncovers early modes of thought rather than impulses; that is, ego functions, as well as id functions, are affected by regression. Inherent in magical thinking is omnipotence of thought. Persons believe that merely by thinking about an event in the external world they can cause the event to occur without intermediate physical actions. This feeling causes them to fear having an aggressive thought.

DIAGNOSIS

As part of the diagnostic criteria for OCD, the text revision of the fourth edition of the *Diagnostic and Statistical Manual of Mental Disorders* (DSM-IV-TR) allows clinicians to specify that patients have the poor insight type of OCD if they generally do not recognize the excessiveness of their obsessions and compulsions (Table 13.4–1).

Table 13.4–1
DSM-IV-TR Diagnostic Criteria for Obsessive-Compulsive Disorder

A. Either obsessions or compulsions:
   Obsessions as defined by (1), (2), (3), and (4):
   (1) recurrent and persistent thoughts, impulses, or images that are experienced, at some time during the disturbance, as intrusive and inappropriate and that cause marked anxiety or distress
   (2) the thoughts, impulses, or images are not simply excessive worries about real-life problems
   (3) the person attempts to ignore or suppress such thoughts, impulses, or images, or to neutralize them with some other thought or action
   (4) the person recognizes that the obsessional thoughts, impulses, or images are a product of his or her own mind (not imposed from without as in thought insertion)
   Compulsions as defined by (1) and (2):
   (1) repetitive behaviors (e.g., hand washing, ordering, checking) or mental acts (e.g., praying, counting, repeating words silently) that the person feels driven to perform in response to an obsession, or according to rules that must be applied rigidly
   (2) the behaviors or mental acts are aimed at preventing or reducing distress or preventing some dreaded event or situation; however, these behaviors or mental acts either are not connected in a realistic way with what they are designed to neutralize or prevent or are clearly excessive
B. At some point during the course of the disorder, the person has recognized that the obsessions or compulsions are excessive or unreasonable. **Note:** This does not apply to children.
C. The obsessions or compulsions cause marked distress, are time-consuming (take more than 1 hour a day), or significantly interfere with the person's normal routine, occupational (or academic) functioning, or usual social activities or relationships.
D. If another Axis I disorder is present, the content of the obsessions or compulsions is not restricted to it (e.g., preoccupation with food in the presence of an eating disorder; hair pulling in the presence of trichotillomania; concern with appearance in the presence of body dysmorphic disorder; preoccupation with drugs in the presence of a substance use disorder; preoccupation with having a serious illness in the presence of hypochondriasis; preoccupation with sexual urges or fantasies in the presence of a paraphilia; or guilty ruminations in the presence of major depressive disorder).
E. The disturbance is not due to the direct physiological effects of a substance (e.g., a drug of abuse, a medication) or a general medical condition.

Specify if:
   With poor insight: if, for most of the time during the current episode, the person does not recognize that the obsessions and compulsions are excessive or unreasonable

From American Psychiatric Association. *Diagnostic and Statistical Manual of Mental Disorders.* 4th ed. Text rev. Washington, DC: American Psychiatric Association; copyright 2000, with permission.

CLINICAL FEATURES

Patients with OCD often take their complaints to physicians other than psychiatrists. Most patients with OCD have both obsessions and compulsions—up to 75 percent in some surveys. Some researchers and clinicians believe that the number may be much closer to 100 percent if patients are carefully assessed for the presence of mental compulsions in addition to behavioral compulsions. For example, an obsession about hurting a child may be followed by a mental compulsion to repeat a specific prayer a specific number of times. Other researchers and clinicians, however, believe that some patients do have only obsessive thoughts without compulsions. Such patients are likely to have repetitious thoughts of a sexual or aggressive act that is reprehensible to them. For clarity, it is best to conceptualize obsessions as thoughts and compulsions as behavior.

Obsessions and compulsions are the essential features of OCD. An idea or an impulse intrudes itself insistently and persistently into a person's conscious awareness. Typical obsessions associated with OCD include thoughts about contamination ("my hands are dirty") or doubts ("I forgot to turn off the stove").

A feeling of anxious dread accompanies the central manifestation, and the key characteristic of a compulsion is that it reduces the anxiety associated with the obsession. The obsession or the compulsion is ego-alien; that is, it is experienced as foreign to the person's experience of himself or herself as a psychological being. No matter how vivid and compelling the obsession or compulsion, the person usually recognizes it as absurd and irrational. The person suffering from obsessions and compulsions usually feels a strong desire to resist them. Nevertheless, about half of all patients offer little resistance to compulsions, although about 80 percent of all patients believe that the compulsion is irrational. Sometimes, patients overvalue obsessions and compulsions—for example, they may insist that compulsive cleanliness is morally correct, even though they have lost their jobs because of time spent cleaning.

Mental Status Examination

On mental status examinations, patients with OCD may show symptoms of depressive disorders. Such symptoms are present in about 50 percent of all patients. Some patients with OCD have character traits suggesting obsessive-compulsive personality disorder (e.g., excessive need for preciseness and neatness), but most do not. Patients with OCD, especially men, have a higher-than-average celibacy rate. Married patients have a greater-than-usual amount of marital discord.

The DSM-IV-TR diagnostic requirement of personal distress and functional impairment differentiates OCD from ordinary or mildly excessive thoughts and habits.

DIFFERENTIAL DIAGNOSIS

Medical Conditions

A number of primary medical disorders can produce syndromes bearing a striking resemblance to OCD. The current conceptualization of OCD as a disorder of the basal ganglia derives from the phenomenological similarity between idiopathic OCD and OCD-like disorders that are associated with basal ganglia diseases, such as Sydenham's chorea and Huntington's disease. Neurological signs of such basal ganglia pathology must be assessed when considering the diagnosis of OCD in a patient presenting for psychiatric treatment. It should also be noted that OCD frequently develops before age 30 years, and new-onset OCD in an older individual should raise questions about potential neurological contributions to the disorder.

Tourette's Disorder

Obsessive-compulsive disorder is closely related to Tourette's syndrome, as the two conditions frequently co-occur, both in individuals over time and within families. About 90 percent of persons with Tourette's disorder have compulsive symptoms, and as many as two thirds meet the diagnostic criteria for OCD.

In its classic form, Tourette's syndrome is associated with a pattern of recurrent vocal and motor tics that bears only a slight resemblance to OCD. The premonitory urges that precede tics often strikingly resemble obsessions, however, and many of the more complicated motor tics are very similar to compulsions.

Other Psychiatric Conditions

Obsessive-compulsive behavior is found in a host of other psychiatric disorders, and the clinician must also rule out these conditions when diagnosing OCD. OCD exhibits a superficial resemblance to obsessive-compulsive personality disorder, which is associated with an obsessive concern for details, perfectionism, and other similar personality traits. The conditions are easily distinguished, in that only OCD is associated with a true syndrome of obsessions and compulsions.

Psychotic symptoms often lead to obsessive thoughts and compulsive behaviors that can be difficult to distinguish from OCD with poor insight, in which obsessions border on psychosis. The keys to distinguishing OCD from psychosis are (1) patients with OCD can almost always acknowledge the unreasonable nature of their symptoms, and (2) psychotic illnesses are typically associated with a host of other features that are not characteristic of OCD. Similarly, OCD can be difficult to differentiate from depression because the two disorders often occur comorbidly, and major depression is often associated with obsessive thoughts that, at times, border on true obsessions such as those that characterize OCD. The two conditions are best distinguished by their courses. Obsessive symptoms associated with depression are only found in the presence of a depressive episode, whereas true OCD persists despite remission of depression.

COURSE AND PROGNOSIS

More than half of all patients with OCD have a sudden onset of symptoms. The onset of symptoms for about 50 to 70 percent of patients occurs after a stressful event, such as a pregnancy, a sexual problem, or the death of a relative. Because many persons manage to keep their symptoms secret, they often delay 5 to 10 years before coming to psychiatric attention, although the delay is probably shortening with increased awareness of the disorder. The course is usually long but variable; some patients experience a fluctuating course, and others experience a constant one.

About 20 to 30 percent of patients have significant improvement in their symptoms, and 40 to 50 percent have moderate improvement. The remaining 20 to 40 percent of patients either remain ill or see their symptoms worsen.

About one third of patients with OCD have major depressive disorder, and suicide is a risk for all patients with OCD. A poor prognosis is indicated by yielding to (rather than resisting) compulsions, childhood onset, bizarre compulsions, the need for hospitalization, a coexisting major depressive disorder, delusional beliefs, the presence of overvalued ideas (i.e., some acceptance of obsessions and compulsions), and the presence of a personality disorder (especially schizotypal personality disorder). A good prognosis is indicated by good social and occupational adjustment, the presence of a precipitating event, and an episodic nature of the symptoms. The obsessional content does not seem to be related to the prognosis.

TREATMENT

With mounting evidence that OCD is largely determined by biological factors, classic psychoanalytic theory has fallen out of favor. Moreover, because OCD symptoms appear to be largely refractory to psychodynamic psychotherapy and psychoanalysis, pharmacological and behavioral treatments have become common. However, psychodynamic factors may be of considerable benefit in understanding what precipitates exacerbations of the disorder and in treating various forms of resistance to treatment, such as noncompliance with medication.

Many patients with OCD tenaciously resist treatment efforts. They may refuse to take medication and may resist carrying out therapeutic homework assignments and other activities prescribed by behavior therapists. The obsessive-compulsive symptoms themselves, no matter how biologically based, may have important psychological meanings that make patients reluctant to give them up. Psychodynamic exploration of a patient's resistance to treatment may improve compliance.

Well-controlled studies have found that pharmacotherapy, behavior therapy, or a combination of both is effective in significantly reducing the symptoms of patients with OCD. The decision about which therapy to use is based on the clinician's judgment and experience and the patient's acceptance of the various modalities.

Pharmacotherapy

The efficacy of pharmacotherapy in OCD has been proved in many clinical trials and is enhanced by the observation that the studies find a placebo response rate of only about 5 percent.

The drugs, some of which are used to treat depressive disorders or other mental disorders, can be given in their usual dose ranges. Initial effects are generally seen after 4 to 6 weeks of treatment, although 8 to 16 weeks are usually needed to obtain maximal therapeutic benefit. Treatment with antidepressant drugs is controversial, and a significant proportion of patients with OCD who respond to treatment with antidepressant drugs seem to relapse if the drug therapy is discontinued.

The standard approach is to start treatment with an SSRI or clomipramine and then move to other pharmacological strategies if the serotonin-specific drugs are not effective. The serotonergic drugs have increased the percentage of patients with OCD who are likely to respond to treatment to the range of 50 to 70 percent.

Serotonin Specific Reuptake Inhibitors. Each of the SSRIs available in the United States—fluoxetine (Prozac), fluvoxamine (Luvox), paroxetine (Paxil), sertraline (Zoloft), citalopram (Celexa)— has been approved by the U.S. Food and Drug Administration (FDA) for the treatment of OCD. Higher doses have often been necessary for a beneficial effect, such as 80 mg a day of fluoxetine. Although the SSRIs can cause sleep disturbance, nausea and diarrhea, headache, anxiety, and restlessness, these adverse effects are often transient and are generally less troubling than the adverse effects associated with tricyclic drugs,

such as clomipramine. The best clinical outcomes occur when SSRIs are used in combination with behavioral therapy.

Clomipramine. Of all the tricyclic and tetracyclic drugs, clomipramine is the most selective for serotonin reuptake versus norepinephrine reuptake and is exceeded in this respect only by the SSRIs. The potency of serotonin reuptake of clomipramine is exceeded only by that of sertraline and paroxetine. Clomipramine was the first drug to be FDA approved for the treatment of OCD. Its dosing must be titrated upward over 2 to 3 weeks to avoid gastrointestinal adverse effects and orthostatic hypotension, and, as with other tricyclic drugs, it causes significant sedation and anticholinergic effects, including dry mouth and constipation. As with SSRIs, the best outcomes result from a combination of drug and behavioral therapy.

Other Drugs. If treatment with clomipramine or an SSRI is unsuccessful, many therapists augment the first drug by the addition of valproate (Depakene), lithium (Eskalith), or carbamazepine (Tegretol). Other drugs that can be tried in the treatment of OCD are venlafaxine (Effexor), pindolol (Visken), and the monoamine oxidase inhibitors, especially phenelzine (Nardil). Other pharmacological agents for the treatment of unresponsive patients include buspirone (BuSpar), 5-hydroxytryptamine, l-tryptophan, and clonazepam (Klonopin). Adding an atypical antipsychotic such as risperidol has helped in some cases.

Behavior Therapy

Although few head-to-head comparisons have been made, behavior therapy is as effective as pharmacotherapies in OCD, and some data indicate that the beneficial effects are longer lasting with behavior therapy. Many clinicians, therefore, consider behavior therapy the treatment of choice for OCD. Behavior therapy can be conducted in both outpatient and inpatient settings. The principal behavioral approaches in OCD are exposure and response prevention. Desensitization, thought stopping, flooding, implosion therapy, and aversive conditioning have also been used in patients with OCD. In behavior therapy, patients must be truly committed to improvement.

Psychotherapy

In the absence of adequate studies of insight-oriented psychotherapy for OCD, any valid generalizations about its effectiveness are hard to make, although there are anecdotal reports of successes. Individual analysts have seen striking and lasting changes for the better in patients with obsessive-compulsive personality disorder, especially when they are able to come to terms with the aggressive impulses underlying their character traits. Likewise, analysts and dynamically oriented psychiatrists have observed marked symptomatic improvement in patients with OCD in the course of analysis or prolonged insight psychotherapy.

Supportive psychotherapy undoubtedly has its place, especially for those patients with OCD who, despite symptoms of varying degrees of severity, are able to work and make social adjustments. With continuous and regular contact with an interested, sympathetic, and encouraging professional person, patients may be able to function by virtue of this help, without which their symptoms would incapacitate them. Occasionally, when obsessional rituals and anxiety reach an intolerable intensity, it is necessary to hospitalize patients until the shelter of an institution and the removal from external environmental stresses diminish symptoms to a tolerable level.

A patient's family members are often driven to the verge of despair by the patient's behavior. Any psychotherapeutic endeavors must include attention to the family members through provision of emotional support, reassurance, explanation, and advice on how to manage and respond to the patient.

Other Therapies

Family therapy is often useful in supporting the family, helping reduce marital discord resulting from the disorder, and building a treatment alliance with the family members for the good of the patient. Group therapy is useful as a support system for some patients.

For extreme cases that are treatment resistant and chronically debilitating, electroconvulsive therapy (ECT) and psychosurgery are considerations. ECT is not as effective as psychosurgery, but it should be tried before surgery. A common psychosurgical procedure for OCD is cingulotomy, which is successful in treating 25 to 30 percent of otherwise treatment-unresponsive patients. Other surgical procedures (e.g., subcaudate tractotomy, also known as *capsulotomy*) have also been used for this purpose. Nonablative surgical techniques involving indwelling electrodes in various basal ganglia nuclei (deep brain stimulation) are under investigation to treat both OCD and Tourette's disorder. All of these are increasingly being performed using MRI-guided stereotactic techniques. The most common complication of psychosurgery is the development of seizures, which are almost always controlled by treatment with phenytoin (Dilantin). Some patients who do not respond to psychosurgery alone and who do not respond to pharmacotherapy or behavior therapy before the operation do respond to pharmacotherapy or behavior therapy after psychosurgery.

▲ 13.5 Posttraumatic Stress Disorder and Acute Stress Disorder

Posttraumatic stress disorder (PTSD) is a condition marked by the development of symptoms after exposure to traumatic life events. The person reacts to this experience with fear and helplessness, persistently relives the event, and tries to avoid being reminded of it. Children who are behaviorally inhibited may be especially susceptible to anxiety or PTSD after threatening events.

To make the diagnosis, the symptoms must last for more than 1 month after the event and must significantly affect important areas of life, such as family and work. The text revision of the fourth edition of the *Diagnostic and Statistical Manual of Mental Disorders* (DSM-IV-TR) defines a disorder that is similar to PTSD called *acute stress disorder*, which occurs earlier than PTSD (within 4 weeks of the event) and remits within 2 days to 4 weeks. If symptoms persist after that time, a diagnosis of PTSD is warranted.

The stressors causing both acute stress disorder and PTSD are sufficiently overwhelming to affect almost anyone. They can arise from experiences in war or as a result of torture, natural catastrophes, assault, rape, and serious accidents, for example, in cars and in burning buildings. Persons reexperience the traumatic event in their dreams and their daily thoughts; they are determined to evade anything that would bring the event to mind, and they undergo a numbing of responsiveness along with a state of hyperarousal. Other symptoms are depression, anxiety, and cognitive difficulties, such as poor concentration.

EPIDEMIOLOGY

The lifetime incidence of PTSD is estimated to be 9 to 15 percent, and the lifetime prevalence of PTSD is estimated to be about 8 percent of the general population, although an additional 5 to 15 percent may experience subclinical forms of the disorder. Among high-risk groups whose members experienced traumatic events, the lifetime prevalence rates range from 5 to 75 percent. About 30 percent of Vietnam veterans have experienced PTSD, and an additional 25 percent have experienced subclinical forms of the disorder. The lifetime prevalence ranges from about 10 to 12 percent among women and from 5 to 6 percent among men. Although PTSD can appear at any age, it is most prevalent in young adults because they tend be more exposed to precipitating situations. Children can also have the disorder (discussed later in this section). Men and women differ in the types of traumas to which they are exposed and their liability to develop PTSD. The lifetime prevalence is significantly higher in women, and a higher proportion of women go on to develop the disorder. Historically, men's trauma was usually combat experience, and women's trauma was most commonly assault or rape. The disorder is most likely to occur in those who are single, divorced, widowed, socially withdrawn, or of low socioeconomic status. The most important risk factors for this disorder, however, are the severity, duration, and proximity of a person's exposure to the trauma. A familial pattern seems to exist for this disorder, and first-degree biological relatives of persons with a history of depression have an increased risk for developing PTSD following a traumatic event.

COMORBIDITY

Comorbidity rates are high among patients with PTSD, with about two thirds having at least two other disorders. Common comorbid conditions include depressive disorders, substance-related disorders, other anxiety disorders, and bipolar disorders. Comorbid disorders make persons more vulnerable to developing PTSD.

ETIOLOGY

Stressor

By definition, a stressor is the prime causative factor in the development of PTSD. Not everyone experiences the disorder after a traumatic event, however. The stressor alone does not suffice to cause the disorder. The response to the traumatic event must involve intense fear or horror. Clinicians must also consider individual preexisting biological and psychosocial factors and events that happened before and after the trauma. For example, a member of a group who lived through a disaster can sometimes deal with trauma because others shared the experience. The stressor's subjective meaning to a person is also important. For example, survivors of a catastrophe may experience guilt feelings (survivor guilt) that can predispose to, or exacerbate, PTSD.

Risk Factors

As mentioned, even when faced with overwhelming trauma, most persons do not experience PTSD symptoms. The National Comorbidity Study found that 60 percent of males and 50 percent of females had experienced some significant trauma, whereas the reported lifetime prevalence of PTSD was only 6.7 percent. Similarly, events that may appear mundane or less than catastrophic to most persons can produce PTSD in some. Evidence indicates a dose–response relationship between the degree of trauma and the likelihood of symptoms.

Psychodynamic Factors

The psychoanalytic model of the PTSD hypothesizes that the trauma has reactivated a previously quiescent yet unresolved psychological conflict. The revival of the childhood trauma results in regression and the use of the defense mechanisms of repression, denial, reaction formation, and undoing. According to Sigmund Freud, a splitting of consciousness occurs in patients who reported a history of childhood sexual trauma. A preexisting conflict might be symbolically reawakened by the new traumatic event. The ego relives and thereby tries to master and reduce the anxiety. Persons who suffer from alexithymia—the inability to identify or verbalize feeling states—are incapable of soothing themselves when under stress.

Cognitive-Behavioral Factors

The cognitive model of PTSD posits that affected persons cannot process or rationalize the trauma that precipitated the disorder. They continue to experience the stress and attempt to avoid experiencing it by avoidance techniques. Consistent with their partial ability to cope cognitively with the event, persons experience alternating periods of acknowledging and blocking the event. The attempt of the brain to process the massive amount of information provoked by the trauma is thought to produce these alternating periods. The behavioral model of PTSD emphasizes two phases in its development. First, the trauma (the unconditioned stimulus) that produces a fear response is paired, through classic conditioning, with a conditioned stimulus (physical or mental reminders of the trauma, such as sights, smells, or sounds). Second, through instrumental learning, the conditioned stimuli elicit the fear response independent of the original unconditioned stimulus, and persons develop a pattern of avoiding both the conditioned stimulus and the unconditioned stimulus. Some persons also receive secondary gains from the external world, commonly monetary compensation, increased attention or sympathy, and the satisfaction of dependency needs. These gains reinforce the disorder and its persistence.

Biological Factors

The biological theories of PTSD have developed both from preclinical studies of animal models of stress and from measures of biological variables in clinical populations with the disorder. Many neurotransmitter systems have been implicated by both sets of data. Preclinical models of learned helplessness, kindling, and sensitization in animals have led to theories about norepinephrine, dopamine, endogenous opioids, and benzodiazepine receptors and the hypothalamic-pituitary-adrenal (HPA) axis. In clinical populations, data have supported hypotheses that the noradrenergic and endogenous opiate systems, as well as the HPA axis, are hyperactive in at least some patients with PTSD. Other major biological findings are increased activity and responsiveness of the autonomic nervous system, as evidenced by elevated heart rates and blood pressure readings and by abnormal sleep architecture (e.g., sleep fragmentation and increased sleep latency). Some researchers have suggested a similarity between PTSD and two other psychiatric disorders, major depressive disorder and panic disorder.

Noradrenergic System. Soldiers with PTSD-like symptoms exhibit nervousness, increased blood pressure and heart rate, palpitations, sweating, flushing, and tremors—symptoms associated with adrenergic drugs. Studies found increased 24-hour urine epinephrine concentrations in veterans with PTSD and increased urine catecholamine concentrations in sexually abused girls. Furthermore, platelet α_2- and lymphocyte β-adrenergic receptors are downregulated in PTSD, possibly in response to chronically elevated catecholamine concentrations. About 30 to 40 percent of patients with PTSD report flashbacks after yohimbine (Yocon) administration. Such findings are strong evidence for altered function in the noradrenergic system in PTSD.

Opioid System. Abnormality in the opioid system is suggested by low plasma β-endorphin concentrations in PTSD. Combat veterans with PTSD demonstrate a naloxone (Narcan)-reversible analgesic response to combat-related stimuli, raising the possibility of opioid system hyperregulation similar to that in the HPA axis. One study showed that nalmefene (Revex), an opioid receptor antagonist, was of use in reducing symptoms of PTSD in combat veterans.

Corticotropin-Releasing Factor and the HPA Axis. Several factors point to dysfunction of the HPA axis. Studies have demonstrated low plasma and urinary free cortisol concentrations in PTSD. More glucocorticoid receptors are found on lymphocytes, and challenge with exogenous corticotropin-releasing factor yields a blunted adrenocorticotropic hormone response. Furthermore, suppression of cortisol by challenge with low-dose dexamethasone (Decadron) is enhanced in PTSD. This indicates hyperregulation of the HPA axis in PTSD. In addition, some studies have revealed cortisol hypersuppression in traumaexposed patients who develop PTSD compared with patients exposed to trauma who do not develop PTSD, indicating that it might be specifically associated with PTSD and not just trauma. Overall, this hyperregulation of the HPA axis differs from the neuroendocrine activity usually seen during stress and in other disorders such as depression. Recently, the role of the hippocampus in PTSD has received increased attention, although the issue remains controversial. Animal studies have shown that stress is associated with structural changes in the hippocampus, and studies of combat veterans with PTSD have revealed a lower average volume in the hippocampal region of the brain. Structural changes in the amygdala, an area of the brain associated with fear, have also been demonstrated.

DIAGNOSIS

The DSM-IV-TR diagnostic criteria for PTSD (Table 13.5–1) specify that the symptoms of experiencing, avoidance, and hyperarousal must have lasted more than 1 month. For patients

Table 13.5–1
DSM-IV-TR Diagnostic Criteria for Posttraumatic Stress Disorder

A. The person has been exposed to a traumatic event in which both of the following were present:

  (1) the person experienced, witnessed, or was confronted with an event or events that involved actual or threatened death or serious injury, or a threat to the physical integrity of self or others
  (2) the person's response involved intense fear, helplessness, or horror. **Note:** In children, this may be expressed instead by disorganized or agitated behavior.

B. The traumatic event is persistently reexperienced in one (or more) of the following ways:

  (1) recurrent and intrusive distressing recollections of the event, including images, thoughts, or perceptions. **Note:** In young children, repetitive play may occur in which themes or aspects of the trauma are expressed.
  (2) recurrent distressing dreams of the event. **Note:** In children, there may be frightening dreams without recognizable content.
  (3) acting or feeling as if the traumatic event were recurring (includes a sense of reliving the experience, illusions, hallucinations, and dissociative flashback episodes, including those that occur on awakening or when intoxicated). **Note:** In young children, trauma-specific reenactment may occur.
  (4) intense psychological distress at exposure to internal or external cues that symbolize or resemble an aspect of the traumatic event
  (5) physiological reactivity on exposure to internal or external cues that symbolize or resemble an aspect of the traumatic event

C. Persistent avoidance of stimuli associated with the trauma and numbing of general responsiveness (not present before the trauma), as indicated by three (or more) of the following:

  (1) efforts to avoid thoughts, feelings, or conversations associated with the trauma
  (2) efforts to avoid activities, places, or people that arouse recollections of the trauma
  (3) inability to recall an important aspect of the trauma
  (4) markedly diminished interest or participation in significant activities
  (5) feeling of detachment or estrangement from others
  (6) restricted range of affect (e.g., unable to have loving feelings)
  (7) sense of a foreshortened future (e.g., does not expect to have a career, marriage, children, or a normal life span)

D. Persistent symptoms of increased arousal (not present before the trauma), as indicated by two (or more) of the following:

  (1) difficulty falling or staying asleep
  (2) irritability or outbursts of anger
  (3) difficulty concentrating
  (4) hypervigilance
  (5) exaggerated startle response

E. Duration of the disturbance (symptoms in Criteria B, C, and D) is more than 1 month.

F. The disturbance causes clinically significant distress or impairment in social, occupational, or other important areas of functioning.

Specify if:

  Acute: if duration of symptoms is less than 3 months
  Chronic: if duration of symptoms is 3 months or more

Specify if:

  With delayed onset: if onset of symptoms is at least 6 months after the stressor

From American Psychiatric Association. *Diagnostic and Statistical Manual of Mental Disorders.* 4th ed. Text rev. Washington, DC: American Psychiatric Association; copyright 2000, with permission.

Table 13.5–2
DSM-IV-TR Diagnostic Criteria for Acute Stress Disorder

A. The person has been exposed to a traumatic event in which both of the following were present:

  (1) the person experienced, witnessed, or was confronted with an event or events that involved actual or threatened death or serious injury, or a threat to the physical integrity of self or others
  (2) the person's response involved intense fear, helplessness, or horror

B. Either while experiencing or after experiencing the distressing event, the individual has three (or more) of the following dissociative symptoms:

  (1) a subjective sense of numbing, detachment, or absence of emotional responsiveness
  (2) a reduction in awareness of his or her surroundings (e.g., "being in a daze")
  (3) derealization
  (4) depersonalization
  (5) dissociative amnesia (i.e., inability to recall an important aspect of the trauma)

C. The traumatic event is persistently reexperienced in at least one of the following ways: recurrent images, thoughts, dreams, illusions, flashback episodes, or a sense of reliving the experience; or distress on exposure to reminders of the traumatic event.

D. Marked avoidance of stimuli that arouse recollections of the trauma (e.g., thoughts, feelings, conversations, activities, places, people).

E. Marked symptoms of anxiety or increased arousal (e.g., difficulty sleeping, irritability, poor concentration, hypervigilance, exaggerated startle response, motor restlessness).

F. The disturbance causes clinically significant distress or impairment in social, occupational, or other important areas of functioning or impairs the individual's ability to pursue some necessary task, such as obtaining necessary assistance or mobilizing personal resources by telling family members about the traumatic experience.

G. The disturbance lasts for a minimum of 2 days and a maximum of 4 weeks and occurs within 4 weeks of the traumatic event.

H. The disturbance is not due to the direct physiological effects of a substance (e.g., a drug of abuse, a medication) or a general medical condition, is not better accounted for by brief psychotic disorder, and is not merely an exacerbation of a preexisting Axis I or Axis II disorder.

From American Psychiatric Association. *Diagnostic and Statistical Manual of Mental Disorders.* 4th ed. Text rev. Washington, DC: American Psychiatric Association; copyright 2000, with permission.

whose symptoms have been present less than 1 month, the appropriate diagnosis may be acute stress disorder (Table 13.5–2). The DSM-IV-TR diagnostic criteria for PTSD allow clinicians to specify whether the disorder is acute (if the symptoms have lasted less than 3 months) or chronic (if the symptoms have lasted 3 months or more). DSM-IV-TR also allows clinicians to specify that the disorder was with delayed onset if the onset of the symptoms was 6 months or more after the stressful event. An example of an acute stress disorder not progressing to PTSD as a result of timely therapy is given in the following vignette.

A 40-year-old man saw the September 11, 2001, terrorist attack on the World Trade Center [discussed later in this section] on television. Immediately thereafter he developed feelings of panic associated with thoughts that he was going to die. The panic disappeared within a few hours; however, for the next few nights he had nightmares with obsessive thoughts about dying. He sought consultation and reported to the psychiatrist that his wife had been killed in a plane crash 10 years earlier. He described having adapted to the loss "normally" and was aware that his current symptoms were probably related to that traumatic event. On further exploration in brief psychotherapy, he realized that his reactions to his wife's death were muted and that his relationship with her was ambivalent. At the time of her death he was contemplating divorce and frequently had wished her dead. He had never fully worked through the mourning process for his wife, and his catastrophic reaction to the terrorist attack was related, in part, to those suppressed feelings. He was able to recognize his feelings of guilt related to his wife and his need for punishment manifested by thinking he was going to die.

CLINICAL FEATURES

The principal clinical features of PTSD are painful reexperiencing of the event, a pattern of avoidance and emotional numbing, and fairly constant hyperarousal. The disorder may not develop until months or even years after the event. The mental status examination often reveals feelings of guilt, rejection, and humiliation. Patients may also describe dissociative states and panic attacks, and illusions and hallucinations may be present. Associated symptoms can include aggression, violence, poor impulse control, depression, and substance-related disorders. Cognitive testing may reveal that patients have impaired memory and attention. Patients have elevated Sc, D, F, and Ps scores on the Minnesota Multiphasic Personality Inventory, and the Rorschach test findings often include aggressive and violent material.

PTSDs in Children and Adolescents

PTSD occurs in children and adolescents, but most studies of the disorder have focused on adults. DSM-IV-TR has little to say about PTSD as it affects young children except to describe symptoms such as repetitive dreams of the event, nightmares of monsters, and the development of physical symptoms such as stomachaches and headaches.

High rates of PTSD have been documented in children exposed to such life-threatening events as combat and other war-related trauma, kidnapping, severe illness or burns, bone marrow transplantation, and a number of natural and human-caused disasters. Studies on young victims or witnesses to criminal assault, domestic violence, and community violence have revealed high psychiatric morbidity following exposure to violence. As might be expected, the prevalence of PTSD is higher in children than in adults exposed to the same stressor. In certain situations, up to 90 percent of children will develop the disorder. In general, PTSD has been underestimated in children and adolescents.

Child risk factors include demographic factors (e.g., age, sex, socioeconomic status), other life events (positive and negative), social and cultural cognitions, psychiatric comorbidity, and inherent coping strategies. Family factors (e.g., parental psychopathology and functioning, marital status, and education) play key roles in determining a child's symptoms. Parents' responses to traumatic events particularly influence young children, who may not completely understand the nature of the trauma or its inherent danger.

Stressor. Stressors in children may be sudden, single-incident trauma or ongoing or chronic trauma, such as physical or sexual abuse. Children also suffer as the result of "indirect" exposure—that is, the unwitnessed death or injury of a loved one, as in situations of disaster, war, or community violence.

Reenactment and Reexperiencing. Children, as with adults, reexperience the traumatic event in the form of distressing, intrusive thoughts or memories, flashbacks, and dreams. Children's nightmares may be linked specifically to a trauma theme or may generalize to other fears. Flashbacks occur in children as well as in their adolescent or adult victim counterparts. "Traumatic play," a specific form of reexperiencing seen in young children, consists of repetitive acting out of the trauma or trauma-related themes in play. Older children may incorporate aspects of the trauma into their lives in a process termed *reenactment*. Fantasized actions of intervention or revenge are common; adolescents should be considered at increased risk for impulsive acting out secondary to anger and revenge fantasies. Related behaviors in child and adolescent victims of trauma include sexual acting out, substance use, and delinquency. Children often withdraw and show reduced interest in previously enjoyable activities. Regressive behaviors, such as enuresis or fear of sleeping alone, may also occur.

Gulf War Syndrome

In the Persian Gulf War against Iraq, which began in 1990 and ended in 1991, approximately 700,000 U.S. soldiers served in the coalition forces. On their return, more than 100,000 U.S. veterans reported a vast array of health problems, including irritability, chronic fatigue, shortness of breath, muscle and joint pain, migraine headaches, digestive disturbances, rash, hair loss, forgetfulness, and difficulty concentrating. Collectively, these symptoms were called the *Gulf War syndrome*. The U.S. Department of Defense acknowledges that up to 20,000 troops serving in the combat area may have been exposed to chemical weapons, and the best evidence indicates that the condition is a disorder that in some cases may have been precipitated by exposure to an unidentified toxin. One study of loss of memory found structural change in the right parietal lobe and damage to the basal ganglia with associated neurotransmitter dysfunction. A significant number of veterans have developed amyotrophic lateral sclerosis, thought to be the result of genetic mutations.

In addition, thousands of Gulf War veterans developed PTSD, and the differentiation between it and Gulf War syndrome has proved difficult. PTSD is caused by psychological stress, and the Gulf War syndrome is presumed to be caused by environmental biological stressors. Signs and symptoms often overlap, and both conditions may exist at the same time.

9/11/01

On September 11, 2001, terrorist activity destroyed the World Trade Center in New York City and damaged the Pentagon in Washington, D.C. It resulted in more than 3,500 deaths and injuries and left many people in need of therapeutic intervention.

One survey found a prevalence rate of 11.4 percent for PTSD and 9.7 percent for depression in U.S. citizens 1 month after 9/11. As of 2004, it was estimated that more than 25,000 people continued to suffer symptoms of PTSD related to the 9/11 attacks beyond the 1-year mark.

Wars in Iraq and Afghanistan

In October 2001, the United States, along with Australia, Canada, and the United Kingdom, began the invasion of Afghanistan in the wake of the September 11, 2001 attacks. On March 20, 2003, U.S. forces, along with allies, invaded Iraq, marking the beginning of the Iraq War.

Both wars are ongoing, and PTSD is a rising problem, with an estimated 17 percent of returning soldiers having PTSD. The rate of PTSD is higher in women soldiers. Women account for 11 percent of those who served in Iraq and Afghanistan and for 14 percent of patients at Veterans Affairs hospitals and clinics. Women soldiers are more likely to seek help than are men soldiers.

Natural Disasters

Tsunami.   On December 26, 2004, a massive tsunami struck the shores of Indonesia, Sri Lanka, South India, and Thailand and caused serious damage and deaths as far west as the eastern coast of Africa and South Africa. The tsunami caused nearly 300,000 deaths and left more than 1 million people without homes. Many survivors continue to live in fear and show signs of PTSD; fishermen fear venturing out to sea, children fear playing at beaches they once enjoyed, and many families have trouble sleeping in fear of another tsunami.

Hurricane.   In August 2005, a category 5 hurricane, Hurricane Katrina, ravaged the Gulf of Mexico, the Bahamas, southern Florida, Louisiana, Mississippi, and Alabama. Its high winds and torrential rainfall breached the levee system that protected New Orleans, Louisiana, causing major flooding. More than 1,300 people were killed, and tens of thousands were stranded.

Earthquake.   On October 8, 2005, a magnitude 7.6 earthquake hit parts of Asia, affecting Pakistan, Afghanistan, and northern India. The area of Kashmir was the worst hit. More than 85,000 casualties occurred. Up to 3 million people were left homeless. Many cases of PTSD developed among those who experienced these disasters.

DIFFERENTIAL DIAGNOSIS

Because patients often exhibit complex reactions to trauma, the clinician must be careful to exclude other syndromes as well when evaluating patients presenting in the wake of trauma. It is particularly important to recognize potentially treatable medical contributors to posttraumatic symptomatology, especially head injury during the trauma. Medical contributors can usually be detected through a careful history and physical examination. Other organic considerations that can both cause and exacerbate the symptoms are epilepsy, alcohol use disorders, and other substance-related disorders. Acute intoxication or withdrawal from some substances may also present a clinical picture that is difficult to distinguish from the disorder until the effects of the substance have worn off.

Symptoms of PTSD can be difficult to distinguish from those of both panic disorder and generalized anxiety disorder because all three syndromes are associated with prominent anxiety and autonomic arousal. Keys to correctly diagnosing PTSD involve a careful review of the time course relating the symptoms to a traumatic event. PTSD is also associated with reexperiencing and avoidance of a trauma, features typically not present in panic or generalized anxiety disorder. Major depression is also a frequent concomitant of PTSD. Although the two syndromes are not usually difficult to distinguish phenomenologically, it is important to note the presence of comorbid depression because this can influence treatment of PTSD. PTSD must be differentiated from a series of related disorders that can exhibit phenomenological similarities, including borderline personality disorder, dissociative disorders, and factitious disorders. Borderline personality disorder can be difficult to distinguish from PTSD. The two disorders can coexist or even be causally related. Patients with dissociative disorders do not usually have the degree of avoidance behavior, the autonomic hyperarousal, or the history of trauma that patients with PTSD report.

COURSE AND PROGNOSIS

PTSD usually develops some time after the trauma. The delay can be as short as 1 week or as long as 30 years. Symptoms can fluctuate over time and may be most intense during periods of stress. Untreated, about 30 percent of patients recover completely, 40 percent continue to have mild symptoms, 20 percent continue to have moderate symptoms, and 10 percent remain unchanged or become worse. After 1 year, about 50 percent of patients recover. A good prognosis is predicted by rapid onset of the symptoms, short duration of the symptoms (less than 6 months), good premorbid functioning, strong social supports, and the absence of other psychiatric, medical, or substance-related disorders or other risk factors.

In general, the very young and the very old have more difficulty with traumatic events than do those in midlife. For example, about 80 percent of young children who sustain a burn injury show symptoms of PTSD 1 or 2 years after the initial injury; only 30 percent of adults who suffer such an injury have a PTSD after 1 year. Presumably, young children do not yet have adequate coping mechanisms to deal with the physical and emotional insults of the trauma. Likewise, older persons are likely to have more rigid coping mechanisms than younger adults and to be less able to muster a flexible approach to dealing with the effects of trauma. Furthermore, the traumatic effects can be exacerbated by physical disabilities characteristic of late life, particularly disabilities of the nervous system and the cardiovascular system, such as reduced cerebral blood flow, failing vision, palpitations, and arrhythmias. Preexisting psychiatric disability, whether a personality disorder or a more serious condition, also increases the effects of particular stressors. PTSD that is comorbid with other disorders is often more severe and perhaps more chronic and may be difficult to treat. The availability of social supports may also influence the development, severity, and duration of PTSD. In general, patients who have a good network of social support are less likely to have the disorder and to experience it in its severe forms and are more likely to recover faster.

TREATMENT

When a clinician is faced with a patient who has experienced a significant trauma, the major approaches are support, encouragement to discuss the event, and education about a variety of coping mechanisms (e.g., relaxation). The use of sedatives and hypnotics can also be helpful. When a patient experienced a traumatic event in the past and now has PTSD, the emphasis should be on education about the disorder and its treatment, both pharmacological and psychotherapeutic. The clinician should also work to destigmatize the notion of mental illness and PTSD. Additional support for the patient and the family can be obtained through local and national support groups for patients with PTSD.

Pharmacotherapy

Selective serotonin reuptake inhibitors (SSRIs), such as sertraline (Zoloft) and paroxetine (Paxil), are considered first-line treatments for PTSD, owing to their efficacy, tolerability, and safety ratings. SSRIs reduce symptoms from all PTSD symptom clusters and are effective in improving symptoms unique to PTSD, not just symptoms similar to those of depression or other anxiety disorders. Buspirone (BuSpar) is serotonergic and may also be of use.

The efficacy of imipramine (Tofranil) and amitriptyline (Elavil), two tricyclic drugs, in the treatment of PTSD is supported by a number of well-controlled clinical trials. Although some trials of the two drugs had negative findings, most of these trials had serious design flaws, including too short a duration. Doses of imipramine and amitriptyline should be the same as those used to treat depressive disorders, and an adequate trial should last at least 8 weeks. Patients who respond well should probably continue the pharmacotherapy for at least 1 year before an attempt is made to withdraw the drug. Some studies indicate that pharmacotherapy is more effective in treating the depression, anxiety, and hyperarousal than in treating the avoidance, denial, and emotional numbing.

Other drugs that may be useful in the treatment of PTSD include the monoamine oxidase inhibitors (e.g., phenelzine [Nardil]), trazodone (Desyrel), and the anticonvulsants (e.g., carbamazepine [Tegretol], valproate [Depakene]). Some studies have also revealed improvement in PTSD in patients treated with reversible monoamine oxidase inhibitors. Use of clonidine (Catapres) and propranolol (Inderal), which are antiadrenergic agents, is suggested by the theories about noradrenergic hyperactivity in the disorder. Almost no positive data concern the use of antipsychotic drugs in the disorder, so the use of drugs such as haloperidol (Haldol) should be reserved for the short-term control of severe aggression and agitation.

Psychotherapy

Psychodynamic psychotherapy may be useful in the treatment of many patients with PTSD. In some cases, reconstruction of the traumatic events with associated abreaction and catharsis may be therapeutic, but psychotherapy must be individualized because reexperiencing the trauma overwhelms some patients.

Psychotherapeutic interventions for PTSD include behavior therapy, cognitive therapy, and hypnosis. Many clinicians advocate time-limited psychotherapy for the victims of trauma. Such therapy usually takes a cognitive approach and also provides support and security. The short-term nature of the psychotherapy minimizes the risk of dependence and chronicity, but issues of suspicion, paranoia, and trust often adversely affect compliance. Therapists should overcome patients' denial of the traumatic event, encourage them to relax, and remove them from the source of the stress. Patients should be encouraged to sleep, using medication if necessary. Support from persons in their environment (e.g., friends and relatives) should be provided. Patients should be encouraged to review and abreact emotional feelings associated with the traumatic event and to plan for future recovery. Abreaction—experiencing the emotions associated with the event—may be helpful for some patients. The amobarbital (Amytal) interview has been used to facilitate this process.

Psychotherapy after a traumatic event should follow a model of crisis intervention with support, education, and the development of coping mechanisms and acceptance of the event. When PTSD has developed, two major psychotherapeutic approaches can be taken. The first is exposure therapy, in which the patient reexperiences the traumatic event through imaging techniques or in vivo exposure. The exposures can be intense, as in implosive therapy, or graded, as in systematic desensitization. The second approach is to teach the patient methods of stress management, including relaxation techniques and cognitive approaches to coping with stress. Some preliminary data indicate that, although stress management techniques are effective more rapidly than exposure techniques, the results of exposure techniques last longer.

Another psychotherapeutic technique that is relatively novel and somewhat controversial is eye movement desensitization and reprocessing (EDMR), in which the patient focuses on the lateral movement of the clinician's finger while maintaining a mental image of the trauma experience. The general belief is that symptoms can be relieved as patients work through the traumatic event while in a state of deep relaxation. Proponents of this treatment state that it is as effective as, and possibly more effective than, other treatments for PTSD and that it is preferred by both clinicians and patients who have tried it.

In addition to individual therapy techniques, group therapy and family therapy have been reported to be effective in cases of PTSD. The advantages of group therapy include sharing of traumatic experiences and support from other group members. Group therapy has been particularly successful with Vietnam veterans and survivors of catastrophic disasters such as earthquakes. Family therapy often helps sustain a marriage through periods of exacerbated symptoms. Hospitalization may be necessary when symptoms are particularly severe or when a risk of suicide or other violence exists.

▲ 13.6 Generalized Anxiety Disorder

Anxiety can be conceptualized as a normal and adaptive response to threat that prepares the organism for flight or fight. Persons who seem to be anxious about almost everything, however, are likely to be classified as having generalized anxiety disorder. The text revision of the fourth edition of the *Diagnostic and*

Statistical Manual of Mental Disorders (DSM-IV-TR) defines generalized anxiety disorder as excessive anxiety and worry about several events or activities for most days during at least a 6-month period. The worry is difficult to control and is associated with somatic symptoms, such as muscle tension, irritability, difficulty sleeping, and restlessness. The anxiety is not focused on features of another Axis I disorder, is not caused by substance use or a general medical condition, and does not occur only during a mood or psychiatric disorder. The anxiety is difficult to control, is subjectively distressing, and produces impairment in important areas of a person's life.

EPIDEMIOLOGY

Generalized anxiety disorder is a common condition; reasonable estimates for its 1-year prevalence range from 3 to 8 percent. The ratio of women to men with the disorder is about 2 to 1, but the ratio of women to men who are receiving inpatient treatment for the disorder is about 1 to 1. Lifetime prevalence is close to 5 percent, with the Epidemiological Catchment Area study suggesting a lifetime prevalence as high as 8 percent. In anxiety disorder clinics, about 25 percent of patients have generalized anxiety disorder. The disorder usually has its onset in late adolescence or early adulthood, although cases are commonly seen in older adults. In addition, some evidence suggests that the prevalence of generalized anxiety disorder is particularly high in primary care settings.

COMORBIDITY

Generalized anxiety disorder is probably the disorder that most often coexists with another mental disorder, usually social phobia, specific phobia, panic disorder, or a depressive disorder. Perhaps 50 to 90 percent of patients with generalized anxiety disorder have another mental disorder. As many as 25 percent of patients eventually experience panic disorder. Generalized anxiety disorder is differentiated from panic disorder by the absence of spontaneous panic attacks. An additional high percentage of patients are likely to have major depressive disorder. Other common disorders associated with generalized anxiety disorder are dysthymic disorder and substance-related disorders.

ETIOLOGY

The cause of generalized anxiety disorder is not known. As currently defined, generalized anxiety disorder probably affects a heterogeneous group of persons. Perhaps because a certain degree of anxiety is normal and adaptive, differentiating normal anxiety from pathological anxiety and differentiating biological causative factors from psychosocial factors are difficult. Biological and psychological factors probably work together.

Biological Factors

The therapeutic efficacies of benzodiazepines and the azaspirones (e.g., buspirone [BuSpar]) have focused biological research efforts on the γ-aminobutyric acid and serotonin neurotransmitter systems. Benzodiazepines (which are benzodiazepine receptor agonists) are known to reduce anxiety, whereas flumazenil (Romazicon) (a benzodiazepine receptor antagonist)

and the β-carbolines (benzodiazepine receptor reverse agonists) are known to induce anxiety. Although no convincing data indicate that the benzodiazepine receptors are abnormal in patients with generalized anxiety disorder, some researchers have focused on the occipital lobe, which has the highest concentrations of benzodiazepine receptors in the brain. Other brain areas hypothesized to be involved in generalized anxiety disorder are the basal ganglia, the limbic system, and the frontal cortex. Because buspirone is an agonist at the serotonin 5-HT$_{1A}$ receptor, there is the hypothesis that the regulation of the serotonergic system in generalized anxiety disorder is abnormal. Other neurotransmitter systems that have been the subject of research in generalized anxiety disorder include the norepinephrine, glutamate, and cholecystokinin systems. Some evidence indicates that patients with generalized anxiety disorder may have subsensitivity of their α_2-adrenergic receptors, as indicated by a blunted release of growth hormone after clonidine (Catapres) infusion.

Brain-imaging studies of patients with generalized anxiety disorder have revealed significant findings. One positron emission tomography study reported a lower metabolic rate in basal ganglia and white matter in patients with generalized anxiety disorder than in normal control subjects. A few genetic studies have also been conducted. One study found that a genetic relation might exist between generalized anxiety disorder and major depressive disorder in women. Another study showed a distinct but difficult-to-quantitate genetic component in generalized anxiety disorder. About 25 percent of first-degree relatives of patients with generalized anxiety disorder are also affected. Male relatives are likely to have an alcohol use disorder. Some twin studies report a concordance rate of 50 percent in monozygotic twins and 15 percent in dizygotic twins. Table 13.6–1 lists relative genetic risks in selected anxiety disorders.

A variety of electroencephalogram (EEG) abnormalities has been noted in alpha rhythm and evoked potentials. Sleep EEG studies have reported increased sleep discontinuity, decreased delta sleep, decreased stage 1 sleep, and reduced rapid eye movement sleep. These changes in sleep architecture differ from the changes seen in depressive disorders.

Psychosocial Factors

The two major schools of thought about psychosocial factors leading to the development of generalized anxiety disorder are the cognitive-behavioral school and the psychoanalytic school. According to the cognitive-behavioral school, patients with generalized anxiety disorder respond to incorrectly and inaccurately perceived dangers. The inaccuracy is generated by selective attention to negative details in the environment, by distortions in information processing, and by an overly negative view of the person's ability to cope. The psychoanalytic school hypothesizes that anxiety is a symptom of unresolved, unconscious conflicts.

Table 13.6–1
Familial Relative Risks in Selected Anxiety Disorders

Disorder	Population Prevalence (%)	Familial Relative Risk[a]
Panic disorder	1–3	2–20
Generalized anxiety disorder	3–5	6
Obsessive-compulsive disorder	1–3	3–5

[a] Ratio of risk to relatives of cases versus risk to relatives of controls.

Table 13.6–2
DSM-IV-TR Diagnostic Criteria for Generalized Anxiety Disorder

A. Excessive anxiety and worry (apprehensive expectation), occurring more days than not for at least 6 months, about a number of events or activities (such as work or school performance).
B. The person finds it difficult to control the worry.
C. The anxiety and worry are associated with three (or more) of the following six symptoms (with at least some symptoms present for more days than not for the past 6 months).
   Note: Only one item is required in children.
   (1) restlessness or feeling keyed up or on edge
   (2) being easily fatigued
   (3) difficulty concentrating or mind going blank
   (4) irritability
   (5) muscle tension
   (6) sleep disturbance (difficulty falling or staying asleep, or restless unsatisfying sleep)
D. The focus of the anxiety and worry is not confined to features of an Axis I disorder, e.g., the anxiety or worry is not about having a panic attack (as in panic disorder), being embarrassed in public (as in social phobia), being contaminated (as in obsessive-compulsive disorder), being away from home or close relatives (as in separation anxiety disorder), gaining weight (as in anorexia nervosa), having multiple physical complaints (as in somatization disorder), or having a serious illness (as in hypochondriasis), and the anxiety and worry do not occur exclusively during posttraumatic stress disorder.
E. The anxiety, worry, or physical symptoms cause clinically significant distress or impairment in social, occupational, or other important areas of functioning.
F. The disturbance is not due to the direct physiological effects of a substance (e.g., a drug of abuse, a medication) or a general medical condition (e.g., hyperthyroidism) and does not occur exclusively during a mood disorder, a psychotic disorder, or a pervasive developmental disorder.

From American Psychiatric Association. *Diagnostic and Statistical Manual of Mental Disorders.* 4th ed. Text rev. Washington, DC: American Psychiatric Association; copyright 2000, with permission.

Table 13.6–3
Physiological Symptoms of Anxiety Disorders Explicitly Mentioned in DSM-IV-TR

Panic disorder
Palpitations, pounding heart, or accelerated heart rate
Sweating
Trembling or shaking
Sensation of shortness of breath or smothering
Feeling of choking
Chest pain or discomfort
Nausea or abdominal distress
Feeling dizzy, unsteady, lightheaded, or faint
Chills or hot flushes
Posttraumatic stress disorder
Physiological reactivity on exposure to trauma-related cues
Difficulties falling asleep or staying asleep
Exaggerated startle response
Generalized anxiety disorder
Muscle tension
Sleep disturbance
Acute stress disorder
Marked symptoms of arousal

Sigmund Freud first presented this psychological theory in 1909 with his description of Little Hans—a boy afraid of horses; before then, Freud had conceptualized anxiety as having a physiological basis.

DIAGNOSIS

Generalized anxiety disorder, according to DSM-IV-TR, is characterized by a pattern of frequent, persistent worry and anxiety that is out of proportion to the impact of the event or circumstance that is the focus of the worry (Table 13.6–2). The distinction between generalized anxiety disorder and normal anxiety is emphasized by the use of the words "excessive" and "difficult to control" in the criteria and by the specification that the symptoms cause significant impairment or distress.

CLINICAL FEATURES

The essential characteristics of generalized anxiety disorder are sustained and excessive anxiety and worry accompanied by a number of physiological symptoms, including motor tension, autonomic hyperactivity, and cognitive vigilance (Table 13.6–3). The anxiety is excessive and interferes with other aspects of a person's life. This pattern must occur more days than not for at least 6 months. The motor tension is most commonly manifested as shakiness, restlessness, and headaches. The autonomic hyperactivity is commonly manifested by shortness of breath, excessive sweating, palpitations, and various gastrointestinal symptoms. The cognitive vigilance is evidenced by irritability and the ease with which patients are startled.

Patients with generalized anxiety disorder usually seek out a general practitioner or internist for help with a somatic symptom. Alternatively, the patients go to a specialist for a specific symptom (e.g., chronic diarrhea). A specific nonpsychiatric medical disorder is rarely found, and patients vary in their doctor-seeking behavior. Some patients accept a diagnosis of generalized anxiety disorder and the appropriate treatment; others seek additional medical consultations for their problems. Generalized anxiety disorders can be disabling, as in the following case.

A 27-year-old married electrician complained of dizziness, sweating palms, heart palpitations, and ringing of the ears of more than 18 months' duration. He also experienced dry mouth and throat, periods of extreme muscle tension, and a constant "edgy" and watchful feeling that had often interfered with his ability to concentrate. These feelings had been present most of the time over the previous 2 years; they had not been limited to discrete periods. Although these symptoms made him feel "discouraged," he denied feeling depressed and continued to enjoy activities with his family.

Because of these symptoms the patient had seen a family practitioner, a neurologist, a neurosurgeon, a chiropractor, and an ear-nose-throat specialist. He had been placed on a hypoglycemic diet, received physiotherapy for a pinched nerve, and been told he might have "an inner ear problem."

He also had many worries. He constantly worried about the health of his parents. His father, in fact, had a myocardial infarction 2 years previously, but is now feeling well. He also worried about whether he is "a good father," whether his wife will ever leave him (there is no indication that she is dissatisfied with the marriage), and whether he is liked by co-workers on the job. Although he recognizes that his worries are often unfounded, he can't stop worrying.

For the past 2 years the patient has had few social contacts because of his nervous symptoms. Although he sometimes had to leave work when the symptoms became intolerable, he continues to work for the same company he joined for his apprenticeship following high school graduation. He tends to hide his symptoms from his wife and children, to whom he wants to appear "perfect." (Adapted from *DSM-IV-TR Casebook*.)

DIFFERENTIAL DIAGNOSIS

As with other anxiety disorders, generalized anxiety disorder must be differentiated from both medical and psychiatric disorders. Neurological, endocrinological, metabolic, and medication-related disorders similar to those considered in the differential diagnosis of panic disorder must be considered in the differential diagnosis of generalized anxiety disorder. Common co-occurring anxiety disorders also must be considered, including panic disorder, phobias, obsessive-compulsive disorder (OCD), and posttraumatic stress disorder. To meet criteria for generalized anxiety disorder, patients must exhibit the full syndrome and their symptoms should not be explainable by the presence of a comorbid anxiety disorder. To diagnose generalized anxiety disorder in the context of other anxiety disorders, it is most important to document anxiety or worry related to circumstances or topics that are either unrelated, or only minimally related, to other disorders. Proper diagnosis involves both definitively establishing the presence of generalized anxiety disorder and properly diagnosing other anxiety disorders. Patients with generalized anxiety disorder frequently develop major depressive disorder. As a result, this condition must also be recognized and distinguished. The key to making a correct diagnosis is documenting anxiety or worry that is unrelated to the depressive disorder.

COURSE AND PROGNOSIS

The age of onset is difficult to specify; most patients with the disorder report that they have been anxious for as long as they can remember. Patients usually come to a clinician's attention in their 20s, although the first contact with a clinician can occur at virtually any age. Only one third of patients who have generalized anxiety disorder seek psychiatric treatment. Many go to general practitioners, internists, cardiologists, pulmonary specialists, or gastroenterologists seeking treatment for the somatic component of the disorder. Because of the high incidence of comorbid mental disorders in patients with generalized anxiety disorder, the clinical course and prognosis of the disorder are difficult to predict. Nonetheless, some data indicate that life events are associated with the onset of generalized anxiety disorder: The occurrence of several negative life events greatly increases the likelihood that the disorder will develop. By definition, generalized anxiety disorder is a chronic condition that may well be lifelong.

TREATMENT

The most effective treatment of generalized anxiety disorder is probably one that combines psychotherapeutic, pharmacotherapeutic, and supportive approaches. The treatment may take a significant amount of time for the involved clinician, whether the clinician is a psychiatrist, a family practitioner, or another specialist.

Psychotherapy

The major psychotherapeutic approaches to generalized anxiety disorder are cognitive-behavioral, supportive, and insight oriented. Data are limited on the relative merits of those approaches, although the most sophisticated studies have examined cognitive-behavioral techniques, which seem to have both short-term and long-term efficacy. Cognitive approaches address patients' hypothesized cognitive distortions directly, and behavioral approaches address somatic symptoms directly. The major techniques used in behavioral approaches are relaxation and biofeedback. Some preliminary data indicate that the combination of cognitive and behavioral approaches is more effective than either technique used alone. Supportive therapy offers patients reassurance and comfort, although its long-term efficacy is doubtful. Insight-oriented psychotherapy focuses on uncovering unconscious conflicts and identifying ego strengths. The efficacy of insight-oriented psychotherapy for generalized anxiety disorder is found in many anecdotal case reports, but large controlled studies are lacking.

Most patients experience a marked lessening of anxiety when given the opportunity to discuss their difficulties with a concerned and sympathetic physician. If clinicians discover external situations that are anxiety provoking, they may be able—alone or with the help of the patients or their families—to change the environment and, thus, reduce the stressful pressures. A reduction in symptoms often allows patients to function effectively in their daily work and relationships and, thus, gain new rewards and gratification that are themselves therapeutic.

In the psychoanalytic perspective, anxiety sometimes signals unconscious turmoil that deserves investigation. The anxiety can be normal, adaptive, maladaptive, too intense, or too mild, depending on the circumstances. Anxiety appears in numerous situations over the course of the life cycle; in many cases, symptom relief is not the most appropriate course of action.

For patients who are psychologically minded and motivated to understand the sources of their anxiety, psychotherapy may be the treatment of choice. Psychodynamic therapy proceeds with the assumption that anxiety can increase with effective treatment. The goal of the dynamic approach may be to increase the patient's anxiety tolerance (a capacity to experience anxiety without having to discharge it) rather than to eliminate anxiety. Empirical research indicates that many patients who have successful psychotherapeutic treatment may continue to experience anxiety after termination of the psychotherapy, but their increased ego mastery allows them to use the anxiety symptoms as a signal to reflect on internal struggles and to expand their insight and understanding. A psychodynamic approach to patients with generalized anxiety disorder involves a search for the patient's underlying fears.

Pharmacotherapy

The decision to prescribe an anxiolytic to patients with generalized anxiety disorder should rarely be made on the first visit. Because of the long-term nature of the disorder, a treatment plan must be carefully thought out. The three major drugs to be considered for the treatment of generalized anxiety disorder are benzodiazepines, the serotonin specific reuptake inhibitors (SSRIs), buspirone (BuSpar), and venlafaxine (Effexor). Other drugs that may be useful are the tricyclic drugs (e.g., imipramine [Tofranil]), antihistamines, and the β-adrenergic antagonists (e.g., propranolol [Inderal]).

Although drug treatment of generalized anxiety disorder is sometimes seen as a 6- to 12-month treatment, some evidence indicates that treatment should be long term, perhaps lifelong. About 25 percent of patients relapse in the first month after the discontinuation of therapy, and 60 to 80 percent relapse over the course of the next year. Although some patients become dependent on the benzodiazepines, tolerance rarely develops to the therapeutic effects of the benzodiazepines, buspirone, venlafaxine, or the SSRIs.

Benzodiazepines.   Benzodiazepines have been the drugs of choice for generalized anxiety disorder. They can be prescribed on an as-needed basis, so that patients take a rapidly acting benzodiazepine when they feel particularly anxious. The alternative approach is to prescribe benzodiazepines for a limited period, during which psychosocial therapeutic approaches are implemented.

Several problems are associated with the use of benzodiazepines in generalized anxiety disorder. About 25 to 30 percent of all patients fail to respond, and tolerance and dependence can occur. Some patients also experience impaired alertness while taking the drugs and, therefore, are at risk for accidents involving automobiles and machinery.

The clinical decision to initiate treatment with a benzodiazepine should be considered and specific. The patient's diagnosis, the specific target symptoms, and the duration of treatment should all be defined, and the information should be shared with the patient. Treatment for most anxiety conditions lasts for 2 to 6 weeks, followed by 1 or 2 weeks of tapering drug use before it is discontinued. The most common clinical mistake with benzodiazepine treatment is routinely to continue treatment indefinitely.

For the treatment of anxiety, it is usual to begin giving a drug at the low end of its therapeutic range and to increase the dose to achieve a therapeutic response. The use of a benzodiazepine with an intermediate half-life (8 to 15 hours) will likely avoid some of the adverse effects associated with the use of benzodiazepines with long half-lives, and the use of divided doses prevents the development of adverse effects associated with high peak plasma levels. The improvement produced by benzodiazepines may go beyond a simple antianxiety effect. For example, the drugs may cause patients to regard various occurrences in a positive light. The drugs can also have a mild disinhibiting action, similar to that observed after ingesting modest amounts of alcohol.

Buspirone.   Buspirone is a 5-HT$_{1A}$ receptor partial agonist and is most likely effective in 60 to 80 percent of patients with generalized anxiety disorder. Data indicate that buspirone is more effective in reducing the cognitive symptoms of generalized anxiety disorder than in reducing the somatic symptoms. Evidence also indicates that patients who have previously had treatment with benzodiazepines are not likely to respond to treatment with buspirone. The lack of response may be caused by the absence, with buspirone treatment, of some of the nonanxiolytic effects of benzodiazepines (e.g., muscle relaxation and the additional sense of well-being). The major disadvantage of buspirone is that its effects take 2 to 3 weeks to become evident, in contrast to the almost immediate anxiolytic effects of the benzodiazepines. One approach is to initiate benzodiazepine and buspirone use simultaneously, then taper off the benzodiazepine use after 2 to 3 weeks, at which point the buspirone should have reached its maximal effects. Some studies have also reported that long-term combined treatment with benzodiazepine and buspirone may be more effective than use of either drug alone. Buspirone is not an effective treatment for benzodiazepine withdrawal.

Venlafaxine.   Venlafaxine is effective in treating the insomnia, poor concentration, restlessness, irritability, and excessive muscle tension associated with generalized anxiety disorder. Venlafaxine is a nonselective inhibitor of the reuptake of three biogenic amines—serotonin, norepinephrine, and, to a lesser extent, dopamine.

Selective Serotonin Reuptake Inhibitors.   SSRIs may be effective, especially for patients with comorbid depression. The prominent disadvantage of SSRIs, especially fluoxetine (Prozac), is that they can transiently increase anxiety and cause agitated states. For this reason, the SSRIs sertraline (Zoloft), citalopram (Celexa), and paroxetine (Paxil) are better choices in patients with high anxiety disorder. It is reasonable to begin treatment with sertraline, citalopram, or paroxetine plus a benzodiazepine and then to taper benzodiazepine use after 2 to 3 weeks. Further studies are needed to determine whether SSRIs are as effective for generalized anxiety disorder as they are for panic disorder and OCD.

Other Drugs.   If conventional pharmacological treatment (e.g., with buspirone or a benzodiazepine) is ineffective or not completely effective, then a clinical reassessment is indicated to rule out comorbid conditions, such as depression, or to better understand the patient's environmental stresses. Other drugs that have proved useful for generalized anxiety disorder include the tricyclic and tetracyclic drugs. The β-adrenergic receptor antagonists may reduce the somatic manifestations of anxiety but not the underlying condition, and their use is usually limited to situational anxieties, such as performance anxiety.

▲ 13.7 Other Anxiety Disorders

ANXIETY DISORDER DUE TO A GENERAL MEDICAL CONDITION

Many medical disorders are associated with anxiety. Symptoms can include panic attacks, generalized anxiety, obsessions and compulsions, and other signs of distress. In all cases, the signs and symptoms will be due to the direct physiological effects of the medical condition.

Epidemiology

The occurrence of anxiety symptoms related to general medical conditions is common, although the incidence of the disorder varies for each specific general medical condition.

Etiology

A wide range of medical conditions can cause symptoms similar to those of anxiety disorders. Hyperthyroidism, hypothyroidism, hypoparathyroidism, and vitamin B$_{12}$ deficiency are frequently associated with anxiety symptoms. A pheochromocytoma produces epinephrine, which can cause paroxysmal episodes of anxiety symptoms. Certain lesions of the brain and post-encephalitic states reportedly produce symptoms identical to those seen in obsessive-compulsive disorder (OCD). Other medical conditions, such as cardiac arrhythmia, can produce physiological symptoms of panic disorder. Hypoglycemia can also mimic the symptoms of an anxiety disorder. The diverse medical conditions that can cause symptoms of anxiety disorder may do so through a common mechanism—the noradrenergic system—although the effects on the serotonergic system are also under study. Each of these conditions is characterized by prominent anxiety that arises as the direct result of some underlying physiological perturbation.

Diagnosis

The text revision of the fourth edition of the *Diagnostic and Statistical Manual of Mental Disorders* (DSM-IV-TR) diagnosis of anxiety disorder due to a general medical condition (Table 13.7–1) requires the presence of symptoms of an anxiety disorder. DSM-IV-TR allows clinicians to specify whether the disorder is characterized by symptoms of generalized anxiety, panic attacks, or obsessive-compulsive symptoms.

Clinicians should have an increased level of suspicion for the diagnosis when chronic or paroxysmal anxiety is associated with a physical disease known to cause such symptoms in some patients. Paroxysmal bouts of hypertension in an anxious patient may indicate that a workup for a pheochromocytoma is appropriate. A general medical workup may reveal diabetes, an adrenal tumor, thyroid disease, or a neurological condition. For example, some patients with complex partial epilepsy have extreme

Table 13.7–1
DSM-IV-TR Diagnostic Criteria for Anxiety Disorder Due to a General Medical Condition

A. Prominent anxiety, panic attacks, or obsessions or compulsions predominate in the clinical picture.
B. There is evidence from the history, physical examination, or laboratory findings that the disturbance is the direct physiological consequence of a general medical condition.
C. The disturbance is not better accounted for by another mental disorder (e.g., adjustment disorder with anxiety in which the stressor is a serious general medical condition).
D. The disturbance does not occur exclusively during the course of a delirium.
E. The disturbance causes clinically significant distress or impairment in social, occupational, or other important areas of functioning.

Specify if:
 With generalized anxiety: if excessive anxiety or worry about a number of events or activities predominates in the clinical presentation
 With panic attacks: if panic attacks predominate in the clinical presentation
 With obsessive-compulsive symptoms: if obsessions or compulsions predominate in the clinical presentation
 Coding note: Include the name of the general medical condition on Axis I, e.g., anxiety disorder due to pheochromocytoma, with generalized anxiety; also code the general medical condition on Axis III.

From American Psychiatric Association. *Diagnostic and Statistical Manual of Mental Disorders.* 4th ed. Text rev. Washington, DC: American Psychiatric Association; copyright 2000, with permission.

episodes of anxiety or fear as their only manifestation of the epileptic activity.

Clinical Features

Panic Attacks.   Patients who have cardiomyopathy may have the highest incidence of panic disorder secondary to a general medical condition. One study reported that 83 percent of patients with cardiomyopathy awaiting cardiac transplantation had panic disorder symptoms. Increased noradrenergic tone in these patients may be the provoking stimulus for the panic attacks. In some studies, about 25 percent of patients with Parkinson's disease and chronic obstructive pulmonary disease have symptoms of panic disorder. Other medical disorders associated with panic disorder include chronic pain, primary biliary cirrhosis, and epilepsy, particularly when the focus is in the right parahippocampal gyrus.

Generalized Anxiety.   A high prevalence of generalized anxiety disorder symptoms has been reported in patients with Sjögren's syndrome, and this rate may be related to the effects of Sjögren's syndrome on cortical and subcortical functions and thyroid function. The highest prevalence of generalized anxiety disorder symptoms in a medical disorder seems to be in Graves' disease (hyperthyroidism), in which as many as two thirds of all patients meet the criteria for generalized anxiety disorder.

Obsessive-Compulsive Symptoms

Reports have associated the development of OCD symptoms with Sydenham's chorea.

A 12-year-old girl had a sudden onset of high fever, lethargy, and sore throat with purulent tonsillar exudate. Streptococci were found in the infected site, and she was treated successfully with penicillin. Following recovery, mild athetoid movements of the upper torso and facial tics were noted and diagnosed as sequelae of the infection. She was kept on antibiotics (to prevent reinfection) until the neurological complication subsided spontaneously after 1 year.

Phobias.   Symptoms of phobias appear to be uncommon, although one study reported a 17 percent prevalence of symptoms of social phobia in patients with Parkinson's disease. Older persons with balance difficulties often complain of a fear of falling, which may express itself by their being unwilling or fearful of walking.

Differential Diagnosis

Anxiety, as a symptom, can be associated with many psychiatric disorders in addition to the anxiety disorders themselves. A mental status examination is necessary to determine the presence of mood symptoms or psychotic symptoms that may suggest another psychiatric diagnosis. For a clinician to conclude that a patient has an anxiety disorder caused by a general medical condition, the patient should clearly have anxiety as the predominant symptom and should have a specific causative nonpsychiatric medical disorder. To ascertain the degree to which a general medical condition is causative for the anxiety, the clinician should know whether the medical condition and the anxiety symptoms have been related closely in the literature, the age of onset (primary anxiety disorders usually have their onset before age 35 years), and the patient's family history of both anxiety disorders and relevant general medical conditions (e.g., hyperthyroidism). A diagnosis of adjustment disorder with anxiety must also be considered in the differential diagnosis.

Course and Prognosis

The unremitting experience of anxiety can be disabling and can interfere with every aspect of life, including social, occupational, and psychological functioning. A sudden increase in anxiety level may prompt an affected person to seek medical or psychiatric help more quickly than when the onset is insidious. The treatment or the removal of the primary medical cause of the anxiety usually initiates a clear course of improvement in the anxiety disorder symptoms. In some cases, however, the anxiety disorder symptoms continue even after the primary medical condition is treated (e.g., after an episode of encephalitis). Some symptoms, particularly OCD symptoms, linger for a longer time than other anxiety disorder symptoms. When anxiety disorder symptoms are present for a significant period after the medical disorder has been treated, the remaining symptoms should probably be treated as if they were primary—that is, with psychotherapy, pharmacotherapy, or both.

Treatment

The primary treatment for anxiety disorder due to a general medical condition is to treat the underlying medical condition. If a patient also has an alcohol or other substance use disorder, this disorder must also be addressed therapeutically to gain control of the anxiety disorder symptoms. If the removal of the primary medical condition does not reverse the anxiety disorder symptoms, treatment of these symptoms should follow the treatment guidelines for the specific mental disorder. In general, behavioral modification techniques, anxiolytic agents, and serotonergic antidepressants have been the most effective treatment modalities.

SUBSTANCE-INDUCED ANXIETY DISORDER

Substance-induced disorder is the direct result of a toxic substance, including drugs of abuse, medication, poison, and alcohol, among others.

Epidemiology

Substance-induced anxiety disorder is common, both as the result of the ingestion of so-called recreational drugs and as the result of prescription drug use.

Etiology

A wide range of substances can cause symptoms of anxiety that can mimic any of the DSM-IV-TR anxiety disorders. Although sympathomimetics, such as amphetamine, cocaine, and caffeine, have been most associated with the production of anxiety disorder symptoms, many serotonergic drugs (e.g., lysergic acid diethylamide and methylenedioxymethamphetamine) can also cause both acute and chronic anxiety syndromes in users. A wide range of prescription medications is also associated with the production of anxiety disorder symptoms in susceptible persons.

Diagnosis

The DSM-IV-TR diagnostic criteria for substance-induced anxiety disorder require the presence of prominent anxiety, panic attacks, obsessions, or compulsions (Table 13.7–2). The DSM-IV-TR guidelines state that the symptoms should have developed during the use of the substance or within 1 month of the cessation of substance use, but DSM-IV-TR encourages clinicians to use appropriate clinical judgment to assess the relation between substance exposure and anxiety symptoms. The structure of the diagnosis includes specification of (1) the substance (e.g., cocaine), (2) the appropriate state during the onset (e.g., intoxication), and (3) the specific symptom pattern (e.g., panic attacks).

Clinical Features

The associated clinical features of substance-induced anxiety disorder vary with the particular substance involved. Even infrequent use of psychostimulants can result in anxiety disorder symptoms in some persons. Cognitive impairments in comprehension, calculation, and memory can be associated with anxiety disorder symptoms. These cognitive deficits are usually reversible when the substance use is stopped.

Virtually everyone who drinks alcohol has used it on at least a few occasions to reduce anxiety, most often social anxiety. In contrast, carefully controlled studies have found that the effects of alcohol on anxiety are variable and can be significantly affected by gender, the amount of alcohol ingested, and cultural attitudes. Nevertheless, alcohol use disorders and other substance-related disorders are commonly associated with anxiety disorders. Alcohol use disorders are about four times more common among patients with panic disorder than among the general population, about three and a half times more common among patients with OCD, and about two and a half times more common among patients with phobias. Several studies have reported data indicating that genetic diatheses for both anxiety disorders and alcohol use disorders can exist in some families.

Differential Diagnosis

The differential diagnosis for substance-induced anxiety disorder includes the primary anxiety disorders, anxiety disorder due to a general medical condition (for which the patient may be receiving an implicated drug), and mood disorders, which are frequently accompanied by symptoms of anxiety disorders. Personality disorders and malingering must be considered in the differential diagnosis, particularly in some urban emergency rooms.

Course and Prognosis

The course and prognosis generally depend on removal of the causally involved substance and the long-term ability of the affected person to limit use of the substance. The anxiogenic effects of most drugs are reversible. When the anxiety does not reverse with cessation of the drug, clinicians should reconsider the

Table 13.7–2
DSM-IV-TR Diagnostic Criteria for
Substance-Induced Anxiety Disorder

A. Prominent anxiety, panic attacks, or obsessions or compulsions predominate in the clinical picture.
B. There is evidence from the history, physical examination, or laboratory findings of either (1) or (2):
   (1) the symptoms in Criterion A developed during, or within 1 month of, substance intoxication or withdrawal
   (2) medication use is etiologically related to the disturbance
C. The disturbance is not better accounted for by an anxiety disorder that is not substance induced. Evidence that the symptoms are better accounted for by an anxiety disorder that is not substance induced might include the following: the symptoms precede the onset of the substance use (or medication use); the symptoms persist for a substantial period of time (e.g., about a month) after the cessation of acute withdrawal or severe intoxication or are substantially in excess of what would be expected given the type or amount of the substance used or the duration of use; or there is other evidence suggesting the existence of an independent non–substance-induced anxiety disorder (e.g., a history of recurrent non–substance-related episodes).
D. The disturbance does not occur exclusively during the course of a delirium.
E. The disturbance causes clinically significant distress or impairment in social, occupational, or other important areas of functioning.
   Note: This diagnosis should be made instead of a diagnosis of substance intoxication or substance withdrawal only when the anxiety symptoms are in excess of those usually associated with the intoxication or withdrawal syndrome and when the anxiety symptoms are sufficiently severe to warrant independent clinical attention.

Code [Specific substance]-induced anxiety disorder: Alcohol; amphetamine (or amphetaminelike substance); caffeine; cannabis; cocaine; hallucinogen; inhalant; phencyclidine (or phencyclidinelike substance); sedative, hypnotic, or anxiolytic; other [or unknown] substance

Specify if:
   With generalized anxiety: if excessive anxiety or worry about a number of events or activities predominates in the clinical presentation
   With panic attacks: if panic attacks predominate in the clinical presentation
   With obsessive-compulsive symptoms: if obsessions or compulsions predominate in the clinical presentation
   With phobic symptoms: if phobic symptoms predominate in the clinical presentation

Specify if:
   With onset during intoxication: if the criteria are met for intoxication with the substance and the symptoms develop during the intoxication syndrome
   With onset during withdrawal: if criteria are met for withdrawal from the substance and the symptoms develop during, or shortly after, a withdrawal syndrome

From American Psychiatric Association. *Diagnostic and Statistical Manual of Mental Disorders.* 4th ed. Text rev. Washington, DC: American Psychiatric Association; copyright 2000, with permission.

diagnosis of substance-induced anxiety disorder or consider the possibility that the substance caused irreversible brain damage.

Treatment

The primary treatment for substance-induced anxiety disorder is the removal of the causally involved substance. Treatment then must focus on finding an alternative treatment if the substance

was a medically indicated drug, on limiting the patient's exposure if the substance was introduced through environmental exposure, or on treating the underlying substance-related disorder. If anxiety disorder symptoms continue even after stopping substance use, treatment of the anxiety disorder symptoms with appropriate psychotherapeutic or pharmacotherapeutic modalities may be appropriate.

ANXIETY DISORDER NOT OTHERWISE SPECIFIED

Some patients have symptoms of anxiety disorders that do not meet the criteria for any specific DSM-IV-TR anxiety disorder or adjustment disorder with anxiety or mixed anxiety and depressed mood. Such patients are most appropriately classified as having anxiety disorder not otherwise specified. DSM-IV-TR includes four examples of conditions that are appropriate for the diagnosis (Table 13.7–3). One of the examples is mixed anxiety-depressive disorder.

MIXED ANXIETY-DEPRESSIVE DISORDER

Mixed anxiety-depressive disorder describes patients with both anxiety and depressive symptoms who do not meet the diagnostic criteria for either an anxiety disorder or a mood disorder. The combination of depressive and anxiety symptoms results in significant functional impairment for the affected person. The condition may be particularly prevalent in primary care practices and outpatient mental health clinics. Opponents have argued that the availability of the diagnosis may discourage clinicians from taking the necessary time to obtain a complete psychiatric

Table 13.7–3
DSM-IV-TR Diagnostic Criteria for Anxiety Disorder Not Otherwise Specified

This category includes disorders with prominent anxiety or phobic avoidance that do not meet criteria for any specific anxiety disorder, adjustment disorder with anxiety, or adjustment disorder with mixed anxiety and depressed mood. Examples include
1. Mixed anxiety-depressive disorder: clinically significant symptoms of anxiety and depression, but the criteria are not met for either a specific mood disorder or a specific anxiety disorder
2. Clinically significant social phobic symptoms that are related to the social impact of having a general medical condition or mental disorder (e.g., Parkinson's disease, dermatological conditions, stuttering, anorexia nervosa, body dysmorphic disorder)
3. Situations in which the disturbance is severe enough to warrant a diagnosis of an anxiety disorder but the individual fails to report enough symptoms for the full criteria for any specific anxiety disorder to have been met; for example, an individual who reports all of the features of panic disorder without agoraphobia except that the panic attacks are all limited-symptom attacks
4. Situations in which the clinician has concluded that an anxiety disorder is present but is unable to determine whether it is primary, due to a general medical condition, or substance induced

From American Psychiatric Association. *Diagnostic and Statistical Manual of Mental Disorders.* 4th ed. Text rev. Washington, DC: American Psychiatric Association; copyright 2000, with permission.

history to differentiate true depressive disorders from true anxiety disorders. In Europe and, especially, in China, many of these patients are given a diagnosis of neurasthenia.

Epidemiology

The coexistence of major depressive disorder and panic disorder is common. As many as two thirds of all patients with depressive symptoms have prominent anxiety symptoms, and one third may meet the diagnostic criteria for panic disorder. Researchers have reported that 20 to 90 percent of all patients with panic disorder have episodes of major depressive disorder. These data suggest that the coexistence of depressive and anxiety symptoms, neither of which meet the diagnostic criteria for other depressive or anxiety disorders, may be common. However, formal epidemiological data on mixed anxiety-depressive disorder are not available. Nevertheless, some clinicians and researchers have estimated that the prevalence of the disorder in the general population is as high as 10 percent and in primary care clinics as high as 50 percent, although conservative estimates suggest a prevalence of about 1 percent in the general population.

Etiology

Four principal lines of evidence suggest that anxiety symptoms and depressive symptoms are causally linked in some affected patients. First, several investigators have reported similar neuroendocrine findings in depressive disorders and anxiety disorders, particularly panic disorder, including blunted cortisol response to adrenocorticotropic hormone, blunted growth hormone response to clonidine (Catapres), and blunted thyroid-stimulating hormone and prolactin responses to thyrotropin-releasing hormone. Second, several investigators have reported data indicating that hyperactivity of the noradrenergic system is causally relevant to some patients with depressive disorders and with panic disorder. Specifically, these studies have found elevated concentrations of the norepinephrine metabolite 3-methoxy-4-hydroxyphenyglycol in the urine, the plasma, or the cerebrospinal fluid of depressed patients and patients with panic disorder who were actively experiencing a panic attack. As with other anxiety and depressive disorders, serotonin and γ-aminobutyric acid may also be causally involved in mixed anxiety-depressive disorder. Third, many studies have found that serotonergic drugs, such as fluoxetine (Prozac) and clomipramine (Anafranil), are useful in treating both depressive and anxiety disorders. Fourth, a number of family studies have reported data indicating that anxiety and depressive symptoms are genetically linked in at least some families.

Diagnosis

The DSM-IV-TR criteria (Table 13.7–4) require the presence of subsyndromal symptoms of both anxiety and depression and the presence of some autonomic symptoms, such as tremor, palpitations, dry mouth, and the sensation of a churning stomach. Some preliminary studies have indicated that the sensitivity of general practitioners to a syndrome of mixed anxiety-depressive disorder is low, although this lack of recognition may reflect the lack of an appropriate diagnostic label for the patients.

Table 13.7–4
DSM-IV-TR Research Criteria for Mixed Anxiety-Depressive Disorder

A. Persistent or recurrent dysphoric mood lasting at least 1 month.
B. The dysphoric mood is accompanied by at least 1 month of four (or more) of the following symptoms:
   (1) difficulty concentrating or mind going blank
   (2) sleep disturbance (difficulty falling or staying asleep, or restless, unsatisfying sleep)
   (3) fatigue or low energy
   (4) irritability
   (5) worry
   (6) being easily moved to tears
   (7) hypervigilance
   (8) anticipating the worst
   (9) hopelessness (pervasive pessimism about the future)
   (10) low self-esteem or feelings of worthlessness
C. The symptoms cause clinically significant distress or impairment in social, occupational, or other important areas of functioning.
D. The symptoms are not due to the direct physiological effects of a substance (e.g., a drug of abuse, a medication) or a general medical condition.
E. All of the following:
   (1) criteria have never been met for major depressive disorder, dysthymic disorder, panic disorder, or generalized anxiety disorder
   (2) criteria are not currently met for any other anxiety or mood disorder (including an anxiety or mood disorder, in partial remission)
   (3) the symptoms are not better accounted for by any other mental disorder

From American Psychiatric Association. *Diagnostic and Statistical Manual of Mental Disorders.* 4th ed. Text rev. Washington, DC: American Psychiatric Association; copyright 2000, with permission.

Clinical Features

The clinical features of mixed anxiety-depressive disorder combine symptoms of anxiety disorders and some symptoms of depressive disorders. In addition, symptoms of autonomic nervous system hyperactivity, such as gastrointestinal complaints, are common and contribute to the high frequency with which the patients are seen in outpatient medical clinics.

Differential Diagnosis

The differential diagnosis includes other anxiety and depressive disorders and personality disorders. Among the anxiety disorders, generalized anxiety disorder is most likely to overlap with mixed anxiety-depressive disorder. Among the mood disorders, dysthymic disorder and minor depressive disorder are most likely to overlap with mixed anxiety-depressive disorder. Among the personality disorders, avoidant, dependent, and obsessive-compulsive personality disorders may have symptoms that resemble those of mixed anxiety-depressive disorder. A diagnosis of a somatoform disorder should also be considered. Only a psychiatric history, a mental status examination, and a working knowledge of the specific DSM-IV-TR criteria can help clinicians differentiate among these conditions. The prodromal signs of schizophrenia may show itself as a mixed picture of mounting anxiety and depression with eventual onset of psychotic symptoms.

Course and Prognosis

On the basis of clinical data, patients seem to be equally likely to have prominent anxiety symptoms, prominent depressive symptoms, or an equal mixture of the two symptoms at onset. During the course of the illness, anxiety or depressive symptoms may alternate in their predominance. The prognosis is not known.

Treatment

Because adequate studies comparing treatment modalities for mixed anxiety-depressive disorder are not available, clinicians are probably most likely to provide treatment based on the symptoms present, their severity, and the clinician's level of experience with various treatment modalities. Psychotherapeutic approaches may involve time-limited approaches, such as cognitive therapy or behavior modification, although some clinicians use a less-structured psychotherapeutic approach, such as insight-oriented psychotherapy. Pharmacotherapy for mixed anxiety-depressive disorder can include antianxiety drugs, antidepressant drugs, or both. Among the anxiolytic drugs, some data indicate that the use of triazolobenzodiazepines (e.g., alprazolam [Xanax]) may be indicated because of their effectiveness in treating depression associated with anxiety. A drug that affects the serotonin 5-HT$_{1A}$ receptor, such as buspirone (BuSpar), may also be indicated. Among the antidepressants, despite the noradrenergic theories linking anxiety disorders and depressive disorders, the serotonergic antidepressants may be most effective in treating mixed anxiety-depressive disorder. Venlafaxine (Effexor) is an effective antidepressant that has been approved by the U.S. Food and Drug Administration for the treatment of depression as well as generalized anxiety disorder and is a drug of choice in the combined disorder.

14 ▲

Somatoform Disorders

Seven somatoform disorders are listed in the text revision of the fourth edition of the *Diagnostic and Statistical Manual of Mental Disorders* (DSM-IV-TR): (1) somatization disorder, characterized by many physical complaints affecting many organ systems; (2) conversion disorder, characterized by one or two neurological complaints; (3) hypochondriasis, characterized less by a focus on symptoms than by patients' beliefs that they have a specific disease; (4) body dysmorphic disorder, characterized by a false belief or exaggerated perception that a body part is defective; (5) pain disorder, characterized by symptoms of pain that are either solely related to, or significantly exacerbated by, psychological factors; (6) undifferentiated somatoform disorder, which includes somatoform disorders not otherwise described that have been present for 6 months or longer; and (7) somatoform disorder not otherwise specified, which is the category for somatoform symptoms that do not meet any of the somatoform disorder diagnoses mentioned previously (Table 14–1).

The term *somatoform* derives from the Greek *soma* for body, and the somatoform disorders are a broad group of illnesses that have bodily signs and symptoms as a major component. These disorders encompass mind–body interactions in which, in ways not well understood, signals within the brain give rise to a patient's awareness of a serious problem in the body. In addition, minor or as yet undetectable changes in neurochemistry, neurophysiology, and neuroimmunology may result from unknown mental or brain mechanisms that cause illness.

SOMATIZATION DISORDER

Somatization disorder is an illness of multiple somatic complaints in multiple organ systems that occurs over a period of several years and results in significant impairment, treatment seeking, or both. Somatization disorder is the prototypic somatoform disorder and has the best evidence of any of the somatoform disorders for being a stable and reliably measured entity over many years in individuals with the disorder. Somatization disorder differs from other somatoform disorders because of the multiplicity of the complaints and the multiple organ systems (e.g., gastrointestinal and neurological) that are affected. The disorder is chronic and is associated with significant psychological distress, impaired social and occupational functioning, and excessive medical-help–seeking behavior.

Somatization disorder has been recognized since the time of ancient Egypt. An early name for somatization disorder was hysteria, a condition incorrectly thought to affect only women. (The word *hysteria* is derived from the Greek word for uterus, *hystera*.) In the 17th century, Thomas Sydenham recognized that psychological factors, which he called "an-

tecedent sorrows," were involved in the pathogenesis of the symptoms. In 1859, Paul Briquet, a French physician, observed the multiplicity of symptoms and affected organ systems and commented on the usually chronic course of the disorder. Because of these clinical observations, the disorder was called *Briquet's syndrome* until the term *somatization disorder* became the standard in the United States.

Epidemiology

The lifetime prevalence of somatization disorder in the general population is estimated to be 0.2 to 2 percent in women and 0.2 percent in men. Women with somatization disorder outnumber men 5 to 20 times, but the highest estimates may be because of the early tendency not to diagnose somatization disorder in male patients. Nevertheless, it is not an uncommon disorder. With a 5:1 female-to-male ratio, the lifetime prevalence of somatization disorder among women in the general population may be 1 or 2 percent. Among patients in the offices of general practitioners and family practitioners, as many as 5 to 10 percent may meet the diagnostic criteria for somatization disorder. The disorder is inversely related to social position and occurs most often among patients who have little education and low incomes. Somatization disorder is defined as beginning before age 30 years; it usually begins during a person's teenage years.

Several studies have noted that somatization disorder commonly coexists with other mental disorders. About two thirds of all patients with somatization disorder have identifiable psychiatric symptoms, and up to half have other mental disorders. Commonly associated personality traits or personality disorders are those characterized by avoidant, paranoid, self-defeating, and obsessive-compulsive features. Two disorders that are not seen more commonly in patients with somatization disorder than in the general population are bipolar I disorder and substance abuse.

Etiology

Psychosocial Factors. The cause of somatization disorder is unknown. Psychosocial formulations of the cause involve interpretations of the symptoms as a social communication whose result is to avoid obligations (e.g., going to a job a person does not like), to express emotions (e.g., anger at a spouse), or to symbolize a feeling or a belief (e.g., a pain in the gut). Strict psychoanalytic interpretations of symptoms rest on the hypothesis that the symptoms substitute for repressed instinctual impulses.

A behavioral perspective on somatization disorder emphasizes that parental teaching, parental example, and ethnic mores may teach some children to somatize more than others. In addition, some patients with somatization disorder come from

Table 14-1
Clinical Features of Somatoform Disorders

Diagnosis	Clinical Presentation	Demographic and Epidemiological Features	Diagnostic Features	Management Strategy	Prognosis	Associated Disturbances	Primary Differential Presentation	Psychological Processes Contributing to Symptoms	Motivation for Symptom Production
Somatization disorder	Polysymptomatic Recurrent and chronic Sickly by history	Young age Female predominance 20 to 1 Familial pattern 5%–10% incidence in primary care populations	Review of systems profusely positive Multiple clinical contacts Polysurgical	Therapeutic alliance Regular appointments Crisis intervention	Poor to fair	Histrionic personality disorder Antisocial personality disorder Alcohol and other substance abuse Many life problems Conversion disorder	Physical disease Depression	Unconscious Cultural and developmental	Unconscious psychological factors
Conversion disorder	Monosymptomatic Mostly acute Simulates disease	Highly prevalent Female predominance Young age Rural and low social class Little-educated and psychologically unsophisticated	Simulation incompatible with known physiological mechanisms or anatomy	Suggestion and persuasion Multiple techniques	Excellent except in chronic conversion disorder	Alcohol and other substance dependence Antisocial personality disorder Somatization disorder Histrionic personality disorder	Depression Schizophrenia Neurological disease	Unconscious Psychological stress or conflict may be present	Unconscious psychological factors
Hypochondriasis	Disease concern or preoccupation	Previous physical disease Middle or old age Male-female ratio equal	Disease conviction amplifies symptoms Obsessional	Document symptoms Psychosocial review Psychotherapeutic	Fair to good Waxes and wanes	Obsessive-compulsive personality disorder Depressive and anxiety disorders	Depression Physical disease Personality disorder Delusional disorder	Unconscious Stress–bereavement Developmental factors	Unconscious psychological factors
Body dysmorphic disorder	Subjective feelings of ugliness or concern with body defect	Adolescence or young adult Female predominance	Pervasive bodily concerns	Therapeutic alliance Stress management Psychotherapies Antidepressant medications	Guarded	Anorexia nervosa Psychosocial distress Plastic surgery addiction	Delusional disorder Depressive disorders Somatization disorder	Unconscious Self-esteem factors	Unconscious psychological factors
Pain disorder	Pain syndrome simulated	Female predominance 2 to 1 Older: 4th or 5th decade Familial pattern Up to 40% of pain populations	Simulation or intensity incompatible with known physiological mechanisms or anatomy	Therapeutic alliance Redefine goals of treatment Antidepressant medications	Guarded, variable	Depressive disorders Alcohol and other substance abuse Dependent or histrionic personality disorder	Depression Psychophysiological Physical disease Malingering and disability syndrome	Unconscious Acute stressor and developmental Physical trauma may predispose	Unconscious psychological factors

(Adapted from Folks DG, Ford CV, Houck CA. Somatoform disorders, factitious disorders, and malingering. In: Stoudemire A, ed. *Clinical Psychiatry for Medical Students.* Philadelphia: JB Lippincott; 1990:233, with permission.)

unstable homes and have been physically abused. Social, cultural, and ethnic factors may also be involved in the development of symptoms.

Biological Factors.   Some studies point to a neuropsychological basis for somatization disorder. These studies propose that the patients have characteristic attention and cognitive impairments that result in the faulty perception and assessment of somatosensory inputs. The reported impairments include excessive distractibility, inability to habituate to repetitive stimuli, grouping of cognitive constructs on an impressionistic basis, partial and circumstantial associations, and lack of selectivity, as indicated in some studies of evoked potentials. A limited number of brain-imaging studies have reported decreased metabolism in the frontal lobes and the nondominant hemisphere.

GENETICS.   Genetic data indicate that in at least some families, the transmission of somatization disorder has genetic components. Somatization disorder tends to run in families and occurs in 10 to 20 percent of the first-degree female relatives of patients with this disorder. Within these families, first-degree male relatives are susceptible to substance abuse and antisocial personality disorder. One study also reported a concordance rate of 29 percent in monozygotic twins and 10 percent in dizygotic twins, an indication of a genetic effect. The male relatives of women with somatization disorder show an increased risk of antisocial personality disorder and substance-related disorders. Having a biological or adoptive parent with any of these three disorders increases the risk of developing antisocial personality disorder, a substance-related disorder, or somatization disorder.

CYTOKINES.   Cytokines are messenger molecules that the immune system uses to communicate within itself and with the nervous system, including the brain. Examples of cytokines are interleukins, tumor necrosis factor, and interferons. Some preliminary experiments indicate that cytokines contribute to some of the nonspecific symptoms of disease, such as hypersomnia, anorexia, fatigue, and depression. The hypothesis that abnormal regulation of the cytokine system may result in some of the symptoms seen in somatoform disorders is under investigation.

Diagnosis

For the diagnosis of somatization disorder, DSM-IV-TR requires onset of symptoms before age 30 years (Table 14–2). During the course of the disorder, patients must have complained of at least four pain symptoms, two gastrointestinal symptoms, one sexual symptom, and one pseudoneurological symptom, none of which is completely explained by physical or laboratory examinations.

Clinical Features

Patients with somatization disorder have many somatic complaints and long, complicated medical histories. Nausea and vomiting (other than during pregnancy), difficulty swallowing, pain in the arms and legs, shortness of breath unrelated to exertion, amnesia, and complications of pregnancy and menstruation are among the most common symptoms. Patients frequently believe that they have been sickly most of their lives. Pseudoneurological symptoms suggest, but are not pathognomonic of, a neurological disorder. According to DSM-IV-TR, they include impaired coordination or balance, paralysis or localized weakness, difficulty swallowing or lump in throat, aphonia, urinary retention, hallucinations, loss of touch or pain sensation, double

Table 14–2
DSM-IV-TR Diagnostic Criteria for Somatization Disorder

A. A history of many physical complaints beginning before age 30 years that occur over a period of several years and result in treatment being sought or significant impairment in social, occupational, or other important areas of functioning.

B. Each of the following criteria must have been met, with individual symptoms occurring at any time during the course of the disturbance:

   (1) four pain symptoms: a history of pain related to at least four different sites or functions (e.g., head, abdomen, back, joints, extremities, chest, rectum, during menstruation, during sexual intercourse, or during urination)

   (2) two gastrointestinal symptoms: a history of at least two gastrointestinal symptoms other than pain (e.g., nausea, bloating, vomiting other than during pregnancy, diarrhea, or intolerance of several different foods)

   (3) one sexual symptom: a history of at least one sexual or reproductive symptom other than pain (e.g., sexual indifference, erectile or ejaculatory dysfunction, irregular menses, excessive menstrual bleeding, vomiting throughout pregnancy)

   (4) one pseudoneurological symptom: a history of at least one symptom or deficit suggesting a neurological condition not limited to pain (conversion symptoms such as impaired coordination or balance, paralysis or localized weakness, difficulty swallowing or lump in throat, aphonia, urinary retention, hallucinations, loss of touch or pain sensation, double vision, blindness, deafness, seizures; dissociative symptoms such as amnesia; or loss of consciousness other than fainting)

C. Either (1) or (2):

   (1) after appropriate investigation, each of the symptoms in Criterion B cannot be fully explained by a known general medical condition or the direct effects of a substance (e.g., a drug of abuse, a medication)

   (2) when there is a related general medical condition, the physical complaints or resulting social or occupational impairment are in excess of what would be expected from the history, physical examination, or laboratory findings

D. The symptoms are not intentionally produced or feigned (as in factitious disorder or malingering).

From American Psychiatric Association. *Diagnostic and Statistical Manual of Mental Disorders.* 4th ed. Text rev. Washington, DC: American Psychiatric Association; copyright 2000, with permission.

vision, blindness, deafness, seizures, or loss of consciousness other than fainting.

Psychological distress and interpersonal problems are prominent; anxiety and depression are the most prevalent psychiatric conditions. Suicide threats are common, but actual suicide is rare. If suicide does occur, it is often associated with substance abuse. Patients' medical histories are often circumstantial, vague, imprecise, inconsistent, and disorganized. Patients classically (but not always) describe their complaints in a dramatic, emotional, and exaggerated fashion, with vivid and colorful language; they may confuse temporal sequences and cannot clearly distinguish current from past symptoms. Female patients with somatization disorder may dress in an exhibitionistic manner. Patients may be perceived as dependent, self-centered, hungry for admiration or praise, and manipulative.

Somatization disorder is commonly associated with other mental disorders, including major depressive disorder, personality disorders, substance-related disorders, generalized anxiety disorder, and phobias. The combination of these disorders and the chronic symptoms results in an increased incidence of marital, occupational, and social problems.

A 34-year-old female temporary clerk presented with chronic and intermittent dizziness, paresthesias, pain in multiple areas of her body, and intermittent nausea and diarrhea. On further history, the patient said that the symptoms had been present most of the time, although they had been undulating since she was approximately 24 years of age. In addition to the symptoms previously mentioned, she had mild depression, was disinterested in many things in life, including sexual activity, and had been to many doctors to try to find out what was wrong with her. Even though she had seen many doctors and had many tests, she stated that "no one can find out what's wrong" with her. She wanted another opinion. She commented that she had been "sick a lot" since childhood and had been on various medications on and off. Physical examination revealed a normotensive, slightly overweight female in no acute distress. She had diffuse and mild abdominal tenderness, without true guarding or rebound tenderness. Her neurological examination was normal. She winced when physical examination was conducted on various parts of her body, although this wincing went away when the physician was speaking with her while conducting the examination. (Courtesy of Michael A. Hollifield, M.D.)

Differential Diagnosis

The three features that most suggest a diagnosis of somatization disorder instead of another medical disorder are (1) the involvement of multiple organ systems, (2) early onset and chronic course without development of physical signs or structural abnormalities, and (3) absence of laboratory abnormalities that are characteristic of the suggested medical condition. In the process of diagnosis, the astute clinician considers other medical disorders that are characterized by vague, multiple, and confusing somatic symptoms, such as thyroid disease, hyperparathyroidism, intermittent porphyria, multiple sclerosis, and systemic lupus erythematosus.

Mood and anxiety disorders often, but not always, have prominent somatic symptoms, which do not exist separately from the mood or anxiety disorder. Somatization disorder may be diagnosed, however, as a comorbid condition with mood and anxiety disorders. Schizophrenia and other psychotic disorders with multiple somatic delusions need to be differentiated from the nondelusional somatic complaints of individuals with somatization disorder. Hallucinations can occur as pseudoneurological symptoms and must be distinguished from the typical hallucinations seen in schizophrenia. Somatization disorder symptoms are usually easier to distinguish from psychotic disorders than is the case for hypochondriasis, the disease fears of which can reach delusional quality.

Course and Prognosis

Somatization disorder is a chronic, undulating, and relapsing disorder that rarely remits completely. It is unusual for the individual with somatization disorder to be free of symptoms for greater than 1 year. Research has indicated that a person diagnosed with somatization disorder has approximately an 80 percent chance of being diagnosed with this disorder 5 years later. Although patients with this disorder consider themselves to be medically ill, good evidence is that they are no more likely to develop another medical illness in the next 20 years than are people without somatization disorder.

Treatment

Somatization disorder is best treated when the patient has a single identified physician as primary caretaker. When more than one clinician is involved, patients have increased opportunities to express somatic complaints. Primary physicians should see patients during regularly scheduled visits, usually at monthly intervals. The visits should be relatively brief, although a partial physical examination should be conducted to respond to each new somatic complaint. Additional laboratory and diagnostic procedures should generally be avoided. Once somatization disorder has been diagnosed, the treating physician should listen to the somatic complaints as emotional expressions rather than as medical complaints. Nevertheless, patients with somatization disorder can also have bona fide physical illnesses; therefore, physicians must always use their judgment about what symptoms to work up and to what extent. A reasonable long-range strategy for a primary care physician who is treating a patient with somatization disorder is to increase the patient's awareness of the possibility that psychological factors are involved in the symptoms until the patient is willing to see a mental health clinician. In complex cases with many medical presentations, a psychiatrist is better able to judge whether to seek a medical or surgical consultation because of his or her medical training; however, a nonmedical mental health professional can explore the psychological antecedents of the disorder as well, especially if he or she consults closely with a physician.

Psychotherapy, both individual and group, decreases these patients' personal health care expenditures by 50 percent, largely by decreasing their rates of hospitalization. In psychotherapy settings, patients are helped to cope with their symptoms, to express underlying emotions, and to develop alternative strategies for expressing their feelings.

Giving psychotropic medications whenever somatization disorder coexists with a mood or anxiety disorder is always a risk, but psychopharmacological treatment, as well as psychotherapeutic treatment, of the coexisting disorder is indicated. Medication must be monitored because patients with somatization disorder tend to use drugs erratically and unreliably. Few available data indicate that pharmacological treatment is effective in patients without coexisting mental disorders.

CONVERSION DISORDER

Conversion disorder is an illness of symptoms or deficits that affect voluntary motor or sensory functions that suggest another medical condition but is judged to be due to psychological factors because the illness is preceded by conflicts or other stressors. The symptoms or deficits of conversion disorder are not intentionally produced, are not due to substances, and are not limited to pain or sexual symptoms, and the gain is primarily psychological and not social, monetary, or legal.

Epidemiology

Some symptoms of conversion disorder that are not severe enough to warrant the diagnosis may occur in up to one third of the general population at some time during their lives. Reported rates of conversion disorder vary from 11 of 100,000 to 300 of 100,000 in general population samples. Among specific populations, the occurrence of conversion disorder may be even higher than that, perhaps making conversion disorder the most common somatoform disorder in some populations. Several studies have reported that 5 to 15 percent of psychiatric consultations in a general hospital and 25 to 30 percent of admissions to a Veterans Administration hospital involve patients with conversion disorder diagnoses.

The ratio of women to men among adult patients is at least 2:1 and as much as 10:1; among children there is an even higher predominance in girls. Symptoms are more common on the left than on the right side of the body in women. Women who present with conversion symptoms are more likely subsequently to develop somatization disorder than women who have not had conversion symptoms. An association exists between conversion disorder and antisocial personality disorder in men. Men with conversion disorder have often been involved in occupational or military accidents.

The onset of conversion disorder is generally from late childhood to early adulthood and is rare before 10 years of age or after 35 years of age, but onset as late as the ninth decade of life has been reported. When symptoms suggest a conversion disorder onset in middle or old age, the probability of an occult neurological or other medical condition is high. Conversion symptoms in children younger than 10 years of age are usually limited to gait problems or seizures.

Data indicate that conversion disorder is most common among rural populations, persons with little education, those with low intelligence quotients, those in low socioeconomic groups, and military personnel who have been exposed to combat situations. Conversion disorder is commonly associated with comorbid diagnoses of major depressive disorder, anxiety disorders, and schizophrenia and shows an increased frequency in relatives of probands with conversion disorder. Limited data suggest that conversion symptoms are more frequent in relatives of people with conversion disorder. An increased risk of conversion disorder in monozygotic, but not dizygotic, twin pairs has been reported.

Comorbidity

Medical and, especially, neurological disorders occur frequently among patients with conversion disorders. What is typically seen in these comorbid neurological or medical conditions is an elaboration of symptoms stemming from the original organic lesion.

Among the Axis I psychiatric conditions, depressive disorders, anxiety disorders, and somatization disorders are especially noted for their association with conversion disorder. Conversion

in schizophrenia is reported, but it is uncommon. Studies of patients admitted to a psychiatric hospital for conversion disorder reveal that on further study, one fourth to one half have a clinically significant mood disorder or schizophrenia.

Personality disorders also frequently accompany conversion disorder, especially the histrionic type (in 5 to 21 percent of cases) and the passive-dependent type (9 to 40 percent of cases). Conversion disorders can occur, however, in persons with no predisposing medical, neurological, or psychiatric disorder.

Etiology

Psychoanalytic Factors.   According to psychoanalytic theory, conversion disorder is caused by repression of unconscious intrapsychic conflict and conversion of anxiety into a physical symptom. The conflict is between an instinctual impulse (e.g., aggression or sexuality) and the prohibitions against its expression. The symptoms allow partial expression of the forbidden wish or urge but disguise it, so that patients can avoid consciously confronting their unacceptable impulses; that is, the conversion disorder symptom has a symbolic relation to the unconscious conflict—for example, vaginismus protects the patient from expressing unacceptable sexual wishes. Conversion disorder symptoms also let patients communicate that they need special consideration and special treatment. Such symptoms may function as a nonverbal means of controlling or manipulating others.

Learning Theory.   In terms of conditioned learning theory, a conversion symptom can be seen as a piece of classically conditioned learned behavior; symptoms of illness, learned in childhood, are called forth as a means of coping with an otherwise impossible situation.

Biological Factors.   Increasing data implicate biological and neuropsychological factors in the development of conversion disorder symptoms. Preliminary brain-imaging studies have found hypometabolism of the dominant hemisphere and hypermetabolism of the nondominant hemisphere and have implicated impaired hemispheric communication in the cause of conversion disorder. The symptoms may be caused by an excessive cortical arousal that sets off negative feedback loops between the cerebral cortex and the brainstem reticular formation. Elevated levels of corticofugal output, in turn, inhibit the patient's awareness of bodily sensation, which may explain the observed sensory deficits in some patients with conversion disorder. Neuropsychological tests sometimes reveal subtle cerebral impairments in verbal communication, memory, vigilance, affective incongruity, and attention in these patients.

Diagnosis

DSM-IV-TR limits the diagnosis of conversion disorder to those symptoms that affect a voluntary motor or sensory function, that is, neurological symptoms (Table 14–3). Physicians cannot explain the neurological symptoms solely on the basis of any known neurological condition.

The diagnosis of conversion disorder requires that clinicians find a necessary and critical association between the cause of the neurological symptoms and psychological factors, although the symptoms cannot result from malingering or factitious

Table 14–3
DSM-IV-TR Diagnostic Criteria for Conversion Disorder

A. One or more symptoms or deficits affecting voluntary motor or sensory function that suggest a neurological or other general medical condition.
B. Psychological factors are judged to be associated with the symptom or deficit because the initiation or exacerbation of the symptom or deficit is preceded by conflicts or other stressors.
C. The symptom or deficit is not intentionally produced or feigned (as in factitious disorder or malingering).
D. The symptom or deficit cannot, after appropriate investigation, be fully explained by a general medical condition, or by the direct effects of a substance, or as a culturally sanctioned behavior or experience.
E. The symptom or deficit causes clinically significant distress or impairment in social, occupational, or other important areas of functioning or warrants medical evaluation.
F. The symptom or deficit is not limited to pain or sexual dysfunction, does not occur exclusively during the course of somatization disorder, and is not better accounted for by another mental disorder.

Specify type of symptom or deficit:
With motor symptom or deficit
With sensory symptom or deficit
With seizures or convulsions
With mixed presentation

From American Psychiatric Association. *Diagnostic and Statistical Manual of Mental Disorders.* 4th ed. Text rev. Washington, DC: American Psychiatric Association; copyright 2000, with permission.

disorder. The diagnosis of conversion disorder also excludes symptoms of pain and sexual dysfunction and symptoms that occur only in somatization disorder. DSM-IV-TR allows specification of the type of symptom or deficit seen in conversion disorder (Table 14–3).

Clinical Features

Paralysis, blindness, and mutism are the most common conversion disorder symptoms. Conversion disorder may be most commonly associated with passive-aggressive, dependent, antisocial, and histrionic personality disorders. Depressive and anxiety disorder symptoms often accompany the symptoms of conversion disorder, and affected patients are at risk for suicide.

Mr. J. is a 28-year-old single man who is employed in a factory. He was brought to an emergency department by his father, complaining that he had lost his vision while sitting in the back seat on the way home from a family gathering. He had been playing volleyball at the gathering but had sustained no significant injury except for the volleyball hitting him in the head a few times. As was usual for this man, he had been reluctant to play volleyball because of the lack of his athletic skills, and was placed on a team at the last moment. He recalls having some problems with seeing during the game, but his vision did not become ablated until he was in the car on the way home. By the time he got to the emergency department, his vision was improving, although he still complained of blurriness and mild diplopia. The double

vision could be attenuated by having him focus on items at different distances.

On examination, Mr. J. was fully cooperative, somewhat uncertain about why this would have occurred, and rather nonchalant. Pupillary, oculomotor, and general sensorimotor examinations were normal. After being cleared medically, the patient was sent to a mental health center for further evaluation.

At the mental health center, the patient recounts the same story as he did in the emergency department, and he was still accompanied by his father. He began to recount how his vision started to return to normal when his father pulled over on the side of the road and began to talk to him about the events of the day. He spoke with his father about how he had felt embarrassed and somewhat conflicted about playing volleyball and how he had felt that he really should play because of external pressures. Further history from the patient and his father revealed that this young man had been shy as an adolescent, particularly around athletic participation. He had never had another episode of visual loss. He did recount feeling anxious and sometimes not feeling well in his body during athletic activities.

Discussion with the patient at the mental health center focused on the potential role of psychological and social factors in acute vision loss. The patient was somewhat perplexed by this but was also amenable to discussion. He stated that he clearly recognized that he began seeing and feeling better when his father pulled off to the side of the road and discussed things with him. Doctors admitted that they did not know the cause of the vision loss and that it would likely not return. The patient and his father were satisfied with the medical and psychiatric evaluation and agreed to return for care if there were any further symptoms. The patient was appointed a follow-up time at the outpatient psychiatric clinic. (Courtesy of Michael A. Hollifield, M.D.)

Sensory Symptoms. In conversion disorder, anesthesia and paresthesia are common, especially of the extremities. All sensory modalities can be involved, and the distribution of the disturbance is usually inconsistent with either central or peripheral neurological disease. Thus, clinicians may see the characteristic stocking-and-glove anesthesia of the hands or feet or the hemianesthesia of the body beginning precisely along the midline.

Conversion disorder symptoms may involve the organs of special sense and can produce deafness, blindness, and tunnel vision. These symptoms may be unilateral or bilateral, but neurological evaluation reveals intact sensory pathways. In conversion disorder blindness, for example, patients walk around without collisions or self-injury, their pupils react to light, and their cortical evoked potentials are normal.

Motor Symptoms. The motor symptoms of conversion disorder include abnormal movements, gait disturbance, weakness, and paralysis. Gross rhythmical tremors, choreiform movements, tics, and jerks may be present. The movements generally worsen when attention is called to them. One gait disturbance seen in conversion disorder is *astasia-abasia*, which is a wildly ataxic, staggering gait accompanied by gross, irregular, jerky truncal movements and thrashing and waving arm movements. Patients with the symptoms rarely fall; if they do, they are generally not injured.

Other common motor disturbances are paralysis and paresis involving one, two, or all four limbs, although the distribution of the involved muscles does not conform to the neural pathways. Reflexes remain normal; the patients have no fasciculations or muscle atrophy (except after long-standing conversion paralysis); electromyography findings are normal.

Seizure Symptoms. Pseudoseizures are another symptom in conversion disorder. Clinicians may find it difficult to differentiate a pseudoseizure from an actual seizure by clinical observation alone. Moreover, about one third of the patient's pseudoseizures also have a coexisting epileptic disorder. Tongue-biting, urinary incontinence, and injuries after falling can occur in pseudoseizures, although these symptoms are generally not present. Pupillary and gag reflexes are retained after pseudoseizure, and patients have no postseizure increase in prolactin concentrations.

Other Associated Features. Several psychological symptoms have also been associated with conversion disorder.

PRIMARY GAIN. Patients achieve primary gain by keeping internal conflicts outside their awareness. Symptoms have symbolic value; they represent an unconscious psychological conflict.

SECONDARY GAIN. Patients accrue tangible advantages and benefits as a result of being sick; for example, being excused from obligations and difficult life situations, receiving support and assistance that might not otherwise be forthcoming, and controlling other persons' behavior.

LA BELLE INDIFFÉRENCE. La belle indifférence is a patient's inappropriately cavalier attitude toward serious symptoms; that is, the patient seems to be unconcerned about what appears to be a major impairment. That bland indifference is also seen in some seriously ill medical patients who develop a stoic attitude. The presence or absence of la belle indifférence is not pathognomonic of conversion disorder, but it is often associated with the condition.

IDENTIFICATION. Patients with conversion disorder may unconsciously model their symptoms on those of someone important to them. For example, a parent or a person who has recently died may serve as a model for conversion disorder. During pathological grief reaction, bereaved persons commonly have symptoms of the deceased.

Differential Diagnosis

One of the major problems in diagnosing conversion disorder is the difficulty of definitively ruling out a medical disorder. Concomitant nonpsychiatric medical disorders are common in hospitalized patients with conversion disorder, and evidence of a current or previous neurological disorder or a systemic disease affecting the brain has been reported in 18 to 64 percent of such patients. An estimated 25 to 50 percent of patients classified as having conversion disorder eventually receive diagnoses of neurological or nonpsychiatric medical disorders that could have caused their earlier symptoms. Thus, a thorough medical and neurological workup is essential in all cases. If the symptoms can be resolved by suggestion, hypnosis, or parenteral amobarbital (Amytal) or lorazepam (Ativan), they are probably the result of conversion disorder.

Neurological disorders (i.e., dementia and other degenerative diseases), brain tumors, and basal ganglia disease must be considered in the differential diagnosis. For example, weakness may be confused with myasthenia gravis, polymyositis, acquired myopathies, or multiple sclerosis. Optic neuritis may be misdiagnosed as conversion disorder blindness. Other diseases that can cause confusing symptoms are Guillain-Barré syndrome, Creutzfeldt-Jakob disease, periodic paralysis, and early neurological manifestations of acquired immunodeficiency syndrome (AIDS). Conversion disorder symptoms occur in schizophrenia, depressive disorders, and anxiety disorders, but these other disorders are associated with their own distinct symptoms that eventually make differential diagnosis possible.

Sensorimotor symptoms also occur in somatization disorder. However, somatization disorder is a chronic illness that begins early in life and includes symptoms in many other organ systems. In hypochondriasis, patients have no actual loss or distortion of function; the somatic complaints are chronic and are not limited to neurological symptoms, and the characteristic hypochondriacal attitudes and beliefs are present. If the patient's symptoms are limited to pain, pain disorder can be diagnosed. Patients whose complaints are limited to sexual function are classified as having a sexual dysfunction rather than conversion disorder.

In both malingering and factitious disorder, the symptoms are under conscious, voluntary control. A malingerer's history is usually more inconsistent and contradictory than that of a patient with conversion disorder, and a malingerer's fraudulent behavior is clearly goal directed.

Course and Prognosis

The onset of conversion disorder is usually acute, but a crescendo of symptomatology may also occur. Symptoms or deficits are usually of short duration, and approximately 95 percent of acute cases remit spontaneously, usually within 2 weeks in hospitalized patients. If symptoms have been present for 6 months or longer, the prognosis for symptom resolution is less than 50 percent and diminishes further the longer that conversion is present. Recurrence occurs in one fifth to one fourth of people within 1 year of the first episode. Thus, one episode is a predictor for future episodes. A good prognosis is heralded by acute onset, presence of clearly identifiable stressors at the time of onset, a short interval between onset and the institution of treatment, and above-average intelligence. Paralysis, aphonia, and blindness are associated with a good prognosis, whereas tremor and seizures are poor prognostic factors.

Treatment

Resolution of the conversion disorder symptom is usually spontaneous, although it is probably facilitated by insight-oriented supportive or behavior therapy. The most important feature of the therapy is a relationship with a caring and confident therapist. With patients who are resistant to the idea of psychotherapy, physicians can suggest that the psychotherapy will focus on issues of stress and coping. Telling such patients that their symptoms are imaginary often makes them worse. Hypnosis, anxiolytics, and behavioral relaxation exercises are effective in some cases. Parenteral amobarbital or lorazepam may be helpful in obtaining additional historic information, especially when a patient has recently experienced a traumatic event. Psychodynamic approaches include psychoanalysis and insight-oriented psychotherapy, in which patients explore intrapsychic conflicts and the symbolism of the conversion disorder symptoms. Brief and direct forms of short-term psychotherapy have also been used to treat conversion disorder. The longer the duration of these patients' sick role and the more they have regressed, the more difficult is the treatment.

HYPOCHONDRIASIS

Hypochondriasis is characterized by 6 months or more of a general and nondelusional preoccupation with fears of having, or the idea that one has, a serious disease based on the person's misinterpretation of bodily symptoms. This preoccupation causes significant distress and impairment in one's life; it is not accounted for by another psychiatric or medical disorder; and a subset of individuals with hypochondriasis has poor insight about the presence of this disorder. The term *hypochondriasis* is derived from the old medical term hypochondrium ("below the ribs") and reflects the common abdominal complaints of many patients with the disorder, but they may occur in any part of the body.

Epidemiology

One recent study reported a 6-month prevalence of hypochondriasis of 4 to 6 percent in a general medical clinic population, but it may be as high as 15 percent. Men and women are equally affected by hypochondriasis. Although the onset of symptoms can occur at any age, the disorder most commonly appears in persons 20 to 30 years of age. Some evidence indicates that the diagnosis is more common among blacks than among whites, but social position, education level, and marital status do not appear to affect the diagnosis. Hypochondriacal complaints reportedly occur in about 3 percent of medical students, usually in the first 2 years, but they are generally transient.

Etiology

Many theories have been postulated as to the cause of hypochondriasis. One theory, based on reasonable data, is that persons with hypochondriasis augment and amplify their somatic sensations; they have low thresholds for, and low tolerance of, physical discomfort. For example, what persons normally perceive as abdominal pressure, persons with hypochondriasis experience as abdominal pain. They may focus on bodily sensations, misinterpret them, and become alarmed by them because of a faulty cognitive scheme.

A second theory is that hypochondriasis is understandable in terms of a social learning model. The symptoms of hypochondriasis are viewed as a request for admission to the sick role made by a person facing seemingly insurmountable and insolvable problems. The sick role offers an escape that allows a patient to avoid noxious obligations, to postpone unwelcome challenges, and to be excused from usual duties and obligations.

A third theory suggests that hypochondriasis is a variant form of other mental disorders, among which depressive disorders and anxiety disorders are most frequently included. An estimated 80 percent of patients with hypochondriasis may have coexisting depressive or anxiety disorders. Patients who meet the diagnostic criteria for hypochondriasis may be somatizing subtypes of these other disorders.

The psychodynamic school of thought has produced a fourth theory of hypochondriasis. According to this theory, aggressive and hostile wishes toward others are transferred (through repression and displacement) into physical complaints. The anger

of patients with hypochondriasis originates in past disappointments, rejections, and losses, but the patients express their anger in the present by soliciting the help and concern of other persons and then rejecting them as ineffective. Hypochondriasis is also viewed as a defense against guilt, a sense of innate badness, an expression of low self-esteem, and a sign of excessive self-concern. Pain and somatic suffering, thus, become means of atonement and expiation (undoing) and can be experienced as deserved punishment for past wrongdoing (either real or imaginary) and for a person's sense of wickedness and sinfulness.

Diagnosis

The DSM-IV-TR diagnostic criteria for hypochondriasis require that patients be preoccupied with the false belief that they have a serious disease based on their misinterpretation of physical signs or sensations (Table 14–4). The belief must last at least 6 months, despite the absence of pathological findings on medical and neurological examinations. The diagnostic criteria also stipulate that the belief cannot have the intensity of a delusion (more appropriately diagnosed as delusional disorder) and cannot be restricted to distress about appearance (more appropriately diagnosed as body dysmorphic disorder). The symptoms of hypochondriasis must be sufficiently intense to cause emotional distress or impair the patient's ability to function in important areas of life. Clinicians may specify the presence of poor insight; patients do not consistently recognize that their concerns about disease are excessive.

Clinical Features

Patients with hypochondriasis believe that they have a serious disease that has not yet been detected, and they cannot be

Table 14–4
DSM-IV-TR Diagnostic Criteria for Hypochondriasis

A. Preoccupation with fears of having, or the idea that one has, a serious disease based on the person's misinterpretation of bodily symptoms.
B. The preoccupation persists despite appropriate medical evaluation and reassurance.
C. The belief in Criterion A is not of delusional intensity (as in delusional disorder, somatic type) and is not restricted to a circumscribed concern about appearance (as in body dysmorphic disorder).
D. The preoccupation causes clinically significant distress or impairment in social, occupational, or other important areas of functioning.
E. The duration of the disturbance is at least 6 months.
F. The preoccupation is not better accounted for by generalized anxiety disorder, obsessive-compulsive disorder, panic disorder, a major depressive episode, separation anxiety, or another somatoform disorder.

Specify if:
With poor insight: if, for most of the time during the current episode, the person does not recognize that the concern about having a serious illness is excessive or unreasonable

From American Psychiatric Association. *Diagnostic and Statistical Manual of Mental Disorders.* 4th ed. Text rev. Washington, DC: American Psychiatric Association; copyright 2000, with permission.

persuaded to the contrary. They may maintain a belief that they have a particular disease, or, as time progresses, they may transfer their belief to another disease. Their convictions persist despite negative laboratory results, the benign course of the alleged disease over time, and appropriate reassurances from physicians. Yet, their beliefs are not sufficiently fixed to be delusions. Hypochondriasis is often accompanied by symptoms of depression and anxiety and commonly coexists with a depressive or anxiety disorder.

Although DSM-IV-TR specifies that the symptoms must be present for at least 6 months, transient hypochondriacal states can occur after major stresses, most commonly the death or serious illness of someone important to the patient, or a serious (perhaps life-threatening) illness that has been resolved but that leaves the patient temporarily hypochondriacal in its wake. Such states that last fewer than 6 months should be diagnosed as somatoform disorder not otherwise specified. Transient hypochondriacal responses to external stress generally remit when the stress is resolved, but they can become chronic if reinforced by persons in the patient's social system or by health professionals.

Differential Diagnosis

Hypochondriasis must be differentiated from nonpsychiatric medical conditions, especially disorders that show symptoms that are not necessarily easily diagnosed. Such diseases include AIDS, endocrinopathies, myasthenia gravis, multiple sclerosis, degenerative diseases of the nervous system, systemic lupus erythematosus, and occult neoplastic disorders.

Hypochondriasis is differentiated from somatization disorder by the emphasis in hypochondriasis on fear of having a disease and emphasis in somatization disorder on concern about many symptoms. Patients with hypochondriasis usually complain about fewer symptoms than patients with somatization disorder. Somatization disorder usually has an onset before age 30 years, whereas hypochondriasis has a less specific age of onset. Patients with somatization disorder are more likely to be women; hypochondriasis is equally distributed among men and women.

Hypochondriasis must also be differentiated from the other somatoform disorders. Conversion disorder is acute and generally transient and usually involves a symptom rather than a particular disease. The presence or absence of la belle indifférence is an unreliable feature with which to differentiate the two conditions. Pain disorder is chronic, as is hypochondriasis, but the symptoms are limited to complaints of pain. Patients with body dysmorphic disorder wish to appear normal but believe that others notice that they are not, whereas those with hypochondriasis seek out attention for their presumed diseases.

Hypochondriacal symptoms can also occur in patients with depressive disorders and anxiety disorders. If a patient meets the full diagnostic criteria for both hypochondriasis and another major mental disorder, such as major depressive disorder or generalized anxiety disorder, the patient should receive both diagnoses, unless the hypochondriacal symptoms occur only during episodes of the other mental disorder. Patients with panic disorder may initially complain that they are affected by a disease (e.g., heart trouble), but careful questioning during the medical history usually uncovers the classic symptoms of a panic attack. Delusional hypochondriacal beliefs occur in schizophrenia and other psychotic disorders but can be differentiated from hypochondriasis by their delusional intensity and by the presence of other psychotic symptoms. In addition, schizophrenic patients' somatic delusions tend to be bizarre, idiosyncratic, and out of keeping with their cultural milieus.

Hypochondriasis is distinguished from factitious disorder with physical symptoms and from malingering in that patients with hypochondriasis actually experience and do not simulate the symptoms they report.

Course and Prognosis

The course of hypochondriasis is usually episodic; the episodes last from months to years and are separated by equally long quiescent periods. There may be an obvious association between exacerbations of hypochondriacal symptoms and psychosocial stressors. Although no well-conducted large outcome studies have been reported, an estimated one third to one half of all patients with hypochondriasis eventually improve significantly. A good prognosis is associated with high socioeconomic status, treatment-responsive anxiety or depression, sudden onset of symptoms, the absence of a personality disorder, and the absence of a related nonpsychiatric medical condition. Most children with hypochondriasis recover by late adolescence or early adulthood.

Treatment

Patients with hypochondriasis usually resist psychiatric treatment, although some accept this treatment if it takes place in a medical setting and focuses on stress reduction and education in coping with chronic illness. Group psychotherapy often benefits such patients, in part because it provides the social support and social interaction that seem to reduce their anxiety. Other forms of psychotherapy, such as individual insight-oriented psychotherapy, behavior therapy, cognitive therapy, and hypnosis, may be useful.

Frequent, regularly scheduled physical examinations help to reassure patients that their physicians are not abandoning them and that their complaints are being taken seriously. Invasive diagnostic and therapeutic procedures should only be undertaken, however, when objective evidence calls for them. When possible, the clinician should refrain from treating equivocal or incidental physical examination findings.

Pharmacotherapy alleviates hypochondriacal symptoms only when a patient has an underlying drug-responsive condition, such as an anxiety disorder or major depressive disorder. When hypochondriasis is secondary to another primary mental disorder, that disorder must be treated in its own right. When hypochondriasis is a transient situational reaction, clinicians must help patients cope with the stress without reinforcing their illness behavior and their use of the sick role as a solution to their problems.

BODY DYSMORPHIC DISORDER

Body dysmorphic disorder is characterized by a preoccupation with an imagined defect in appearance that causes clinically significant distress or impairment in important areas of functioning.

If a slight physical anomaly is actually present, the person's concern with the anomaly is excessive and bothersome.

The disorder was recognized and named *dysmorphophobia* more than 100 years ago by Emil Kraepelin, who considered it a compulsive neurosis; Pierre Janet called it *obsession de la honte du corps* (obsession with shame of the body). Freud wrote about the condition in his description of the Wolf-Man, who was excessively concerned about his nose. Although dysmorphophobia was widely recognized and studied in Europe, it was not until the publication of DSM-III in 1980 that dysmorphophobia, as an example of a typical somatoform disorder, was specifically mentioned in the U.S. diagnostic criteria. In DSM-IV-TR, the condition is known as body dysmorphic disorder because the DSM editors believed that the term *dysmorphophobia* inaccurately implied the presence of a behavioral pattern of phobic avoidance.

Epidemiology

Body dysmorphic disorder is a poorly studied condition, partly because patients are more likely to go to dermatologists, internists, or plastic surgeons than to psychiatrists. One study of a group of college students found that more than 50 percent had at least some preoccupation with a particular aspect of their appearance, and in about 25 percent of the students, the concern had at least some significant effect on their feelings and functioning.

Data indicate that the most common age of onset is between 15 and 30 years and that women are affected somewhat more often than men. Affected patients are also likely to be unmarried. Body dysmorphic disorder commonly coexists with other mental disorders. One study found that more than 90 percent of patients with body dysmorphic disorder had experienced a major depressive episode in their lifetimes, about 70 percent had experienced an anxiety disorder, and about 30 percent had experienced a psychotic disorder.

Etiology

The cause of body dysmorphic disorder is unknown. The high comorbidity with depressive disorders, a higher-than-expected family history of mood disorders and obsessive-compulsive disorder (OCD), and the reported responsiveness of the condition to serotonin-specific drugs indicate that in at least some patients, the pathophysiology of the disorder may involve serotonin and may be related to other mental disorders. Stereotyped concepts of beauty emphasized in certain families and within the culture at large may significantly affect patients with body dysmorphic disorder. In psychodynamic models, body dysmorphic disorder is seen as reflecting the displacement of a sexual or emotional conflict onto a nonrelated body part. Such an association occurs through the defense mechanisms of repression, dissociation, distortion, symbolization, and projection.

Diagnosis

The DSM-IV-TR diagnostic criteria for body dysmorphic disorder stipulate preoccupation with an imagined defect in appearance or overemphasis of a slight defect (Table 14–5). The preoccupation causes patients significant emotional distress or markedly impairs their ability to function in important areas.

Table 14–5
DSM-IV-TR Diagnostic Criteria for Body Dysmorphic Disorder

A. Preoccupation with an imagined defect in appearance. If a slight physical anomaly is present, the person's concern is markedly excessive.
B. The preoccupation causes clinically significant distress or impairment in social, occupational, or other important areas of functioning.
C. The preoccupation is not better accounted for by another mental disorder (e.g., dissatisfaction with body shape and size in anorexia nervosa).

From American Psychiatric Association. *Diagnostic and Statistical Manual of Mental Disorders*. 4th ed. Text rev. Washington, DC: American Psychiatric Association; copyright 2000, with permission.

Clinical Features

The most common concerns involve facial flaws, particularly those involving specific parts (e.g., the nose). Sometimes the concern is vague and difficult to understand, such as extreme concern over a "scrunchy" chin. One study found that, on average, patients had concerns about four body regions during the course of the disorder. Other body parts of concern are hair, breasts, and genitalia. A proposed variant of dysmorphic disorder among men is the desire to "bulk up" and develop large muscle mass, which can interfere with ordinary living, holding a job, or staying healthy. The specific body part may change during the time a patient is affected with the disorder. Common associated symptoms include ideas or frank delusions of reference (usually about persons' noticing the alleged body flaw), either excessive mirror checking or avoidance of reflective surfaces, and attempts to hide the presumed deformity (with makeup or clothing). The effects on a person's life can be significant; almost all affected patients avoid social and occupational exposure. As many as one third of the patients may be housebound because of worry about being ridiculed for the alleged deformities, and approximately one fifth of patients attempt suicide. As discussed previously, comorbid diagnoses of depressive disorders and anxiety disorders are common, and patients may also have traits of obsessive-compulsive, schizoid, and narcissistic personality disorders.

Differential Diagnosis

The diagnosis of body dysmorphic disorder should not be made if the excessive bodily preoccupation is better accounted for by another psychiatric disorder. Individuals with avoidant personality disorder or social phobia may worry about being embarrassed by imagined or real defects in appearance, but this concern is usually not prominent, persistent, distressing, or impairing. Taijin kyofu-sho, a diagnosis in Japan, is similar to social phobia but has some features that are more consistent with body dysmorphic disorder, such as the belief that the person has an offensive odor or body parts that are offensive to others. Although individuals with body dysmorphic disorder have obsessional preoccupations about their appearance and may have associated compulsive behaviors (e.g., mirror checking), a separate or additional diagnosis of OCD is made only when the obsessions or compulsions are not restricted to concerns about appearance and are ego-dystonic. An additional diagnosis of delusional disorder, somatic type, can be made in people with body dysmorphic disorder only if their preoccupation with the imagined defect in appearance is held with a delusional intensity. Unlike normal concerns about appearance, the preoccupation with appearance and specific imagined defects in body dysmorphic disorder and the changed behavior because of the preoccupation are excessively time consuming and are associated with significant distress or impairment.

Course and Prognosis

Body dysmorphic disorder usually begins during adolescence, although it may begin later after a protracted dissatisfaction with the body. Age of onset is not well understood because of a variably long delay between symptom onset and treatment seeking. The onset can be gradual or abrupt. The disorder usually has a long and undulating course with few symptom-free intervals. The part of the body on which concern is focused may remain the same or may change over time.

Treatment

Treatment of patients with body dysmorphic disorder with surgical, dermatological, dental, and other medical procedures to address the alleged defects is almost invariably unsuccessful. Although tricyclic drugs, monoamine oxidase inhibitors, and pimozide (Orap) have reportedly been useful in individual cases, a larger body of data indicates that serotonin-specific drugs—for example, clomipramine (Anafranil) and fluoxetine (Prozac)—reduce symptoms in at least 50 percent of patients. In any patient with a coexisting mental disorder, such as a depressive disorder or an anxiety disorder, the coexisting disorder should be treated with the appropriate pharmacotherapy and psychotherapy. How long treatment should be continued after the symptoms of body dysmorphic disorder have remitted is unknown. Augmentation of the selective serotonin reuptake inhibitor (SSRI) with clomipramine (Anafranil), buspirone (BuSpar), lithium (Eskalith), methylphenidate (Ritalin), or antipsychotics may improve the response rate.

Relation to Plastic Surgery

Few data exist about the number of patients seeking plastic surgery who have body dysmorphic disorder. One study found that only 2 percent of the patients in a plastic surgery clinic had the diagnosis. The overall percentage may be much higher, however. Surgical requests are varied: removal of facial sags, jowls, wrinkles, or puffiness; rhinoplasty; breast reduction or enhancement; and penile enlargement. Men who request penile enlargements and women who request cosmetic surgery of the labia of the vagina or the lips of the mouth often are suffering from this disorder. Commonly associated with the belief about appearance is an unrealistic expectation of the extent to which surgery will correct the defect. As reality sets in, the person realizes that life's problems are not solved by altering the perceived cosmetic defect. Ideally, such patients will seek out psychotherapy to understand the true nature of their neurotic feelings of inadequacy. Absent that, patients may take out their anger by suing their plastic surgeons—who have one of highest malpractice-suit rates of any specialty—or by developing a clinical depression.

PAIN DISORDER

A pain disorder is characterized by the presence of, and focus on, pain in one or more body sites and is severe enough to come to clinical attention. Psychological factors are necessary in the genesis, severity, or maintenance of the pain, which causes significant distress or impairment, or both. The physician does not have to judge the pain to be "inappropriate" or "in excess of what would be expected." Rather, the phenomenological and diagnostic focus is on the importance of psychological factors and the degree of impairment caused by the pain. The disorder has been called somatoform pain disorder, psychogenic pain disorder, idiopathic pain disorder, and atypical pain disorder.

Epidemiology

Pain disorder appears to be common. Recent work indicates that the 6-month and lifetime prevalences are approximately 5 and 12 percent, respectively. It has been estimated that 10 to 15 percent of adults in the United States have some form of work disability due to back pain alone in any year. Approximately 3 percent of people in a general practice have persistent pain, with at least 1 day per month of activity restriction due to the pain.

Pain disorder can begin at any age. The gender ratio is unknown. Pain disorder is associated with other psychiatric disorders, especially affective and anxiety disorders. Chronic pain appears to be most frequently associated with depressive disorders, and acute pain appears to be more commonly associated with anxiety disorders. The associated psychiatric disorders may precede the pain disorder, may co-occur with it, or may result from it. Depressive disorders, alcohol dependence, and chronic pain may be more common in relatives of individuals with chronic pain disorder. Individuals whose pain is associated with severe depression and those whose pain is related to a terminal illness, such as cancer, are at increased risk for suicide. Differences may exist in how various ethnic and cultural groups respond to pain, but the usefulness of cultural factors for the clinician remains obscure to the treatment of individuals with pain disorder because of a lack of good data and because of high individual variability.

Etiology

Psychodynamic Factors. Patients who experience bodily aches and pains without identifiable and adequate physical causes may be symbolically expressing an intrapsychic conflict through the body. Patients suffering from alexithymia, who are unable to articulate their internal feeling states in words, express their feelings with their bodies. Other patients may unconsciously regard emotional pain as weak and somehow lacking legitimacy. By displacing the problem to the body, they may feel that they have a legitimate claim to the fulfillment of their dependency needs. The symbolic meaning of body disturbances may also relate to atonement for perceived sin, to expiation of guilt, or to suppressed aggression. Many patients have intractable and unresponsive pain because they are convinced that they deserve to suffer.

Pain can function as a method of obtaining love, a punishment for wrongdoing, and a way of expiating guilt and atoning for an innate sense of badness. Among the defense mechanisms used by patients with pain disorder are displacement, substitution, and repression. Identification plays a part when a patient takes on the role of an ambivalent love object who also has pain, such as a parent.

Behavioral Factors.   Pain behaviors are reinforced when rewarded and are inhibited when ignored or punished. For example, moderate pain symptoms may become intense when followed by the solicitous and attentive behavior of others, by monetary gain, or by the successful avoidance of distasteful activities.

Interpersonal Factors.   Intractable pain has been conceptualized as a means for manipulation and gaining advantage in interpersonal relationships, for example, to ensure the devotion of a family member or to stabilize a fragile marriage. Such secondary gain is most important to patients with pain disorder.

Biological Factors.   The cerebral cortex can inhibit the firing of afferent pain fibers. Serotonin is probably the main neurotransmitter in the descending inhibitory pathways, and endorphins also play a role in the central nervous system modulation of pain. Endorphin deficiency seems to correlate with augmentation of incoming sensory stimuli. Some patients may have pain disorder rather than another mental disorder because of sensory and limbic structural or chemical abnormalities that predispose them to experience pain.

Diagnosis

The DSM-IV-TR diagnostic criteria for pain disorder require the presence of clinically significant complaints of pain (Table 14–6). The complaints of pain must be judged to be significantly affected by psychological factors, and the symptoms must result in a patient's significant emotional distress or functional impairment (e.g., social or occupational). DSM-IV-TR requires that the pain disorder be associated primarily with psychological factors or with both psychological factors and a general medical condition. DSM-IV-TR further specifies that pain disorder associated solely with a general medical condition be diagnosed as an Axis III condition; it also allows clinicians to specify whether the pain disorder is acute or chronic, depending on whether the duration of symptoms has been 6 months or more.

Clinical Features

Patients with pain disorder are not a uniform group but comprise a heterogeneous collection of persons with low back pain, headache, atypical facial pain, chronic pelvic pain, and other kinds of pain. A patient's pain may be posttraumatic, neuropathic, neurological, iatrogenic, or musculoskeletal; to meet a diagnosis of pain disorder, however, the disorder must have a psychological factor judged to be significantly involved in the pain symptoms and their ramifications.

Patients with pain disorder often have long histories of medical and surgical care. They visit many physicians, request many medications, and may be especially insistent in their desire for surgery. Indeed, they can be completely preoccupied with their pain and cite it as the source of all their misery. Such patients often deny any other sources of emotional dysphoria and insist that their lives are blissful except for their pain. Their clinical picture can be complicated by substance-related disorders because these patients attempt to reduce the pain through the use of alcohol and other substances.

At least one study has correlated the number of pain symptoms with the likelihood and severity of symptoms of somatization disorder, depressive disorders, and anxiety disorders. Major depressive disorder is present in about 25 to 50 percent of patients with pain disorder, and dysthymic disorder or depressive disorder symptoms are reported in 60 to 100 percent of the patients. Some investigators believe that chronic pain is almost always a variant of a depressive disorder, a masked or somatized

Table 14–6
DSM-IV-TR Diagnostic Criteria for Pain Disorder

A. Pain in one or more anatomical sites is the predominant focus of the clinical presentation and is of sufficient severity to warrant clinical attention.
B. The pain causes clinically significant distress or impairment in social, occupational, or other important areas of functioning.
C. Psychological factors are judged to have an important role in the onset, severity, exacerbation, or maintenance of the pain.
D. The symptom or deficit is not intentionally produced or feigned (as in factitious disorder or malingering).
E. The pain is not better accounted for by a mood, anxiety, or psychotic disorder and does not meet criteria for dyspareunia.

Code as follows:
  Pain disorder associated with psychological factors: psychological factors are judged to have the major role in the onset, severity, exacerbation, or maintenance of the pain. (If a general medical condition is present, it does not have a major role in the onset, severity, exacerbation, or maintenance of the pain.) This type of pain disorder is not diagnosed if criteria are also met for somatization disorder.

Specify if:
  Acute: duration of less than 6 months
  Chronic: duration of 6 months or longer
  Pain disorder associated with both psychological factors and a general medical condition: both psychological factors and a general medical condition are judged to have important roles in the onset, severity, exacerbation, or maintenance of the pain. The associated general medical condition or anatomical site of the pain (see below) is coded on Axis III.

Specify if:
  Acute: duration of less than 6 months
  Chronic: duration of 6 months or longer
  Note: The following is not considered to be a mental disorder and is included here to facilitate differential diagnosis.
  Pain disorder associated with a general medical condition: a general medical condition has a major role in the onset, severity, exacerbation, or maintenance of the pain. (If psychological factors are present, they are not judged to have a major role in the onset, severity, exacerbation, or maintenance of the pain.) The diagnostic code for the pain is selected based on the associated general medical condition if one has been established or on the anatomical location of the pain if the underlying general medical condition is not yet clearly established—for example, low back, sciatic, pelvic, headache, facial, chest, joint, bone, abdominal, breast, renal, ear, eye, throat, tooth, and urinary.

From American Psychiatric Association. *Diagnostic and Statistical Manual of Mental Disorders.* 4th ed. Text rev. Washington, DC: American Psychiatric Association; copyright 2000, with permission.

form of depression. The most prominent depressive symptoms in patients with pain disorder are anergia, anhedonia, decreased libido, insomnia, and irritability; diurnal variation, weight loss, and psychomotor retardation appear to be less common.

Differential Diagnosis

Purely physical pain can be difficult to distinguish from purely psychogenic pain, especially because the two are not mutually exclusive. Physical pain fluctuates in intensity and is highly sensitive to emotional, cognitive, attentional, and situational influences. Pain that does not vary and is insensitive to any of these factors is likely to be psychogenic. When pain does not wax and wane and is not even temporarily relieved by distraction or analgesics, clinicians can suspect an important psychogenic component.

Pain disorder must be distinguished from other somatoform disorders, although some somatoform disorders can coexist. Patients with hypochondriacal preoccupations may complain of pain, and aspects of the clinical presentation of hypochondriasis, such as bodily preoccupation and disease conviction, can also be present in patients with pain disorder. Patients with hypochondriasis tend to have many more symptoms than patients with pain disorder, and their symptoms tend to fluctuate more than those of patients with pain disorder. Conversion disorder is generally short lived, whereas pain disorder is chronic. In addition, pain is, by definition, not a symptom in conversion disorder. Malingering patients consciously provide false reports, and their complaints are usually connected to clearly recognizable goals.

The differential diagnosis can be difficult because patients with pain disorder often receive disability compensation or a litigation award. Muscle contraction (tension) headaches, for example, have a pathophysiological mechanism to account for the pain and so are not diagnosed as pain disorder. However, patients with pain disorder are not pretending to be in pain. As in all of the somatoform disorders, symptoms are not imaginary.

Course and Prognosis

The pain in pain disorder generally begins abruptly and increases in severity for a few weeks or months. The prognosis varies, although pain disorder can often be chronic, distressful, and completely disabling. Acute pain disorders have a more favorable prognosis than chronic pain disorders. There is a wide range of variability in the onset and course of chronic pain disorder. In many cases, the pain has been present for many years by the time the individual comes to psychiatric care, owing to the reluctance of patient and physician to see pain as a psychiatric disorder. People with pain disorder who resume participation in regularly scheduled activities despite the pain have a more favorable prognosis than people who allow the pain to become the determining factor in their lifestyle.

Treatment

Because it may not be possible to reduce the pain, the treatment approach must address rehabilitation. Clinicians should discuss the issue of psychological factors early in treatment and should frankly tell patients that such factors are important in the cause and consequences of both physical and psychogenic pain. Ther-

apists should also explain how various brain circuits that are involved with emotions (e.g., the limbic system) may influence the sensory pain pathways. For example, persons who hit their head while happy at a party can seem to experience less pain than when they hit their head while angry and at work. Nevertheless, therapists must fully understand that the patient's experiences of pain are real.

Pharmacotherapy.   Analgesic medications do not generally benefit most patients with pain disorder. In addition, substance abuse and dependence are often major problems for such patients who receive long-term analgesic treatment. Sedatives and antianxiety agents are not especially beneficial and are also subject to abuse, misuse, and adverse effects.

Antidepressants, such as tricyclics and SSRIs, are the most effective pharmacological agents. Whether antidepressants reduce pain through their antidepressant action or exert an independent, direct analgesic effect (possibly by stimulating efferent inhibitory pain pathways) remains controversial. The success of SSRIs supports the hypothesis that serotonin is important in the pathophysiology of the disorder. Amphetamine, which has analgesic effects, may benefit some patients, especially when used as an adjunct to SSRIs, but doses must be monitored carefully.

Psychotherapy.   Some outcome data indicate that psychodynamic psychotherapy benefits patients with pain disorder. The first step in psychotherapy is to develop a solid therapeutic alliance by empathizing with the patient's suffering. Clinicians should not confront somatizing patients with comments such as "This is all in your head." For the patient, the pain is real, and clinicians must acknowledge the reality of the pain, even as they understand that it is largely intrapsychic in origin. A useful entry point into the emotional aspects of the pain is to examine its interpersonal ramifications in the patient's life. In marital therapy, for example, the psychotherapist may soon get to the source of the patient's psychological pain and the function of the physical complaints in significant relationships. Cognitive therapy has been used to alter negative thoughts and to foster a positive attitude.

Other Therapies.   Biofeedback can be helpful in the treatment of pain disorder, particularly with migraine pain, myofascial pain, and muscle tension states, such as tension headaches. Hypnosis, transcutaneous nerve stimulation, and dorsal column stimulation also have been used. Nerve blocks and surgical ablative procedures are effective for some patients with pain disorder, but these procedures must be repeated because the pain returns after 6 to 18 months.

Pain Control Programs.   Sometimes it may be necessary to remove patients from their usual settings and place them in a comprehensive inpatient or outpatient pain control program or clinic. Multidisciplinary pain units use many modalities, such as cognitive, behavior, and group therapies. They provide extensive physical conditioning through physical therapy and exercise and offer vocational evaluation and rehabilitation. Concurrent mental disorders are diagnosed and treated, and patients who are dependent on analgesics and hypnotics are detoxified. Inpatient multimodal treatment programs generally report encouraging results.

Table 14–7
DSM-IV-TR Diagnostic Criteria for
Undifferentiated Somatoform Disorder

A. One or more physical complaints (e.g., fatigue, loss of appetite, gastrointestinal or urinary complaints).
B. Either (1) or (2):
   (1) after appropriate investigation, the symptoms cannot be fully explained by a known general medical condition or the direct effects of a substance (e.g., a drug of abuse, a medication)
   (2) when there is a related general medical condition, the physical complaints or resulting social or occupational impairment is in excess of what would be expected from the history, physical examination, or laboratory findings
C. The symptoms cause clinically significant distress or impairment in social, occupational, or other important areas of functioning.
D. The duration of the disturbance is at least 6 months.
E. The disturbance is not better accounted for by another mental disorder (e.g., another somatoform disorder, sexual dysfunction, mood disorder, anxiety disorder, sleep disorder, or psychotic disorder).
F. The symptom is not intentionally produced or feigned (as in factitious disorder or malingering).

From American Psychiatric Association. *Diagnostic and Statistical Manual of Mental Disorders.* 4th ed. Text rev. Washington, DC: American Psychiatric Association; copyright 2000, with permission.

UNDIFFERENTIATED SOMATOFORM DISORDER

Undifferentiated somatoform disorder is characterized by one or more unexplained physical symptoms of at least 6 months' duration that are below the threshold for a diagnosis of somatization disorder (Table 14–7). These symptoms are not caused, or fully explained, by another medical, psychiatric, or substance abuse disorder, and they cause clinically significant distress or impairment.

Two types of symptom patterns may be seen in patients with undifferentiated somatoform disorder: those involving the autonomic nervous system and those involving sensations of fatigue or weakness. In what is sometimes referred to as *autonomic arousal disorder*, some patients are affected with somatoform disorder symptoms that are limited to bodily functions innervated by the autonomic nervous system. Such patients have complaints involving the cardiovascular, respiratory, gastroin-

Table 14–8
DSM-IV-TR Diagnostic Criteria for Somatoform Disorder Not Otherwise Specified

This category includes disorders with somatoform symptoms that do not meet the criteria for any specific somatoform disorder. Examples include
1. Pseudocyesis: a false belief of being pregnant that is associated with objective signs of pregnancy, which may include abdominal enlargement (although the umbilicus does not become everted), reduced menstrual flow, amenorrhea, subjective sensation of fetal movement, nausea, breast engorgement and secretions, and labor pains at the expected date of delivery. Endocrine changes may be present, but the syndrome cannot be explained by a general medical condition that causes endocrine changes (e.g., a hormone-secreting tumor).
2. A disorder involving nonpsychotic hypochondriacal symptoms of less than 6 months' duration.
3. A disorder involving unexplained physical complaints (e.g., fatigue or body weakness) of less than 6 months' duration that are not due to another mental disorder.

From American Psychiatric Association. *Diagnostic and Statistical Manual of Mental Disorders.* 4th ed. Text rev. Washington, DC: American Psychiatric Association; copyright 2000, with permission.

testinal, urogenital, and dermatological systems. Other patients complain of mental and physical fatigue, physical weakness and exhaustion, and inability to perform many everyday activities because of their symptoms. Some clinicians believe this syndrome is neurasthenia, a diagnosis used primarily in Europe and Asia. The syndrome may overlap chronic fatigue syndrome, which various research reports have hypothesized to involve psychiatric, virological, and immunological factors.

SOMATOFORM DISORDER NOT OTHERWISE SPECIFIED

The DSM-IV-TR diagnostic category of somatoform disorder not otherwise specified (Table 14–8) is a residual category for patients who have symptoms suggesting a somatoform disorder but do not meet the specific diagnostic criteria for other somatoform disorders. Such patients may have a symptom not covered in the other somatoform disorders (e.g., pseudocyesis) or may not have met the 6-month criterion of the other somatoform disorders.

15 ▲

Factitious Disorders

Persons with factitious disorder fake illness. They simulate, induce, or aggravate illness, often inflicting painful, deforming, or even life-threatening injury on themselves or those under their care. Unlike malingerers, who have material goals, such as monetary gain or avoidance of duties, patients with factitious disorder undertake these tribulations primarily to gain the emotional care and attention that comes with playing the role of the patient. In doing so, they practice artifice and art, creating hospital drama that often causes frustration and dismay. The disorders have a compulsive quality, but the behaviors are considered voluntary in that they are deliberate and purposeful, even if they cannot be controlled. Clinicians can assess whether a symptom is intentional both by direct evidence and by excluding other causes.

In a 1951 article in *Lancet*, Richard Asher coined the term "Munchausen's syndrome" to refer to a syndrome in which patients embellish their personal history, chronically fabricate symptoms to gain hospital admission, and move from hospital to hospital. The syndrome was named after Baron Karl Friedrich Hieronymus Freiherr von Munchausen (1720–1791), a German cavalry officer who was known for humorously exaggerated tales of his adventures.

EPIDEMIOLOGY

No comprehensive epidemiological data on factitious disorder exist. Limited studies indicate that factitious disorder patients may comprise approximately 0.8 to 1.0 percent of psychiatric consultation patients. According to the text revision of the fourth edition of the *Diagnostic and Statistical Manual of Mental Disorders* (DSM-IV-TR), factitious disorder is diagnosed in about 1 percent of patients who are seen in psychiatric consultation in general hospitals. The prevalence appears to be greater in highly specialized treatment settings. Cases of feigned psychological signs and symptoms are reported much less commonly than those of physical signs and symptoms. A data bank of persons who feign illness has been established to alert hospitals about such patients, many of whom travel from place to place, seek admission under different names, or simulate different illnesses.

Approximately two thirds of patients with Munchausen's syndrome are male. They tend to be white, middle-aged, unemployed, unmarried, and without significant social or family attachments. Patients diagnosed with factitious disorders with physical signs and symptoms are mostly women, who outnumber men 3 to 1. They are usually 20 to 40 years of age with a history of employment or education in nursing or a health care occupation. Factitious physical disorders usually begin for pa-

tients in their 20s or 30s, although the literature contains cases ranging from 4 to 79 years of age.

Factitious disorder by proxy (discussed separately later) is most commonly perpetrated by mothers against infants or young children. Rare or underrecognized, it accounts for less than 0.04 percent, or 1,000 of 3 million cases, of child abuse reported in the United States each year. Good epidemiological data are lacking, however.

COMORBIDITY

Many persons diagnosed with factitious disorder have comorbid psychiatric diagnoses (e.g., mood disorders, personality disorders, or substance-related disorders).

ETIOLOGY

Psychosocial Factors

The psychodynamic underpinnings of factitious disorders are poorly understood because the patients are difficult to engage in an exploratory psychotherapy process. They may insist that their symptoms are physical and that psychologically oriented treatment is therefore useless. Anecdotal case reports indicate that many of the patients suffered childhood abuse or deprivation, resulting in frequent hospitalizations during early development. In such circumstances, an inpatient stay may have been regarded as an escape from a traumatic home situation, and the patient may have found a series of caretakers (such as doctors, nurses, and hospital workers) to be loving and caring, in contrast to their families of origin, which may have included a rejecting mother or an absent father. The usual history reveals that the patient perceives one or both parents as rejecting figures who are unable to form close relationships. The facsimile of genuine illness, therefore, is used to recreate the desired positive parent–child bond. The disorders are a form of repetitional compulsion, repeating the basic conflict of needing and seeking acceptance and love while expecting that they will not be forthcoming. Hence, the patient transforms the physicians and staff members into rejecting parents.

Patients who seek out painful procedures, such as surgical operations and invasive diagnostic tests, may have a masochistic personality makeup in which pain serves as punishment for past sins, imagined or real. Some patients may attempt to master the past and the early trauma of serious medical illness or hospitalization by assuming the role of the patient and reliving the painful and frightening experience over and over again through multiple hospitalizations. Patients who feign psychiatric illness may

287

have had a relative who was hospitalized with the illness they are simulating. Through identification, patients hope to reunite with the relative in a magical way.

Many patients have the poor identity formation and disturbed self-image that is characteristic of someone with borderline personality disorder. Some patients are *as-if personalities* who have assumed the identities of those around them. If these patients are health professionals, they are often unable to differentiate themselves from the patients with whom they come in contact. The cooperation or encouragement of other persons in simulating a factitious illness occurs in a rare variant of the disorder. Although most patients act alone, friends or relatives participate in fabricating the illness in some instances.

Significant defense mechanisms are repression, identification with the aggressor, regression, and symbolization.

Some researchers have proposed that brain dysfunction may be a factor in factitious disorders. It has been hypothesized that impaired information processing contributes to *pseudologia fantastica* and aberrant behavior of patients with Munchausen's disorder; however, no genetic patterns have been established, and electroencephalographic studies noted no specific abnormalities in patients with factitious disorders.

DIAGNOSIS AND CLINICAL FEATURES

The diagnostic criteria for factitious disorder in DSM-IV-TR are given in Table 15–1. The psychiatric examination should emphasize securing information from any available friends, relatives, or other informants because interviews with reliable outside sources often reveal the false nature of the patient's illness. Although time consuming and tedious, verifying all the facts presented by the patient about previous hospitalizations and medical care is essential.

Psychiatric evaluation is requested on a consultation basis in about 50 percent of cases, usually after a simulated illness is suspected. The psychiatrist is often asked to confirm the diagnosis of factitious disorder. Under these circumstances, it is necessary

Table 15–1
DSM-IV-TR Diagnostic Criteria for Factitious Disorder

A. Intentional production or feigning of physical or psychological signs or symptoms.
B. The motivation for the behavior is to assume the sick role.
C. External incentives for the behavior (such as economic gain, avoiding legal responsibility, or improving physical well-being, as in malingering) are absent.

Code based on type:
   With predominantly psychological signs and symptoms: if psychological signs and symptoms predominate in the clinical presentation
   With predominantly physical signs and symptoms: if physical signs and symptoms predominate in the clinical presentation
   With combined psychological and physical signs and symptoms: if both psychological and physical signs and symptoms are present but neither predominates in the clinical presentation

From American Psychiatric Association. *Diagnostic and Statistical Manual of Mental Disorders.* 4th ed. Text rev. Washington, DC: American Psychiatric Association; copyright 2000, with permission.

to avoid pointed or accusatory questioning that may provoke truculence, evasion, or flight from the hospital. A danger may exist of provoking frank psychosis if vigorous confrontation is used; in some instances, the feigned illness serves an adaptive function and is a desperate attempt to ward off further disintegration.

Factitious Disorder with Predominantly Psychological Signs and Symptoms

Some patients show psychiatric symptoms judged to be feigned. This determination can be difficult and is often made only after a prolonged investigation (Table 15–1). The feigned symptoms frequently include depression, hallucinations, dissociative and conversion symptoms, and bizarre behavior. Because the patient's condition does not improve after routine therapeutic measures are administered, he or she may receive large doses of psychoactive drugs and may undergo electroconvulsive therapy.

Factitious psychological symptoms resemble the phenomenon of pseudomalingering, conceptualized as satisfying the need to maintain an intact self-image, which would be marred by admitting psychological problems that are beyond the person's capacity to master through conscious effort. In this case, deception is a transient ego-supporting device.

Recent findings indicate that factitious psychotic symptoms are more common than had previously been suspected. The presence of simulated psychosis as a feature of other disorders, such as mood disorders, indicates a poor overall prognosis.

Inpatients who are psychotic and found to have factitious disorder with predominantly psychological signs and symptoms—that is, exclusively simulated psychotic symptoms—generally have a concurrent diagnosis of borderline personality disorder. In these cases, the outcome appears to be worse than that that of bipolar I disorder or schizoaffective disorder.

Patients may appear depressed and may explain their depression by offering a false history of the recent death of a significant friend or relative. Elements of the history that may suggest factitious bereavement include a violent or bloody death, a death under dramatic circumstances, and the dead person's being a child or a young adult. Other patients may describe either recent and remote memory loss or both auditory and visual hallucinations. According to DSM-IV-TR,

The individual may surreptitiously use psychoactive substances for the purpose of producing symptoms that suggest a mental disorder (e.g., stimulants to produce restlessness or insomnia, hallucinogens to induce altered perceptual states, analgesics to induce euphoria, and hypnotics to induce lethargy). Combinations of psychoactive substances can produce very unusual presentations.

Other symptoms, which also appear in the physical type of factitious disorder, include pseudologia fantastica and impostorship. In pseudologia fantastica, limited factual material is mixed with extensive and colorful fantasies. The listener's interest pleases the patient and, thus, reinforces the symptom. The history or the symptoms are not the only distortions of truth. Patients often give false and conflicting accounts about other areas of their lives (e.g., they may claim the death of a parent, to play on the sympathy of others). Imposture is commonly related to lying in these cases. Many patients assume the identity of a prestigious person. Men, for example, report being war heroes and attribute their surgical scars to wounds received during battle or in other dramatic and dangerous exploits. Similarly, they may say that they have ties to accomplished or renowned figures.

Ms. M. A. was 24 years of age when she first presented in 1973 after an overdose. She gave a history of recurrent overdoses and wrist-slashing attempts since 1969, and, on admission, she stated that she was controlled by her dead sister who kept telling her to take her own life. Her family history was negative.

She was found to be carrying a list of schneiderian first-rank symptoms in her handbag; she behaved bizarrely, picking imaginary objects out of the wastepaper basket and opening imaginary doors in the waiting room. She admitted to visual hallucinations and offered four of the first-rank symptoms on her list, but her mental state reverted to normal after 2 days. When she was presented at a case conference, the consensus view was that she had been simulating schizophrenia but had a gross personality disorder; however, the consultant in charge dissented from that general view, feeling that she was genuinely psychotic.

On follow-up, this turned out to be the case. She was readmitted in 1975 and was mute, catatonic, grossly thought disordered, and the diagnosis was changed to that of a schizophrenic illness. She has been followed up regularly since, and now presents the picture of a mild schizophrenic defect state; she takes regular depot medication but still complains of auditory hallucinations, hearing her dead sister's voice. She is a day patient. (Courtesy of Dora Wang, M.D., Deepa N. Nadiga, M.D., and James J. Jenson, M.D.)

Chronic Factitious Disorder with Predominantly Physical Signs and Symptoms (Munchausen's Syndrome)

Factitious disorder with predominantly physical signs and symptoms is the best-known type of Munchausen's syndrome. The disorder has also been called hospital addiction, polysurgical addiction—producing the so-called washboard abdomen—and professional patient syndrome, among others.

The essential feature of patients with the disorder is their ability to present physical symptoms so well that they can gain admission to, and stay in, a hospital (Table 15–1). To support their history, these patients may feign symptoms suggesting a disorder involving any organ system. They are familiar with the diagnoses of most disorders that usually require hospital admission or medication and can give excellent histories capable of deceiving even experienced clinicians. Clinical presentations are myriad and include hematoma, hemoptysis, abdominal pain, fever, hypoglycemia, lupus-like syndromes, nausea, vomiting, dizziness, and seizures. Urine is contaminated with blood or feces; anticoagulants are taken to simulate bleeding disorders; insulin is used to produce hypoglycemia; and so on. Such patients often insist on surgery and claim adhesions from previous surgical procedures. They may acquire a "gridiron" or washboard-like abdomen from multiple procedures. Complaints of pain, especially that simulating renal colic, are common, with the patients wanting narcotics.

In about half of the reported cases, these patients demand treatment with specific medications, usually analgesics. Once in the hospital, they continue to be demanding and difficult. As each test is returned with a negative result, they may accuse doctors of incompetence, threaten litigation, and become generally abusive. Some may sign out abruptly shortly before they believe they are going to be confronted with their factitious behavior. They then go to another hospital in the same or another city and begin the cycle again. Specific predisposing factors are true physical disorders during childhood leading to extensive medical treatment, a grudge against the medical profession, employment as a medical paraprofessional, and an important relationship with a physician in the past.

Factitious Disorder with Combined Psychological and Physical Signs and Symptoms

In combined forms of factitious disorder, both psychological and physical signs and symptoms are present. If neither type predominates in the clinical presentation, a diagnosis of factitious disorder with combined psychological and physical signs and symptoms should be made (see Table 15–1). In one representative report a patient alternated among feigned dementia, bereavement, rape, and seizures.

Mr. M. T. was a man who appeared to be middle-aged but who arrived at a children's psychiatric hospital claiming to be 17 years of age and suicidal. As he held a gun to his head, staff called security officers who promptly recognized him as the Munchausen syndrome patient who arrived in early May each year. He was denied admission.

Late that evening, he presented to the ER of the main hospital claiming that he was diabetic, dizzy, and weak. Intern physicians found his blood glucose to be low and immediately admitted him. Hospital staff on the wards recognized him as "that Munchausen syndrome patient," and a psychiatric consultation was requested. The patient continued to insist that he was 17 years of age and that he was the son of famous golfer Lee Trevino. Hospital legal counsel revealed that he used at least two other pseudonyms and social security numbers and was wanted for health insurance fraud in at least two other states.

When the psychiatry consultants greeted him with familiarity, the patient immediately claimed suicidal tendency, but, when denied psychiatric admission, he left the hospital against medical advice. An inquisitive medical student called local pharmacies, which informed him that, if a customer claimed to be diabetic, traveling, and without insulin, they would give the customer insulin even without a prescription to avoid liability. In this manner, Mr. M. T. could have procured insulin to induce hypoglycemia.

At a care conference, a psychiatry consultant expressed that, in the past, common practice was to call ERs in town to alert them to Munchausen syndrome patients, giving all possibly helpful descriptions and information. However, because of heightened attention to confidentiality rights, she now instead advocated calling ERs and simply warning them about the possible appearance of a patient with factitious hypoglycemia. An ER physician, however, stated that he would go ahead and give a detailed description of the patient to friends in each ER in town. The May of the following year, the patient failed to appear for the first time in several years. (Courtesy of Dora Wang, M.D., Deepa N. Nadiga, M.D., and James J. Jenson, M.D.)

Factitious Disorder Not Otherwise Specified

Some patients with factitious signs and symptoms do not meet the DSM-IV-TR criteria for a specific factitious disorder and should be classified as having factitious disorder not otherwise specified (Table 15–2). The most notable example of the diagnosis is factitious disorder by proxy, which is also included in a DSM-IV-TR appendix (Table 15–3). In this diagnosis, a person intentionally produces physical signs or symptoms in another person who is under the first person's care. One apparent purpose of the behavior is for the caretaker to indirectly assume the sick role; another is to be relieved of the caretaking role by having the child hospitalized. The most common case of factitious disorder by proxy involves a mother who deceives medical personnel into believing that her child is ill. The deception may involve a false medical history, contamination of laboratory samples, alteration of records, or induction of injury and illness in the child.

PATHOLOGY AND LABORATORY EXAMINATION

Psychological testing may reveal specific underlying pathology in individual patients. Features that are overrepresented in patients with factitious disorder include normal or above-average intelligence quotient; absence of a formal thought disorder; poor sense of identity, including confusion over sexual identity; poor sexual adjustment; poor frustration tolerance; strong dependence needs; and narcissism. An invalid test profile and elevations of all clinical scales on the Minnesota Multiphasic Personality Inventory-2 indicate an attempt to appear more disturbed than is the case ("fake bad").

No specific laboratory tests are available for factitious disorders. Certain tests (e.g., drug screening), however, may help confirm or rule out specific mental or medical disorders.

Table 15–2
DSM-IV-TR Diagnostic Criteria for Factitious Disorder Not Otherwise Specified

This category includes disorders with factitious symptoms that do not meet the criteria for factitious disorder. An example is factitious disorder by proxy: the intentional production or feigning of physical or psychological signs or symptoms in another person who is under the individual's care for the purpose of indirectly assuming the sick role (see Table 15-3 for suggested research criteria).

From American Psychiatric Association. *Diagnostic and Statistical Manual of Mental Disorders.* 4th ed. Text rev. Washington, DC: American Psychiatric Association; copyright 2000, with permission.

Table 15–3
DSM-IV-TR Research Criteria for Factitious Disorder by Proxy

A. Intentional production or feigning of physical or psychological signs or symptoms in another person who is under the individual's care.
B. The motivation for the perpetrator's behavior is to assume the sick role by proxy.
C. External incentives for the behavior (such as economic gain) are absent.
D. The behavior is not better accounted for by another mental disorder.

From American Psychiatric Association. *Diagnostic and Statistical Manual of Mental Disorders.* 4th ed. Text rev. Washington, DC: American Psychiatric Association; copyright 2000, with permission.

DIFFERENTIAL DIAGNOSIS

Any disorder in which physical signs and symptoms are prominent should be considered in the differential diagnosis, and the possibility of authentic or concomitant physical illness must always be explored. In addition, a history of many surgeries in patients with factious disorder may predispose such patients to complications or actual diseases, necessitating even further surgery. Factitious disorder is on a continuum between somatoform disorders and malingering, the goal being to assume the sick role. On one hand it is unconscious and nonvolitional (somatoform), and on the other hand it is conscious and willful (malingering).

Somatoform Disorders

A factitious disorder is differentiated from somatization disorder (Briquet's syndrome) by the voluntary production of factitious symptoms, the extreme course of multiple hospitalizations, and the seeming willingness of patients with a factitious disorder to undergo an extraordinary number of mutilating procedures. Patients with conversion disorder are not usually conversant with medical terminology and hospital routines, and their symptoms have a direct temporal relation or symbolic reference to specific emotional conflicts.

Hypochondriasis differs from factitious disorder in that the hypochondriacal patient does not voluntarily initiate the production of symptoms, and hypochondriasis typically has a later age of onset. As with somatization disorder, patients with hypochondriasis do not usually submit to potentially mutilating procedures. (Somatoform disorders are discussed in Chapter 14.)

Personality Disorders

Because of their pathological lying, lack of close relationships with others, hostile and manipulative manner, and associated substance abuse and criminal history, patients with factitious disorder are often classified as having antisocial personality disorder. Antisocial persons, however, do not usually volunteer for invasive procedures or resort to a way of life marked by repeated or long-term hospitalization.

Because of attention seeking and an occasional flair for the dramatic, patients with factitious disorder may be classified as having histrionic personality disorder. Not all such patients have a dramatic flair, however, and many are withdrawn and bland.

Consideration of the patient's chaotic lifestyle, history of disturbed interpersonal relationships, identity crisis, substance abuse, self-damaging acts, and manipulative tactics may lead to the diagnosis of borderline personality disorder. Persons with factitious disorder usually do not have the eccentricities of dress, thought, or communication that characterize schizotypal personality disorder patients. (Personality disorders are discussed in Chapter 23.)

Schizophrenia

The diagnosis of schizophrenia is often based on patients' admittedly bizarre lifestyles, but patients with factitious disorder do not usually meet the diagnostic criteria for schizophrenia unless they have the fixed delusion that they are actually ill and act on this belief by seeking hospitalization. Such a practice seems to be the exception; few patients with factitious disorder show evidence of a severe thought disorder or bizarre delusions.

Malingering

Factitious disorders must be distinguished from malingering. Malingerers have an obvious, recognizable environmental goal in producing signs and symptoms. They may seek hospitalization to secure financial compensation, evade the police, avoid work, or merely obtain free bed and board for the night, but they always have some apparent end for their behavior. Moreover, these patients can usually stop producing their signs and symptoms when they are no longer considered profitable or when the risk becomes too great. (Malingering is discussed in Chapter 29.)

Substance Abuse

Although patients with factitious disorders may have a complicating history of substance abuse, they should be considered not merely as substance abusers but as having coexisting diagnoses.

Ganser's Syndrome

Ganser's syndrome, a controversial condition most typically associated with prison inmates, is characterized by the use of approximate answers. Persons with the syndrome respond to simple questions with astonishingly incorrect answers. For example, when asked about the color of a blue car, the person answers "red," or when asked a simple arithmetic question, answers "2 plus 2 equals 5." Ganser's syndrome may be a variant of malingering, in that the patients avoid punishment or responsibility for their actions. Ganser's syndrome is classified in DSM-IV-TR as a dissociative disorder not otherwise specified. Patients with factitious disorder with predominantly psychological signs and symptoms may intentionally give approximate answers, however. (See Chapter 16, Dissociative Disorders, for a further discussion.)

COURSE AND PROGNOSIS

Factitious disorders typically begin in early adulthood, although they can appear during childhood or adolescence. The onset of

the disorder or of discrete episodes of seeking treatment may follow real illness, loss, rejection, or abandonment. Usually, the patient or a close relative had a hospitalization in childhood or early adolescence for a genuine physical illness. Thereafter, a long pattern of successive hospitalizations begins insidiously and evolves. As the disorder progresses, the patient becomes knowledgeable about medicine and hospitals. The onset of the disorder in patients who had early hospitalizations for actual illness is earlier than generally reported.

Factitious disorders are incapacitating to the patient and often produce severe trauma or untoward reactions related to treatment. A course of repeated or long-term hospitalization is obviously incompatible with meaningful vocational work and sustained interpersonal relationships. The prognosis in most cases is poor. A few patients occasionally spend time in jail, usually for minor crimes, such as burglary, vagrancy, and disorderly conduct. Patients may also have a history of intermittent psychiatric hospitalization.

Although no adequate data are available about the ultimate outcome for these patients, a few of them probably die as a result of needless medication, instrumentation, or surgery. In view of the patients' often expert simulation and the risks that they take, some may die without the disorder being suspected. Possible features that indicate a favorable prognosis are (1) the presence of a depressive-masochistic personality; (2) functioning at a borderline, not a continuously psychotic, level; and (3) the attributes of an antisocial personality disorder with minimal symptoms.

TREATMENT

No specific psychiatric therapy has been effective in treating factitious disorders. It is a clinical paradox that patients with the disorders simulate serious illness and seek and submit to unnecessary treatment while they deny to themselves and others their true illness and thus avoid possible treatment for it. Ultimately, the patients elude meaningful therapy by abruptly leaving the hospital or failing to keep follow-up appointments.

Treatment, thus, is best focused on management rather than on cure. The three major goals in the treatment and management of factitious disorders are (1) to reduce the risk of morbidity and mortality, (2) to address the underlying emotional needs or psychiatric diagnosis underlying factitious illness behavior, and (3) to be mindful of legal and ethical issues. Perhaps the most important factor in successful management is a physician's early recognition of the disorder. In this way, physicians can forestall a multitude of painful and potentially dangerous diagnostic procedures for these patients. Good liaison between psychiatrists and the medical or surgical staff is strongly advised. Although a few cases of individual psychotherapy have been reported in the literature, no consensus exists about the best approach. In general, working in concert with the patient's primary care physician is more effective than working with the patient in isolation.

The personal reactions of physicians and staff members are of great significance in treating and establishing a working alliance with the patients, who invariably evoke feelings of futility, bewilderment, betrayal, hostility, and even contempt. In essence, staff members are forced to abandon a basic element of their relationship with patients—accepting the truthfulness of the patients' statements. One appropriate psychiatric intervention is to suggest to the staff ways of remaining aware that even though the patient's illness is factitious, the patient is ill.

Physicians should try not to feel resentment when patients humiliate their diagnostic prowess, and they should avoid any unmasking ceremony that sets up the patients as adversaries and precipitates their flight from the hospital. The staff should not perform unnecessary procedures or discharge patients abruptly, both of which are manifestations of anger.

Clinicians who find themselves involved with patients suffering from factitious disorders often become enraged at the patients for lying and deceiving them. Hence, therapists must be mindful of countertransference whenever they suspect factitious disorder. Often, the diagnosis is unclear because a definitive physical cause cannot be entirely ruled out. Although the use of confrontation is controversial, at some point in the treatment, patients must be made to face reality. Most patients simply leave treatment when their methods of gaining attention are identified and exposed. In some cases, clinicians should reframe the factitious disorder as a cry for help, so that patients do not view the clinicians' responses as punitive. A major role for psychiatrists working with factitious disorder patients is to help other staff members in the hospital deal with their own sense of outrage at having been duped. Education about the disorder and some attempt to understand the patient's motivations may help staff members maintain their professional conduct in the face of extreme frustration.

In cases of factitious disorder by proxy, legal intervention has been obtained in several instances, particularly when children are involved. The senselessness of the disorder and the denial of false action by parents are obstacles to successful court action and often make conclusive proof unobtainable. In such cases, the child welfare services should be notified and arrangements made for ongoing monitoring of the children's health.

Pharmacotherapy of factitious disorders is of limited use. Comorbid Axis I disorder (e.g., schizophrenia) will respond to antipsychotic medication, but in all cases medication should be administered carefully because of the potential for abuse. Selective serotonin reuptake inhibitors may be useful in decreasing impulsive behavior when that is a major component in acting-out factitious behavior.

16 ▲

Dissociative Disorders

According to the text revision of the fourth edition of the *Diagnostic and Statistical Manual of Mental Disorders* (DSM-IV-TR), "the essential feature of the dissociative disorders is a disruption in the usually integrated functions of consciousness, memory, identity, or perception of the environment. The disturbance may be sudden or gradual, transient or chronic." The DSM-IV-TR dissociative disorders are dissociative identity disorder, depersonalization disorder, dissociative amnesia, dissociative fugue, and dissociative disorder not otherwise specified (NOS).

DISSOCIATIVE AMNESIA

According to DSM-IV-TR (Table 16–1), the essential feature of dissociative amnesia is an inability to recall important personal information, usually of a traumatic or stressful nature, that is too extensive to be explained by normal forgetfulness. The disturbance does not occur exclusively during the course of dissociative identity disorder, dissociative fugue, posttraumatic stress disorder (PTSD), acute stress disorder, or somatization disorder and does not result from the direct physiological effects of a substance or a neurological or other general medical condition. This disturbance may be based on neurobiological changes in the brain caused by traumatic stress.

A 45-year-old, divorced, left-handed, male bus dispatcher was seen in psychiatric consultation on a medical unit. He had been admitted with an episode of chest discomfort, light headedness, and left-arm weakness. He had a history of hypertension and had a medical admission in the past year for ischemic chest pain, although he had not suffered a myocardial infarction. Psychiatric consultation was called, as the patient complained of memory loss for the previous 12 years, behaving and responding to the environment as if it were 12 years previously (e.g., he didn't recognize his 8-year-old son, insisted that he was unmarried, and denied recollection of current events, such as the current president). Physical and laboratory findings were unchanged from the patient's usual baseline. Brain computed tomography scan was normal.

On mental status examination, the patient displayed intact intellectual function but insisted that the date was 12 years earlier, denying recall of his entire subsequent personal history and of current events for the last 12 years. He was perplexed by the contradiction between his memory and current circumstances. The patient described a family history

of brutal beatings and physical discipline. He was a decorated combat veteran, although he described amnestic episodes for some of his combat experiences. In the military, he had been a champion Golden Glove boxer noted for his powerful left hand.

He was educated about his disorder and given the suggestion that his memory could return as he could tolerate it, perhaps overnight during sleep or perhaps over a longer time. If this strategy was unsuccessful, hypnosis or an amobarbital interview was proposed. (Adapted from a case of Richard J. Loewenstein, M.D., and Frank W. Putnam, M.D.)

Epidemiology

Dissociative amnesia has been reported in approximately 6 percent of the general population. No difference is seen in incidence between men and women. Cases generally begin to be reported in late adolescence and adulthood. Dissociative amnesia can be especially difficult to assess in preadolescent children because of their more limited ability to describe subjective experience.

Etiology

Amnesia and Extreme Intrapsychic Conflict. In many cases of acute dissociative amnesia, the psychosocial environment out of which the amnesia develops is massively conflictual, with the patient experiencing intolerable emotions of shame, guilt, despair, rage, and desperation. These usually result from conflicts over unacceptable urges or impulses, such as intense sexual, suicidal, or violent compulsions.

Betrayal Trauma. *Betrayal trauma* attempts to explain amnesia by the intensity of trauma and by the extent that a negative event represents a betrayal by a trusted, needed other. This betrayal is thought to influence the way in which the event is processed and remembered. Information about the abuse is not linked to mental mechanisms that control attachment and attachment behavior.

Diagnosis and Clinical Features

Classic Presentation. The classic disorder is an overt, florid, dramatic clinical disturbance that frequently results in the patient being brought quickly to medical attention specifically for symptoms related to the dissociative disorder. It is frequently found in those who have experienced extreme acute trauma. It

293

Epidemiology

Transient experiences of depersonalization and derealization are extremely common in normal and clinical populations. They are the third most commonly reported psychiatric symptoms, after depression and anxiety. One survey found a 1-year prevalence of 19 percent in the general population. It is common in seizure patients and migraine sufferers; they can also occur with use of psychedelic drugs, especially marijuana, lysergic acid diethylamide, and mescaline, and less frequently as a side effect of some medications, such as anticholinergic agents. They have been described after certain types of meditation, deep hypnosis, extended mirror or crystal gazing, and sensory deprivation experiences. They are also common after mild to moderate head injury, wherein little or no loss of consciousness occurs, but they are significantly less likely if unconsciousness lasts for more than 30 minutes. They are also common after life-threatening experiences, with or without serious bodily injury. Depersonalization is found two to four times more frequently in women than in men.

Etiology

Psychodynamic.   Traditional psychodynamic formulations have emphasized the disintegration of the ego or have viewed depersonalization as an affective response in defense of the ego. These explanations stress the role of overwhelming painful experiences or conflictual impulses as triggering events.

Traumatic Stress.   A substantial proportion, typically one third to one half, of patients in clinical depersonalization case series report histories of significant trauma. Several studies of accident victims find as much as 60 percent of those with a life-threatening experience report at least transient depersonalization during the event or immediately thereafter. Military training studies find that symptoms of depersonalization and derealization are commonly evoked by stress and fatigue and are inversely related to performance.

Neurobiological Theories.   The association of depersonalization with migraines and marijuana, its generally favorable response to selective serotonin reuptake inhibitor (SSRI) drugs, and the increase in depersonalization symptoms seen with the depletion of L-tryptophan, a serotonin precursor, point to serotoninergic involvement. Depersonalization is the primary dissociative symptom elicited by the drug-challenge studies described in the section on neurobiological theories of dissociation. These studies strongly implicate the N-methyl-D-aspartate subtype of the glutamate receptor as central to the genesis of depersonalization symptoms.

Diagnosis and Clinical Features

A number of distinct components comprise the experience of depersonalization, including a sense of (1) bodily changes, (2) duality of self as observer and actor, (3) being cut off from others, and (4) being cut off from one's emotions. Patients experiencing depersonalization often have great difficulty expressing what they are feeling. Trying to express their subjective suffering with banal phrases such as "I feel dead," "nothing seems real," or

"I'm standing outside of myself," depersonalized patients may not adequately convey to the examiner the distress they experience. While complaining bitterly about how this is ruining their life, they may nonetheless appear remarkably undistressed.

Ms. R was a 27-year-old unmarried graduate student with a master's in biology. She complained about intermittent episodes of "standing back," usually associated with anxiety-provoking social situations. When asked about a recent episode, she described presenting in a seminar course. "All of a sudden, I was talking, but it didn't feel like it was me talking. It was very disconcerting. I had this feeling, 'who's doing the talking?' I felt like I was just watching someone else talk. Listening to words come out of my mouth, but I wasn't saying them. It wasn't me. It went on for a while. I was calm, even sort of peaceful. It was as if I was very far away. In the back of the room somewhere—just watching myself. But the person talking didn't even seem like me really. It was like I was watching someone else." The feeling lasted the rest of that day and persisted into the next, during which time it gradually dissipated. She thought that she remembered having similar experiences during high school but was certain that they occurred at least once a year during college and graduate school.

As a child, Ms. R reported frequent intense anxiety due to overhearing or witnessing the frequent violent arguments and periodic physical fights between her parents. In addition, the family was subject to many unpredictable dislocations and moves owing to the patient's father's intermittent difficulties with finances and employment. The patient's anxieties did not abate when the parents divorced when she was a late adolescent. Her father moved away and had little further contact with her. Her relationship with her mother became increasingly angry, critical, and contentious. She was unsure if she experienced depersonalization during childhood while listening to her parents' fights. (Adapted from a case of Richard J. Loewenstein, M.D., and Frank W. Putnam, M.D.)

Differential Diagnosis

The variety of conditions associated with depersonalization complicates the differential diagnosis of depersonalization disorder. Depersonalization can result from a medical condition or neurological condition, from intoxication or withdrawal from illicit drugs, or as a side effect of medications, and it can be associated with panic attacks, phobias, PTSD, acute stress disorder, schizophrenia, or another dissociative disorder. A thorough medical and neurological evaluation is essential, including standard laboratory studies, an EEG, and any indicated drug screens. Drug-related depersonalization is typically transient, but persistent depersonalization can follow an episode of intoxication with a variety of substances, including marijuana, cocaine, and other psychostimulants. A range of neurological conditions, including seizure disorders, brain tumors, postconcussive syndrome, metabolic abnormalities, migraine, vertigo, and Ménière's disease, have been reported as causes. Depersonalization caused by organic conditions tends to be primarily sensory without the elaborated descriptions and personalized meanings common to psychiatric etiologies.

Course and Prognosis

Depersonalization after traumatic experiences or intoxications commonly remits spontaneously after removal from the traumatic circumstances or ending of the episode of intoxication. Depersonalization accompanying mood, psychotic, or other anxiety disorders commonly remits with definitive treatment of these conditions.

Depersonalization disorder itself may have an episodic, relapsing and remitting, or chronic course. Many patients with chronic depersonalization may have a course characterized by severe impairment in occupational, social, and personal functioning. Mean age of onset is thought to be in late adolescence or early adulthood in most cases.

Treatment

Clinicians working with patients with depersonalization often find them to be a singularly clinically refractory group. Some systematic evidence indicates that SSRI antidepressants, such as fluoxetine (Prozac), may be helpful to patients with depersonalization. Two recent double-blind, placebo-controlled studies, however, found no efficacy for fluoxetine (Luvox) and lamotrigine, respectively, for depersonalization disorder. Some depersonalization patients respond at best sporadically and partially to the usual groups of psychiatric medications, singly or in combination: antidepressants, mood stabilizers, typical and atypical neuroleptics, anticonvulsants, and so forth.

Many different types of psychotherapy have been used with depersonalization patients: psychodynamic, cognitive, cognitive-behavioral, hypnotherapeutic, and supportive. Many depersonalization patients do not have a robust response to these specific types of standard psychotherapy. Stress management strategies, distraction techniques, reduction of sensory stimulation, relaxation training, and physical exercise may be somewhat helpful in some patients.

DISSOCIATIVE FUGUE

The essential feature of dissociative fugue (Table 16–3) is described as sudden, unexpected travel away from home or one's customary place of daily activities, with inability to recall some or all of one's past. This is accompanied by confusion about personal identity or even the assumption of a new identity. The disturbance does not occur exclusively during the course of dissociative identity disorder and is not due to the direct physiological effects of a substance or a general medical condition. The symptoms must cause clinically significant distress or impairment in social, occupational, or other important areas of functioning.

Epidemiology

Dissociative fugue is thought to be more common during natural disasters, wartime, or times of major social dislocation and violence, although no systematic data exist on this point. No adequate data exist to demonstrate a gender bias to this disor-

Table 16–3
DSM-IV-TR Diagnostic Criteria for Dissociative Fugue

A. The predominant disturbance is sudden, unexpected travel away from home or one's customary place of work, with inability to recall one's past.
B. Confusion about personal identity or assumption of a new identity (partial or complete).
C. The disturbance does not occur exclusively during the course of dissociative identity disorder and is not due to the direct physiological effects of a substance (e.g., a drug of abuse, a medication) or a general medical condition (e.g., temporal lobe epilepsy).
D. The symptoms cause clinically significant distress or impairment in social, occupational, or other important areas of functioning.

From American Psychiatric Association. *Diagnostic and Statistical Manual of Mental Disorders.* 4th ed. Text rev. Washington, DC: American Psychiatric Association; copyright 2000, with permission.

der; however, most cases describe men, primarily in the military. Dissociative fugue is usually described in adults.

Etiology

Traumatic circumstances (i.e., combat, rape, recurrent childhood sexual abuse, massive social dislocations, natural disasters), leading to an altered state of consciousness dominated by a wish to flee, are the underlying cause of most fugue episodes. In some cases, a similar antecedent history is seen, although a psychological trauma is not present at the onset of the fugue episode. In these cases, instead of, or in addition to, external dangers or traumas, the patients are usually struggling with extreme emotions or impulses (i.e., overwhelming fear, guilt, shame, or intense incestuous, sexual, suicidal, or violent urges) that are in conflict with the patient's conscience or ego ideals.

Diagnosis and Clinical Features

Dissociative fugues have been described to last from minutes to months. Some patients report multiple fugues. In most cases in which this was described, a more chronic dissociative disorder, such as dissociative identity disorder, was not ruled out.

In some extremely severe cases of PTSD, nightmares may be terminated by a waking fugue in which the patient runs to another part of the house or runs outside. Children or adolescents may be more limited than adults in their ability to travel. Thus, fugues in this population may be brief and involve only short distances.

A teenage girl was continually sexually abused by her alcoholic father and another family friend. She was threatened with perpetration of sexual abuse on her younger siblings if she told anyone about the abuse. The girl became suicidal but felt that she had to stay alive to protect her siblings. She precipitously ran away from home after being raped by her father and several of his friends as a "birthday present" for one of them. She traveled to a part of the city where she had lived previously with the idea that she would find her grandmother with whom she had lived before the abuse began. She traveled by public transportation and walked the streets, undifferentiated somatoform disorder, somatoform pain disorder, or conversion disorder, or a combination of these.

Obsessive-compulsive personality traits are common in dissociative identity disorder, and intercurrent obsessive-compulsive disorder (OCD) symptoms are regularly found in dissociative identity disorder patients, with a subgroup manifesting severe OCD symptoms. OCD symptoms commonly have a posttraumatic quality: repeatedly checking to be sure that no one can enter the house or the bedroom, compulsively washing to relieve a feeling of being dirty because of abuse, and repetitively counting or singing in the mind to distract from anxiety over being abused, for example.

Child and Adolescent Presentations.

Children and adolescents manifest the same core dissociative symptoms and secondary clinical phenomena as adults. Age-related differences in autonomy and lifestyle, however, may significantly influence the clinical expression of dissociative symptoms in youth. Younger children, in particular, have a less linear and less continuous sense of time and are often not able to self-identify dissociative discontinuities in their behavior. Often, additional informants, such as teachers and relatives, are available to help document dissociative behaviors.

A number of normal childhood phenomena, such as imaginary companionship and elaborated daydreams, must be carefully differentiated from pathological dissociation in younger children. The clinical presentation may be that of an elaborated or autonomous imaginary companionship, with the imaginary companions taking control of the child's behavior, often experienced through passive influence experiences or auditory pseudohallucinations, or both, that command the child to behave in certain ways.

Differential Diagnosis

Indicators of falsified or *imitative dissociative identity disorder* are reported to include those typical of other factitious or malingering presentations. These include symptom exaggeration, lies, use of symptoms to excuse antisocial behavior (e.g., amnesia only for bad behavior), amplification of symptoms when under observation, refusal to allow collateral contacts, legal problems, and pseudologia fantastica. Patients with genuine dissociative identity disorder are usually confused, conflicted, ashamed, and distressed by their symptoms and trauma history. Those with nongenuine disorder frequently show little dysphoria about their disorder.

Course and Prognosis

Little is known about the natural history of untreated dissociative identity disorder. Some individuals with untreated dissociative identity disorder are thought to continue involvement in abusive relationships or violent subcultures, or both, that may result in the traumatization of their children, with the potential for additional family transmission of the disorder. Many authorities believe that some percentage of patients with undiagnosed or untreated dissociative identity disorder die by suicide or as a result of their risk-taking behaviors.

Prognosis is poorer in patients with comorbid organic mental disorders, psychotic disorders (*not* dissociative identity disorder pseudopsychosis), and severe medical illnesses. Refractory substance abuse and eating disorders also suggest a poorer progno-

sis. Other factors that usually indicate a poorer outcome include significant antisocial personality features, current criminal activity, ongoing perpetration of abuse, and current victimization, with refusal to leave abusive relationships. Repeated adult traumas with recurrent episodes of acute stress disorder may severely complicate clinical course.

Treatment

Psychotherapy. Successful psychotherapy for the dissociative identity disorder patient requires the clinician to be comfortable with a range of psychotherapeutic interventions and a willingness actively to work to structure the treatment. These modalities include psychoanalytic psychotherapy, cognitive therapy, behavioral therapy, hypnotherapy, and a familiarity with the psychotherapy and psychopharmacological management of the traumatized patient. Comfort with family treatment and systems theory is helpful in working with a patient who subjectively experiences himself or herself as a complex system of selves with alliances, family-like relationships, and intragroup conflict. A grounding in work with patients with somatoform disorders may also be helpful in sorting through the plethora of somatic symptoms with which these patients commonly present.

Psychopharmacological Interventions. Antidepressant medications are often important in the reduction of depression and stabilization of mood. Clinicians report some success with SSRI, tricyclic, and monoamine oxidase antidepressants, β-blockers, clonidine (Catapres), anticonvulsants, and benzodiazepines in reducing intrusive symptoms, hyperarousal, and anxiety in dissociative identity disorder patients. Recent research suggests that the α_1-adrenergic antagonist prazosin (Minipress) may be helpful for nightmares. Case reports suggest that aggression may respond to carbamazepine in some individuals if EEG abnormalities are present. Patients with obsessive-compulsive symptoms may respond to antidepressants with antiobsessive efficacy. Open-label studies suggest that naltrexone (ReVia) may be helpful for amelioration of recurrent self-injurious behaviors in a subset of traumatized patients. The use of antipsychotic medications is rarely indicated.

DISSOCIATIVE DISORDER NOT OTHERWISE SPECIFIED

The category of dissociative disorder NOS covers all of the conditions characterized by a primary dissociative response that do not meet diagnostic criteria for one of the other DSM-IV-TR dissociative disorders (Table 16–5). Dissociative disorder NOS cases must also fail to exclusively meet diagnostic criteria for acute stress disorder, PTSD, or somatization disorder, which all include dissociative symptoms among their criteria.

Dissociative Trance Disorder

Dissociative trance disorder is manifest by a temporary, marked alteration in the state of consciousness or by loss of the customary sense of personal identity without the replacement by an alternate sense of identity (Table 16–6). A variant of this, possession trance, involves single or episodic alternations in the state of consciousness, characterized by the exchange of the person's customary identity by a new identity usually attributed

Table 16–5
DSM-IV-TR Diagnostic Criteria for Dissociative Disorder Not Otherwise Specified

This category is included for disorders in which the predominant feature is a dissociative symptom (i.e., a disruption in the usually integrated functions of consciousness, memory, identity, or perception of the environment) that does not meet the criteria for any specific dissociative disorder. Examples include the following:

(1) Clinical presentations similar to dissociative identity disorder that fail to meet full criteria for this disorder. Examples include presentations in which (a) there are not two or more distinct personality states or (b) amnesia for important personal information does not occur.
(2) Derealization unaccompanied by depersonalization in adults.
(3) States of dissociation that occur in individuals who have been subjected to periods of prolonged and intense coercive persuasion (e.g., brainwashing, thought reform, or indoctrination while captive).
(4) Dissociative trance disorder: single or episodic disturbances in the state of consciousness, identity, or memory that are indigenous to particular locations and cultures. Dissociative trance involves narrowing of awareness of immediate surroundings or stereotyped behaviors or movements that are experienced as being beyond one's control. Possession trance involves replacement of the customary sense of personal identity by a new identity, attributed to the influence of a spirit, power, deity, or other person and associated with stereotyped involuntary movements or amnesia, and is perhaps the most common dissociative disorder in Asia. Examples include *amok* (Indonesia), *bebainan* (Indonesia), *latah* (Malaysia), *pibloktoq* (Arctic), *ataque de nervios* (Latin America), and possession (India). The dissociative or trance disorder is not a normal part of a broadly accepted collective cultural or religious practice.
(5) Loss of consciousness, stupor, or coma not attributable to a general medical condition.
(6) Ganser syndrome: the giving of approximate answers to questions (e.g., 2 + 2 = 5) when not associated with dissociative amnesia or dissociative fugue.

From American Psychiatric Association. *Diagnostic and Statistical Manual of Mental Disorders.* 4th ed. Text rev. Washington, DC: American Psychiatric Association; copyright 2000, with permission.

Table 16–6
DSM-IV-TR Research Criteria for Dissociative Trance Disorder

A. Either (1) or (2):
  (1) Trance, that is, temporary marked alteration in the state of consciousness or loss of customary sense of personal identity without replacement by an alternate identity, associated with at least one of the following:
    (a) Narrowing of awareness of immediate surroundings or unusually narrow and selective focusing on environmental stimuli
    (b) Stereotyped behaviors or movements that are experienced as being beyond one's control
  (2) Possession trance, a single or episodic alteration in the state of consciousness characterized by the replacement of customary sense of personal identity by a new identity. This is attributed to the influence of a spirit, power, deity, or other person, as evidenced by one or more of the following:
    (a) Stereotyped and culturally determined behaviors or movements that are experienced as being controlled by the possessing agent
    (b) Full or partial amnesia for the event
B. The trance or possession trance state is not accepted as a normal part of a collective cultural or religious practice.
C. The trance or possession trance state causes clinically significant distress or impairment in social, occupational, or other important areas of functioning.
D. The trance or possession trance state does not occur exclusively during the course of a psychotic disorder (including mood disorder with psychotic features and brief psychotic disorder) or dissociative identity disorder and is not due to the direct physiological effects of a substance or a general medical condition.

From American Psychiatric Association. *Diagnostic and Statistical Manual of Mental Disorders.* 4th ed. Text rev. Washington, DC: American Psychiatric Association; copyright 2000, with permission.

to a spirit, divine power, deity, or another person. In this possessed state, the individual exhibits stereotypical and culturally determined behaviors or experiences being controlled by the possessing entity. There must be partial or full amnesia for the event. The trance or possession state must not be a normally accepted part of a cultural or religious practice and must cause significant distress or functional impairment in one or more of the usual domains. Finally, the dissociative trance state must not occur exclusively during the course of a psychotic disorder and not be the result of any substance or general medical condition.

Brainwashing

DSM-IV-TR describes this dissociative disorder as "states of dissociation that occur in individuals who have been subjected to periods of prolonged and intense coercive persuasion (e.g., brainwashing, thought reform, or indoctrination while captive)." Brainwashing occurs largely in the setting of political reform, as has been described at length with the Cultural Revolution in Communist China, war imprisonment, torture of political dissidents, terrorist hostages, and, more familiarly in Western culture, totalitarian cult indoctrination. It implies that under conditions of adequate stress and duress, individuals can be made to comply with

the demands of those with power, thereby undergoing major changes in their personality, beliefs, and behaviors. Persons submitted to such conditions can undergo considerable harm, including loss of health and life, and they typically manifest a variety of posttraumatic and dissociative symptoms.

The treatment of the victims of coercion can vary considerably, depending on their particular background, the circumstances involved, and the setting in which help is sought. Although there are no systematic studies in this domain, basic principles involve validation of the traumatic experience and coercive techniques used, cognitive reframing of the events that occurred, exploration of preexisting psychopathology and vulnerabilities (when applicable), and general techniques used in treating posttraumatic and dissociative states. In addition, family interventions and therapy may be required, at least in cases of cult indoctrination, because significant family duress and disruption commonly occur.

Recovered Memory Syndrome

Under hypnosis or during psychotherapy, a patient may recover a memory of a painful experience or conflict—particularly of sexual or physical abuse—that is etiologically significant. When the repressed material is brought back to consciousness, the person not only may recall the experience, but he or she may relive it, accompanied by the appropriate affective response (a process called *abreaction*). If the event recalled never really happened but the person believes it to be true and reacts accordingly, it is known as *false memory syndrome*.

unplanned learning, (2) explicit instruction and inculcation, and (3) spontaneously putting two and two together to make sometimes four and sometimes five. The usual outcome is a congruence of gender identity and gender role. Although biological attributes are significant, the major factor in achieving the role appropriate to a person's sex is learning.

Research on sex differences in children's behavior reveals more psychological similarities than differences. Girls, however, are found to be less susceptible to tantrums after the age of 18 months than are boys, and boys generally are more physically and verbally aggressive than are girls from age 2 years onward. Little girls and little boys are similarly active, but boys are more easily stimulated to sudden bursts of activity when they are in groups. Some researchers speculate that, although aggression is a learned behavior, male hormones may have sensitized boys' neural organizations to absorb these lessons more easily than do those of girls.

Persons' gender roles can seem to be opposed to their gender identities. Persons may identify with their own sex and yet adopt the dress, hairstyle, or other characteristics of the opposite sex. Or, they may identify with the opposite sex and yet for expediency adopt many behavioral characteristics of their own sex. A further discussion of gender issues appears in Chapter 18.

SEXUAL ORIENTATION

Sexual orientation describes the object of a person's sexual impulses: heterosexual (opposite sex), homosexual (same sex), or bisexual (both sexes). A group of people have defined themselves as "asexual" and assert this as a positive identity. Some researchers believe this lack of attraction to any object is a manifestation of a desire disorder.

SEXUAL BEHAVIOR

Physiological Responses

Sexual response is a true psychophysiological experience. Arousal is triggered by both psychological and physical stimuli; levels of tension are experienced both physiologically and emotionally; and, with orgasm, normally a subjective perception of a peak of physical reaction and release occurs. Psychosexual development, psychological attitudes toward sexuality, and attitudes toward one's sexual partner are directly involved with, and affect, the physiology of human sexual response.

Normally, men and women experience a series of physiological responses to sexual stimulation. In the first detailed description of these responses, William Masters and Virginia Johnson observed that the physiological process involves increasing levels of vasocongestion and myotonia (tumescence) and the subsequent release of the vascular activity and muscle tone as a result of orgasm (detumescence). The text revision of the fourth edition of *Diagnostic and Statistical Manual of Mental Disorders* (DSM-IV-TR) defines a four-phase response cycle: phase 1, desire; phase 2, excitement; phase 3, orgasm; phase 4, resolution. However, the sexes differ, with men responding in sequential fashion, whereas women may respond out of sequence (e.g., arousal may precede desire) and their response phases may overlap. It is important to remember that the sequence of responses can overlap and fluctuate. In addition, a person's subjective experiences are as important to sexual satisfaction as the objective physiologic response.

Phase 1: Desire.   The classification of the desire (or appetitive) phase, which is distinct from any phase identified solely through physiology, reflects the psychiatric concern with motivations, drives, and personality. The phase is characterized by sexual fantasies and the desire to have sexual activity.

Phase 2: Excitement.   The excitement and arousal phase, brought on by psychological stimulation (fantasy or the presence of a love object) or physiological stimulation (stroking or kissing) or a combination of the two, consists of a subjective sense of pleasure. During this phase, penile tumescence leads to erection in men and vaginal lubrication occurs in women. The nipples of both sexes become erect, although nipple erection is more common in women than in men. A woman's clitoris becomes hard and turgid, and her labia minora become thicker as a result of venous engorgement. Initial excitement may last from several minutes to several hours. With continued stimulation, a man's testes increase 50 percent in size and elevate. A woman's vaginal barrel shows a characteristic constriction along the outer third, known as the orgasmic platform. The clitoris elevates and retracts behind the symphysis pubis, and as a result is not easily accessible. Stimulation of the area, however, causes traction on the labia minora and the prepuce and intrapreputial movement of the clitoral shaft. Women's breast size increases 25 percent. Continued engorgement of the penis and the vagina produces color changes, particularly in the labia minora, which become bright or deep red. Voluntary contractions of large muscle groups occur, heartbeat and respiration rates increase, and blood pressure rises. Heightened excitement lasts from 30 seconds to several minutes.

Phase 3: Orgasm.   The orgasm phase consists of a peaking of sexual pleasure, with the release of sexual tension and the rhythmic contraction of the perineal muscles and the pelvic reproductive organs. A subjective sense of ejaculatory inevitability triggers men's orgasms. The forceful emission of semen follows. The male orgasm is also associated with four to five rhythmic spasms of the prostate, seminal vesicles, vas, and urethra. In women, orgasm is characterized by 3 to 15 involuntary contractions of the lower third of the vagina and by strong sustained contractions of the uterus, flowing from the fundus downward to the cervix. Both men and women have involuntary contractions of the internal and external anal sphincters. These and the other contractions during orgasm occur at 0.8-second intervals. Other manifestations include voluntary and involuntary movements of the large muscle groups, including facial grimacing and carpopedal spasm. Blood pressure rises 20 to 40 mm Hg (both systolic and diastolic), and the heart rate increases up to 160 beats per minute. Orgasm lasts from 3 to 25 seconds and is associated with a slight clouding of consciousness.

Phase 4: Resolution.   Resolution consists of the disgorgement of blood from the genitalia (detumescence), which brings the body back to its resting state. If orgasm occurs, resolution is rapid and is characterized by a subjective sense of well-being, general relaxation, and muscular relaxation. If orgasm does not occur, resolution may take from 2 to 6 hours and may be associated with irritability and discomfort. After orgasm, men have a refractory period that may last from several minutes to many hours; in that period they cannot be stimulated to further orgasm. Women do not have a refractory period and are capable of multiple and successive orgasms.

HORMONES AND SEXUAL BEHAVIOR

In general, substances that increase dopamine levels in the brain increase desire, whereas substances that augment serotonin decrease desire. Testosterone increases libido in both men and women, although estrogen is a key factor in the lubrication involved in female arousal and may increase sensitivity in the woman to stimulation. Progesterone mildly depresses desire in men and women, as do excessive prolactin and cortisol. Oxytocin is involved in pleasurable sensations during sex and is found in higher levels in men and women following orgasm.

MASTURBATION

Masturbation is usually a normal precursor of object-related sexual behavior. No other form of sexual activity has been more frequently discussed, more roundly condemned, and more universally practiced than masturbation. Research by Alfred Kinsey into the prevalence of masturbation indicated that nearly all men and three fourths of all women masturbate sometime during their lives.

Longitudinal studies of development show that sexual self-stimulation is common in infancy and childhood. Just as infants learn to explore the functions of their fingers and mouths, they learn to do the same with their genitalia. At about 15 to 19 months of age, both sexes begin genital self-stimulation. Pleasurable sensations result from any gentle touch to the genital region. Those sensations, coupled with the ordinary desire for exploration of the body, produce a normal interest in masturbatory pleasure at that time. Children also develop an increased interest in the genitalia of others—parents, children, and even animals. As youngsters acquire playmates, the curiosity about their own and others' genitalia motivates episodes of exhibitionism or genital exploration. Such experiences, unless blocked by guilty fear, contribute to continued pleasure from sexual stimulation.

With the approach of puberty, the upsurge of sex hormones, and the development of secondary sex characteristics, sexual curiosity intensifies, and masturbation increases. Adolescents are physically capable of coitus and orgasm, but are usually inhibited by social restraints. The dual and often conflicting pressures of establishing their sexual identities and controlling their sexual impulses produce a strong physiological sexual tension in teenagers that demands release, and masturbation is a normal way to reduce sexual tensions. In general, males learn to masturbate to orgasm earlier than females and masturbate more frequently. An important emotional difference between the adolescent and the youngster of earlier years is the presence of coital fantasies during masturbation in the adolescent. These fantasies are an important adjunct to the development of sexual identity; in the comparative safety of the imagination, the adolescent learns to perform the adult sex role. This autoerotic activity is usually maintained into the young adult years, when it is normally replaced by coitus.

Couples in a sexual relationship do not abandon masturbation entirely. When coitus is unsatisfactory or is unavailable because of illness or the absence of the partner, self-stimulation often serves an adaptive purpose, combining sensual pleasure and tension release. Kinsey reported that when women masturbate, most prefer clitoral stimulation. Masters and Johnson stated that women prefer the shaft of the clitoris to the glans because the glans is hypersensitive to intense stimulation. Most men masturbate by vigorously stroking the penile shaft and glans.

Moral taboos against masturbation have generated myths that masturbation causes mental illness or decreased sexual potency. No scientific evidence supports such claims. Masturbation is a psychopathological symptom only when it becomes a compulsion beyond a person's willful control. Then, it is a symptom of emotional disturbance, not because it is sexual but because it is compulsive. Masturbation is probably a universal aspect of psychosexual development and, in most cases, it is adaptive.

Several studies found that in men, orgasm from masturbation raised the serum prostate-specific antigen (PSA) significantly. Male patients scheduled for PSA tests should be advised not to masturbate (or have coitus) for at least 7 days prior to the examination.

HOMOSEXUALITY

In 1973 homosexuality was eliminated as a diagnostic category by the American Psychiatric Association, and in 1980, it was removed from DSM. The 10th revision of the *International Statistical Classification of Diseases and Related Health Problems* (ICD-10) states "Sexual orientation alone is not to be regarded as a disorder." This change reflects a change in the understanding of homosexuality, which is now considered to occur with some regularity as a variant of human sexuality, not as a pathological disorder. As David Hawkins wrote, "The presence of homosexuality does not appear to be a matter of choice; the expression of it is a matter of choice."

Definition

The term *homosexuality* often describes a person's overt behavior, sexual orientation, and sense of personal or social identity. Many persons prefer to identify sexual orientation by using terms such as *lesbians* and *gay men* rather than *homosexual*, which may imply pathology and etiology based on its origin as a medical term, and refer to sexual behavior with terms such as *same sex* and *male–female*. Hawkins wrote that the terms *gay* and *lesbian* refer to a combination of self-perceived identity and social identity; they reflect a person's sense of belonging to a social group that is similarly labeled. Homophobia is a negative attitude toward, or fear of, homosexuality or homosexuals. Heterosexism is the belief that a heterosexual relationship is preferable to all others; it implies discrimination against those practicing other forms of sexuality.

Coming Out

According to Rochelle Klinger and Robert Cabaj, coming out is a "process by which an individual acknowledges his or her sexual orientation in the face of societal stigma and with successful resolution accepts himself or herself." The authors wrote

> Successful coming out involves the individual accepting his or her sexual orientation and integrating it into all spheres (e.g., social, vocational, and familial). Another milestone that individuals and couples must eventually confront is the degree of disclosure of sexual orientation to the external world. Some degree of disclosure is probably necessary for successful coming out.

Difficulty in negotiating coming out and disclosure is a common cause of relationship difficulties. For each person, problems resolving the coming-out process can contribute to poor self-esteem caused by internalized homophobia and lead to deleterious effects on the person's ability to function in the relationship. Conflict can also arise within a relationship when partners disagree on the degree of disclosure.

LOVE AND INTIMACY

Sigmund Freud postulated that psychological health could be determined by a person's ability to function well in two spheres, work and love. A person able to give and receive love with a minimum of fear and conflict has the capacity to develop genuinely intimate relationships with others. A desire to maintain closeness to the love object typifies being in love. Mature love is marked by the intimacy that is a special attribute of the relationship between two persons. When involved in an intimate relationship, the person actively strives for the growth and happiness of the loved person. Sex frequently acts as a catalyst in forming and maintaining intimate relationships. The quality of intimacy in a mature sexual relationship is what Rollo May called "active receiving," in which a person, while loving, permits himself or herself to be loved. May describes the value of sexual love as an expansion of self-awareness, the experience of tenderness, an increase of self-affirmation and pride, and sometimes, at the moment of orgasm, loss of feeling of separateness. In that setting, sex and love are reciprocally enhancing and healthily fused.

Some persons suffer from conflicts that prevent them from fusing tender and passionate impulses. This can inhibit the expression of sexuality in a relationship, interfere with feelings of closeness to another person, and diminish a person's sense of adequacy and self-esteem. When these problems are severe, they may prevent the formation of, or commitment to, an intimate relationship.

▲ 17.2 Abnormal Sexuality and Sexual Dysfunctions

In the text revision of the fourth edition of the *Diagnostic and Statistical Manual of Mental Disorders* (DSM-IV-TR), sexual dysfunctions are categorized as Axis I disorders. The syndromes listed are correlated with the sexual physiological response, which is divided into the four phases as described in the preceding section. The essential feature of the sexual dysfunctions is inhibition in one or more of the phases, including disturbance in the subjective sense of pleasure or desire or in the objective performance. Either type of disturbance can occur alone or in combination with others. Sexual dysfunctions are diagnosed only when they are a major part of the clinical picture. They can be lifelong or acquired, generalized or situational, and result from psychological factors, physiological factors, or combined factors. If they are attributable entirely to a general medical condition, substance use, or adverse effects of medication, then sexual dysfunction due to a general medical condition or substance-induced sexual dysfunction is diagnosed.

Seven major categories of sexual dysfunction are listed in DSM-IV-TR: sexual desire disorders, sexual arousal disorders, orgasm disorders, sexual pain disorders, sexual dysfunction caused by a general medical condition, substance-induced sexual dysfunction, and sexual dysfunction not otherwise specified.

Sexual dysfunctions can be symptomatic of biological (biogenic) problems or intrapsychic or interpersonal (psychogenic) conflicts or a combination of these factors. Sexual function can be adversely affected by stress of any kind, by emotional disorders, or by ignorance of sexual function and physiology.

In considering each of the disorders, clinicians need to rule out an acquired medical condition and the use of a pharmacological substance that could account for, or contribute to, the dysfunction. If the disorder is biogenic, it is coded on Axis III unless substantial evidence indicates dysfunctional episodes apart from the onset of physiological or pharmacological influences.

In some cases, a patient has more than one dysfunction—for example, premature ejaculation and male erectile disorder.

SEXUAL DESIRE DISORDERS

Sexual desire disorders are divided into two classes: hypoactive sexual desire disorder, characterized by a deficiency or absence of sexual fantasies and desire for sexual activity (Table 17.2–1), and sexual aversion disorder, characterized by an aversion to, and avoidance of, genital sexual contact with a sexual partner or by masturbation (Table 17.2–2). The former condition is more common than the latter and more common among women than among men. Minimal spontaneous sexual thinking or minimal desire for sex ahead of sexual experiences does not necessarily constitute a desire disorder in women, particularly if desire is triggered during the sexual encounter. Low desire has been reported by 10 to 15 percent of women in various countries. In the United States, an estimated 20 percent of persons have hypoactive sexual desire disorder.

A variety of causative factors are associated with sexual desire disorders. Patients with desire problems often use inhibition of desire defensively, to protect against unconscious fears about sex. Sigmund Freud conceptualized low sexual desire as the result of inhibition during the phallic psychosexual phase of development and of unresolved oedipal conflicts. Some men, fixated at the phallic state of development, are fearful of the vagina and believe that they will be castrated if they approach it. Freud called this concept *vagina dentata*; because men unconsciously believe that the vagina has teeth, they avoid contact with the female genitalia. Equally, women may suffer from unresolved developmental conflicts that inhibit desire. Lack of desire can also result from chronic stress, anxiety, or depression.

Table 17.2–1
DSM-IV-TR Diagnostic Criteria for Hypoactive Sexual Desire Disorder

A. Persistently or recurrently deficient (or absent) sexual fantasies and desire for sexual activity. The judgment of deficiency or absence is made by the clinician, taking into account factors that affect sexual functioning, such as age and the context of the person's life.

B. The disturbance causes marked distress or interpersonal difficulty.

C. The sexual dysfunction is not better accounted for by another Axis I disorder (except another sexual dysfunction) and is not due exclusively to the direct physiological effects of a substance (e.g., a drug of abuse, a medication) or a general medical condition.

Specify type:
Lifelong type
Acquired type

Specify type:
Generalized type
Situational type

Specify:
Due to psychological factors
Due to combined factors

Table 17.2–2
DSM-IV-TR Diagnostic Criteria for Sexual Aversion Disorder

A. Persistent or recurrent extreme aversion to, and avoidance of, all (or almost all) genital sexual contact with a sexual partner.
B. The disturbance causes marked distress or interpersonal difficulty.
C. The sexual dysfunction is not better accounted for by another Axis I disorder (except another sexual dysfunction).

Specify type:
  Lifelong type
  Acquired type
Specify type:
  Situational type
  Generalized type
Specify:
  Due to psychological factors
  Due to combined factors

From American Psychiatric Association. *Diagnostic and Statistical Manual of Mental Disorders*. 4th ed. Text rev. Washington, DC: American Psychiatric Association; copyright 2000, with permission.

Table 17.2–3
DSM-IV-TR Diagnostic Criteria for Female Sexual Arousal Disorder

A. Persistent or recurrent inability to attain, or to maintain until completion of the sexual activity, an adequate lubrication-swelling response of sexual excitement.
B. The disturbance causes marked distress or interpersonal difficulty.
C. The sexual dysfunction is not better accounted for by another Axis I disorder (except another sexual dysfunction) and is not due exclusively to the direct physiological effects of a substance (e.g., a drug of abuse, a medication) or a general medical condition.

Specify type:
  Lifelong type
  Acquired type
Specify type:
  Generalized type
  Situational type
Specify:
  Due to psychological factors
  Due to combined factors

From American Psychiatric Association. *Diagnostic and Statistical Manual of Mental Disorders*. 4th ed. Text rev. Washington, DC: American Psychiatric Association; copyright 2000, with permission.

Abstinence from sex for a prolonged period sometimes results in suppression of sexual impulses. Loss of desire may also be an expression of hostility to a partner or the sign of a deteriorating relationship. In one study of young married couples who ceased having sexual relations for 2 months, marital discord was the reason most frequently given for the cessation or inhibition of sexual activity.

The presence of desire depends on several factors: biological drive, adequate self-esteem, the ability to accept oneself as a sexual person, previous good experiences with sex, the availability of an appropriate partner, and a good relationship in nonsexual areas with a partner. Damage to, or absence of, any of these factors can diminish desire.

In making the diagnosis, clinicians must evaluate a patient's age, general health, and life stresses and must attempt to establish a baseline of sexual interest before the disorder began. The need for sexual contact and satisfaction varies among persons and over time in any given person. In a group of 100 couples with stable marriages, 8 percent reported having intercourse less than once a month. In another group of couples, one third reported episodic lack of sexual relations for periods averaging 8 weeks. Married couples have coitus three times a month, on average. The diagnosis should not be made unless the lack of desire is a source of distress to a patient.

SEXUAL AROUSAL DISORDERS

The sexual arousal disorders are divided by DSM-IV-TR into female sexual arousal disorder, characterized by the persistent or recurrent partial or complete failure to attain or maintain the lubrication-swelling response of sexual excitement until the completion of the sexual act (Table 17.2–3), and male erectile disorder, characterized by the recurrent and persistent partial or complete failure to attain or maintain an erection to perform the sex act (Table 17.2–4). The diagnosis takes into account the focus, intensity, and duration of the sexual activity in which patients engage. If sexual stimulation is inadequate in focus, intensity, or duration, the diagnosis should not be made.

Female Sexual Arousal Disorder

The DSM-IV-TR defines female sexual arousal disorder in terms of the physiological arousal response. A subjective sense of arousal is often poorly correlated, however, with genital lubrication in both dysfunctional and normal women. A woman complaining of lack of arousal may lubricate vaginally but may not experience a subjective sense of excitement. Some studies using functional magnetic resonance imaging have revealed a low correlation between brain activation in areas controlling genital response and simultaneous ratings of subjective arousal.

Table 17.2–4
DSM-IV-TR Diagnostic Criteria for Male Erectile Disorder

A. Persistent or recurrent inability to attain, or to maintain until completion of the sexual activity, an adequate erection.
B. The disturbance causes marked distress or interpersonal difficulty.
C. The erectile dysfunction is not better accounted for by another Axis I disorder (other than a sexual dysfunction) and is not due exclusively to the direct physiological effects of a substance (e.g., a drug of abuse, a medication) or a general medical condition.

Specify type:
  Lifelong type
  Acquired type
Specify type:
  Generalized type
  Situational type
Specify:
  Due to psychological factors
  Due to combined factors

From American Psychiatric Association. *Diagnostic and Statistical Manual of Mental Disorders*. 4th ed. Text rev. Washington, DC: American Psychiatric Association; copyright 2000, with permission.

Physiological studies of sexual dysfunctions indicate that a hormonal pattern may contribute to responsiveness in women who have excitement-phase dysfunction. William Masters and Virginia Johnson found that women were particularly desirous of sex before the onset of the menses. Other women report feeling the greatest sexual excitement immediately after the menses or at the time of ovulation. Alterations in testosterone, estrogen, prolactin, and thyroxin levels have been implicated in female sexual arousal disorder. In addition, medications with antihistaminic or anticholinergic properties cause a decrease in vaginal lubrication.

Male Erectile Disorder

Male erectile disorder is also called *erectile dysfunction* and *impotence*. A man with lifelong male erectile disorder has never been able to obtain an erection sufficient for vaginal insertion. In acquired male erectile disorder, a man has successfully achieved vaginal penetration at some time in his sexual life but is later unable to do so. In situational male erectile disorder, a man is able to have coitus in certain circumstances but not in others; for example, he may function effectively with a prostitute but be impotent with his wife.

Acquired male erectile disorder has been reported in 10 to 20 percent of all men. Freud declared it common among his patients. Impotence is the chief complaint of more than 50 percent of all men treated for sexual disorders. Lifelong male erectile disorder is rare; it occurs in about 1 percent of men under age 35 years, but the incidence increases with age. It has been reported in about 8 percent of the young adult population. Alfred Kinsey reported that 75 percent of all men were impotent at age 80 years. Masters and Johnson reported that men older than 40 years of age have a fear of impotence, which the researchers believed reflects the masculine fear of loss of virility with advancing age. Male erectile disorder, however, is not universal in aging men; having an available sex partner is related to continuing potency, as is a history of consistent sexual activity and the absence of vascular disease.

Male erectile disorder can be organic or psychological or a combination of both, but in young and middle-aged men the cause is usually psychological. A good history is of primary importance in determining the cause of the dysfunction. If a man reports having spontaneous erections at times when he does not plan to have intercourse, having morning erections, or having good erections with masturbation or with partners other than his usual one, the organic causes of his impotence can be considered negligible, and costly diagnostic procedures can be avoided. Male erectile disorder caused by a general medical condition or a pharmacological substance is discussed later in this section.

Freud ascribed one type of impotence to an inability to reconcile feelings of affection toward a woman with feelings of desire for her. Men with such conflicting feelings can function only with women whom they see as degraded (Madonna–Putana complex). Other factors that have been cited as contributing to impotence include a punitive superego, an inability to trust, and feelings of inadequacy or a sense of being undesirable as a partner. A man may be unable to express a sexual impulse because of fear, anxiety, anger, or moral prohibition. In an ongoing relationship, impotence may reflect difficulties between the partners, particularly when a man cannot communicate his needs or his anger in a direct and constructive way. In addition, episodes of impotence are reinforcing, with the man becoming increasingly anxious before each sexual encounter.

ORGASM DISORDERS

Female Orgasmic Disorder

Female orgasmic disorder, sometimes called *inhibited female orgasm* or *anorgasmia*, is defined as the recurrent or persistent inhibition of female orgasm, as manifested by the recurrent delay in, or absence of, orgasm after a normal sexual excitement phase that a clinician judges to be adequate in focus, intensity, and duration—in short, a woman's inability to achieve orgasm by masturbation or coitus (Table 17.2–5). Women who can achieve orgasm by one of these methods are not necessarily categorized as anorgasmic, although some sexual inhibition may be postulated.

Research on the physiology of the female sexual response has shown that orgasms caused by clitoral stimulation and those caused by vaginal stimulation are physiologically identical. Freud's theory that women must give up clitoral sensitivity for vaginal sensitivity to achieve sexual maturity is now considered misleading, but some women report that they gain a special sense of satisfaction from an orgasm precipitated by coitus. Some researchers attribute this satisfaction to the psychological feeling of closeness engendered by the act of coitus, but others maintain that the coital orgasm is a physiologically different experience. Many women achieve orgasm during coitus by a combination of manual clitoral stimulation and penile vaginal stimulation.

A woman with lifelong female orgasmic disorder has never experienced orgasm by any kind of stimulation. A woman with acquired orgasmic disorder has previously experienced at least one orgasm, regardless of the circumstances or means of stimulation, whether by masturbation or while dreaming during sleep. Kinsey found that only 5 percent of married women older than

Table 17.2–5
DSM-IV-TR Diagnostic Criteria for Female Orgasmic Disorder

A. Persistent or recurrent delay in, or absence of, orgasm following a normal sexual excitement phase. Women exhibit wide variability in the type or intensity of stimulation that triggers orgasm. The diagnosis of female orgasmic disorder should be based on the clinician's judgment that the woman's orgasmic capacity is less than would be reasonable for her age, sexual experience, and the adequacy of sexual stimulation she receives.

B. The disturbance causes marked distress or interpersonal difficulty.

C. The orgasmic dysfunction is not better accounted for by another Axis I disorder (except another sexual dysfunction) and is not due exclusively to the direct physiological effects of a substance (e.g., a drug of abuse, a medication) or a general medical condition.

Specify type:
   Lifelong type
   Acquired type
Specify type:
   Generalized type
   Situational type
Specify:
   Due to psychological factors
   Due to combined factors

From American Psychiatric Association. *Diagnostic and Statistical Manual of Mental Disorders.* 4th ed. Text rev. Washington, DC: American Psychiatric Association; copyright 2000, with permission.

35 years of age had never achieved orgasm by any means. The incidence of orgasm increases with age. According to Kinsey, the first orgasm occurs during adolescence in about 50 percent of women as a result of masturbation or genital caressing with a partner; the rest usually experience orgasm as they get older. Lifelong female orgasmic disorder is more common among unmarried women than married women. Increased orgasmic potential in women older than 35 years of age has been explained on the basis of less psychological inhibition, greater sexual experience, or both.

Acquired female orgasmic disorder is a common complaint in clinical populations. One clinical treatment facility reported having about four times as many nonorgasmic women in its practice as patients with all other sexual disorders. In another study, 46 percent of women complained of difficulty reaching orgasm. The true prevalence of problems maintaining excitement is not known, but inhibition of excitement and orgasmic problems often occur together. The overall prevalence of female orgasmic disorder from all causes is estimated to be 30 percent. A recent twin study suggests that orgasmic dysfunction in some females has a genetic basis and cannot be attributed solely to cultural differences. That study demonstrated an estimated heritability for difficulty reaching orgasm with intercourse of 34 percent and an estimated heritability in women who could not climax with masturbation of 45 percent.

Numerous psychological factors are associated with female orgasmic disorder. They include fears of impregnation, rejection by a sex partner, and damage to the vagina; hostility toward men; and feelings of guilt about sexual impulses. Some women equate orgasm with loss of control or with aggressive, destructive, or violent impulses; their fear of these impulses may be expressed through inhibition of excitement or orgasm. Cultural expectations and social restrictions on women are also relevant. Many women have grown up to believe that sexual pleasure is not a natural entitlement for so-called decent women. Nonorgasmic women may be otherwise symptom free or may experience frustration in a variety of ways; they may have such pelvic complaints as lower abdominal pain, itching, and vaginal discharge, as well as increased tension, irritability, and fatigue.

Male Orgasmic Disorder

In male orgasmic disorder, sometimes called *inhibited orgasm* or *retarded ejaculation*, a man achieves ejaculation during coitus with great difficulty, if at all (Table 17.2–6). A man with lifelong orgasmic disorder has never been able to ejaculate during coitus. The disorder is diagnosed as acquired if it develops after previously normal functioning. Some researchers think that orgasm and ejaculation should be differentiated, especially in the case of men who ejaculate but complain of a decreased or absent subjective sense of pleasure during the orgasmic experience (orgasmic anhedonia).

The incidence of male orgasmic disorder is much lower than the incidence of premature ejaculation or impotence. Masters and Johnson reported an incidence of male orgasmic disorder of only 3.8 percent in one group of 447 men with sexual dysfunctions. A general prevalence of 5 percent has been reported.

Lifelong male orgasmic disorder indicates severe psychopathology. A man may come from a rigid, puritanical background; he may perceive sex as sinful and the genitals as dirty; and he may have conscious or unconscious incest wishes and guilt. He usually has difficulty with closeness in areas beyond those of sexual relations. In a few cases, the condition is aggravated by an attention-deficit disorder. A man's distractibility prevents sufficient arousal for climax to occur.

Table 17.2–6
DSM-IV-TR Diagnostic Criteria for Male Orgasmic Disorder

A. Persistent or recurrent delay in, or absence of, orgasm following a normal sexual excitement phase during sexual activity that the clinician, taking into account the person's age, judges to be adequate in focus, intensity, and duration.
B. The disturbance causes marked distress or interpersonal difficulty.
C. The orgasmic dysfunction is not better accounted for by another Axis I disorder (except another sexual dysfunction) and is not due exclusively to the direct physiological effects of a substance (e.g., a drug of abuse, a medication) or a general medical condition.

Specify type:
   Lifelong type
   Acquired type
Specify type:
   Generalized type
   Situational type
Specify:
   Due to psychological factors
   Due to combined factors

From American Psychiatric Association. *Diagnostic and Statistical Manual of Mental Disorders.* 4th ed. Text rev. Washington, DC: American Psychiatric Association; copyright 2000, with permission.

In an ongoing relationship, acquired male orgasmic disorder frequently reflects interpersonal difficulties. The disorder may be a man's way of coping with real or fantasized changes in a relationship, such as plans for pregnancy about which the man is ambivalent, the loss of sexual attraction to the partner, or demands by the partner for greater commitment as expressed by sexual performance. In some men, the inability to ejaculate reflects unexpressed hostility toward a woman. The problem is more common among men with obsessive-compulsive disorder than among others.

Premature Ejaculation

In premature ejaculation, men persistently or recurrently achieve orgasm and ejaculation before they wish to. No definite time-frame exists within which to define the dysfunction; the diagnosis is made when a man regularly ejaculates before or immediately after entering the vagina. Clinicians need to consider factors that affect the duration of the excitement phase, such as age, the novelty of the sex partner, and the frequency and duration of coitus (Table 17.2–7). Masters and Johnson conceptualized the disorder in terms of the couple and considered a man a premature ejaculator if he could not control ejaculation sufficiently long enough during intravaginal containment to satisfy his partner in at least half their episodes of coitus. This definition assumes that the female partner is capable of an orgasmic response. As with the other sexual dysfunctions, premature ejaculation is not diagnosed when it is caused exclusively by organic factors or when it is not symptomatic of any other clinical psychiatric syndrome.

Premature ejaculation is more commonly reported among college-educated men than among men with less education. The complaint is thought to be related to their concern for partner satisfaction, but the true cause of this increased frequency has not been determined. Premature ejaculation is the chief complaint of about 35 to 40 percent of men treated for sexual disorders. Some researchers divide men who experience premature ejaculation into two groups: those who are physiologically

Table 17.2–7
DSM-IV-TR Diagnostic Criteria for
Premature Ejaculation

A. Persistent or recurrent ejaculation with minimal sexual stimulation before, on, or shortly after penetration and before the person wishes it. The clinician must take into account factors that affect duration of the excitement phase, such as age, novelty of the sexual partner or situation, and recent frequency of sexual activity.
B. The disturbance causes marked distress or interpersonal difficulty.
C. The premature ejaculation is not due exclusively to the direct effects of a substance (e.g., withdrawal from opioids).

Specify type:
    Lifelong type
    Acquired type
Specify type:
    Generalized type
    Situational type
Specify:
    Due to psychological factors
    Due to combined factors

From American Psychiatric Association. *Diagnostic and Statistical Manual of Mental Disorders.* 4th ed. Text rev. Washington, DC: American Psychiatric Association; copyright 2000, with permission.

Table 17.2–8
DSM-IV-TR Diagnostic Criteria for Dyspareunia

A. Recurrent or persistent genital pain associated with sexual intercourse in either a male or a female.
B. The disturbance causes marked distress or interpersonal difficulty.
C. The disturbance is not caused exclusively by vaginismus or lack of lubrication, is not better accounted for by another Axis I disorder (except another sexual dysfunction), and is not due exclusively to the direct physiological effects of a substance (e.g., a drug of abuse, a medication) or a general medical condition.

Specify type:
    Lifelong type
    Acquired type
Specify type:
    Generalized type
    Situational type
Specify:
    Due to psychological factors
    Due to combined factors

From American Psychiatric Association. *Diagnostic and Statistical Manual of Mental Disorders.* 4th ed. Text rev. Washington, DC: American Psychiatric Association; copyright 2000, with permission.

predisposed to climax quickly because of shorter nerve latency time and those with a psychogenic or behaviorally conditioned cause. Difficulty in ejaculatory control can be associated with anxiety regarding the sex act, with unconscious fears about the vagina, or with negative cultural conditioning. Men whose early sexual contacts occurred largely with prostitutes who demanded that the sex act proceed quickly or whose sexual contacts took place in situations in which discovery would be embarrassing (e.g., in the back seat of a car or in the parental home) might have been conditioned to achieve orgasm rapidly. With young, inexperienced men, who are more likely to have the problem, it may resolve in time. In ongoing relationships, the partner has a great influence on a premature ejaculator, and a stressful marriage exacerbates the disorder. The developmental background and the psychodynamics found in premature ejaculation and in impotence are similar.

SEXUAL PAIN DISORDERS

Dyspareunia

Dyspareunia is recurrent or persistent genital pain occurring in either men or women before, during, or after intercourse. Much more common in women than in men, dyspareunia is related to, and often coincides with, vaginismus. Repeated episodes of vaginismus can lead to dyspareunia and vice versa; in either case, somatic causes must be ruled out. Dyspareunia should not be diagnosed when an organic basis for the pain is found or when, in a woman, it is caused exclusively by vaginismus or by a lack of lubrication (Table 17.2–8). The incidence of dyspareunia is unknown.

In most cases, dynamic factors are considered causative. Chronic pelvic pain is a common complaint in women with a history of rape or childhood sexual abuse. Painful coitus can result from tension and anxiety about the sex act that cause women to involuntarily contract their vaginal muscles. The pain is real and makes intercourse unpleasant or unbearable. Anticipation of further pain may cause women to avoid coitus altogether. If a partner proceeds with intercourse regardless of a woman's state of readiness, the condition is aggravated. Dyspareunia can also

occur in men, but it is uncommon and is usually associated with an organic condition, such as herpes, prostatitis, or Peyronie's disease, which consists of sclerotic plaques on the penis that cause penile curvature.

Vaginismus

Vaginismus is an involuntary muscle constriction of the outer third of the vagina that interferes with penile insertion and intercourse. This response may occur during a gynecological examination when involuntary vaginal constriction prevents the introduction of the speculum into the vagina. The diagnosis is not made when the dysfunction is caused exclusively by organic factors or when it is symptomatic of another Axis I mental disorder (Table 17.2–9).

Table 17.2–9
DSM-IV-TR Diagnostic Criteria for Vaginismus

A. Recurrent or persistent involuntary spasm of the musculature of the outer third of the vagina that interferes with sexual intercourse.
B. The disturbance causes marked distress or interpersonal difficulty.
C. The disturbance is not better accounted for by another Axis I disorder (e.g., somatization disorder) and is not due exclusively to the direct physiological effects of a general medical condition.

Specify type:
    Lifelong type
    Acquired type
Specify type:
    Generalized type
    Situational type
Specify:
    Due to psychological factors
    Due to combined factors

From American Psychiatric Association. *Diagnostic and Statistical Manual of Mental Disorders.* 4th ed. Text rev. Washington, DC: American Psychiatric Association; copyright 2000, with permission.

Vaginismus is less prevalent than female orgasmic disorder. It most often afflicts highly educated women and those in high socioeconomic groups. Women with vaginismus may consciously wish to have coitus but unconsciously wish to keep a penis from entering their bodies. A sexual trauma, such as rape, may cause vaginismus; women with psychosexual conflicts may perceive the penis as a weapon. In some cases, pain or the anticipation of pain at the first coital experience causes vaginismus. Clinicians have noted that a strict religious upbringing in which sex is associated with sin is frequent in these patients. Other women have problems in dyadic relationships; if women feel emotionally abused by their partners, they may protest in this nonverbal fashion.

SEXUAL DYSFUNCTION DUE TO A GENERAL MEDICAL CONDITION

The category sexual dysfunction due to a general medical condition covers sexual dysfunction that results in marked distress and interpersonal difficulty; the history, physical examination, or laboratory findings must provide evidence of a general medical condition judged to be causally related to the sexual dysfunction (Table 17.2–10).

Table 17.2–10
DSM-IV-TR Diagnostic Criteria for Sexual Dysfunction Due to a General Medical Condition

A. Clinically significant sexual dysfunction that results in marked distress or interpersonal difficulty predominates in the clinical picture.
B. There is evidence from the history, physical examination, or laboratory findings that the sexual dysfunction is fully explained by the direct physiological effects of a general medical condition.
C. The disturbance is not better accounted for by another mental disorder (e.g., major depressive disorder).

Select code and term based on the predominant sexual dysfunction:

Female hypoactive sexual desire disorder due to ... [indicate the general medical condition]: if deficient or absent sexual desire is the predominant feature
Male hypoactive sexual desire disorder due to ... [indicate the general medical condition]: if deficient or absent sexual desire is the predominant feature
Male erectile disorder due to ... [indicate the general medical condition]: if male erectile dysfunction is the predominant feature
Female dyspareunia due to ... [indicate the general medical condition]: if pain associated with intercourse is the predominant feature
Male dyspareunia due to ... [indicate the general medical condition]: if pain associated with intercourse is the predominant feature
Other female sexual dysfunction due to ... [indicate the general medical condition]: if some other feature is predominant (e.g., orgasmic disorder) or no feature predominates
Other male sexual dysfunction due to ... [indicate the general medical condition]: if some other feature is predominant (e.g., orgasmic disorder) or no feature predominates
Coding note: Include the name of the general medical condition on Axis I, e.g., male erectile disorder due to diabetes mellitus; also code the general medical condition on Axis III.

From American Psychiatric Association. *Diagnostic and Statistical Manual of Mental Disorders.* 4th ed. Text rev. Washington, DC: American Psychiatric Association; copyright 2000, with permission.

Male Erectile Disorder Due to a General Medical Condition

The incidence of psychological, as opposed to organic, male erectile disorder has been the focus of many studies. Statistics indicate that 20 to 50 percent of men with erectile disorder have an organic basis for the disorder. Side effects of medication can impair male sexual functioning in a variety of ways. Castration (removal of the testes) does not always lead to sexual dysfunction, because erection may still occur. A reflex arc, fired when the inner thigh is stimulated, passes through the sacral cord erectile center to account for the phenomenon.

A number of procedures, benign and invasive, are used to help differentiate organically caused impotence from functional impotence. The procedures include monitoring nocturnal penile tumescence (erections that occur during sleep), normally associated with rapid eye movement; monitoring tumescence with a strain gauge; measuring blood pressure in the penis with a penile plethysmograph or an ultrasound (Doppler) flowmeter, both of which assess blood flow in the internal pudendal artery; and measuring pudendal nerve latency time. Other diagnostic tests that delineate organic bases for impotence include glucose tolerance tests, plasma hormone assays, liver and thyroid function tests, prolactin and follicle-stimulating hormone determinations, and cystometric examinations. Invasive diagnostic studies include penile arteriography, infusion cavernosonography, and radioactive xenon penography. Invasive procedures require expert interpretation and are used only for patients who are candidates for vascular reconstructive procedures.

Dyspareunia Due to a General Medical Condition

An estimated 30 percent of all surgical procedures on the female genital area result in temporary dyspareunia. In addition, 30 to 40 percent of women with the complaint who are seen in sex therapy clinics have pelvic pathology. Organic abnormalities leading to dyspareunia and vaginismus include irritated or infected hymenal remnants, episiotomy scars, Bartholin's gland infection, various forms of vaginitis and cervicitis, and endometriosis. Postcoital pain has been reported by women with myomata and endometriosis and is attributed to the uterine contractions during orgasm. Postmenopausal women may have dyspareunia resulting from thinning of the vaginal mucosa and reduced lubrication.

Two conditions not readily apparent on physical examination that produce dyspareunia are vulvar vestibulitis and interstitial cystitis. The former may present with chronic vulvar pain and the latter produces pain most intensely following orgasm. Dyspareunia can also occur in men, but it is uncommon and is usually associated with an organic condition, such as Peyronie's disease, which consists of sclerotic plaques on the penis that cause penile curvature.

Hypoactive Sexual Desire Disorder Due to a General Medical Condition

Sexual desire commonly decreases after major illness or surgery, particularly when the body image is affected after such procedures as mastectomy, ileostomy, hysterectomy, and prostatectomy. Illnesses that deplete a person's energy, chronic conditions that require physical and psychological adaptation, and serious illnesses that can cause a person to become depressed can all markedly lessen sexual desire in both men and women.

In some cases, biochemical correlates are associated with hypoactive sexual desire disorder. A recent study found markedly lower levels of serum testosterone in men complaining of low desire than in normal controls in a sleep-laboratory situation. Drugs that depress the central nervous system (CNS) or decrease testosterone production can decrease desire.

Other Male Sexual Dysfunction Due to a General Medical Condition

When another dysfunctional feature is predominant (e.g., orgasmic disorder) or when no feature predominates, the category other male sexual dysfunction due to a general medical condition is used.

Male orgasmic disorder can have physiological causes and can occur after surgery on the genitourinary tract, such as prostatectomy. It may also be associated with Parkinson's disease and other neurological disorders involving the lumbar or sacral sections of the spinal cord. The antihypertensive drug guanethidine monosulfate (Ismelin), methyldopa (Aldomet), the phenothiazines, the tricyclic drugs, and the selective serotonin reuptake inhibitors (SSRIs), among others, have been implicated in retarded ejaculation. Male orgasmic disorder must also be differentiated from retrograde ejaculation, in which ejaculation occurs but the seminal fluid passes backward into the bladder. Retrograde ejaculation always has an organic cause. It can develop after genitourinary surgery and is also associated with medications that have anticholinergic adverse effects, such as the phenothiazines, especially thioridazine (Mellaril).

Other Female Sexual Dysfunction Due to a General Medical Condition

Some medical conditions—specifically, endocrine diseases such as hypothyroidism, diabetes mellitus, and primary hyperprolactinemia—can affect a woman's ability to have orgasms. Several drugs also affect some women's capacity to have orgasms. Antihypertensive medications, CNS stimulants, tricyclic drugs, SSRIs, and, frequently, monoamine oxidase inhibitors (MAOIs) have interfered with female orgasmic capacity. One study of women taking MAOIs, however, found that after 16 to 18 weeks of pharmacotherapy, the adverse effect of the medication disappeared and the women were able to reexperience orgasms, although they continued taking an undiminished dose of the drug.

SUBSTANCE-INDUCED SEXUAL DYSFUNCTION

The diagnosis of substance-induced sexual dysfunction is used when evidence of substance intoxication or withdrawal is apparent from the history, physical examination, or laboratory findings. Distressing sexual dysfunction occurs within 1 month of significant substance intoxication or withdrawal (Table 17.2–11). Specified substances include alcohol, amphetamines or related substances, cocaine, opioids, sedatives, hypnotics, or anxiolytics, and other or unknown substances.

Abused recreational substances affect sexual function in various ways. In small doses, many substances enhance sexual performance by decreasing inhibition or anxiety or by causing a temporary elation of mood. With continued use, however, erectile engorgement and orgasmic and ejaculatory capacities become impaired. The abuse of sedatives, anxiolytics, hypnotics, and particularly opiates and opioids nearly always depresses desire. Alcohol may foster the initiation of sexual ac-

**Table 17.2–11
DSM-IV-TR Diagnostic Criteria for
Substance-Induced Sexual Dysfunction**

A. Clinically significant sexual dysfunction that results in marked distress or interpersonal difficulty predominates in the clinical picture.
B. There is evidence from the history, physical examination, or laboratory findings that the sexual dysfunction is fully explained by substance use as manifested by either (1) or (2):
  (1) the symptoms in Criterion A developed during, or within a month of, substance intoxication
  (2) medication use is etiologically related to the disturbance
C. The disturbance is not better accounted for by a sexual dysfunction that is not substance induced. Evidence that the symptoms are better accounted for by a sexual dysfunction that is not substance induced might include the following: the symptoms precede the onset of the substance use or dependence (or medication use); the symptoms persist for a substantial period of time (e.g., about a month) after the cessation of intoxication, or are substantially in excess of what would be expected given the type or amount of the substance used or the duration of use; or there is other evidence that suggests the existence of an independent non–substance-induced sexual dysfunction (e.g., a history of recurrent non–substance-related episodes).

Note: This diagnosis should be made instead of a diagnosis of substance intoxication only when the sexual dysfunction is in excess of that usually associated with the intoxication syndrome and when the dysfunction is sufficiently severe to warrant independent clinical attention.

Code [Specific substance]-induced sexual dysfunction: Alcohol; amphetamine [or amphetamine-like substance]; cocaine; opioid; sedative, hypnotic, or anxiolytic; other [or unknown] substance

Specify if:
  With impaired desire
  With impaired arousal
  With impaired orgasm
  With sexual pain
Specify if:
  With onset during intoxication: if the criteria are met for intoxication with the substance and the symptoms develop during the intoxication syndrome

From American Psychiatric Association. *Diagnostic and Statistical Manual of Mental Disorders.* 4th ed. Text rev. Washington, DC: American Psychiatric Association; copyright 2000, with permission.

tivity by removing inhibition, but it also impairs performance. Cocaine and amphetamines produce similar effects. Although no direct evidence indicates that sexual drive is enhanced, users initially have feelings of increased energy and may become sexually active. Ultimately, dysfunction occurs. Men usually go through two stages: an experience of prolonged erection without ejaculation, then a gradual loss of erectile capability.

Patients recovering from substance dependency may need therapy to regain sexual function, partly because of psychological readjustment to a nondependent state. Many substance abusers have always had difficulty with intimate interactions. Others who spent their crucial developmental years under the influence of a substance have missed the experiences that would have enabled them to learn social and sexual skills.

PHARMACOLOGICAL AGENTS IMPLICATED IN SEXUAL DYSFUNCTION

Almost every pharmacological agent, particularly those used in psychiatry, has been associated with an effect on sexuality. In men, these effects include decreased sex drive, erectile failure (impotence), decreased volume of ejaculate, and delayed or retrograde ejaculation. In women, decreased sex drive, decreased vaginal lubrication, inhibited or delayed orgasm, and decreased or absent vaginal contractions may occur. Drugs may also enhance the sexual responses and increase the sex drive, but this is less common than adverse effects.

Psychoactive Drugs

Antipsychotic Drugs.   Most antipsychotic drugs are dopamine receptor antagonists that also block adrenergic and cholinergic receptors, thus accounting for adverse sexual effects. Chlorpromazine (Thorazine), thioridazine, and trifluoperazine (Stelazine) are potent anticholinergics that impair erection and ejaculation; the seminal fluid backs up into the bladder rather than being propelled through the penile urethra. Patients still have a pleasurable sensation, but the orgasm is dry. When urinating after orgasm, the urine may be milky white because it contains the ejaculate. The condition is startling but harmless and may occur in up to 50 percent of patients taking the drug. Paradoxically, some rare cases of priapism have been reported with antipsychotics.

Antidepressant Drugs.   The tricyclic and tetracyclic antidepressants have anticholinergic effects that interfere with erection and delay ejaculation. Because the anticholinergic effects vary among the cyclic antidepressants, those with the fewest side effects (e.g., desipramine [Norpramin]) produce the fewest sexual adverse effects. The effects of the tricyclics and tetracyclics have not been documented sufficiently in women; however, few women seem to complain of any effects.

Some men report increased sensitivity of the glans that is pleasurable and that does not interfere with erection, although it delays ejaculation. In some cases, however, the tricyclic causes painful ejaculation, perhaps as the result of interference with seminal propulsion caused by interference with, in turn, urethral, prostatic, vas, and epididymal smooth muscle contractions. Clomipramine (Anafranil) has been reported to increase sex drive in some persons. Selegiline (Deprenyl), a selective MAO type B (MAO$_B$) inhibitor, and bupropion (Wellbutrin) have also been reported to increase sex drive, possibly by dopaminergic activity and increased production of norepinephrine.

Venlafaxine (Effexor) and the SSRIs most often have adverse effects because of the rise in serotonin levels. A lowering of the sex drive and difficulty reaching orgasm occur in both sexes. Reversal of those negative effects has been achieved with cyproheptadine (Periactin), an antihistamine with antiserotonergic effects, and with methylphenidate (Ritalin), which has adrenergic effects. Trazodone (Desyrel) is associated with the rare occurrence of priapism, the symptom of prolonged erection in the absence of sexual stimuli. That symptom appears to result from the α_2-adrenergic antagonism of trazodone.

The MAOIs affect biogenic amines broadly. Accordingly, they produce impaired erection, delayed or retrograde ejaculation, vaginal dryness, and inhibited orgasm. Tranylcypromine (Parnate) has a paradoxical sexually stimulating effect in some persons, possibly as a result of its amphetamine-like properties.

Lithium.   Lithium (Eskalith) regulates mood and, in the manic state, may reduce hypersexuality, possibly by a dopamine antagonist activity. In some patients, impaired erection has been reported.

Sympathomimetics.   Psychostimulants, which are sometimes used in the treatment of depression, include amphetamines, methylphenidate, and pemoline (Cylert), which raise the plasma levels of norepinephrine and dopamine. Libido is increased; however, with prolonged use, men may experience a loss of desire and erections.

α-Adrenergic and β-Adrenergic Receptor Antagonists. α-Adrenergic and β-adrenergic receptor antagonists are used in the treatment of hypertension, angina, and certain cardiac arrhythmias. They diminish tonic sympathetic nerve outflow from vasomotor centers in the brain. As a result, they can cause impotence, decrease the volume of ejaculate, and produce retrograde ejaculation. Changes in libido have been reported in both sexes.

Suggestions have been made to use the side effects of drugs therapeutically. Thus, a drug that delays or interferes with ejaculation (e.g., fluoxetine [Prozac]) might be used to treat premature ejaculation.

Anticholinergics.   The anticholinergics block cholinergic receptors and include such drugs as amantadine (Symmetrel) and benztropine (Cogentin). They produce dryness of the mucous membranes (including those of the vagina) and impotence. However, amantadine may reverse SSRI-induced orgasmic dysfunction through its dopaminergic effect.

Antihistamines.   Drugs such as diphenhydramine (Benadryl) have anticholinergic activity and are mildly hypnotic. They may inhibit sexual function as a result. Cyproheptadine, although an antihistamine, also has potent activity as a serotonin antagonist. It is used to block the serotonergic sexual adverse effects produced by SSRIs, such as delayed orgasm and impotence.

Antianxiety Agents.   The major class of anxiolytics is the benzodiazepines (e.g., diazepam [Valium]). They act on the γ-aminobutyric acid receptors, which are believed to be involved in cognition, memory, and motor control. Because they decrease plasma epinephrine concentrations, they diminish anxiety, and as a result they improve sexual function in persons inhibited by anxiety.

Alcohol.   Alcohol suppresses CNS activity generally and can produce erectile disorders in men as a result. Alcohol has a direct gonadal effect that decreases testosterone levels in men; paradoxically, it can produce a slight rise in testosterone levels in women. The latter finding may account for women reporting increased libido after drinking small amounts of alcohol. The long-term use of alcohol reduces the ability of the liver to metabolize estrogenic compounds. In men, that produces signs of feminization (such as gynecomastia as a result of testicular atrophy).

Opioids.   Opioids, such as heroin, have adverse sexual effects, such as erectile failure and decreased libido. The alteration of consciousness may enhance the sexual experience in occasional users.

Hallucinogens.   The hallucinogens include lysergic acid diethylamide, phencyclidine, psilocybin (from some mushrooms), and mescaline (from peyote cactus). In addition to inducing hallucinations, the drugs cause loss of contact with reality and an expanding and heightening of consciousness. Some users report that the sexual experience is similarly enhanced, but others experience anxiety, delirium, or psychosis, which clearly interferes with sexual function.

Cannabis.   The altered state of consciousness produced by cannabis may enhance sexual pleasure for some persons. Its prolonged use depresses testosterone levels.

Barbiturates and Similarly Acting Drugs.   Barbiturates and similarly acting sedative-hypnotic drugs may enhance sexual responsiveness in persons who are sexually unresponsive as a result of anxiety. They have no direct effect on the sex organs; however, they do produce an alteration in consciousness that some persons find pleasurable. They are subject to abuse and can be fatal when combined with alcohol or other CNS depressants.

Table 17.2–12
DSM-IV-TR Diagnostic Criteria for Sexual Dysfunction Not Otherwise Specified

This category includes sexual dysfunctions that do not meet criteria for any specific sexual dysfunction. Examples include:

1. No (or substantially diminished) subjective erotic feelings despite otherwise normal arousal and orgasm
2. Situations in which the clinician has concluded that a sexual dysfunction is present but is unable to determine whether it is primary, due to a general medical condition, or substance induced

From American Psychiatric Association. *Diagnostic and Statistical Manual of Mental Disorders*. 4th ed. Text rev. Washington, DC: American Psychiatric Association; copyright 2000, with permission.

Methaqualone (Quaalude) acquired a reputation as a sexual enhancer, which had no biological basis in fact. It is no longer marketed in the United States.

SEXUAL DYSFUNCTION NOT OTHERWISE SPECIFIED

The category sexual dysfunction not otherwise specified covers sexual dysfunctions that cannot be classified under the categories described previously (Table 17.2–12). Examples include persons who experience the physiological components of sexual excitement and orgasm but report no erotic sensation or even anesthesia (orgasmic anhedonia). Women with conditions analogous to premature ejaculation in men are classified here. Orgasmic women who desire but have not experienced multiple orgasms can be classified under this heading as well. In addition, disorders of excessive, rather than inhibited, dysfunction, such as compulsive masturbation or coitus (sex addiction), or those with genital pain occurring during masturbation may be classified here. Other unspecified disorders are found in persons who have one or more sexual fantasies about which they feel guilty or otherwise dysphoric, but the range of common sexual fantasies is broad.

Female Premature Orgasm

Data on female premature orgasm are lacking; no separate category of premature orgasm for women is included in DSM-IV-TR. A case of multiple spontaneous orgasms without sexual stimulation was seen in a woman; the cause was an epileptogenic focus in the temporal lobe. Instances have been reported of women taking antidepressants (e.g., fluoxetine and clomipramine) who experience spontaneous orgasm associated with yawning.

Postcoital Headache

Postcoital headache, characterized by headache immediately after coitus, may last for several hours. It is usually described as throbbing and is localized in the occipital or frontal area. The cause is unknown. There may be vascular, muscle-contraction (tension), or psychogenic causes. Coitus may precipitate migraine or cluster headaches in predisposed persons.

Orgasmic Anhedonia

Orgasmic anhedonia is a condition in which a person has no physical sensation of orgasm, even though the physiological component (e.g., ejaculation) remains intact. Organic causes, such as sacral and cephalic lesions that interfere with afferent pathways from the genitalia to the cortex, must be ruled out. Psychiatric causes usually relate to extreme guilt about experiencing sexual pleasure. These feelings produce a dissociative response that isolates the affective component of the orgasmic experience from consciousness.

Masturbatory Pain

Persons may experience pain during masturbation. Organic causes should always be ruled out; a small vaginal tear or early Peyronie's disease can produce a painful sensation. The condition should be differentiated from compulsive masturbation. Persons may masturbate to the extent that they do physical damage to their genitals and eventually experience pain during subsequent masturbatory acts. Such cases constitute a separate sexual disorder and should be so classified.

Certain masturbatory practices have resulted in what has been called autoerotic asphyxiation. The practices involve persons masturbating while hanging by the neck to heighten the erotic sensations and the orgasm's intensity through the mechanism of mild hypoxia. Although the persons intend to release themselves from the noose after orgasm, an estimated 500 to 1,000 persons a year accidentally kill themselves by hanging. Most who indulge in the practice are male; transvestism is often associated with the habit, and most deaths occur among adolescents. Such masochistic practices are usually associated with severe mental disorders, such as schizophrenia and major mood disorders.

TREATMENT

Before 1970, the most common treatment of sexual dysfunctions was individual psychotherapy. Classic psychodynamic theory holds that sexual inadequacy has its roots in early developmental conflicts, and the sexual disorder is treated as part of a pervasive emotional disturbance. Treatment focuses on the exploration of unconscious conflicts, motivation, fantasy, and various interpersonal difficulties. One of the assumptions of therapy is that removal of the conflicts allows the sexual impulse to become structurally acceptable to the ego, and thereby the patient finds appropriate means of satisfaction in the environment. The symptoms of sexual dysfunctions, however, frequently become secondarily autonomous and continue to persist, even when other problems evolving from the patients' pathology have been resolved. The addition of behavioral techniques is often necessary to cure the sexual problem.

Dual-Sex Therapy

The theoretical basis of dual-sex therapy is the concept of the marital unit or dyad as the object of therapy. The methodology was originated and developed by Masters and Johnson. In dual-sex therapy, treatment is based on a concept that the couple must be treated when a dysfunctional person is in a relationship. Because both are involved in a sexually distressing situation, both must participate in the therapy program. The sexual problem often reflects other areas of disharmony or misunderstanding in the marriage so that the entire marital relationship is treated, with emphasis on sexual functioning as a part of the relationship.

The keystone of the program is the roundtable session in which a male and female therapy team clarifies, discusses, and works through problems with the couple. The four-way sessions require active participation by the patients. Therapists and patients discuss the psychological and physiological aspects of sexual functioning, and therapists have an educative attitude.

Therapists suggest specific sexual activities, which the couple follow in the privacy of their home. The aim of the therapy is to establish or reestablish communication within the marital unit. Sex is emphasized as a natural function that flourishes in the appropriate domestic climate, and improved communication is encouraged toward that end. In a variation of this therapy that has proved effective, one therapist may treat the couple. Treatment is short term and behaviorally oriented. The therapists attempt to reflect the situation as they see it, rather than interpret underlying dynamics. An undistorted picture of the relationship presented by the therapists often corrects the myopic, narrow view held by each marriage partner. This new perspective can interrupt the couple's destructive pattern of relating and can encourage improved, more effective communication. Specific exercises are prescribed for the couple to treat their particular problems. Sexual inadequacy often involves lack of information, misinformation, and performance fear. Therefore, the couple are specifically prohibited from any sexual play other than that prescribed by the therapists. Beginning exercises usually focus on heightening sensory awareness to touch, sight, sound, and smell. Initially, intercourse is interdicted, and the couple learns to give and receive bodily pleasure without the pressure of performance or penetration. At the same time, they learn how to communicate nonverbally in a mutually satisfactory way, and they learn that sexual foreplay is an enjoyable alternative to intercourse and orgasm.

During the sensate focus exercises, the couple receive much reinforcement to reduce their anxiety. They are urged to use fantasies to distract them from obsessive concerns about performance (spectatoring). The needs of both the dysfunctional partner and the nondysfunctional partner are considered. If either partner becomes sexually excited by the exercises, the other is encouraged to bring him or her to orgasm by manual or oral means. Open communication between the partners is urged, and the expression of mutual needs is encouraged. Resistances, such as claims of fatigue or not enough time to complete the exercises, are common and must be dealt with by the therapists. Issues of body image, fear of being touched, and difficulty touching oneself arise frequently. Genital stimulation is eventually added to general body stimulation. The couple is instructed sequentially to try various positions for intercourse, without necessarily completing the act, and to use varieties of stimulating techniques before they are instructed to proceed with intercourse.

Psychotherapy sessions follow each new exercise period, and problems and satisfactions, both sexual and in other areas of the couple's lives, are discussed. Specific instructions and the introduction of new exercises geared to the individual couple's progress are reviewed in each session. Gradually, the couple gains confidence and learns to communicate, verbally and sexually. Dual-sex therapy is most effective when the sexual dysfunction exists apart from other psychopathology.

Specific Techniques and Exercises

Various techniques are used to treat the various sexual dysfunctions. These can be prescribed for members of a couple or for unpartnered patients. In cases of vaginismus, a woman is advised to dilate her vaginal opening with her fingers or with size-graduated dilators. Dilators are also used to treat cases of dyspareunia. Sometimes, treatment is coordinated with specially trained physiotherapists who work with the patients to help them relax the perineal muscles.

In cases of premature ejaculation, an exercise known as the squeeze technique is used to raise the threshold of penile excitability. In this exercise, the man or the woman stimulates the erect penis until the earliest sensations of impending ejaculation are felt. At this point, the woman forcefully squeezes the coronal ridge of the glans, the erection is diminished, and ejaculation is inhibited. The exercise program eventually raises the threshold of the sensation of ejaculatory inevitability and allows the man to focus on sensations of arousal without anxiety and develop confidence in his sexual performance. A variant of the exercise is the stop-start technique developed by James H. Semans, in which the woman stops all stimulation of the penis when the man first senses an impending ejaculation. No squeeze is used. Research has shown that the presence or absence of circumcision has no bearing on a man's ejaculatory control; the glans is equally sensitive in the two states. Sex therapy has been most successful in the treatment of premature ejaculation.

A man with a sexual desire disorder or male erectile disorder is sometimes told to masturbate to prove that full erection and ejaculation are possible. Male orgasmic disorder is managed initially by extravaginal ejaculation and then by gradual vaginal entry after stimulation to a point near ejaculation. Most importantly, the early exercises forbid ejaculation to remove the pressure to climax and allow the man to immerse himself in sexual pleasuring.

In cases of lifelong female orgasmic disorder, the woman is directed to masturbate, sometimes using a vibrator. The shaft of the clitoris is the masturbatory site most preferred by women, and orgasm depends on adequate clitoral stimulation. An area on the anterior wall of the vagina has been identified in some women as a site of sexual excitation, known as the *G-spot*, but reports of an ejaculatory phenomenon at orgasm in women following the stimulation of the G-spot have not been satisfactorily verified.

Hypnotherapy

Hypnotherapists focus specifically on the anxiety-producing situation—that is, the sexual interaction that results in dysfunction. The successful use of hypnosis enables patients to gain control over the symptom that has been lowering self-esteem and disrupting psychological homeostasis. The patient's cooperation is first obtained and encouraged during a series of nonhypnotic sessions with the therapist. Those discussions permit the development of a secure doctor–patient relationship, a sense of physical and psychological comfort on the part of the patient, and the establishment of mutually desired treatment goals. During this time, the therapist assesses the patient's capacity for the trance experience. The nonhypnotic sessions also permit the clinician to take a psychiatric history and perform a mental status examination before beginning hypnotherapy. The focus of treatment is on symptom removal and attitude alteration. The patient is instructed in developing alternative means of dealing with the anxiety-provoking situation, the sexual encounter.

Patients are also taught relaxation techniques to use on themselves before sexual relations. With these methods to alleviate anxiety, the physiological responses to sexual stimulation can readily result in pleasurable excitation and discharge. Psychological impediments to vaginal lubrication, erection, and orgasms are removed, and normal sexual functioning ensues. Hypnosis may be added to a basic individual psychotherapy program to accelerate the effects of psychotherapeutic intervention.

Behavior Therapy

Behavioral approaches were initially designed for the treatment of phobias but are now used to treat other problems as well.

Behavior therapists assume that sexual dysfunction is learned maladaptive behavior, which causes patients to be fearful of sexual interaction. Using traditional techniques, therapists set up a hierarchy of anxiety-provoking situations, ranging from least threatening (e.g., the thought of kissing) to most threatening (the thought of penile penetration). The behavior therapist enables the patient to master the anxiety through a standard program of systematic desensitization, which is designed to inhibit the learned anxious response by encouraging behaviors antithetical to anxiety. The patient first deals with the least-anxiety-producing situation in fantasy and progresses by steps to the most-anxiety-producing situation. Medication, hypnosis, and special training in deep muscle relaxation are sometimes used to help with the initial mastery of anxiety.

Assertiveness training is helpful in teaching patients to express sexual needs openly and without fear. Exercises in assertiveness are given in conjunction with sex therapy; patients are encouraged to make sexual requests and to refuse to comply with requests perceived as unreasonable. Sexual exercises may be prescribed for patients to perform at home, and a hierarchy may be established, starting with those activities that have proved most pleasurable and successful in the past.

One treatment variation involves the participation of the patient's sexual partner in the desensitization program. The partner, rather than the therapist, presents items of increasing stimulation value to the patient. A cooperative partner is necessary to help the patient carry gains made during treatment sessions to sexual activity at home.

Group Therapy

Group therapy has been used to examine both intrapsychic and interpersonal problems in patients with sexual disorders. A therapy group provides a strong support system for a patient who feels ashamed, anxious, or guilty about a particular sexual problem. It is a useful forum in which to counteract sexual myths, correct misconceptions, and provide accurate information about sexual anatomy, physiology, and varieties of behavior.

Groups for the treatment of sexual disorders can be organized in several ways. Members may all share the same problem, such as premature ejaculation; members may all be of the same sex with different sexual problems; or groups may be composed of both men and women who are experiencing a variety of sexual problems. Group therapy can be an adjunct to other forms of therapy or the prime mode of treatment. Groups organized to treat a particular dysfunction are usually behavioral in approach.

Groups composed of married couples with sexual dysfunctions have also been effective. A group provides the opportunity to gather accurate information, offers consensual validation of individual preferences, and enhances self-esteem and self-acceptance. Techniques, such as role playing and psychodrama, may be used in treatment. Such groups are not indicated for couples when one partner is uncooperative, when a patient has a severe depressive disorder or psychosis, when a patient finds explicit sexual audiovisual material repugnant, or when a patient fears or dislikes groups.

Analytically Oriented Sex Therapy

One of the most effective treatment modalities is the use of sex therapy integrated with psychodynamic and psychoanalytically oriented psychotherapy. The sex therapy is conducted over a longer period than usual, which allows learning or relearning of sexual satisfaction under the realities of patients' day-to-day lives. The addition of psychodynamic conceptualizations to behavioral techniques used to treat sexual dysfunctions allows the treatment of patients with sexual disorders associated with other psychopathology.

The material and dynamics that emerge in patients in analytically oriented sex therapy are the same as those in psychoanalytic therapy, such as dreams, fear of punishment, aggressive feelings, difficulty trusting a partner, fear of intimacy, oedipal feelings, and fear of genital mutilation. The combined approach of analytically oriented sex therapy is used by the general psychiatrist who carefully judges the optimal timing of sex therapy and the ability of patients to tolerate the directive approach that focuses on their sexual difficulties.

Biological Treatments

Biological treatments, including pharmacotherapy, surgery, and mechanical devices, are used to treat specific cases of sexual disorder. Most of the recent advances involve male sexual dysfunction. Studies are underway to test biological treatment of sexual dysfunction in women.

Pharmacotherapy. The major new medications to treat sexual dysfunction are sildenafil (Viagra) and its congeners; oral phentolamine (Vasomax); alprostadil (Caverject), an injectable prostaglandin; and a transurethral alprostadil (MUSE), all used to treat erectile disorder.

Sildenafil is a nitric oxide enhancer that facilitates the inflow of blood to the penis necessary for an erection. The drug takes effect about 1 hour after ingestion, and its effect can last up to 4 hours. Sildenafil is not effective in the absence of sexual stimulation. The most common adverse events associated with its use are headaches, flushing, and dyspepsia. The use of sildenafil is contraindicated for persons taking organic nitrates. The concomitant action of the two drugs can result in large, sudden, and sometimes fatal drops in systemic blood pressure. Sildenafil is not effective in all cases of erectile dysfunction. It fails to produce an erection rigid enough for penetration in about 50 percent of men who have had radical prostate surgery or in those with long-standing insulin-dependent diabetes. It is also ineffective in certain cases of nerve damage.

A small number of patients developed nonarteritic ischemic optic neuropathy (NAION) soon after use of sildenafil. Six patients had vision loss within 24 hours after use of the agent. Both eyes were affected in one individual. All affected individuals had preexisting hypertension, diabetes, elevated cholesterol, or hyperlipidemia. Although very rare, sildenafil may provoke NAION in individuals with an arteriosclerotic risk profile.

Sildenafil use in women results in vaginal lubrication but not in increased desire. Anecdotal reports, however, describe individual women who have experienced intensified excitement with sildenafil.

Oral phentolamine and apomorphine are not U.S. Food and Drug Administration approved but have proved effective as potency enhancers in men with minimal erectile dysfunction. Phentolamine reduces sympathetic tone and relaxes corporeal smooth muscle. Adverse events include hypotension, tachycardia, and dizziness. Apomorphine effects are mediated by the autonomic nervous system and result in vasodilation that facilitates the inflow of blood to the penis. Adverse events include nausea and sweating.

In contrast to the oral medications, injectable and transurethral alprostadil act locally on the penis and can produce erections in the absence of sexual stimulation. Alprostadil contains a naturally occurring form of prostaglandin E, a vasodilating agent. Alprostadil may be administered by direct injection into the corpora cavernosa or by intraurethral insertion of a pellet through a cannula. The firm erection produced within 2 to 3 minutes after administration of the drug may last as long as 1 hour. Infrequent and reversible adverse effects of injections include penile bruising and changes in liver function test results. Possible hazardous sequelae exist, including priapism and sclerosis of the small veins of the penis. Users of transurethral alprostadil sometimes complain of burning sensations in the penis.

Two small trials found different topical agents effective in alleviating erectile dysfunction. One cream consists of three vasoactive substances known to be absorbed through the skin: aminophylline, isosorbide dinitrate, and co-dergocrine mesylate, which is a mixture of ergot alkaloids. The other is a gel containing alprostadil and an additional ingredient, which temporarily makes the outer layer of the skin more permeable.

A cream incorporating alprostadil also has been developed to treat female sexual arousal disorder. The initial results are promising. In addition, vaginally applied phentolamine mesylate, an α-receptor antagonist, significantly increased vasocongestion and a subjective sense of arousal in a trial of postmenopausal women with arousal problems who were already on hormonal therapy. A nasal inhalant, bremekinotide, set to enter phase 3 of clinical trials, affects the brain and has been shown to activate the same neural circuitry that is activated when a person feels desire. If approved, it will be offered as a stimulant of desire to both men and women.

The pharmacological treatments described here are useful in the treatment of arousal dysfunction of various causes: neurogenic, arterial insufficiency, venous leakage, psychogenic, and mixed. When coupled with insight-oriented or behavioral sex therapy, the use of medications can reverse psychogenic arousal disorder resistant to psychotherapy alone, the ultimate goal being pharmacologically unassisted sexual functioning.

Other Pharmacological Agents

Numerous other pharmacological agents have been used to heal the various sexual disorders. Intravenous methohexital sodium (Brevital) has been used in desensitization therapy. Antianxiety agents may have some application in tense patients, although these drugs can also interfere with the sexual response. The side effects of antidepressants, in particular the SSRIs and tricyclic drugs, have been used to prolong the sexual response in patients with premature ejaculation. This approach is particularly useful in patients refractory to behavioral techniques who may fall into the category of physiologically disposed premature ejaculators. The use of antidepressants has also been advocated in treatment for patients who are phobic of sex and in those with a posttraumatic stress disorder following rape. Trazodone is an antidepressant that improves nocturnal erections. The risks of taking such medications must be carefully weighed against their possible benefits. Bromocriptine (Parlodel) is used in the treatment of hyperprolactinemia, which is frequently associated with hypogonadism. In such patients, it is necessary to rule out pituitary tumors. Bromocriptine, a dopamine agonist, may improve sexual function impaired by hyperprolactinemia.

A number of substances have popular standing as aphrodisiacs; for example, ginseng root and yohimbine (Yocon). Studies, however, have not confirmed any aphrodisiac properties. Yohimbine, an α-receptor antagonist, may cause dilation of the penile artery; however the American Urologic Association does not recommend its use to treat organic erectile dysfunction. Many recreational drugs, including cocaine, amphetamines, alcohol, and cannabis, are considered enhancers of sexual performance. Although they may provide the user with an initial benefit because of their tranquilizing, disinhibiting, or mood-elevating effects, consistent or prolonged use of any of these substances impairs sexual functioning.

Dopaminergic agents have been reported to increase libido and improve sex function. Those drugs include L-dopa, a dopamine precursor, and bromocriptine, a dopamine agonist. The antidepressant bupropion has dopaminergic effects and has increased sex drive in some patients. Selegiline, an MAOI, is selective for MAO_B and is dopaminergic. It improves sexual functioning in older persons. Drugs to enhance arousal, including melanin-stimulating drugs and vasointestinal polypeptides. are in trial.

Hormone Therapy.   Androgens increase the sex drive in women and in men with low testosterone concentrations. Women may experience virilizing effects, some of which are irreversible (e.g., deepening of the voice). In men, prolonged use of androgens produces hypertension and prostatic enlargement. Testosterone is most effective when given parenterally; however, effective oral and transdermal preparations are available.

Women who use estrogens for replacement therapy or for contraception may report decreased libido; in such cases, a combined preparation of estrogen and testosterone has been used effectively. Estrogen itself prevents thinning of the vaginal mucous membrane and facilitates lubrication. Two new forms of estrogen, vaginal rings and vaginal tablets, provide alternate administration routes to treat women with arousal problems or genital atrophy. Because tablets and rings do not significantly increase circulating estrogen levels, these devices may be considered for patients with breast cancer with arousal problems.

Antiandrogens and Antiestrogens.   Estrogens and progesterone are antiandrogens that have been used to treat compulsive sexual behavior in men, usually in sex offenders. Clomiphene (Clomid) and tamoxifen (Nolvadex) are both antiestrogens, and both stimulate gonadotropin-releasing hormone secretion and increase testosterone concentrations, thereby increasing libido. Women being treated for breast cancer with tamoxifen report an increased libido. However, tamoxifen may cause uterine cancer.

Mechanical Treatment Approaches

In male patients with arteriosclerosis (especially of the distal aorta, known as Leriche's syndrome), the erection may be lost during active pelvic thrusting. The need for increased blood in the gluteal muscles and others served by the ilial or hypogastric arteries takes blood away (steals) from the pudendal artery and, thus, interferes with penile blood flow. Relief may be obtained by decreasing pelvic thrusting, which is also aided by the woman's superior coital position.

Vacuum Pump.   Vacuum pumps are mechanical devices that patients without vascular disease can use to obtain erections. The blood drawn into the penis following the creation of the vacuum is kept there by a ring placed around the base of the penis. This device has no adverse effects, but it is cumbersome, and partners must be willing to accept its use. Some women complain that the penis is redder and cooler than when erection is produced by natural circumstances, and they find the process and the result objectionable.

A similar device, called EROS, has been developed to create clitoral erections in women. EROS is a small suction cup that fits over the clitoral region and draws blood into the clitoris. Studies have reported its success in treating female sexual arousal disorder. Vibrators used to stimulate the clitoral area have been successful in treating anorgasmic women.

Surgical Treatment

Male Prostheses.   Surgical treatment is infrequently advocated, but penile prosthetic devices are available for men with inadequate erectile responses who are resistant to other treatment methods or who have medically caused deficiencies. The two main types of prostheses are (1) a semirigid rod prosthesis that produces a permanent erection that can be positioned close to the body for concealment and (2) an inflatable type that is implanted with its own reservoir and pump for inflation and deflation. The latter type is designed to mimic normal physiological functioning.

Vascular Surgery.   When vascular insufficiency is present due to atherosclerosis or other blockage, bypass surgery of penile arteries has been attempted in selected cases with some success.

Outcome

Demonstrating the effectiveness of traditional outpatient psychotherapy is just as difficult when therapy is oriented to sexual problems as it is in general. The more severe the psychopathology associated with a problem of long duration, the more adverse the outcome is likely to be. The results of different treatment methods have varied considerably since Masters and Johnson first reported positive results for their treatment approach in 1970. Masters and Johnson studied the failure rates of their patients (defined as the failure to initiate reversal of the basic symptom of the presenting dysfunction). They compared initial failure rates with 5-year follow-up findings for the same couples. Although some have criticized their definition of the percentage of presumed successes, other studies have confirmed the effectiveness of their approach.

The more difficult treatment cases involve couples with severe marital discord. Desire disorders are particularly difficult to treat. They require longer, more intensive therapy than some other disorders, and their outcomes vary greatly.

When behavioral approaches are used, empirical criteria that predict outcome are more easily isolated. Based on these criteria, for instance, couples who regularly practice assigned exercises appear to have a much greater likelihood of success than do more resistant couples or those whose interaction involves sadomasochistic or depressive features or mechanisms of blame and projection. Attitude flexibility is also a positive prognostic factor. Overall, younger couples tend to complete sex therapy more often than older couples. Couples whose interactional difficulties center on their sex problems, such as inhibition, frustration,

or fear of performance failure, are also likely to respond well to therapy.

Although most therapists prefer to treat a couple for sexual dysfunction, treatment of individual persons has also been successful. In general, methods that have proved effective singly or in combination include training in behavioral sexual skills, systematic desensitization, directive marital counseling, traditional psychodynamic approaches, group therapy, and pharmacotherapy.

▲ 17.3 Paraphilias and Sexual Disorder Not Otherwise Specified

PARAPHILIAS

Paraphilias or perversions are sexual stimuli or acts that are deviations from normal sexual behaviors but are necessary for some persons to experience arousal and orgasm. These individuals can experience sexual pleasure but are inhibited from responding to stimuli that are normally considered erotic. The paraphiliac's sexuality is restricted to specific deviant stimuli or acts. Persons that occasionally experiment with paraphiliac behavior (e.g., infrequent episode of bondage or dressing in costumes) but are capable of responding to more typical erotic stimuli are not diagnosed as suffering from paraphilias.

Paraphilias can range from nearly normal behavior to behavior that is destructive or hurtful only to a person's self or to a person's self and partner, and finally to behavior that is deemed destructive or threatening to the community at large. The text revision of the fourth edition of the *Diagnostic and Statistical Manual of Mental Disorders* (DSM-IV-TR) addresses these differences by designating impulses toward pedophilia, frotteurism, voyeurism, exhibitionism, and sexual sadism clinically significant if the person has acted on these fantasies or if these fantasies cause marked distress or interpersonal difficulty. The remaining paraphilias, such as transvestic fetishism, sexual masochism, or those not otherwise specified (e.g., zoophilia), meet the criteria for clinical significance only if they cause marked distress or impairment in social, occupational, or other important areas of functioning, even if the urges have been expressed behaviorally.

Epidemiology

Paraphilias are practiced by only a small percentage of the population, but the insistent, repetitive nature of the disorders results in a high frequency of such acts. Thus, a large proportion of the population has been victimized by persons with paraphilias. DSM-IV-TR suggests that the prevalence of paraphilias is significantly higher than the number of cases diagnosed in general clinical facilities, based on the large commercial market in paraphilic pornography and paraphernalia.

Among legally identified cases of paraphilias, pedophilia is most common. Of all children, 10 to 20 percent have been molested by age 18 years. Because a child is the object, the act is taken more seriously, and greater effort is spent tracking down the culprit than in other paraphilias. Persons with exhibitionism who publicly display themselves to young children are also commonly apprehended. Those with voyeurism may be apprehended, but their risk is not great. Of adult females, 20 percent have been the targets of persons with exhibitionism or voyeurism. Sexual masochism and sexual sadism are underrepresented in any prevalence estimates. Sexual sadism usually comes to attention only in sensational cases of rape, brutality, and lust murder. The excretory paraphilias are scarcely reported because activity usually takes place between consenting adults or between prostitute and client. Persons with fetishism rarely become entangled in the legal system. Those with transvestic fetishism may be arrested occasionally for disturbing the peace or on other misdemeanor charges if they are obviously men dressed in women's clothes, but arrest is more common among those with gender identity disorders. Zoophilia as a true paraphilia is rare.

As usually defined, the paraphilias seem to be largely male conditions. Fetishism almost always occurs in men. More than 50 percent of all paraphilias have their onset before age 18 years. Patients with paraphilia frequently have three to five paraphilias, either concurrently or at different times in their lives. This pattern of occurrence is especially the case with exhibitionism, fetishism, sexual masochism, sexual sadism, transvestic fetishism, voyeurism, and zoophilia. The occurrence of paraphiliac behavior peaks between ages 15 and 25 years and gradually declines; in men aged 50 years, criminal paraphiliac acts are rare. Those that occur are practiced in isolation or with a cooperative partner.

Etiology

Psychosocial Factors.   In the classic psychoanalytic model, persons with a paraphilia have failed to complete the normal developmental process toward heterosexual adjustment, but the model has been modified by new psychoanalytic approaches. What distinguishes one paraphilia from another is the method chosen by a person (usually male) to cope with the anxiety caused by the threat of castration by the father and separation from the mother. However bizarre its manifestation, the resulting behavior provides an outlet for the sexual and aggressive drives that would otherwise have been channeled into normal sexual behavior.

Failure to resolve the oedipal crisis by identifying with the father-aggressor (for boys) or mother-aggressor (for girls) results either in improper identification with the opposite-sex parent or in an improper choice of object for libido cathexis. Classic psychoanalytic theory holds that transsexualism and transvestic fetishism are disorders because each involves identification with the opposite-sex parent instead of the same-sex parent; for instance, a man dressing in women's clothes is believed to identify with his mother. Exhibitionism and voyeurism may be attempts to calm anxiety about castration because the reaction of the victim or the arousal of the voyeur reassures the paraphiliac that the penis is intact. Fetishism is an attempt to avoid anxiety by displacing libidinal impulses to inappropriate objects. A person with a shoe fetish unconsciously denies that women have lost their penises through castration by attaching libido to a phallic object, the shoe, which symbolizes the female penis. Persons with pedophilia and sexual sadism have a need to dominate and

control their victims to compensate for their feelings of powerlessness during the oedipal crisis. Some theorists believe that choosing a child as a love object is a narcissistic act. Persons with sexual masochism overcome their fear of injury and their sense of powerlessness by showing that they are impervious to harm. Another theory proposes that the masochist directs the aggression inherent in all paraphilias toward herself or himself. Although recent developments in psychoanalysis place more emphasis on treating defense mechanisms than on oedipal traumas, psychoanalytic therapy for patients with a paraphilia remains consistent with Sigmund Freud's theory.

Other theories attribute the development of a paraphilia to early experiences that condition or socialize children into committing a paraphiliac act. The first shared sexual experience can be important in that regard. Molestation as a child can predispose a person to accept continued abuse as an adult or, conversely, to become an abuser of others. In addition, early experiences of abuse that is not specifically sexual, such as spanking, enemas, or verbal humiliation, can be sexualized by a child and can form the basis for a paraphilia. Such experiences can result in the development of an *eroticized child*. The onset of paraphiliac acts can result from persons' modeling their behavior on the behavior of others who have carried out paraphiliac acts, mimicking sexual behavior depicted in the media, or recalling emotionally laden events from the past, such as their own molestation. Learning theory indicates that because the fantasizing of paraphiliac interests begins at an early age and because personal fantasies and thoughts are not shared with others (who could block or discourage them), the use and misuse of paraphiliac fantasies and urges continue uninhibited until late in life. Only then do persons begin to realize that such paraphiliac interests and urges are inconsistent with societal norms. By that time, however, the repetitive use of such fantasies has become ingrained, and the sexual thoughts and behaviors have become associated with, or conditioned to, paraphiliac fantasies.

Biological Factors.   Several studies have identified abnormal organic findings in persons with paraphilias. None has used random samples of such persons; instead, they have extensively investigated patients with paraphilia who were referred to large medical centers. Among these patients, those with positive organic findings included 74 percent with abnormal hormone levels, 27 percent with hard or soft neurological signs, 24 percent with chromosomal abnormalities, 9 percent with seizures, 9 percent with dyslexia, 4 percent with abnormal electroencephalograms, 4 percent with major mental disorders, and 4 percent with mental handicaps. The question is whether these abnormalities are causally related to paraphiliac interests or are incidental findings that bear no relevance to the development of paraphilia.

Psychophysiological tests have been developed to measure penile volumetric size in response to paraphiliac and nonparaphiliac stimuli. The procedures may be of use in diagnosis and treatment but are of questionable diagnostic validity because some men are able to suppress their erectile responses.

Diagnosis and Clinical Features

In DSM-IV-TR, the diagnostic criteria for paraphilias include the presence of a pathognomonic fantasy and an intense urge to

Table 17.3–1
DSM-IV-TR Diagnostic Criteria for Exhibitionism

A. Over a period of at least 6 months, recurrent, intense sexually arousing fantasies, sexual urges, or behaviors involving the exposure of one's genitals to an unsuspecting stranger.

B. The person has acted on these sexual urges, or the sexual urges or fantasies cause marked distress or interpersonal difficulty.

From American Psychiatric Association. *Diagnostic and Statistical Manual of Mental Disorders.* 4th ed. Text rev. Washington, DC: American Psychiatric Association; copyright 2000, with permission.

act out the fantasy or its behavior elaboration. The fantasy, which may distress a patient, contains unusual sexual material that is relatively fixed and shows only minor variations. Arousal and orgasm depend on the mental elaboration or the behavioral playing out of the fantasy. Sexual activity is ritualized or stereotyped and makes use of degraded, reduced, or dehumanized objects.

Exhibitionism.   Exhibitionism is the recurrent urge to expose the genitals to a stranger or to an unsuspecting person (Table 17.3–1). Sexual excitement occurs in anticipation of the exposure, and orgasm is brought about by masturbation during or after the event. In almost 100 percent of cases, those with exhibitionism are men exposing themselves to women. The dynamic of men with exhibitionism is to assert their masculinity by showing their penises and by watching the victims' reactions—fright, surprise, and disgust. In this situation, men unconsciously feel castrated and impotent. Wives of men with exhibitionism often substitute for the mothers to whom the men were excessively attached during childhood. In other related paraphilias, the central themes involve derivatives of looking or showing.

Fetishism.   In fetishism the sexual focus is on objects (e.g., shoes, gloves, pantyhose, and stockings) that are intimately associated with the human body (Table 17.3–2). The particular fetish is linked to someone closely involved with a patient during childhood and has a quality associated with this loved, needed, or even traumatizing person. Usually, the disorder begins by adolescence, although the fetish may have been established in childhood. Once established, the disorder tends to be chronic.

Sexual activity may be directed toward the fetish itself (e.g., masturbation with or into a shoe), or the fetish may be incorporated into

Table 17.3–2
DSM-IV-TR Diagnostic Criteria for Fetishism

A. Over a period of at least 6 months, recurrent, intense sexually arousing fantasies, sexual urges, or behaviors involving the use of nonliving objects (e.g., female undergarments).

B. The fantasies, sexual urges, or behaviors cause clinically significant distress or impairment in social, occupational, or other important areas of functioning.

C. The fetish objects are not limited to articles of female clothing used in cross-dressing (as in transvestic fetishism) or devices designed for the purpose of tactile genital stimulation (e.g., a vibrator).

From American Psychiatric Association. *Diagnostic and Statistical Manual of Mental Disorders.* 4th ed. Text rev. Washington, DC: American Psychiatric Association; copyright 2000, with permission.

sexual intercourse (e.g., the demand that high-heeled shoes be worn). The disorder is almost exclusively found in men. According to Freud, the fetish serves as a symbol of the phallus to persons with unconscious castration fears. Learning theorists believe that the object was associated with sexual stimulation at an early age.

A single, 32-year-old male freelance photographer presented with the chief complaint of "abnormal sex drive." The patient related that although he was somewhat sexually attracted by women, he was far more attracted by "their panties."

To the best of the patient's memory, sexual excitement began at about age 7, when he came upon a pornographic magazine and felt stimulated by pictures of partially nude women wearing "panties." His first ejaculation occurred at age 13 via masturbation to fantasies of women wearing panties. He masturbated into his older sister's panties, which he had stolen without her knowledge. Subsequently he stole panties from her friends and from other women he met socially. He found pretexts to "wander" into the bedrooms of women during social occasions, and would quickly rummage through their possessions until he found a pair of panties to his satisfaction. He later used these to masturbate into and then "saved them" in a "private cache." The pattern of masturbating into women's underwear had been his preferred method of achieving sexual excitement and orgasm from adolescence until the present consultation.

The patient first had sexual intercourse at age 18. Since then he had had intercourse on many occasions, and his preferred partner was a prostitute paid to wear panties, with the crotch area cut away, during the act. On less common occasions when sexual activity was attempted with a partner who did not wear panties, his sexual excitement was sometimes weak.

The patient felt uncomfortable dating "nice women" as he felt that friendliness might lead to sexual intimacy and that they would not understand his sexual needs. He avoided socializing with friends who might introduce him to such women. He recognized that his appearance, social style, and profession all resulted in his being perceived as a highly desirable bachelor. He felt anxious and depressed because his social life was limited by his sexual preference.

The patient sought consultation shortly after his mother's sudden and unexpected death. Despite the fact that he complained of loneliness, he admitted that the pleasure he experienced from his unusual sexual activity made him unsure about whether or not he wished to give it up. (Reprinted with permission from *DSM-IV-TR Casebook.*)

Frotteurism.   Frotteurism is usually characterized by a man's rubbing his penis against the buttocks or other body parts of a fully clothed woman to achieve orgasm (Table 17.3–3). At other times, he may use his hands to rub an unsuspecting victim. The acts usually occur in crowded places, particularly in subways and buses. Those with frotteurism are extremely passive and isolated, and frottage is often their only source of sexual gratification. The expression of aggression in this paraphilia is readily apparent.

Pedophilia.   Pedophilia involves recurrent intense sexual urges toward, or arousal by, children 13 years of age or younger, over a period of

Table 17.3–3
DSM-IV-TR Diagnostic Criteria for Frotteurism

A. Over a period of at least 6 months, recurrent, intense sexually arousing fantasies, sexual urges, or behaviors involving touching and rubbing against a nonconsenting person.
B. The person has acted on these sexual urges, or the sexual urges or fantasies cause marked distress or interpersonal difficulty.

From American Psychiatric Association. *Diagnostic and Statistical Manual of Mental Disorders.* 4th ed. Text rev. Washington, DC: American Psychiatric Association; copyright 2000, with permission.

at least 6 months. Persons with pedophilia are at least 16 years of age and at least 5 years older than the victims (Table 17.3–4). When a perpetrator is a late adolescent involved in an ongoing sexual relationship with a 12- or 13-year-old, the diagnosis is not warranted.

Most child molestations involve genital fondling or oral sex. Vaginal or anal penetration of children occurs infrequently, except in cases of incest. Although most child victims coming to public attention are girls, this finding appears to be a product of the referral process. Offenders report that when they touch a child, most (60 percent) of the victims are boys. This figure is in sharp contrast to the figure for nontouching victimization of children, such as window peeping and exhibitionism; 99 percent of all such cases are perpetrated against girls. Of those with pedophilia, 95 percent are heterosexual, and 50 percent have consumed alcohol to excess at the time of the incident. In addition to their pedophilia, a significant number of the perpetrators are concomitantly or have previously been involved in exhibitionism, voyeurism, or rape.

Incest is related to pedophilia by the frequent selection of an immature child as a sex object, the subtle or overt element of coercion, and occasionally the preferential nature of the adult–child liaison.

Table 17.3–4
DSM-IV-TR Diagnostic Criteria for Pedophilia

A. Over a period of at least 6 months, recurrent, intense sexually arousing fantasies, sexual urges, or behaviors involving sexual activity with a prepubescent child or children (generally age 13 years or younger).
B. The person has acted on these sexual urges, or the sexual urges or fantasies cause marked distress or interpersonal difficulty.
C. The person is at least age 16 years and at least 5 years older than the child or children in Criterion A.

Note: Do not include an individual in late adolescence involved in an ongoing sexual relationship with a 12- or 13-year-old.

Specify if:
 Sexually attracted to males
 Sexually attracted to females
 Sexually attracted to both

Specify if:
 Limited to incest

Specify type:
 Exclusive type (attracted only to children)
 Nonexclusive type

From American Psychiatric Association. *Diagnostic and Statistical Manual of Mental Disorders.* 4th ed. Text rev. Washington, DC: American Psychiatric Association; copyright 2000, with permission.

Dr. C, a single, 35-year-old child psychiatrist, had been arrested and convicted of fondling several neighborhood boys, ages 6 to 12. Friends and colleagues were shocked and dismayed, as he had been considered by all to be particularly caring and supportive of children. Not only had he chosen a profession involving their care, but he had been a Cub Scout leader for many years and also a member of the local Big Brothers.

Dr. C was from a stable family. His father, who had also been a physician, was described as a workaholic, spending little time with his three children. Dr. C never married and, when interviewed by a psychiatrist as part of his presentence investigation, admitted that he experienced little, if any, sexual attraction toward females, either adults or children. He also denied sexual attraction toward adult men. In presenting the history of his psychosexual development, he reported that he had become somewhat dismayed as a child when his boyfriends began expressing rudimentary awareness of an attraction toward girls. His "secret" at the time was that he was attracted more to other boys, eventually progressing to mutual masturbation with some of his boyfriends.

His first sexual experience was at age 6, when a 15-year-old male camp counselor performed fellatio on him several times over the course of the summer—an experience that he had always kept to himself. As he reached his teenage years, he began to suspect that he was homosexual. As he grew older, he was surprised to notice that the age range of males who attracted him sexually did not change, and he continued to have recurrent erotic urges and fantasies about boys between the ages of 6 and 12. Whenever he masturbated, he would fantasize about a boy in that age range, and on a couple of occasions over the years had felt himself to be in love with such a youngster.

Intellectually, Dr. C knew that others would disapprove of his many sexual involvements with young boys. He never believed, however, that he had caused any of these youngsters harm, feeling instead that they were simply sharing pleasurable feelings together. He yearned to be able to experience the same sort of feelings toward women, but he never was able to do so. He frequently prayed for help and that his actions would go undetected. He kept promising himself that he would stop, but he could not. He was so fearful of destroying his reputation, his friendships, and his career that he had never been able to bring himself to tell anyone about his problem. (Reprinted with permission from *DSM-IV-TR Casebook.*)

Sexual Masochism.   Masochism takes its name from the activities of Leopold von Sacher-Masoch, a 19th-century Austrian novelist whose characters derived sexual pleasure from being abused and dominated by women. According to DSM-IV-TR, persons with sexual masochism have a recurrent preoccupation with sexual urges and fantasies involving the act of being humiliated, beaten, bound, or otherwise made to suffer (Table 17.3–5). In some cases, persons can allow themselves to experience sexual feelings only when punishment for the feelings follows. Persons with sexual masochism may have had childhood experiences that convinced them that pain is a prerequisite for sexual pleasure. About 30 percent of those with sexual masochism also have sadistic fantasies. Moral masochism involves a need to suffer but is not accompanied by sexual fantasies.

Table 17.3–5
DSM-IV-TR Diagnostic Criteria for Sexual Masochism

A. Over a period of at least 6 months, recurrent, intense sexually arousing fantasies, sexual urges, or behaviors involving the act (real, not simulated) of being humiliated, beaten, bound, or otherwise made to suffer.
B. The fantasies, sexual urges, or behaviors cause clinically significant distress or impairment in social, occupational, or other important areas of functioning.

From American Psychiatric Association. *Diagnostic and Statistical Manual of Mental Disorders*. 4th ed. Text rev. Washington, DC: American Psychiatric Association; copyright 2000, with permission.

Table 17.3–6
DSM-IV-TR Diagnostic Criteria for Sexual Sadism

A. Over a period of at least 6 months, recurrent, intense sexually arousing fantasies, sexual urges, or behaviors involving acts (real, not simulated) in which the psychological or physical suffering (including humiliation) of the victim is sexually exciting to the person.
B. The person has acted on these sexual urges with a nonconsenting person, or the sexual urges or fantasies cause marked distress or interpersonal difficulty.

From American Psychiatric Association. *Diagnostic and Statistical Manual of Mental Disorders*. 4th ed. Text rev. Washington, DC: American Psychiatric Association; copyright 2000, with permission.

A 25-year-old female graduate student asked for a consultation because of depression and marital discord. The patient had been married for 5 years, during which time both she and her husband were in school. For the past 3 years, her academic performance had been consistently better than his, and she attributed their frequent, intense arguments to this. She noted that she experienced a feeling of sexual excitement when her husband screamed at her or hit her in rage. Sometimes she would taunt him until he had sexual intercourse with her in a brutal fashion, as if she were being raped. She experienced the brutality and sense of being punished as sexually exciting.

One year before the consultation, the patient had found herself often ending arguments by storming out of the house. On one such occasion she went to a "singles bar," picked up a man, and got him to slap her as part of their sexual activity. She found the "punishment" sexually exciting and subsequently fantasized about being beaten during masturbation to orgasm. The patient then discovered that she enjoyed receiving physical punishment at the hands of strange men more than any other type of sexual stimulus. In a setting in which she could be whipped or beaten, all aspects of sexual activity, including the quality of orgasms, were far in excess of anything she had previously experienced.

This sexual preference was not the reason for the consultation, however. She complained that she could not live without her husband, yet could not live with him. She had suicidal fantasies stemming from the fear that he would leave her.

She recognized that her sexual behavior was dangerous to herself and felt mildly ashamed of it. She was unaware of any possible reasons for its emergence and was not sure she wished treatment for "it," because it gave her so much pleasure. (Reprinted with permission from *DSM-IV-TR Casebook*.)

quis de Sade, an 18th-century French author and military officer who was repeatedly imprisoned for his violent sexual acts against women. Sexual sadism is related to rape, although rape is more aptly considered an expression of power. Some sadistic rapists, however, kill their victims after having sex (so-called lust murders). In many cases, these persons have underlying schizophrenia. John Money believes that lust murderers have dissociative identity disorder and perhaps a history of head trauma. He lists five contributory causes of sexual sadism: hereditary predisposition, hormonal malfunctioning, pathological relationships, a history of sexual abuse, and the presence of other mental disorders.

A controlling, narcissistic physician, raised alone by his widowed mother since age 2, has been preoccupied with spanking's erotic charge for him since age 6. Socially awkward during adolescence and his 20s, he married the first woman he dated and gradually introduced her to his secret arousal pattern of imagining himself spanking women. Although horrified, she episodically agreed to indulge him on an infrequent schedule to supplement their frequent ordinary sexual behavior. He ejaculated only when imagining spanking. Following her sixth episode of anxious, sullen depression in 20 years of marriage, her psychologist instructed her to tell him "No more." He fell into despair, was diagnosed with a major depressive disorder, and wrote a long letter to her about why he was entitled to spank her. He claimed to have had little idea that her participation in this humiliation was negatively affecting her mental health ("She even had orgasms sometimes after I spanked her!"). He became suicidal as a solution to the dilemma of choosing between his or her happiness and becoming conscious that what he was asking was abusive. He was shocked to discover that she had long considered suicide as a solution to her marital trap of loving an otherwise good husband and father who had an unexplained sick sexual need.

Sexual Sadism. The DSM-IV-TR diagnostic criteria for sexual sadism are presented in Table 17.3–6. The onset of the disorder is usually before the age of 18 years, and most persons with sexual sadism are male. According to psychoanalytic theory, sadism is a defense against fears of castration; persons with sexual sadism do to others what they fear will happen to them and derive pleasure from expressing their aggressive instincts. The disorder was named after the Mar-

Voyeurism. Voyeurism, also known as *scopophilia*, is the recurrent preoccupation with fantasies and acts that involve observing persons who are naked or engaged in grooming or sexual activity (Table 17.3–7). Masturbation to orgasm usually accompanies or follows the event. The first voyeuristic act usually occurs during childhood, and the paraphilia is most common in men. When persons with voyeurism are apprehended, the charge is usually loitering.

Table 17.3–7
DSM-IV-TR Diagnostic Criteria for Voyeurism

A. Over a period of at least 6 months, recurrent, intense sexually arousing fantasies, sexual urges, or behaviors involving the act of observing an unsuspecting person who is naked, in the process of disrobing, or engaging in sexual activity.
B. The person has acted on these sexual urges, or the sexual urges or fantasies cause marked distress or interpersonal difficulty.

From American Psychiatric Association. *Diagnostic and Statistical Manual of Mental Disorders.* 4th ed. Text rev. Washington, DC: American Psychiatric Association; copyright 2000, with permission.

One man, best described as polymorphous perverse, spent the early years of his marriage avoiding sex with his wife while sneaking glances of a woman across the courtyard dressing and undressing. This man, as with many other voyeurs, had a number of coexisting paraphilias; he preferred watching his spouse insert the tube of an enema bag into her vagina, so as to masturbate rather than having intercourse with her. He associated this preference to having once seen his mother naked in her bathroom, holding a douche bag or an enema bag. In his therapy sessions, he frequently closed his eyes. He eventually disclosed that, during such moments, he had flash fantasies in which he visualized women in a number of erotic poses. (Courtesy of Ethel Spector Person, M.D.)

Transvestic Fetishism.
Transvestic fetishism is described as fantasies and sexual urges to dress in opposite gender clothing as a means of arousal and as an adjunct to masturbation or coitus (Table 17.3–8). Transvestic fetishism typically begins in childhood or early adolescence. As years pass, some men with transvestic fetishism want to dress and live permanently as women. More rarely, women want to dress and live as men. These persons are classified in DSM-IV-TR as persons with transvestic fetishism and gender dysphoria. Usually, a person wears more than one article of opposite-sex clothing; frequently, an entire wardrobe is involved. When a man with transvestic fetishism is cross-dressed, the appearance of femininity may be striking, although not usually to the degree found in transsexualism. When not dressed in women's clothes, men with transvestic fetishism may be hypermasculine in appearance and occupation. Cross-dressing can be graded from solitary, depressed,

Table 17.3–8
DSM-IV-TR Diagnostic Criteria for Transvestic Fetishism

A. Over a period of at least 6 months, in a heterosexual male, recurrent, intense sexually arousing fantasies, sexual urges, or behaviors involving cross-dressing.
B. The fantasies, sexual urges, or behaviors cause clinically significant distress or impairment in social, occupational, or other important areas of functioning.

Specify if:
  With gender dysphoria: if the person has persistent discomfort with gender role or identity

From American Psychiatric Association. *Diagnostic and Statistical Manual of Mental Disorders.* 4th ed. Text rev. Washington, DC: American Psychiatric Association; copyright 2000, with permission.

Table 17.3–9
DSM-IV-TR Diagnostic Criteria for Paraphilia Not Otherwise Specified

This category is included for coding paraphilias that do not meet the criteria for any of the specific categories. Examples include, but are not limited to, telephone scatologia (obscene phone calls), necrophilia (corpses), partialism (exclusive focus on part of body), zoophilia (animals), coprophilia (feces), klismaphilia (enemas), and urophilia (urine).

From American Psychiatric Association. *Diagnostic and Statistical Manual of Mental Disorders.* 4th ed. Text rev. Washington, DC: American Psychiatric Association; copyright 2000, with permission.

guilt-ridden dressing to ego-syntonic, social membership in a transvestite subculture.

The overt clinical syndrome of transvestic fetishism may begin in latency, but is more often seen around pubescence or in adolescence. Frank dressing in opposite-sex clothing usually does not begin until mobility and relative independence from parents are well established.

Paraphilia Not Otherwise Specified.
The classification of paraphilia not otherwise specified includes various paraphilias that do not meet the criteria for any of the aforementioned categories (Table 17.3–9).

TELEPHONE AND COMPUTER SCATOLOGIA. Telephone scatologia is characterized by obscene phone calling and involves an unsuspecting partner. Tension and arousal begin in anticipation of phoning; the recipient of the call listens while the telephoner (usually male) verbally exposes his preoccupations or induces her to talk about her sexual activity. The conversation is accompanied by masturbation, which is often completed after the contact is interrupted.

Persons also use interactive computer networks, sometimes compulsively, to send obscene messages by electronic mail and to transmit sexually explicit messages and video images. Because of the anonymity of the users in chat rooms who use aliases, on-line or computer sex (cybersex) allows some persons to play the role of the opposite sex ("genderbending"), which represents an alternative method of expressing transvestic or transsexual fantasies. A danger of on-line cybersex is that pedophiles often make contact with children or adolescents who are lured into meeting them and are then molested. Many on-line contacts develop into off-line liaisons. Although some persons report that the off-line encounters develop into meaningful relationships, most such meetings are filled with disappointment and disillusionment as the fantasized person fails to meet unconscious expectations of perfection. In other situations, when adults meet, rape or even homicide may occur.

NECROPHILIA. Necrophilia is an obsession with obtaining sexual gratification from cadavers. Most persons with this disorder find corpses in morgues, but some have been known to rob graves or even to murder to satisfy their sexual urges. In the few cases studied, those with necrophilia believed that they were inflicting the greatest conceivable humiliation on their lifeless victims. According to Richard von Krafft-Ebing, the diagnosis of psychosis is, under all circumstances, justified.

PARTIALISM. Persons with the disorder of partialism concentrate their sexual activity on one part of the body to the exclusion of all others. Mouth–genital contact—such as cunnilingus (oral contact with a woman's external genitals), fellatio (oral contact with the penis), and anilingus (oral contact with the anus)—is normally associated with foreplay; Freud recognized the mucosal surfaces of the body as erotogenic and capable of producing pleasurable sensation. But when a person uses these activities as the sole source of sexual gratification and cannot have or refuses to have coitus, a paraphilia exists. It is also known as *oralism.*

ZOOPHILIA. In zoophilia, animals—which may be trained to participate—are preferentially incorporated into arousal fantasies or sexual activities, including intercourse, masturbation, and oral–genital contact. Zoophilia as an organized paraphilia is rare. For many persons, animals are the major source of relatedness, so it is not surprising that a broad variety of domestic animals are used sensually or sexually.

Sexual relations with animals may occasionally be an outgrowth of availability or convenience, especially in parts of the world where rigid convention precludes premarital sexuality and in situations of enforced isolation. Because masturbation is also available in such situations, however, a predilection for animal contact is probably present in opportunistic zoophilia.

COPROPHILIA AND KLISMAPHILIA. Coprophilia is sexual pleasure associated with the desire to defecate on a partner, to be defecated on, or to eat feces (coprophagia). A variant is the compulsive utterance of obscene words (coprolalia). These paraphilias are associated with fixation at the anal stage of psychosexual development. Similarly, klismaphilia, the use of enemas as part of sexual stimulation, is related to anal fixation.

UROPHILIA. Urophilia, a form of urethral eroticism, is interest in sexual pleasure associated with the desire to urinate on a partner or to be urinated on. In both men and women, the disorder may be associated with masturbatory techniques involving the insertion of foreign objects into the urethra for sexual stimulation.

HYPOXYPHILIA. Hypoxyphilia is the desire to achieve an altered state of consciousness secondary to hypoxia while experiencing orgasm. Persons may use a drug (e.g., a volatile nitrite or nitrous oxide) to produce hypoxia. Autoerotic asphyxiation is also associated with hypoxic states, but it should be classified as a form of sexual masochism. (A discussion of autoerotic asphyxiation appears in Section 17.2.)

Differential Diagnosis

Clinicians must differentiate a paraphilia from an experimental act that is not recurrent or compulsive and that is done for its novelty. Paraphiliac activity most likely begins during adolescence. Some paraphilias (especially the bizarre types) are associated with other mental disorders, such as schizophrenia. Brain diseases can also release perverse impulses.

Course and Prognosis

The difficulty in controlling or curing paraphilias rests in the fact that it is hard for people to give up sexual pleasure with no assurance that new routes to sexual gratification will be secured. A poor prognosis for paraphilias is associated with an early age of onset, a high frequency of acts, no guilt or shame about the act, and substance abuse. The course and the prognosis are better when patients have a history of coitus in addition to the paraphilia and when they are self-referred rather than referred by a legal agency.

Treatment

Five types of psychiatric interventions are used to treat persons with paraphilias: external control, reduction of sexual drives, treatment of comorbid conditions (e.g., depression or anxiety), cognitive-behavioral therapy, and dynamic psychotherapy.

Prison is an external control mechanism for sexual crimes that usually does not contain a treatment element. When victimization occurs in a family or work setting, the external control comes from informing supervisors, peers, or other adult family members of the problem and advising them about eliminating opportunities for the perpetrator to act on urges.

Drug therapy, including antipsychotic or antidepressant medication, is indicated for the treatment of schizophrenia or depressive disorders if the paraphilia is associated with these disorders. Antiandrogens, such as cyproterone acetate in Europe and medroxyprogesterone acetate (depo-Provera) in the United States, may reduce the drive to behave sexually by decreasing serum testosterone levels to subnormal concentrations. Serotonergic agents, such as fluoxetine (Prozac), have been used with limited success in some patients with paraphilia.

Cognitive-behavioral therapy is used to disrupt learned paraphiliac patterns and modify behavior to make it socially acceptable. The interventions include social skills training, sex education, cognitive restructuring (confronting and destroying the rationalizations used to support victimization of others), and development of victim empathy. Imaginal desensitization, relaxation technique, and learning what triggers the paraphiliac impulse so that such stimuli can be avoided are also taught. In modified aversive behavior rehearsal, perpetrators are videotaped acting out their paraphilia with a mannequin. Then the patient with paraphilia is confronted by a therapist and a group of other offenders who ask questions about feelings, thoughts, and motives associated with the act and repeatedly try to correct cognitive distortions and point out lack of victim empathy to the patient.

Insight-oriented psychotherapy is a long-standing treatment approach. Patients have the opportunity to understand their dynamics and the events that caused the paraphilia to develop. In particular, they become aware of the daily events that cause them to act on their impulses (e.g., a real or fantasized rejection). Treatment helps them deal with life stresses better and enhances their capacity to relate to a life partner. Psychotherapy also allows patients to regain self-esteem, which in turn allows them to approach a partner in a more normal sexual manner. Sex therapy is an appropriate adjunct to the treatment of patients who suffer from specific sexual dysfunctions when they attempt nondeviant sexual activities.

Good prognostic indicators include the presence of only one paraphilia, normal intelligence, the absence of substance abuse, the absence of nonsexual antisocial personality traits, and the presence of a successful adult attachment. Paraphilias, however, remain significant treatment challenges even under these circumstances.

SEXUAL DISORDER NOT OTHERWISE SPECIFIED

Many sexual disorders are not classifiable as sexual dysfunctions or as paraphilias. These unclassified disorders are rare, poorly documented, not easily classified, or not specifically described in DSM-IV-TR (Table 17.3–10). The 10th revision of the *International Statistical Classification of Diseases and Related Health Problems* has a similar residual category for problems related to sexual development or preference.

Postcoital Dysphoria

Not listed in DSM-IV-TR, postcoital dysphoria occurs during the resolution phase of sexual activity, when persons normally experience a sense of general well-being and muscular and psychological relaxation. Some

Table 17.3–10
DSM-IV-TR Diagnostic Criteria for Sexual Disorder Not Otherwise Specified

This category is included for coding a sexual disturbance that does not meet the criteria for any specific sexual disorder and is neither a sexual dysfunction nor a paraphilia. Examples include

1. Marked feelings of inadequacy concerning sexual performance or other traits related to self-imposed standards of masculinity or femininity
2. Distress about a pattern of repeated sexual relationships involving a succession of lovers who are experienced by the individual only as things to be used
3. Persistent and marked distress about sexual orientation

From American Psychiatric Association. *Diagnostic and Statistical Manual of Mental Disorders.* 4th ed. Text rev. Washington, DC: American Psychiatric Association; copyright 2000, with permission.

persons, however, undergo postcoital dysphoria at this time and, after an otherwise satisfactory sexual experience, become depressed, tense, anxious, and irritable and show psychomotor agitation. They often want to get away from their partners and may become verbally or even physically abusive. The incidence of the disorder is unknown, but it is more common in men than in women. The causes relate to the person's attitude toward sex in general and toward the partner in particular. The disorder may occur in adulterous sex and in contacts with prostitutes. The fear of acquired immune deficiency syndrome causes some persons to experience postcoital dysphoria. Treatment requires insight-oriented psychotherapy to help patients understand the unconscious antecedents to their behavior and attitudes.

Couple Problems

At times, a complaint arises from the spousal unit or the couple rather than from an individual dysfunction. For example, one partner may prefer morning sex, but the other partner may function more readily at night, or the partners may have unequal frequencies of desire.

Unconsummated Marriage

A couple involved in an unconsummated marriage have never had coitus and are typically uninformed and inhibited about sexuality. Their feelings of guilt, shame, or inadequacy are increased by their problem, and they experience conflict between their need to seek help and their need to conceal their difficulty. Couples may seek help for the problem after having been married several months or several years. William Masters and Virginia Johnson reported one unconsummated marriage of 17 years' duration.

Body Image Problems

Some persons are ashamed of their bodies and experience feelings of inadequacy related to self-imposed standards of masculinity or femininity. They may insist on sex only during total darkness, not allow certain body parts to be seen or touched, or seek unnecessary operative procedures to deal with their imagined inadequacies. Body dysmorphic disorder should be ruled out.

Sex Addiction and Compulsivity

The concept of sex addiction developed over the past two decades to refer to persons who compulsively seek out sexual experiences and whose behavior becomes impaired if they are unable to gratify their sexual impulses. The concept of sex addiction derived from the model of addiction to such drugs as heroin or addiction to behavioral patterns, such as gambling. Addiction implies psychological dependence, physical dependence, and the presence of a withdrawal syndrome if the substance (e.g., the drug) is unavailable or the behavior (e.g., gambling) is frustrated.

In DSM-IV-TR the term *sex addiction* is not used, nor is it a disorder that is universally recognized or accepted. Nevertheless, the phenomenon of a person whose entire life revolves around sex-seeking behavior and activities, who spends an excessive amount of time in such behavior, and who often tries to stop such behavior but is unable to do so is well known to clinicians. Such persons show repeated and increasingly frequent attempts to have a sexual experience, deprivation of which gives rise to symptoms of distress. Sex addiction is a useful concept heuristically, in that it can alert the clinician to seek an underlying cause for the manifest behavior.

Persistent and Marked Distress about Sexual Orientation

Distress about sexual orientation is characterized by dissatisfaction with sexual arousal patterns and it is usually applied to dissatisfaction with homosexual arousal patterns, a desire to increase heterosexual arousal, and strong negative feelings about being homosexual. Occasional statements to the effect that life would be easier if the speaker were not homosexual do not constitute persistent and marked distress about sexual orientation.

Treatment of sexual orientation distress is controversial. One study reported that with a minimum of 350 hours of psychoanalytic therapy, about one third of 100 bisexual and gay men achieved a heterosexual reorientation at a 5-year follow-up; this study has been challenged, however. Behavior therapy and avoidance conditioning techniques have also been used, but these techniques may change behavior only in the laboratory setting. Prognostic factors weighing in favor of heterosexual reorientation for men include being under 35 years of age, having some experience of heterosexual arousal, and feeling highly motivated to reorient.

Another and more prevalent style of intervention is directed at enabling persons with persistent and marked distress about sexual orientation to live comfortably with homosexuality without shame, guilt, anxiety, or depression. Gay counseling centers are engaged with patients in such treatment programs. Outcome studies of such centers have not been reported in detail.

Few data are available about the treatment of women with persistent and marked distress about sexual orientation, and these are primarily from single-case studies with variable outcomes. (Section 17.1 presents a further discussion of sexual orientation, homosexuality, and coming out.)

18 ▲

Gender Identity Disorders

Gender identity refers to the sense one has of being male or being female, which corresponds, normally, to the person's anatomical sex. The text revision of the fourth edition of the *Diagnostic and Statistical Manual of Mental Disorders* (DSM-IV-TR) defines *gender identity disorders* as a group whose common feature is a strong, persistent preference for living as a person of the other sex. The affective component of gender identity disorders is gender dysphoria—discontent with one's designated birth sex and a desire to have the body of the other sex and to be regarded socially as a person of the other sex. Gender identity disorder in adults was referred to in early versions of the DSM as *transsexualism*.

In DSM-IV-TR, no distinction is made for the overriding diagnostic term *gender identity disorder* as a function of age. In children, it can manifest as statements of wanting to be the other sex and as a broad range of sex-typed behaviors conventionally shown by children of the other sex. Gender identity crystallizes in most persons by age 2 or 3 years.

EPIDEMIOLOGY

Children

Most children with gender identity disorder are referred for clinical evaluation in early grade school years. Parents, however, typically report that the cross-gender behaviors were apparent before 3 years of age. Among a sample of boys younger than age 12 years referred for a range of clinical problems, the reported desire to be the opposite sex was 10 percent. For clinically referred girls younger than age 12 years, the reported desire to be the opposite sex was 5 percent.

The sex ratio of referred children is four to five boys for each girl.

Adults

The best estimate of gender identity disorder or transsexualism in adults comes from Europe, with a prevalence of 1 in 30,000 men and 1 in 100,000 women. Most clinical centers report a sex ratio of three to five male patients for each female patient. Many adults with gender identity disorder may well have qualified for gender identity disorder in childhood. Most adults with gender identity disorder report having felt different from other children of their same sex, although, in retrospect, many could not identify the source of that difference. Many report feeling extensively cross-gender identified from the earliest years, with the cross-gender identification becoming more profound in adolescence and young adulthood.

ETIOLOGY

Biological Factors

For mammals, the resting state of tissue is initially female; as the fetus develops, a male is produced only if androgen (coded for by a region of the Y chromosome, which is responsible for testicular development) is introduced. Without testes and androgen, female external genitalia develop. Thus, maleness and masculinity depend on fetal and perinatal androgens. The sexual behavior of animals lower on the evolutionary tree is governed by sex steroids, but this effect diminishes as one ascends the evolutionary tree. Sex steroids influence the expression of sexual behavior in mature men and women; that is, testosterone can increase libido and aggressiveness in women, and estrogen can decrease libido and aggressiveness in men. However, masculinity, femininity, and gender identity result more from postnatal life events than from prenatal hormonal organization.

The same principle of masculinization or feminization has been applied to the brain. Testosterone affects brain neurons that contribute to the masculinization of the brain in such areas as the hypothalamus. Whether testosterone contributes to so-called masculine or feminine behavioral patterns in gender identity disorders remains a controversial issue.

Psychosocial Factors

Children usually develop a gender identity consonant with their sex of rearing (also known as *assigned sex*). The formation of gender identity is influenced by the interaction of children's temperament and parents' qualities and attitudes. Culturally acceptable gender roles exist: Boys are not expected to be effeminate, and girls are not expected to be masculine. There are boys' games (e.g., cops and robbers) and girls' toys (e.g., dolls and dollhouses). These roles are learned, although some investigators believe that some boys are temperamentally delicate and sensitive and that some girls are aggressive and energized—traits that are stereotypically known in today's culture as feminine and masculine, respectively. However, greater tolerance for mild cross-gender activity in children has developed in the past few decades.

The quality of the mother–child relationship in the first years of life is paramount in establishing gender identity. During this period, mothers normally facilitate their children's awareness of, and pride in, their gender: Children are valued as little boys and girls, but devaluing, hostile mothering can result in gender problems. At the same time, the separation-individuation process is unfolding. When gender problems become associated with separation-individuation problems, the result can be the use of sexuality to remain in relationships characterized by shifts between a desperate infantile closeness and a hostile, devaluing distance.

Some children are given the message that they would be more valued if they adopted the gender identity of the opposite sex. Rejected or abused children may act on such a belief. Gender identity problems can also be triggered by a mother's death, extended absence, or depression, to which a young boy may react by totally identifying with her—that is, by becoming a mother to replace her.

The father's role is also important in the early years, and his presence normally helps the separation-individuation process. Without a father, mother and child may remain overly close. For a girl, the father is normally the prototype of future love objects; for a boy, the father is a model for male identification.

DIAGNOSIS AND CLINICAL FEATURES

Current diagnostic criteria for children and adults are organized under two main groupings: *cross-gender identification* and *discomfort with assigned gender role*. For children, this includes the intense desire to participate in the games and pastimes of the other sex and may include rejection of gender-conventional toys and games. The essential features, for all ages, are a persistent and intense distress about his or her assigned sex and a desire to be of the other sex. Table 18–1 lists the DSM-IV-TR criteria for the disorder.

Children

At the extreme of gender identity disorder in children are boys who, by the standards of their cultures, are as feminine as the most feminine of girls and girls who are as masculine as the most masculine of boys. No sharp line can be drawn on the continuum of gender identity disorder between children who should receive a formal diagnosis and those who should not. Girls with the disorder regularly have male companions and an avid interest in sports and rough-and-tumble play; they show no interest in dolls or playing house (unless they play the father or another male role). They may refuse to urinate in a sitting position, claim that they have or will grow a penis and do not want to grow breasts or to menstruate, and assert that they will grow up to become a man (not merely to play a man's role).

Boys with the disorder are usually preoccupied with stereotypically female activities. They may have a preference for dressing in girls' or women's clothes or may improvise such items from available material when the genuine articles are not available. (The cross-dressing typically does not cause sexual excitement, as in transvestic fetishism.) They often have a compelling desire to participate in the games and pastimes of girls. Female dolls are often their favorite toys, and girls are regularly their preferred playmates. When playing house, they take a girl's role. Their gestures and actions are often judged to be feminine, and they are usually subjected to male peer group teasing and rejection, a phenomenon that rarely occurs with boyish girls until adolescence. Boys with the disorder may assert that they will grow up to become a woman (not merely in role). They may claim that their penis or testes are disgusting or will disappear or that it would be better not to have a penis or testes. Some children refuse to attend school because of teasing or the pressure to

Table 18–1
DSM-IV-TR Diagnostic Criteria for Gender Identity Disorder

A. A strong and persistent cross-gender identification (not merely a desire for any perceived cultural advantages of being the other sex).
   In children, the disturbance is manifested by four (or more) of the following:
   (1) repeatedly stated desire to be, or insistence that he or she is, the other sex
   (2) in boys, preference for cross-dressing or simulating female attire; in girls, insistence on wearing only stereotypical masculine clothing
   (3) strong and persistent preferences for cross-sex roles in make-believe play or persistent fantasies of being the other sex
   (4) intense desire to participate in the stereotypical games and pastimes of the other sex
   (5) strong preference for playmates of the other sex
       In adolescents and adults, the disturbance is manifested by symptoms such as a stated desire to be the other sex, frequent passing as the other sex, desire to live or be treated as the other sex, or the conviction that he or she has the typical feelings and reactions of the other sex.

B. Persistent discomfort with his or her sex or sense of inappropriateness in the gender role of that sex.
   In children, the disturbance is manifested by any of the following: in boys, assertion that his penis or testes are disgusting or will disappear or assertion that it would be better not to have a penis, or aversion toward rough-and-tumble play and rejection of male stereotypical toys, games, and activities; in girls, rejection of urinating in a sitting position, assertion that she has or will grow a penis, or assertion that she does not want to grow breasts or menstruate, or marked aversion toward normative feminine clothing.
   In adolescents and adults, the disturbance is manifested by symptoms such as preoccupation with getting rid of primary and secondary sex characteristics (e.g., request for hormones, surgery, or other procedures to physically alter sexual characteristics to simulate the other sex) or belief that he or she was born the wrong sex.

C. The disturbance is not concurrent with a physical intersex condition.

D. The disturbance causes clinically significant distress or impairment in social, occupational, or other important areas of functioning.

Code based on current age:
   Gender identity disorder in children
   Gender identity disorder in adolescents or adults
Specify if (for sexually mature individuals):
   Sexually attracted to males
   Sexually attracted to females
   Sexually attracted to both
   Sexually attracted to neither

From American Psychiatric Association. *Diagnostic and Statistical Manual of Mental Disorders.* 4th ed. Text rev. Washington, DC: American Psychiatric Association; copyright 2000, with permission.

dress in attire stereotypical of their assigned sex. Most children deny being disturbed by the disorder, except that it brings them into conflict with the expectations of their families or peers.

The parents of a 7-year-old boy came for consultation because the boy had told his parents on several occasions that he would like to be a girl. From 2 to 3 years of age, he showed interest in dressing in his older sister's clothing. Initially, both parents thought that their son's interest in his sister's and, occasionally, his mother's clothes was cute. They were reassured of its transient nature by their family doctor. Preschool teachers told them that many boys dress up and that it was normal. When his parents kept the clothes from him, he would improvise with a towel for long hair and a large t-shirt for a dress. When playing mother–father games, he would be mother, and he imitated female characters from children's stories. Most of his playmates were girls. He played often with his sister's discarded dolls and did not like sports. At school, he was teased by age-mates, notably boys, for cross-gender activities. At consultation, the father was concerned that his son would grow up to be gay. Mother was less concerned with this potential but was more worried that he was becoming a loner and unhappy at school in consequence of peer stigma. (Adapted from a case of Richard Green, M.D.)

Differential Diagnosis of Children.

Children with a gender identity disorder must be distinguished from other gender-atypical children. For girls, tomboys without gender identity disorder prefer functional and gender-neutral clothing. By contrast, gender identity-disordered girls adamantly refuse to wear girls' clothes and reject gender-neutral clothes. They make repeated statements of being or wanting to be a boy and wanting to grow up to be a man, along with repeated cross-sex fantasy play, so that, in mother–father games or other games imitating characters from mass media, they are male. This accompanies a marked aversion to traditionally feminine activities.

For boys, the differential diagnosis must distinguish those who do not conform to traditional masculine sex-typed expectations but do not show extensive cross-gender identification and are not discontent with being male. It is not uncommon for boys to reject rough-and-tumble play or sports and to prefer nonathletic activities or occasionally to role play as a girl, to play with a doll, or to dress up in girl's or women's costumes. Such boys do not necessarily have a gender identity disorder. Boys who do have a gender identity disorder state a preference for being a girl and for growing up to become a woman, along with repeated cross-sex fantasy play, as in mother–father games, a strong preference for traditionally female-typed activities, cross-dressing, and a female peer group.

Because the diagnosis of gender identity disorder excludes children with anatomical intersex, a medical history needs to be taken with the focus on any suggestion of hermaphroditism in the child. With doubt, referral to a pediatric endocrinologist is indicated.

Adolescents and Adults

Similar signs and symptoms are seen in adolescents and adults. Adolescents and adults with the disorder manifest a stated desire to be the other sex; they frequently try to pass as a member of the other sex, and they desire to live or to be treated as the other sex. In addition, they find their genitals repugnant, and they desire to acquire the sex characteristics of the opposite sex. This desire may override all other wishes. They may believe that they were born the wrong sex and may make such characteristic statements as "I feel that I'm a woman trapped in a male body" or vice versa.

Adolescents and adults frequently request medical or surgical procedures to alter their physical appearance. Although the term transsexual is not used in DSM-IV-TR, many clinicians find the term useful and will probably continue to use it. In addition, transsexualism appears in the 10th revision of *International Statistical Classification of Diseases and Related Health Problems*, and such persons refer to themselves as transsexuals.

Most retrospective studies of transsexuals report gender identity problems during childhood, but prospective studies of children with gender identity disorders indicate that few become transsexuals and want to change their sex. The disorder is much more common in men (1 per 30,000) than in women (1 per 100,000).

Men take estrogen to create breasts and other feminine contours, have electrolysis to remove their male hair, and have surgery to remove the testes and the penis and to create an artificial vagina. Women bind their breasts or have a double mastectomy, a hysterectomy, and an oophorectomy; they take testosterone to build up muscle mass and deepen the voice and have surgery in which an artificial phallus is created. These procedures may make a person indistinguishable from members of the other sex.

A 27-year-old anatomical woman referred to a gender identity clinic reported having felt different as a child from other girls, although unable then to identify its source. As a young girl, she enjoyed playing sports with girls and boys, but generally preferred the companionship of boys. She preferred wearing unisex or boyish clothes and resisted wearing a skirt or dress. Everyone referred to her as a tomboy. She tried to hide her breast development by wearing loose-fitting tops and stooping forward. Menses were embarrassing and poignantly reminded her of her femaleness, which was becoming increasingly alienating. As sexual attractions evolved, they were exclusively directed to female partners. In her late teens, she had one sexual experience with a man, and it was aversive. She began socializing in lesbian circles, but did not feel comfortable there and did not consider herself a lesbian, but more a man. For sexual partners, she wanted heterosexual women and wanted to be considered by the partner as a man. As gender dysphoric feelings became increasingly pronounced, she consulted transsexual sites on the Internet and contacted a female-to-male transsexual community support group. She then set into motion the process of clinical referral. She transitioned to living as a man, had a name change, and was administered androgen injections. Voice deepened, facial and body hair grew, menses stopped, and sex drive increased, along with clitoral hypertrophy. After 2 years, the patient underwent bilateral mastectomy and is on the wait list for phalloplasty and hysterectomy-ovariectomy. Employment as a man continues, as does a 3-year relationship with a female partner. The partner has a child from a previous marriage. (Adapted from a case of Richard Green, M.D.)

Gender identity disorders can be associated with other diagnoses. Although some patients with gender identity disorder have a history of major psychosis, including schizophrenia or major affective disorder, most do not. When a diagnosis of gender identity disorder is made, as well as another DSM Axis I diagnosis, it is necessary to consider whether the diagnoses are distinct. A variety of Axis II personality disorders may be found in patients with gender identity disorder, particularly borderline personality, but none is specific. A proportion of nonhomosexual men with gender identity disorder report a history of erotic arousal in association with cross-dressing, and some would still qualify for a concurrent diagnosis of fetishistic transvestism. Some are more sexually aroused by imagining themselves with a female body or by seeing themselves cross-dressed in a mirror (autogynephilia) than by items of women's clothing per se.

COURSE AND PROGNOSIS

Children

Boys begin to have the disorder before the age of 4 years, and peer conflict develops during the early school years, at about the age of 7 or 8 years. Grossly feminine mannerisms may lessen as boys grow older, especially if attempts are made to discourage such behavior. Cross-dressing may be part of the disorder, and 75 percent of boys who cross-dress begin to do so before age 4 years. The age of onset is also early for girls, but most give up masculine behavior by adolescence.

In both sexes, homosexuality is likely to develop in one third to two thirds of all cases, although, for reasons that are unclear, fewer girls than boys have a homosexual orientation. Steven Levine reported that follow-up studies of gender-disturbed boys consistently indicated that homosexual orientation was the usual adolescent outcome.

Adults

Adult male patients who are gender dysphoric and sexually attracted to male partners may have a continuous development of gender dysphoria from childhood. Some manifestations of their gender dysphoria may be driven underground, however, in an effort, during their teens and, perhaps, early 20s, to merge with the larger community. They may also hope or think that their gender dysphoria will disappear. Sexual interest in male partners begins in early puberty, and some may consider themselves to be homosexual. They find, however, that they do not integrate effectively into the gay community. Approximately two thirds of adult men with gender identity disorder are sexually attracted to men only.

Gender identity disorders in men sexually attracted to female partners may be characterized as more-progressive disorders with insidious onset. The course is fairly continuous in some cases; in others, the intensity of symptoms fluctuates. Some experience a lifelong struggle with feminine identification that changes in intensity from time to time and may temporarily recede in the face of conflicting desires, such as those for marriage and family. In most cases, the first outward manifestation is cross-dressing in childhood—dressing in mother's or sister's clothing—and many patients report that they first began wishing to be female during that period. The extent of their cross-gender behavior in childhood does not usually warrant diagnosis of gender identity disorder, however.

Female patients may experience adolescence in which they initially consider themselves lesbian because of sexual attraction to female partners. They come to define themselves as distinct from lesbians, however, because they consider themselves to be men in their relationships with women. They insist that their partners treat them as men and that the partners are heterosexual women. Female patients are often, more often than male patients, in a romantic or sexual relationship at the time of initial clinical assessment.

In earlier clinical experience, it was the rare female-to-male transsexual who reported sexual attractions to male partners. This has changed. Some gender identity clinics report that approximately one tenth of patients born female have a sexual partner orientation to men and consider themselves to be gay men.

TREATMENT

Children

No convincing evidence indicates that psychiatric or psychological intervention for children with gender identity disorder affects the direction of subsequent sexual orientation. The treatment of gender identity disorder in children is directed largely at developing social skills and comfort in the sex role expected by birth anatomy. To the extent that treatment is successful, transsexual development may be interrupted. The low prevalence of transsexualism in the general population, however, even in the special population of cross-gender children, thwarts the testing of this assumption.

No hormonal or psychopharmacological treatments for gender identity disorder in childhood have been identified.

Adolescents

Adolescents whose gender identity disorder has persisted beyond puberty present unique treatment problems. One is how to manage the rapid emergence of unwanted secondary sex characteristics. Thus, a new area of treatment management has evolved with respect to slowing down or stopping pubertal changes expected by anatomical birth sex and then implementing cross-sex body changes with cross-sex hormones.

Young persons whose previous gender identity disorder has remitted may experience new conflicts should homosexual feelings emerge. This may be a source of anxiety in the adolescent and may cause conflict within the family. Teenagers should be reassured about the prevalence and nonpathological aspects of a same-sex partner preference. Parents must also be informed of the nonpathological nature of same-sex orientation. The goal of family intervention is to keep the family stable and to provide a supportive environment for the teenager.

Adults

Adult patients coming to a gender identity clinic usually present with straightforward requests for hormonal and surgical sex reassignment. No drug treatment has been shown to be effective in reducing cross-gender desires per se. When patient gender dysphoria is severe and intractable, sex reassignment may be the best solution.

Sex-Reassignment Surgery. Sex-reassignment surgery for a person born anatomically male consists principally in removal of the penis, scrotum, and testes, construction of labia, and vaginoplasty. Some clinicians attempt to construct a neoclitoris from the former frenulum of the penis. The neoclitoris may have erotic sensation. Postoperative complications include urethral strictures, rectovaginal fistulas, vaginal stenosis, and inadequate width or depth.

Some male patients who do not have adequate breast development from years of hormone treatment may elect augmentation mammoplasty. Some also have thyroid cartilage shaved to reduce the male-appearing thyroid cartilage. Patients need to undergo vocal retraining, and those who do not have a fully effective response may undergo a cricothyroid approximation procedure, which can raise vocal pitch. The results of these operations are variable.

Female-to-male patients typically may undergo bilateral mastectomy and construction of a neophallus. Because of increased technical skills in phalloplasty, more female-to-male patients are now electing these procedures.

Uncertainty and controversy exist with respect to the capacity for sexual arousal by the patient postsurgery. Some patients maintain that they are orgasmic. They describe the sensation of orgasm as more gradual and attenuated than their orgasms preoperatively. On the other hand, some patients report little sexual responsivity postsurgery. No adequate assessments have been made of the physiological functioning of postoperative male-to-female transsexuals with respect to the human sexual response cycle. Many patients, however, report satisfaction with being able to have vaginal intercourse with a male partner.

Hormonal Treatment

Persons born male are typically treated with daily doses of oral estrogen. This may be conjugated equine estrogens or ethinylestradiol or estrogen patches. These hormones produce breast enlargement, the amount being largely determined by genetic predisposition, which continues for approximately 2 years. Other major effects of estrogen treatment are testicular atrophy, decreased libido, and diminished erectile capacity. In addition, a decrease occurs in the density of body hair and, perhaps, an arrest of male pattern baldness. Side effects of endocrine treatment can be elevated levels of prolactin, blood lipids, fasting blood sugar, and hepatic enzymes. Patients should be monitored with appropriate blood tests. Smoking is a contraindication of endocrine treatment because it increases the risk of deep vein thrombosis and pulmonary embolism. There is no effect on voice. Facial hair removal is required by laser treatment or electrolysis.

Biological women are treated with monthly or three-weekly injections of testosterone. Because the effects of exogenous testosterone are more profound than those of estrogen, clinicians should be more cautious about commencing female patients on hormone treatment. The pitch of the voice drops permanently into the male range as the vocal cords thicken. The clitoris enlarges to two or three times its pretreatment length and is often accompanied by increased libido. Hair growth changes to the male pattern, and a full complement of facial hair may grow. Menses cease. Male pattern baldness may develop, and acne may be a complication.

Ethinylestradiol in male-to-female transsexuals increases regional fat depots and thigh muscle mass. Conversely, female-to-male transsexuals receiving testosterone may have increased thigh muscle and reduced subcutaneous fat deposition. Thus, cross-sex steroid hormones affect general body fat and muscle distribution, as well as promote breast development in patients born male.

GENDER IDENTITY DISORDER NOT OTHERWISE SPECIFIED

The diagnosis of gender identity disorder not otherwise specified is reserved for persons who cannot be classified as having a gender identity disorder with the characteristics described previously (Table 18–2). Three examples are listed in DSM-IV-TR: persons with intersex conditions and gender dysphoria; adults with transient, stress-related cross-dressing behavior; and persons who have a persistent preoccupation with castration or penectomy without a desire to acquire the sex characteristics of the other sex.

Intersex Conditions

Intersex conditions include a variety of syndromes in which persons have gross anatomical or physiological aspects of the opposite sex.

Congenital Virilizing Adrenal Hyperplasia.

Congenital virilizing adrenal hyperplasia was formerly called *the adrenogenital syndrome*. An enzymatic defect in the production of adrenal cortisol, beginning prenatally, leads to overproduction of adrenal androgens and virilization of the female fetus. Postnatally, excessive adrenal androgen can be controlled by steroid administration.

The androgenization can range from mild clitoral enlargement to external genitals that look like a normal scrotal sac, testes, and a penis, but hidden behind these external genitals are a vagina and a uterus. The patients are otherwise normally female. At birth, if the genitals look male, children are assigned to the male sex and so reared; the result is usually a clear sense of maleness and unremarkable masculinity. If the children are assigned to the female sex and so reared, a sense of femaleness and femininity usually results. If the parents are uncertain about the sex of their child, a hermaphroditic identity results. The resultant gender identity usually reflects the rearing practices, but androgens may help determine behavior. Children raised unequivocally as girls have a more intense tomboy quality than that found in a control group. The girls most often have a heterosexual orientation. Some of these children experience gender identity conflicts and do not feel comfortable in the sex of assignment. Higher rates of bisexual or homosexual behavior in adulthood have been reported.

Table 18–2
DSM-IV-TR Diagnostic Criteria for Gender Identity Disorder Not Otherwise Specified

This category is included for coding disorders in gender identity that are not classifiable as a specific gender identity disorder. Examples include
1. Intersex conditions (e.g., partial androgen insensitivity syndrome or congenital adrenal hyperplasia) and accompanying gender dysphoria
2. Transient, stress-related cross-dressing behavior
3. Persistent preoccupation with castration or penectomy without a desire to acquire the sex characteristics of the other sex

From American Psychiatric Association. *Diagnostic and Statistical Manual of Mental Disorders.* 4th ed. Text rev. Washington, DC: American Psychiatric Association; copyright 2000, with permission.

Androgen Insensitivity Syndrome.

Androgen insensitivity syndrome was formerly called *testicular feminization*. In these persons with the XY karyotype, tissue cells are unable to use testosterone or other androgens. Therefore, the person appears to be a normal female at birth and is raised as a girl. She is later found to have cryptorchid testes, which produce the testosterone to which the tissues do not respond, and minimal or absent internal sexual organs. Secondary sex characteristics at puberty are female because of the small, but sufficient, amount of estrogens, which results from the conversion of testosterone into estradiol. The patients usually sense themselves as females and are feminine. However, some experience gender conflicts and distress.

TURNER'S SYNDROME.

In Turner's syndrome, one sex chromosome is missing, such that the sex karyotype is simply X. Children have female genitalia, are short, and, possibly, have anomalies such as a shield-shaped chest and a webbed neck. As a consequence of dysfunctional ovaries, they require exogenous estrogen to develop female secondary sex characteristics. Gender identity is female.

KLINEFELTER'S SYNDROME.

An extra X chromosome is present in Klinefelter's syndrome, such that the karyotype is XXY. At birth, patients appear to be normal males. Excessive gynecomastia may occur in adolescence. Testes are small, usually without sperm production. Such persons are tall, and body habitus is eunuchoid. Reports suggest a higher rate of gender identity disorder.

5-α-Reductase Deficiency.

In 5-α-reductase deficiency, an enzymatic defect prevents the conversion of testosterone to dihydrotestosterone, which is required for prenatal virilization of the genitalia. At birth, the affected person appears to be female, although some anomaly is visible. In earlier generations, before childhood identification of the disorder was common, these persons, raised as girls, virilized at puberty and changed their gender identity to male. Later generations were expected to virilize and, thus, may have been raised with ambiguous gender. Recently, there are reports of a small number of patients for whom early removal of the testes and socialization as girls have resulted in a female gender identity.

Pseudohermaphroditism.

Infants born with ambiguous genitals are pseudohermaphrodites. True hermaphroditism is characterized by the presence of both testes and ovaries in the same person. It is a rare condition. Sex assignment based on the genitals' appearance at birth determines gender identity, which is male, female, or hermaphroditic, depending on the family's conviction about the child's sex. Recently, treatment has changed, postponing sex assignment based on the appearance of the genitalia at birth to adolescence, when the child is included in the decision-making process. Male pseudohermaphroditism is incomplete differentiation of the external genitalia even though a Y chromosome is present; testes are present but rudimentary. Female pseudohermaphroditism is the presence of virilized genitals in a person who is XX, the most common cause being the adrenogenital syndrome described previously.

Treatment.

Because intersex conditions are present at birth, treatment must be timely, and some physicians believe the conditions to be true medical emergencies. The appearance of the genitalia in diverse conditions is often ambiguous, and a decision must be made about the assigned sex (boy or girl) and how the child should be reared.

Problems should be addressed as early as possible, so that the entire family can regard the child in a consistent, relaxed manner. This is particularly important because intersex patients may have gender identity problems because of complicated biological influences and familial confusion about their actual sex. When intersex conditions are discovered, a panel of pediatric, urological, and psychiatric experts usually determines the sex of rearing on the basis of clinical examination, urological studies, buccal smears, chromosomal analyses, and assessment of the parental wishes.

Education of parents and presentation of the range of options open to them is essential because parents respond to the infant's genitalia in ways that promote the formation of gender identity. One option is for parents to decide against immediate surgery for ambiguous genitalia but assign the label of boy or girl to the infant on the basis of chromosomal and urological examination. They can then react to the child according to sex-role assignment with leeway to adjust the sex assignment should the child act definitively as a member of the sex opposite to the one designated.

If the parents decide on surgery to normalize genital appearance, it is generally undertaken before the age of 3 years. It is easier to assign a child to be female than to assign one to be male because male-to-female genital surgical procedures are far more advanced than female-to-male procedures. That is an insufficient reason, however, to assign a chromosomal male to be female.

Some groups oppose surgical interventions on principle. The Intersex Society of North America, one such group, proposes that change is cosmetic at best and at worst may interfere with later sexual functioning. Some advocate that the U.S. Congress pass laws prohibiting doctors from performing such surgery, especially because the infant cannot consent. The goal of treatment, however, is to have genitals concordant with chromosomal, biological, physiological, and other genetic antecedents, thus allowing the development of a person with healthy gender identity. If this cannot be determined with certainty, then treatment can and should wait.

Cross-Dressing

The DSM-IV-TR lists cross-dressing—dressing in clothes of the opposite sex—as a gender identity disorder if it is transient and related to stress. If the disorder is not stress related, persons who cross-dress are classified as having transvestic fetishism, which is described as a paraphilia in DSM-IV-TR (see Section 17.3 on Paraphilias). An essential feature of transvestic fetishism is that it produces sexual excitement. Stress-related cross-dressing may sometimes produce sexual excitement, but it also reduces a patient's tension and anxiety. Patients may harbor fantasies of cross-dressing but act them out only under stress. Male adult cross-dressers may have the fantasy that they are female, in whole or in part.

Cross-dressing is commonly known as *transvestism* and the cross-dresser as a *transvestite*. Cross-dressing phenomena range from the occasional solitary wearing of clothes of the other sex to extensive feminine identification in men and masculine identification in women, with involvement in a transvestic subculture. More than one article of clothing of the other sex is involved, and a person may dress entirely as a member of the opposite sex. The degree to which a cross-dressed person appears as a member of the other sex varies, depending on mannerisms, body habitus, and cross-dressing skill. When not cross-dressed, these persons usually appear as unremarkable members of their assigned sex. Cross-dressing can coexist with paraphilias, such as sexual sadism, sexual masochism, and pedophilia.

Cross-dressing differs from transsexualism in that the patients have no persistent preoccupation with getting rid of their primary and secondary sex characteristics and acquiring the sex characteristics of the other sex. Some persons with the disorder once had transvestic fetishism but no longer become sexually aroused by cross-dressing. Other persons with the disorder are homosexual men and women who cross-dress. The disorder is most common among female impersonators.

Treatment.   A combined approach, using psychotherapy and pharmacotherapy, is often useful in the treatment of cross-dressing. The stress factors that precipitate the behavior are identified in therapy. The goal is to help patients cope with the stressors appropriately and, if possible, eliminate them. Intrapsychic dynamics about attitudes toward men and women are examined, and unconscious conflicts are identified. Medication, such as antianxiety and antidepressant agents, is used to treat the symptoms. Because cross-dressing can occur impulsively, medications that reinforce impulse control may be helpful, such as fluoxetine (Prozac). Behavior therapy, aversive conditioning, and hypnosis are alternative methods that may be of use in selected patients.

Preoccupation with Castration

The category of preoccupation with castration, that is, removal of ovaries or testes, is reserved for men and women who have a persistent preoccupation with castration or penectomy without a desire to acquire the sex characteristics of the opposite sex. They are clearly uncomfortable with their assigned sex, and their lives are driven by the fantasy of what it would be like to be a different gender. They may be asexual and lack sexual interest in either men or women.

A 45-year-old married male was admitted to the hospital after amputating the glans of his penis with a carving knife. He claimed that he heard voices telling him to carry out the act. He had been diagnosed with schizophrenia at age 25 after an episode of paranoid ideation in which he felt that persons were going to harm him. Although married, he had had repeated homosexual encounters since adolescence. He was able to function in the community when taking antipsychotic medications, but at the time of the event, he had not taken medication for more than 1 year.

19 ▲

Eating Disorders

▲ 19.1 Anorexia Nervosa

The term *anorexia nervosa* is derived from the Greek term *anorexia* for "loss of appetite" and the Latin word *nervosa* implying nervous origin. Anorexia nervosa is a syndrome characterized by three essential criteria: (1) a self-induced starvation to a significant degree, (2) a relentless drive for thinness or a morbid fear of fatness, and (3) the presence of medical signs and symptoms resulting from starvation. Anorexia nervosa is often associated with disturbances of body image—the perception that one is distressingly large despite obvious thinness. In the text revision of the fourth edition of the *Diagnostic and Statistical Manual of Mental Disorders* (DSM-IV-TR), anorexia nervosa is characterized as a disorder in which persons refuse to maintain a minimally normal weight, intensely fear gaining weight, and significantly misinterpret their body and its shape. DSM-IV-TR also notes that the term anorexia is misleading because loss of appetite rarely occurs in the early stage of the disorder.

EPIDEMIOLOGY

Eating disorders of various kinds have been reported in up to 4 percent of adolescent and young adult students. Anorexia nervosa is much more prevalent in females than in males. The most common ages of onset of anorexia nervosa are the midteens, but up to 5 percent of anorectic patients have the onset of the disorder in their early 20s. According to DSM-IV-TR, the most common age of onset is between 14 and 18 years. Anorexia nervosa is estimated to occur in about 0.5 to 1 percent of adolescent girls. It occurs 10 to 20 times more often in females than in males. The prevalence of young women with some symptoms of anorexia nervosa who do not meet the diagnostic criteria is estimated to be close to 5 percent. Although the disorder was initially reported most often among those of higher socioeconomic status, recent epidemiological surveys do not show that distribution. It seems to be most frequent in developed countries, and it may be seen with greatest frequency among young women in professions that require thinness, such as modeling and ballet.

COMORBIDITY

Anorexia nervosa is associated with depression in 65 percent of cases, social phobia in 34 percent of cases, and obsessive-compulsive disorder in 26 percent of cases.

ETIOLOGY

Biological, social, and psychological factors are implicated in the causes of anorexia nervosa. Some evidence points to higher concordance rates in monozygotic twins than in dizygotic twins. Sisters of patients with anorexia nervosa are likely to be afflicted, but this association may reflect social influences more than genetic factors. Major mood disorders are more common in family members than in the general population. Neurochemically, diminished norepinephrine turnover and activity are suggested by reduced 3-methoxy-4-hydroxyphenylglycol (MHPG) levels in the urine and the cerebrospinal fluid (CSF) of some patients with anorexia nervosa. An inverse relation is seen between MHPG and depression in these patients; an increase in MHPG is associated with a decrease in depression.

Biological Factors

Endogenous opioids may contribute to the denial of hunger in patients with anorexia nervosa. Preliminary studies show dramatic weight gains in some patients given opiate antagonists. Starvation results in many biochemical changes, some of which are also present in depression, such as hypercortisolemia and nonsuppression by dexamethasone. Thyroid function is suppressed as well. These abnormalities are corrected by realimentation. Starvation produces amenorrhea, which reflects lowered hormonal levels (luteinizing, follicle-stimulating, and gonadotropin-releasing hormones). Some patients with anorexia nervosa, however, become amenorrheic before significant weight loss. Several computed tomographic studies reveal enlarged CSF spaces (enlarged sulci and ventricles) in anorectic patients during starvation, a finding that is reversed by weight gain. In one positron emission tomographic scan study, caudate nucleus metabolism was higher in the anorectic state than after realimentation.

Some authors have proposed a hypothalamic-pituitary axis (neuroendocrine) dysfunction. Some studies have shown evidence for dysfunction in serotonin, dopamine, and norepinephrine, three neurotransmitters involved in regulating eating behavior in the paraventricular nucleus of the hypothalamus. Other humoral factors that may be involved include corticotropin-releasing factor, neuropeptide Y, gonadotropin-releasing hormone, and thyroid-stimulating hormone.

Social Factors

Patients with anorexia nervosa find support for their practices in society's emphasis on thinness and exercise. No family constellations are specific to anorexia nervosa, but some evidence indicates that these patients have close but troubled relationships with their parents. Families of children who present with eating disorders, especially binge-eating or purging subtypes, may exhibit high levels of hostility, chaos, and isolation and low levels of nurturance and empathy. An adolescent with a severe eating disorder may tend to draw attention away from strained marital relationships.

Vocational and avocational interests interact with other vulnerability factors to increase the probability of developing eating disorders. In young women, participation in strict ballet schools increases the probability of developing anorexia nervosa at least sevenfold. In high school boys, wrestling is associated with a prevalence of full or partial eating-disordered syndromes during wrestling season of approximately 17 percent, with a minority developing an eating disorder and not improving spontaneously at the end of training.

A gay orientation in men is a proved predisposing factor, not because of sexual orientation or sexual behavior per se, but because norms for slimness, albeit muscular slimness, are very strong in the gay community, only slightly lower than for heterosexual women. In contrast, a lesbian orientation may be slightly protective because lesbian communities may be more tolerant of higher weights and a more normative natural distribution of body shapes than their heterosexual female counterparts.

Psychological and Psychodynamic Factors

Anorexia nervosa appears to be a reaction to the demand that adolescents behave more independently and increase their social and sexual functioning. Patients with the disorder substitute their preoccupations, which are similar to obsessions, with eating and weight gain for other, normal adolescent pursuits. These patients typically lack a sense of autonomy and selfhood. Many experience their bodies as somehow under the control of their parents, so that self-starvation may be an effort to gain validation as a unique and special person. Only through acts of extraordinary self-discipline can an anorectic patient develop a sense of autonomy and selfhood.

Psychoanalytic clinicians who treat patients with anorexia nervosa generally agree that these young patients have been unable to separate psychologically from their mothers. The body may be perceived as though it were inhabited by the introject of an intrusive and unempathic mother. Starvation may unconsciously mean arresting the growth of this intrusive internal object and thereby destroying it. Often, a projective identification process is involved in the interactions between the patient and the patient's family. Many anorectic patients feel that oral desires are greedy and unacceptable; therefore, these desires are projectively disavowed. Other theories have focused on fantasies of oral impregnation. Parents respond to the refusal to eat by becoming frantic about whether the patient is actually eating. The patient can then view the parents as the ones who have unacceptable desires and can projectively disavow them; that is, others may be voracious and ruled by desire, but not the patient.

DIAGNOSIS AND CLINICAL FEATURES

The onset of anorexia nervosa usually occurs between the ages of 10 and 30 years. It is present when (1) an individual voluntarily reduces and maintains an unhealthy degree of weight loss

**Table 19.1–1
DSM-IV-TR Diagnostic Criteria for
Anorexia Nervosa**

A. Refusal to maintain body weight at or above a minimally normal weight for age and height (e.g., weight loss leading to maintenance of body weight less than 85% of that expected; or failure to make expected weight gain during period of growth, leading to body weight less than 85% of that expected).

B. Intense fear of gaining weight or becoming fat, even though underweight.

C. Disturbance in the way in which one's body weight or shape is experienced, undue influence of body weight or shape on self-evaluation, or denial of the seriousness of the current low body weight.

D. In postmenarcheal females, amenorrhea, i.e., the absence of at least three consecutive menstrual cycles. (A woman is considered to have amenorrhea if her periods occur only following hormone, e.g., estrogen, administration.)

Specify type:
 Restricting type: during the current episode of anorexia nervosa, the person has not regularly engaged in binge-eating or purging behavior (i.e., self-induced vomiting or the misuse of laxatives, diuretics, or enemas)
 Binge-eating/purging type: during the current episode of anorexia nervosa, the person has regularly engaged in binge-eating or purging behavior (i.e., self-induced vomiting or the misuse of laxatives, diuretics, or enemas)

From American Psychiatric Association. *Diagnostic and Statistical Manual of Mental Disorders.* 4th ed. Text rev. Washington, DC: American Psychiatric Association; copyright 2000, with permission.

or fails to gain weight proportional to growth; (2) an individual experiences an intense fear of becoming fat, has a relentless drive for thinness despite obvious medical starvation, or both; (3) an individual experiences significant starvation-related medical symptomatology, often, but not exclusively, abnormal reproductive hormone functioning, but also hypothermia, bradycardia, orthostasis, and severely reduced body fat stores; and (4) the behaviors and psychopathology are present for at least 3 months. The DSM-IV-TR diagnostic criteria for anorexia nervosa are given in Table 19.1–1.

An intense fear of gaining weight and becoming obese is present in all patients with the disorder and undoubtedly contributes to their lack of interest in, and even resistance to, therapy. Most aberrant behavior directed toward losing weight occurs in secret. Patients with anorexia nervosa usually refuse to eat with their families or in public places. They lose weight by drastically reducing their total food intake, with a disproportionate decrease in high-carbohydrate and fatty foods.

As mentioned, the term *anorexia* is a misnomer because loss of appetite is usually rare until late in the disorder. Evidence that patients are constantly thinking about food is their passion for collecting recipes and for preparing elaborate meals for others. Some patients cannot continuously control their voluntary restriction of food intake and so have eating binges. These binges usually occur secretly and often at night and are frequently followed by self-induced vomiting. Patients abuse laxatives and even diuretics to lose weight, and ritualistic exercising and extensive cycling, walking, jogging, and running are common activities.

Patients with the disorder exhibit peculiar behavior about food. They hide food all over the house and frequently carry large quantities of candies in their pockets and purses. While eating meals, they try to dispose of food in their napkins or hide it in their pockets. They cut their meat into very small pieces and spend a great deal of time rearranging the pieces on their plates. If the patients are confronted with their peculiar behavior, they often deny that their behavior is unusual or flatly refuse to discuss it.

Obsessive-compulsive behavior, depression, and anxiety are other psychiatric symptoms of anorexia nervosa most frequently noted in the literature. Patients tend to be rigid and perfectionist, and somatic complaints, especially epigastric discomfort, are usual. Compulsive stealing, usually of candies and laxatives but occasionally of clothes and other items, is common.

Poor sexual adjustment is frequently described in patients with the disorder. Many adolescent patients with anorexia nervosa have delayed psychosocial sexual development; in adults, a markedly decreased interest in sex often accompanies onset of the disorder. An unusual minority of anorectic patients have a premorbid history of promiscuity, substance abuse, or both and during the disorder do not show a decreased interest in sex.

Patients usually come to medical attention when their weight loss becomes apparent. As the weight loss grows profound, physical signs such as hypothermia (as low as 35°C), dependent edema, bradycardia, hypotension, and lanugo (the appearance of neonatal-like hair) appear, and patients show a variety of metabolic changes. Some female patients with anorexia nervosa come to medical attention because of amenorrhea, which often appears before their weight loss is noticeable. Some patients induce vomiting or abuse purgatives and diuretics; such behavior causes concern about hypokalemic alkalosis. Impaired water diuresis may be noted.

Electrocardiographic (ECG) changes, such as T-wave flattening or inversion, ST-segment depression, and lengthening of the QT interval, have been noted in the emaciated stage of anorexia nervosa. ECG changes may also result from potassium loss, which can lead to death. Gastric dilation is a rare complication of anorexia nervosa. In some patients, aortography has shown a superior mesenteric artery syndrome.

Subtypes

Anorexia nervosa has been divided into two subtypes—the food-restricting category and the binge-eating or purging category. In the food-restricting category, present in approximately 50 percent of cases, food intake is highly restricted (usually with attempts to consume fewer than 300 to 500 calories per day and no fat grams), and the patient may be relentlessly and compulsively overactive, with overuse athletic injuries. In the binge-eating or purging subtype, patients alternate attempts at rigorous dieting with intermittent binge or purge episodes, with the binges, if present, being either subjective (more than the patient intended, or because of social pressure, but not enormous) or objective. Purging represents a secondary compensation for the unwanted calories, most often accomplished by self-induced vomiting, frequently by laxative abuse, less frequently by diuretics, and occasionally with emetics. Sometimes, repetitive purging occurs without prior binge eating, after ingesting only relatively few calories. Both may be socially isolated and have depressive disorder symptoms and diminished sexual interest. Overexercising and perfectionistic traits are common in both types.

Those who practice binge eating and purging share many features with persons who have bulimia nervosa without anorexia nervosa. Those who binge eat and purge tend to have families in which some members are obese, and they themselves have histories of heavier body weights before the disorder than do persons with the restricting type. Binge eating–purging persons are likely to be associated with substance abuse, impulse control disorders, and personality disorders. Persons with restricting anorexia nervosa often have obsessive-compulsive traits with respect to food and other matters. Some persons with anorexia nervosa may purge but not binge.

Persons with anorexia nervosa have high rates of comorbid major depressive disorders; major depressive disorder or dysthymic disorder has been reported in up to 50 percent of patients with anorexia nervosa. The suicide rate is higher in persons with the binge eating–purging type of anorexia nervosa than in those with the restricting type.

Patients with anorexia nervosa are often secretive, deny their symptoms, and resist treatment. In almost all cases, relatives or intimate acquaintances must confirm a patient's history. The mental status examination usually shows a patient who is alert and knowledgeable on the subject of nutrition and who is preoccupied with food and weight.

A patient must have a thorough general physical and neurological examination. If the patient is vomiting, a hypokalemic alkalosis may be present. Because most patients are dehydrated, serum electrolyte levels must be determined initially and periodically during hospitalization.

When Peggy was first evaluated for admission to an inpatient eating disorder program, she was a 20-year-old woman who had difficulty supporting her 5′3″ body with a weight of only 67 pounds. She had begun to lose weight 4 years earlier, initially dieting to lose an unwanted 6 pounds. Encouraged by compliments on her new body, she proceeded to lose 8 more pounds. Over the next 2 years she continued to lose weight, increased her physical activity until her weight reached a low of 64 pounds, and stopped menstruating. She was admitted to a medical unit, treated for peptic ulcer disease, and discharged, only to be admitted 3 months thereafter to the psychiatric unit of a general hospital. During that 8-week hospitalization, she went from 84 pounds to 100 pounds. She did well until she went off to college, where, with increased academic and social demands, she again began to diet until she weighed only 67 pounds. Her eating habits were ritualized: she cut food into very small pieces, moved them around on the plate, and ate very slowly. She resisted eating foods with high fat and carbohydrate content. She was troubled by the changes in her body, and became increasingly anxious as her figure developed. She was forced to drop out of school and to accept another hospitalization.

Peggy was motivated to comply with treatment, but her fears of gaining weight and becoming obese affected her progress. She was expected to gain a minimum of 2 pounds every week, and she was restricted to bed rest if she failed to gain sufficient weight. In psychotherapy Peggy was gradually guided to discuss her feelings and to actually look at herself in the mirror. She was initially instructed to look at one part of her body for a minimum of 10 seconds, and the time was progressively increased until she could look at her whole body without any anxiety. Her menses returned at a weight of 93 pounds. After 7 months of individual and family treatment, she was discharged at a weight of 100 pounds. Peggy returned to college, worked part time, and lived with her parents. (Reprinted with permission from the *DSM-IV Casebook*.)

PATHOLOGY AND LABORATORY EXAMINATION

A complete blood count often reveals leukopenia with a relative lymphocytosis in emaciated patients with anorexia nervosa. If binge eating and purging are present, serum electrolyte determination reveals hypokalemic alkalosis. Fasting serum glucose concentrations are often low during the emaciated phase, and serum salivary amylase concentrations are often elevated if the patient is vomiting. The ECG may show ST-segment and T-wave changes, which are usually secondary to electrolyte disturbances; emaciated patients have hypotension and bradycardia. Young girls may have a high serum cholesterol level. All of these values revert to normal with nutritional rehabilitation and cessation of purging behaviors. Endocrine changes that occur, such as amenorrhea, mild hypothyroidism, and hypersecretion of corticotrophin-releasing hormone, are caused by the underweight condition and revert to normal with weight gain.

DIFFERENTIAL DIAGNOSIS

The differential diagnosis of anorexia nervosa is complicated by patients' denial of the symptoms, the secrecy surrounding their bizarre eating rituals, and their resistance to seeking treatment. Thus, it may be difficult to identify the mechanism of weight loss and the patient's associated ruminative thoughts about distortions of body image.

Clinicians must ascertain that a patient does not have a medical illness that can account for the weight loss (e.g., a brain tumor or cancer). Weight loss, peculiar eating behaviors, and vomiting can occur in several mental disorders. Depressive disorders and anorexia nervosa have several features in common, such as depressed feelings, crying spells, sleep disturbance, obsessive ruminations, and occasional suicidal thoughts. The two disorders, however, have several distinguishing features. Generally, a patient with a depressive disorder has decreased appetite, whereas a patient with anorexia nervosa claims to have normal appetite and to feel hungry; only in the severe stages of anorexia nervosa do patients actually have decreased appetite. In contrast to depressive agitation, the hyperactivity seen in anorexia nervosa is planned and ritualistic. The preoccupation with recipes, the caloric content of foods, and the preparation of gourmet feasts is typical of patients with anorexia nervosa but is absent in patients with a depressive disorder. In depressive disorders, patients have no intense fear of obesity or disturbance of body image.

Weight fluctuations, vomiting, and peculiar food handling may occur in somatization disorder. On rare occasions, a patient fulfills the diagnostic criteria for both somatization disorder and anorexia nervosa; in such a case, both diagnoses should be made. Generally, the weight loss in somatization disorder is not as severe as that in anorexia nervosa, nor does a patient with somatization disorder express a morbid fear of becoming overweight, as is common in those with anorexia nervosa. Amenorrhea for 3 months or longer is unusual in somatization disorder.

In patients with schizophrenia, delusions about food are seldom concerned with caloric content. More likely, they believe the food to be poisoned. Patients with schizophrenia are rarely preoccupied with a fear of becoming obese and do not have the hyperactivity that is seen in patients with anorexia nervosa. Patients with schizophrenia have bizarre eating habits but not the entire syndrome of anorexia nervosa.

Anorexia nervosa must be differentiated from bulimia nervosa, a disorder in which episodic binge eating, followed by depressive moods, self-deprecating thoughts, and often self-induced vomiting, occurs while patients maintain their weight within a normal range. Patients with bulimia nervosa seldom lose 15 percent of their weight, but the two conditions frequently coexist.

Rare conditions of unknown etiology are seen in which hyperactivity of the vagus nerve causes changes in eating patterns that are associated with weight loss, sometimes of severe degree. In such cases bradycardia, hypotension, and other parasympathomimetic signs and symptoms are seen. Because the vagus nerve relates to the enteric nervous system, eating may be associated with gastric distress such as nausea or bloating. Patients do not generally lose their appetite. Treatment is symptomatic, and anticholinergic drugs can reverse hypotension and bradycardia, which may be life threatening.

COURSE AND PROGNOSIS

The course of anorexia nervosa varies greatly—spontaneous recovery without treatment, recovery after a variety of treatments, a fluctuating course of weight gains followed by relapses, and a gradually deteriorating course resulting in death caused by complications of starvation. A recent study reviewing subtypes of anorectic patients found that restricting-type anorectic patients seemed less likely to recover than those of the binge eating–purging type. The short-term response of patients to almost all hospital treatment programs is good. Those who have regained sufficient weight, however, often continue their preoccupation with food and body weight, have poor social relationships, and exhibit depression. In general, the prognosis is not good. Studies have shown a range of mortality rates from 5 to 18 percent.

Indicators of a favorable outcome are admission of hunger, lessening of denial and immaturity, and improved self-esteem. Such factors as childhood neuroticism, parental conflict, bulimia nervosa, vomiting, laxative abuse, and various behavioral manifestations (e.g., obsessive-compulsive, hysterical, depressive, psychosomatic, neurotic, and denial symptoms) have been related to poor outcome in some studies but not in others.

Ten-year outcome studies in the United States have shown that about one fourth of patients recover completely and another one half are markedly improved and functioning fairly well. The other one fourth includes an overall 7 percent mortality rate and those who are functioning poorly with a chronic underweight condition. Swedish and English studies over 20- and 30-year periods show a mortality rate of 18 percent. About half of patients with anorexia nervosa eventually have the symptoms of bulimia, usually within the first year after the onset of anorexia nervosa.

TREATMENT

In view of the complicated psychological and medical implications of anorexia nervosa, a comprehensive treatment plan, including hospitalization when necessary and both individual and family therapy, is recommended. Behavioral, interpersonal, and cognitive approaches and, in some cases, medication should be considered.

Hospitalization

The first consideration in the treatment of anorexia nervosa is to restore patients' nutritional state; dehydration, starvation, and electrolyte imbalances can seriously compromise health and, in some cases, lead to death. The decision to hospitalize a patient is based on the patient's medical condition and the amount of structure needed to ensure patient cooperation. In general, patients with anorexia nervosa who are 20 percent below the expected weight for their height are recommended for inpatient programs, and patients who are 30 percent below their expected weight require psychiatric hospitalization for 2 to 6 months.

Inpatient psychiatric programs for patients with anorexia nervosa generally use a combination of a behavioral management approach, individual psychotherapy, family education and therapy, and, in some cases, psychotropic medications. Successful treatment is promoted by the ability of staff members to maintain a firm yet supportive approach to patients, often through a combination of positive reinforcers (praise) and negative reinforcers (restriction of exercise and purging behavior). The program must have some flexibility for individualizing treatment to meet patients' needs and cognitive abilities. Patients must become willing participants for treatment to succeed in the long run.

Most patients are uninterested in psychiatric treatment and even resist it; they are brought to a doctor's office unwillingly by agonizing relatives or friends. The patients rarely accept the recommendation of hospitalization without arguing about and criticizing the proposed program. Emphasizing the benefits, such as relief of insomnia and depressive signs and symptoms, may help persuade the patients to admit themselves willingly to the hospital. Relatives' support and confidence in the physicians and treatment team are essential when firm recommendations must be carried out. Patients' families should be warned that the patients will resist admission and, for the several weeks of treatment, will make many dramatic pleas for the family's support to obtain release from the hospital program. Compulsory admission or commitment should be obtained only when the risk of death from the complications of malnutrition is likely. On rare occasions, patients prove that doctor's statements about the probable failure of outpatient treatment are wrong. Some patients may gain a specified amount of weight by the time of each outpatient visit, but such behavior is uncommon, and a period of inpatient care is usually necessary.

The following considerations apply to the general management of patients with anorexia nervosa during a hospitalized treatment program. Patients should be weighed daily, early in the morning after emptying the bladder. The daily fluid intake and urine output should be recorded. If vomiting is occurring, hospital staff members must monitor serum electrolyte levels regularly and watch for the development of hypokalemia. Because food is often regurgitated after meals, the staff may be able to control vomiting by making the bathroom inaccessible for at least 2 hours after meals or by having an attendant in the bathroom to prevent vomiting. Constipation in these patients is relieved when they begin to eat normally. Stool softeners may occasionally be given, but never laxatives. If diarrhea occurs, it usually means that patients are surreptitiously taking laxatives. Because of the rare complication of stomach dilation and the possibility of circulatory overload when patients immediately start eating an enormous number of calories, the hospital staff should give patients about 500 calories over the amount required to maintain their present weight (usually 1,500 to 2,000 calories a day). It is wise to give these calories in six equal feedings throughout the day, so that patients need not eat a large amount of food at one sitting. Giving patients a liquid food supplement such as Sustagen may be advisable because they may be less apprehensive about gaining weight slowly with the formula than by eating food. After patients are discharged from the hospital, clinicians usually find it necessary to continue outpatient supervision of the problems identified in the patients and their families.

Psychotherapy

Cognitive-Behavioral Therapy.

Cognitive and behavioral therapy principles can be applied in both inpatient and outpatient settings. Behavior therapy has been found effective for inducing weight gain; no large, controlled studies of cognitive therapy with behavior therapy in patients with anorexia nervosa have been reported. Monitoring is an essential component of cognitive-behavioral therapy. Patients are taught to monitor their food intake, their feelings and emotions, their binging and purging behaviors, and their problems in interpersonal relationships. Patients are taught cognitive restructuring to identify automatic thoughts and to challenge their core beliefs. Problem solving is a specific method whereby patients learn how to think through and devise strategies to cope with their food-related and interpersonal problems. Patients' vulnerability to rely on anorectic behavior as a means of coping can be addressed if they can learn to use these techniques effectively.

Dynamic Psychotherapy.

Dynamic expressive-supportive psychotherapy is sometimes used in the treatment of patients with anorexia nervosa, but their resistance may make the process difficult and painstaking. Because patients view their symptoms as constituting the core of their specialness, therapists must avoid excessive investment in trying to change their eating behavior. The opening phase of the psychotherapy process must be geared to building a therapeutic alliance. Patients may experience early interpretations as though someone else were telling them what they really feel and thereby minimizing and invalidating their own experiences. Therapists who empathize with patients' points of view and take an active interest in what their patients think and feel, however, convey to patients that their autonomy is respected. Above all, psychotherapists must be flexible, persistent, and durable in the face of patients' tendencies to defeat any efforts to help them.

Family Therapy.

A family analysis should be done for all patients with anorexia nervosa who are living with their families, as a basis for a clinical judgment on what type of family therapy or counseling is advisable. In some cases, family therapy is not possible; however, issues of family relationships can then be addressed in individual therapy. Sometimes, brief counseling sessions with immediate family members is the extent of family therapy required. In one controlled family therapy study in London, anorectic patients younger than the age of 18 years benefited from family therapy, whereas patients older than the age of 18 years did worse in family therapy than with the control therapy. No controlled studies have been reported on the combination of individual and family therapy; however, in practice, most clinicians provide individual therapy and some form of family counseling in managing patients with anorexia nervosa.

Pharmacotherapy

Pharmacological studies have not yet identified any medication that yields definitive improvement of the core symptoms of anorexia nervosa. Some reports support the use of cyproheptadine (Periactin), a drug with antihistaminic and antiserotonergic properties, for patients with the restricting type of anorexia nervosa. Amitriptyline (Elavil) has also been reported to have some benefit. Concern exists about the use of tricyclic drugs in low-weight, depressed patients with anorexia nervosa, who may be vulnerable to hypotension, cardiac arrhythmia, and dehydration. Once an adequate nutritional status has been attained, the risk of serious adverse effects from the tricyclic drugs may decrease; in some patients, the depression improves with weight gain and normalized nutritional status.

Other medications that have been tried by patients with anorexia nervosa with variable results include clomipramine, pimozide (Orap), and chlorpromazine (Thorazine). Trials of fluoxetine have resulted in some reports of weight gain, and serotonergic agents may yield positive responses in the future. In patients with anorexia nervosa and coexisting depressive disorders, the depressive condition should be treated.

▲ 19.2 Bulimia Nervosa and Eating Disorder Not Otherwise Specified

BULIMIA NERVOSA

In many ways, bulimia nervosa represents a failed attempt at anorexia nervosa; these patients share the goal of becoming very thin but are less able to sustain prolonged semistarvation or severe hunger as consistently as classic restricting anorexia nervosa patients. These eating binges provoke panic as individuals feel that their eating has been out of control. The unwanted binges lead to secondary attempts to avoid the feared weight gain by a variety of compensatory behaviors, such as purging or excessive exercise.

In the text revision of the fourth edition of the *Diagnostic and Statistical Manual of Mental Disorders* (DSM-IV-TR), bulimia nervosa is defined as binge eating combined with inappropriate ways of stopping weight gain. Social interruption or physical discomfort—that is, abdominal pain or nausea—terminates the binge eating, which is often followed by feelings of guilt, depression, or self-disgust. Unlike patients with anorexia nervosa, those with bulimia nervosa may maintain a normal body weight.

Epidemiology

Bulimia nervosa is more prevalent than anorexia nervosa. Estimates of bulimia nervosa range from 2 to 4 percent of young women. As with anorexia nervosa, bulimia nervosa is significantly more common in women than in men, but its onset is often later in adolescence than that of anorexia nervosa. According to DSM-IV-TR, the rate of occurrence in males is one tenth of that in females. The onset may even occur in early adulthood. Approximately 20 percent of college women experience transient bulimic symptoms at some point during their college years. Although bulimia nervosa is often present in normal-weight young women, they sometimes have a history of obesity. In industrialized countries, the prevalence is about 1 percent of the general population.

Etiology

Biological Factors.   Some investigators have attempted to associate cycles of binging and purging with various neurotransmitters. Because antidepressants often benefit patients with bulimia nervosa and because serotonin has been linked to satiety, serotonin and norepinephrine have been implicated. Because plasma endorphin levels are raised in some bulimia nervosa patients who vomit, the feeling of well-being after vomiting that some of these patients experience may be mediated by raised endorphin levels. According to DSM-IV-TR, increased frequency of bulimia nervosa is found in first-degree relatives of persons with the disorder.

Social Factors.   Patients with bulimia nervosa, as with those with anorexia nervosa, tend to be high achievers and to respond to societal pressures to be slender. As with anorexia nervosa patients, many patients with bulimia nervosa are depressed and have increased familial depression, but the families of patients with bulimia nervosa are generally less close and more conflictual than the families of those with anorexia nervosa. Patients with bulimia nervosa describe their parents as neglectful and rejecting.

Psychological Factors.   Patients with bulimia nervosa, as with those with anorexia nervosa, have difficulties with adolescent demands, but patients with bulimia nervosa are more outgoing, angry, and impulsive than those with anorexia nervosa. Alcohol dependence, shoplifting, and emotional lability (including suicide attempts) are associated with bulimia nervosa. These patients generally experience their uncontrolled eating as more ego-dystonic than do patients with anorexia nervosa and so seek help more readily.

Patients with bulimia nervosa lack superego control and the ego strength of their counterparts with anorexia nervosa. Their difficulties controlling their impulses are often manifested by substance dependence and self-destructive sexual relationships in addition to the binge eating and purging that characterize the disorder. Many patients with bulimia nervosa have histories of difficulties separating from caretakers, as manifested by the absence of transitional objects during their early childhood years. Some clinicians have observed that patients with bulimia nervosa use their own bodies as transitional objects. The struggle for separation from a maternal figure is played out in the ambivalence toward food; eating may represent a wish to fuse with the caretaker, and regurgitating may unconsciously express a wish for separation.

Diagnosis and Clinical Features

According to DSM-IV-TR, bulimia nervosa is present when (1) episodes of binge eating occur relatively frequently (twice a week or more) for at least 3 months; (2) compensatory behaviors are practiced after binge eating to prevent weight gain—primarily self-induced vomiting, laxative abuse, diuretics, or abuse of emetics (80 percent of cases), and, less commonly, severe dieting and strenuous exercise (20 percent of cases); (3) weight is not severely lowered as in anorexia nervosa; and (4) the patient has a morbid fear of fatness, a relentless drive for thinness, or both and a disproportionate amount of self-evaluation depends on body weight and shape (Table 19.2–1). When making a diagnosis of bulimia nervosa, clinicians should explore the possibility that the patient has experienced a brief or prolonged prior bout of anorexia nervosa, which is present in approximately half of those with bulimia nervosa. Binging usually precedes vomiting by about 1 year.

Vomiting is common and is usually induced by sticking a finger down the throat, although some patients are able to vomit at will. Vomiting decreases the abdominal pain and the feeling of being bloated and allows patients to continue eating without fear of gaining weight. Depression, sometimes called *postbinge anguish*, often follows the episode. During binges, patients eat food that is sweet, high in calories, and generally soft or smooth textured, such as cakes and pastry. Some patients prefer bulky foods without regard to taste. The food is eaten secretly and rapidly and is sometimes not even chewed.

Most patients with bulimia nervosa are within their normal weight range, but some may be underweight or overweight. These patients are concerned about their body image and their appearance, worry about how others see them, and are concerned about their sexual attractiveness. Most are sexually active, compared with anorexia nervosa patients, who are not interested in sex. Pica and struggles during meals are sometimes revealed in the histories of patients with bulimia nervosa.

Bulimia nervosa occurs in persons with high rates of mood disorders and impulse control disorders. Bulimia nervosa is also reported to occur in those at risk for substance-related disorders and a variety of personality disorders. Patients with bulimia nervosa also have increased rates of anxiety disorders, bipolar I disorder, and dissociative disorders and histories of sexual abuse.

Subtypes. Evidence indicates that bulimic persons who purge differ from binge eaters who do not purge in that the latter tend to have less body-image disturbance and less anxiety concerning eating. Those with bulimia nervosa who do not purge tend to be obese. Distinct physiological differences also exist between patients with bulimia who purge and those who do not. Because of all these differences, the diagnosis of bulimia nervosa is subtyped into a purging type, for those who regularly engage in self-induced vomiting or the use of laxatives or diuretics, and a nonpurging type, for those who use strict dieting, fasting, or vigorous exercise but do not regularly engage in purging.

Patients with the purging type of bulimia nervosa may be at risk for certain medical complications, such as hypokalemia from vomiting or laxative abuse and hypochloremic alkalosis. Those who vomit repeatedly are at risk for gastric and esophageal tears, although these complications are rare. Patients who purge may have a different course from that of patients who binge and then diet or exercise.

Pathology and Laboratory Examinations

Bulimia nervosa can result in electrolyte abnormalities and various degrees of starvation, although it may not be as obvious as in low-weight patients with anorexia nervosa. Thus, even normal-weight patients with bulimia nervosa should have laboratory studies of electrolytes and metabolism. In general, thyroid function remains intact in bulimia nervosa, but patients may show nonsuppression on the dexamethasone-suppression test. Dehydration and electrolyte disturbances are likely to occur in patients with bulimia nervosa who purge regularly. These patients commonly exhibit hypomagnesemia and hyperamylasemia. Although not a core diagnostic feature, many patients with bulimia nervosa have menstrual disturbances. Hypotension and bradycardia occur in some patients.

Differential Diagnosis

The diagnosis of bulimia nervosa cannot be made if the binge-eating and purging behaviors occur exclusively during episodes of anorexia nervosa. In such cases, the diagnosis is anorexia nervosa, binge eating–purging type.

Clinicians must ascertain that patients have no neurological disease, such as epileptic-equivalent seizures, central nervous system tumors, Klüver-Bucy syndrome, or Kleine-Levin syndrome. The pathological features manifested by Klüver-Bucy syndrome are visual agnosia, compulsive licking and biting, examination of objects by the mouth, inability to ignore any stimulus, placidity, altered sexual behavior (hypersexuality), and altered dietary habits, especially hyperphagia. The syndrome is

Table 19.2–1
DSM-IV-TR Diagnostic Criteria for Bulimia Nervosa

A. Recurrent episodes of binge eating. An episode of binge eating is characterized by both of the following:
  (1) eating, in a discrete period of time (e.g., within any 2-hour period), an amount of food that is definitely larger than most people would eat during a similar period of time and under similar circumstances
  (2) a sense of lack of control over eating during the episode (e.g., a feeling that one cannot stop eating or control what or how much one is eating)
B. Recurrent inappropriate compensatory behavior in order to prevent weight gain, such as self-induced vomiting; misuse of laxatives, diuretics, enemas, or other medications; fasting; or excessive exercise.
C. The binge eating and inappropriate compensatory behaviors both occur, on average, at least twice a week for 3 months.
D. Self-evaluation is unduly influenced by body shape and weight.
E. The disturbance does not occur exclusively during episodes of anorexia nervosa.
Specify type:
  Purging type: during the current episode of bulimia nervosa, the person has regularly engaged in self-induced vomiting or the misuse of laxatives, diuretics, or enemas
  Nonpurging type: during the current episode of bulimia nervosa, the person has used other inappropriate compensatory behaviors, such as fasting or excessive exercise, but has not regularly engaged in self-induced vomiting or the misuse of laxatives, diuretics, or enemas

From American Psychiatric Association. *Diagnostic and Statistical Manual of Mental Disorders.* 4th ed. Text rev. Washington, DC: American Psychiatric Association; copyright 2000, with permission.

exceedingly rare and is unlikely to cause a problem in differential diagnosis. Kleine-Levin syndrome consists of periodic hypersomnia lasting for 2 to 3 weeks and hyperphagia. As in bulimia nervosa, the onset is usually during adolescence, but the syndrome is more common in men than in women.

Patients with bulimia nervosa who have concurrent seasonal affective disorder and patterns of atypical depression (with overeating and oversleeping in low-light months) may manifest seasonal worsening of both bulimia nervosa and depressive features. In these cases, binges are typically much more severe during winter months. Bright-light therapy (10,000 lux for 30 minutes in the early morning at 18 to 22 inches from the eyes) may be a useful component of comprehensive treatment of an eating disorder with seasonal affective disorder.

Some patients with bulimia nervosa—perhaps 15 percent—have multiple comorbid impulsive behaviors, including substance abuse, and lack of ability to control themselves in such diverse areas as money management (resulting in impulse buying and compulsive shopping) and sexual relationships (often resulting in brief, passionate attachments and promiscuity). They exhibit self-mutilation, chaotic emotions, and chaotic sleeping patterns. They often meet criteria for borderline personality disorder and other mixed personality disorders and, not infrequently, bipolar II disorder.

Course and Prognosis

Bulimia nervosa is characterized by higher rates of partial and full recovery compared with anorexia nervosa. As noted in the treatment section, those treated fare much better than those untreated. Untreated patients tend to remain chronic or may show small but generally unimpressive degrees of improvement with time. In a 10-year follow-up study of patients who had previously participated in treatment programs, the number of women who continued to meet full criteria for bulimia nervosa declined as the duration of follow-up increased. Approximately 30 percent continued to engage in recurrent binge-eating or purging behaviors. A history of substance use problems and a longer duration of the disorder at presentation predicted worse outcome. Depending on definitions, 38 to 47 percent of women were fully recovered at follow-up.

Treatment

Most patients with uncomplicated bulimia nervosa do not require hospitalization. In general, patients with bulimia nervosa are not as secretive about their symptoms as patients with anorexia nervosa. Therefore, outpatient treatment is usually not difficult, but psychotherapy is frequently stormy and may be prolonged. Some obese patients with bulimia nervosa who have had prolonged psychotherapy do surprisingly well. In some cases—when eating binges are out of control, outpatient treatment does not work, or a patient exhibits such additional psychiatric symptoms as suicidality and substance abuse—hospitalization may become necessary. In addition, electrolyte and metabolic disturbances resulting from severe purging may necessitate hospitalization.

Psychotherapy

COGNITIVE-BEHAVIORAL THERAPY. Cognitive-behavioral therapy (CBT) should be considered the benchmark, first-line treatment for bulimia nervosa. The data supporting the efficacy of CBT are based on strict adherence to rigorously implemented, highly detailed, manual-guided treatments that include about 18 to 20 sessions over 5 to 6 months. CBT implements a number of cognitive and behavioral procedures to (1) interrupt the self-maintaining behavioral cycle of bingeing and dieting and (2) alter the individual's dysfunctional cognitions; beliefs about food, weight, body image; and overall self-concept.

DYNAMIC PSYCHOTHERAPY. Psychodynamic treatment of patients with bulimia nervosa has revealed a tendency to concretize introjective and projective defense mechanisms. In a manner analogous to splitting, patients divide food into two categories: items that are nutritious and those that are unhealthy. Food that is designated nutritious may be ingested and retained because it unconsciously symbolizes good introjects. But junk food is unconsciously associated with bad introjects and, therefore, is expelled by vomiting, with the unconscious fantasy that all destructiveness, hate, and badness are being evacuated. Patients can temporarily feel good after vomiting because of the fantasized evacuation, but the associated feeling of "being all good" is short lived because it is based on an unstable combination of splitting and projection.

PHARMACOTHERAPY. Antidepressant medications have been shown to be helpful in treating bulimia. This includes the selective serotonin reuptake inhibitors, such as fluoxetine. This may be based on elevating central 5-hydroxytryptamine levels. Antidepressant medications can reduce binge eating and purging independent of the presence of a mood disorder. Thus, antidepressants have been used successfully for particularly difficult binge–purge cycles that do not respond to psychotherapy alone. Imipramine (Tofranil), desipramine (Norpramin), trazodone (Desyrel), and monoamine oxidase inhibitors have been helpful. In general, most of the antidepressants have been

Table 19.2–2
DSM-IV-TR Diagnostic Criteria for Eating Disorder Not Otherwise Specified

The eating disorder not otherwise specified category is for disorders of eating that do not meet the criteria for any specific eating disorder. Examples include

1. For females, all of the criteria for anorexia nervosa are met except that the individual has regular menses.
2. All of the criteria for anorexia nervosa are met except that, despite significant weight loss, the individual's current weight is in the normal range.
3. All of the criteria for bulimia nervosa are met except that the binge eating and inappropriate compensatory mechanisms occur at a frequency of less than twice a week or for a duration of less than 3 months.
4. The regular use of inappropriate compensatory behavior by an individual of normal body weight after eating small amounts of food (e.g., self-induced vomiting after the consumption of two cookies).
5. Repeatedly chewing and spitting out, but not swallowing, large amounts of food.
6. Binge-eating disorder: recurrent episodes of binge eating in the absence of the regular use of inappropriate compensatory behaviors characteristic of bulimia nervosa.

From American Psychiatric Association. *Diagnostic and Statistical Manual of Mental Disorders.* 4th ed. Text rev. Washington, DC: American Psychiatric Association; copyright 2000, with permission.

effective at doses usually given in the treatment of depressive disorders. Doses of fluoxetine that are effective in decreasing binge eating, however, may be higher (60 to 80 mg a day) than those used for depressive disorders. Medication is helpful in patients with comorbid depressive disorders and bulimia nervosa. Carbamazepine (Tegretol) and lithium (Eskalith) have not shown impressive results as treatments for binge eating, but they have been used in the treatment of patients with bulimia nervosa with comorbid mood disorders, such as bipolar I disorder. Evidence indicates that the use of antidepressants alone results in a 22 percent rate of abstinence from bingeing and purging; other studies show that CBT and medication is the most effective combination.

EATING DISORDER NOT OTHERWISE SPECIFIED

The DSM-IV-TR diagnostic classification eating disorder not otherwise specified is a residual category used for eating disorders that do not meet the criteria for a specific eating disorder (Table 19.2–2). Binge-eating disorder—that is, recurrent episodes of binge eating in the absence of the inappropriate compensatory behaviors characteristic of bulimia nervosa (Table 19.2–3)—falls into this category. Such patients are not fixated on body shape and weight.

Table 19.2–3
DSM-IV-TR Research Criteria for Binge-Eating Disorder

A. Recurrent episodes of binge eating. An episode of binge eating is characterized by both of the following:
  (1) eating, in a discrete period of time (e.g., within any 2-hour period), an amount of food that is definitely larger than what most people would eat in a similar period of time under similar circumstances
  (2) a sense of lack of control over eating during the episode (e.g., a feeling that one cannot stop eating or control what or how much one is eating)
B. The binge-eating episodes are associated with three (or more) of the following:
  (1) eating much more rapidly than normal
  (2) eating until feeling uncomfortably full
  (3) eating large amounts of food when not feeling physically hungry
  (4) eating alone because of being embarrassed by how much one is eating
  (5) feeling disgusted with oneself, depressed, or very guilty after overeating
C. Marked distress regarding binge eating is present.
D. The binge eating occurs, on average, at least 2 days a week for 6 months.
  Note: The method of determining frequency differs from that used for bulimia nervosa; future research should address whether the preferred method of setting a frequency threshold is counting the number of days on which binges occur or counting the number of episodes of binge eating.
E. The binge eating is not associated with the regular use of inappropriate compensatory behaviors (e.g., purging, fasting, excessive exercise) and does not occur exclusively during the course of anorexia nervosa or bulimia nervosa.

From American Psychiatric Association. *Diagnostic and Statistical Manual of Mental Disorders.* 4th ed. Text rev. Washington, DC: American Psychiatric Association; copyright 2000, with permission.

▲ 19.3 Obesity

Obesity is a complex syndrome resulting from a combination of genetic susceptibility, increased availability of high-energy foods, and decreased requirement for physical activity in modern society. The prevalence of obesity has reached epidemic proportions in industrialized countries and is now considered the leading cause of preventable death in the United States. Because it is associated with significant increases in morbidity and mortality, the health care costs directly attributable to obesity also have dramatically increased over the past few decades.

Obesity refers to an excess of body fat. In healthy individuals, body fat accounts for approximately 25 percent of body weight in women and 18 percent in men. Overweight refers to weight above some reference norm, typically standards derived from actuarial or epidemiological data. In most cases, increasing weight reflects increasing obesity, but not always. Muscular individuals might be overweight (weight might be high for height) but not obese, and a person might have normal weight but have high body fat.

Indexes have been developed using height and weight to estimate level of obesity. The most common of these is the body mass index (BMI). BMI is calculated by dividing weight in kilograms by height in meters squared. Although there is debate about the ideal BMI, it is generally thought that a BMI of 20 to 25 kg/m^2 represents healthy weight, a BMI of 25 to 27 kg/m^2 is associated with somewhat elevated risk, a BMI above 27 kg/m^2 represents clearly increased risk, and a BMI above 30 kg/m^2 carries greatly increased risk.

EPIDEMIOLOGY

Obesity rates continue to grow at epidemic proportions in the United States and other industrialized nations, representing a serious public health threat to millions of people. In the United States, 34 percent of the population is overweight (defined as a BMI of 25.0 to 29.9 kg/m^2), whereas 30 percent is obese (defined as a BMI >30 kg/m^2). Obesity (BMI >30 kg/m^2) among adults increased from 30 percent in 2000 to 32.2 percent in 2004. Extreme obesity (BMI $\geq$40 kg/m^2) also increased significantly during the same time period and now is 2.8 percent in men and 6.9 percent in women.

The prevalence of obesity is highest in minority populations, particularly among non-Hispanic black women. More than one half of these individuals 40 years of age or older are obese and more than 80 percent are overweight. The prevalence of overweight and obesity in children and adolescents in the United States has also increased substantially, from about 15 percent in 2000 to about 18 percent in 2004. About 10 percent of 2- to 5-year-olds are overweight.

ETIOLOGY

Persons accumulate fat by eating more calories than are expended as energy; thus, intake of energy exceeds its dissipation. If fat is to be removed from the body, fewer calories must be put in or more calories must be taken out than are put in. An error of no more than 10 percent in either intake or output would lead to a 30-pound change in body weight in 1 year.

Satiety

Satiety is the feeling that results when hunger is satisfied. Persons stop eating at the end of a meal because they have replenished nutrients that had been depleted. Persons become hungry again when nutrients restored by earlier meals are once again depleted. It seems reasonable that a metabolic signal derived from food that has been absorbed is carried by the blood to the brain, where the signal activates receptor cells, probably in the hypothalamus, to produce satiety. Some studies have shown evidence for dysfunction in serotonin, dopamine, and norepinephrine involvement in regulating eating behavior through the hypothalamus. Other hormonal factors that may be involved include corticotrophin releasing factor, neuropeptide Y, gonadotropin-releasing hormone, and thyroid-stimulating hormone. A new substance, obestatin, made in the stomach, is a hormone that in animal experiments produces satiety and may have potential use as a weight loss agent in humans. Hunger results from a decrease in the strength of metabolic signals secondary to the depletion of critical nutrients.

Cannabinoid receptors are related to appetite and are stimulated with cannabis (marijuana). A cannabinoid inverse antagonist has been developed that blocks appetite.

Satiety occurs soon after the beginning of a meal and before the total caloric content of the meal has been absorbed; therefore satiety is only one regulatory mechanism controlling food intake. Appetite, defined as the desire for food, is also involved. A hungry person may eat to full satisfaction when food is available, but appetite can also induce a person to overeat past the point of satiety. Appetite may be increased by psychological factors such as thoughts or feelings, and an abnormal appetite may result in an abnormal increase in food intake. Eating is also affected by cannabinoid receptors, which, when stimulated, increases appetite. Marijuana acts on that receptor, which accounts for the "munchies" associated with marijuana use. The drug rimonabant is an inverse agonist to the cannabidiol receptor, meaning that it blocks appetite. It may have clinical use.

The olfactory system may play a role in satiety. Experiments have shown that strong stimulation of the olfactory bulbs in the nose with food odors by use of an inhaler saturated with a particular smell produces satiety for that food. This may have implications for therapy of obesity.

Genetic Factors

The existence of numerous forms of inherited obesity in animals and the ease with which adiposity can be produced by selective breeding make it clear that genetic factors can play a role in obesity. These factors must also be presumed to be important in human obesity.

About 80 percent of patients who are obese have a family history of obesity. This fact can be accounted for not only by genetic factors but also in part by identification with fat parents and by learned oral methods for coping with anxiety. Nonetheless, studies show that identical twins raised apart can both be obese, an observation that suggests a hereditary role. No specific genetic marker of obesity has been found.

Developmental Factors

Early in life, adipose tissue grows by increases in both cell number and cell size. Once the number of adipocytes has been established, it does not seem to be susceptible to change. Obesity that begins early in life is characterized by adipose tissue with an increased number of adipocytes of increased size. Obesity that begins in adult life, on the other hand, results solely from an increase in the size of the adipocytes. In both instances, weight reduction produces a decrease in cell size. The greater number and size of adipocytes in patients with juvenile-onset diabetes may be a factor in their widely recognized difficulties with weight reduction and the persistence of their obesity.

The distribution and amount of fat vary in individuals, and fat in different body areas has different characteristics. Fat cells around the waist, flanks, and abdomen (the so-called potbelly) are more active metabolically than those in the thighs and buttocks. The former pattern is more common in men and has a higher correlation with cardiovascular disease than does the latter pattern. Women, whose fat distribution is in the thighs and buttocks, may become obsessed with nostrums that are advertised to reduce fat in these areas (so-called cellulite, which is not a medical term), but no externally applied preparation to reduce this fat pattern exists. Men with abdominal fat may attempt to reduce their girth with machines that exercise the abdominal muscles, but exercise has no effect on fat loss.

A hormone called leptin, made by fat cells, acts as a fat thermostat. When the blood level of leptin is low, more fat is consumed; when high, less fat is consumed. Further research is needed to determine whether this might lead to new ways of managing obesity.

Physical Activity Factors

The marked decrease in physical activity in affluent societies seems to be the major factor in the rise of obesity as a public health problem. Physical inactivity restricts energy expenditure and may contribute to increased food intake. Although food intake increases with increasing energy expenditure over a wide range of energy demands, intake does not decrease proportionately when physical activity falls below a certain minimum level.

Brain-Damage Factors

Destruction of the ventromedial hypothalamus can produce obesity in animals, but this is probably a very rare cause of obesity in humans. There is evidence that the central nervous system, particularly in the lateral and ventromedial hypothalamic areas, adjusts to food intake in response to changing energy requirements so as to maintain fat stores at a baseline determined by a specific set point. This set point varies from one person to another and depends on height and body build.

Health Factors

In only a small number of cases is obesity the consequence of identifiable illness. Such cases include a variety of rare genetic disorders, such as Prader-Willi syndrome, as well as neuroendocrine abnormalities. Hypothalamic obesity results from damage to the ventromedial region of the hypothalamus (VMH), which has been studied extensively in laboratory animals and is a known center of appetite and weight regulation. In humans, damage to the VMH may result from trauma, surgery, malignancy, or inflammatory disease.

Some forms of depression, particularly seasonal affective disorder, are associated with weight gain. Most persons who live in seasonal climates report increases in appetite and weight during the fall and winter months, with decreases in the spring and summer. Depressed patients usually lose weight, but some gain weight.

Other Clinical Factors

A variety of clinical disorders are associated with obesity. Cushing's disease is associated with a characteristic fat distribution and moon-like face. Myxedema is associated with weight gain, although not invariably. Other neuroendocrine disorders include adiposogenital dystrophy (Fröhlich's syndrome), which is characterized by obesity and sexual and skeletal abnormalities.

Psychotropic Drugs

Long-term use of steroid medications is associated with significant weight gain, as is the use of several psychotropic agents. Patients treated for major depression, psychotic disturbances, and bipolar disorder typically gain 3 to 10 kg, with even larger gains with chronic use. This can produce the so-called metabolic syndrome discussed later.

Psychological Factors

Although psychological factors are evidently crucial to the development of obesity, how such psychological factors result in obesity is not known. The food-regulating mechanism is susceptible to environmental influence, and cultural, family, and psychodynamic factors have all been shown to contribute to the development of obesity. Although many investigators have proposed that specific family histories, precipitating factors, personality structures, or unconscious conflicts cause obesity, overweight persons may suffer from any conceivable psychiatric disorder and come from a variety of disturbed backgrounds. Many obese patients are emotionally disturbed persons who, because of the availability of the overeating mechanism in their environments, have learned to use hyperphagia as a means of coping with psychological problems. Some patients may show signs of serious mental disorder when they attain normal weight because they no longer have that coping mechanism.

DIAGNOSIS AND CLINICAL FEATURES

The diagnosis of obesity, if done in a sophisticated way, involves the assessment of body fat. Because this is rarely practical, the use of height and weight to calculate BMI is recommended.

In most cases of obesity, it is not possible to identify the precise etiology, given the multitude of possible causes and their interactions. Instances of secondary obesity are rare but should not be overlooked.

The habitual eating patterns of many obese persons often seem similar to patterns found in experimental obesity. Impaired satiety is a particularly important problem. Obese persons seem inordinately susceptible to food cues in their environment, to the palatability of foods, and to the inability to stop eating if food is available. Obese persons are usually susceptible to all kinds of external stimuli to eating, but they remain relatively unresponsive to the usual internal signals of hunger. Some are unable to distinguish between hunger and other kinds of dysphoria.

DIFFERENTIAL DIAGNOSIS

Other Syndromes

The night-eating syndrome, in which persons eat excessively after they have had their evening meal, seems to be precipitated by stressful life circumstances and, once present, tends to recur daily until the stress is alleviated. Night-eating may also occur as a result of using sedatives to sleep that may produce sleep-walking and eating. This has been reported with the use of Zolpidem (Ambien) in patients.

The binge-eating syndrome (bulimia) is characterized by sudden, compulsive ingestion of very large amounts of food in a short time, usually with great subsequent agitation and self-condemnation. Binge eating also appears to represent a reaction to stress. In contrast to the night-eating syndrome, however, these bouts of overeating are not periodic, and they are far more often linked to specific precipitating circumstances. (See Section 19.2 for a complete discussion of bulimia.) The Pickwickian syndrome is said to exist when a person is 100 percent over desirable weight and has associated respiratory and cardiovascular pathology.

Body Dysmorphic Disorder (Dysmorphophobia)

Some obese persons feel that their bodies are grotesque and loathsome and that others view them with hostility and contempt. This feeling is closely associated with self-consciousness and impaired social functioning. Emotionally healthy obese persons have no body image disturbances, and only a minority of neurotic obese persons have such disturbances. The disorder is confined mainly to persons who have been obese since childhood; even among them, less than half suffer from it. (Body dysmorphic disorder is discussed further in Chapter 14 on Somatoform Disorders.)

Metabolic Syndrome

The metabolic syndrome consists of a cluster of metabolic abnormalities associated with obesity and that contribute to an increased risk of cardiovascular disease and type II diabetes. The syndrome is diagnosed when a patient has three or more of the following five risk factors: (1) abdominal obesity, (2) high triglyceride level, (3) low high-density lipoprotein (HDL) cholesterol level, (4) hypertension, and (5) an elevated fasting blood glucose level. The syndrome is believed to occur in about 30 percent of the U.S. population, but it is also well known in other industrialized countries around the world.

The cause of the syndrome is unknown, but obesity, insulin resistance, and a genetic vulnerability are involved. Treatment involves weight loss, exercise, and the use of statins and antihypertensives as needed to lower lipid levels and blood pressure. Because of the increased risk of mortality, it is important that the syndrome be recognized early and treated.

Second-generation (atypical) antipsychotic medication has been implicated as a cause of metabolic syndrome. In patients with schizophrenia, treatment with these medications can cause a rapid increase in body weight in the first few months of therapy that may continue for more than 1 year. In addition, insulin resistance leading to type II diabetes has been associated with an artherogenic lipid profile.

Clozapine and olanzapine (Zyprexa) are the two drugs most implicated, but other atypical antipsychotics may also be involved.

Patients prescribed second-generation antipsychotic medication should be monitored periodically with fasting blood glucose levels at the beginning of treatment and during its course. Lipid profiles should also be obtained.

Psychological reactions to the metabolic syndrome depend on the signs and symptoms experienced by the patient. Those who suffer primarily from obesity must deal with self-esteem issues from being overweight as well as the stress of participating in weight loss programs. In many cases of obesity, eating is a way of satisfying deep-seated dependency needs. As weight is lost, some patients become depressed or anxious. Cases of psychosis have been reported in a few markedly obese patients during or after the process of losing a vast amount of weight. Other metabolic discrepancies, particularly variations in blood sugar, may be accompanied by irritability or other mood changes. Finally, fatigue is a common occurrence in patients with this syndrome. As the condition improves, especially if exercise is part of the regimen, fatigue eventually diminishes, but patients may be misdiagnosed as having a dysthymic disorder or chronic fatigue syndrome if metabolic causes of fatigue are not considered.

COURSE AND PROGNOSIS

Effects on Health

Obesity has adverse effects on health and is associated with a broad range of illnesses. There is a strong correlation between obesity and cardiovascular disorders. Hypertension (blood pressure >160/95 mm Hg) is three times higher for persons who are overweight, and hypercholesterolemia (blood cholesterol >250 mg/dL) is twice as common. Studies show that blood pressure and cholesterol levels can be reduced by weight reduction. Diabetes, which has clear genetic determinations, can often be reversed with weight reduction, especially type II diabetes (mature-onset or non–insulin-dependent diabetes mellitus).

According to National Institutes of Health data, obese men, regardless of smoking habits, have a higher mortality from colon, rectal, and prostate cancer than men of normal weight. Obese women have a higher mortality from cancer of the gallbladder, biliary passages, breast (postmenopause), uterus (including cervix and endometrium), and ovaries than women of normal weight.

Longevity

Reliable studies indicate that the more overweight a person is, the higher is that person's risk for death. A person who reduces weight to acceptable levels has a mortality decline to normal rates. Weight reduction may be lifesaving for patients with extreme obesity, defined as weight that is twice the desirable weight. Such patients may have cardiorespiratory failure, especially when asleep (sleep apnea).

A number of studies have demonstrated that decreasing caloric intake by 30 percent or more in young or middle-aged laboratory animals prevents or retards age-related chronic diseases and significantly prolongs maximal life span. The mechanisms through which this effect is mediated are not known, but they may include reductions in metabolic rate, oxidative stress and inflammation, improved insulin sensitivity, and changes in neuroendocrine and sympathetic nervous system function. Whether long-term calorie restriction with adequate nutrition slows aging in humans is not yet known.

Prognosis

The prognosis for weight reduction is poor, and the course of obesity tends toward inexorable progression. Of patients who

lose significant amounts of weight, 90 percent regain it eventually. The prognosis is particularly poor for those who become obese in childhood. Juvenile-onset obesity tends to be more severe, more resistant to treatment, and more likely to be associated with emotional disturbance than is adult obesity.

Discrimination toward the Obese. Overweight and obese individuals are subject to significant prejudice and discrimination in the United States and other industrialized nations. In a culture in which beauty ideals include highly unrealistic thinness, overweight people are blamed for their condition and are the subject of teasing, bias, and discrimination (sometimes called "fatism"). Income and earning power are reduced in overweight people, and untoward social conditions, such as absence of romantic relationships, are more common. Furthermore, obese individuals face limited access to health care and may receive biased diagnoses and treatment from medical and mental health providers.

TREATMENT

As mentioned, many patients routinely treated for obesity may develop anxiety or depression. A high incidence of emotional disturbances has been reported among obese persons undergoing long-term, in-hospital treatment by fasting or severe calorie restriction. Obese persons with extensive psychopathology, those with a history of emotional disturbance during dieting, and those in the midst of a life crisis should attempt weight reduction, if at all, cautiously and under careful supervision.

Diet

The basis of weight reduction is simple—establish a caloric deficit by bringing intake below output. The simplest way to reduce caloric intake is by means of a low-calorie diet. The best long-term effects are achieved with a balanced diet that contains readily available foods. For most persons, the most satisfactory reducing diet consists of their usual foods in amounts determined with the aid of tables of food values that are available in standard books on dieting. Such a diet gives the best chance of long-term maintenance of weight loss. Total unmodified fasts are used for short-term weight loss, but they have associated morbidity including orthostatic hypotension, sodium diuresis, and impaired nitrogen balance.

Ketogenic diets are high-protein, high-fat diets used to promote weight loss. They have high cholesterol content and produce ketosis, which is associated with nausea, hypotension, and lethargy. Many obese persons find it tempting to use a novel or even bizarre diet. Whatever effectiveness these diets may have in large part results from their monotony. When a dieter stops the diet and returns to the usual fare, the incentives to overeat are multiplied.

In general, the best method of weight loss is a balanced diet of 1,100 to 1,200 calories. Such a diet can be followed for long periods but should be supplemented with vitamins, particularly iron, folic acid, zinc, and vitamin B_6.

Exercise

Increased physical activity is an important part of a weight-reduction regimen. Because caloric expenditure in most forms of physical activity is directly proportional to body weight, obese persons expend more calories than persons of normal weight with the same amount of activity. Furthermore, increased physical activity may actually decrease food intake by formerly sedentary persons. This combination of increased caloric expenditure and decreased food intake makes an increase in physical activity a highly desirable feature of any weight-reduction program. Exercise also helps maintain weight loss. It is essential in the treatment of the metabolic syndrome.

Pharmacotherapy

Various drugs, some more effective than others, are used to treat obesity. Drug treatment is effective because it suppresses appetite, but tolerance to this effect may develop after several weeks of use. An initial trial period of 4 weeks with a specific drug can be used; then, if the patient responds with weight loss, the drug can be continued to see whether tolerance develops. If a drug remains effective, it can be dispensed for a longer time until the desired weight is achieved.

One weight-loss medication approved by the Food and Drug Administration (FDA) for long-term use (in 1999) is orlistat (Xenical), which is a selective gastric and pancreatic lipase inhibitor that reduces the absorption of dietary fat (which is then excreted in stool). In clinical trials, orlistat (120 mg, three times a day), in combination with a low-calorie diet, induced losses of approximately 10 percent of initial weight in the first 6 months, which were generally well maintained for periods up to 24 months. Because of its peripheral mechanism of action, orlistat is generally free of the central nervous system effects (i.e., increased pulse, dry mouth, insomnia, etc.) that are associated with most weight-loss medications. The principal adverse effects of orlistat are gastrointestinal; patients must consume 30 percent or fewer calories from fat to prevent adverse events that include oily stool, flatulence with discharge, and fecal urgency. Another medication, Sibutramine (Meridia) is a β-phenylethylamine that inhibits the reuptake of serotonin and norepinephrine (and dopamine to a limited extent). It was approved by the FDA in 1997 for weight loss and the maintenance of weight loss (i.e., long-term use).

Rimonabant. Dopamine receptor agonists, or sympathomimetics, are among the most widely used appetite suppressants. An alternative to psychostimulants, rimonabant has a unique mechanism of action: It is a selective cannabinoid-1 receptor blocker. Rimonabant has been shown to reduce body weight and improve cardiovascular risk factors in obese patients. The effects of rimonabant on metabolic risk factors have been studied in clinical trials of high-risk patients who are overweight or obese and have dyslipidemia. At a dose of 20 mg, rimonabant causes significant weight loss, reduction in waist circumference, increase in HDL cholesterol, and reduction in triglycerides. At that dose it also increases plasma levels of adiponectin, a protein hormone that modulates glucose regulation and fatty acid catabolism. Adiponectin is exclusively secreted from adipose tissue, and its plasma levels are inversely correlated with body BMI. It appears to help suppress metabolic abnormalities that lead to type II diabetes, obesity, and atherosclerosis. Rimonabant has not been studied in patients with psychiatric disorders. It should thus be used with caution in that population because the most frequent adverse events resulting in discontinuation of the drug in clinical trials were nausea, depression, and anxiety. However, because weight gain is such a common side effect of many psychiatric drugs, the use of rimonabant to mitigate drug-induced metabolic disturbances may be justified in some patients.

Surgery

Surgical methods that cause malabsorption of food or reduce gastric volume have been used in persons who are markedly obese. *Gastric bypass* is a procedure in which the stomach is made smaller by transecting or stapling one of the stomach curvatures. In *gastroplasty* the size of the stomach stoma is reduced so that the passage of food slows. Results are successful, although vomiting, electrolyte imbalance, and obstruction may occur. A syndrome called dumping, which consists of palpitations, weakness, and sweating, may follow surgical procedures in some patients if they ingest large amounts of carbohydrates in a single meal. The surgical removal of fat (lipectomy) has no effect on weight loss in the long run nor does liposuction, which has value only for cosmetic reasons. Bariatric surgery is now recommended in individuals who have serious obesity-related health complications and a BMI of greater than 35 kg/m^2 (or a BMI >40 kg/m^2 in the absence of major health complications). Before surgery, candidates should have tried to lose weight using the safer, more traditional options of diet, exercise, and weight loss medication.

Psychotherapy

The psychological problems of obese persons vary, and there is no particular personality type that is obese. Some patients may respond to insight-oriented psychodynamic therapy with weight loss, but this treatment has not had much success. Uncovering the unconscious causes of overeating may not alter the behavior of persons who overeat in response to stress, although it may serve to augment other treatment methods. Years after successful psychotherapy, many persons who overeat under stress continue to do so. Obese persons seem particularly vulnerable to overdependency on a therapist, and the inordinate regression that may occur during the uncovering psychotherapies should be carefully monitored.

Behavior modification has been the most successful of the therapeutic approaches for obesity and is considered the method of choice. Patients are taught to recognize external cues that are associated with eating and to keep diaries of foods consumed in particular circumstances, such as at the movies or while watching television, or during certain emotional states, such as anxiety or depression. Patients are also taught to develop new eating patterns, such as eating slowly, chewing food well, not reading while eating, and not eating between meals or when not seated. Operant conditioning therapies that use rewards such as praise or new clothes to reinforce weight loss have also been successful. Group therapy helps to maintain motivation, to promote identification among members who have lost weight, and to provide education about nutrition.

Sleep-Wake Rhythm

Without external clues, the natural body clock follows a 25-hour cycle. The influence of external factors—such as the light-dark cycle, daily routines, meal periods, and other external synchronizers—entrain persons to the 24-hour clock. Sleep is also influenced by biological rhythms. Within a 24-hour period, adults sleep once, sometimes twice. This rhythm is not present at birth but develops over the first 2 years of life. Some women exhibit sleep pattern changes during the phases of the menstrual cycle. Naps taken at different times of the day differ greatly in their proportions of REM and NREM sleep. In a normal night-time sleeper, a nap taken in the morning or at noon includes a great deal of REM sleep, whereas a nap taken in the afternoon or the early evening has much less REM sleep. A circadian cycle apparently affects the tendency to have REM sleep. Sleep patterns are not physiologically the same when persons sleep in the daytime or during the time when they are accustomed to being awake; the psychological and behavioral effects of sleep differ as well. In a world of industry and communications that often functions 24 hours a day, these interactions are becoming increasingly significant. Even in persons who work at night, interference with the various rhythms can produce problems. The best-known example is jet lag, in which, after flying east to west, persons try to convince their bodies to go to sleep at a time that is out of phase with some body cycles. Most persons adapt within a few days, but some require more time. Conditions in these persons' bodies apparently involve long-term cycle disruption and interference.

▲ 20.2 Sleep Disorders

The text revision of the fourth edition of the *Diagnostic and Statistical Manual of Mental Disorders* (DSM-IV-TR) divides primary sleep disorders into *dyssomnias* and *parasomnias*. The dyssomnias—disorders of quantity or timing of sleep—are divided into *insomnia* and *hypersomnia*. Insomnia is a perceived disturbance in the quantity or quality of sleep, which, depending on the specific condition, may be associated with disturbances in objectively measured sleep. Forms of insomnia include the primary insomnias and circadian rhythm sleep disturbances. Hypersomnias represent conditions that are clinically expressed as excessive sleepiness. Parasomnias are abnormal behaviors during sleep or the transition between sleep and wakefulness. Often, they reflect the appearance of normal sleep processes at inappropriate times. The symptoms often overlap and are described in this section.

INSOMNIA

Insomnia is difficulty initiating or maintaining sleep. It is the most common sleep complaint and may be transient or persistent. Population surveys show a 1-year prevalence rate of 30 to 45 percent in adults.

A brief period of insomnia is most often associated with anxiety, either as a sequela to an anxious experience or in anticipation of an anxiety-provoking experience (e.g., an examination or an impending job interview). In some persons, transient insomnia of this kind may be related to grief, loss, or almost any life change

or stress. The condition is not likely to be serious, although a psychotic episode or a severe depression sometimes begins with acute insomnia. Specific treatment for the condition is usually not required. When treatment with hypnotic medication is indicated, both the physician and the patient should be clear that the treatment is of short duration and that some symptoms, including a brief recurrence of the insomnia, may be expected when the medication is discontinued.

Persistent insomnia is composed of a fairly common group of conditions in which the problem is most often difficulty falling asleep rather than remaining asleep. This insomnia involves two sometimes separable but often intertwined problems: somatized tension and anxiety, and a conditioned associative response. Patients often have no clear complaint other than insomnia. They may not experience anxiety per se but discharge the anxiety through physiological channels; they may complain chiefly of apprehensive feeling or ruminative thoughts that appear to keep them from falling asleep. Sometimes (but not always) a patient describes the condition's exacerbation at times of stress at work or at home and its remission during vacations.

HYPERSOMNIA

Hypersomnia manifests as excessive amounts of sleep, excessive daytime sleepiness (somnolence), or sometimes both. The term *somnolence* should be reserved for patients who complain of sleepiness and have a clearly demonstrable tendency to fall asleep suddenly in the waking state, who have sleep attacks, and who cannot remain awake; it should not be used for persons who are simply physically tired or weary. The distinction, however, is not always clear. Complaints of hypersomnia are much less frequent (5 percent of adults) than complaints of insomnia, but they are by no means rare if clinicians are alert to them. More than 100,000 persons with narcolepsy are estimated to live in the United States, and narcolepsy is just one well-known condition that clearly produces hypersomnia. If substance-related conditions are included, hypersomnia is a common symptom.

As with insomnia, hypersomnia is associated with conditions that are hard to classify and idiopathic cases. According to a recent survey, the most common conditions responsible for hypersomnia sufficiently severe to be evaluated by all-night recordings at a sleep disorders center were sleep apnea and narcolepsy.

Transient and situational hypersomnia is a disruption of the normal sleep-wake pattern; it is marked by excessive difficulty in remaining awake and a tendency to remain in bed for unusually long periods or to return to bed to nap frequently during the day. The pattern is experienced suddenly in response to an identifiable recent life change, conflict, or loss and is much less common than insomnia. It is seldom marked by definite sleep attacks or unavoidable sleep but, rather, is characterized by tiredness or by falling asleep sooner than usual and by difficulty arising in the morning.

PARASOMNIA

Parasomnia is an unusual or undesirable phenomenon that appears suddenly during sleep or that occurs at the threshold between waking and sleeping. Parasomnia usually occurs in stages 3 and 4 and, thus, is associated with poor recall of the disturbance.

Sleep-Wake Schedule Disturbance

Sleep-wake schedule disturbance involves the displacement of sleep from its desired circadian period. Patients commonly cannot sleep when they wish to sleep, although they are able to sleep at other times. Correspondingly, they cannot be fully awake when they want to be fully awake, but they are able to be awake at other times. The disturbance does not precisely produce insomnia or somnolence, although the initial complaint is often either insomnia or somnolence; the inabilities to sleep and be awake are elicited only on careful questioning. Sleep-wake schedule disturbance can be considered a misalignment between sleep and wake behaviors. A sleep history questionnaire is helpful in diagnosing a patient's sleep disorder.

CLASSIFICATION

DSM-IV-TR

The DSM-IV-TR classifies sleep disorders on the basis of clinical diagnostic criteria and presumed etiology. The three major categories of sleep disorders in DSM-IV-TR are primary sleep disorders, sleep disorders related to another mental disorder, and other sleep disorders (due to a general medical condition or are substance induced). The disorders described in DSM-IV-TR are only a fraction of the known sleep disorders; they provide a framework for clinical assessment.

PRIMARY SLEEP DISORDERS

The DSM-IV-TR defines primary sleep disorders as those not caused by another mental disorder, a physical condition, or a substance but, rather, are caused by an abnormal sleep-wake mechanism and often by conditioning. The two main primary sleep disorders are dyssomnias and parasomnias. Dyssomnias are a heterogeneous group of sleep disorders that includes primary insomnia, primary hypersomnia, narcolepsy, breathing-related sleep disorder, circadian rhythm sleep disorder (sleep-wake schedule disorder), and dyssomnia not otherwise specified. Parasomnias include nightmare disorder (dream anxiety disorder), sleep terror disorder, sleepwalking disorder, and parasomnia not otherwise specified.

Dyssomnias

Primary Insomnia. Primary insomnia is diagnosed when the chief complaint is nonrestorative sleep or difficulty in initiating or maintaining sleep and the complaint continues for at least 1 month (Table 20.2–1). (According to the tenth revision of the *International Statistical Classification of Diseases and Related Health Problems*, the disturbance must occur at least three times a week for a month.) The term *primary* indicates that the insomnia is independent of any known physical or mental condition. Primary insomnia is often characterized both by difficulty falling asleep and by repeated awakening. Increased nighttime physiological or psychological arousal and negative conditioning for sleep are frequently evident. Patients with primary insomnia are generally preoccupied with getting enough sleep. The more they try to sleep, the greater the sense of frustration and distress and the more elusive sleep becomes.

TREATMENT. Treatment of primary insomnia is among the most difficult problems in sleep disorders. When the conditioned com-

Table 20.2–1
DSM-IV-TR Diagnostic Criteria for Primary Insomnia

A. The predominant complaint is difficulty initiating or maintaining sleep, or nonrestorative sleep, for at least 1 month.
B. The sleep disturbance (or associated daytime fatigue) causes clinically significant distress or impairment in social, occupational, or other important areas of functioning.
C. The sleep disturbance does not occur exclusively during the course of narcolepsy, breathing-related sleep disorder, circadian rhythm sleep disorder, or a parasomnia.
D. The disturbance does not exclusively occur during the course of another mental disorder (e.g., major depressive disorder, generalized anxiety disorder, a delirium).
E. The disturbance is not due to the direct physiological effects of a substance (e.g., a drug of abuse, a medication) or a general medical condition.

From American Psychiatric Association. *Diagnostic and Statistical Manual of Mental Disorders.* 4th ed. Text rev. Washington, DC: American Psychiatric Association; copyright 2000, with permission.

ponent is prominent, a deconditioning technique may be useful. Patients are asked to use their beds for sleeping and for nothing else; if they are not asleep after 5 minutes in bed, they are instructed simply to get up and do something else. Sometimes, changing to another bed or to another room is useful. When somatized tension or muscle tension is prominent, relaxation tapes, meditation, and practicing the relaxation response and biofeedback are occasionally helpful. Psychotherapy has not been very useful in the treatment of primary insomnia. Satisfying sexual experiences promote sleep, more so in men than in women.

DRUG THERAPY. Primary insomnia is commonly treated with benzodiazepines, zolpidem, zaleplon (Sonata), and other hypnotics. Hypnotic drugs should be used with care. Over-the-counter sleep aids have limited effectiveness. Long-acting sleep medications (e.g., flurazepam [Dalmane], quazepam [Doral]) are best for middle-of-the-night insomnia; short-acting drugs (e.g., zolpidem, triazolam [Halcion]) are useful for persons who have difficulty falling asleep. In general, sleep medications should not be prescribed for more than 2 weeks because tolerance and withdrawal may result.

Some dietary supplements used for insomnia include melatonin and L-tryptophan. Melatonin is an endogenous hormone produced by the pineal gland, which is linked to the regulation of sleep. Administration of exogenous melatonin has yielded mixed results, however, in clinical research. Melatonin's precursor, L-tryptophan, was used previously with the same rationale; however, in addition to having uncertain efficacy, it was found to be contaminated with a substance causing eosinophilic myalgia, a possibly deadly dyscrasia. These substances are available worldwide, however, and may be obtained by patients in the United States. Other concerns with L-tryptophan include serotonin syndrome if used in conjunction with a selective serotonin reuptake inhibitor (SSRI). Dietary supplement use has increased during the past decade.

Other drugs used for insomnia, although off-label, are mirtazapim (Remeron) 15 mg nightly, nefazadone (Trazadone) 25 mg nightly, and quetiapine (Seroquel) 25 mg nightly. These drugs have sedation as a side effect that can help relieve insomnia in some patients.

Various nonspecific measures—so-called sleep hygiene—can help improve sleep. Physicians must reassure patients with insomnia that their health is not at risk if they do not get 6 to 8 hours of sleep.

INADEQUATE SLEEP HYGIENE. A common finding is that a patient's lifestyle leads to sleep disturbance. This is usually phrased whereas CSA is manifest as insomnia, but later case series have emphasized that either symptom may appear in either disorder. The polysomnogramic features of CSA are similar to those of OSA, except that, during the periods of apnea, a cessation of respiratory effort is seen in the abdominal and chest expansion leads.

Several features of OSA and CSA are significant in psychiatric practice. These include decreased ability to concentrate, decreased libido, memory complaints, and deficits in neuropsychological testing. Many or even most patients have dysthymic features and, although many patients manifest OSA and major depression, it is not certain that they occur more often than would be seen by chance. One study indicated that, among patients with OSA, those with a history of treatment for affective disorder show greater decrements in ventilatory measurements. Although systematic data are minimal, many clinicians believe that if OSA is found and treated in cases of refractory depression, the depressive symptoms may improve. Neuropsychological testing indicates that most, but not all, deficits can be relieved by treatment.

Patients sometimes awaken from apneas with a sensation of being unable to breathe, and these episodes need to be distinguished from nocturnal panic attacks. In taking a history, it should be noted that perhaps one third of patients with daytime panic attacks also have these episodes during sleep, but it is rare to have panic attacks purely at night. Similar awakenings can occur in cases of paradoxical vocal cord movement: In this situation, however, there is usually a history of trauma or surgery of the neck. Sleep apnea episodes also need to be distinguished from nocturnal laryngospasm, in which patients report that they are unable to speak or can only whisper for a few minutes after awakening.

Nasal continuous positive airway pressure is the treatment of choice for OSA. Other procedures include weight loss, nasal surgery, tracheostomy, and uvulopalatoplasty. Some medications may normalize sleep in patients with apnea. SSRIs and heterocyclic antidepressant drugs sometimes help treat sleep apnea by decreasing the amount of time spent in REM sleep, the stage of sleep in which apneic episodes occur most often. In addition, theophylline has been shown to decrease the number of episodes of apnea; however, it may interfere with the overall quality of sleep, limiting its general utility. When sleep apnea is established or suspected, patients must avoid the use of sedative medication, including alcohol, because it can considerably exacerbate the condition, which may then become life threatening.

Central Alveolar Hypoventilation.

Central alveolar hypoventilation refers to several conditions marked by impaired ventilation in which the respiratory abnormality appears or greatly worsens only during sleep and in which no significant apneic episodes are present. The ventilatory dysfunction is characterized by inadequate tidal volume or respiratory rate during sleep. Death may occur during sleep (Ondine's curse). Central alveolar hypoventilation is treated with some form of mechanical ventilation (e.g., nasal ventilation).

Circadian Rhythm Sleep Disorder.

Circadian rhythm sleep disorder includes a wide range of conditions involving a misalignment between desired and actual sleep periods. DSM-IV-TR lists four types of circadian rhythm sleep disorders: de-

Table 20.2–5
DSM-IV-TR Diagnostic Criteria for Circadian Rhythm Sleep Disorder

A. A persistent or recurrent pattern of sleep disruption leading to excessive sleepiness or insomnia that is due to a mismatch between the sleep-wake schedule required by a person's environment and his or her circadian sleep-wake pattern.
B. The sleep disturbance causes clinically significant distress or impairment in social, occupational, or other important areas of functioning.
C. The disturbance does not occur exclusively during the course of another sleep disorder or other mental disorder.
D. The disturbance is not due to the direct physiological effects of a substance (e.g., a drug of abuse, a medication) or a general medical condition.

Specify type:
  Delayed sleep phase type: a persistent pattern of late sleep onset and late awakening times, with an inability to fall asleep and awaken at a desired earlier time
  Jet lag type: sleepiness and alertness that occur at an inappropriate time of day relative to local time, occurring after repeated travel across more than one time zone
  Shift work type: insomnia during the major sleep period or excessive sleepiness during the major awake period associated with night shift work or frequently changing shift work
Unspecified type

From American Psychiatric Association. *Diagnostic and Statistical Manual of Mental Disorders.* 4th ed. Text rev. Washington, DC: American Psychiatric Association; copyright 2000, with permission.

layed sleep-phase type, jet lag type, shift work type, and unspecified (Table 20.2–5).

DELAYED SLEEP-PHASE TYPE. In delayed sleep-phase syndrome, the circadian system is operating in a delayed but stable relationship to the day–night cues of the external world. It is marked by sleep and wake times that are intractably later than desired, actual sleep times at virtually the same daily clock hour, no reported difficulty in maintaining sleep once begun, and an inability to advance the sleep phase by enforcing conventional sleep and wake times. The patients' major complaint is often the difficulty of falling asleep at a desired conventional time, and their disorder may appear to be similar to sleep-onset insomnia. Daytime sleepiness often occurs secondary to sleep loss.

The first major therapy for delayed sleep-phase syndrome is chronotherapy, in which the patient is instructed to shift his or her hours of sleep and waking progressively later each night until he or she has moved around the clock to a point at which he or she has a more traditional bedtime. An alternative approach is bright-light therapy in which the patient is exposed to bright artificial light in the early morning.

JET LAG TYPE. Depending on the length of the east-to-west trip and individual sensitivity, jet lag sleep disorder usually disappears spontaneously in 2 to 7 days; no specific treatment is required. Some persons find that they can prevent the symptoms by altering their mealtimes and sleep times in an appropriate direction before traveling. Others find that what appear to be symptoms of jet lag (fatigue and so on) are actually associated with sleep deprivation and that simply obtaining enough sleep helps. Melatonin taken orally at prescribed times is useful for some persons. Maximizing light exposure during the new daytime and minimizing light during the new nighttime are also helpful.

SHIFT WORK TYPE. Shift work can induce sleep disturbances, as well as other difficulties, including accidents because of sleepiness during nighttime working hours and, in more extreme cases, a *shift-work syndrome* characterized by gastrointestinal and cardiovascular disorders.

A common experience among night shift workers is to come home in the early morning, go to bed feeling exhausted, sleep only 2 to 3 hours, and awaken feeling unrefreshed but unable to continue sleeping. The treatments for this type of sleep disorder are complex and vary with the type of work schedule. Various strategies, including napping before going into work in the evening or taking a scheduled nap during nighttime work hours, may be helpful. Using bright light at night and avoiding light during the day have been proposed. It may be helpful, for instance, for a night-shift worker driving home in the morning to wear sunglasses, so as not to get a large light exposure immediately before going to bed. It has been demonstrated that using circadian principles to design industrial work schedules can reduce absenteeism and medical difficulties. Treatment with melatonin has been found to be less successful than timed bright-light exposure in aiding adjustment to shift work.

A particular problem occurs in the training of physicians, who are often required to work 36 to 48 hours without sleeping. This condition is dangerous to both doctors and their patients. It behooves medical educators to develop more shifts for doctors in training.

Unspecified

ADVANCED SLEEP-PHASE SYNDROME. The advanced sleep-phase syndrome is characterized by sleep onsets and wake times that are intractably earlier than desired, actual sleep times at virtually the same daily clock hour, no reported difficulty in maintaining sleep once begun, and an inability to delay the sleep phase by enforcing conventional sleep and wake times. Unlike delayed sleep-phase type, the condition does not interfere with the work or school day. The major presenting complaint is the inability to stay awake in the evening and to sleep in the morning until desired conventional times. It is particularly common in the elderly, who have a phase advance of approximately 1 hour in terms of their temperature and melatonin rhythms. This condition can be treated by administering bright light in the early evening, resulting in a phase delay of the pacemaker, such that the sleep-wake signal is in closer concert with traditional hours for bedtime and arising.

DISORGANIZED SLEEP-WAKE PATTERN. *Disorganized sleep-wake pattern* is defined as irregular, variable sleep and waking behavior that disrupts the regular sleep-wake pattern. The condition is associated with frequent daytime naps at irregular times and excessive bed rest. Sleep at night is not adequately long, and the condition may seem to be insomnia, although the total amount of sleep in 24 hours is normal for the patient's age.

Dyssomnia Not Otherwise Specified. According to DSM-IV-TR, dyssomnia not otherwise specified includes insomnias, hypersomnias, and circadian rhythm disturbances that do not meet the criteria for any specific dyssomnia (Table 20.2–6).

PERIODIC LIMB MOVEMENT SYNDROME. Periodic limb movement syndrome (PLMS) (also known as *nocturnal myoclonus*) consists of highly stereotyped abrupt contractions of certain leg

Table 20.2–6
DSM-IV-TR Diagnostic Criteria for Dyssomnia Not Otherwise Specified

The dyssomnia not otherwise specified category is for insomnias, hypersomnias, or circadian rhythm disturbances that do not meet criteria for any specific dyssomnia. Examples include

1. Complaints of clinically significant insomnia or hypersomnia that are attributable to environmental factors (e.g., noise, light, frequent interruptions).
2. Excessive sleepiness that is attributable to ongoing sleep deprivation.
3. "Restless legs syndrome": This syndrome is characterized by a desire to move the legs or arms, associated with uncomfortable sensations typically described as creeping, crawling, tingling, burning, or itching. Frequent movements of the limbs occur in an effort to relieve the uncomfortable sensations. Symptoms are worse when the individual is at rest and in the evening or night, and they are relieved temporarily by movement. The uncomfortable sensations and limb movements can delay sleep onset, awaken the individual from sleep, and lead to daytime sleepiness or fatigue. Sleep studies demonstrate involuntary periodic limb movements during sleep in a majority of individuals with restless legs syndrome. A minority of individuals have evidence of anemia or reduced serum iron stores. Peripheral nerve electrophysiological studies and gross brain morphology are usually normal. Restless legs syndrome can occur in an idiopathic form, or it can be associated with general medical or neurological conditions, including normal pregnancy, renal failure, rheumatoid arthritis, peripheral vascular disease, or peripheral nerve dysfunction. Phenomenologically, the two forms are indistinguishable. The onset of restless legs syndrome is typically in the second or third decade, although up to 20% of individuals with this syndrome may have symptoms before age 10. The prevalence of restless legs syndrome is between 2% and 10% in the general population and as high as 30% in general medical populations. Prevalence increases with age and is equal in males and females. Course is marked by stability or worsening of symptoms with age. There is a positive family history in 50%–90% of individuals. The major differential diagnoses include medication-induced akathisia, peripheral neuropathy, and nocturnal leg cramps. Worsening at night and periodic limb movements are more common in restless legs syndrome than in medication-induced akathisia or peripheral neuropathy. Unlike restless legs syndrome, nocturnal leg cramps do not present with the desire to move the limbs nor are there frequent limb movements.
4. Periodic limb movements: Periodic limb movements are repeated low-amplitude brief limb jerks, particularly in the lower extremities. These movements begin near sleep onset and decrease during stage 3 or 4 non-rapid eye movement (NREM) and rapid eye movement (REM) sleep. Movements usually occur rhythmically every 20–60 seconds and are associated with repeated, brief arousals. Individuals are often unaware of the actual movements, but may complain of insomnia, frequent awakenings, or daytime sleepiness if the number of movements is very large. Individuals may have considerable variability in the number of periodic limb movements from night to night. Periodic limb movements occur in the majority of individuals with restless legs syndrome, but they may also occur without the other symptoms of restless legs syndrome. Individuals with normal pregnancy or with conditions such as renal failure, congestive heart failure, and posttraumatic stress disorder may also develop periodic limb movements. Although typical age at onset and prevalence in the general population are unknown, periodic limb movements increase with age and may occur in more than one-third of individuals over age 65. Men are more commonly affected than women.
5. Situations in which the clinician has concluded that a dyssomnia is present but is unable to determine whether it is primary, due to a general medical condition, or substance induced.

From American Psychiatric Association. *Diagnostic and Statistical Manual of Mental Disorders.* 4th ed. Text rev. Washington, DC: American Psychiatric Association; copyright 2000, with permission.

muscles during sleep. These movements include extension of the toes, as well as flexion of the ankle and knee. The patient is usually unaware that these movements occur, although the bed partner may be only too aware. The result of these events is usually insomnia, although hypersomnia may also appear. The condition is associated with renal disease, as well as iron and vitamin B_{12} anemia; some investigators believe that it is exacerbated by tricyclic antidepressants, although there are differing views regarding this issue. The disorder tends to be a problem of middle age in both sexes, with increasing frequency with advancing age.

On the polysomnogram, periodic limb movements are 0.5 to 5.0 seconds in duration and occur every 20 to 40 seconds during periods of NREM sleep. Often, they are accompanied by a K-complex or brief arousal signal in the EEG channels of a polysomnogram. Clinicians differ on whether to count only those that are accompanied by EEG evidence of arousal or to count all periodic limb movements regardless of EEG consequences. A diagnosis of PLMS requires a periodic limb movement index of at least five per hour. No treatment for nocturnal myoclonus is universally effective. Treatments that may be useful include benzodiazepines, levodopa (Larodopa), quinine, and, in rare cases, opioids.

RESTLESS LEGS SYNDROME.   Restless limbs syndrome (RLS) (also known as Ekbom's syndrome) is an uncomfortable, subjective sensation of the limbs, usually the legs, sometimes described as a "creepy crawly" feeling or as the sensation of ants walking on the skin. It tends to be worse at night, and is relieved by walking or moving about. It appears as a cause of sleep initiation insomnia because the patient may find it difficult to lie still in bed, needing to get up to relieve the discomfort. The cause is unknown, but it appears often in pregnancy, iron or vitamin B_{12} deficiency anemia, and renal disease.

The first step in treatment is to look for anemia and treat it, if found. Benzodiazepines are relatively ineffective. The off-label use of L-dopa and carbidopa (Sinemet), bromocriptine (Parlodel), and pergolide (Permax) is often helpful. In rare patients who are severely affected, the off-label use of narcotic analgesics can help when other treatments have been tried and have failed. Ropinirole (Requip), a dopamine agonist available for treatment of Parkinson's disease, is the first drug approved by the FDA for treatment of moderate to severe RLS.

KLEINE-LEVIN SYNDROME.   Kleine-Levin syndrome is a relatively rare condition consisting of recurrent periods of prolonged sleep (from which patients may be aroused) with intervening periods of normal sleep and alert waking. During the hypersomniac episodes, wakeful periods are usually marked by withdrawal from social contacts and return to bed at the first opportunity; patients may also display apathy, irritability, confusion, voracious eating, loss of sexual inhibitions, delusions, hallucinations, frank disorientation, memory impairment, incoherent speech, excitation or depression, and truculence. Unexplained fevers have occurred in a few such patients.

MENSTRUAL-ASSOCIATED SYNDROME.   Some women experience intermittent marked hypersomnia, altered behavioral patterns, and voracious eating at, or shortly before, the onset of their menses. Nonspecific EEG abnormalities similar to those associated with Kleine-Levin syndrome have been documented in several instances. Endocrine factors are probably involved, but no specific abnormalities in laboratory endocrine measures have been reported. Increased cerebrospinal fluid serotonin levels were found in one patient.

SLEEP DISTURBANCE IN PREGNANCY.   Sleep disturbance is common in pregnant women. Several hormonal factors contribute to this disturbance, including changes in levels of estrogen, progesterone, cortisol, and melatonin from baseline. In addition, changes in maternal respiratory physiology and body habitus and, in the third trimester, movements of the fetus can all act to diminish the quantity and quality of sleep.

INSUFFICIENT SLEEP.   Insufficient sleep is defined as an earnest complaint of daytime sleepiness and associated waking symptoms by a person who persistently fails to obtain sufficient daily sleep to support alert wakefulness. The person is voluntarily, but often unwittingly, chronically sleep deprived. The diagnosis can usually be made on the basis of the history, including a sleep log. Some persons, especially students and shift workers, who want to maintain an active daytime life and perform their nighttime jobs may seriously deprive themselves of sleep and, thus, produce somnolence during waking hours.

SLEEP DRUNKENNESS.   Sleep drunkenness is an abnormal form of awakening in which the lack of a clear sensorium in the transition from sleep to full wakefulness is prolonged and exaggerated. A confusional state develops that often leads to individual or social inconvenience and sometimes to criminal acts. The diagnosis requires the absence of sleep deprivation. It is a rare condition, and there may be a familial tendency. Before making the diagnosis, clinicians should examine patients' sleep and rule out such conditions as apnea, nocturnal myoclonus, narcolepsy, and excessive use of alcohol and other substances.

Parasomnias

Nightmare Disorder.

Nightmares are vivid dreams that become progressively more anxiety producing, ultimately resulting in an awakening (Table 20.2–7). As with other dreams, nightmares almost always occur during REM sleep and usually after a long REM period late in the night. Some persons have frequent nightmares as a lifelong condition; others experience them predominantly at times of stress and illness. About 50 percent of the adult population may report occasional nightmares. No specific treatment is usually required for nightmare disorder. Agents that suppress REM sleep, such as tricyclic drugs, may reduce the

Table 20.2–7
DSM-IV-TR Diagnostic Criteria for Nightmare Disorder

A. Repeated awakenings from the major sleep period or naps with detailed recall of extended and extremely frightening dreams, usually involving threats to survival, security, or self-esteem. The awakenings generally occur during the second half of the sleep period.

B. On awakening from the frightening dreams, the person rapidly becomes oriented and alert (in contrast to the confusion and disorientation seen in sleep terror disorder and some forms of epilepsy).

C. The dream experience, or the sleep disturbance resulting from the awakening, causes clinically significant distress or impairment in social, occupational, or other important areas of functioning.

D. The nightmares do not occur exclusively during the course of another mental disorder (e.g., a delirium, posttraumatic stress disorder) and are not due to the direct physiological effects of a substance (e.g., a drug of abuse, a medication) or a general medical condition.

From American Psychiatric Association. *Diagnostic and Statistical Manual of Mental Disorders.* 4th ed. Text rev. Washington, DC: American Psychiatric Association; copyright 2000, with permission.

Table 20.2–8
DSM-IV-TR Diagnostic Criteria for Sleep Terror Disorder

A. Recurrent episodes of abrupt awakening from sleep, usually occurring during the first third of the major sleep episode and beginning with a panicky scream.
B. Intense fear and signs of autonomic arousal, such as tachycardia, rapid breathing, and sweating, during each episode.
C. Relative unresponsiveness to efforts of others to comfort the person during the episode.
D. No detailed dream is recalled and there is amnesia for the episode.
E. The episodes cause clinically significant distress or impairment in social, occupational, or other important areas of functioning.
F. The disturbance is not due to the direct physiological effects of a substance (e.g., a drug of abuse, a medication) or a general medical condition.

From American Psychiatric Association. *Diagnostic and Statistical Manual of Mental Disorders*. 4th ed. Text rev. Washington, DC: American Psychiatric Association; copyright 2000, with permission.

Table 20.2–9
DSM-IV-TR Diagnostic Criteria for Sleepwalking Disorder

A. Repeated episodes of rising from bed during sleep and walking about, usually occurring during the first third of the major sleep episode.
B. While sleepwalking, the person has a blank, staring face, is relatively unresponsive to the efforts of others to communicate with him or her, and can be awakened only with great difficulty.
C. On awakening (either from the sleepwalking episode or the next morning), the person has amnesia for the episode.
D. Within several minutes after awakening from the sleepwalking episode, there is no impairment of mental activity or behavior (although there may initially be a short period of confusion or disorientation).
E. The sleepwalking causes clinically significant distress or impairment in social, occupational, or other important areas of functioning.
F. The disturbance is not due to the direct physiological effects of a substance (e.g., a drug of abuse, a medication) or a general medical condition.

From American Psychiatric Association. *Diagnostic and Statistical Manual of Mental Disorders*. 4th ed. Text rev. Washington, DC: American Psychiatric Association; copyright 2000, with permission.

frequency of nightmares, and benzodiazepines have also been used. Contrary to popular belief, no harm results from awakening a person who is having a nightmare.

Sleep Terror Disorder.   Sleep terror disorder is an arousal in the first third of the night during deep NREM (stages 3 and 4) sleep. It is almost invariably inaugurated by a piercing scream or cry and accompanied by behavioral manifestations of intense anxiety bordering on panic (Table 20.2–8).

Typically, patients sit up in bed with a frightened expression, scream loudly, and sometimes awaken immediately with a sense of intense terror. Patients may remain awake in a disoriented state, but more often fall asleep, and, as with sleepwalking, they forget the episodes. A night terror episode after the original scream frequently develops into a sleepwalking episode. Polygraphic recordings of night terrors are somewhat like those of sleepwalking; in fact, the two conditions appear to be closely related. Night terrors, as isolated episodes, are especially frequent in children. About 1 to 6 percent of children have the disorder, which is more common in boys than in girls and tends to run in families.

Night terrors may reflect a minor neurological abnormality, perhaps in the temporal lobe or underlying structures, because when night terrors begin in adolescence and young adulthood, they turn out to be the first symptom of temporal lobe epilepsy. In a typical case of night terrors, however, no signs of temporal lobe epilepsy or other seizure disorders are seen, either clinically or on EEG recordings.

Although night terrors are closely related to sleepwalking and are occasionally related to enuresis, they differ from nightmares. Night terrors are associated with simply awakening in terror. Patients generally have no dream recall but may occasionally recall a single frightening image.

Specific treatment for night terror disorder is seldom required. Investigation of stressful family situations may be important, and individual or family therapy is sometimes useful. In the rare cases in which medication is required, diazepam (Valium) in small doses at bedtime improves the condition and sometimes completely eliminates the attacks.

Sleepwalking Disorder.   Sleepwalking, also known as *somnambulism*, consists of a sequence of complex behaviors that are initiated in the first third of the night during deep NREM (stage 3 and 4) sleep and frequently, although not always, progress—without full consciousness or later memory of the episode—to leaving bed and walking about (Table 20.2–9).

Patients sit up and sometimes perform preservative motor acts, such as walking, dressing, going to the bathroom, talking, screaming, and even driving. The behavior occasionally terminates in awakening, with several minutes of confusion; more frequently, the person returns to sleep without any recollection of the sleepwalking event. An artificially induced arousal from stage 4 sleep can sometimes produce the condition. For instance, in children, especially those with a history of sleepwalking, an attack can sometimes be provoked by standing them on their feet and thus producing a partial arousal during stage 4 sleep.

Sleepwalking usually begins between the ages of 4 and 8 years and tends to dissipate in adolescence. Peak prevalence is at about 12 years of age. The disorder is more common in boys than in girls, and about 15 percent of children have an occasional episode. It tends to run in families. A minor neurological abnormality probably underlies the condition; the episodes should not be considered purely psychogenic, although stressful periods are associated with increased sleepwalking in affected persons. Extreme tiredness or previous sleep deprivation exacerbates attacks. The disorder is occasionally dangerous because of the possibility of accidental injury. Treatment consists primarily in educating and reassuring the parents. Although it can be exacerbated by periods of stress or sleep deprivation, in childhood it is not associated with psychiatric illness. Some cases of sleepwalking can be induced by medication. Medical intervention is rarely needed for typical night terrors or sleepwalking. In difficult cases, some clinicians try the off-label use of benzodiazepines, which decrease slow-wave sleep. Recent reports of sleepwalking associated with the use of the sedative zolpidem (Ambien) require further study.

An 11-year-old girl asked her mother to take her to a psychiatrist because she feared she might be "going crazy." Several times during the last 2 months she had awakened confused about where she was until she realized she was on the living room couch or in her little sister's bed, even though she went to bed in her own room. When she recently woke up in her older brother's bedroom, she became very concerned and felt quite guilty about it. Her younger sister said that she had seen the patient walking during the night, looking like a "zombie," that she didn't answer when she called her, and that the patient had done that several times, but usually went back to her bed. The patient feared she might have "amnesia" because she had no memory of anything happening during the night.

There is no history of seizures or of similar episodes during the day. An EEG and physical examination proved normal. The patient's mental status was unremarkable except for some anxiety about her symptoms and the usual early adolescent concerns. School and family functioning were excellent. (Reprinted with permission from *DSM-IV Casebook*.)

Parasomnia Not Otherwise Specified.   The diagnostic criteria for parasomnia not otherwise specified are given in Table 20.2–10.

SLEEP-RELATED BRUXISM.   Bruxism—tooth grinding—occurs throughout the night, most prominently in stage 2 sleep. According to dentists, 5 to 10 percent of the population has sufficient bruxism to produce noticeable damage to teeth. The condition often goes unnoticed by the sleepers, except for an occasional jaw ache in the morning, but bed partners and roommates are consistently awakened by the sound.

Table 20.2–10
DSM-IV-TR Diagnostic Criteria for Parasomnia Not Otherwise Specified

The parasomnia not otherwise specified category is for disturbances that are characterized by abnormal behavioral or physiological events during sleep or sleep-wake transitions, but that do not meet criteria for a more specific parasomnia. Examples include

1. REM sleep behavior disorder: motor activity, often of a violent nature, that arises during rapid eye movement (REM) sleep. Unlike sleepwalking, these episodes tend to occur later in the night and are associated with vivid dream recall.

2. Sleep paralysis: an inability to perform voluntary movement during the transition between wakefulness and sleep. The episodes may occur at sleep onset (hypnagogic) or with awakening (hypnopompic). The episodes are usually associated with extreme anxiety and, in some cases, fear of impending death. Sleep paralysis occurs commonly as an ancillary symptom of narcolepsy and, in such cases, should not be coded separately.

3. Situations in which the clinician has concluded that a parasomnia is present but is unable to determine whether it is primary, due to a general medical condition, or substance induced.

From American Psychiatric Association. *Diagnostic and Statistical Manual of Mental Disorders.* 4th ed. Text rev. Washington, DC: American Psychiatric Association; copyright 2000, with permission.

Treatment consists in using a dental bite plate and corrective orthodontic procedures.

REM SLEEP BEHAVIOR DISORDER.   REM behavior disorder is characterized by episodes of complex, often violent behavior and is thought to represent a patient acting out his or her dreams. It is more common in older men, and often a history exists of a small stroke or other CNS insult in recent months or last year. It can also appear as an early event in the evolution of Parkinson's disease. If an episode is captured on the polygraph, it shows motor artifact appearing out of REM sleep. If a patient with REM behavior disorder does not have an episode while in the laboratory, the sleep study may show a failure of the normal hypotonia of the weight-bearing muscles during REM sleep. In cats, a syndrome that is suggestive of REM behavior disorder can be induced by lesions of the areas surrounding the locus ceruleus, a brainstem noradrenergic center. The initial view was that the clinical disorder represents a malfunction of the descending pathway to the spinal cord, which produces atonia during REM; its prevalence in the elderly and in patients with Parkinson's disease has suggested a more complex etiology involving alteration of function in pontine areas, including the nucleus pedunculopontine, where integration of sleep-wake regulation with locomotor systems takes place. The most widely used treatment for REM behavior disorder is the off-label administration of clonazepam (Klonopin), 0.5 to 2.0 mg a day. Carbamazepine, 100 mg three times a day, is also effective in controlling the disorder.

SLEEPTALKING (SOMNILOQUY).   Sleeptalking is common in children and adults. It has been studied extensively in the sleep laboratory and is found in all stages of sleep. The talking usually involves a few words that are difficult to distinguish. Long episodes of talking involve the sleeper's life and concerns, but sleeptalkers do not relate their dreams during sleep, nor do they often reveal deep secrets. Episodes of sleeptalking sometimes accompany night terrors and sleepwalking. Sleeptalking alone requires no treatment.

SLEEP-RELATED HEAD BANGING (JACTATIO CAPITIS NOCTURNA).   Sleep-related head banging is the term for a sleep behavior consisting chiefly in rhythmic to-and-fro head rocking (less commonly, total body rocking) occurring just before or during sleep. Usually, it is observed in the immediate presleep period and is sustained into light sleep. It uncommonly persists into, or occurs in, deep NREM sleep. Treatment consists in using measures to prevent injury.

SLEEP PARALYSIS.   Familial sleep paralysis is characterized by a sudden inability to execute voluntary movements, either just at the onset of sleep or on awakening during the night or in the morning.

SLEEP DISORDERS RELATED TO ANOTHER MENTAL DISORDER. DSM-IV-TR defines a sleep disorder related to another mental disorder as a complaint of sleep disturbance caused by a diagnosable mental disorder but sufficiently severe to merit clinical attention on its own.

Insomnia Related to Axis I or Axis II Disorder

Insomnia that occurs for at least 1 month and is clearly related to the psychological and behavioral symptoms of the clinically well-known mental disorders is classified here (Table 20.2–11). The category consists of a heterogeneous group of conditions. The sleep problem is usually, but not always, difficulty falling asleep secondary to anxiety that is part of any of the various mental disorders listed. The insomnia is more common in women than in men. In clear-cut cases in which the anxiety has psychological roots, psychiatric treatment of the anxiety (e.g., individual psychotherapy, group psychotherapy, or family therapy) often relieves the insomnia.

Table 20.2–11
DSM-IV-TR Diagnostic Criteria for Insomnia Related to Another Mental Disorder

A. The predominant complaint is difficulty initiating or maintaining sleep, or nonrestorative sleep, for at least 1 month that is associated with daytime fatigue or impaired daytime functioning.
B. The sleep disturbance (or daytime sequelae) causes clinically significant distress or impairment in social, occupational, or other important areas of functioning.
C. The insomnia is judged to be related to another Axis I or Axis II disorder (e.g., major depressive disorder, generalized anxiety disorder, adjustment disorder with anxiety) but is sufficiently severe to warrant independent clinical attention.
D. The disturbance is not better accounted for by another sleep disorder (e.g., narcolepsy, breathing-related sleep disorder, a parasomnia).
E. The disturbance is not due to the direct physiological effects of a substance (e.g., a drug of abuse, a medication) or a general medical condition.

From American Psychiatric Association. *Diagnostic and Statistical Manual of Mental Disorders.* 4th ed. Text rev. Washington, DC: American Psychiatric Association; copyright 2000, with permission.

The insomnia associated with major depressive disorder involves relatively normal sleep onset but repeated awakenings during the second half of the night and premature morning awakening, usually with an uncomfortable mood in the morning. (Morning is the worst time of day for many patients with major depressive disorder.) Polysomnography shows reduced stage 3 and 4 sleep, often a short REM latency, and a long first REM period. The use of partial or total sleep deprivation can accelerate the response to antidepressant medication.

B.A. awoke in the middle of the night gasping for breath, sweating, shaking, and experiencing palpitations. He felt his pulse; it was 120. He thought, "I could be dying." It was his third attack of the week and at least his tenth that month that had awakened him from sleep. The problem, which had begun 2 years previously when he turned 50, was getting much worse: not only was he having trouble staying asleep because of similar attacks, but after such nights he felt tired all day. He decided to take a friend's advice and seek help from the psychiatrist who specialized in sleep problems.

The psychiatrist elicited this additional history. Attacks of panic occurring during the day had begun at age 12 and had recurred every few months since that time. They did not begin to occur during sleep until the patient turned 50, 2 years earlier. A few months ago the attacks had become much rarer, after the patient had discontinued drinking the 8 to 10 beers he had drunk every weekend for most of his adult life. His weight had fallen from 227 pounds to a mildly overweight 181 pounds, and the mild hypertension he had had for several years disappeared.

In addition to the recurrent attacks, for most of his life the patient had also felt anxious in anticipation of particular situations, including being shut inside airplanes or elevators or traveling in the middle lane of a road. On a turnpike he counted the exits until he could leave, fearing that he would have a panic attack.

He described a fear of falling apart if he ever got too far from his "support system," his term for a beer cooler, which he carried with him always, although he rarely drank the beer. In anticipation of an airplane flight, however, he would drink six to eight beers. He almost always had a company employee, his son, or a friend accompany him, and particularly disliked plane flights when he was not with a familiar person. The night after he drank, the anxiety almost always occurred, awakening him from sleep.

Mr. A ran a successful auto parts business and consulted for several others. Recently, however, anxiety had prevented his accepting a huge government contract to set up an international distribution system for retail stores on military bases. He felt he would be too exposed to scrutiny and would therefore fail. He also worried that some long plane rides would be unavoidable.

During the interview Mr. A was highly verbal, informative, cheerful, friendly, and engaging. He talked about uncomfortable subjects frankly and productively. He had two sisters and two daughters who had "agoraphobia"; one of the daughters was housebound.

Initially, the patient was thought to have sleep apnea (recurrent periods of not breathing during sleep), on the basis of the loud snoring that he reported and the awakening provoked by drinking alcohol, relieved by weight loss, and the presence of mild hypertension. (Reprinted with permission from *DSM-IV-TR Casebook.*)

Panic disorder may be associated with paroxysmal awakenings or with entering stage 3 and 4 sleep. The emotional and cognitive symptoms of a panic attack are present, along with tachycardia and increased respiratory rate. Patients with manic episodes and bipolar II disorder appear to be extreme cases of short sleepers. They sometimes appear to have difficulty falling asleep but most often do not complain of sleep problems. They awaken refreshed after 2 to 4 hours of sleep and appear to have a true reduction in their need for sleep during the course of the manic or hypomanic episode. In schizophrenia, total sleep time and slow-wave sleep are reduced. REM sleep is often reduced early during an exacerbation. Other conditions associated with insomnia include posttraumatic stress disorder (nightmares), obsessive-compulsive disorder (rituals), and eating disorders. Attention-deficit/hyperactivity disorder has been linked to higher-than-normal rates of sleep disturbance (usually difficulty falling asleep). At times, this can be exacerbated by the patient's schedule of stimulant administration; special care should be taken when designing a medication regimen.

Hypersomnia Related to Axis I or Axis II Disorder

Hypersomnia that occurs for at least 1 month and is associated with a mental disorder is found in a variety of conditions, including mood disorders. Excessive daytime sleepiness may be reported in the initial stages of many mild depressive disorders and characteristically in the depressed phase of bipolar I disorder. For a few weeks, hypersomnia sometimes is associated with uncomplicated grief. Other mental disorders—such as personality disorders, dissociative disorders, somatoform disorders,

Table 20.2–12
DSM-IV-TR Diagnostic Criteria for Hypersomnia
Related to Another Mental Disorder

A. The predominant complaint is excessive sleepiness for at least 1 month as evidenced by either prolonged sleep episodes or daytime sleep episodes that occur almost daily.
B. The excessive sleepiness causes clinically significant distress or impairment in social, occupational, or other important areas of functioning.
C. The hypersomnia is judged to be related to another Axis I or Axis II disorder (e.g., major depressive disorder, dysthymic disorder) but is sufficiently severe to warrant independent clinical attention.
D. The disturbance is not better accounted for by another sleep disorder (e.g., narcolepsy, breathing-related sleep disorder, a parasomnia) or by an inadequate amount of sleep.
E. The disturbance is not due to the direct physiological effects of a substance (e.g., a drug of abuse, a medication) or a general medical condition.

From American Psychiatric Association. *Diagnostic and Statistical Manual of Mental Disorders.* 4th ed. Text rev. Washington, DC: American Psychiatric Association; copyright 2000, with permission.

dissociative fugue, and amnestic disorders—can produce hypersomnia (Table 20.2–12). Treatment of the primary disorder should resolve the hypersomnia.

OTHER SLEEP DISORDERS

The DSM-IV-TR defines a sleep disorder caused by a medical condition as a complaint of sleep disturbance produced by a physiological effect of the medical condition on the sleep-wake system. A substance-induced sleep disorder arises from the use, or the recently discontinued use, of a substance.

Sleep Disorder Due to a General Medical Condition

Any sleep disturbance (e.g., insomnia, hypersomnia, parasomnia, or a combination) can be caused by a general medical condition (Table 20.2–13). Almost any medical condition associated with pain and discomfort (e.g., arthritis or angina) can produce insomnia. Some conditions are associated with insomnia even when pain and discomfort are not specifically present. These conditions include neoplasms, vascular lesions, infections, and degenerative and traumatic conditions. Other conditions, especially endocrine and metabolic diseases, frequently involve some sleep disturbance.

Being aware of the possibility of such conditions and obtaining a good medical history usually lead to a correct diagnosis. The treatment, when possible, is treatment of the underlying medical condition.

Sleep-Related Epileptic Seizures.   The relation of sleep and epilepsy is complex. Sleep disorders (sleep apnea, in particular) can exacerbate seizures. Seizures, in turn, can disrupt sleep structure, particularly REM sleep. When seizures occur almost exclusively during sleep, the condition is called *sleep epilepsy.*

Sleep-Related Cluster Headaches and Chronic Paroxysmal Hemicrania.   Sleep-related cluster headaches are agonizingly severe unilateral headaches that often appear during sleep and are

Table 20.2–13
DSM-IV-TR Diagnostic Criteria for Sleep Disorder
Due to a General Medical Condition

A. A prominent disturbance in sleep that is sufficiently severe to warrant independent clinical attention.
B. There is evidence from the history, physical examination, or laboratory findings that the sleep disturbance is the direct physiological consequence of a general medical condition.
C. The disturbance is not better accounted for by another mental disorder (e.g., an adjustment disorder in which the stressor is a serious medical illness).
D. The disturbance does not occur exclusively during the course of a delirium.
E. The disturbance does not meet the criteria for breathing-related sleep disorder or narcolepsy.
F. The sleep disturbance causes clinically significant distress or impairment in social, occupational, or other important areas of functioning.

Specify type:
   Insomnia type: if the predominant sleep disturbance is insomnia
   Hypersomnia type: if the predominant sleep disturbance is hypersomnia
   Parasomnia type: if the predominant sleep disturbance is a parasomnia
   Mixed type: if more than one sleep disturbance is present and none predominates
Coding note: Include the name of the general medical condition on Axis I, e.g., sleep disorder due to chronic obstructive pulmonary disease, insomnia type; also code the general medical condition on Axis III.

From American Psychiatric Association. *Diagnostic and Statistical Manual of Mental Disorders.* 4th ed. Text rev. Washington, DC: American Psychiatric Association; copyright 2000, with permission.

marked by an on-off pattern of attacks. Chronic paroxysmal hemicrania is a similar unilateral headache that occurs every day with more frequent but short-lived onsets that are without a preponderant sleep distribution. Both types of vascular headaches are examples of sleep-exacerbated conditions and appear in association with REM sleep periods; paroxysmal hemicrania is virtually REM sleep locked.

Sleep-Related Abnormal Swallowing Syndrome.   Abnormal swallowing syndrome is a condition during sleep in which inadequate swallowing results in aspiration of saliva, coughing, and choking. It is intermittently associated with brief arousals or awakenings.

Sleep-Related Asthma.   Asthma that is exacerbated by sleep in some persons can result in significant sleep disturbances.

Sleep-Related Cardiovascular Symptoms.   Sleep-related cardiovascular symptoms derive from disorders of cardiac rhythm, myocardial incompetence, coronary artery insufficiency, and blood pressure variability, which may be induced or exacerbated by sleep-altered or sleep-state-modified cardiovascular physiology.

Sleep-Related Gastroesophageal Reflux.   Sleep-related gastroesophageal reflux is a disorder in which patients awaken from sleep with burning, substernal pain or a feeling of general pain or tightness in the chest or a sour taste in the mouth. Coughing, choking, and vague respiratory discomfort may also occur repeatedly.

Sleep-Related Hemolysis (Paroxysmal Nocturnal Hemoglobinuria).   Paroxysmal nocturnal hemoglobinuria is a rare, acquired, chronic hemolytic anemia in which intravascular hemolysis results in hemoglobinemia and hemoglobinuria. The hemolysis and consequent hemoglobinuria are accelerated during sleep, and the morning urine is brownish red. Hemolysis is linked to the sleep period, even when the period is shifted.

Substance-Induced Sleep Disorder

Any sleep disturbance (e.g., insomnia, hypersomnia, parasomnia, or a combination) can be caused by a substance (Table 20.2–14). According to DSM-IV-TR, clinicians should also specify whether the onset of the disorder occurred during intoxication or withdrawal.

Somnolence related to tolerance or withdrawal from a CNS stimulant is common in persons withdrawing from amphetamines, cocaine, caffeine, and related substances. The somnolence may be associated with severe depression, which occasionally reaches suicidal proportions. Sustained use of a CNS depressant, such as alcohol, can cause somnolence. Heavy alcohol use in the evening produces sleepiness and difficulty arising the next day. This reaction may present a diagnostic problem when patients do not admit alcohol abuse.

Insomnia is associated with tolerance to, or withdrawal from, sedative-hypnotic drugs, such as benzodiazepines, barbiturates, and chloral hydrate. With the sustained use of such agents—usually undertaken to treat insomnia arising from a different source—tolerance increases, and the drugs lose their sleep-inducing effects; patients then often increase the dose. On sudden discontinuation of the drug, severe sleeplessness supervenes, often accompanied by the general features of substance withdrawal. Typically, patients experience a temporary increase in the severity of the insomnia.

Long-term use (more than 30 days) of a hypnotic agent is well tolerated by some patients, but others begin to complain of sleep disturbance, most often multiple brief awakenings during the night. Recordings show a disruption of sleep architecture, reduced stage 3 and 4 sleep, increased stage 1 and 2 sleep, and fragmentation of sleep throughout the night.

Clinicians should be aware of CNS stimulants as a possible cause of insomnia and should remember that various medications for weight reduction, beverages containing caffeine, and, occasionally, adrenergic drugs taken by asthmatic patients may all produce this insomnia. Alcohol may help induce sleep but frequently results in nocturnal awakening. Alcohol use during the cocktail hour can produce difficulty falling asleep later in the evening.

For reasons that are not always clear, a wide variety of drugs occasionally produce sleep problems as a side effect. These drugs include antimetabolites and other cancer chemotherapeutic agents, thyroid preparations, anticonvulsant agents, antidepressant drugs, adrenocorticotropic hormone–like drugs, oral contraceptives, α-methyldopa, and β-adrenergic receptor antagonists.

Other agents do not produce sleep disturbance while being used but may have this effect after withdrawal. Almost any sedating or tranquilizing agent, including at times the benzodiazepines, the phenothiazines, the sedating tricyclic drugs, and various street drugs, including marijuana and opioids, can have this effect.

Alcohol is a CNS depressant and produces the serious problems of other CNS depressants, both during administration—perhaps related to the development of tolerance—and after withdrawal. The insomnia after long-term alcohol consumption is sometimes severe and lasts for weeks or longer. Clinicians should not give potentially addicting medications to patients who have

Table 20.2–14
DSM-IV-TR Diagnostic Criteria for Substance-Induced Sleep Disorder

A. A prominent disturbance in sleep that is sufficiently severe to warrant independent clinical attention.
B. There is evidence from the history, physical examination, or laboratory findings of either (1) or (2):
   (1) the symptoms in Criterion A developed during, or within a month of, substance intoxication or withdrawal
   (2) medication use is etiologically related to the sleep disturbance
C. The disturbance is not better accounted for by a sleep disorder that is not substance induced. Evidence that the symptoms are better accounted for by a sleep disorder that is not substance induced might include the following: the symptoms precede the onset of the substance use (or medication use); the symptoms persist for a substantial period of time (e.g., about a month) after the cessation of acute withdrawal or severe intoxication or are substantially in excess of what would be expected given the type or amount of the substance used or the duration of use; or there is other evidence that suggests the existence of an independent non–substance-induced sleep disorder (e.g., a history of recurrent non–substance-related episodes).
D. The disturbance does not occur exclusively during the course of a delirium.
E. The sleep disturbance causes clinically significant distress or impairment in social, occupational, or other important areas of functioning.

Note: This diagnosis should be made instead of a diagnosis of substance intoxication or substance withdrawal only when the sleep symptoms are in excess of those usually associated with the intoxication or withdrawal syndrome and when the symptoms are sufficiently severe to warrant independent clinical attention.

Code [Specific substance]-induced sleep disorder:
   Alcohol; amphetamine; caffeine; cocaine; opioid; sedative, hypnotic, or anxiolytic; other [or unknown] substance

Specify type:
   Insomnia type: if the predominant sleep disturbance is insomnia
   Hypersomnia type: if the predominant sleep disturbance is hypersomnia
   Parasomnia type: if the predominant sleep disturbance is a parasomnia
   Mixed type: if more than one sleep disturbance is present and none predominates

Specify if:
   With onset during intoxication: if the criteria are met for intoxication with the substance and the symptoms develop during the intoxication syndrome
   With onset during withdrawal: if criteria are met for withdrawal from the substance and the symptoms develop during, or shortly after, a withdrawal syndrome

From American Psychiatric Association. *Diagnostic and Statistical Manual of Mental Disorders.* 4th ed. Text rev. Washington, DC: American Psychiatric Association; copyright 2000, with permission.

just recovered from an addiction; if possible, sleeping medications should be avoided.

Among cigarette smokers, the combination of a relaxing ritual and the tendency of low doses of nicotine to cause sedation may actually help sleep, but high doses of nicotine can interfere with sleep, particularly sleep onset. Cigarette smokers typically sleep less than nonsmokers. Nicotine withdrawal can cause drowsiness or arousal.

21

Impulse-Control Disorders Not Elsewhere Classified

Six conditions comprise the category of impulse-control disorders not elsewhere specified. They include (1) intermittent explosive disorder, (2) kleptomania, (3) pyromania, (4) pathological gambling, (5) trichotillomania, and (6) impulse-control disorder not otherwise specified (NOS). Each disorder is characterized by the inability to resist an intense impulse, drive, or temptation to perform a particular act that is obviously harmful to self or others, or both. Before the event, the individual usually experiences mounting tension and arousal, sometimes—but not consistently—mingled with conscious anticipatory pleasure. Completing the action brings immediate gratification and relief. Within a variable time afterward, the individual experiences a conflation of remorse, guilt, self-reproach, and dread. These feelings may stem from obscure unconscious conflicts or awareness of the deed's impact on others (including the possibility of serious legal consequences in syndromes such as kleptomania). Shameful secretiveness about the repeated impulsive activity frequently expands to pervade the individual's entire life, often significantly delaying treatment.

ETIOLOGY

Psychodynamic, psychosocial, and biological factors all play an important role in impulse-control disorders; however, the primary causal factor remains unknown. Some impulse-control disorders may have common underlying neurobiological mechanisms. Fatigue, incessant stimulation, and psychic trauma can lower a person's resistance to control impulses.

Psychodynamic Factors

An impulse is a disposition to act to decrease heightened tension caused by the buildup of instinctual drives or by diminished ego defenses against the drives. The impulse disorders have in common an attempt to bypass the experience of disabling symptoms or painful affects by acting on the environment. In his work with adolescents who were delinquent, August Aichhorn described impulsive behavior as related to a weak superego and weak ego structures associated with psychic trauma produced by childhood deprivation.

Otto Fenichel linked impulsive behavior to attempts to master anxiety, guilt, depression, and other painful affects by means of action. He thought that such actions defend against internal danger and that they produce a distorted aggressive or sexual gratification. To observers, impulsive behaviors may appear irrational and motivated by greed, but they may actually be endeavors to find relief from pain.

Heinz Kohut considered many forms of impulse-control problems, including gambling, kleptomania, and some paraphiliac behaviors, to be related to an incomplete sense of self. He observed that when patients do not receive the validating and affirming responses that they seek from persons in significant relationships with them, the self might fragment. As a way of dealing with this fragmentation and regaining a sense of wholeness or cohesion in the self, persons may engage in impulsive behaviors that to others appear self-destructive. Kohut's formulation has some similarities to Donald Winnicott's view that impulsive or deviant behavior in children is a way for them to try to recapture a primitive maternal relationship. Winnicott saw such behavior as hopeful in that the child searches for affirmation and love from the mother rather than abandoning any attempt to win her affection.

Patients attempt to master anxiety, guilt, depression, and other painful affects by means of actions, but such actions aimed at obtaining relief seldom succeed even temporarily.

Psychosocial Factors

Psychosocial factors implicated causally in impulse-control disorders are related to early-life events. The growing child may have had improper models for identification, such as parents who had difficulty controlling impulses. Other psychosocial factors associated with the disorders include exposure to violence in the home, alcohol abuse, promiscuity, and antisocial behavior.

Biological Factors

Many investigators have focused on possible organic factors in the impulse-control disorders, especially for patients with overtly violent behavior. Experiments have shown that impulsive and violent activity is associated with specific brain regions, such as the limbic system, and that the inhibition of such behaviors is associated with other brain regions. A relation has been found between low cerebrospinal fluid (CSF) levels of 5-hydroxyindoleacetic acid (5-HIAA) and impulsive aggression. Certain hormones, especially testosterone, have also been associated with violent and aggressive behavior. Some reports have described a relation between temporal lobe epilepsy and certain impulsive violent behaviors, as well as an association of aggressive behavior in patients who have histories of head trauma with increased numbers of emergency room visits and other potential organic antecedents. A high incidence of mixed cerebral dominance may be found in some violent populations.

Considerable evidence indicates that the serotonin neurotransmitter system mediates symptoms evident in impulse-control disorders. Brainstem and CSF levels of 5-HIAA are decreased and serotonin-binding sites are increased in persons who have committed suicide. The dopaminergic and noradrenergic systems have also been implicated in impulsivity.

Impulse-control disorder symptoms can continue into adulthood in persons whose disorder has been diagnosed as childhood attention-deficit/hyperactivity disorder (ADHD). Lifelong or acquired mental deficiency, epilepsy, and even reversible brain syndromes have long been implicated in lapses in impulse control.

INTERMITTENT EXPLOSIVE DISORDER

Intermittent explosive disorder manifests as discrete episodes of losing control of aggressive impulses; these episodes can result in serious assault or the destruction of property. The aggressiveness expressed is grossly out of proportion to any stressors that may have helped elicit the episodes. The symptoms, which patients may describe as spells or attacks, appear within minutes or hours and, regardless of duration, remit spontaneously and quickly. After each episode, patients usually show genuine regret or self-reproach, and signs of generalized impulsivity or aggressiveness are absent between episodes. The diagnosis of intermittent explosive disorder should not be made if the loss of control can be accounted for by schizophrenia, antisocial or borderline personality disorder, ADHD, conduct disorder, or substance intoxication.

Epidemiology

Intermittent explosive disorder is underreported. The disorder appears to be more common in men than in women. The men are likely to be found in correctional institutions and the women in psychiatric facilities. In one study, about 2 percent of all persons admitted to a university hospital psychiatric service had disorders that were diagnosed as intermittent explosive disorder; 80 percent were men.

Evidence indicates that intermittent explosive disorder is more common in first-degree biological relatives of persons with the disorder than in the general population. Many factors other than a simple genetic explanation may be responsible.

Comorbidity

High rates of fire setting in patients with intermittent explosive disorder have been reported. Other disorders of impulse control and substance use and mood, anxiety, and eating disorders have also been associated with intermittent explosive disorder.

Etiology

Psychodynamic Factors. Psychoanalysts have suggested that explosive outbursts occur as a defense against narcissistic injurious events. Rage outbursts serve as interpersonal distance and protect against any further narcissistic injury.

Psychosocial Factors. Typical patients have been described as physically large but dependent men whose sense of masculine identity is

poor. A sense of being useless and impotent or of being unable to change the environment often precedes an episode of physical violence, and a high level of anxiety, guilt, and depression usually follows an episode.

An unfavorable childhood environment often filled with alcohol dependence, beatings, and threats to life is usual in these patients. Predisposing factors in infancy and childhood include perinatal trauma, infantile seizures, head trauma, encephalitis, minimal brain dysfunction, and hyperactivity. Workers who have concentrated on psychogenesis as causing episodic explosiveness have stressed identification with assaultive parental figures as symbols of the target for violence. Early frustration, oppression, and hostility have been noted as predisposing factors. Situations that are directly or symbolically reminiscent of early deprivations (e.g., persons who directly or indirectly evoke the image of the frustrating parent) become targets for destructive hostility.

Biological Factors. Some investigators suggest that disordered brain physiology, particularly in the limbic system, is involved in most cases of episodic violence. Compelling evidence indicates that serotonergic neurons mediate behavioral inhibition. Decreased serotonergic transmission, which can be induced by inhibiting serotonin synthesis or by antagonizing its effects, decreases the effect of punishment as a deterrent to behavior. The restoration of serotonin activity by administering serotonin precursors such as L-tryptophan or drugs that increase synaptic serotonin levels restores the behavioral effect of punishment, and appears to restore control of episodic violent tendencies. Low levels of CSF 5-HIAA have been correlated with impulsive aggression. High CSF testosterone concentrations are correlated with aggressiveness and interpersonal violence in men. Antiandrogenic agents have been shown to decrease aggression.

Familial and Genetic Factors. First-degree relatives of patients with intermittent explosive disorder have higher rates of impulse-control disorders, depressive disorders, and substance use disorders than the general population. Biological relatives of patients with the disorder were more likely to have histories of temper or explosive outbursts than the general population.

Diagnosis and Clinical Features

The diagnosis of intermittent explosive disorder should be the result of history taking that reveals several episodes of loss of control associated with aggressive outbursts (Table 21–1). One

Table 21–1
DSM-IV-TR Diagnostic Criteria for Intermittent Explosive Disorder

A. Several discrete episodes of failure to resist aggressive impulses that result in serious assaultive acts or destruction of property.
B. The degree of aggressiveness expressed during the episodes is grossly out of proportion to any precipitating psychosocial stressors.
C. The aggressive episodes are not better accounted for by another mental disorder (e.g., antisocial personality disorder, borderline personality disorder, a psychotic disorder, a manic episode, conduct disorder, or attention-deficit/hyperactivity disorder) and are not due to the direct physiological effects of a substance (e.g., a drug of abuse, a medication) or a general medical condition (e.g., head trauma, Alzheimer's disease).

From American Psychiatric Association. *Diagnostic and Statistical Manual of Mental Disorders.* 4th ed. Text rev. Washington, DC: American Psychiatric Association; copyright 2000, with permission.

Jane was a 42-year-old, highly successful, single executive from a wealthy background. She called herself a "shop-'til-you-drop type" and had always been able to afford the expensive designer clothing that she loved. Since college, her "legit" shopping had been paralleled by "boosting" cheap panties and brassieres from discount stores. She did not wear the stolen items; indeed, she considered them "sleazy." She could never bring herself to get rid of them either and kept boxes filled with pilfered lingerie in a storage facility.

Jane talked or bought her way out of trouble until her 30s, when she was arrested while stealing pantyhose from the same K-Mart for the third time in as many months. As a condition of probation, she was ordered to see a psychiatrist. Her attendance was sporadic, and several more thefts occurred over the next 2 years. She also experienced substantial depression, which she tried to alleviate by heavy drinking.

Jane finally began taking her problem seriously after yet another arrest precipitated a suicidal gesture. She began keeping appointments regularly and consented to taking citalopram (Celexa) and naltrexone (ReVia). She believes that her participation in an AA (Alcoholics Anonymous) group for high-pressured executives has been at least as effective—if not more so—in controlling her stealing. (Courtesy of Harvey Roy Greenberg, M.D.)

Differential Diagnosis

Episodes of theft occasionally occur during psychotic illness, for example, acute mania, major depression with psychotic features, or schizophrenia. Psychotic stealing is obviously a product of pathological elevation or depression of mood or command hallucinations or delusions. Theft in individuals with antisocial personality disorder is deliberately undertaken for personal gain, with some degree of premeditation and planning, often executed with others. Antisocial stealing regularly involves the threat of harm or actual violence, particularly to elude capture. Guilt and remorse are distinctively lacking, or patients are patently insincere. Shoplifting has become a national epidemic. Few shoplifters have true kleptomania; most are teenagers and young adults who "boost" in pairs or small groups for "kicks," as well as goods, and do not have a major psychiatric disorder. Acute intoxication with drugs or alcohol may precipitate theft in an individual with another psychiatric disorder or without significant psychopathology. Patients with Alzheimer's disease or other dementing organic illness may leave a store without paying due to forgetfulness rather than larcenous intent. Malingering kleptomania is common in apprehended antisocial types, as well as nonantisocial youthful shoplifters. Given a sufficiently intelligent perpetrator, the fictive version can be difficult to distinguish from the genuine disorder.

Course and Prognosis

Kleptomania may begin in childhood, although most children and adolescents who steal do not become kleptomaniac adults. The onset of the disorder generally is late adolescence. Women are more likely to present for psychiatric evaluation or treatment than are men. Men are more likely to be sent to prison. Men tend to present with the disorder at about 50 years of age and women at about 35 years of age. In quiescent cases, new bouts of the disorder may be precipitated by loss or disappointment.

The course of the disorder waxes and wanes, but it tends to be chronic. Persons sometimes have bouts of being unable to resist the impulse to steal, followed by free periods that last for weeks or months. Its spontaneous recovery rate is unknown.

Serious impairment and complications are usually secondary to being caught, particularly to being arrested. Many persons seem never consciously to have considered the possibility of facing the consequences of their acts, a feature that agrees with some descriptions of patients with kleptomania (sometimes, as persons who feel wronged and therefore entitled to steal). Often, the disorder in no way impairs a person's social or work functioning.

The prognosis with treatment can be good, but few patients come for help of their own accord.

Treatment

Because true kleptomania is rare, reports of treatment tend to be individual case descriptions or a short series of cases. Insight-oriented psychotherapy and psychoanalysis have been successful, but depend on patients' motivations. Those who feel guilt and shame may be helped by insight-oriented psychotherapy because of their increased motivation to change their behavior.

Behavior therapy, including systematic desensitization, aversive conditioning, and a combination of aversive conditioning and altered social contingencies, has been reported successful, even when motivation was lacking. The reports cite follow-up studies of up to 2 years. SSRIs, such as fluoxetine (Prozac) and fluvoxamine (Luvox), appear to be effective in some patients with kleptomania. Case reports indicated successful treatment with tricyclic drugs, trazodone, lithium, valproate, naltrexone, and electroconvulsive therapy.

PYROMANIA

Pyromania is the recurrent, deliberate, and purposeful setting of fires. Associated features include tension or affective arousal before setting the fires; fascination with, interest in, curiosity about, or attraction to fire and the activities and equipment associated with firefighting; and pleasure, gratification, or relief when setting fires or when witnessing or participating in their aftermath. Patients may make considerable advance preparations before starting a fire. Pyromania differs from arson in that the latter is done for financial gain, revenge, or other reasons and is planned beforehand.

Epidemiology

No information is available on the prevalence of pyromania, but only a small percentage of adults who set fires can be classified as having pyromania. The disorder is found far more often in men than in women, with a male to female ratio of approximately 8:1. More than 40 percent of arrested arsonists are younger than 18 years of age.

Comorbidity

Pyromania is significantly associated with substance abuse disorder (especially alcoholism); affective disorders, depressive or bipolar; other impulse control disorders, such as kleptomania in female fire setters; and various personality disturbances, such as inadequate and borderline personality disorders. Attention-deficit disorder and learning disabilities may be conspicuously associated with childhood pyromania; this constellation frequently persists into adulthood. Persons who set fires are more likely to have mild retardation than are those in the general population. Some studies have noted an increased incidence of alcohol use disorders in persons who set fires. Fire setters also tend to have a history of antisocial traits, such as truancy, running away from home, and delinquency. Enuresis has been considered a common finding in the history of fire setters, although controlled studies have failed to confirm this. Studies, however, have found an association between cruelty to animals and fire setting. Childhood and adolescent fire setting is often associated with ADHD or adjustment disorders.

Etiology

Psychosocial. Sigmund Freud saw fire as a symbol of sexuality. He believed the warmth radiated by fire evokes the same sensation that accompanies a state of sexual excitation, and a flame's shape and movements suggest a phallus in activity. Other psychoanalysts have associated pyromania with an abnormal craving for power and social prestige. Some patients with pyromania are volunteer firefighters who set fires to prove themselves brave, to force other firefighters into action, or to demonstrate their power to extinguish a blaze. The incendiary act is a way to vent accumulated rage over frustration caused by a sense of social, physical, or sexual inferiority. Several studies have noted that the fathers of patients with pyromania were absent from the home. Thus, one explanation of fire setting is that it represents a wish for the absent father to return home as a rescuer, to put out the fire, and to save the child from a difficult existence.

Female fire setters, in addition to being much fewer in number than male fire setters, do not start fires to put firefighters into action as men frequently do. Frequently noted delinquent trends in female fire setters include promiscuity without pleasure and petty stealing, often approaching kleptomania.

Biological Factors. Significantly low CSF levels of 5-HIAA and 3-methoxy-4-hydroxyphenylglycol (MHPG) have been found in fire setters, which suggests possible serotonergic or adrenergic involvement. The presence of reactive hypoglycemia, based on blood glucose concentrations on glucose tolerance tests, has been put forward as a cause of pyromania. Further studies are needed, however.

Diagnosis and Clinical Features

Persons with pyromania often regularly watch fires in their neighborhoods, frequently set off false alarms, and show interest in firefighting paraphernalia (Table 21–3). Their curiosity is evident, but they show no remorse and may be indifferent to the consequences for life or property. Fire setters may gain satisfaction from the resulting destruction; frequently they leave obvious

Table 21–3
DSM-IV-TR Diagnostic Criteria for Pyromania

A. Deliberate and purposeful fire setting on more than one occasion.
B. Tension or affective arousal before the act.
C. Fascination with, interest in, curiosity about, or attraction to fire and its situational contexts (e.g., paraphernalia, uses, consequences).
D. Pleasure, gratification, or relief when setting fires, or when witnessing or participating in their aftermath.
E. The fire setting is not done for monetary gain, as an expression of sociopolitical ideology, to conceal criminal activity, to express anger or vengeance, to improve one's living circumstances, in response to a delusion or hallucination, or as a result of impaired judgment (e.g., in dementia, mental retardation, substance intoxication).
F. The fire setting is not better accounted for by conduct disorder, a manic episode, or antisocial personality disorder.

From American Psychiatric Association. *Diagnostic and Statistical Manual of Mental Disorders.* 4th ed. Text rev. Washington, DC: American Psychiatric Association; copyright 2000, with permission.

clues. Commonly associated features include alcohol intoxication, sexual dysfunctions, below-average intelligence quotient, chronic personal frustration, and resentment toward authority figures. Some fire setters become sexually aroused by the fire.

Differential Diagnosis

Clinicians should have little trouble distinguishing between pyromania and the fascination of many young children with matches, lighters, and fire as part of the normal investigation of their environments. Pyromania must also be separated from incendiary acts of sabotage carried out by dissident political extremists or by paid torches, termed arsonists in the legal system.

When fire setting occurs in conduct disorder and antisocial personality disorder, it is a deliberate act, not a failure to resist an impulse. Fires may be set for profit, sabotage, or retaliation. Patients with schizophrenia or mania may set fires in response to delusions or hallucinations. Patients with brain dysfunction (e.g., dementia), mental retardation, or substance intoxication may set fires because of a failure to appreciate the consequences of the act.

Course and Prognosis

Although fire setting often begins in childhood, the typical age of onset of pyromania is unknown. When the onset is in adolescence or adulthood, the fire setting tends to be deliberately destructive. Fire setting in pyromania is episodic and may wax and wane in frequency. The prognosis for treated children is good, and complete remission is a realistic goal. The prognosis for adults is guarded because they frequently deny their actions, refuse to take responsibility, are dependent on alcohol, and lack insight.

Treatment

Little has been written about the treatment of pyromania, and treating fire setters has been difficult because of their lack of motivation. No single treatment has been proved effective; thus alimentary tract from hair pulling and swallowing—was described in the late 18th century. The term *trichotillomania* was coined by a French dermatologist, Francois Hallopeau, in 1889.

Trichotillomania was once deemed rare, and little about it was described beyond phenomenology. The condition is now regarded as more common. With a substantial increase in research, treatment has greatly improved since the 1980s.

Epidemiology

The prevalence of trichotillomania may be underestimated because of accompanying shame and secretiveness. The diagnosis encompasses at least two categories of hair pullers differing in incidence, severity, age of presentation, and gender ratio. Other subsets may exist.

The potentially most serious, chronic form of the disorder usually begins in early to mid-adolescence, with a lifetime prevalence ranging from 0.6 percent to as high as 3.4 percent in general populations and with a female to male ratio as high as 9:1. The number of men may actually be higher because men are even more likely than women to conceal hair pulling. A patient with chronic trichotillomania is likely to be the only or oldest child in the family.

A childhood type of trichotillomania occurs approximately equally in girls and boys. It is said to be more common than the adolescent or young adult syndrome and is generally far less serious dermatologically and psychologically.

An estimated 33 to 40 percent of patients with trichotillomania chew or swallow the hair that they pull out at one time or another. Of this group, approximately 37.5 percent develop potentially hazardous bezoars.

Comorbidity

Significant comorbidity is found between trichotillomania and OCD (as well as other anxiety disorders); Tourette's syndrome; affective illness, especially depressive conditions; eating disorders; and various personality disorders—particularly obsessive-compulsive, borderline, and narcissistic personality disorders. Comorbid substance abuse disorder is not encountered as frequently as it is in pathological gambling, kleptomania, and other disorders.

Etiology

Although trichotillomania is regarded as multidetermined, its onset has been linked to stressful situations in more than one fourth of all cases. Disturbances in mother–child relationships, fear of being left alone, and recent object loss are often cited as critical factors contributing to the condition. Substance abuse may encourage development of the disorder. Depressive dynamics are often cited as predisposing factors, but no particular personality trait or disorder characterizes patients. Some see self-stimulation as the primary goal of hair pulling.

Trichotillomania is increasingly being viewed as having a biologically determined substrate that may reflect inappropriately released motor activity or excessive grooming behaviors. Biological theories have also pointed to metabolic differences in the serotonin and opioid systems. Family members of trichotillomania patients often have a history of tics, impulse-control disorders, and obsessive-compulsive symptoms, further supporting a possible genetic predisposition.

Table 21–5
DSM-IV-TR Diagnostic Criteria for Trichotillomania

A. Recurrent pulling out of one's hair resulting in noticeable hair loss.
B. An increasing sense of tension immediately before pulling out the hair or when attempting to resist the behavior.
C. Pleasure, gratification, or relief when pulling out the hair.
D. The disturbance is not better accounted for by another mental disorder and is not due to a general medical condition (e.g., a dermatological condition).
E. The disturbance causes clinically significant distress or impairment in social, occupational, or other important areas of functioning.

From American Psychiatric Association. *Diagnostic and Statistical Manual of Mental Disorders.* 4th ed. Text rev. Washington, DC: American Psychiatric Association; copyright 2000, with permission.

Diagnosis and Clinical Features

Before engaging in the behavior, patients with trichotillomania experience an increasing sense of tension and achieve a sense of release or gratification from pulling out their hair (Table 21–5). All areas of the body may be affected, most commonly the scalp. Other areas involved are eyebrows, eyelashes, and beard; trunk, armpits, and pubic area are less commonly involved. Hair loss is often characterized by short, broken strands appearing together with long, normal hairs in the affected areas. No abnormalities of the skin or scalp are present. Hair pulling is not reported to be painful, although pruritus and tingling may occur in the involved area. Trichophagy, mouthing of the hair, may follow the hair plucking. Complications of trichophagy include trichobezoars, malnutrition, and intestinal obstruction. Patients usually deny the behavior and often try to hide the resultant alopecia. Head banging, nail biting, scratching, gnawing, excoriation, and other acts of self-mutilation may be present.

Kathy was a 24-year-old editor who had suffered from trichotillomania since 17 years of age. Typical hair-pulling behavior began during junior year at a highly competitive private high school in the setting of increasing torment by ruminations about not getting into the "right" college. She plucked, chewed, and swallowed hair from the top and sides of her scalp, as well as her eyebrows. She concealed hair pulling from her family and friends, because she thought "I was going nuts." She finally blurted out her symptoms to a trusted pediatrician during a routine office visit.

Kathy's parents were professionals who made intense academic demands on all of their children; family life was otherwise not notably problematic. As a child, she was extremely critical of herself and afraid of failure. Her father experienced mild periodic depression since college. One brother developed obsessions and compulsions during his late teens. Both responded well to fluoxetine (Prozac).

Kathy had received analytic psychotherapy, behavioral therapy, and medication (recently fluoxetine and clomipramine) elsewhere. Although she made reasonably good progress psychologically, she was never able to stop pulling her hair long enough for it to grow back. She had a wide circle of friends but still kept romance at arm's length, fearing that a potential lover would be frightened off if he found out her "secret." She could not bring herself to replace the "ratty" wig that she had been wearing since her late teens. "It makes me look dowdy," she said, "but buying a new one would be like telling myself I'll never get better."

Kathy sought treatment chiefly for regulation of her medication but quickly proved amenable to weekly psychotherapy sessions. Her clomipramine was increased, while she explored the sense of damage and "freakiness" that made her fend off men who liked her. She was much helped by weekly meetings at a trichotillomania support group. After 6 months, her self-esteem had improved, she had fewer bouts of hair pulling and had begun dating hesitantly. She arrived at her last session displaying an attractive new wig, stating ironically: "It isn't my real hair yet, but at least it's better than my old rug." (Courtesy of Harvey Roy Greenberg, M.D.)

Pathology and Laboratory Examination

If necessary, the clinical diagnosis of trichotillomania can be confirmed by punch biopsy of the scalp. In patients with a trichobezoar, blood count may reveal a mild leukocytosis and hypochromic anemia due to blood loss. Appropriate chemistries and radiological studies should also be performed, depending on the bezoar's suspected location and impact on the gastrointestinal tract.

Differential Diagnosis

Hair pulling may be a wholly benign condition or it may occur in the context of several mental disorders. The phenomenologies of trichotillomania and OCD overlap. As with OCD, trichotillomania is often chronic and recognized by patients as undesirable. Unlike those with OCD, patients with trichotillomania do not experience obsessive thoughts, and the compulsive activity is limited to one act, hair pulling. Patients with factitious disorder with predominantly physical signs and symptoms actively seek medical attention and the patient role and deliberately simulate illness toward these ends. Patients who malinger or who have factitious disorder may mutilate themselves to get medical attention, but they do not acknowledge the self-inflicted nature of the lesions. Patients with stereotypic movement disorder have stereotypical and rhythmic movements, and they usually do not seem distressed by their behavior. A biopsy may be necessary to distinguish trichotillomania from alopecia areata and tinea capitis.

Course and Prognosis

The mean age at onset of trichotillomania is in the early teens, most frequently before age 17 years, but onsets have been reported much later in life. The course of the disorder is not well known; both chronic and remitting forms occur. An early onset (before age 6 years) tends to remit more readily and responds to suggestion, support, and behavioral strategies. Late onset (after age 13 years) is associated with an increased likelihood of chronicity and poorer prognosis than the early-onset form. About one third of persons presenting for treatment report a duration of 1 year or less, whereas in some cases, the disorder has persisted for more than two decades.

Treatment

No consensus exists on the best treatment modality for trichotillomania. Treatment usually involves psychiatrists and dermatologists in a joint endeavor. Psychopharmacological methods that have been used to treat psychodermatological disorders include topical steroids and hydroxyzine hydrochloride (Vistaril), an anxiolytic with antihistamine properties; antidepressants; serotonergic agents; and antipsychotics. Whether depression is present or not, antidepressant agents can lead to dermatological improvement. Current evidence strongly points to the efficacy of drugs that alter central serotonin turnover. Patients who respond poorly to SSRIs may improve with augmentation with pimozide (Orap), a dopamine receptor antagonist. A report of successful lithium treatment for trichotillomania cited the possible effect of the drug on aggression, impulsivity, and mood instability as an explanation. Lithium also possesses serotonergic activity. Case reports indicate successful treatment with buspirone, clonazepam (Klonopin), and trazodone. In one placebo-controlled study, patients taking naltrexone had a reduction in symptom severity.

Successful behavioral treatments, such as biofeedback, self-monitoring, covert desensitization, and habit reversal, have been reported, but most studies have been based on individual cases or a small series of cases with relatively short follow-up periods. Further controlled study of the treatments is warranted. Chronic trichotillomania has been treated successfully with insight-oriented psychotherapy. Hypnotherapy and behavior therapy have been mentioned as potentially effective in the treatment of dermatological disorders in which psychological factors may be involved; the skin has been shown to be susceptible to hypnotic suggestion.

IMPULSE-CONTROL DISORDER NOT OTHERWISE SPECIFIED

The DSM-IV-TR diagnostic category of impulse-control disorder not otherwise specified (Table 21–6) is a residual category for disorders of impulse control that do not meet the criteria for a specific impulse-control disorder.

Table 21–6
DSM-IV-TR Diagnostic Criteria for Impulse-Control Disorder Not Otherwise Specified

This category is for disorders of impulse control (e.g., skin picking) that do not meet the criteria for any specific impulse-control disorder or for another mental disorder having features involving impulse control described elsewhere in the manual (e.g., substance dependence, a paraphilia).

From American Psychiatric Association. *Diagnostic and Statistical Manual of Mental Disorders.* 4th ed. Text rev. Washington, DC: American Psychiatric Association; copyright 2000, with permission.

Table 21–7
Diagnostic Criteria for Compulsive Buying

A. Maladaptive preoccupation with buying or shopping, or maladaptive buying or shopping impulses or behavior, as indicated by at least one of the following:
  1. Frequent preoccupation with buying or impulses to buy that are experienced as irresistible, intrusive, and/or senseless.
  2. Frequent buying of more than can be afforded, frequent buying of items that are not needed, or shopping for longer periods of time than intended.
B. The buying preoccupations, impulses, or behaviors cause marked distress, are time consuming, significantly interfere with social or occupational functioning, or result in financial problems (e.g., indebtedness or bankruptcy).
C. The excessive buying or shopping behavior does not occur exclusively during periods of hypomania or mania.

From McElroy SL, Keck PE Jr, Pope HG Jr, Smith JM, Strakowski SM. Compulsive buying: A report of 20 cases. *J Clin Psychiatry*. 1994;55:242, with permission.

Compulsive Buying

Originally referred to as *oniomania* and recognized by Emil Kraepelin and Eugen Bleuler, compulsive buying is not listed as a separate diagnostic category in DSM-IV-TR. Proposed diagnostic criteria are listed in Table 21–7. Compulsive buying is estimated to affect 1.1 to 5.9 percent of the general population. It is more common in women than in men.

The cause of the disorder is unknown. Psychodynamic theories have implicated low self-esteem, anxiety, and the need to reduce stress. Co-morbid conditions include other disorders of impulse control (e.g., kleptomania), mood disorders, and OCD. A diagnosis of compulsive buying should not be made if the behavior occurs as part of a hypomanic or manic episode.

Internet Compulsion

Also called *Internet addiction*, persons with this condition spend almost all of their waking hours at the computer terminal. Their patterns of use are repetitive and constant, and they are unable to resist strong urges to use the computer or to "surf the Web." Internet addicts may gravitate to certain sites that meet specific needs (e.g., shopping, sex, and interactive games, among others). Video game compulsive behavior is a variant behavioral pattern.

Cellular or Mobile Phone Compulsion

Some persons compulsively use mobile phones to call others—friends, acquaintances, or business associates. They justify their need to contact others by giving plausible reasons for calling; but underlying conflicts may be expressed in the behavior, such as fear of being alone, the need to satisfy unconscious dependency needs, or undoing a hostile wish toward a loved one, among others (e.g., "I just want to make sure you are OK").

Compulsive Sexual Behavior

Some persons repeatedly seek out sexual gratification, often in perverse ways (e.g., exhibitionism). They are unable to control their behavior and may not experience feelings of guilt after an episode of acting-out behavior. Sometimes called *sexual addiction*, this condition is discussed in Chapter 17, Human Sexuality.

22

Adjustment Disorders

The adjustment disorders make up a diagnostic category characterized by an emotional response to a stressful event. Typically, the stressor involves financial issues, a medical illness, or a relationship problem. The symptom complex that develops may involve anxious or depressive affect or may present with a disturbance of conduct. By definition, the symptoms must begin within 3 months of the stressor and must remit within 6 months of removal of the stressor. A variety of subtypes of adjustment disorder are identified in the text revision of the fourth edition of the *Diagnostic and Statistical Manual of Mental Disorders* (DSM-IV-TR), varying according to the particular predominant affective presentation. These include adjustment disorder with depressed mood, anxious mood, mixed anxiety and depressed mood, disturbance of conduct, and mixed disturbance of emotions and conduct and of unspecified type.

EPIDEMIOLOGY

According to DSM-IV-TR, the prevalence of the disorder is estimated to be from 2 to 8 percent of the general population. Women are diagnosed with the disorder twice as often as men, and single women are generally overly represented as most at risk. In children and adolescents, boys and girls are equally diagnosed with adjustment disorders. The disorders can occur at any age but are most frequently diagnosed in adolescents. Among adolescents of either sex, common precipitating stresses are school problems, parental rejection and divorce, and substance abuse. Among adults, common precipitating stresses are marital problems, divorce, moving to a new environment, and financial problems.

Adjustment disorders are among the most common psychiatric diagnoses for disorders of patients hospitalized for medical and surgical problems. In one study, 5 percent of persons admitted to a hospital over a 3-year period were classified as having an adjustment disorder. Up to 50 percent of persons with specific medical problems or stressors have been diagnosed with adjustment disorders. Furthermore, 10 to 30 percent of mental health outpatients and up to 12 percent of general hospital inpatients referred for mental health consultations have been diagnosed with adjustment disorders.

ETIOLOGY

By definition, an adjustment disorder is precipitated by one or more stressors. The severity of the stressor or stressors does not always predict the severity of the disorder; the stressor severity is a complex function of degree, quantity, duration, reversibility, environment, and personal context. For example, the loss of a parent is different for a child 10 years of age than for a person 40 years of age. Personality organization and cultural or group norms and values also contribute to the disproportionate responses to stressors.

Stressors may be single, such as a divorce or the loss of a job, or multiple, such as the death of a person important to a patient that coincides with the patient's own physical illness and loss of a job. Stressors may be recurrent, such as seasonal business difficulties, or continuous, such as chronic illness or poverty. A discordant intrafamilial relationship can produce an adjustment disorder that affects the entire family system, or the disorder may be limited to a patient who was perhaps the victim of a crime or who has a physical illness. Sometimes, adjustment disorders occur in a group or community setting and the stressors affect several persons, as in a natural disaster or in racial, social, or religious persecution. Specific developmental stages, such as beginning school, leaving home, getting married, becoming a parent, failing to achieve occupational goals, having the last child leave home, and retiring, are often associated with adjustment disorders.

Psychodynamic Factors

Pivotal to understanding adjustment disorders is an understanding of three factors: the nature of the stressor, the conscious and unconscious meanings of the stressor, and the patient's preexisting vulnerability. A concurrent personality disorder or organic impairment may make a person vulnerable to adjustment disorders. Vulnerability is also associated with the loss of a parent during infancy or being reared in a dysfunctional family. Actual or perceived support from key relationships can affect behavioral and emotional responses to stressors.

Several psychoanalytic researchers have pointed out that the same stress can produce a range of responses in various persons. Throughout his life, Sigmund Freud remained interested in why the stresses of ordinary life produce illness in some and not in others, why an illness takes a particular form, and why some experiences and not others predispose a person to psychopathology. He gave considerable weight to constitutional factors and viewed them as interacting with a person's life experiences to produce fixation.

Psychoanalytic research has emphasized the role of the mother and the rearing environment in a person's later capacity to respond to stress. Particularly important was Donald Winnicott's concept of the good-enough mother, a person who adapts to the infant's needs and provides sufficient support to enable the growing child to tolerate the frustrations in life.

Clinicians must undertake a detailed exploration of a patient's experience of the stressor. Certain patients commonly place all the blame on a particular event when a less obvious event may have had more significant psychological meaning for the patient. Current events may reawaken past traumas or disappointments from childhood, so patients should be encouraged to think about how the current situation relates to similar past events.

Throughout early development, each child develops a unique set of defense mechanisms to deal with stressful events. Because of greater amounts of trauma or greater constitutional vulnerability, some children have less-mature defensive constellations than other children. This disadvantage may cause them as adults to react with substantially impaired functioning when they are faced with a loss, a divorce, or a financial setback; those who have developed mature defense mechanisms are less vulnerable and bounce back more quickly from the stressor. Resilience is also crucially determined by the nature of children's early relationships with their parents. Studies of trauma repeatedly indicate that supportive, nurturant relationships prevent traumatic incidents from causing permanent psychological damage.

Psychodynamic clinicians must consider the relation between a stressor and the human developmental life cycle. When adolescents leave home for college, for example, they are at high developmental risk for reacting with a temporary symptomatic picture. Similarly, if the young person who leaves home is the last child in the family, the parents may be particularly vulnerable to a reaction of adjustment disorder. Moreover, middle-aged persons who are confronting their mortality may be especially sensitive to the effects of loss or death.

Family and Genetic Factors

Some studies suggest that certain persons appear to be at increased risk both for the occurrence of these adverse life events and for the development of pathology once they occur. Findings from a study of more than 2,000 twin pairs indicate that life events and stressors are modestly correlated in twin pairs, with monozygotic twins showing greater concordance than dizygotic twins. Family environmental and genetic factors each accounted for approximately 20 percent of the variance in that study. Another twin study that examined genetic contributions to the development of posttraumatic stress disorder (PTSD) symptoms (not necessarily at the level of full disorder and, therefore, relevant to adjustment disorders) also concluded that the likelihood of developing symptoms in response to traumatic life events is partially under genetic control.

DIAGNOSIS AND CLINICAL FEATURES

Although by definition adjustment disorders follow a stressor, the symptoms do not necessarily begin immediately. Up to 3 months may elapse between a stressor and the development of symptoms. Symptoms do not always subside as soon as the stressor ceases; if the stressor continues, the disorder may be chronic. The disorder can occur at any age, and its symptoms vary considerably, with depressive, anxious, and mixed features most common in adults. Physical symptoms, which are most common in children and the elderly, can occur in any age group. Manifestations may also include assaultive behavior and reckless driving, excessive drinking, defaulting on legal responsibilities, withdrawal, vegetative signs, insomnia, and suicidal behavior.

The clinical presentations of adjustment disorder can vary widely. DSM-IV-TR lists six adjustment disorders, including an unspecified category (Table 22–1).

Adjustment Disorder with Depressed Mood

In adjustment disorder with depressed mood, the predominant manifestations are depressed mood, tearfulness, and hopeless-

Table 22–1
DSM-IV-TR Diagnostic Criteria for Adjustment Disorders

A. The development of emotional or behavioral symptoms in response to an identifiable stressor(s) occurring within 3 months of the onset of the stressor(s).
B. These symptoms or behaviors are clinically significant as evidenced by either of the following:
　(1) marked distress that is in excess of what would be expected from exposure to the stressor
　(2) significant impairment in social or occupational (academic) functioning
C. The stress-related disturbance does not meet the criteria for another specific Axis I disorder and is not merely an exacerbation of a preexisting Axis I or Axis II disorder.
D. The symptoms do not represent bereavement.
E. Once the stressor (or its consequences) has terminated, the symptoms do not persist for more than an additional 6 months.

Specify if:
　Acute: if the disturbance lasts less than 6 months
　Chronic: if the disturbance lasts for 6 months or longer
　Adjustment disorders are coded based on the subtype, which is selected according to the predominant symptoms. The specific stressor(s) can be specified on Axis IV.
　With depressed mood
　With anxiety
　With mixed anxiety and depressed mood
　With disturbance of conduct
　With mixed disturbance of emotions and conduct
　Unspecified

From American Psychiatric Association. *Diagnostic and Statistical Manual of Mental Disorders.* 4th ed. Text rev. Washington, DC: American Psychiatric Association; copyright 2000.

ness. This type must be distinguished from major depressive disorder and uncomplicated bereavement. Adolescents with this type of adjustment disorder are at increased risk for major depressive disorder in young adulthood.

Adjustment Disorder with Anxiety

Symptoms of anxiety, such as palpitations, jitteriness, and agitation, are present in adjustment disorder with anxiety, which must be differentiated from anxiety disorders.

Adjustment Disorder with Mixed Anxiety and Depressed Mood

In adjustment disorder with mixed anxiety and depressed mood, patients exhibit features of both anxiety and depression that do not meet the criteria for an already established anxiety disorder or depressive disorder.

A 48-year-old married woman, in good health, with no previous psychiatric difficulties, presented to the emergency room reporting that she had overdosed on a handful of antihistamines shortly before she arrived. She described her problems as having started 2 months earlier, soon after her husband unexpectedly requested a divorce. She felt betrayed after having devoted much of her 20-year marriage to being a wife, mother, and homemaker. She was sad and tearful at times, and she occasionally had difficulty sleeping. Otherwise, she had no vegetative symptoms and enjoyed time with family and friends. She felt desperate and suicidal after she realized that "he no longer loved me." After crisis intervention in the emergency setting, she responded well to individual psychotherapy over a 3-month period. She occasionally required benzodiazepines for anxiety during the period of treatment. By the time of discharge, she had returned to her baseline function. She came to terms with the possibility of life after divorce and was exploring her best options under the circumstances. (Courtesy of Jeffrey William Katz, M.D., and Oladapo Tomori, M.D.)

Adjustment Disorder with Disturbance of Conduct

In adjustment disorder with disturbance of conduct, the predominant manifestation involves conduct in which the rights of others are violated or age-appropriate societal norms and rules are disregarded. Examples of behavior in this category are truancy, vandalism, reckless driving, and fighting. The category must be differentiated from conduct disorder and antisocial personality disorder.

Adjustment Disorder with Mixed Disturbance of Emotions and Conduct

A combination of disturbances of emotions and of conduct sometimes occurs. Clinicians are encouraged to try to make one or the other diagnosis in the interest of clarity.

Adjustment Disorder Unspecified

Adjustment disorder unspecified is a residual category for atypical maladaptive reactions to stress. Examples include inappropriate responses to the diagnosis of physical illness, such as massive denial, severe noncompliance with treatment, and social withdrawal, without significant depressed or anxious mood.

DIFFERENTIAL DIAGNOSIS

Although uncomplicated bereavement often produces temporarily impaired social and occupational functioning, the person's dysfunction remains within the expectable bounds of a reaction to the loss of a loved one and, thus, is not considered adjustment disorder. Other disorders from which adjustment disorder must be differentiated include major depressive disorder, brief psychotic disorder, generalized anxiety disorder, somatization disorder, substance-related disorder, conduct disorder, academic problem, occupational problem, identity problem, and PTSD. These diagnoses should be given precedence in all cases that meet their criteria, even in the presence of a stressor or group of stressors that served as a precipitant. Patients with an adjustment disorder are impaired in social or occupational functioning and show symptoms beyond the normal and expectable reaction to the stressor. Because no absolute criteria help to distinguish an adjustment disorder from another condition, clinical judgment is necessary. Some patients may meet the criteria for both an adjustment disorder and a personality disorder. If the adjustment disorder follows a physical illness, the clinician must make sure that the symptoms are not a continuation or another manifestation of the illness or its treatment.

Acute and Posttraumatic Stress Disorders

The presence of a stressor is a requirement in the diagnosis of adjustment disorder, PTSD, and acute stress disorder. In PTSD and acute stress disorder the nature of the stressor is better characterized, and they include a defined constellation of affective and autonomic symptoms. In contrast, the stressor in adjustment disorder can be of any severity, with a wide range of possible symptoms. When the response to an extreme stressor does not meet the acute stress or posttraumatic disorder threshold, the adjustment disorder diagnosis would be appropriate. PTSD is discussed fully in Chapter 13.5.

COURSE AND PROGNOSIS

With appropriate treatment, the overall prognosis of an adjustment disorder is generally favorable. Most patients return to their previous level of functioning within 3 months. Some persons (particularly adolescents) who receive a diagnosis of an adjustment disorder later have mood disorders or substance-related disorders. Adolescents usually require a longer time to recover than adults.

TREATMENT

Psychotherapy

Psychotherapy remains the treatment of choice for adjustment disorders. Group therapy can be particularly useful for patients who have had similar stresses—for example, a group of retired persons or patients having renal dialysis. Individual psychotherapy offers the opportunity to explore the meaning of the stressor to the patient so that earlier traumas can be worked through. After successful therapy, patients sometimes emerge from an adjustment disorder stronger than in the premorbid period, although no pathology was evident during that period. Because a stressor can be clearly delineated in adjustment disorders, it is often believed that psychotherapy is not indicated and that the disorder will remit spontaneously. This viewpoint, however, ignores the fact that many persons exposed to the same stressor experience different symptoms, and in adjustment disorders, the response is pathological. Psychotherapy can help persons adapt to stressors that are not reversible or time limited and can serve as a preventive intervention if the stressor does remit. Psychiatrists treating adjustment disorders must be particularly aware of problems of secondary gain. The illness role may be rewarding to some normally healthy persons who have had little experience with illness's capacity to free them from responsibility. Thus, patients can find therapists' attention, empathy, and understanding, which are necessary for success, rewarding in their own right, and therapists may thereby reinforce patients' symptoms. Such

Table 23–1
DSM-IV-TR General Diagnostic Criteria for a Personality Disorder

A. An enduring pattern of inner experience and behavior that deviates markedly from the expectations of the individual's culture. This pattern is manifested in two (or more) of the following areas:
  (1) cognition (i.e., ways of perceiving and interpreting self, other people, and events)
  (2) affectivity (i.e., the range, intensity, lability, and appropriateness of emotional response)
  (3) interpersonal functioning
  (4) impulse control
B. The enduring pattern is inflexible and pervasive across a broad range of personal and social situations.
C. The enduring pattern leads to clinically significant distress or impairment in social, occupational, or other important areas of functioning.
D. The pattern is stable and of long duration, and its onset can be traced back at least to adolescence or early adulthood.
E. The enduring pattern is not better accounted for as a manifestation or consequence of another mental disorder.
F. The enduring pattern is not due to the direct physiological effects of a substance (e.g., a drug of abuse, a medication) or a general medical condition (e.g., head trauma).

From American Psychiatric Association. *Diagnostic and Statistical Manual of Mental Disorders.* 4th ed. Text rev. Washington, DC: American Psychiatric Association; copyright 2000, with permission.

Smooth Pursuit Eye Movements.   Smooth pursuit eye movements are saccadic (i.e., jumpy) in persons who are introverted, who have low self-esteem and tend to withdraw, and who have schizotypal personality disorder.

Neurotransmitters.   Endorphins have effects similar to those of exogenous morphine, such as analgesia and the suppression of arousal. High endogenous endorphin levels may be associated with persons who are phlegmatic. Studies of personality traits and the dopaminergic and serotonergic systems indicate an arousal-activating function for these neurotransmitters. Levels of 5-hydroxyindoleacetic acid, a metabolite of serotonin, are low in persons who attempt suicide and in patients who are impulsive and aggressive.

Raising serotonin levels with serotonergic agents such as fluoxetine (Prozac) can produce dramatic changes in some character traits of personality. In many persons, serotonin reduces depression, impulsiveness, and rumination and can produce a sense of general well-being. Increased dopamine concentrations in the central nervous system produced by certain psychostimulants (e.g., amphetamines) can induce euphoria. The effects of neurotransmitters on personality traits have generated much interest and controversy about whether personality traits are inborn or acquired.

Electrophysiology.   Changes in electrical conductance on the electroencephalogram (EEG) occur in some patients with personality disorders—most commonly antisocial and borderline types; these changes appear as slow-wave activity on EEGs.

Psychoanalytic Factors

Sigmund Freud suggested that personality traits are related to a fixation at one psychosexual stage of development. For example, individuals with an oral character are passive and dependent because they are fixated at the oral stage, when the dependence on others for food is prominent. Individuals with an anal character are stubborn, parsimonious, and highly conscientious because of struggles over toilet training during the anal period.

Wilhelm Reich subsequently coined the term *character armor* to describe persons' characteristic defensive styles for protecting themselves from internal impulses and from interpersonal anxiety in significant relationships. Reich's theory has had a broad influence on contemporary concepts of personality and personality disorders. For example, each human being's unique stamp of personality is considered largely determined by his or her characteristic defense mechanisms. Each personality disorder in Axis II has a cluster of defenses that help psychodynamic clinicians recognize the type of character pathology present. Persons with paranoid personality disorder, for instance, use projection, whereas schizoid personality disorder is associated with withdrawal.

When defenses work effectively, persons with personality disorders master feelings of anxiety, depression, anger, shame, guilt, and other affects. They often view their behavior as egosyntonic; that is, it creates no distress for them, even though it may adversely affect others. They may also be reluctant to engage in a treatment process; because their defenses are important in controlling unpleasant affects, they are not interested in surrendering them.

In addition to characteristic defenses in personality disorders, another central feature is internal object relations. During development, particular patterns of self in relation to others are internalized. Through introjection, children internalize a parent or another significant person as an internal presence that continues to feel like an object rather than a self. Through identification, children internalize parents and others in such a way that the traits of the external object are incorporated into the self and the child "owns" the traits. These internal self-representations and object representations are crucial in developing the personality and, through externalization and projective identification, are played out in interpersonal scenarios in which others are coerced into playing a role in the person's internal life. Hence, persons with personality disorders are also identified by particular patterns of interpersonal relatedness that stem from these internal object relations patterns.

Defense Mechanisms.   To help those with personality disorders, psychiatrists must appreciate patients' underlying defenses—the unconscious mental processes that the ego uses to resolve conflicts among the four lodestars of the inner life: instinct (wish or need), reality, important persons, and conscience. When defenses are most effective, especially in those with personality disorders, they can abolish anxiety and depression. Thus, abandoning a defense increases conscious anxiety and depression—a major reason that those with personality disorders are reluctant to alter their behavior.

PARANOID PERSONALITY DISORDER

Persons with paranoid personality disorder are characterized by long-standing suspiciousness and mistrust of persons in general. They refuse responsibility for their feelings and assign responsibility to others. They are often hostile, irritable, and angry.

Bigots, injustice collectors, pathologically jealous spouses, and litigious cranks often have paranoid personality disorder.

Epidemiology

The prevalence of paranoid personality disorder is 0.5 to 2.5 percent of the general population. Those with the disorder rarely seek treatment themselves; when referred to treatment by a spouse or an employer, they can often pull themselves together and appear undistressed. Relatives of patients with schizophrenia show a higher incidence of paranoid personality disorder than controls. The disorder is more common in men than in women and does not appear to have a familial pattern. The prevalence among persons who are homosexual is no higher than usual, as was once thought, but it is believed to be higher among minority groups, immigrants, and persons who are deaf than it is in the general population.

Diagnosis

On psychiatric examination, patients with paranoid personality disorder may be formal in manner and act baffled about having to seek psychiatric help. Muscular tension, an inability to relax, and a need to scan the environment for clues may be evident, and the patient's manner is often humorless and serious. Although some premises of their arguments may be false, their speech is goal directed and logical. Their thought content shows evidence of projection, prejudice, and occasional ideas of reference. The DSM-IV-TR diagnostic criteria are listed in Table 23–2.

Clinical Features

The hallmarks of paranoid personality disorder are excessive suspiciousness and distrust of others expressed as a pervasive tendency to interpret actions of others as deliberately demeaning, malevolent, threatening, exploiting, or deceiving. This tendency begins by early adulthood and appears in a variety of contexts. Almost invariably, those with the disorder expect to be exploited or harmed by others in some way. They frequently dispute, without any justification, friends' or associates' loyalty or trustworthiness. Such persons are often pathologically jealous and, for no reason, question the fidelity of their spouses or sexual partners. Persons with this disorder externalize their emotions and use the defense of projection; they attribute to others the impulses and thoughts that they cannot accept in themselves. Ideas of reference and logically defended illusions are common.

Persons with paranoid personality disorder are affectively restricted and appear to be unemotional. They pride themselves on being rational and objective, but such is not the case. They lack warmth and are impressed with, and pay close attention to, power and rank. They express disdain for those they see as weak, sickly, impaired, or in some way defective. In social situations, persons with paranoid personality disorder may appear business-like and efficient, but they often generate fear or conflict in others.

Differential Diagnosis

Paranoid personality disorder can usually be differentiated from delusional disorder by the absence of fixed delusions. Unlike persons with paranoid schizophrenia, those with personality disorders have no hallucinations or formal thought disorder. Paranoid personality disorder can be distinguished from borderline personality disorder because patients who are paranoid are rarely capable of overly involved, tumultuous relationships with others. Patients with paranoia lack the long history of antisocial behavior of persons with antisocial character. Persons with schizoid personality disorder are withdrawn and aloof and do not have paranoid ideation.

Course and Prognosis

No adequate, systematic long-term studies of paranoid personality disorder have been conducted. In some, paranoid personality disorder is lifelong; in others, it is a harbinger of schizophrenia. In still others, paranoid traits give way to reaction formation, appropriate concern with morality, and altruistic concerns as they mature or as stress diminishes. In general, however, those with paranoid personality disorder have lifelong problems working and living with others. Occupational and marital problems are common.

Treatment

Psychotherapy.   Psychotherapy is the treatment of choice for paranoid personality disorder. Therapists should be straightforward in all their dealings with these patients. If a therapist is accused of inconsistency or a fault, such as lateness for an

Table 23–2
DSM-IV-TR Diagnostic Criteria for Paranoid Personality Disorder

A. A pervasive distrust and suspiciousness of others such that their motives are interpreted as malevolent, beginning by early adulthood and present in a variety of contexts, as indicated by four (or more) of the following:

(1) suspects, without sufficient basis, that others are exploiting, harming, or deceiving him or her

(2) is preoccupied with unjustified doubts about the loyalty or trustworthiness of friends or associates

(3) is reluctant to confide in others because of unwarranted fear that the information will be used maliciously against him or her

(4) reads hidden demeaning or threatening meanings into benign remarks or events

(5) persistently bears grudges, i.e., is unforgiving of insults, injuries, or slights

(6) perceives attacks on his or her character or reputation that are not apparent to others and is quick to react angrily or to counterattack

(7) has recurrent suspicions, without justification, regarding fidelity of spouse or sexual partner

B. Does not occur exclusively during the course of schizophrenia, a mood disorder with psychotic features, or another psychotic disorder and is not due to the direct physiological effects of a general medical condition.

Note: If criteria are met prior to the onset of schizophrenia, add "premorbid," e.g., "paranoid personality disorder (premorbid)."

From American Psychiatric Association. *Diagnostic and Statistical Manual of Mental Disorders.* 4th ed. Text rev. Washington, DC: American Psychiatric Association; copyright 2000, with permission.

appointment, honesty and an apology are preferable to a defensive explanation. Therapists must remember that trust and toleration of intimacy are troubled areas for patients with this disorder. Individual psychotherapy, thus, requires a professional and not overly warm style from therapists. Clinicians' overzealous use of interpretation—especially interpretation about deep feelings of dependence, sexual concerns, and wishes for intimacy—increase patients' mistrust significantly. Patients who are paranoid usually do not do well in group psychotherapy, although it can be useful for improving social skills and diminishing suspiciousness through role playing. Many cannot tolerate the intrusiveness of behavior therapy, also used for social skills training.

Pharmacotherapy.   Pharmacotherapy is useful in dealing with agitation and anxiety. In most cases, an antianxiety agent such as diazepam (Valium) suffices. It may be necessary, however, to use an antipsychotic such as haloperidol (Haldol) in small doses and for brief periods to manage severe agitation or quasi-delusional thinking. The antipsychotic drug pimozide (Orap) has successfully reduced paranoid ideation in some patients.

SCHIZOID PERSONALITY DISORDER

Schizoid personality disorder is diagnosed in patients who display a lifelong pattern of social withdrawal. Their discomfort with human interaction, their introversion, and their bland, constricted affect are noteworthy. Persons with schizoid personality disorder are often seen by others as eccentric, isolated, or lonely.

Epidemiology

The prevalence of schizoid personality disorder is not clearly established, but the disorder may affect 7.5 percent of the general population. The sex ratio of the disorder is unknown; some studies report a 2:1 male-to-female ratio. Persons with the disorder tend to gravitate toward solitary jobs that involve little or no contact with others. Many prefer night work to day work, so that they need not deal with many persons.

Diagnosis

On an initial psychiatric examination, patients with schizoid personality disorder may appear ill at ease. They rarely tolerate eye contact, and interviewers may surmise that such patients are eager for the interview to end. Their affect may be constricted, aloof, or inappropriately serious, but underneath the aloofness, sensitive clinicians can recognize fear. These patients find it difficult to be lighthearted: Their efforts at humor may seem adolescent and off the mark. Their speech is goal directed, but they are likely to give short answers to questions and to avoid spontaneous conversation. They may occasionally use unusual figures of speech, such as an odd metaphor, and may be fascinated with inanimate objects or metaphysical constructs. Their mental content may reveal an unwarranted sense of intimacy with persons they do not know well or whom they have not seen for a long time. Their sensorium is intact, their memory functions well,

Table 23–3
DSM-IV-TR Diagnostic Criteria for Schizoid Personality Disorder

A. A pervasive pattern of detachment from social relationships and a restricted range of expression of emotions in interpersonal settings, beginning by early adulthood and present in a variety of contexts, as indicated by four (or more) of the following:
  (1) neither desires nor enjoys close relationships, including being part of a family
  (2) almost always chooses solitary activities
  (3) has little, if any, interest in having sexual experiences with another person
  (4) takes pleasure in few, if any, activities
  (5) lacks close friends or confidants other than first-degree relatives
  (6) appears indifferent to the praise or criticism of others
  (7) shows emotional coldness, detachment, or flattened affectivity
B. Does not occur exclusively during the course of schizophrenia, a mood disorder with psychotic features, another psychotic disorder, or a pervasive developmental disorder and is not due to the direct physiological effects of a general medical condition.
  Note: If criteria are met prior to the onset of schizophrenia, add "premorbid," e.g., "schizoid personality disorder (premorbid)."

From American Psychiatric Association. *Diagnostic and Statistical Manual of Mental Disorders.* 4th ed. Text rev. Washington, DC: American Psychiatric Association; copyright 2000, with permission.

and their proverb interpretations are abstract. The DSM-IV-TR diagnostic criteria are listed in Table 23–3.

Clinical Features

Persons with schizoid personality disorder seem to be cold and aloof; they display a remote reserve and show no involvement with everyday events and the concerns of others. They appear quiet, distant, seclusive, and unsociable. They may pursue their lives with remarkably little need or longing for emotional ties, and they are the last to be aware of changes in popular fashion.

The life histories of such persons reflect solitary interests and success at noncompetitive, lonely jobs that others find difficult to tolerate. Their sexual lives may exist exclusively in fantasy, and they may postpone mature sexuality indefinitely. Men may not marry because they are unable to achieve intimacy; women may passively agree to marry an aggressive man who wants the marriage. Persons with schizoid personality disorder usually reveal a lifelong inability to express anger directly. They can invest enormous affective energy in interests in which the human element can be abstracted, such as mathematics and astronomy, and they may be very attached to animals. Dietary and health fads, philosophical movements, and social improvement schemes, especially those that require no personal involvement, often engross them.

Although persons with schizoid personality disorder appear self-absorbed and lost in daydreams, they have a normal capacity to recognize reality. Because aggressive acts are rarely included in their repertoire of usual responses, most threats, real or imagined, are dealt with by fantasized omnipotence or resignation. They are often seen as aloof, yet such persons can sometimes conceive, develop, and give to the world genuinely original, creative ideas.

Differential Diagnosis

Schizoid personality disorder is distinguished from schizophrenia, delusional disorder, and affective disorder with psychotic features based on periods with positive psychotic symptoms, such as delusions and hallucinations in the latter. Although patients with paranoid personality disorder share many traits with those with schizoid personality disorder, the former exhibit more social engagement, a history of aggressive verbal behavior, and a greater tendency to project their feelings onto others. If just as emotionally constricted, patients with obsessive-compulsive and avoidant personality disorders experience loneliness as dysphoric, possess a richer history of past object relations, and do not engage as much in autistic reverie. Theoretically, the chief distinction between a patient with schizotypal personality disorder and one with schizoid personality disorder is that the patient who is schizotypal is more similar to a patient with schizophrenia in oddities of perception, thought, behavior, and communication. Patients with avoidant personality disorder are isolated but strongly wish to participate in activities, a characteristic absent in those with schizoid personality disorder. Schizoid personality disorder is distinguished from autistic disorder and Asperger's syndrome by more severely impaired social interactions and stereotypical behaviors and interests than in those two disorders.

Course and Prognosis

The onset of schizoid personality disorder usually occurs in early childhood. As with all personality disorders, schizoid personality disorder is long lasting but not necessarily lifelong. The proportion of patients who incur schizophrenia is unknown.

Treatment

Psychotherapy. The treatment of patients with schizoid personality disorder is similar to that of those with paranoid personality disorder. Patients who are schizoid tend toward introspection; however, these tendencies are consistent with psychotherapists' expectations, and such patients may become devoted, if distant, patients. As trust develops, patients who are schizoid may, with great trepidation, reveal a plethora of fantasies, imaginary friends, and fears of unbearable dependence—even of merging with the therapist.

In group therapy settings, patients with schizoid personality disorder may be silent for long periods; nonetheless, they do become involved. The patients should be protected against aggressive attack by group members for their proclivity to be silent. With time, the group members become important to patients who are schizoid and may provide the only social contact in their otherwise isolated existence.

Pharmacotherapy. Pharmacotherapy with small doses of antipsychotics, antidepressants, and psychostimulants has benefited some patients. Serotonergic agents may make patients less sensitive to rejection. Benzodiazepines may help diminish interpersonal anxiety.

SCHIZOTYPAL PERSONALITY DISORDER

Persons with schizotypal personality disorder are strikingly odd or strange, even to laypersons. Magical thinking, peculiar notions, ideas of reference, illusions, and derealization are part of a schizotypal person's everyday world.

Epidemiology

Schizotypal personality disorder occurs in about 3 percent of the population. The sex ratio is unknown. A greater association of cases exists among the biological relatives of patients with schizophrenia than among controls, and a higher incidence among monozygotic twins than among dizygotic twins (33 percent vs. 4 percent in one study).

Diagnosis

Schizotypal personality disorder is diagnosed on the basis of the patients' peculiarities of thinking, behavior, and appearance. Taking a history may be difficult because of the patients' unusual way of communicating. The DSM-IV-TR diagnostic criteria for schizotypal personality disorder are given in Table 23–4.

Table 23–4
DSM-IV-TR Diagnostic Criteria for Schizotypal Personality Disorder

A. A pervasive pattern of social and interpersonal deficits marked by acute discomfort with, and reduced capacity for, close relationships as well as by cognitive or perceptual distortions and eccentricities of behavior, beginning by early adulthood and present in a variety of contexts, as indicated by five (or more) of the following:

(1) ideas of reference (excluding delusions of reference)
(2) odd beliefs or magical thinking that influences behavior and is inconsistent with subcultural norms (e.g., superstitiousness, belief in clairvoyance, telepathy, or "sixth sense"; in children and adolescents, bizarre fantasies or preoccupations)
(3) unusual perceptual experiences, including bodily illusions
(4) odd thinking and speech (e.g., vague, circumstantial, metaphorical, overelaborate, or stereotyped)
(5) suspiciousness or paranoid ideation
(6) inappropriate or constricted affect
(7) behavior or appearance that is odd, eccentric, or peculiar
(8) lack of close friends or confidants other than first-degree relatives
(9) excessive social anxiety that does not diminish with familiarity and tends to be associated with paranoid fears rather than negative judgments about self

B. Does not occur exclusively during the course of schizophrenia, a mood disorder with psychotic features, another psychotic disorder, or a pervasive developmental disorder.

Note: If criteria are met prior to the onset of schizophrenia, add "premorbid," e.g., "schizotypal personality disorder (premorbid)."

From American Psychiatric Association. *Diagnostic and Statistical Manual of Mental Disorders.* 4th ed. Text rev. Washington, DC: American Psychiatric Association; copyright 2000, with permission.

Clinical Features

Patients with schizotypal personality disorder exhibit disturbed thinking and communicating. Although frank thought disorder is absent, their speech may be distinctive or peculiar, may have meaning only to them, and often needs interpretation. As with patients with schizophrenia, those with schizotypal personality disorder may not know their own feelings and yet are exquisitely sensitive to, and aware of, the feelings of others, especially negative affects such as anger. These patients may be superstitious or claim powers of clairvoyance and may believe that they have other special powers of thought and insight. Their inner world may be filled with vivid imaginary relationships and child-like fears and fantasies. They may admit to perceptual illusions or macropsia and confess that other persons seem wooden and all the same.

Because persons with schizotypal personality disorder have poor interpersonal relationships and may act inappropriately, they are isolated and have few, if any, friends. Patients may show features of borderline personality disorder, and indeed, both diagnoses can be made. Under stress, patients with schizotypal personality disorder may decompensate and have psychotic symptoms, but these are usually brief. Patients with severe cases of the disorder may exhibit anhedonia and severe depression.

Differential Diagnosis

Theoretically, persons with schizotypal personality disorder can be distinguished from those with schizoid and avoidant personality disorders by the presence of oddities in their behavior, thinking, perception, and communication and perhaps by a clear family history of schizophrenia. Patients with schizotypal personality disorder can be distinguished from those with schizophrenia by their absence of psychosis. If psychotic symptoms do appear, they are brief and fragmentary. Some patients meet the criteria for both schizotypal personality disorder and borderline personality disorder. Patients with paranoid personality disorder are characterized by suspiciousness but lack the odd behavior of patients with schizotypal personality disorder.

Course and Prognosis

A long-term study by Thomas McGlashan reported that 10 percent of those with schizotypal personality disorder eventually committed suicide. Retrospective studies have shown that many patients thought to have had schizophrenia actually had schizotypal personality disorder, and, according to current clinical thinking, the schizotype is the premorbid personality of the patient with schizophrenia. Some, however, maintain a stable schizotypal personality throughout their lives and marry and work, despite their oddities.

Treatment

Psychotherapy.   The principles of treatment of schizotypal personality disorder do not differ from those of schizoid personality disorder, but clinicians must deal sensitively with the former. These patients have peculiar patterns of thinking, and some are involved in cults, strange religious practices, and the occult. Therapists must not ridicule such activities or be judgmental about these beliefs or activities.

Pharmacotherapy.   Antipsychotic medication may be useful in dealing with ideas of reference, illusions, and other symptoms of the disorder and can be used in conjunction with psychotherapy. Antidepressants are useful when a depressive component of the personality is present.

ANTISOCIAL PERSONALITY DISORDER

Antisocial personality disorder is an inability to conform to the social norms that ordinarily govern many aspects of a person's adolescent and adult behavior. Although characterized by continual antisocial or criminal acts, the disorder is not synonymous with criminality.

Epidemiology

The prevalence of antisocial personality disorder is 3 percent in men and 1 percent in women. It is most common in poor urban areas and among mobile residents of these areas. Boys with the disorder come from larger families than girls with the disorder. The onset of the disorder is before the age of 15 years. Girls usually have symptoms before puberty, and boys even earlier. In prison populations, the prevalence of antisocial personality disorder may be as high as 75 percent. A familial pattern is present; the disorder is five times more common among first-degree relatives of men with the disorder than among controls.

Diagnosis

Patients with antisocial personality disorder can fool even the most experienced clinicians. In an interview, patients can appear composed and credible, but beneath the veneer (or, to use Hervey Cleckley's term, *the mask of sanity*) lurks tension, hostility, irritability, and rage. A stress interview, in which patients are vigorously confronted with inconsistencies in their histories, may be necessary to reveal the pathology.

A diagnostic workup should include a thorough neurological examination. Because patients often show abnormal EEG results and soft neurological signs suggesting minimal brain damage in childhood, these findings can be used to confirm the clinical impression. The DSM-IV-TR diagnostic criteria are listed in Table 23–5.

Clinical Features

Patients with antisocial personality disorder can often seem to be normal and even charming and ingratiating. Their histories, however, reveal many areas of disordered life functioning. Lying, truancy, running away from home, thefts, fights, substance abuse, and illegal activities are typical experiences that patients report as beginning in childhood. These patients often impress opposite-sex clinicians with the colorful, seductive aspects of their personalities, but same-sex clinicians may regard them as manipulative and demanding. Patients with antisocial personality disorder exhibit no anxiety or depression, a lack that may seem grossly incongruous with their situations, although suicide threats and somatic preoccupations may be common. Their

Table 23–5
DSM-IV-TR Diagnostic Criteria for Antisocial Personality Disorder

A. There is a pervasive pattern of disregard for and violation of the rights of others occurring since age 15 years, as indicated by three (or more) of the following:

  (1) failure to conform to social norms with respect to lawful behaviors as indicated by repeatedly performing acts that are grounds for arrest
  (2) deceitfulness, as indicated by repeated lying, use of aliases, or conning others for personal profit or pleasure
  (3) impulsivity or failure to plan ahead
  (4) irritability and aggressiveness, as indicated by repeated physical fights or assaults
  (5) reckless disregard for safety of self or others
  (6) consistent irresponsibility, as indicated by repeated failure to sustain consistent work behavior or honor financial obligations
  (7) lack of remorse) as indicated by being indifferent to or rationalizing having hurt, mistreated, or stolen from another

B. The individual is at least age 18 years.
C. There is evidence of conduct disorder with onset before age 15 years.
D. The occurrence of antisocial behavior is not exclusively during the course of schizophrenia or a manic episode.

From American Psychiatric Association. *Diagnostic and Statistical Manual of Mental Disorders.* 4th ed. Text rev. Washington, DC: American Psychiatric Association; copyright 2000, with permission.

explanations of their antisocial behavior make it seem mindless, but their mental content reveals the complete absence of delusions and other signs of irrational thinking. In fact, they frequently have a heightened sense of reality testing and often impress observers as having good verbal intelligence.

Persons with antisocial personality disorder are highly representative of so-called con men. They are extremely manipulative and can frequently talk others into participating in schemes for easy ways to make money or to achieve fame or notoriety. These schemes may eventually lead the unwary to financial ruin or social embarrassment or both. Those with this disorder do not tell the truth and cannot be trusted to carry out any task or adhere to any conventional standard of morality. Promiscuity, spousal abuse, child abuse, and drunk driving are common events in their lives. A notable finding is a lack of remorse for these actions; that is, they appear to lack a conscience.

Differential Diagnosis

Antisocial personality disorder can be distinguished from illegal behavior in that antisocial personality disorder involves many areas of a person's life. When antisocial behavior is the only manifestation, patients are classified in the DSM-IV-TR category of additional conditions that may be a focus of clinical attention—specifically, adult antisocial behavior. Dorothy Lewis found that many of these persons have a neurological or mental disorder that has been either overlooked or undiagnosed. More difficult is the differentiation of antisocial personality disorder from substance abuse. When both substance abuse and antisocial behavior begin in childhood and continue into adult life, both disorders should be diagnosed. When, however, the antisocial behavior is clearly secondary to premorbid alcohol abuse or other substance abuse, the diagnosis of antisocial personality disorder is not warranted.

In diagnosing antisocial personality disorder, clinicians must adjust for the distorting effects of socioeconomic status, cultural background, and sex. Furthermore, the diagnosis of antisocial personality disorder is not warranted when mental retardation, schizophrenia, or mania can explain the symptoms.

Course and Prognosis

Once an antisocial personality disorder develops, it runs an unremitting course, with the height of antisocial behavior usually occurring in late adolescence. The prognosis varies. Some reports indicate that symptoms decrease as persons grow older. Many patients have somatization disorder and multiple physical complaints. Depressive disorders, alcohol use disorders, and other substance abuse are common.

Treatment

Psychotherapy.   If patients with antisocial personality disorder are immobilized (e.g., placed in hospitals), they often become amenable to psychotherapy. When patients feel that they are among peers, their lack of motivation for change disappears. Perhaps for this reason, self-help groups have been more useful than jails in alleviating the disorder.

Before treatment can begin, firm limits are essential. Therapists must find ways of dealing with patients' self-destructive behavior. In addition, to overcome patients' fear of intimacy, therapists must frustrate patients' desire to run from honest human encounters. In doing so, a therapist faces the challenge of separating control from punishment and of separating help and confrontation from social isolation and retribution.

Pharmacotherapy.   Pharmacotherapy is used to deal with incapacitating symptoms such as anxiety, rage, and depression, but because patients are often substance abusers, drugs must be used judiciously. If a patient shows evidence of attention-deficit/hyperactivity disorder, psychostimulants such as methylphenidate (Ritalin) may be useful. Attempts have been made to alter catecholamine metabolism with drugs and to control impulsive behavior with antiepileptic drugs, for example, carbamazepine (Tegretol) or valproate (Depakote), especially if abnormal waveforms are noted on an EEG. β-Adrenergic receptor antagonists have been used to reduce aggression.

BORDERLINE PERSONALITY DISORDER

Patients with borderline personality disorder stand on the border between neurosis and psychosis and they are characterized by extraordinarily unstable affect, mood, behavior, object relations, and self-image. The disorder has also been called *ambulatory schizophrenia, as-if personality* (a term coined by Helene Deutsch), *pseudoneurotic schizophrenia* (described by Paul Hoch and Phillip Politan), and *psychotic character disorder* (described by John Frosch).

Epidemiology

No definitive prevalence studies are available, but borderline personality disorder is thought to be present in about 1 to 2 percent of the population and is twice as common in women as in men. An increased prevalence of major depressive disorder, alcohol use disorders, and substance abuse is found in first-degree relatives of persons with borderline personality disorder.

Diagnosis

According to DSM-IV-TR, the diagnosis of borderline personality disorder can made by early adulthood when patients show at least five of the criteria listed in Table 23–6. Biological studies may aid in the diagnosis; some patients with borderline personality disorder show shortened REM latency and sleep continuity disturbances, abnormal DST results, and abnormal thyrotropin-releasing hormone test results. Those changes, however, are also seen in some patients with depressive disorders.

Clinical Features

Persons with borderline personality disorder almost always appear to be in a state of crisis. Mood swings are common. Patients can be argumentative at one moment, depressed the next, and later complain of having no feelings. Patients can have short-lived psychotic episodes (so-called *micropsychotic episodes*) rather than full-blown psychotic breaks, and the psychotic symptoms of these patients are almost always circumscribed, fleeting, or doubtful. The behavior of patients with borderline personality disorder is highly unpredictable, and their achievements are

Table 23–6
DSM-IV-TR Diagnostic Criteria for Borderline Personality Disorder

A pervasive pattern of instability of interpersonal relationships, self-image, and affects, and marked impulsivity beginning by early adulthood and present in a variety of contexts, as indicated by five (or more) of the following:

  (1) frantic efforts to avoid real or imagined abandonment.
    Note: Do not include suicidal or self-mutilating behavior covered in Criterion 5.
  (2) a pattern of unstable and intense interpersonal relationships characterized by alternating between extremes of idealization and devaluation
  (3) identity disturbance: markedly and persistently unstable self-image or sense of self
  (4) impulsivity in at least two areas that are potentially self-damaging (e.g., spending, sex, substance abuse, reckless driving, binge eating). **Note:** Do not include suicidal or self-mutilating behavior covered in Criterion 5.
  (5) recurrent suicidal behavior, gestures, or threats, or self-mutilating behavior
  (6) affective instability due to a marked reactivity of mood (e.g., intense episodic dysphoria, irritability, or anxiety usually lasting a few hours and only hours and only rarely more than a few days)
  (7) chronic feelings of emptiness
  (8) inappropriate, intense anger or difficulty controlling anger (e.g., frequent displays of temper, constant anger, recurrent physical fights)
  (9) transient, stress-related paranoid ideation or severe dissociative symptoms

From American Psychiatric Association. *Diagnostic and Statistical Manual of Mental Disorders.* 4th ed. Text rev. Washington, DC: American Psychiatric Association; copyright 2000, with permission.

rarely at the level of their abilities. The painful nature of their lives is reflected in repetitive self-destructive acts. Such patients may slash their wrists and perform other self-mutilations to elicit help from others, to express anger, or to numb themselves to overwhelming affect.

Because they feel both dependent and hostile, persons with this disorder have tumultuous interpersonal relationships. They can be dependent on those with whom they are close and, when frustrated, can express enormous anger toward their intimate friends. Patients with borderline personality disorder cannot tolerate being alone, and they prefer a frantic search for companionship, no matter how unsatisfactory, to their own company. To assuage loneliness, if only for brief periods, they accept a stranger as a friend or behave promiscuously. They often complain about chronic feelings of emptiness and boredom and the lack of a consistent sense of identity (identity diffusion); when pressed, they often complain about how depressed they usually feel, despite the flurry of other affects.

Otto Kernberg described the defense mechanism of projective identification that occurs in patients with borderline personality disorder. In this primitive defense mechanism, intolerable aspects of the self are projected onto another; the other person is induced to play the projected role, and the two persons act in unison. Therapists must be aware of this process so that they can act neutrally toward such patients.

Most therapists agree that these patients show ordinary reasoning abilities on structured tests, such as the Wechsler Adult Intelligence Scale, and show deviant processes only on unstructured projective tests, such as the Rorschach test.

Functionally, patients with borderline personality disorder distort their relationships by considering each person to be either all good or all bad. They see persons as either nurturing attachment figures or as hateful, sadistic figures who deprive them of security needs and threaten them with abandonment whenever they feel dependent. As a result of this splitting, the good person is idealized, and the bad person is devalued. Shifts of allegiance from one person or group to another are frequent. Some clinicians use the concepts of panphobia, pananxiety, panambivalence, and chaotic sexuality to delineate these patients' characteristics.

Differential Diagnosis

The disorder is differentiated from schizophrenia on the basis that the patient with borderline personality lacks prolonged psychotic episodes, thought disorder, and other classic schizophrenic signs. Patients with schizotypal personality disorder show marked peculiarities of thinking, strange ideation, and recurrent ideas of reference. Those with paranoid personality disorder are marked by extreme suspiciousness. Patients with borderline personality disorder generally have chronic feelings of emptiness and short-lived psychotic episodes; they act impulsively and demand extraordinary relationships; they may mutilate themselves and make manipulative suicide attempts.

Course and Prognosis

Borderline personality disorder is fairly stable; patients change little over time. Longitudinal studies show no progression toward schizophrenia, but patients have a high incidence of major depressive disorder episodes. The diagnosis is usually made before the age of 40 years, when patients are attempting to make occupational, marital, and other choices and are unable to deal with the normal stages of the life cycle.

Treatment

Psychotherapy.   Psychotherapy for patients with borderline personality disorder is an area of intensive investigation and has been the treatment of choice. For best results, pharmacotherapy has been added to the treatment regimen.

Psychotherapy is difficult for patient and therapist alike. Patients regress easily, act out their impulses, and show labile or fixed negative or positive transferences, which are difficult to analyze. Projective identification may also cause countertransference problems when therapists are unaware that patients are unconsciously trying to coerce them to act out a particular behavior. The splitting defense mechanism causes patients to alternately love and hate therapists and others in the environment. A reality-oriented approach is more effective than in-depth interpretations of the unconscious.

Therapists have used behavior therapy to control patients' impulses and angry outbursts and to reduce their sensitivity to criticism and rejection. Social skills training, especially with videotape playback, helps patients to see how their actions affect others and thereby improve their interpersonal behavior.

Patients with borderline personality disorder often do well in a hospital setting in which they receive intensive psychotherapy on both an individual and a group basis. In a hospital, they can also interact with trained staff members from a variety of disciplines and can be provided with occupational, recreational, and vocational therapy. Such programs are especially helpful when the home environment is detrimental to a patient's rehabilitation because of intrafamilial conflicts or other stresses, such as parental abuse. Within the protected environment of the hospital, patients who are excessively impulsive, self-destructive, or self-mutilating can be given limits, and their actions can be observed. Under ideal circumstances, patients remain in the hospital until they show marked improvement, up to 1 year in some cases. Patients can then be discharged to special support systems, such as day hospitals, night hospitals, and halfway houses.

A particular form of psychotherapy called dialectical behavior therapy (DBT) has been used for patients with borderline personality disorder, especially those with parasuicidal behavior, such as frequent cutting. (For further discussion of DBT see Section 31.5 in Chapter 31.)

Pharmacotherapy.   Pharmacotherapy is useful in dealing with specific personality features that interfere with patients' overall functioning. Antipsychotics have been used to control anger, hostility, and brief psychotic episodes. Antidepressants improve the depressed mood common in patients with borderline personality disorder. The MAO inhibitors have successfully modulated impulsive behavior in some patients. Benzodiazepines, particularly alprazolam (Xanax), help anxiety and depression, but some patients show a disinhibition with this class of drugs. Anticonvulsants, such as carbamazepine, may improve global functioning for some patients. Serotonergic agents such as selective serotonin reuptake inhibitors have been helpful in some cases.

HISTRIONIC PERSONALITY DISORDER

Persons with histrionic personality disorder are excitable and emotional and behave in a colorful, dramatic, extroverted fashion. Accompanying their flamboyant aspects, however, is often an inability to maintain deep, long-lasting attachments.

Epidemiology

According to DSM-IV-TR, limited data from general population studies suggest a prevalence of histrionic personality disorder of about 2 to 3 percent. Rates of about 10 to 15 percent have been reported in inpatient and outpatient mental health settings when structured assessment is used. The disorder is diagnosed more frequently in women than in men. Some studies have found an association with somatization disorder and alcohol use disorders.

Diagnosis

In interviews, patients with histrionic personality disorder are generally cooperative and eager to give a detailed history. Gestures and dramatic punctuation in their conversations are common; they may make frequent slips of the tongue, and their language is colorful. Affective display is common, but, when pressed to acknowledge certain feelings (e.g., anger, sadness, and sexual wishes), they may respond with surprise, indignation, or denial. The results of the cognitive examination are usually normal, although a lack of perseverance may be shown on arithmetic or concentration tasks, and the patients' forgetfulness of affect-laden material may be astonishing. The DSM-IV-TR diagnostic criteria are listed in Table 23–7.

Clinical Features

Persons with histrionic personality disorder show a high degree of attention-seeking behavior. They tend to exaggerate their

Table 23–7
DSM-IV-TR Diagnostic Criteria for Histrionic Personality Disorder

A pervasive pattern of excessive emotionality and attention seeking, beginning by early adulthood and present in a variety of contexts, as indicated by five (or more) of the following:

(1) is uncomfortable in situations in which he or she is not the center of attention
(2) interaction with others is often characterized by inappropriate sexually seductive or provocative behavior
(3) displays rapidly shifting and shallow expression of emotions
(4) consistently uses physical appearance to draw attention to self
(5) has a style of speech that is excessively impressionistic and lacking in detail
(6) shows self-dramatization, theatricality, and exaggerated expression of emotion
(7) is suggestible, i.e., easily influenced by others or circumstances
(8) considers relationships to be more intimate than they actually are

thoughts and feelings and make everything sound more important than it really is. They display temper tantrums, tears, and accusations when they are not the center of attention or are not receiving praise or approval.

Seductive behavior is common in both sexes. Sexual fantasies about persons with whom patients are involved are common, but patients are inconsistent about verbalizing these fantasies and may be coy or flirtatious rather than sexually aggressive. In fact, histrionic patients may have a psychosexual dysfunction; women may be anorgasmic, and men may be impotent. Their need for reassurance is endless. They may act on their sexual impulses to reassure themselves that they are attractive to the other sex. Their relationships tend to be superficial, however, and they can be vain, self-absorbed, and fickle. Their strong dependence needs make them overly trusting and gullible.

The major defenses of patients with histrionic personality disorder are repression and dissociation. Accordingly, such patients are unaware of their true feelings and cannot explain their motivations. Under stress, reality testing easily becomes impaired.

Differential Diagnosis

Distinguishing between histrionic personality disorder and borderline personality disorder is difficult, but in borderline personality disorder, suicide attempts, identity diffusion, and brief psychotic episodes are more likely. Although both conditions may be diagnosed in the same patient, clinicians should separate the two. Somatization disorder (Briquet's syndrome) may occur in conjunction with histrionic personality disorder. Patients with brief psychotic disorder and dissociative disorders may warrant a coexisting diagnosis of histrionic personality disorder.

Course and Prognosis

With age, persons with histrionic personality disorder show fewer symptoms, but because they lack the energy of earlier years, the difference in number of symptoms may be more apparent than real. Persons with this disorder are sensation seekers, and they may get into trouble with the law, abuse substances, and act promiscuously.

Treatment

Psychotherapy.   Patients with histrionic personality disorder are often unaware of their real feelings; clarification of their inner feelings is an important therapeutic process. Psychoanalytically oriented psychotherapy, whether group or individual, is probably the treatment of choice for histrionic personality disorder.

Pharmacotherapy.   Pharmacotherapy can be adjunctive when symptoms are targeted (e.g., the use of antidepressants for depression and somatic complaints, antianxiety agents for anxiety, and antipsychotics for derealization and illusions).

NARCISSISTIC PERSONALITY DISORDER

Persons with narcissistic personality disorder are characterized by a heightened sense of self-importance and grandiose feelings of uniqueness.

Epidemiology

According to DSM-IV-TR, estimates of the prevalence of narcissistic personality disorder range from 2 to 16 percent in the clinical population and less than 1 percent in the general population. Persons with the disorder may impart an unrealistic sense of omnipotence, grandiosity, beauty, and talent to their children; thus, offspring of such parents may have a higher than usual risk for developing the disorder themselves. The number of cases of narcissistic personality disorder reported is increasing steadily.

Diagnosis

Table 23–8 gives the DSM-IV-TR diagnostic criteria for narcissistic personality disorder.

Clinical Features

Persons with narcissistic personality disorder have a grandiose sense of self-importance; they consider themselves special and expect special treatment. Their sense of entitlement is striking. They handle criticism poorly and may become enraged when someone dares to criticize them, or they may appear completely indifferent to criticism. Persons with this disorder want their own way and are frequently ambitious to achieve fame and fortune. Their relationships are fragile, and they can make others furious by their refusal to obey conventional rules of behavior. Interpersonal exploitiveness is commonplace. They cannot show empathy, and they feign sympathy only to achieve their selfish ends. Because of their fragile self-esteem, they are susceptible to depression. Interpersonal difficulties, occupational problems, rejection, and loss are among the stresses that narcissists

Table 23–8
DSM-IV-TR Diagnostic Criteria for Narcissistic Personality Disorder

A pervasive pattern of grandiosity (in fantasy or behavior), need for admiration, and lack of empathy, beginning by early adulthood and present in a variety of contexts, as indicated by five (or more) of the following:

(1) has a grandiose sense of self-importance (e.g., exaggerates achievements and talents, expects to be recognized as superior without commensurate achievements)

(2) is preoccupied with fantasies of unlimited success, power, brilliance, beauty, or ideal love

(3) believes that he or she is "special" and unique and can only be understood by, or should associate with, other special or high-status people (or institutions)

(4) requires excessive admiration

(5) has a sense of entitlement, i.e., unreasonable expectations of especially favorable treatment or automatic compliance with his or her expectations

(6) is interpersonally exploitative, i.e., takes advantage of others to achieve his or her own ends

(7) lacks empathy: is unwilling to recognize or identify with the feelings and needs of others

(8) is often envious of others or believes that others are envious of him or her

(9) shows arrogant, haughty behaviors or attitudes

From American Psychiatric Association. *Diagnostic and Statistical Manual of Mental Disorders.* 4th ed. Text rev. Washington, DC: American Psychiatric Association; copyright 2000, with permission.

commonly produce by their behavior—stresses they are least able to handle.

Differential Diagnosis

Borderline, histrionic, and antisocial personality disorders often accompany narcissistic personality disorder, so a differential diagnosis is difficult. Patients with narcissistic personality disorder have less anxiety than those with borderline personality disorder; their lives tend to be less chaotic, and they are less likely to attempt suicide. Patients with antisocial personality disorder have a history of impulsive behavior, often associated with alcohol or other substance abuse, which frequently gets them into trouble with the law. Patients with histrionic personality disorder show features of exhibitionism and interpersonal manipulativeness that resemble those of patients with narcissistic personality disorder.

Course and Prognosis

Narcissistic personality disorder is chronic and difficult to treat. Patients with the disorder must constantly deal with blows to their narcissism resulting from their behavior or from life experience. Aging is handled poorly; patients value beauty, strength, and youthful attributes, to which they cling inappropriately. They may be more vulnerable, therefore, to midlife crises than are other groups.

Treatment

Psychotherapy.   Because patients must renounce their narcissism to make progress, the treatment of narcissistic personality disorder is difficult. Psychiatrists such as Kernberg and Heinz Kohut have advocated using psychoanalytic approaches to effect change, but much research is required to validate the diagnosis and to determine the best treatment. Some clinicians advocate group therapy for their patients so they can learn how to share with others and, under ideal circumstances, can develop an empathic response to others.

Pharmacotherapy.   Lithium (Eskalith) has been used with patients whose clinical picture includes mood swings. Because patients with narcissistic personality disorder tolerate rejection poorly and are susceptible to depression, antidepressants, especially serotonergic drugs, may also be of use.

AVOIDANT PERSONALITY DISORDER

Persons with avoidant personality disorder show extreme sensitivity to rejection and may lead a socially withdrawn life. Although shy, they are not asocial and show a great desire for companionship, but they need unusually strong guarantees of uncritical acceptance. Such persons are commonly described as having an inferiority complex.

Epidemiology

Avoidant personality disorder is common. The prevalence of the disorder is 1 to 10 percent of the general population. No information is available on sex ratio or familial pattern. Infants clas-

sified as having a timid temperament may be more susceptible to the disorder than those who score high on activity-approach scales.

Diagnosis

In clinical interviews, patients' most striking aspect is anxiety about talking with an interviewer. Their nervous and tense manner appears to wax and wane with their perception of whether an interviewer likes them. They seem vulnerable to the interviewer's comments and suggestions and may regard a clarification or interpretation as criticism. The DSM-IV-TR diagnostic criteria for avoidant personality disorder are listed in Table 23–9.

Clinical Features

Hypersensitivity to rejection by others is the central clinical feature of avoidant personality disorder, and patients' main personality trait is timidity. These persons desire the warmth and security of human companionship, but justify their avoidance of relationships by their alleged fear of rejection. When talking with someone, they express uncertainty, show a lack of self-confidence, and may speak in a self-effacing manner. Because they are hypervigilant about rejection, they are afraid to speak up in public or to make requests of others. They are apt to misinterpret other persons' comments as derogatory or ridiculing. The refusal of any request leads them to withdraw from others and to feel hurt.

In the vocational sphere, patients with avoidant personality disorder often take jobs on the sidelines. They rarely attain much personal advancement or exercise much authority but seem shy and eager to please. These persons are generally unwilling to enter relationships unless they are given an unusually strong guarantee of uncritical acceptance. Consequently, they often have no close friends or confidants.

Table 23–9
DSM-IV-TR Diagnostic Criteria for Avoidant Personality Disorder

A pervasive pattern of social inhibition, feelings of inadequacy, and hypersensitivity to negative evaluation, beginning by early adulthood and present in a variety of contexts, as indicated by four (or more) of the following:

(1) avoids occupational activities that involve significant interpersonal contact, because of fears of criticism, disapproval, or rejection
(2) is unwilling to get involved with people unless certain of being liked
(3) shows restraint within intimate relationships because of the fear of being shamed or ridiculed
(4) is preoccupied with being criticized or rejected in social situations
(5) is inhibited in new interpersonal situations because of feelings of inadequacy
(6) views self as socially inept, personally unappealing, or inferior to others
(7) is unusually reluctant to take personal risks or to engage in any new activities because they may prove embarrassing

From American Psychiatric Association. *Diagnostic and Statistical Manual of Mental Disorders.* 4th ed. Text rev. Washington, DC: American Psychiatric Association; copyright 2000, with permission.

Differential Diagnosis

Patients with avoidant personality disorder desire social interaction, unlike patients with schizoid personality disorder, who want to be alone. Patients with avoidant personality disorder are not as demanding, irritable, or unpredictable as those with borderline and histrionic personality disorders. Avoidant personality disorder and dependent personality disorder are similar. Patients with dependent personality disorder are presumed to have a greater fear of being abandoned or unloved than those with avoidant personality disorder, but the clinical picture may be indistinguishable.

Course and Prognosis

Many persons with avoidant personality disorder are able to function in a protected environment. Some marry, have children, and live surrounded only by family members. Should their support system fail, however, they are subject to depression, anxiety, and anger. Phobic avoidance is common, and patients with the disorder may give histories of social phobia or incur social phobia in the course of their illness.

Treatment

Psychotherapy.   Psychotherapeutic treatment depends on solidifying an alliance with patients. As trust develops, a therapist must convey an accepting attitude toward the patient's fears, especially the fear of rejection. The therapist eventually encourages a patient to move out into the world to take what are perceived as great risks of humiliation, rejection, and failure. But therapists should be cautious when giving assignments to exercise new social skills outside therapy; failure can reinforce a patient's already poor self-esteem. Group therapy may help patients understand how their sensitivity to rejection affects them and others. Assertiveness training is a form of behavior therapy that may teach patients to express their needs openly and to enlarge their self-esteem.

Pharmacotherapy.   Pharmacotherapy has been used to manage anxiety and depression when they are associated with the disorder. Some patients are helped by β-adrenergic receptor antagonists, such as atenolol (Tenormin), to manage autonomic nervous system hyperactivity, which tends to be high in patients with avoidant personality disorder, especially when they approach feared situations. Serotonergic agents may help rejection sensitivity. Theoretically, dopaminergic drugs might engender novelty-seeking behavior in these patients; however, the patient must be psychologically prepared for any new experience that might result.

DEPENDENT PERSONALITY DISORDER

Persons with dependent personality disorder subordinate their needs to those of others, get others to assume responsibility for major areas of their lives, lack self-confidence, and may experience intense discomfort when alone for more than a brief period. The disorder has been called *passive-dependent personality*. Freud described an oral-dependent personality dimension characterized by dependence, pessimism, fear of sexuality, self-

doubt, passivity, suggestibility, and lack of perseverance; his description is similar to the DSM-IV-TR categorization of dependent personality disorder.

Epidemiology

Dependent personality disorder is more common in women than in men. One study diagnosed 2.5 percent of all personality disorders as falling into this category. It is more common in young children than in older ones. Persons with chronic physical illness in childhood may be most susceptible to the disorder.

Diagnosis

In interviews, patients appear compliant. They try to cooperate, welcome specific questions, and look for guidance. The DSM-IV-TR diagnostic criteria for dependent personality disorder are listed in Table 23–10.

Clinical Features

Dependent personality disorder is characterized by a pervasive pattern of dependent and submissive behavior. Persons with the disorder cannot make decisions without an excessive amount of advice and reassurance from others. They avoid positions of responsibility and become anxious if asked to assume a leadership role. They prefer to be submissive. When on their own, they find it difficult to persevere at tasks, but they may find it easy to perform these tasks for someone else.

Table 23–10
DSM-IV-TR Diagnostic Criteria for Dependent Personality Disorder

A pervasive and excessive need to be taken care of that leads to submissive and clinging behavior and fears of separation, beginning by early adulthood and present in a variety of contexts, as indicated by five (or more) of the following:

(1) has difficulty making everyday decisions without an excessive amount of advice and reassurance from others
(2) needs others to assume responsibility for most major areas of his or her life
(3) has difficulty expressing disagreement with others because of fear of loss of support or approval. **Note:** Do not include realistic fears of retribution.
(4) has difficulty initiating projects or doing things on his or her own (because of a lack of self-confidence in judgment or abilities rather than a lack of motivation or energy)
(5) goes to excessive lengths to obtain nurturance and support from others, to the point of volunteering to do things that are unpleasant
(6) feels uncomfortable or helpless when alone because of exaggerated fears of being unable to care for himself or herself
(7) urgently seeks another relationship as a source of care and support when a close relationship ends
(8) is unrealistically preoccupied with fears of being left to take care of himself or herself

Because persons with the disorder do not like to be alone, they seek out others on whom they can depend; their relationships, thus, are distorted by their need to be attached to another person. In folie à deux (shared psychotic disorder), one member of the pair usually has dependent personality disorder; the submissive partner takes on the delusional system of the more aggressive, assertive partner on whom he or she depends.

Pessimism, self-doubt, passivity, and fears of expressing sexual and aggressive feelings all typify the behavior of persons with dependent personality disorder. An abusive, unfaithful, or alcoholic spouse may be tolerated for long periods to avoid disturbing the sense of attachment.

Differential Diagnosis

The traits of dependence are found in many psychiatric disorders, so differential diagnosis is difficult. Dependence is a prominent factor in patients with histrionic and borderline personality disorders, but those with dependent personality disorder usually have a long-term relationship with one person rather than a series of persons on whom they are dependent, and they do not tend to be overtly manipulative. Patients with schizoid and schizotypal personality disorders may be indistinguishable from those with avoidant personality disorder. Dependent behavior can occur in patients with agoraphobia, but these patients tend to have a high level of overt anxiety or even panic.

Course and Prognosis

Little is known about the course of dependent personality disorder. Occupational functioning tends to be impaired because persons with the disorder cannot act independently and without close supervision. Social relationships are limited to those on whom they can depend, and many suffer physical or mental abuse because they cannot assert themselves. They risk major depressive disorder if they lose the person on whom they depend, but, with treatment, the prognosis is favorable.

Treatment

Psychotherapy.   The treatment of dependent personality disorder is often successful. Insight-oriented therapies enable patients to understand the antecedents of their behavior, and, with the support of a therapist, patients can become more independent, assertive, and self-reliant. Behavioral therapy, assertiveness training, family therapy, and group therapy have all been used, with successful outcomes in many cases.

A pitfall may arise in treatment when a therapist encourages a patient to change the dynamics of a pathological relationship (e.g., supports a physically abused wife in seeking help from the police). At this point, patients may become anxious and unable to cooperate in therapy; they may feel torn between complying with the therapist and losing a pathological external relationship. Therapists must show great respect for these patients' feelings of attachment, no matter how pathological these feelings may seem.

Pharmacotherapy.   Pharmacotherapy has been used to deal with specific symptoms, such as anxiety and depression, which are common associated features of dependent personality disorder. Patients who experience panic attacks or who have high levels of separation anxiety may be helped by imipramine (Tofranil). Benzodiazepines and serotonergic agents have also been useful. If a patient's depression or withdrawal symptoms respond to psychostimulants, they may be used.

OBSESSIVE-COMPULSIVE PERSONALITY DISORDER

Obsessive-compulsive personality disorder is characterized by emotional constriction, orderliness, perseverance, stubbornness, and indecisiveness. The essential feature of the disorder is a pervasive pattern of perfectionism and inflexibility.

Epidemiology

The prevalence of obsessive-compulsive personality disorder is unknown. It is more common in men than in women and is diagnosed most often in oldest children. The disorder also occurs more frequently in first-degree biological relatives of persons with the disorder than in the general population. Patients often have backgrounds characterized by harsh discipline. Freud hypothesized that the disorder is associated with difficulties in the anal stage of psychosexual development, generally around the age of 2 years, but various studies have failed to validate this theory.

Diagnosis

In interviews, patients with obsessive-compulsive personality disorder may have a stiff, formal, and rigid demeanor. Their affect is not blunted or flat but can be described as constricted. They lack spontaneity, and their mood is usually serious. Such patients may be anxious about not being in control of the interview. Their answers to questions are unusually detailed. The defense mechanisms they use are rationalization, isolation, intellectualization, reaction formation, and undoing. The DSM-IV-TR diagnostic criteria for obsessive-compulsive personality disorder are listed in Table 23–11.

Clinical Features

Persons with obsessive-compulsive personality disorder are preoccupied with rules, regulations, orderliness, neatness, details, and the achievement of perfection. These traits account for the general constriction of the entire personality. They insist that rules be followed rigidly and cannot tolerate what they consider infractions. Accordingly, they lack flexibility and are intolerant. They are capable of prolonged work, provided it is routinized and does not require changes to which they cannot adapt.

Persons with obsessive-compulsive personality disorder have limited interpersonal skills. They are formal and serious and often lack a sense of humor. They alienate persons, are unable to compromise, and insist that others submit to their needs. They are eager to please those whom they see as more powerful than they are, however, and they carry out these persons' wishes in an authoritarian manner. Because they fear making mistakes, they are indecisive and ruminate about making decisions. Although a stable marriage and occupational adequacy are common,

Table 23–11
DSM-IV-TR Diagnostic Criteria for Obsessive-Compulsive Personality Disorder

A pervasive pattern of preoccupation with orderliness, perfectionism, and mental and interpersonal control, at the expense of flexibility, openness, and efficiency, beginning by early adulthood and present in a variety of contexts, as indicated by four (or more) of the following:

(1) is preoccupied with details, rules, lists, order, organization, or schedules to the extent that the major point of the activity is lost
(2) shows perfectionism that interferes with task completion (e.g., is unable to complete a project because his or her own overly strict standards are not met)
(3) is excessively devoted to work and productivity to the exclusion of leisure activities and friendships (not accounted for by obvious economic necessity)
(4) is overconscientious, scrupulous, and inflexible about matters of morality, ethics, or values (not accounted for by cultural or religious identification)
(5) is unable to discard worn-out or worthless objects even when they have no sentimental value
(6) is reluctant to delegate tasks or to work with others unless they submit to exactly his or her way of doing things
(7) adopts a miserly spending style toward both self and others; money is viewed as something to be hoarded for future catastrophes
(8) shows rigidity and stubbornness

From American Psychiatric Association. *Diagnostic and Statistical Manual of Mental Disorders.* 4th ed. Text rev. Washington, DC: American Psychiatric Association; copyright 2000, with permission.

persons with obsessive-compulsive personality disorder have few friends. Anything that threatens to upset their perceived stability or the routine of their lives can precipitate much anxiety otherwise bound up in the rituals that they impose on their lives and try to impose on others.

The patient was a 45-year-old lawyer who sought treatment at his wife's insistence. She was fed up with their marriage; she could no longer tolerate his emotional coldness, rigid demands, bullying behavior, sexual disinterest, long work hours, and frequent business trips. The patient felt no particular distress in his marriage and had agreed to the consultation only to humor his wife.

It soon developed, however, that the patient was troubled by problems at work. He was known as that hardest-driving member of a hard-driving law firm. He was the youngest full partner in the firm's history and is famous for being able to handle many cases at the same time. Lately, he found himself increasingly unable to keep up. He was too proud to turn down a new case and too much of a perfectionist to be satisfied with the quality of work performed by his assistants. Displeased by their writing style and sentence structure, he found himself constantly correcting their briefs and, therefore, unable to stay abreast of his schedule. People at work complained that his attention to detail and inability to delegate responsibility were reducing his efficiency. He has had two or three secretaries a year for 15 years. No one could tolerate working for him for very long because he was so critical of any mistakes made by others. When assignments got backed up, he could not decide which to address first,

started making schedules for himself and his staff, but then was unable to meet them and worked 15 hours a day. He found it difficult to be decisive now that his work had expanded beyond his own direct control.

The patient discussed his children as if they were mechanical dolls, but also with a clear underlying affection. He described his wife as a "suitable mate" and had trouble understanding why she was dissatisfied. He was punctilious in his manners and dress and slow and ponderous in his speech, dry and humorless, with a stubborn determination to get his point across.

The patient was the son of two upwardly mobile, extremely hardworking parents. He grew up feeling that he was never working hard enough, that he had much to achieve and very little time. He was a superior student, a "bookworm," awkward and unpopular in adolescent social pursuits. He had always been competitive and a high achiever. He had trouble relaxing on vacations, developed elaborate activity schedules for every family member, and became impatient and furious if they refused to follow his plans. He liked sports but had little time for them and refused to play if he couldn't be at the top of his form. He was a ferocious competitor on the tennis courts and a poor loser. (Reprinted with permission from the *DSM-IV-TR Casebook.*)

Differential Diagnosis

When recurrent obsessions or compulsions are present, obsessive-compulsive disorder should be noted on Axis I. Perhaps the most difficult distinction is between outpatients with some obsessive-compulsive traits and those with obsessive-compulsive personality disorder. The diagnosis of personality disorder is reserved for those with significant impairments in their occupational or social effectiveness. In some cases, delusional disorder coexists with personality disorders and should be noted.

Course and Prognosis

The course of obsessive-compulsive personality disorder is variable and unpredictable. From time to time, persons may develop obsessions or compulsions in the course of their disorder. Some adolescents with obsessive-compulsive personality disorder evolve into warm, open, and loving adults; in others, the disorder can be either the harbinger of schizophrenia or—decades later and exacerbated by the aging process—major depressive disorder.

Persons with obsessive-compulsive personality disorder may flourish in positions demanding methodical, deductive, or detailed work, but they are vulnerable to unexpected changes, and their personal lives may remain barren. Depressive disorders, especially those of late onset, are common.

Treatment

Psychotherapy.   Unlike patients with the other personality disorders, those with obsessive-compulsive personality disorder are often aware of their suffering, and they seek treatment on their own. Overtrained and oversocialized, these patients value free association and non-directive therapy highly. Treatment, however, is often long and complex, and countertransference problems are common.

Group therapy and behavior therapy occasionally offer certain advantages. In both contexts, it is easy to interrupt the patients in the midst of their maladaptive interactions or explanations. Preventing the completion of their habitual behavior raises patients' anxiety and leaves them susceptible to learning new coping strategies. Patients can also receive direct rewards for change in group therapy, something less often possible in individual psychotherapies.

Pharmacotherapy.   Clonazepam (Klonopin), a benzodiazepine with anticonvulsant use, has reduced symptoms in patients with severe obsessive-compulsive disorder. Whether it is of use in the personality disorder is unknown. Clomipramine (Anafranil) and such serotonergic agents as fluoxetine, usually at doses of 60 to 80 mg a day, may be useful if obsessive-compulsive signs and symptoms break through. Nefazodone (Serzone) may benefit some patients.

PERSONALITY DISORDER NOT OTHERWISE SPECIFIED

In DSM-IV-TR, the category personality disorder not otherwise specified is reserved for disorders that do not fit into any of the personality disorder categories described previously. Passive-aggressive personality disorder and depressive personality disorder are now listed as examples of personality disorder not otherwise specified. A narrow spectrum of behavior or a particular trait—such as oppositionalism, sadism, or masochism—can also be classified in this category. A patient with features of more than one personality disorder but without the complete criteria of any one disorder can be assigned this classification. The DSM-IV-TR criteria for personality disorder not otherwise specified are presented in Table 23–12.

Passive-Aggressive Personality Disorder

Persons with passive-aggressive personality disorder are characterized by covert obstructionism, procrastination, stubbornness, and inefficiency. Such behavior is a manifestation of passively

Table 23–12
DSM-IV-TR Diagnostic Criteria for Personality Disorder Not Otherwise Specified

This category is for disorders of personality functioning that do not meet criteria for any specific personality disorder. An example is the presence of features of more than one specific personality disorder that do not meet the full criteria for any one personality disorder ("mixed personality"), but that together cause clinically significant distress or impairment in one or more important areas of functioning (e.g., social or occupational). This category can also be used when the clinician judges that a specific personality disorder that is not included in the classification is appropriate. Examples include depressive personality disorder and passive-aggressive personality disorder.

From American Psychiatric Association. *Diagnostic and Statistical Manual of Mental Disorders.* 4th ed. Text rev. Washington, DC: American Psychiatric Association; copyright 2000, with permission.

Table 23–13
DSM-IV-TR Research Criteria for Passive-Aggressive Personality Disorder

A. A pervasive pattern of negativistic attitudes and passive resistance to demands for adequate performance, beginning by early adulthood and present in a variety of contexts, as indicated by four (or more) of the following:
    (1) passively resists fulfilling routine social and occupational tasks
    (2) complains of being misunderstood and unappreciated by others
    (3) is sullen and argumentative
    (4) unreasonably criticizes and scorns authority
    (5) expresses envy and resentment toward those apparently more fortunate
    (6) voices exaggerated and persistent complaints of personal misfortune
    (7) alternates between hostile defiance and contrition
B. Does not occur exclusively during major depressive episodes and is not better accounted for by dysthymic disorder.

From American Psychiatric Association. *Diagnostic and Statistical Manual of Mental Disorders.* 4th ed. Text rev. Washington, DC: American Psychiatric Association; copyright 2000, with permission.

expressed underlying aggression. In DSM-IV-TR, the disorder is also called *negativistic personality disorder*.

Epidemiology.   No data are available about the epidemiology of the disorder. Sex ratio, familial patterns, and prevalence have not been adequately studied.

Diagnosis.   The criteria for passive-aggressive personality disorder are presented in Table 23–13.

Clinical Features.   Patients with passive-aggressive personality disorder characteristically procrastinate, resist demands for adequate performance, find excuses for delays, and find fault with those on whom they depend; yet they refuse to extricate themselves from the dependent relationships. They usually lack assertiveness and are not direct about their needs and wishes. They fail to ask needed questions about what is expected of them and may become anxious when forced to succeed or when their usual defense of turning anger against themselves is removed.

Differential Diagnosis.   Passive-aggressive personality disorders must be differentiated from histrionic and borderline personality disorders. Patients with passive-aggressive personality disorder, however, are less flamboyant, dramatic, affective, and openly aggressive than those with histrionic and borderline personality disorders.

Course and Prognosis.   In a follow-up study averaging 11 years of 100 inpatients with passive-aggressive disorder, Ivor Small found that the primary diagnosis in 54 was passive-aggressive personality disorder; 18 were also alcohol abusers, and 30 could be clinically labeled as depressed. Of the 73 former patients located, 58 (79 percent) had persistent psychiatric difficulties, and 9 (12 percent) were considered symptom free. Most seemed irritable, anxious, and depressed; somatic complaints were numerous. Only 32 (44 percent) were employed full time as workers or homemakers. Although neglect of responsibility and suicide attempts were common, only 1 patient had committed suicide in the interim. Twenty-eight (38 percent) had been readmitted to a hospital, but only 3 had been diagnosed as having schizophrenia.

Treatment.   Patients with passive-aggressive personality disorder who receive supportive psychotherapy have good outcomes, but psychotherapy for these patients has many pitfalls. Fulfilling their demands often supports their pathology, but refusing their demands rejects them. Therapy sessions, thus, can become a battleground on which a patient expresses feelings of resentment against a therapist on whom the patient wishes to become dependent. With these patients, clinicians must treat suicide gestures like any covert expression of anger and not like object loss in major depressive disorder. Therapists must point out the probable consequences of passive-aggressive behaviors as they occur. Such confrontations may be more helpful than a correct interpretation in changing patients' behavior.

Antidepressants should be prescribed only when clinical indications of depression and the possibility of suicide exist. Depending on the clinical features, some patients have responded to benzodiazepines and psychostimulants.

Depressive Personality Disorder

Persons with depressive personality disorder are characterized by lifelong traits that fall along the depressive spectrum. They are pessimistic, anhedonic, duty bound, self-doubting, and chronically unhappy. The disorder is newly classified in DSM-IV-TR, but melancholic personality was described by early 20th-century European psychiatrists such as Ernst Kretschmer.

Epidemiology.   Because depressive personality disorder is a new category, no epidemiological data are available. On the basis of the prevalence of depressive disorders in the overall population, however, depressive personality disorder seems to be common, to occur equally in men and women, and to occur in families in which depressive disorders are found.

Etiology.   The cause of depressive personality disorder is unknown, but the same factors involved in dysthymic disorder and major depressive disorder may be at work. Psychological theories involve early loss, poor parenting, punitive superegos, and extreme feelings of guilt. Biological theories involve the hypothalamic-pituitary-adrenal-thyroid axis, including the noradrenergic and serotonergic amine systems. Genetic predisposition, as indicated by Stella Chess's studies of temperament, may also play a role.

Diagnosis and Clinical Features.   More recently, Hagop Akiskal described seven groups of depressive traits: quiet, introverted, passive, and nonassertive; gloomy, pessimistic, serious, and incapable of fun; self-critical, self-reproachful, and self-derogatory; skeptical, critical of others, and hard to please; conscientious, responsible, and self-disciplined; brooding and given to worry; and preoccupied with negative events, feelings of inadequacy, and personal shortcomings.

Patients with depressive personality disorder complain of chronic feelings of unhappiness. They admit to low self-esteem and difficulty finding anything in their lives about which they are

Table 23–14
DSM-IV-TR Research Criteria for Depressive Personality Disorder

A. A pervasive pattern of depressive cognitions and behaviors beginning by early adulthood and present in a variety of contexts, as indicated by five (or more) of the following:
   (1) usual mood is dominated by dejection, gloominess, cheerlessness, joylessness, unhappiness
   (2) self-concept centers around beliefs of inadequacy, worthlessness, and low self-esteem
   (3) is critical, blaming, and derogatory toward self
   (4) is brooding and given to worry
   (5) is negativistic, critical, and judgmental toward others
   (6) is pessimistic
   (7) is prone to feeling guilty or remorseful
B. Does not occur exclusively during major depressive episodes and is not better accounted for by dysthymic disorder.

From American Psychiatric Association. *Diagnostic and Statistical Manual of Mental Disorders.* 4th ed. Text rev. Washington, DC: American Psychiatric Association; copyright 2000, with permission.

joyful, hopeful, or optimistic. They are self-critical and derogatory and are likely to denigrate their work, themselves, and their relationships with others. Their physiognomy often reflects their mood—poor posture, depressed facies, hoarse voice, and psychomotor retardation. The DSM-IV-TR criteria are listed in Table 23–14.

Differential Diagnosis.   Dysthymic disorder is a mood disorder characterized by greater fluctuation in mood than occurs in depressive personality disorder. The personality disorder is chronic and lifelong, whereas dysthymic disorder is episodic, can occur at any time, and usually has a precipitating stressor. The depressive personality can be conceptualized as part of a spectrum of affective conditions in which dysthymic disorder and major depressive disorder are more severe variants. Patients with avoidant personality disorder are introverted and dependent, but they tend to be more anxious than depressed, compared with persons with depressive personality disorder.

Course and Prognosis.   Persons with depressive personality disorder may be at great risk for dysthymic disorder and major depressive disorder. In a recent study by Donald Klein and Gregory Mills, subjects with depressive personality exhibited significantly higher rates of current mood disorder, lifetime mood disorder, major depression, and dysthymia than subjects without depressive personality.

Treatment.   Psychotherapy is the treatment of choice for depressive personality disorder. Patients respond to insight-oriented psychotherapy, and because their reality testing is good, they can gain insight into the psychodynamics of their illness and appreciate its effects on their interpersonal relationships. Treatment is likely to be long term. Cognitive therapy helps patients understand the cognitive manifestations of their low self-esteem and pessimism. Group psychotherapy and interpersonal therapy are also useful. Some persons respond to self-help measures.

Psychopharmacological approaches include the use of antidepressant medications, especially such serotonergic agents as sertraline (Zoloft), 50 mg a day. Some patients respond to small doses of psychostimulants, such as amphetamine, 5 to 15 mg a day. In all cases, psychopharmacological agents should be combined with psychotherapy to achieve maximum effects.

Sadomasochistic Personality Disorder

Some personality types are characterized by elements of sadism or masochism or a combination of both. Sadomasochistic personality disorder is listed here because it is of major clinical and historical interest in psychiatry. It is not an official diagnostic category in DSM-IV-TR or its appendix, but it can be diagnosed as personality disorder not otherwise classified.

Sadism is the desire to cause others pain by being either sexually abusive or generally physically or psychologically abusive. It is named for the Marquis de Sade, a late 18th-century writer of erotica describing persons who experience sexual pleasure while inflicting pain on others. Freud believed that sadists ward off castration anxiety and are able to achieve sexual pleasure only when they can do to others what they fear will be done to them.

Masochism, named for Leopold von Sacher-Masoch, a 19th-century German novelist, is the achievement of sexual gratification by inflicting pain on the self. So-called moral masochists generally seek humiliation and failure rather than physical pain. Freud believed that masochists' ability to achieve orgasm is disturbed by anxiety and guilt feelings about sex, which are alleviated by suffering and punishment.

Clinical observations indicate that elements of both sadistic and masochistic behavior are usually present in the same person. Treatment with insight-oriented psychotherapy, including psychoanalysis, has been effective in some cases. As a result of therapy, patients become aware of the need for self-punishment secondary to excessive unconscious guilt and also come to recognize their repressed aggressive impulses, which originate in early childhood.

PERSONALITY CHANGE DUE TO A GENERAL MEDICAL CONDITION

Personality change due to a general medical condition (see Table 7.5–8) deserves some discussion here. The tenth revision of the *International Statistical Classification of Diseases and Related Health Problems* includes the category personality and behavioral disorders due to brain disease, damage, and dysfunction, which includes organic personality disorder, postencephalitic syndrome, and postconcussional syndrome. Personality change due to a general medical condition is characterized by a marked change in personality style and traits from a previous level of functioning. Patients must show evidence of a causative organic factor antedating the onset of the personality change.

Etiology

Structural damage to the brain is usually the cause of the personality change, and head trauma is probably the most common cause. Cerebral neoplasms and vascular accidents, particularly of the temporal and frontal lobes, are also common causes.

Diagnosis and Clinical Features

A change in personality from previous patterns of behavior or an exacerbation of previous personality characteristics is notable. Impaired control of the expression of emotions and impulses is a cardinal feature. Emotions are characteristically labile and shallow, although euphoria or apathy may be prominent. The euphoria may mimic hypomania, but true elation is absent, and patients may admit to not really feeling happy. There is a hollow and silly ring to their excitement and facile jocularity, particularly when the frontal lobes are involved. Also associated with damage to the frontal lobes, the so-called frontal lobe syndrome, is prominent indifference and apathy, characterized by a lack of concern for events in the immediate environment. Temper outbursts, which can occur with little or no provocation, especially after alcohol ingestion, can result in violent behavior. The expression of impulses may be manifested by inappropriate jokes, a coarse manner, improper sexual advances, and antisocial conduct resulting in conflicts with the law, such as assaults on others, sexual misdemeanors, and shoplifting. Foresight and the ability to anticipate the social or legal consequences of actions are typically diminished. Persons with temporal lobe epilepsy characteristically show humorlessness, hypergraphia, hyperreligiosity, and marked aggressiveness during seizures.

Persons with personality change due to a general medical condition have a clear sensorium. Mild disorders of cognitive function often coexist but do not amount to intellectual deterioration. Patients may be inattentive, which may account for disorders of recent memory. With some prodding, however, patients are likely to recall what they claim to have forgotten. The diagnosis should be suspected in patients who show marked changes in behavior or personality involving emotional lability and impaired impulse control, who have no history of mental disorder, and whose personality changes occur abruptly or over a relatively brief time. The DSM-IV-TR diagnostic criteria are given in Table 7.5–8.

Anabolic Steroids. An increasing number of high school and college athletes and bodybuilders are using anabolic steroids as a shortcut to maximize physical development. Anabolic steroids include oxymetholone (Anadrol), somatropin (Humatrope), stanozolol (Winstrol), and testosterone.

DSM-IV-TR does not include a diagnostic category for substance-induced personality disorder, so it is unclear whether a personality change caused by steroid abuse is better diagnosed as personality change due to a general medical condition or as one of the other (or unknown) substance use disorders. It is mentioned here because anabolic steroids can cause persistent alterations of personality and behavior. Anabolic steroid abuse is discussed in Section 9.13.

Differential Diagnosis

Dementia involves global deterioration in intellectual and behavioral capacities, of which personality change is just one category. A personality change may herald a cognitive disorder that eventually will evolve into dementia. In these cases, as deterioration begins to encompass significant memory and cognitive deficits, the diagnosis of the disorder changes from personality change caused by a general medical condition to dementia. In differentiating the specific syndrome from other disorders in which personality change may occur—such as schizophrenia, delusional disorder, mood disorders, and impulse control disorders—physicians must consider the most important factor—the presence in personality change disorder of a specific organic causative factor.

Course and Prognosis

Both the course and the prognosis of personality change due to a general medical condition depend on its cause. If the disorder results from structural damage to the brain, the disorder tends to persist. The disorder may follow a period of coma and delirium in cases of head trauma or vascular accident and may be permanent. The personality change can evolve into dementia in cases of brain tumor, multiple sclerosis, and Huntington's disease. Personality changes produced by chronic intoxication, medical illness, or drug therapy (such as levodopa [Larodopa]

for parkinsonism) may be reversed if the underlying cause is treated. Some patients require custodial care or at least close supervision to meet their basic needs, avoid repeated conflicts with the law, and protect themselves and their families from the hostility of others and from destitution resulting from impulsive and ill-considered actions.

Treatment

Management of personality change disorder involves treatment of the underlying organic condition when possible. Psychopharmacological treatment of specific symptoms may be indicated in some cases, such as imipramine or fluoxetine for depression.

Patients with severe cognitive impairment or weakened behavioral controls may need counseling to help avoid difficulties at work or to prevent social embarrassment. As a rule, patients' families need emotional support and concrete advice on how to help minimize patients' undesirable conduct. Alcohol should be avoided, and social engagements should be curtailed when patients tend to act in a grossly offensive manner.

24

Psychosomatic Medicine

Psychosomatic (psychophysiological) medicine has been a specific area of study within the field of psychiatry for more than 75 years. It is informed by two basic assumptions: There is a unity of mind and body (reflected in the term mind-body medicine); and psychological factors must be taken into account when considering all disease states.

No classification for psychosomatic disease is listed in the text revision of the fourth edition of the *Diagnostic and Statistical Manual of Mental Disorders* (DSM-IV-TR). The concepts of psychosomatic medicine are subsumed in the diagnostic entity called Psychological Factors Affecting Medical Conditions. This category covers physical disorders caused by emotional or psychological factors. It also applies to mental or emotional disorders caused or aggravated by physical illness.

CLASSIFICATION

The DSM-IV-TR diagnostic criteria for psychological factors affecting medical condition are presented in Table 24–1. Excluded are (1) classic mental disorders that have physical symptoms as part of the disorder (e.g., conversion disorder, in which a physical symptom is produced by psychological conflict); (2) somatization disorder, in which the physical symptoms are not based on organic pathology; (3) hypochondriasis, in which patients have an exaggerated concern with their health; (4) physical complaints that are frequently associated with mental disorders (e.g., dysthymic disorder, which usually has such somatic accompaniments as muscle weakness, asthenia, fatigue, and exhaustion); and (5) physical complaints associated with substance-related disorders (e.g., coughing associated with nicotine dependence).

STRESS THEORY

Stress can be described as a circumstance that disturbs, or is likely to disturb, the normal physiological or psychological functioning of a person. In the 1920s, Walter Cannon (1875–1945) conducted the first systematic study of the relation of stress to disease. He demonstrated that stimulation of the autonomic nervous system, particularly the sympathetic system, readied the organism for the "fight or flight" response characterized by hypertension, tachycardia, and increased cardiac output. This was useful in the animal who could fight or flee; but in the person who could do neither by virtue of being civilized, the ensuing stress resulted in disease (e.g., produced a cardiovascular disorder).

Hans Selye (1907–1982) developed a model of stress that he called the *general adaptation syndrome*. It consisted of three phases: (1) the alarm reaction, (2) the stage of resistance, in which adaptation is ideally achieved, and (3) the stage of exhaustion, in which acquired adaptation or resistance may be lost. He considered stress a nonspecific bodily response to any demand caused by either pleasant or unpleasant conditions. Selye believed that stress, by definition, need not always be unpleasant. He called unpleasant stress distress. Accepting both types of stress requires adaptation.

The body reacts to stress—in this sense defined as anything (real, symbolic, or imagined) that threatens an individual's survival—by putting into motion a set of responses that seeks to diminish the impact of the stressor and restore homeostasis. Much is known about the physiological response to acute stress, but considerably less is known about the response to chronic stress. Many stressors occur over a prolonged period of time or have long-lasting repercussions. For example, the loss of a spouse may be followed by months or years of loneliness, and a violent sexual assault may be followed by years of apprehension and worry. Neuroendocrine and immune responses to such events help explain why and how stress can have deleterious effects.

Neurotransmitter Responses to Stress

Stressors activate noradrenergic systems in the brain (most notably in the locus ceruleus) and cause release of catecholamines from the autonomic nervous system. Stressors also activate serotonergic systems in the brain, as evidenced by increased serotonin turnover. Recent evidence suggests that, although glucocorticoids tend to enhance overall serotonin functioning, differences may exist in glucocorticoid regulation of serotonin-receptor subtypes, which can have implications for serotonergic functioning in depression and related illnesses. For example, glucocorticoids can increase serotonin 5-hydroxytryptamine–mediated actions, thus contributing to the intensification of actions of these receptor types, which have been implicated in the pathophysiology of major depressive disorder. Stress also increases dopaminergic neurotransmission in mesoprefrontal pathways.

Endocrine Responses to Stress

In response to stress, corticotropin-releasing factor (CRF) is secreted from the hypothalamus into the hypophysial-pituitary-portal system. CRF acts at the anterior pituitary to trigger release of adrenocorticotropic hormone (ACTH). Once ACTH is released, it acts at the adrenal cortex to stimulate the synthesis and release of glucocorticoids. Glucocorticoids themselves have myriad effects within the body, but their actions can be summarized in the short term as promoting energy use,

Table 24–1
DSM-IV-TR Diagnostic Criteria for Psychological Factors Affecting General Medical Condition

A. A general medical condition (coded on Axis III) is present.
B. Psychological factors adversely affect the general medical condition in one of the following ways:

(1) the factors have influenced the course of the general medical condition as shown by a close temporal association between the psychological factors and the development or exacerbation of, or delayed recovery from, the general medical condition
(2) the factors interfere with the treatment of the general medical condition
(3) the factors constitute additional health risks for the individual
(4) stress-related physiological responses precipitate or exacerbate symptoms of the general medical condition

Choose name based on the nature of the psychological factors (if more than one factor is present, indicate the most prominent):

Mental disorder affecting ... [indicate the general medical condition] (e.g., an Axis I disorder such as major depressive disorder delaying recovery from a myocardial infarction)
Psychological symptoms affecting ... [indicate the general medical condition] (e.g., depressive symptoms delaying recovery from surgery; anxiety exacerbating asthma)
Personality traits or coping style affecting ... [indicate the general medical condition] (e.g., pathological denial of the need for surgery in a patient with cancer; hostile, pressured behavior contributing to cardiovascular disease)
Maladaptive health behaviors affecting ... [indicate the general medical condition] (e.g., overeating; lack of exercise; unsafe sex)
Stress-related physiological response affecting ... [indicate the general medical condition] (e.g., stress-related exacerbations of ulcer, hypertension, arrhythmia, or tension headache)
Other or unspecified psychological factors affecting ... [indicate the general medical condition] (e.g., interpersonal, cultural, or religious factors)

From American Psychiatric Association. *Diagnostic and Statistical Manual of Mental Disorders.* 4th ed. Text rev. Washington, DC: American Psychiatric Association; copyright 2000, with permission.

increasing cardiovascular activity (in the service of the "flight or fight" response), and inhibiting functions such as growth, reproduction, and immunity.

Immune Response to Stress

Part of the stress response consists of the inhibition of immune functioning by glucocorticoids. This inhibition may reflect a compensatory action of the hypothalamic-pituitary-adrenal axis to mitigate other physiological effects of stress. Conversely, stress can also cause immune activation through a variety of pathways. CRF itself can stimulate norepinephrine release via CRF receptors located on the locus ceruleus, which activates the sympathetic nervous system, both centrally and peripherally, and increases epinephrine release from the adrenal medulla. In addition, direct links of norepinephrine neurons synapse on immune target cells. Thus, in the face of stressors, profound immune activation also occurs, including the release of humoral immune factors (cytokines) such as interleukin-1 (IL-1) and IL-6. These

cytokines can themselves cause further release of CRF, which in theory serves to increase glucocorticoid effects and thereby self-limit the immune activation.

Life Events

A life event or situation, favorable or unfavorable (Selye's distress), often occurring by chance, generates challenges to which the person must adequately respond. Thomas Holmes and Richard Rahe constructed a social readjustment rating scale after asking hundreds of persons from varying backgrounds to rank the relative degree of adjustment required by changing life events. Holmes and Rahe listed 43 life events associated with varying amounts of disruption and stress in average persons' lives and assigned each of them a certain number of units: for example, the death of a spouse, 100 life-change units; divorce, 73 units; marital separations, 65 units; and the death of a close family member, 63 units. Accumulation of 200 or more life-change units in a single year increases the risk of developing a psychosomatic disorder in that year. Of interest, persons who face general stresses optimistically rather than pessimistically are less apt to experience psychosomatic disorders; if they do, they are more apt to recover easily.

Specific versus Nonspecific Stress Factors

In addition to life stresses such as a divorce or the death of a spouse, some investigators have suggested that specific personalities and conflicts are associated with certain psychosomatic diseases. A specific personality or a specific unconscious conflict may contribute to the development of a specific psychosomatic disorder. Researchers first identified specific personality types in connection with coronary disease. An individual with a coronary personality is a hard-driving, competitive, aggressive person who is predisposed to coronary artery disease. Meyer Friedman and Ray Rosenman first defined two types of personalities: (1) type A, similar to the coronary personality, and (2) type B, calm, relaxed, and not susceptible to coronary disease (see later discussion).

Franz Alexander was a major proponent of the theory that specific unconscious conflicts are associated with specific psychosomatic disorders. For example, persons susceptible to having a peptic ulcer were believed to have strong ungratified dependency needs. Persons with essential hypertension were considered to have hostile impulses about which they felt guilty. Patients with bronchial asthma had issues with separation anxiety. The specific psychic stress theory is no longer considered a reliable indicator of who will develop which disorder; the nonspecific stress theory is more acceptable to most workers in the field today. Nevertheless, chronic stress, usually with the intervening variable of anxiety, predisposes certain persons to psychosomatic disorders. The vulnerable organ may be anywhere in the body. Some persons are "stomach reactors," whereas others are "cardiovascular reactors," "skin reactors," and so on. The diathesis or susceptibility of an organ system to react to stress is probably of genetic origin, but it may also result from acquired vulnerability (e.g., lungs weakened by smoking). According to psychoanalytic theory, the choice of the afflicted region is determined by unconscious factors, a concept known as *somatic compliance*. For example, Freud reported on a male patient with fears of homosexual impulses who developed *pruritis ani* and a woman with guilt over masturbation who developed vulvodynia.

Another nonspecific factor is the concept of alexithymia, developed by Peter Sifneos and John Nemiah, in which persons cannot express feelings because they are unaware of their mood. Such patients develop tension states that leave them susceptible to develop somatic diseases.

SPECIFIC ORGAN SYSTEMS

Gastrointestinal System

Gastrointestinal (GI) disorders rank high in medical illnesses associated with psychiatric consultation. This ranking reflects the high prevalence of GI disorders and the link between psychiatric disorders and GI somatic symptoms.

The following case history is presented to illustrate the relationship between psychiatric illness, GI disease, and GI disorders.

A freshman, male, college cross-country athlete was referred for psychiatric consultation with complaints of frequent belching and anxiety. The patient had been a successful high school runner, but had struggled in his early adjustment to college athletics. His performance was below that of his high school level. Consultation with a gastroenterologist failed to find a physical cause for his complaints.

On psychiatric consultation, the patient noted anxiety about his ability to compete at the college level. Many more talented runners were in practice and meets than he had previously experienced. He reported an urge to belch frequently and feelings of abdominal fullness. When he tried to run, he reported difficulty breathing, and feeling excess gas in his stomach prohibited him from taking a full breath. He reported significant worry with insomnia and feeling "edgy" during the day. There was no history of alcohol or drug use and no previous psychiatric history.

Further interview information was consistent with aerophagia and adjustment disorder with anxious mood. He was referred for relaxation training and brief psychotherapy to address his target anxiety symptoms. The therapy focused on reducing his fear of failing as a college athlete and reducing dysfunctional cognitions about his performance. The therapist advised the coaching staff that performance anxiety significantly contributed to the patient's symptoms. Suggestions to reduce performance anxiety in this athlete were made to the coaching staff. Citalopram (Celexa), 20 mg, was prescribed.

Over the next 6 weeks, the patient reported significant improvement in his breathing, feelings of fullness, anxiety, and sleep disturbance. His running began to improve, but had not yet returned to the expected level of performance. His coaches, however, were happy with his improvement and optimistic about his probability of eventually making a contribution to the team. (Courtesy of William R. Yates, M.D.)

Acute stress can induce physiological responses in several GI target organs. In the esophagus, acute stress increases resting tone of the upper esophageal sphincter and increases contraction amplitude in the distal esophagus. Such physiological responses may result in symptoms that are consistent with globus or esophageal spasm syndrome. In the stomach, acute stress induces decreased antral motor activity, potentially producing functional nausea and vomiting. In the small intestine, reduced migrating motor function can occur, whereas in the large intestine, myoelectrical and motility activity can be increased under acute stress. These effects in the small and large intestine may be responsible for bowel symptoms associated with irritable bowel syndrome.

Patients with contraction abnormalities and functional esophageal syndromes demonstrate high rates of psychiatric comorbidity. Functional esophageal symptoms include globus, dysphagia, chest pain, and regurgitation. Such symptoms can occur in conjunction with esophageal smooth muscle contraction abnormalities in the esophagus. Not all patients with functional esophageal symptoms display contraction abnormalities. Anxiety disorders ranked highest in a study of psychiatric comorbidity in functional esophageal spasm, being present in 67 percent of subjects referred to a GI motility laboratory for testing. Generalized anxiety disorder topped the list of anxiety disorder diagnoses in this series. Many patients in this study had anxiety disorder symptoms before the onset of esophageal symptoms. This suggests that anxiety disorder may induce physiological changes in the esophagus that can produce functional esophageal symptoms.

Peptic Ulcer Disease. Early studies of peptic ulcer disease suggested a role of psychological factors in the production of ulcer vulnerability. This effect was believed to be mediated through the increased gastric acid excretion associated with psychological stress. Studies of prisoners of war during World War II documented rates of peptic ulcer formation twice as high as those in controls. Evidence for a primary role of *Helicobacter pylori* in peptic ulcer initiation suggests that psychosocial factors may play primarily a role in the clinical expression of symptoms. Stressful life events may also reduce immune responses, resulting in a higher vulnerability to infection with *H. pylori*. No consensus exists on specific psychiatric disorders being related to peptic ulcer disease.

Cardiovascular Disorders

Cardiovascular disorders are the leading cause of death in the United States and the industrialized world. Depression, anxiety, type A behavior, hostility, anger, and acute mental stress have been evaluated as risk factors for the development and expression of coronary disease. Negative affect in general, low socioeconomic status, and low social support have been shown to have significant relationships with each of these individual psychological factors, and some investigators have proposed these latter characteristics as more promising indices of psychological risk. Data from the Normative Aging Study on 498 men with a mean age of 60 years demonstrate a dose-response relationship between negative emotions, a combination of anxiety and depression symptoms, and the incidence of coronary disease. At present, however, the strongest evidence available pertains to depression.

Type A Behavior Pattern, Anger, and Hostility. The relationship between a behavior pattern characterized by easily aroused anger, impatience, aggression, competitive striving, and time urgency (type A) and coronary artery disease (CAD) found the type A pattern to be associated with a nearly twofold increased risk of incident myocardial infarction (MI) and CAD-related mortality. Group therapy to modify a type A behavior pattern was associated with reduced reinfarction and mortality in a 4.5-year study of patients with prior MI. Type A behavior modification therapy has also been demonstrated to reduce episodes of silent ischemia seen on ambulatory electrocardiographic (ECG) monitoring.

Hostility is a core component of the type A concept. Low hostility is associated with low CAD risk in studies of workplace populations. High hostility is associated with increased risk of death in 16-year follow-up of survivors of a previous MI. In addition, hostility is associated with several physiological processes that, in turn, are associated with CAD, such as reduced parasympathetic modulation of heart rate, increased circulating catecholamines, increased coronary calcification, and increased lipid levels during interpersonal conflict. Conversely, submissiveness has been found to be protective against CAD risk in women. Adrenergic receptor function is downregulated in hostile men, presumably an adaptive response to heightened sympathetic drive and chronic overproduction of catecholamines caused by chronic and frequent anger.

Stress Management.   Psychosocial treatment has a positive impact on CAD. Individuals who undergo relaxation training, stress management, and group social support have greater reductions in emotional distress, systolic blood pressure, heart rate, and blood cholesterol level than comparison subjects. Cardiac rehabilitation itself may reduce high levels of hostility, as well as anxiety and depression symptoms, in patients after MI. A meta-analytical review of psychoeducational programs for patients with CAD concluded that they led to a substantial improvement in blood pressure, cholesterol, body weight, smoking behavior, physical exercise, and eating habits and to a 29 percent reduction in MI and 34 percent reduction in mortality, without achieving significant effects on mood and anxiety. These programs included health education and stress management components.

Cardiac Arrhythmias and Sudden Cardiac Death.
Because autonomic cardiac modulation is profoundly sensitive to acute emotional stress, such as intense anger, fear, or sadness, it is not surprising that acute emotions can stimulate arrhythmias. Indeed, instances of sudden cardiac death related to sudden emotional distress have been noted throughout history in all cultures. Two studies have demonstrated that, in addition to depression, a high level of anxiety symptoms raises the risk of further coronary events in patients after MI by two to five times that for nonanxious comparison patients. High anxiety symptom levels are associated with a tripling of risk of sudden cardiac death.

Heart Transplantation.   Heart transplantation is available to approximately 2,500 patients annually in the United States. It provides approximately 75 percent 5-year survival for patients with severe heart failure, who would otherwise have a 2-year survival of less than 50 percent. Candidates for heart transplantation typically experience a series of adaptive challenges as they proceed through the process of evaluation, waiting, perioperative management, postoperative recuperation, and long-term adaptation to life with a transplant. These stages of adaptation typically elicit anxiety, depression, elation, and working through of grief. Mood disorders are common in transplant recipients, in part because of chronic prednisone therapy.

Hypertension.   Hypertension is a disease characterized by an elevated blood pressure of 160/95 mm Hg or above. It is primary (essential hypertension of unknown etiology) or secondary to a known medical illness. Some patients have labile blood pressure (e.g., "white coat" hypertension, in which elevations occur only in a physician's office and are related to anxiety). Personality profiles associated with essential hypertension include persons who have a general readiness to be aggressive, which they try to control, albeit unsuccessfully. The psychoanalyst Otto Fenichel observed that the increase in essential hypertension is probably connected to the mental situation of persons who have learned that aggressiveness is bad and must live in a world for which an enormous amount of aggressiveness is required.

Respiratory System

Asthma.   Asthma is a chronic, episodic illness characterized by extensive narrowing of the tracheobronchial tree. Although patients with asthma are characterized as having excessive dependency needs, no specific personality type has been identified; however, up to 30 percent of persons with asthma meet the criteria for panic disorder or agoraphobia. The fear of dyspnea can directly trigger asthma attacks, and high levels of anxiety are associated with increased rates of hospitalization and asthma-associated mortality. Certain personality traits in patients with asthma are associated with greater use of corticosteroids and bronchodilators and longer hospitalizations than would be predicted from pulmonary function alone. These traits include intense fear, emotional lability, sensitivity to rejection, and lack of persistence in difficult situations.

Hyperventilation Syndrome.   Patients with hyperventilation syndrome breathe rapidly and deeply for several minutes, often unaware that they are doing so. They soon complain of feelings of suffocation, anxiety, giddiness, and lightheadedness. Tetany, palpitations, chronic pain, and paresthesias about the mouth and in the fingers and toes are associated symptoms. Finally, syncope may occur. The symptoms are caused by an excessive loss of carbon dioxide resulting in respiratory alkalosis. Cerebral vasoconstriction results from low cerebral tissue partial pressure of carbon dioxide (PCO_2).

The attack can be aborted by having patients breathe into a paper (not plastic) bag or hold their breath for as long as possible, which raises the plasma PCO_2. Another useful treatment technique is to have patients deliberately hyperventilate for 1 or 2 minutes and then describe the syndrome to them. This can also be reassuring to patients who fear they have a progressive, if not fatal, disease.

Endocrine System

Hyperthyroidism.   Hyperthyroidism, or thyrotoxicosis, results from overproduction of thyroid hormone by the thyroid gland. The most common cause is exophthalmic goiter, also called Graves' disease. Toxic nodular goiter causes another 10 percent of cases among middle-aged and elderly patients. Physical signs of hyperthyroidism include increased pulse, arrhythmias, elevated blood pressure, fine tremor, heat intolerance, excessive sweating, weight loss, tachycardia, menstrual irregularities, muscle weakness, and exophthalmos. Psychiatric features include nervousness, fatigue, insomnia, mood lability, and dysphoria. Speech may be pressured, and patients may exhibit a heightened activity level. Cognitive symptoms include a short attention span, impaired recent memory, and an exaggerated startle response. Patients with severe hyperthyroidism may exhibit visual hallucinations, paranoid ideation, and delirium. Although some symptoms of hyperthyroidism resemble those of a manic episode, an association between hyperthyroidism and mania has rarely been observed; however, both disorders may exist in the same patient.

Hypothyroidism.   Hypothyroidism results from inadequate synthesis of thyroid hormone and is categorized as either overt or subclinical. In overt hypothyroidism, thyroid hormone concentrations are abnormally low, thyroid-stimulating hormone (TSH) levels are elevated, and patients are symptomatic; in subclinical hypothyroidism, patients have normal thyroid hormone concentrations but elevated TSH levels.

Psychiatric symptoms of hypothyroidism include depressed mood, apathy, impaired memory, and other cognitive defects. In addition, hypothyroidism can contribute to treatment-refractory depression. A psychotic syndrome of auditory hallucinations and paranoia, named "myxedema madness," has been described in some patients. Urgent psychiatric treatment is necessary for patients presenting with severe psychiatric symptoms (e.g., psychosis or suicidal depression). Psychotropic agents should be given at low doses initially because the reduced metabolic rate of patients with hypothyroidism may reduce breakdown and result in higher concentrations of medications in blood, as in the following case.

Mr. DS was a 52-year-old white man who was admitted for melancholia after a suicide attempt. On admission, he acknowledged having a negative mood and poor memory for 1 year. These symptoms worsened after he was fired from his job. Mental status examination revealed time disorientation, poor memory of recent events, and inability to perform simple calculations. Laboratory tests were as follows: computed axial tomography (CAT) scan was negative, electroencephalogram (EEG) showed diffuse slowing, lumbar puncture was normal, TSH and other thyroid indices were within normal limits. Medical history was remarkable for a thyroid ablation for Graves' disease 4 years earlier, after which Mr. DS had not received thyroid replacement. He began doxepin 300 mg per day and T4 [thyroxine] 250 μg per day and, within 4 weeks, experienced marked improvement in mood, sleep, energy, and cognition. Six weeks after initiation of thyroid hormone, his TSH level was normal at 4.5 mIU/L. (Courtesy of Natalie L. Rasgon, M.D., Ph.D., Victoria C. Hendrick, M.D., and Thomas R. Garrick, M.D.)

Adrenal Disorders

Cushing's Syndrome.   Spontaneous Cushing's syndrome results from adrenocortical hyperfunction and can develop from either excessive secretion of ACTH (which stimulates the adrenal gland to produce cortisol) or from adrenal pathology (e.g., a cortisol-producing adrenal tumor). Cushing's disease, the most common form of spontaneous Cushing's syndrome, results from excessive pituitary secretion of ACTH, usually from a pituitary adenoma.

The clinical features of Cushing's disease include a characteristic "moon facies," or rounded face, from accumulation of adipose tissue around the zygomatic arch. Truncal obesity—a "buffalo hump" appearance—results from cervicodorsal adipose tissue deposition. The catabolic effects of cortisol on protein produce muscle wasting, slow wound healing, easy bruising, and thinning of the skin leading to abdominal striae. Bones become osteoporotic, sometimes resulting in pathological fractures and loss of height. Psychiatric symptoms are common and vary from severe depression to elation with or without evidence of psychotic features.

The treatment of pituitary ACTH-producing tumors involves surgical resection or pituitary irradiation. Medications that antagonize cortisol production (e.g., metyrapone) or suppress ACTH (e.g., serotonin antagonists such as cyproheptadine [Periactin]) are sometimes used but have met with limited success.

Hypercortisolism.   Psychiatric symptoms are myriad. Most patients experience fatigue and approximately 75 percent report depressed mood. Of these, approximately 60 percent experience moderate or severe depression. Depression severity does not appear to be influenced by the etiology underlying the Cushing's syndrome. Depressive symptoms occur more commonly in female patients than in male patients with Cushing's syndrome.

The withdrawal of steroids can also produce psychiatric disturbances, particularly depression, weakness, anorexia, and arthralgia. Other steroid-induced withdrawal symptoms include emotional lability, memory impairment, and delirium. Withdrawal symptoms have been noted to persist for as long as 8 weeks after corticosteroid withdrawal.

Patients presenting with mood lability or depression in association with muscle weakness, obesity, diabetes, easy bruising, cutaneous striae, acne, hypertension, and, in women, hirsutism and oligomenorrhea or amenorrhea benefit from an endocrinological evaluation.

Ms. TS was a 40-year-old white woman who was diagnosed with membranoproliferative glomerulonephritis and began treatment with prednisone, 20 mg per day. Within 10 days of beginning the steroid treatment, her mood became elevated, her speech was pressured, her sleep diminished from 8 to 6 hours a night, and her activity level was heightened. She reported that her house "has never been so clean!" Within 2 weeks of discontinuing the prednisone, her mental state returned to baseline. (Courtesy of Natalie L. Rasgon, M.D., Ph.D., Victoria C. Hendrick, M.D., and Thomas R. Garrick, M.D.)

Skin Disorders   Psychocutaneous disorders encompass a wide variety of dermatological diseases that may be affected by the presence of psychiatric symptoms or stress and psychiatric illnesses in which the skin is the target of disordered thinking, behavior, or perception. Although the link between stress and several dermatological disorders has been suspected for years, few well-controlled studies of treatments of dermatological disorders have assessed whether stress reduction or treatment of psychiatric comorbidity improves their outcome. Although evidence of interactions among the nervous, immune, and endocrine systems has improved the understanding of psychocutaneous disorders, more study of these often disabling disorders and their treatment is needed.

Psychogenic Excoriation. Psychogenic excoriations (also called *psychogenic pruritus*) are lesions caused by scratching or picking in response to an itch or other skin sensation or because of an urge to remove an irregularity on the skin from preexisting dermatoses, such as acne. Lesions are typically found in areas that the patient can easily reach (e.g., the face, upper back, and the upper and lower extremities) and are a few millimeters in diameter and weeping, crusted, or scarred, with occasional postinflammatory hypopigmentation or hyperpigmentation. The behavior in psychogenic excoriation sometimes resembles obsessive-compulsive disorder in that it is repetitive, ritualistic, and tension reducing, and patients attempt (often unsuccessfully) to resist excoriating. The skin is an important erogenous zone, and Freud believed it susceptible to unconscious sexual impulses.

Musculoskeletal System

The musculoskeletal disorders are a diverse group of syndromes and diseases that have the presence of muscle and joint symptoms as their common denominator. The relevance of these disorders to the psychiatrist is the consistently observed correlation with psychiatric illness. Many patients with a musculoskeletal disorder exhibit additional symptoms and signs suggesting the presence of an accompanying psychiatric disorder. These comorbid psychiatric conditions may be a result of the patient's psychological response to the loss and discomfort imposed by the disease or may be produced by the effect of the disease process on the central nervous system.

Rheumatoid Arthritis. Stress can predispose patients to rheumatoid arthritis and other autoimmune diseases by immune suppression. Depression is comorbid with rheumatoid arthritis in about 20 percent of individuals. Those who get depressed are more likely to be unmarried, have a longer duration of illness, and have a higher occurrence of medical comorbidity. Individuals with rheumatoid arthritis and depression commonly demonstrate poorer functional status, and they report more of the following: painful joints, pronounced experience of pain, health care use, bed days, and inability to work than do patients with similar objective measures of arthritic activity without depression.

Low Back Pain. Low back pain affects almost 15 million Americans and is one of the major reasons for days lost from work and for disability claims paid to workers by insurance companies. Signs and symptoms vary from patient to patient, most often consisting of excruciating pain, restricted movement, paresthesias, and weakness or numbness, all of which may be accompanied by anxiety, fear, or even panic. The areas most affected are the lower lumbar, lumbosacral, and sacroiliac regions. It is often accompanied by sciatica, with pain radiating down one or both buttocks or following the distribution of the sciatic nerve. Although low back pain can be caused by a ruptured intervertebral disk, a fracture of the back, congenital defects of the lower spine, or a ligamentous muscle strain, many instances are psychosomatic. Examining physicians should be particularly alert to patients who give a history of minor back trauma followed by

severe disabling pain. Patients with low back pain often report that the pain began at a time of psychological trauma or stress, but others (perhaps 50 percent) develop pain gradually over a period of months. Patients' reaction to the pain is disproportionately emotional, with excessive anxiety and depression. Furthermore, the pain distribution rarely follows a normal neuroanatomical distribution and may vary in location and intensity.

Fibromyalgia. Fibromyalgia is characterized by pain and stiffness of the soft tissues, such as muscles, ligaments, and tendons. Local areas of tenderness are referred to as "trigger points." The cervical and thoracic areas are affected most often, but the pain may be located in the arms, shoulders, low back, or legs. It is more common in women than in men. The etiology is unknown; however, it is often precipitated by stress that causes localized arterial spasm that interferes with perfusion of oxygen in the affected areas. Pain results, with associated symptoms of anxiety, fatigue, and inability to sleep because of the pain. There are no pathognomonic laboratory findings. The diagnosis is made after excluding rheumatic disease or hypothyroidism.

Headaches

Headaches are the most common neurological symptom and one of the most common medical complaints. Every year about 80 percent of the population has at least one headache, and 10 to 20 percent go to physicians with headache as their primary complaint. Headaches are also a major cause of absenteeism from work and avoidance of social and personal activities.

Most headaches are not associated with significant organic disease; many persons are susceptible to headaches at times of emotional stress. Moreover, in many psychiatric disorders, including anxiety and depressive disorders, headache is frequently a prominent symptom. Patients with headaches are often referred to psychiatrists by primary care physicians and neurologists after extensive biomedical workups, which often include magnetic resonance imaging of the head. Most workups for common headache complaints have negative findings, and such results may be frustrating for both patient and physician. Physicians not well versed in psychological medicine may attempt to reassure such patients by telling them that they have no disease. This reassurance may have the opposite effect, however—it may increase patients' anxiety and even escalate into a disagreement about whether the pain is real or imagined. Psychological stress usually exacerbates headaches, whether their primary underlying cause is physical or psychological.

TREATMENT OF PSYCHOSOMATIC DISORDERS

A major role of psychiatrists and other physicians working with patients with psychosomatic disorders is mobilizing the patient to change behavior in ways that optimize the process of healing. This may require a general change in lifestyle (e.g., taking vacations) or a more specific behavioral change (e.g., giving up smoking). Whether or not this occurs depends in large measure on the quality of the relationship between doctor and patient. Failure of the physician to establish good rapport accounts for much of the ineffectiveness in getting patients to change.

Ideally, both physician and patient collaborate and decide on a course of action. At times this may resemble a negotiation in which doctor and patient discuss various options and reach a compromise about an agreed-on goal.

Stress Management and Relaxation Therapy

Cognitive-behavioral therapy methods are increasingly used to help individuals better manage their responses to stressful life events. These treatment methods are based on the notion that cognitive appraisals about stressful events and the coping efforts related to these appraisals play a major role in determining stress responding. Cognitive-behavioral therapy approaches to stress management have three major aims: (1) to help individuals become more aware of their cognitive appraisals of stressful events, (2) to educate individuals about how their appraisals of stressful events can influence negative emotional and behavioral responses and to help them reconceptualize their abilities to alter these appraisals, and (3) to teach individuals how to develop and maintain the use of a variety of effective cognitive and behavioral stress management skills.

Stress-Management Training.   Five skills form the core of almost all stress-management programs: self-observation, cognitive restructuring, relaxation training, time management, and problem-solving.

SELF-OBSERVATION.   A daily diary format is used, with patients being asked to keep a record of how they responded to challenging or stressful events that occurred each day. A particular stress (e.g., argument with spouse) may precipitate a sign or symptom (e.g., pain in the neck).

COGNITIVE RESTRUCTURING.   Helping participants become aware of, and change, their maladaptive thoughts, beliefs, and expectations. Patients are taught to substitute negative assumptions with positive assumptions.

RELAXATION EXERCISES

Relaxation Techniques.   Edmund Jacobson in 1938 developed a method called *progressive muscle relaxation* to teach relaxation without using instrumentation as is used in biofeedback. Patients were taught to relax muscle groups, such as those involved in "tension headaches." When they encountered, and were aware of, situations that caused tension in their muscles, the patients were trained to relax. This method is a type of systematic desensitization—a type of behavior therapy.

Herbert Benson in 1975 used concepts developed from meditation in which a patient maintained a more passive attitude, allowing relaxation to occur on its own. Benson derived his techniques from various Eastern religions and practices, such as yoga. All of these techniques have in common a position of comfort, a peaceful environment, a passive approach, and a pleasant mental image on which to concentrate.

HYPNOSIS.   Hypnosis is effective in smoking cessation and dietary change augmentation. It is used in combination with aversive imagery (e.g., cigarettes taste obnoxious). Some patients exhibit a moderately high relapse rate and may require repeated programs of hypnotic therapy (usually three to four sessions).

BIOFEEDBACK.   Neal Miller in 1969 published his pioneering paper "Learning of Visceral and Glandular Responses," in which he reported that, in animals, various visceral responses regulated by the involuntary autonomic nervous system could be modified by learning accomplished through operant conditioning carried out in the laboratory. This led to humans being able to learn to control certain involuntary physiological responses (called *biofeedback*) such as blood vessel vasoconstriction, cardiac rhythm, and heart rate. These physiological changes seem to play a significant role in the development and treatment or cure of certain psychosomatic disorders. Such studies, in fact, confirmed that conscious learning could control heart rate and systolic pressure in humans.

Biofeedback and related techniques have been useful in tension headaches, migraine headaches, and Raynaud's disease. Although biofeedback techniques initially produced encouraging results in treating essential hypertension, relaxation therapy has produced more significant long-term effects than biofeedback.

TIME MANAGEMENT.   Time-management methods are designed to help individuals restore a sense of balance to their lives. The first step in training in time-management skills is designed to enhance awareness of current patterns of time use. To accomplish this goal, individuals might be asked to keep a record of how they spend their time each day, noting the amount of time spent in important categories, such as work, family, exercise, or leisure activities. Alternatively, they may be asked to list the important areas in their lives and then be asked to provide two time estimates: (1) the amount of time they spend engaging in these activities and (2) the amount of time they would like to spend engaging in these activities. Frequently, a substantial difference is seen in the amount of time individuals would like to spend on important activities and the amount of time they actually spend on them. With awareness of this difference comes increased motivation to make changes.

25

Consultation-Liaison Psychiatry

Consultation-liaison (C-L) psychiatry is the study, practice, and teaching of the relation between medical and psychiatric disorders. In C-L psychiatry, psychiatrists serve as consultants to medical colleagues (either another psychiatrist or, more commonly, a nonpsychiatric physician) or to other mental health professionals (psychologist, social worker, or psychiatric nurse). In addition, C-L psychiatrists consult regarding patients in medical or surgical settings and provide follow-up psychiatric treatment as needed. C-L psychiatry is associated with all the diagnostic, therapeutic, research, and teaching services that psychiatrists perform in the general hospital and serves as a bridge between psychiatry and other specialties.

In the medical wards of the hospital, C-L psychiatrists must play many roles: skillful and brief interviewer, good psychiatrist and psychotherapist, teacher, and knowledgeable physician who understands the medical aspects of the case. The C-L is part of the medical team and makes a unique contribution to the patient's total medical treatment.

DIAGNOSIS

Knowledge of psychiatric diagnosis is essential to C-L psychiatrists. Both dementia and delirium frequently complicate medical illness, especially among hospital patients. Delirium occurs in 15 to 30 percent of hospitalized patients. Psychoses and other mental disorders often complicate the treatment of medical illness, and deviant illness behavior, such as suicide, is a common problem in patients who are organically ill. C-L psychiatrists must be aware of the many medical illnesses that can have psychiatric symptoms. Lifetime prevalence of mental illness in chronically physically ill patients is more than 40 percent, particularly substance abuse and mood and anxiety disorders. Interviews and serial clinical observations are the C-L psychiatrist's tools for diagnosis. The purposes of the diagnosis are to identify (1) mental disorders and psychological responses to physical illness, (2) patients' personality features, and (3) patients' characteristic coping techniques to recommend the most appropriate therapeutic intervention for patients' needs.

TREATMENT

The C-L psychiatrists' principal contribution to medical treatment is a comprehensive analysis of a patient's response to illness, psychological and social resources, coping style, and psychiatric illness, if any. This assessment is the basis of the patient treatment plan. In discussing the plan, C-L psychiatrists provide their patient assessment to nonpsychiatric health professionals.

Psychiatrists' recommendations should be clear, concrete guidelines for action. A C-L psychiatrist may recommend a specific therapy, suggest areas for further medical inquiry, inform doctors and nurses of their roles in the patient's psychosocial care, recommend a transfer to a psychiatric facility for long-term psychiatric treatment, or suggest or undertake brief psychotherapy with the patient on the medical ward.

The C-L psychiatrists must deal with a broad range of psychiatric disorders, the most common symptoms being anxiety, depression, and disorientation. Treatment problems account for 50 percent of the consultation requests made of psychiatrists.

Common Consultation-Liaison Problems

Suicide Attempt or Threat.   Suicide rates are higher in persons with medical illness than in those without medical or surgical problems. High-risk factors for suicide are being a man over 45 years of age, having no social support, having an alcohol dependence, having made a previous attempt, and having a incapacitating or catastrophic medical illness, especially if accompanied by severe pain. If suicide risk is present, the patient should be transferred to a psychiatric unit or started on 24-hour nursing care.

Depression.   As mentioned, suicidal risk must be assessed in every depressed patient. Depression without suicidal ideation is not uncommon in hospitalized patients, and treatment with antidepressant medication can be started if necessary. A careful assessment of drug–drug interactions must be made before prescribing, which should be undertaken in collaboration with the patient's primary physician. Antidepressants should be used cautiously in cardiac patients because of conduction side effects and orthostatic hypotension.

Agitation.   Agitation is often related to the presence of a cognitive disorder or associated with withdrawal from drugs (e.g., opioids, alcohol, sedative-hypnotics). Antipsychotic medications (e.g., haloperidol [Haldol]) are very useful drugs for excessive agitation. Physical restraints should be used with great caution and only as a last resort. The patient should be examined for command hallucinations or paranoid ideation to which he or she is responding in an agitated manner. Toxic reactions to medications that cause agitation should always be ruled out.

Hallucinations.   The most common cause of hallucinations is delirium tremens, which usually begins 3 to 4 days after hospitalization. Patients in intensive care units who experience sensory isolation may respond with hallucinatory activity. Conditions such as brief psychotic disorder, schizophrenia, and cognitive disorders are associated with hallucinations, and they respond rapidly to antipsychotic medication. Formication, in which the patient believes that bugs are crawling over the skin, is often associated with cocainism.

Sleep Disorder.   A common cause of insomnia in hospitalized patients is pain, which, when treated, solves the sleep problem. Early-morning awakening is associated with depression, and difficulty falling asleep is associated with anxiety. Depending on the cause, antianxiety or antidepressant agents may be prescribed. Early substance withdrawal as a cause of insomnia should be considered in the differential diagnosis.

Confusion.   Delirium is the most common cause of confusion or disorientation among hospitalized patients in general hospitals. The causes are myriad and relate to metabolic status, neurological findings, substance abuse, and mental illness, among many others. Small doses of antipsychotics may be used when major agitation occurs in conjunction with the confused state; however, sedatives, such as benzodiazepines, can worsen the condition and cause sundowner syndrome (ataxia, disorientation). If sensory deprivation is a contributing factor, the environment can be modified so that the patient has sensory cues (e.g., radio, clock, no curtains around the bed).

Noncompliance or Refusal to Consent to Procedure.
Issues such as noncompliance and refusal to consent to a procedure can sometimes be traced to the relationship between the patient and his or her treating doctor, which should be explored. A negative transference toward the physician is a common cause of noncompliance. Patients who fear medication or who fear a procedure often respond well to education and reassurance. Patients whose refusal to give consent is related to impaired judgment can be declared incompetent, but only by a judge. Cognitive disorder is the main cause of impaired judgment in hospitalized patients.

No Organic Basis for Symptoms.   The C-L psychiatrist is often called in when the physician cannot find evidence of medical or surgical disease to account for the patient's symptoms. In these instances, several psychiatric conditions must be considered, including conversion disorder, somatization disorder, factitious disorders, and malingering. Glove and stocking anesthesia with autonomic nervous system symptoms is seen in conversion disorder; multiple bodily complaints are present in somatization disorder; the wish to be in the hospital occurs in factitious disorder; and obvious secondary gain is observed in patients who are malingering (e.g., compensation cases).

C-L Psychiatry in Special Situations

Intensive Care Units (ICUs).   All ICUs deal with patients who experience anxiety, depression, and delirium. ICUs also impose extraordinarily high stress on staff and patients, which is related to the intensity of the problems they encounter. Patients and staff members alike frequently observe cardiac arrests, deaths, and medical disasters, which leave them all autonomically aroused and psychologically defensive. ICU nurses and their patients experience particularly high levels of anxiety and depression. As a result, nurse burnout and high turnover rates are common.

The problem of stress among ICU staff receives much attention, especially in the nursing literature. Much less attention is given to the house staff, especially those on the surgical services. All persons in ICUs must be able to deal directly with their feelings about their extraordinary experiences and difficult emotional and physical circumstances. Regular support groups in which persons can discuss their feelings are important to the ICU staff and the house staff. Such support groups protect staff members from the otherwise predictable psychiatric morbidity that some may experience and also protect their patients from the loss of concentration, decreased energy, and psychomotor-

retarded communications that some staff members otherwise exhibit.

Hemodialysis Units.   Hemodialysis units present a paradigm of complex modern medical treatment settings. Patients are coping with lifelong, debilitating, and limiting disease; they are totally dependent on a multiplex group of caretakers for access to a machine controlling their well-being. Dialysis is scheduled three times a week and takes 4 to 6 hours; thus, it disrupts patient's previous living routines.

In this context, patients first and foremost fight the disease. Invariably, however, they also must come to terms with a level of dependence on others that they probably not experienced since childhood. Predictably, patients entering dialysis struggle for their independence; regress to childhood states; show denial by acting out against doctor's orders, by breaking their diet, or by missing sessions; show anger directed against staff members; and bargain and plead or become infantilized and obsequious. Most often, however, they are accepting and courageous. The determinants of patients' responses on entering dialysis include personality styles and previous experiences with this or another chronic illness. Patients who have had time to react and adapt to their chronic renal failure face less new psychological work of adaptation than those with recent renal failure and machine dependence.

Although little has been written about social factors, the effects of culture in reaction to dialysis and the management of the dialysis unit are known to be important. Units run with a firm hand, which is consistent in dealing with patients; clear contingencies that are in place for behavioral failures; and adequate psychological support available for staff members tend to produce the best results.

Complications of dialysis treatment can include psychiatric problems, such as depression, and suicide is not rare. Sexual problems can be neurogenic, psychogenic, or related to gonadal dysfunction and testicular atrophy. Dialysis dementia is a rare condition that evidences loss of memory, disorientation, dystonias, and seizures. The disorder occurs in patients who have been receiving dialysis treatment for many years. The cause is unknown.

The psychological treatment of dialysis patients falls into two areas. First, careful preparation before dialysis, including the work of adaptation to chronic illness, is important, especially in dealing with denial and unrealistic expectations. Predialysis, all patients should have a psychosocial evaluation. Second, once in a dialysis program, patients need periodic specific inquiries about adaptation that do not encourage dependence or the sick role. Staff members should be sensitive to the likelihood of depression and sexual problems. Group sessions function well for support, and patient self-help groups restore a useful social network, self-esteem, and self-mastery. When needed, tricyclic drugs or phenothiazines can be used for dialysis patients. Psychiatric care is most effective when brief and problem oriented.

The use of home dialysis units has improved treatment attitude. Patients treated at home can integrate the treatment into their daily lives more easily, and they feel more autonomous and less dependent on others for their care than do those who are treated in the hospital.

Surgical Units.   Some surgeons believe that patients who expect to die during surgery are more likely to do so. This belief now seems less superstitious than it once did. Chase Patterson Kimball and others have studied the premorbid psychological adjustment of patients scheduled for surgery and have shown that those who show evident depression or anxiety and deny it have a higher risk for morbidity and mortality than those who, given similar depression or anxiety, can express it. Even better results occur in those with a positive attitude toward impending surgery. The factors that contribute to an improved outcome for surgery are informed consent and education so that patients know what they can expect to feel, where they will be (e.g., it is useful to show patients the recovery room), what loss of function to expect, what tubes and gadgets will be in place, and how to cope with the anticipated pain. If patients will not be able to talk or see after surgery, it is helpful to explain before surgery what they can do to compensate for these losses. If postoperative states such as confusion, delirium, and pain can be predicted, they should be discussed with patients in advance so they do not experience them as unwarranted or as signs of danger. Constructive family support members can help both before and after surgery.

Transplantation Issues.   Transplantation programs have expanded over the past decade, and C-L psychiatrists play an important role in helping patients and their families deal with the many psychosocial issues involved: (1) which and when patients on a waiting list will receive organs, (2) anxiety about the procedure, (3) fear of death, (4) organ rejection, and (5) adaptation to life after successful transplantation. After transplant, patients require complex aftercare, and achieving compliance with medication may be difficult without supportive psychotherapy. This is particularly relevant to patients who have received liver transplants as a result of hepatitis C brought on by promiscuous sexual behavior and to drug addicts who use contaminated needles.

Group therapy with patients who have had similar transplantation procedures benefits members who can support one another and share information and feelings about particular stressors related to their disease. Groups may be conducted or supervised by the psychiatrist. Psychiatrists must be especially concerned about psychiatric complication. Within 1 year of transplant, almost 20 percent of patients experience a major depression or an adjustment disorder with depressed mood. In such cases, evaluation for suicidal ideation and risk is important. In addition to depression, another 10 percent of patients experience signs of posttraumatic stress disorder, with nightmares and anxiety attacks related to the procedure. Other issues concern whether or not the transplanted organ came from a cadaver or from a living donor who may or may not be related to the patient. Pretransplant consulting sessions with potential organ donors helps to deal with fears about surgery and concerns about who will receive the donated organ. Sometimes, both the recipient and donor may be counseled together, as in cases where one sibling is donating a kidney to another. Peer support groups with both donors and recipients have also been used to facilitate coping with transplantation issues.

PSYCHO-ONCOLOGY

Psycho-oncology seeks to study both the impact of cancer on psychological functioning and the role that psychological and behavioral variables may play in cancer risk and survival. A hallmark of psycho-oncology research has been intervention studies that attempt to influence the course of illness in patients with cancer. A landmark study by David Spiegel found that women with metastatic breast cancer who received weekly group psychotherapy survived an average of 18 months longer than control patients randomly assigned to routine care; in a review of his study he questioned that finding, but confirmed that the quality of life of the group participants was greatly improved. In another study, patients with malignant melanoma who received structured group intervention exhibited a statistically significant lower recurrence of cancer and a lower mortality rate than patients who did not receive such therapy. Patients with malignant melanoma who received the group intervention also exhibited significantly more large granular lymphocytes and natural killer (NK) cells as well as indications of increased NK cell activity, suggesting an increased immune response. Another study used a group behavioral intervention (relaxation, guided imagery, and biofeedback training) for patients with breast cancer, who demonstrated higher NK cell activity and lymphocyte mitogen responses than the controls.

Because new treatment protocols, in many cases, have transformed cancer from an incurable to frequently chronic and often curable disease, the psychiatric aspects of cancer—the reactions to both the diagnosis and the treatment—are increasingly important. At least half of the persons who contract cancer in the United States each year are alive 5 years later. Currently, an estimated 3 million cancer survivors have no evidence of the disease.

About half of all cancer patients have mental disorders. The largest groups are those with adjustment disorder (68 percent), and major depressive disorder (13 percent) and delirium (8 percent) are the next most common diagnoses. Most of these disorders are thought to be reactive to the knowledge of having cancer.

When persons learn that they have cancer, their psychological reactions include fear of death, disfigurement, and disability; fear of abandonment and loss of independence; fear of disruption in relationships, role functioning, and financial standings; and denial, anxiety, anger, and guilt. Although suicidal thoughts and wishes are frequent in persons with cancer, the actual incidence of suicide is only slightly higher than that in the general population.

Psychiatrists should make a careful assessment of psychiatric and medical issues in every patient. Special attention should be given to family factors, in particular, preexisting intrafamily conflicts, family abandonment, and family exhaustion.

26 ◣◢

Psychiatry and Reproductive Medicine

Reproductive events and processes have profound psychological effects, some of which can progress to overt psychopathological states. This section addresses such events, including pregnancy, infertility, abortion, menopause, and sterilization, among others.

PSYCHOLOGY OF PREGNANCY

Pregnant women undergo marked psychological changes. Their attitudes toward pregnancy reflect deeply felt beliefs about all aspects of reproduction, including whether the pregnancy was planned and whether the baby is wanted. The relationship with the infant's father, the age of the mother, and her sense of identity also affect a woman's reaction to prospective motherhood. Prospective fathers also face psychological challenges.

Psychologically healthy women often find pregnancy to be a means of self-realization. Many women report that being pregnant is a creative act gratifying a fundamental need. Other women use pregnancy to diminish self-doubts about femininity or to reassure themselves that they can function as women in the most basic sense. Still others view pregnancy negatively; they may fear childbirth or feel inadequate about mothering.

During early stages of their development, women must undergo the experience of separating from their mothers and of establishing an independent identity; this experience later affects their success at mothering. If a woman's mother was a poor role model, a woman's sense of maternal competence may be impaired, and she may lack confidence before and after her baby's birth. Women's unconscious fears and fantasies during early pregnancy often center on the idea of fusion with their mothers.

Psychological attachment to the fetus begins in utero, and, by the beginning of the second trimester, most women have a mental picture of the infant. Even before being born, the fetus is viewed as a separate being, endowed with a prenatal personality. Many mothers talk to their unborn children. Recent evidence suggests that emotional talk with the fetus is related not only to early mother–infant bonding, but also to the mother's efforts to have a healthy pregnancy, for example, by giving up cigarettes and caffeine. According to psychoanalytic theorists, the child-to-be is a blank screen on which a mother projects her hopes and fears. In rare instances, these projections account for postpartum pathological states, such as a mother's desire to harm her infant, whom she views as a hated part of herself. Normally, however, giving birth to a child fulfills a woman's need to create and nurture life.

Fathers are also profoundly affected by pregnancy. Impending parenthood demands a synthesis of such developmental issues as gender role and identity, separation-individuation from a man's father, sexuality, and, as Erik Erikson proposed, generativity. Pregnancy fantasies in men and wishes to give birth in boys reflect early identification with their mothers as well as the wish to be as powerful and creative as they perceive mothers to be. For some men, getting a woman pregnant is proof of their potency, a dynamic that plays a large part in adolescent fatherhood.

Marriage and Pregnancy

The prospective mother–wife and father–husband must redefine their roles as a couple and as individuals. They face readjustments in their relationships with friends and relatives and must deal with new responsibilities as caretakers of the newborn and each other. Both parents may experience anxiety about their adequacy as parents; one or both partners may be consciously or unconsciously ambivalent about the addition of the child to the family and about the effects on the dyadic (two-person) relationship. A husband may feel guilty about his wife's discomfort during pregnancy and parturition, and some men experience jealousy or envy of the experience of pregnancy. Accustomed to gratifying each other's dependency needs, the couple must attend to the unremitting needs of a new infant and a developing child. Although most couples respond positively to these demands, some do not. Under ideal conditions, the decision to become a parent and have a child should be agreed on by both partners, but sometimes parenthood is rationalized as a way to achieve intimacy in a conflicted marriage or to avoid having to deal with other life circumstance problems.

Research is underway about the psychology of pregnancy in non-married couples or in otherwise committed relationships; one would expect that many of the observations described above would also apply in those situations.

Attitudes toward the Pregnant Woman

In general, others' attitudes toward a pregnant woman reflect a variety of factors: intelligence, temperament, cultural practices, and myths of the society and the subculture into which the person was born. Married men's responses to pregnancy are generally positive. For some men, however, reactions vary from a misplaced sense of pride that they are able to impregnate the woman to fear of increased responsibility and subsequent termination of the relationship. A woman's risk of abuse by her husband or boyfriend increases during pregnancy, particularly during the first trimester. One study found that 6 percent of pregnant women are abused. Domestic abuse adds significantly to the cost of health care during pregnancy, and abused women are more likely than nonabused controls to have histories of miscarriage, abortion, and neonatal death. The reasons for abuse vary. Some men fear being neglected and not having excessive dependency needs gratified; others may see the fetus as a rival. In most cases, however, one finds a history of abuse before the woman was pregnant.

Alternative Lifestyle Pregnancy

Some lesbian couples decide that one partner should become pregnant through artificial insemination. Societal attitudes may put stress on this arrangement, but if the two women have a secure relationship, they tend to bond strongly together as a family unit. Men in committed gay relationships are fathering children through artificial insemination with surrogate mothers. Recent studies show that children raised in same-sex-couple households are not measurably different from children raised by heterosexual parents with respect to personality development, psychological development, and gender identity. These children are also not more likely to be gay or lesbian themselves.

Some single, never-married women who do not wish to marry but do want to become pregnant may do so through artificial or natural insemination. Such women constitute a group who believe that motherhood is the fulfillment of female identity, without which they view their lives to be incomplete. Most of these women have considered the consequence of single parenthood and feel able to rise to the challenges.

Sexual Behavior

The effects of pregnancy on sexual behavior vary. Some women experience an increased sex drive as pelvic vasocongestion produces a more sexually responsive state. Others are more responsive than before the pregnancy because they no longer fear becoming pregnant. Some have diminished desire or lose interest in sexual activity altogether. Libido may be decreased because of higher estrogen levels or feelings of unattractiveness. Avoidance of sex may also result from physical discomfort or an association of motherhood with asexuality. Men with a Madonna complex view pregnant women as sacred and not to be defiled by the sexual act. Either a man or a woman may erroneously consider intercourse potentially harmful to the developing fetus and, thus, something to be avoided. Men who have extramarital affairs during their wives' pregnancies usually do so during the last trimester.

Coitus. Most obstetricians place no prohibitions on coitus during pregnancy. Some suggest that sexual intercourse cease 4 to 5 weeks antepartum. If bleeding occurs early in pregnancy, an obstetrician may prohibit coitus temporarily as a therapeutic measure. Bleeding in the first 20 days of pregnancy occurs in 20 to 25 percent of women, and approximately half of that group experience spontaneous abortion. Maternal death resulting from forcibly blowing air into the vagina during cunnilingus has been reported; the deaths presumably result from air emboli in the placental–maternal circulation.

Parturition

Fears regarding pain and bodily harm during delivery are universal and, to some extent, warranted. Preparation for childbirth affords a sense of familiarity and can ease anxieties, which facilitates delivery. Continuous emotional support during labor reduces the rate of cesarean section and forceps deliveries, the need for anesthesia, the use of oxytocin, and the duration of labor. A technically difficult or even painful delivery, however, does not appear to influence the decision to bear additional children.

Men's responses to pregnancy and labor have not been well studied, but the recent trend toward inclusion of fathers in the birth process eases their anxieties and elicits a fuller sense of participation. Fathers do not parent the same way as mothers, and new mothers often need to be encouraged to respect these differences and view them positively.

Lamaze Method. Also known as natural childbirth, the Lamaze method originated with the French obstetrician Fernand Lamaze. In this method, women are fully conscious during labor and delivery, and no analgesic or anesthetic is used. The expectant mother and father attend special classes, during which they are taught relaxation and breathing exercises designed to facilitate the birth process. Women who have such training often report minimal pain during labor and delivery. Participating in the birth process may help a fearful or ambivalent father bond to his newborn infant.

Prenatal Screening

Prenatal screening for potential or actual fetal malformation is conducted in most pregnant women. Sonograms are noninvasive and can detect structural fetal abnormalities. Maternal α-fetoprotein (AFP) is measured between 15 and 20 weeks, screening for neural tube defects and Down syndrome. The sensitivity of Down syndrome testing is increased when a triple screen is done (AFP, human chorionic gonadotropin, and estriol). Amniocentesis is indicated for women older than 35 years of age, those with a sibling or parent with a known chromosome anomaly, and those with abnormal AFP or any other risk for severe genetic disorder. Amniocentesis is usually done between 16 and 18 weeks and carries a risk that 1 in 300 women will miscarry after the procedure. In the first trimester, chorionic villus sampling (CVS) can be done, which reveals the same information concerning chromosomal status, enzyme levels, and deoxyribonucleic acid patterns. With CVS, there is a risk that 1 in 100 women will have a spontaneous abortion after the procedure.

Screening in the first trimester allows women to choose early termination, which may be physically and emotionally easier on the woman. Profound ethical questions are involved in whether or not to abort a fetus with a known defect. Some women choose not to terminate and report a strong loving bond that lasts throughout the life of the child, who usually predeceases the parent.

Lactation

Lactation occurs because of a complex psychoneuroendocrine cascade that is triggered by the abrupt decline in estrogen and progesterone concentrations at parturition. In general, babies should be fed as needed rather than by schedule. Breast-feeding has many benefits. The composition of breast milk supports timely neuronal development, confers passive immunity, and reduces food allergies in the child. In subsistence-level cultures in which children are allowed to nurse as long as they want (a practice supported by La Leche League, a breast-feeding advocacy group), most babies will wean themselves between ages 3 and 5 years if not encouraged by the mother to do so earlier. Women who decide to breast-feed need good teaching and social support, which, if lacking, may lead to frustration and feelings of inadequacy. Women must not feel pressured or coerced into breast-feeding if they are opposed to or ambivalent about it. In the long term, no discernible difference exists between bottle-fed and breast-fed children as adults.

An incidental finding about lactation is that some women experience sexual sensations during lactation, which in rare cases can lead to orgasm. In the early 1990s a woman who called a help line about such feelings was put in jail and had her infant taken from her on allegations of sexual abuse. Common sense ultimately prevailed, however, and mother and infant were reunited.

Perinatal Death

Perinatal death, defined as death sometime between the 20th week of gestation and the first month of life, includes spontaneous abortion (miscarriage), fetal demise, stillbirth, and neonatal death. In previous years, the intense bond between the expectant or new parent and the fetus or neonate was underestimated, but perinatal loss is now recognized as a significant trauma for both parents. Parents who experience such a loss go through a period of mourning much as that experienced when any loved one is lost.

Intrauterine fetal death, which can occur at any time during the pregnancy, is an emotionally traumatic experience. In the early months of pregnancy, a woman is usually unaware of fetal death and learns of it only from her doctor. Later in pregnancy, after fetal movements and heart tones have been experienced, a woman may be able to detect fetal demise. When given the diagnosis of fetal death, most women want the dead fetus removed; depending on the trimester, labor may be induced, or the woman may have to wait for spontaneous expulsion of the uterine contents. Many couples consider sexual relations during the period of waiting not only undesirable but psychologically unacceptable as well.

A sense of loss also accompanies the birth of a stillborn child and induced abortion of an abnormal fetus detected by antenatal diagnosis. As mentioned, attachment to an unborn child begins before birth, and grief and mourning occur after a loss at any time. The grief experienced after a third-trimester loss, however, is generally greater than that experienced after a first-trimester loss. Some parents do not wish to view a stillborn child, and their wishes should be respected. Others wish to hold the stillborn, and this act can assist the mourning process. A subsequent pregnancy may diminish overt feelings of grief, but it does not eliminate the need to mourn. So-called replacement children are at risk for overprotection and future emotional problems.

CONCEPTION

Infertility

Infertility is the inability of a couple to conceive after 1 year of coitus without the use of a contraceptive. In the United States, about 15 percent of married couples are unable to have children. Until recently, women were blamed when couples did not have children, and feelings of guilt, depression, and inadequacy frequently accompanied the perception of being barren. Today, causes of infertility are attributed to disorders in women in 40 percent of cases, disorders in men in 40 percent, and disorders of

both in 20 percent. Tests in an infertility workup usually reveal the specific cause; however, 10 to 20 percent of couples have no identifiable cause.

The inability to have a child can produce severe psychological stress on one or both partners in a marriage. Self-blame increases the likelihood of psychological problems. Women—but not men—are at increased risk for psychological distress if they are older and do not already have biological children. If one or both partners are unwilling to take advantage of assisted reproductive techniques, the marriage may falter. A psychiatric evaluation of the couple may be advisable. Marital disharmony or emotional conflicts about intimacy, sexual relations, or parenting roles can directly affect endocrine function and such physiological processes as erection, ejaculation, and ovulation. No evidence exists, however, for any simple, causal relation between stress and infertility.

When preexisting conflict gives rise to problems of identity, self-esteem, and guilt, the disturbance may be severe and may manifest through regression; extreme dependence on a physician, mate, or parent; diffuse anger; impulsive behavior; or depression. The problem is further complicated when hormone therapy is used to treat the infertility, because the therapy may temporarily increase depression in some patients. Mood and cognition can be altered by pharmacological agents used to treat disorders of ovulation or to hyperstimulate the ovaries.

Persons who have difficulty conceiving may experience shock, disbelief, and a general sense of helplessness, and they develop an understandable preoccupation with the problem. Involvement in the infertility workup and the development of expertise about infertility can be a constructive defense against feelings of inadequacy and the humiliating, sometimes painful aspects of the workup itself. Worries about attractiveness and sexual desirability are common. Partners may feel ugly or impotent, and episodes of sexual dysfunction and loss of desire are reported. These problems are aggravated when a couple is scheduling sexual relations according to temperature charts or ovulatory cycles. Treatments for infertility are expensive and consume much time and energy. Both men and women can be overwhelmed by complexity, cost, invasiveness, and uncertainty associated with medical intervention.

Single persons who are aware of their infertility may shy away from relationships for fear of being rejected once their "defect" is known. Persons who are infertile may have particular difficulty in their adult relationships with their parents. The identification and equality that come from sharing the experience of parenthood must be replaced by internal reserves and other generative aspects of their lives.

Professional intervention may be necessary to help infertile couples ventilate their feelings and go through the process of mourning for their lost biological functions and the children they cannot have. Couples who remain infertile must cope with an actual loss. Couples who decide not to pursue parenthood may develop a renewed sense of love, dedication, and identity as a pair. Others may need help in exploring the options of husband or donor insemination, laboratory implantation, and adoption.

FAMILY PLANNING AND CONTRACEPTION

Family planning is the process of choosing when, and if, to bear children. One form of family planning is contraception, the prevention of fecundation, or fertilization of the ovum. The choice of a contraceptive method is a complex decision involving both women and their partners. Factors influencing the decision include a woman's age and medical condition, her access to medical care, the couple's religious beliefs, and the need for coital spontaneity. The woman and her partner can weigh the risks and benefits of the various forms of contraception and make their decision on the basis of their current lifestyle and other factors. The success of contraceptive technology has enabled career-minded couples to delay child-bearing into their 30s and 40s. Such a delay, however, may increase infertility problems. Consequently, many women with careers feel their biological clocks ticking and plan to have children while in their early 30s to avoid the risk of not being able to have them at all.

Sterilization

Sterilization is a procedure that prevents a man or a woman from producing offspring. In a woman, the procedure is usually salpingectomy—ligation of the fallopian tubes—a procedure with low morbidity and low mortality. A man is usually sterilized by vasectomy—excision of part of the vas deferens—which is a simpler procedure than salpingectomy and can be performed in a physician's office. Voluntary sterilization, especially vasectomy, has become the most popular form of birth control in couples married for more than 10 years.

A small proportion of patients who elect sterilization may suffer a neurotic poststerilization syndrome, which can manifest through hypochondriasis, pain, loss of libido, sexual unresponsiveness, depression, and concerns about masculinity or femininity. One study of a group of women who regretted sterilization reported they had chosen the procedure while in poor relationships, frequently with abusive partners. Regret is most prevalent when a woman forms a new relationship and wishes to have a child with a new partner. Psychiatric consultation may be necessary to separate persons seeking sterilization for irrational or psychotic reasons from those who have made the decision after some time and thought.

Abortion

Induced abortion is the planned termination of a pregnancy. About 1.3 million abortions are performed in the United States each year—246 abortions for every 1,000 live births. Over the last decade, the number of abortions has declined by about 15 percent. Family planning experts believe that more sex education and greater availability of contraceptive devices keep the number of abortions down. In Western countries, most women who obtain abortions are young, unmarried, and primiparous; in emerging countries, abortion is most common among married women with two or more children.

Of abortions, 60 percent are performed before 8 weeks of gestation, 88 percent are performed before 13 weeks, and 4.1 percent are performed between 16 and 20 weeks, with 1.4 percent occurring after 21 weeks.

Psychological Reactions to Abortion.   Recent studies demonstrate that most women who have an abortion for an unwanted pregnancy (i.e., induced abortion) were satisfied with their decision, with few, if any, negative psychological sequelae. Women who had miscarriages however (i.e., spontaneous abortion), reported a high rate of dysphoric reactions. The difference can be explained, in part, by the fact that most women who induced abortion did so because they did not want the child. Women who spontaneously miscarried presumably wanted their babies. In the long term, however, women who had induced abor-

tion were more likely to be upset about the procedure than women who had a miscarriage.

Second-trimester abortions are more psychologically traumatic than first-trimester abortions. The most common reason for late abortions is the discovery (via amniocentesis or ultrasound) of an abnormal karyotype or fetal anomaly. Thus, late abortions usually involve the loss of a wanted child with whom the mother has already formed a bond.

Before the legalization of abortion in the United States in 1973, many women sought illegal abortions, often performed by untrained practitioners under nonsterile conditions. Considerable morbidity and mortality were associated with these abortions, and women who were denied abortion sometimes chose suicide over continuation of an unwanted pregnancy. When a woman is forced to carry a fetus to term, the risk increases of infanticide, abandonment, and neglect of the unwanted newborn.

Abortion can also be a significant experience for men. If a man has a close relationship with the woman, he may wish to play an active role in the abortion by accompanying her to the hospital or abortion clinic and providing emotional support. Fathers may experience considerable grief over the termination of a wanted pregnancy.

Reproductive Senescence

Both men and women age and experience an age-related decline in reproductive capacity, but only women experience complete gonadal cessation. Loss of reproductive capacity may present a psychological challenge to those who are not reconciled to the loss of fertility. Even with gonadal failure, however, the availability of donor oocytes and sperm means that pregnancy can be initiated in a menopausal woman with an intact uterus who elects to pursue that option. Studies have shown that older men may develop a genetic sperm mutation giving rise to a higher incidence of autistic or schizophrenic offspring.

Menopause

Menopause—the cessation of ovulation—generally occurs between 47 and 53 years of age. The hypoestrogenism that follows can lead to hot flashes, sleep disturbances, vaginal atrophy and dryness, and cognitive and affective disturbances. Women are at increased risk for osteoporosis, dementia, and cardiovascular disease. Depression at menopause has been attributed to the "empty nest syndrome." Many women, however, report an enhanced sense of well-being and enjoy opportunities to pursue goals postponed because of child rearing.

PSYCHIATRIC CONDITIONS OF PREGNANCY
Postpartum Depression

Many women experience some affective symptoms during the postpartum period, 4 to 6 weeks following delivery. Most of these women report symptoms consistent with "baby blues," a transient mood disturbance characterized by mood lability, sadness, dysphoria, subjective confusion, and tearfulness. These feelings, which may last several days, have been ascribed to rapid changes in women's hormonal levels, the stress of childbirth, and the awareness of the increased responsibility that motherhood brings. No professional treatment is required other than education and support for the new mother. If the symptoms persist longer than 2 weeks, evaluation is indicated for postpartum depression.

Postpartum depression is characterized by a depressed mood, excessive anxiety, insomnia, and change in weight. The onset is generally within 12 weeks after delivery. No conclusive evidence indicates that "baby blues" will lead to a subsequent episode of depression. Several studies do indicate that an episode of postpartum depression increases the risk of lifetime episodes of major depression. Treatment of postpartum depression is not well studied because of the risk of transmitting antidepressants to newborns during lactation.

A syndrome described in fathers is characterized by mood changes during their wives' pregnancies or after the babies are born. These fathers are affected by several factors: added responsibility, diminished sexual outlet, decreased attention from his wife, and the belief that the child is a binding force in an unsatisfactory marriage.

Postpartum Psychosis

Postpartum psychosis (sometimes called *puerperal psychosis*) is an example of psychotic disorder not otherwise specified that occurs in women who have recently delivered a baby. The syndrome is often characterized by the mother's depression, delusions, and thoughts of harming either herself or her infant. Such ideation of suicide or infanticide must be carefully monitored; although rare, some mothers have acted on these ideas. Most data suggest a close relation between postpartum psychosis and mood disorders, particularly bipolar disorder and major depressive disorder.

The incidence of postpartum psychosis is about 1 to 2 per 1,000 childbirths. About 50 to 60 percent of affected women have just had their first child, and about 50 percent of cases involve deliveries associated with nonpsychiatric perinatal complications. About 50 percent of the affected women have a family history of mood disorders. The most robust data indicate that an episode of postpartum psychosis is essentially an episode of a mood disorder, usually a bipolar disorder but possibly a depressive disorder. Relatives of those with postpartum psychosis have an incidence of mood disorders that is similar to the incidence in relatives of persons with mood disorders. As many as two thirds of the patients have a second episode of an underlying affective disorder during the year after the baby's birth. The delivery process may best be seen as a nonspecific stress that causes the development of an episode of a major mood disorder, perhaps through a major hormonal mechanism.

The symptoms of postpartum psychosis can often begin within days of the delivery, although the mean time to onset is within 2 to 3 weeks and almost always within 8 weeks of delivery. Characteristically, patients begin to complain of fatigue, insomnia, and restlessness, and they may have episodes of tearfulness and emotional lability. Later, suspiciousness, confusion, incoherence, irrational statements, and obsessive concerns about the baby's health and welfare may be present. Delusional material may involve the idea that the baby is dead or defective. Patients may deny the birth and express thoughts of being unmarried, virginal, persecuted, influenced, or perverse. Hallucinations with similar content may involve voices telling the patient to kill the baby or herself. Complaints regarding the inability to move, stand, or walk are also common.

The onset of florid psychotic symptoms is usually preceded by prodromal signs such as insomnia, restlessness, agitation, lability of mood, and mild cognitive deficits. Once the psychosis occurs, the patient may be a danger to herself or to her newborn, depending on the content of her delusional system and her degree of agitation. In one study, 5 percent of patients committed suicide and 4 percent committed infanticide. A favorable outcome is associated with a good premorbid adjustment and a supportive family network. Subsequent pregnancies are associated with an increased risk of another episode, sometimes as high as 50 percent.

As with any psychotic disorder, clinicians should consider the possibility of either a psychotic disorder caused by a general medical condition or a substance-induced psychotic disorder. Potential general medical conditions include hypothyroidism and Cushing's syndrome. Substance-induced psychotic disorder can be associated with the use of pain medications such as pentazocine (Talwin) or of antihypertensive drugs during pregnancy. Other potential medical causes include infections, toxemia, and neoplasms.

Postpartum psychosis is a psychiatric emergency. Antipsychotic medications and lithium (Eskalith), often in combination with an antidepressant, are the treatments of choice. No pharmacological agents should be prescribed to a woman who is breastfeeding. Suicidal patients may require transfer to a psychiatric unit to help prevent a suicide attempt.

The mother is usually helped by contact with her baby if she so desires, but the visits must be closely supervised, especially if the mother is preoccupied with harming the infant. Psychotherapy is indicated after the period of acute psychosis, and therapy is usually directed at helping the patient accept and be at ease with the mothering role. Changes in environmental factors may also be indicated, such as increased support from the husband and others in the environment. Most studies report high rates of recovery from the acute illness.

Mrs. Z is a 30-year-old high school teacher living in Lagos, Nigeria. She is married and has five children. The birth of her last child was complicated by hemorrhage and sepsis, and she was still hospitalized on the gynecology service for 13 days after delivery when her gynecologist requested a psychiatric consultation. Mrs. Z was agitated and seemed to be in a daze. She said to the psychiatrist: "I am a sinner. I have to die. My time is past. I cannot be a good Christian again. I need to be reborn. Jesus Christ should help me. He is not helping me." A diagnosis of postpartum psychosis was made. An antipsychotic drug, chlorpromazine (Thorazine), was prescribed, and Mrs. Z was soon well enough to go home. Three weeks later, she was readmitted, this time to the psychiatric ward, claiming she "had had a vision of the spirits" and was "wrestling with the spirits." Her relatives reported that at home she had been fasting and "keeping a vigil" through the nights and was not sleeping. She had complained to the neighbors that there was a witch in her house. The witch turned out to be her mother. Mrs. Z's husband, who was studying engineering in Europe, hurriedly returned and took over the running of the household, sending his mother-in-law away and supervising Mrs. Z's treatment himself. She improved rapidly on an antidepressant medication and was discharged in 2 weeks. Her improvement, however, was short-lived. She threw away her medications and began to attend mass whenever one was given, pursuing the priests to ask questions about scriptures. Within 1 week, she was readmitted. On the ward, she accused the psychiatrist of shining powerful torch-lights on her and taking pictures of her, opening her chest, using her as a guinea pig, poisoning her food, and planning to bury her alive. She claimed to receive messages from Mars and Jupiter and announced that there was a riot in town. She clutched her Bible to her breast and accused all the doctors of being "idol worshippers," calling down the wrath of her god on all of them. After considerable resistance, Mrs. Z was finally convinced to accept electroconvulsive treatment, and she became symptom free after six treatments. At this point, she attributed her illness to a difficult childbirth, the absence of her husband, and her unreasonable mother. She saw no fur-ther role for doctors, called for her priest, and began to speak of her illness as a religious experience that was similar to the experience of religious leaders throughout history. However, her symptoms did not return, and she was discharged after 6 weeks of hospitalization. (Courtesy of Bushra Naz, M.D., Laura J. Fochtmann, M.D., and Evelyn J. Bromet, Ph.D.)

Psychotropic Medications in Pregnancy

No definitive answers exist to the questions of which psy-chotropic medications are safest during pregnancy and lactation. In patients with worsening psychiatric illness during pregnancy, outpatient psychotherapy, hospitalization, and milieu therapy should be attempted before routine use of psychotropic medi-cation. The risks and benefits of treatment with psychotropics versus maternal psychiatric illness must be carefully evaluated on an individual basis. If the patient, her psychiatrist, and her obstetrician decide to continue psychiatric medications through-out pregnancy, the dose should be calibrated to the physiological changes each trimester. Although no antidepressant medications have been associated with intrauterine death or major birth de-fects, both selective serotonin reuptake inhibitors (SSRIs) and tricyclic antidepressants are associated with a transient perinatal syndrome. Studies demonstrate that fluoxetine (Prozac) has been found in amniotic fluid. Mood stabilizers are associated with more-consequential teratogenic risks, namely cardiac anomalies and neural tube defects, but women with bipolar disorder are at a significant risk of relapse without medication maintenance. Lithium has been associated with an increased risk of Ebstein's anomaly, a congenital downward displacement of the tricuspid valve into the right ventricle. In general, all medications that are not absolutely essential should be avoided during pregnancy.

Premenstrual Dysphoric Disorder (PMDD)

Premenstrual dysphoric disorder is a somatopsychic illness trig-gered by changing levels of sex steroids that accompany an ovu-latory menstrual cycle. It occurs about 1 week before the onset of menses and is characterized by irritability, emotional lability, headache, anxiety, and depression. Somatic symptoms include edema, weight gain, breast pain, syncope, and paresthesias. Ap-proximately 5 percent of women have the disorder. Treatment is symptomatic and includes analgesics for pain and sedatives for anxiety and insomnia. Some patients respond to short courses of SSRIs. Fluid retention is relieved with diuretics.

An appendix in the text revision of the fourth edition of the *Diagnos-tic and Statistical Manual of Mental Disorders* (DSM-IV-TR) includes suggested diagnostic criteria for PMDD to help researchers and clini-cians evaluate the validity of the diagnosis (Table 26–1). Nevertheless, the generally recognized syndrome involves mood symptoms (e.g., labil-ity), behavior symptoms (e.g., changes in eating patterns), and physical symptoms (e.g., breast tenderness, edema, and headaches). This pattern of symptoms occurs at a specific time during the menstrual cycle, and the symptoms resolve for some period of time between menstrual cy-cles. The hormonal changes occurring during the menstrual cycle are probably involved in producing symptoms, although the exact etiology is unknown.

Because of the absence of generally agreed-on diagnostic criteria, the epidemiology of premenstrual dysphoria is not known with certainty. Up to 80 percent of all women experience some alteration in mood, sleep, or

Table 26–1
DSM-IV-TR Research Criteria for Premenstrual Dysphoric Disorder

A. In most menstrual cycles during the past year, five (or more) of the following symptoms were present for most of the time during the last week of the luteal phase, began to remit within a few days after the onset of the follicular phase, and were absent in the week postmenses, with at least one of the symptoms being either (1), (2), (3), or (4):

  (1) markedly depressed mood, feelings of hopelessness, or self-deprecating thoughts
  (2) marked anxiety, tension, feelings of being "keyed up," or "on edge"
  (3) marked affective lability (e.g., feeling suddenly sad or tearful or increased sensitivity to rejection)
  (4) persistent and marked anger or irritability or increased interpersonal conflicts
  (5) decreased interest in usual activities (e.g., work, school, friends, hobbies)
  (6) subjective sense of difficulty in concentrating
  (7) lethargy, easy fatigability, or marked lack of energy
  (8) marked change in appetite, overeating, or specific food cravings
  (9) hypersomnia or insomnia
  (10) a subjective sense of being overwhelmed or out of control
  (11) other physical symptoms, such as breast tenderness or swelling, headaches, joint or muscle pain, a sensation of "bloating," weight gain

  Note: In menstruating females, the luteal phase corresponds to the period between ovulation and the onset of menses, and the follicular phase begins with menses. In nonmenstruating females (e.g., those who have had a hysterectomy), the timing of luteal and follicular phases may require measurement of circulating reproductive hormones.

B. The disturbance markedly interferes with work or school or with usual social activities and relationships with others (e.g., avoidance of social activities, decreased productivity and efficiency at work or school).

C. The disturbance is not merely an exacerbation of the symptoms of another disorder, such as major depressive disorder, panic disorder, dysthymic disorder, or a personality disorder (although it may be superimposed on any of these disorders).

D. Criteria A, B, and C must be confirmed by prospective daily ratings during at least two consecutive symptomatic cycles. (The diagnosis may be made provisionally prior to this confirmation.)

From American Psychiatric Association. *Diagnostic and Statistical Manual of Mental Disorders.* 4th ed. Text rev. Washington, DC: American Psychiatric Association; copyright 2000, with permission.

somatic symptoms during the premenstrual period, and about 40 percent of these women have at least mild to moderate premenstrual symptoms prompting them to seek medical advice. Only 3 to 7 percent of women have symptoms that meet the full diagnostic criteria for PMDD.

Given that most women who experience changes in affect or somatic symptoms during the premenstrual period are not severely functionally impaired, it is important to distinguish these women from those who are diagnosed with PMDD. Premenstrual syndrome (PMS) is distinguished from PMDD by the severity and number of symptoms, as well as the degree to which function is impaired.

The course and the prognosis of PMDD have not been studied sufficiently to reach any reasonable conclusions. Anecdotally, the symptoms tend to be chronic unless effective treatment is initiated. Treatment of PMDD includes support for the patient about the presence and recogni-tion of the symptoms. SSRIs—for example, fluoxetine and alprazolam (Xanax)—have all been reported to be effective, although no treatment has been conclusively demonstrated to be effective in multiple, well-controlled trials. If symptoms are present throughout the menstrual cy-cle, with no intercycle symptom relief, clinicians should consider one of the nonmenstrual cycle–related mood disorders and anxiety disorders. The presence of especially severe symptoms, even if cyclical, should prompt clinicians to consider other mood disorders and anxiety disorder. A thorough medical workup is necessary to rule out medical or surgical conditions to account for symptoms (e.g., endometriosis). Recently the U.S. Food and Drug Administration approved YAZ (3 mg drospirenone plus 20 mg ethinyl estradiol) in a 24-day active pill regimen as effective in treating emotional and physical symptoms of PMDD in addition to using it for birth control.

27

Relational Problems

An adult's psychological health and sense of well-being depend to a significant degree on the quality of his or her important relationships—that is, on patterns of interaction with a partner and children, parents and siblings, and friends and colleagues. Problems in the interaction between any of these significant others can lead to clinical symptoms and impaired functioning among one or more members of the relational unit. Relational problems may be a focus of clinical attention (1) when a relational unit is distressed and dysfunctional or threatened with dissolution and (2) when the relational problems precede, accompany, or follow other psychiatric or medical disorders.

DEFINITION

According to the text revision of the fourth edition of the *Diagnostic and Statistical Manual of Mental Disorders* (DSM-IV-TR), relational problems are patterns of interaction between members of a relational unit that are associated with symptoms or significantly impaired functioning in one or more individual members or with significantly impaired functioning of the relational unit itself. DSM-IV-TR distinguishes five categories of relational problems: (1) relational problem related to a mental or general medical condition; (2) parent–child relational problem; (3) partner relational problem; (4) sibling relational problem; and (5) relational problem not otherwise specified.

EPIDEMIOLOGY

No reliable figures are available on the prevalence of relational problems. They can be assumed to be ubiquitous; however, most relational problems resolve without professional intervention. The nature, frequency, and effects of the problem on those involved are elements that must be considered before a diagnosis of relational problem is made. For example, divorce, which occurs in just less than 50 percent of marriages, is a problem between partners that is resolved through the legal remedy of divorce and need not be diagnosed as a relational problem. If the persons cannot resolve their disputation and continue to live together in a sadomasochistic or pathologically depressed relationship with unhappiness and abuse, then they should be so labeled. Relationship problems between involved persons that cannot be resolved by friends, family, or clergy require professional intervention by psychiatrists, clinical psychologists, social workers, and other mental health professionals.

RELATIONAL PROBLEM RELATED TO A MENTAL DISORDER OR GENERAL MEDICAL CONDITION

According to DSM-IV-TR, the category of relational problem related to a mental disorder or general medical condition "should be used when the focus of clinical attention is a pattern of impaired interaction associated with a psychiatric disorder or a general medical condition in a family member."

Studies indicate that satisfying relationships may have a health-protective influence, whereas relationship distress tends to be associated with an increased incidence of illness. The influence of relational systems on health has been explained through psychophysiological mechanisms that link the intense emotions generated in human attachment systems to vascular reactivity and immune processes. Thus, stress-related psychological or physical symptoms can be an expression of family dysfunction.

Adults must often assume responsibility for caring for aging parents while they are still caring for their own children, and this dual obligation can create stress. When adults take care of their parents, both parties must adapt to a reversal of their former roles, and the caretakers not only face the potential loss of their parents, but also must cope with evidence of their own mortality.

Some caretakers abuse their aging parents—a problem that is now receiving attention. Abuse is most likely to occur when the caretaking offspring have substance abuse problems, are under economic stress, and have no relief from their caretaking duties, or when the parent is bedridden or has a chronic illness requiring constant nursing attention. More women are abused than men, and most abuse occurs in persons older than the age of 75 years.

The development of a chronic illness in a family member stresses the family system and requires adaptation by both the sick person and the other family members. The person who has become sick must frequently face a loss of autonomy, an increased sense of vulnerability, and sometimes a taxing medical regimen. The other family members must experience the loss of the person as he or she was before the illness, and they usually have substantial caretaking responsibility—for example, in debilitating neurological diseases, including dementia of the Alzheimer's type, and in diseases such as acquired immunodeficiency syndrome and cancer. In these cases, the whole family must deal with the stress of prospective death as well as the current illness. Some families use the anger engendered by such situations to create support organizations, increase public awareness of the disease, and rally around the sick member. But chronic illness frequently produces depression in family members and can cause them to withdraw from or attack one another. The burden of caring for ill family members falls disproportionately on the women in a family—mothers, daughters, and daughters-in-law.

Chronic emotional illness also requires major adaptations by families. For instance, family members may react with chaos or fear to the psychotic productions of a family member with schizophrenia. The regression, exaggerated emotions, frequent hospitalizations, and economic and social dependence of a person with schizophrenia can stress the family system. Family members may react with hostile feelings (referred to as expressed emotion) that are associated with a poor prognosis for the person who is sick. Similarly, a family member with bipolar I disorder can disrupt a family, particularly during manic episodes.

Family devastation can occur when (1) illness suddenly strikes a previously healthy person, (2) illness occurs earlier than expected in the life cycle (some impairment of physical capacities is expected in old age, although many older persons are healthy), (3) illness affects the economic stability of the family, and (4) little can be done to improve or ease the condition of the sick family member.

PARENT–CHILD RELATIONAL PROBLEM

Parents differ widely in sensing the needs of their infants. Some quickly note their child's moods and needs; others are slow to respond. Parental responsiveness interacts with the child's temperament to affect the quality of the attachment between child and parent. According to DSM-IV-TR, the diagnosis of parent–child relational problem applies when the focus of clinical attention is a pattern of interaction between parent and child that is associated with clinically significant impairment in individual or family functioning or with clinically significant symptoms. Examples include impaired communication, overprotection, and inadequate discipline.

Research on parenting skills has isolated two major dimensions: (1) a permissive-restrictive dimension and (2) a warm-and-accepting versus cold-and-hostile dimension. A typology that separates parents on these dimensions distinguishes between *authoritarian* (restrictive and cold), *permissive* (minimally restrictive and accepting), and *authoritative* (restrictive as needed, but also warm and accepting) parenting styles. Children of authoritarian parents tend to be withdrawn or conflicted; those of permissive parents are likely to be more aggressive, impulsive, and low achievers; and children of authoritative parents seem to function at the highest level, socially and cognitively. Yet, switching from an authoritarian to a permissive mode may create a negative reinforcement pattern.

Difficulties in many situations impose stress on the usual parent–child interaction. Substantial evidence indicates that marital discord leads to problems in children, from depression and withdrawal to conduct disorder and poor performance at school. This negative effect may be partly mediated through *triangulation* of the parent–child relationships, which is a process in which conflicted parents attempt to win the sympathy and support of their child, who is recruited by one parent as an ally in the struggle with the partner. Divorces and remarriages impose stress on the parent–child relationship and may create painful loyalty conflicts. Stepparents often find it difficult to assume a parental role and may resent the special relationship that exists between their new marital partner and the children from that partner's previous marriage(s). The resentment of a stepparent by a stepchild and the favoring of a natural child are usual reactions in

a new family's initial phases of adjustment. When a second child is born, both familial stress and happiness may result, although happiness is the dominant emotion in most families. The birth of a child can also be troublesome when parents had adopted a child in the belief that they were infertile. Single-parent families usually consist of a mother and children, and their relationship is often affected by financial and emotional problems.

Other situations that can produce a parent–child problem are the development of fatal, crippling, or chronic illness, such as leukemia, epilepsy, sickle-cell anemia, or spinal cord injury, in either parent or child. The birth of a child with congenital defects, such as cerebral palsy, blindness, and deafness, may also produce parent–child problems. These situations, which are not rare, challenge the emotional resources of those involved. Parents and child must face present and potential loss and must adjust their day-to-day lives physically, economically, and emotionally. These situations can strain the healthiest families and produce parent–child problems not only with the sick person but also with the unaffected family members. In a family with a severely sick child, parents may resent, prefer, or neglect the other children because the ill child requires so much time and attention.

Parents with children who have emotional disorders face particular problems, depending on the child's illness. In families with a child with schizophrenia, family treatment is beneficial and improves the social adjustment of the patient. Similarly, family therapy is useful when a child has a mood disorder. In families with a substance-abusing child or adolescent, family involvement is crucial to help control the drug-seeking behavior and to allow family members to verbalize the feelings of frustration and anger that are invariably present.

Normal developmental crises can also be related to parent–child problems. For instance, adolescence is a time of frequent conflict as the adolescent resists rules and demands increasing autonomy while at the same time eliciting protective control by displaying immature and dangerous behavior.

The parents of sons aged 18, 15, and 11 years, respectively, presented with distress about the behavior of their middle child. The family had been cohesive with satisfactory relationships among all members until 6 months before this consultation. At that time, the 15-year-old began seeing a girl from a comparatively unsupervised household. Frequent arguments had developed between parents and son regarding going out on school nights, curfews, and neglect of schoolwork. The son's combativeness and lowered academic achievement upset his parents a great deal. They had not experienced similar conflicts with their oldest child. The adolescent, however, maintained a good relationship with his siblings and friends, was not a behavior problem at school, continued to participate on the school basketball team, and was not a substance user.

Day Care Centers

Quality of care during the first 3 years of life is crucial to neuropsychological development. A 1997 study from the National Institute of Child Health and Human Development indicated that day care was not harmful to children when the caregivers and day care teachers provided consistent, empathetic, nurturing care. Not all day care centers can meet that level of care, however, especially those located in poor urban areas. Children receiving less-than-optimal caring exhibit decreased intellectual and verbal skills that indicate delayed neurocognitive development. They may also become irritable, anxious, or depressed, which interferes with the parent–child bonding experience, and they are less assertive and less effectively toilet trained by the age of 5 years.

More than 55 percent of women are in the work force, many of whom have no choice but to place their children in day care centers. Approximately 40 percent of entering medical students are women; few medical centers, however, make adequate provisions for on-site day care centers for their students or staff. Similarly, corporations need to provide on-site, high-quality care for the children of their employees. Not only will that approach benefit the children, but in addition corporate economic benefits will accrue as a result of reduced absenteeism, increased productivity, and happier working mothers. Such programs have the added benefit of decreasing stresses on marriages.

PARTNER RELATIONAL PROBLEM

According to DSM-IV-TR, clinicians should use the category partner relational problem when the focus of clinical attention is a pattern of interaction between the spouses or partners. These patterns are characterized by negative communication (e.g., criticisms), distorted communication (e.g., unrealistic expectations), or noncommunication (e.g., withdrawal), associated with clinically significant impairment in individual or family functioning or symptoms in one or both partners.

When persons have partner relational problems, psychiatrists must assess whether a patient's distress arises from the relationship or from a mental disorder. Mental disorders are more common in single persons—those who never married or who are widowed, separated, or divorced—than among married persons. Clinicians should evaluate developmental, sexual, and occupational and relationship histories for purposes of diagnosis. (Couples therapy is discussed in Chapter 31, Section 31.4.)

Marriage demands a sustained level of adaptation from both partners. In a troubled marriage, a therapist can encourage the partners to explore areas such as the extent of communication between the partners, their ways of solving disputes, their attitudes toward child-bearing and child-rearing, their relationships with their in-laws, their attitudes toward social life, their handling of finances, and their sexual interaction. The birth of a child, an abortion or miscarriage, economic stresses, moves to new areas, episodes of illness, major career changes, and any situations that involve a significant change in marital roles can precipitate stressful periods in a relationship. Illness in a child exerts the greatest strain on a marriage, and marriages in which a child has died through illness or accident more often than not end in divorce. Complaints of lifelong anorgasmia or impotence by marital partners usually indicate intrapsychic problems, although sexual dissatisfaction is involved in many cases of marital maladjustment.

Adjustment to marital roles can be a problem when partners are from different backgrounds and have grown up with different value systems. For example, many members of low socioeconomic status groups perceive a wife as making most of the decisions in the family, and they accept physical punishment as a way to discipline children. Many middle-class persons perceive family decision-making processes as shared, with the husband often being the final arbiter, and they prefer to discipline children

verbally. Problems involving conflicts in values, adjustment to new roles, and poor communication are handled most effectively when therapist and partners examine the couple's relationship, as in marital therapy.

Epidemiological surveys show that unhappy marriages are a risk factor for major depressive disorder. Marital discord also affects physical health. For example, in a study of women aged 30 to 65 years with coronary artery disease, marital stress worsened the prognosis 2.9 times for recurrent coronary events. Marital conflict was also associated with a 46 percent higher relative death risk among female patients having hemodialysis and with elevations in serum epinephrine, norepinephrine, and corticotrophin levels in both men and women. In one study, high levels of hostile marital behavior were associated with slower healing of wounds, lower production of proinflammatory cytokines, and higher cytokine production in peripheral blood. Overall, women show greater psychological and physiological responsiveness to conflict than men.

SIBLING RELATIONAL PROBLEM

According to DSM-IV-TR, the category of sibling relational problem "should be used when the focus of clinical attention is a pattern of interaction between siblings, associated with clinically significant impairment of family functioning, or symptoms in one or more of the siblings."

Sibling relationships tend to be characterized by competition, comparison, and cooperation. Intense sibling rivalry can occur with the birth of a child and can persist as the children grow up, compete for parental approval, and measure their accomplishments against one another. Alliances between siblings are equally common. Siblings may learn to protect one another against parental control or aggression. In households with three children, one pair tends to become closely involved with one another, leaving the extra child in the position of outsider.

Relational problems can arise when siblings are not treated equally—for instance, when one child is idealized, whereas another is cast in the role of the family scapegoat. Differences in gender roles and expectations expressed by the parents can underlie sibling rivalry. Parent–child relationships also are dependent on personality interactions. A child's resentment directed at a parental figure or a child's disavowed dark emotions can be projected onto a sibling and can fuel an intense hate relationship.

A child's general, other medical or psychiatric condition always imposes stress on the sibling relationships. Parental concern and attention to the sick child can elicit envy in the siblings. In addition, chronic disability can leave the sick child feeling devalued and rejected by siblings, and the latter may develop a sense of superiority and may feel embarrassed about having a disabled sister or brother.

RELATIONAL PROBLEM NOT OTHERWISE SPECIFIED

According to DSM-IV-TR, the category of relational problem not otherwise specified "should be used when the focus of clinical attention is on relational problems not classifiable by any of the specific problems above (e.g., difficulties with superiors and coworkers)."

Persons, across the life cycle, may become involved in relational problems with leaders and others in their community at large. In such relationships, conflicts are common and can bring about stress-related symptoms. Many relational problems of children occur in the school setting and involve peers. Impaired peer relationships can be the chief complaint in attention-deficit or conduct disorders, as well as in depressive and other psychiatric disorders of childhood, adolescence, and adulthood.

Racial, ethnic, and religious prejudices and ignorance cause problems in interpersonal relationships. In the workplace and in communities at large, sexual harassment is often a combination of inappropriate sexual interactions, inappropriate displays of abuse of power and dominance, and expressions of negative gender stereotypes, primarily toward women and gay men, although also toward children and adolescents of both sexes.

28

Problems Related to Abuse or Neglect

The text revision of the fourth edition of *Diagnostic and Statistical Manual of Mental Disorders* (DSM-IV-TR) specifies five problems related to abuse or neglect: (1) physical abuse of child, (2) sexual abuse of child, (3) neglect of child, (4) physical abuse of adult, and (5) sexual abuse of adult (Table 28–1). Physical abuse of an adult includes spouse or partner abuse and abuse of elderly persons. Sexual abuse of an adult includes rape, sexual coercion, and sexual harassment.

CHILD ABUSE AND NEGLECT

Physical and sexual abuse occurs in girls and boys of all ages, in all ethnic groups, and at all socioeconomic levels. The abuses vary widely with respect to severity and duration, but any form of continued abuse constitutes an emergency situation for the child. Fear, guilt, anxiety, depression, and ambivalence regarding disclosure commonly surround the child who has been abused.

In child neglect, a child's physical, mental, or emotional condition has been impaired because of a parent's or caretaker's inability to provide adequate food, shelter, education, or supervision. In its extreme form, neglect can contribute to failure to thrive. Failure to thrive typically occurs under circumstances in which adequate nourishment is available, yet a disturbance within the relationship between the caretaker and the child results in a child who does not eat enough to grow and develop. For a further discussion of failure to thrive, see Section 30.2.

Epidemiology

The Department of Health and Human Services estimated that, in 2004, approximately 3 million alleged victims were reported to child protective services. Of those reports, more than 870,000 were substantiated; this represents 2.03 of every 1,000 children. The substantiated cases were distributed as follows: neglect, 62 percent; physical abuse, 18 percent; sexual abuse, 10 percent; and emotional abuse, 7 percent. The Children's Bureau estimated that 1,400 children died as the result of abuse or neglect in 2004: 36 percent from neglect and 28 percent from physical abuse. Approximately 81 percent of these deaths were of children younger than 4 years of age.

The data were analyzed for patterns of maltreatment by the sex and age of victims. Rates of many types of maltreatment were similar for boys and girls, but the sexual abuse rate for girls was higher than the sexual abuse rate for boys. Examining the age distribution of victims, the age group from 0 to 3 years of age had the highest victimization rate, and the rate of victimization declined as the age of the victims increased. For example, the rate for infants (0 to 3 years of age) was 16 per 1,000, whereas the rate for adolescents (16 to 17 years of age) was 6 per 1,000. Regarding the perpetrators of abuse, it was reported that, overall, 58 percent were female and 42 percent were male.

Diagnosis and Clinical Features

Physical Abuse of Child. Clinicians must always consider physical abuse when a child shows bruises or injuries that cannot be adequately explained or that are incompatible with the history that the parent gives. Suspicious physical indicators are bruises and marks that form symmetrical patterns, such as injuries to both sides of the face and regular patterns on the back, buttocks, and thighs; accidental injuries are unlikely to result in symmetrical patterns. Bruises may have the shape of the instrument used to make them, such as a belt buckle or a cord. Burns by cigarettes result in symmetrical, round scars, and immersions in boiling water produce burns that look like socks or gloves or that are doughnut shaped. Physical aggression can cause multiple and spiral fractures, especially in a young baby; retinal hemorrhages in an infant may result from shaking.

Children repeatedly brought to hospitals for treatment of peculiar or puzzling problems by overly cooperative parents may be victims of Munchausen's syndrome by proxy, that is, factitious disorder. In this abuse scenario, a parent repeatedly inflicts illness on, or causes injury to, a child—by injecting toxins or by inducing the child to ingest drugs or toxins to cause diarrhea, dehydration, or other symptoms—and then eagerly seeks medical attention. Because the pathological parents are stealthy and superficially compliant, this is a difficult diagnosis to make.

In hospital emergency rooms, severely abused children show external evidence of body trauma, bruises, abrasions, cuts, lacerations, burns, soft tissue swellings, and hematomas. Hypernatremic dehydration, after periodic water deprivation of children by mothers who are usually psychotic, is another form of child abuse. Inability to move certain extremities because of dislocations and fractures associated with neurological signs of intracranial damage can also indicate inflicted trauma. Other clinical signs and symptoms attributed to inflicted abuse may include injury to the viscera. Abdominal trauma can result in unexplained ruptures of the stomach, the bowel, the liver, or the pancreas, with manifestations of an injured abdomen. Children with the most severe maltreatment injuries arrive at the hospital

Table 28–1
DSM-IV-TR Problems Related to Abuse or Neglect

Physical abuse of child
This category should be used when the focus of clinical attention is physical abuse of a child.
Sexual abuse of child
This category should be used when the focus of clinical attention is sexual abuse of a child.
Neglect of child
This category should be used when the focus of clinical attention is child neglect.
Physical abuse of adult
This category should be used when the focus of clinical attention is physical abuse of an adult (e.g., spouse beating, abuse of elderly parent).
Sexual abuse of adult
This category should be used when the focus of clinical attention is sexual abuse of an adult (e.g., sexual coercion, rape).

From American Psychiatric Association. *Diagnostic and Statistical Manual of Mental Disorders.* 4th ed. Text rev. Washington, DC: American Psychiatric Association; copyright 2000, with permission.

or physician's office in a coma or in convulsions; some arrive dead.

Behaviorally, abused children may appear withdrawn and frightened or may show aggressive behavior and labile mood. They often exhibit depression, poor self-esteem, and anxiety. They may try physically to cover up injuries and are usually reticent to disclose the abuse for fear of retaliation. Abused children often show some delay in developmental milestones; they may have difficulties with peer relationships and may engage in self-destructive or suicidal behaviors.

Carol, 4 years of age, had a change in her behavior at preschool approximately 3 months after the birth of her sister. Her teacher saw Carol push other children and hit a classmate with a wooden block, causing a laceration of the child's lip. When Carol's teacher took her aside to talk about her behavior, she noticed what seemed to be belt marks on Carol's abdomen and forehead. The teacher reported possible child abuse to protective services. Also, the family was referred for psychiatric evaluation.

Carol's baby sister was colicky and slept only for short periods of time throughout the day and night. She stopped crying only when her mother held her. Her mother, therefore, had little time for Carol, and Carol's father took over her care on evenings after day care and on weekends. He began to drink more than usual and became increasingly irritable. The parents argued over the mother's attention to the infant and the requirement that the father take care of Carol. Carol, who was a bright, curious, and talkative child, constantly asked questions and often asked to carry the baby. When refused, she would lie on the floor and have a tantrum. She also began to have difficulty falling asleep and awoke repeatedly during the night. Carol's father was unable to cope with her requests for attention and often told her to shut up and slapped her when she continued her demands. On many occasions, he responded to her tantrums or repeated questions by hitting her with his belt.

While protective services monitored the situation, Carol and her parents began a family therapy program that included parenting training and behavioral therapy for Carol, which was coordinated with the preschool. Carol's father attended Alcoholics Anonymous (AA) meetings and stopped drinking. He was able to control his anger at his daughter. Six months later, Carol's aggressive behavior ceased. She was doing well with peers, was sleeping through the night, and stopped having temper tantrums. (Courtesy of William Bernet, M.D.)

Sexual Abuse of Child. Adults within the immediate or extended family of a child perpetrate most child sexual abuse. Thus, children commonly know the sexual abuser, who is often a highly trusted family member with a position of authority and with wide access to the child. Most cases of sexual abuse involving children are never revealed because of the victim's feelings of guilt, shame, ignorance, and tolerance, compounded by some physicians' reluctance to recognize and report sexual abuse, the court's insistence on strict rules of evidence, and families' fears of dissolution if the sexual abuse is discovered. Despite their familial roles, sexual abusers often threaten to hurt, kill, or abandon the children if the events are disclosed.

The incidence of sexual abuse and of child pornography, which is a form of sexual abuse, is much higher than had been previously assumed. Children may be sexually abused as early as infancy and as late as adolescence. Sexual abuse has been reported in schools, day care centers, and group homes, where adult caretakers are the major offenders.

The overwhelming fear, shame, and guilt that contribute to a child's reticence to disclose sexual abuse also complicate identifying the abuse. Most often, no definitive physical evidence can prove the occurrence of sexual abuse. Physical indicators of sexual abuse include bruises, pain, and itching in the genital region. Genital or rectal bleeding may be a sign of sexual molestation. Recurrent urinary tract infections and vaginal discharges may be related to abuse. Sexually transmitted diseases and difficulty walking and sitting raise suspicions of sexual abuse.

No specific behavioral manifestations prove that sexual abuse has taken place, but children may exhibit many possible significant behaviors. Young children who have a detailed knowledge of sexual acts have usually witnessed or participated in sexual behavior. Young sexually abused children often exhibit their sexual knowledge through play and may initiate sexual behaviors with their peers. Aggressive behavior is common among abused children. Children who are extremely fearful of adults, particularly men, may have been subjected to sexual abuse. Clinicians should listen carefully to children who report sexual assaults even when parts of their stories are not consistent. When a child begins to disclose information about sexual assaults, retractions and contradictions are typical, and anxiety may prevent full disclosure.

The diagnosis of sexual abuse in children is full of pitfalls. An estimated 2 to 8 percent of allegations of sexual abuse are false. A much higher percentage of reports cannot be substantiated. Many investigations are done hastily or are carried out by inexperienced evaluators. In custody cases, an allegation of sexual abuse can be a maneuver to limit a parent's visitation rights. Alleged sexual abuse of a pre–school-aged child is particularly difficult to evaluate because of the child's immature cognitive and language development. The use of anatomically correct dolls has grown in popularity but is controversial. Patient and careful evaluations by experienced, objective professionals are necessary, and leading questions must be avoided. Children younger than the age of 3 years are unlikely to produce a verbal memory of past trauma or abuses, but their experience may be reflected in play or fantasies. Some abused children meet the DSM-IV-TR diagnostic criteria for posttraumatic stress disorder (PTSD).

No specific psychiatric symptom results universally from sexual abuse. Vulnerability to the sequelae of sexual abuse depends on the type of abuse, its chronicity, the age of the child, and the overall relationship of the victim and the abuser. The psychological and physical effects of sexual abuse can be devastating and long lasting. Children who are sexually stimulated by an adult feel anxiety and overexcitement, lose confidence in themselves, and become mistrustful of adults. Seduction, incest, and rape are important predisposing factors to later symptom formations, such as phobias, anxiety, and depression. Abused children tend to be hyperalert to external aggression as shown by an inability to deal with their aggressive impulses toward others or with others' hostility directed toward them.

Depressive feelings, usually combined with shame, guilt, and a sense of permanent damage, are commonly reported among children who have been sexually abused. Adolescents who have undergone sexual abuse are said to show high rates of poor impulse control and self-destructive and suicidal behaviors. PTSD and dissociative disorders are common in adults who have been sexually abused as children. Sexual abuse is a common preexisting factor in the development of dissociative identity disorder (also known as *multiple personality disorder*). Signs of dissociation include periods in which the children are amnestic, do not feel the pain, or feel that they are somewhere else. Borderline personality disorder has been reported in some patients with histories of sexual abuse. Substance abuse has also been reported with high frequency among adolescents and adults who were sexually abused as children.

INCEST.   *Incest* is defined as the occurrence of sexual relations between close blood relatives. A broader definition describes incest as sexual intercourse between participants who are related to each other by a formal or informal kinship bond that is culturally regarded as a bar to sexual relations. For example, sexual relations between stepparents and stepchildren or among stepsiblings are usually considered incestuous, even though no blood relationships exist.

Sociologists have underlined the role of incest prohibitions as socialization factors, and biological factors also support the taboo. Inbreeding groups risk unmasking lethal or detrimental recessive genes, and the progeny of inbred groups are generally less fit than less closely related offspring. Anthropologists have observed that different cultures have different types of incest taboos. In *Totem and Taboo*, Sigmund Freud developed the concept of the primal horde, in which young men collectively murdered the group's patriarch, who had kept all the women to himself. According to Freud, the incest taboo arose both from guilt about the murder and from a group's desire to prevent a repetition of the act, further rivalry after the murder, and subsequent disintegration of the horde.

Fathers, stepfathers, uncles, and older siblings most commonly abuse children. A passive, sick, absent, or somehow incapacitated mother, a daughter who takes on a maternal role in the family, a father who abuses alcohol, and overcrowding are features of father–daughter incest common in many homes. Mother–son incest is the strongest and most nearly universal taboo and is the rarest form of incest. Such behavior usually indicates more severe psychopathology in the participants than is the case in father–daughter and sibling incest.

Accurate figures on the incidence of incest are difficult to obtain because of families' shame and embarrassment. Girls are victims more often than are boys; in the United States, about 15 million women have

been the objects of incestuous attention, and one third of all sexually abused persons were molested before the age of 9 years.

Incestuous behavior is reported much more frequently among families of low socioeconomic status than among other families. This difference may be caused by greater contact with reporting officials, such as welfare workers, public health personnel, and law enforcement agents and does not truly reflect a higher incidence in these families. Incest is more easily hidden by economically stable families than by those of low socioeconomic status.

Social, cultural, physiological, and psychological factors all contribute to the breakdown of the incest taboo. Incestuous behavior has been associated with alcohol abuse, overcrowding, increased physical proximity, and rural isolation that prevents adequate extrafamilial contacts. Some communities are more tolerant of incestuous behavior than is the whole of society. Major mental disorders and intellectual deficiencies can contribute to clinical incest. Some family therapists view incest as a defense designed to maintain a dysfunctional family unit. The older and stronger participant in incestuous behavior is usually male. Thus, incest may be viewed as a form of child abuse, a pedophilia, or a variant of rape.

About 75 percent of reported cases involve father–daughter incest, but parents often deny the occurrence of sibling incest. Other instances of sibling incest involve nearly normal interaction of prepubertal sexual play and exploration. In many cases of father–daughter incest, the daughter has had a close relationship with her father throughout her childhood and may appear to be pleased when he approaches her sexually. The incestuous behavior usually begins when the daughter is 10 years of age. As the behavior continues, however, the abused daughter becomes bewildered, confused, and frightened, and when she nears adolescence, she undergoes physiological changes that add to her confusion. She never knows whether her father is a parent or sexual partner. Her mother may be alternately caring and competitive and may often refuse to believe her daughter's reports or to confront her husband with her suspicion. The daughter's relationships with her siblings are also affected; they sense her special position with her father and treat her as an outsider. The father, fearing that his daughter may expose their relationship and often jealously possessive of her, interferes with her development of normal peer relationships.

Physicians must be aware that intrafamilial sexual abuse can cause a wide variety of emotional and physical symptoms, including abdominal pain, genital irritations, separation anxiety disorder, phobias, nightmares, and school problems. When incest is suspected, clinicians must interview the child apart from the rest of the family.

HOMOSEXUAL INCEST.   Father–son and mother–daughter incest are rarely reported, but a family in which same-sex incest occurs is usually highly disturbed, with a violent, alcohol-dependent, or antisocial father; a dependent or disabled mother who is unable to protect her children; and an absence of the usual family roles and individual identities. A son involved in father–son incest is frequently the eldest child, and, if there is a daughter, the father often sexually abuses her as well. Fathers in this situation do not necessarily have any other history of homosexual behavior. Sons may experience homicidal or suicidal ideation and may first consult or be sent to a psychiatrist because of self-destructive behavior.

STATUTORY RAPE.   Intercourse is unlawful between a man older than16 years of age and a woman under the age of consent, which varies from 14 to 21 years, depending on the jurisdiction. Thus, an 18-year-old man and a 15-year-old girl may have consensual intercourse, yet the man may be held for statutory rape. Statutory rape can vary dramatically from other types of rape in being nonassaultive and nonviolent, and it is not a deviant act unless the age discrepancy is sufficiently large for the man to be defined as a pedophile—that is, when the girl is less than 13 years of age. Parents of a consenting girl, rather than the girl herself, usually press charges of statutory rape.

Neglect of Child.   A maltreated child often shows no obvious signs of being battered but has multiple minor physical evidences of emotional and, at times, nutritional deprivation, neglect, and abuse. A maltreated child, often brought to a hospital or to a private physician, has a history of failure to thrive, malnutrition, poor skin hygiene, irritability, withdrawal, and other signs of psychological and physical neglect.

Children who have been neglected may show overt failure to thrive at less than 1 year of age. Their physical and emotional development is drastically impaired; they may be physically small and unable to display appropriate social interaction. Hunger, chronic infections, poor hygiene, inappropriate dress, and eventual malnutrition may all be evident. Behaviorally, children who are chronically neglected can be indiscriminately affectionate, even with strangers, or socially unresponsive, even in familiar situations. Neglected children may be runaways or exhibit conduct disorder.

An extreme form of failure to thrive in children 5 years of age or older is psychosocial dwarfism, in which a chronically deprived child does not grow and develop, even when offered adequate amounts of food. Such children have normal proportions but are exceedingly small for their age. They often have reversible endocrinological changes resulting in decreased growth hormone, and they cease to grow for a time. Children with this disorder exhibit bizarre eating behaviors and disturbed social relationships. Binge eating, ingestion of garbage or inedible substances, drinking of toilet water, and induced vomiting have been reported.

Parents who neglect their children are often overwhelmed, depressed, isolated, and impoverished. Unemployment, the absence of a two-parent family, and substance abuse can exacerbate the situation. There are several possible prototypes of neglectful mothers. Some young, inexperienced, socially isolated, and ignorant mothers may temporarily be unable to care for their children. Other neglectful mothers are chronically passive and withdrawn women who may have been raised in chaotic, abusive, and neglectful homes. In these cases, once the situation comes to the attention of a child protective agency, the mother often accepts help. Mothers with major mental disorders who view their children as evil or as purposely driving them crazy are difficult to help.

Differential Diagnosis

Parental feuding and custody disputes are among the factors that complicate identifying and substantiating abuse and neglect situations. When marital discord is severe, children are often caught in the line of fire. A mother who is overwhelmingly hostile toward a separated father may be convinced and may convince a child that the father is abusive. In some cases, parents have gone so far as to fabricate entire abuse scenarios and coach children to repeat them. In other instances, parents may refuse to accept the possibility that a spouse or close relative is the perpetrator of abuse, and they may repeatedly insist that a child stop telling lies and coerce a child into retracting the disclosures. In either scenario, the child suffers profoundly, and the alleged abuse situation is never disentangled.

When a child speaks in a manner consistent with his or her language development stage, does not sound rehearsed, and does not use adult-like phrasing, the abuse allegations may be true. Distress, the display of precocious sexual behavior, and a knowledge of, or preoccupation with, sexual material also support the possibility of sexual abuse. A child who has not been abused but who is coached to report sexual or physical abuse is also placed under unbearable duress. Therefore, clinicians must recognize that severe chronic parental conflict in which a child is caught can be as destructive as physical and sexual abuse.

Controversies are now arising in the courts because children are accusing caretakers and teachers of sexual abuse, and the children's veracity is being challenged. See Chapter 16 for a discussion of the recovered or false memory syndrome.

Course and Prognosis

The outcome of child physical and sexual abuse and neglect is multifactorial, depending on the severity, duration, and nature of the abuse and the child's vulnerabilities. Children who already suffer from mental retardation, pervasive developmental disorders, physical disabilities, disruptive behavior, and attention-deficit disorders are likely to have a poorer outcome than children who are unhampered by mental or physical disorders. Children who are abused for long periods, from the time they are babies or toddlers into adolescence, are likely to be more profoundly damaged than those who have experienced only brief episodes of abuse. The development of mental disorders—such as major depressive disorder, suicidal behavior, PTSD, dissociative identity disorder, and substance abuse—further complicates the long-term prognosis, as does the nature of the relationship between victim and abuser and the adult support figures available to children after disclosure. The best outcomes occur when children are cognitively intact, the abuse is recognized and interrupted in an early phase, and the entire family is capable of participating in treatment.

Treatment

Child.   The first part of treating child abuse and neglect is to ensure the child's safety and well-being. Children may need to be removed from abusive or neglectful families to ensure their protection; yet, on an emotional level, a child may feel additionally vulnerable in an unfamiliar setting. Because of the high risk for psychiatric symptoms in abused and neglected children, a comprehensive psychiatric evaluation is in order. Next, along with providing specific treatments for any mental disorders present, a therapist may have to deal with the immediate situation and the long-term implications of the abuse or neglect. Therapists must address several psychotherapeutic issues: dealing with the child's fears, anxieties, and self-esteem; building a trusting adult relationship in which the child is not exploited or betrayed; and ultimately gaining a helpful perspective on the factors contributing to the child's victimization at home.

Ideally, each abused and neglected child should receive an intervention plan based on the assessment of the factors responsible for the parental psychopathology. The plan should include an overall prognosis for parents' achieving adequate parenting skills; the time estimated to achieve meaningful change in their ability to parent; an estimate of whether the parental dysfunction is confined to this child or involves other children and, if that is the case, whether the parents' overall malfunctioning is short term or long term, and whether a mother's malfunctioning is confined to infants as opposed to older children (i.e., when the incidence of abuse is inversely related to a child's age); willingness of those involved to participate in the intervention plan; the availability of personnel and physical resources to implement the various intervention strategies; and the risk of the child sustaining additional physical or sexual abuse by remaining in the home.

Parents.   On the basis of the information obtained, several options can be selected to improve parental functioning: (1) eliminate or diminish the social or environmental stresses; (2) lessen the adverse psychological effects of social factors on the parents; (3) reduce the demands on the mother to a level within her capacity through day care placement of the child or provision of a housekeeper or baby-sitter; (4) provide emotional support, encouragement, sympathy, stimulation, instruction in maternal care, and aid in learning to plan for, assess, and meet the needs of the infant (supportive casework); and (5) resolve or diminish the parents' inner psychic conflicts (psychotherapy). Some clinics provide group counseling for nonoffending parents.

INCESTUOUS BEHAVIOR.   The first step in the treatment of incestuous behavior is its disclosure. Once a breakthrough of family members' denial, collusion, and fear has been achieved, incest is unlikely to recur. When the participants have severe psychopathology, treatment must be directed toward the underlying illness. Family therapy is useful to reestablish the group as a functioning unit and to develop healthier role definitions for each member. While the participants are learning to develop internal restraints and appropriate ways to gratify their needs, the external control provided by therapy helps prevent further incestuous behavior. At times, legal agencies must help enforce external controls.

Reporting.   In cases of suspected child abuse and neglect, physicians should diagnose the suspected maltreatment; secure the child's safety by admitting the child to a hospital or arranging out-of-home placement; report the case to the appropriate social service department, child protection unit, or central registry; make an assessment with the help of a history, a physical examination, a skeletal survey, and photographs; request a social worker's report and appropriate surgical and medical consultations; confer with members of a child abuse committee within 72 hours; arrange a program of care for the child and the parents; and arrange for social service follow-up. Among those generally included as mandated child-abuse reporters are physicians, psychologists, school officials, police officers, hospital personnel engaged in the treatment of patients, district attorneys, and providers of child day care and foster care.

Prevention.   To prevent child abuse and neglect, clinicians must identify those families at high risk and intervene before a child becomes a victim. Once high-risk families have been identified, a comprehensive program should include psychiatric monitoring of the families, including the identified high-risk child. Families can be educated to recognize when they are being neglectful or abusive, and alternative coping strategies can be suggested.

In general, child abuse and neglect prevention and treatment programs should try to prevent the separation of parents and children if possible, prevent the placement of children in institutions, encourage parental attainment of self-care status, and encourage the family's attainment of self-sufficiency. As a last resort and to prevent further abuse and neglect, children may have to be removed from families who are unwilling or unable to profit from the treatment program. In cases of sexual abuse, the licensing of day care centers and the psychological screening of persons who work in them should be mandatory to prevent further abuses. Education of the medical profession, members of allied health fields, and all who come in contact with children aid in early detection. Providing support services to stressed families helps to prevent the problem in the first place.

PHYSICAL ABUSE OF ADULT

Spouse Abuse

Spouse abuse (also known as *domestic violence*) is defined as physical assault within the home in which one spouse is repeatedly assaulted by the other. Spouse abuse is estimated to occur in 2 to 12 million families in the United States. This aspect of domestic violence has been recognized as a severe problem largely because of recent cultural emphasis on civil rights and the work of feminist groups, but the problem is long-standing.

The major problem in spouse abuse is wife abuse. One study estimated that 1.8 million wives are battered in the United States, excluding divorced women and women battered on dates. Wife beating occurs in families of every racial and religious background and in all socioeconomic strata. It is most frequent in families with problems of substance abuse, particularly alcohol and crack abuse. Behavioral, cultural, intrapsychic, and interpersonal factors all contribute to the problem. Abusive men are likely to have come from violent homes where they witnessed wife beating or were abused as children. The act itself is reinforcing; once a man has beaten his wife, he is likely to do so again. Abusive husbands tend to be immature, dependent, and nonassertive and to suffer from strong feelings of inadequacy.

The husbands' aggression is bullying behavior designed to humiliate their wives and to build up their own low self-esteem. Impatient, impulsive, abusive husbands physically displace aggression provoked by others onto their wives. The abuse most likely occurs when a man feels threatened or frustrated at home, at work, or with his peers. The dynamics include identification with an aggressor (father, boss), testing behavior (Will she stay with me, no matter how I treat her?), distorted desires to express manhood, and dehumanization of women. As in rape, aggression is deemed permissible when a woman is perceived as property. About 50 percent of battered wives grew up in violent homes, and their most common trait is dependence.

The Surgeon General's office has identified pregnancy as a high-risk period for battering; 15 to 25 percent of pregnant women are physically abused while pregnant, and the abuse often results in birth defects. Hot lines, emergency shelters for women, and other organizations (e.g., the National Coalition Against Domestic Violence) have been established to aid battered wives and to educate the public. One major problem of abused women is finding a place to go when they leave home, frequently in fear of their lives.

Battering is often severe, involving broken limbs, broken ribs, internal bleeding, and brain damage. When an abused wife tries to leave her husband, he often becomes doubly intimidating and threatens to "get" her. If the woman has small children to care for, her problem is compounded. The abusive husband wages a conscious campaign to isolate his wife and make her feel worthless. Women face risks when they leave an abusive husband; they have a 75 percent greater chance of being killed by their batterers than women who stay. New York State has prepared a physician reference card to alert and guide doctors about domestic violence.

Some men feel remorse and guilt after an episode of violent behavior and so become particularly loving. If this behavior gives the wife hope, she remains until the next, inevitable cycle of violence.

When a man is convinced that a woman will no longer tolerate the situation and when she begins to exert control over his behavior, change is initiated. By leaving for a prolonged period, if she is physically and economically able to do so, and by making therapy for the man a condition of return, a woman can begin a cycle of improvement. Family therapy is effective in treating the problem, usually in conjunction with social and legal agencies. With men who are relatively less impulsive, external controls, such as calling the neighbors or the police, may suffice to stop the behavior.

Some husband-beating wives have been also reported. Husbands complain of fear of ridicule if they expose the problem; they fear charges of counterassault and often feel unable to leave the situation because of financial difficulties. Husband abuse has also been reported when a frail, elderly man is married to a much younger woman.

Elder Abuse

Elder abuse is discussed in Chapter 50.

SEXUAL ABUSE OF ADULT

Rape

Rape is the forceful coercion of an unwilling victim to engage in a sexual act, usually sexual intercourse, although anal intercourse and fellatio can also be acts of rape. Using this definition, one survey found that 1 of 6 women and 1 of 33 men have experienced an attempted or completed rape as a child or as an adult in the United States. Rape can occur between married partners and between persons of the same sex. The crime of rape requires only slight penile penetration of the victim's outer vulva; full erection and ejaculation are unnecessary for defining the crime. Forced acts of fellatio and anal penetration, although they frequently accompany rape, are legally considered sodomy. As noted later, in most states, male rape is legally defined as sodomy.

The problem of rape is most appropriately discussed under the heading of aggression. Rape is an act of violence and humiliation that happens to be expressed through sexual means. Rape expresses power or anger; sex is rarely the dominant issue, because sexuality is used in the service of nonsexual needs.

Rape of Women.   Between 680,000 and 1.5 million women are raped annually in the United States. One of every eight adult women, or at least 12.1 million American women, is estimated to become the victim of forcible rape sometime in her lifetime. The male rapist can be categorized into separate groups: sexual sadists, who are aroused by the pain of their victims; exploitive

predators, who use their victims as objects for their gratification in an impulsive way; inadequate men, who believe that no woman would voluntarily sleep with them and who are obsessed with fantasies about sex; and men for whom rape is a displaced expression of anger and rage. Some believe that the anger was originally directed toward a wife or mother, but feminist theory proposes that a woman serves as an object for the displacement of aggression that a rapist cannot express directly toward other men. Women are considered men's property or vulnerable possessions, a rapist's instrument for revenge against other men.

Rape often accompanies another crime. Rapists always threaten their victims, with fists, a knife, or a gun, and frequently harm them in nonsexual ways as well. Victims can be beaten, wounded, and killed.

Statistics show that most men who commit rapes are between 25 and 44 years of age; 51 percent are white and tend to rape white victims, 47 percent are black and tend to rape black victims, and the remaining 2 percent come from all other races. Alcohol is involved in 34 percent of all forcible rapes. A composite characterization of the archetypal rapist drawn from police statistics portrays a single 19-year-old man from a low socioeconomic group who has a police record of acquisitive offenses.

According to the Federal Bureau of Investigation (FBI), 97,464 forcible rapes were reported to law enforcement in the United States in 1995. Rape, however, is a highly underreported crime: An estimated four to five of ten rapes are reported. The underreporting is attributed to victims' feelings of shame and to the belief that there is no recourse through the legal system. According to the FBI Uniform Crime Reporting program, in 1995, 72 of every 100,000 females in the United States were reported rape victims.

Persons who are raped can be of any age. Cases have been reported in which the victims were as young as 15 months and as old as 82 years, but women ages 16 to 24 years are at highest risk. Rape most commonly occurs in a woman's neighborhood, frequently inside or near her home. Most rapes are premeditated; about half are committed by strangers and half by men known, to varying degrees, by the victims. Seven percent of all rapes are perpetrated by close relatives of the victim; 10 percent of rapes involve more than one attacker.

A woman being raped is frequently in a life-threatening situation. During the rape, she experiences shock and fright approaching panic; her prime motivation is to stay alive. In most cases, rapists choose victims slightly smaller than themselves. Rapists may urinate or defecate on their victims, ejaculate into their faces and hair, force anal intercourse, and insert foreign objects into their vaginas and rectums.

After a rape, a woman often experiences shame, humiliation, confusion, fear, and rage. The type and duration of the reactions vary, but women report that the effects last for a year or longer. Many women experience the symptoms of PTSD. Some women, particularly those who have always felt sexually adequate, are able to resume sexual relations with men, but others become phobic about sexual interaction or exhibit such symptoms as vaginismus. Few women emerge from the assault completely unscathed. The manifestations and the degree of damage depend on the violence of the attack, the vulnerability of the woman, and the support system available to her immediately after the attack.

A rape victim fares best when she receives immediate support and can ventilate her fear and rage to loving family members, sympathetic physicians, and law enforcement officials. Knowing that she has socially acceptable means of recourse, such as the arrest and conviction of the rapist, can help a rape victim.

Unless a woman has a severe underlying disorder, therapy usually has a supportive approach and focuses on restoring a victim's sense of adequacy and control over her life; it also aims to relieve feelings of helplessness, dependence, and obsession with the assault, which frequently follow the rape. Group therapy with homogeneous groups of persons who have been raped is a particularly effective form of treatment.

In addition to the physical and psychological trauma experienced when they are assaulted, until recently rape victims also faced skepticism from those to whom they reported the crime (if they had sufficient strength to do so) or accusations of having provoked or desired the assault. In reality, the National Commission on the Causes and Prevention of Violence found discernible victim participation in rape in only 4.4 percent of all cases. This statistic is lower than that of any other crime of violence. Educating police officers and assigning policewomen to deal with rape victims have helped increase reporting of the crime. Rape crisis centers and telephone hot lines are available for immediate aid and information for victims. Volunteer groups work in emergency rooms in hospitals and with physician education programs to assist in the treatment of victims.

Legally, women no longer must prove in court that they actively struggled against a rapist, and testimony about a victim's previous sexual history has been declared inadmissible as evidence in several states. Because penalties for first-time rapists have been reduced, juries are likely to consider a conviction. In some states, wives can now prosecute husbands for rape.

In her book *Against Our Will: Men, Women, and Rape*, feminist writer and historian Susan Brownmiller theorized that rape is a conscious process of intimidation to keep a group of people in fear. She suggested that the crime can be eliminated "when men cease aggression and when women cease to identify their femininity with submission and passivity."

DATE RAPE.   *Date rape* and *acquaintance rape* are terms applied to rapes in which the rapist is known to the victim. The assault can occur on a first date or after the man and woman have known each other for many months. Considerable data on date rape have been gathered from college populations. In one study, 38 percent of male students said that they would commit rape if they thought they could get away with it, and 11 percent stated that they had committed rape; 16 percent of female students said that they had been raped by men they knew or were dating. In addition to suffering the symptoms of all rape survivors, victims of date rape berate themselves for exercising poor judgment in their choice of male friends and are more likely to blame themselves for provoking the rapist than are other victims. Many colleges and universities have set up programs for rape prevention and for counseling those who have been assaulted.

RAPE OF MEN.   In some states the definition of rape is being changed to substitute the word *person* for *female*. In most states, male rape is legally defined as sodomy. Homosexual rape is much more frequent among men than among women and occurs frequently in closed institutions such as prisons and maximum-security hospitals.

29

Additional Conditions That May Be a Focus of Clinical Attention

As defined in the text revision of the fourth edition of *Diagnostic and Statistical Manual of Mental Disorders* (DSM-IV-TR), conditions that may be a focus of clinical attention have led to contact with the mental health care system but without sufficient evidence to justify a diagnosis of a mental disorder. In some instances, one of these conditions will be noted during the course of a psychiatric evaluation, although no mental disorder has been found. In other instances, the diagnostic evaluation reveals no mental disorder, but a need is seen to note the primary reason for contact with the mental health care system.

Thirteen conditions make up the diagnostic category of additional disorders that may be a focus of clinical attention. Nine of these conditions are discussed in this chapter: malingering, bereavement, occupational problems, adult antisocial behavior, religious or spiritual problem, acculturation problem, phase of life problem, noncompliance with treatment for a mental disorder, and age-associated memory decline. (Four other conditions included in the DSM-IV-TR are discussed in Chapter 48: borderline intellectual functioning, academic problem, childhood or adolescent antisocial behavior, and identity problem.)

MALINGERING

According to the DSM-IV-TR,

The essential feature of Malingering is the intentional production of false or grossly exaggerated physical or psychological symptoms, motivated by external incentives such as avoiding military duty, avoiding work, obtaining financial compensation, evading criminal prosecution, or obtaining drugs. Under some circumstances, malingering may represent adaptive behavior—for example, feigning illness while a captive of the enemy during wartime.

Malingering should be strongly suspected if any combination of the following is noted: (1) medicolegal context of presentation (e.g., the person is referred by an attorney to the clinician for examination or is incarcerated), (2) evident discrepancy between the individual's claimed stress or disability and the objective findings, (3) lack of cooperation during the diagnostic evaluation and in complying with the prescribed treatment regimen, and (4) the presence of Antisocial Personality Disorder.

Epidemiology

A 1 percent prevalence of malingering has been estimated among mental health patients in civilian clinical practice, with the estimate rising to 5 percent in the military. In a litigious context, during interviews of criminal defendants, the estimated prevalence of malingering is much higher—between 10 and 20 percent.

Approximately 50 percent of children presenting with conduct disorders are described as having serious lying-related issues.

Although no familial or genetic patterns have been reported and no clear sex bias or age at onset has been delineated, malingering does appear to be highly prevalent in certain military, prison, and litigious populations and, in Western society, in men from youth through middle age. Associated disorders include conduct disorder and anxiety disorders in children and antisocial, borderline, and narcissistic personality disorders in adults.

Etiology

Although no biological factors have been found to be causally related to malingering, its frequent association with antisocial personality disorder raises the possibility that hypoarousability may be an underlying metabolic factor. Still, no predisposing genetic, neurophysiological, neurochemical, or neuroendocrinological forces are known.

Diagnosis and Clinical Features

Avoidance of Criminal Responsibility, Trial, and Punishment.
Criminals may pretend to be incompetent to avoid standing trial; they may feign insanity at the time of perpetration of the crime, malinger symptoms to receive a less harsh penalty, or attempt to act too incapacitated (incompetent) to be executed.

Avoidance of Military Service or of Particularly Hazardous Duties.
Persons may malinger to avoid conscription into the armed forces, and, once conscripted, they may feign illness to escape from particularly onerous or hazardous duties.

Financial Gain.
Malingerers may seek financial gain in the form of undeserved disability insurance, veterans' benefits, workers' compensation, or tort damages for purported psychological injury.

Avoidance of Work, Social Responsibility, and Social Consequences.
Individuals may malinger to escape from unpleasant vocational or social circumstances or to avoid the social and litigation-related consequences of vocational or social improprieties.

Facilitation of Transfer from Prison to Hospital.
Prisoners may malinger (fake bad) with the goal of obtaining a transfer to a psychiatric hospital from which they may hope to escape or in which they expect to do "easier time." The prison context may also give rise to dissimulation (faking good), however; the prospect of an indeterminate

number of days on a mental health ward may prompt an inmate with true psychiatric symptoms to make every effort to conceal them.

Admission to a Hospital.

In this era of deinstitutionalization and homelessness, individuals may malinger in an effort to gain admission to a psychiatric hospital. Such institutions may be seen as providing free room and board, a safe haven from the police, or refuge from rival gang members or disgruntled drug cronies who have made street life even more unbearable and hazardous than it usually is.

Drug-Seeking.

Malingerers may feign illness in an effort to obtain favored medications, either for personal use or, in a prison setting, as currency to barter for cigarettes, protection, or other inmate-provided favors.

The plaintiff, a woman in her late 20s, was injured while dancing at a club. Although her claim initially appeared bona fide, subsequent investigation cast doubt on the mechanism of injury that she claimed—namely, that a misplaced electrical cord under a carpet caused her to slip. This was true, she claimed, despite that she had to be dancing in a particularly jerky manner that could have easily caused problems without tripping.

Subsequently, she sought medical and surgical treatment for torn cartilage in her injured knee. Despite that the initial surgery went well, she kept reinjuring the knee with various "slips." As a result, she requested narcotic analgesics. A careful medical record review revealed that she was obtaining such medications from multiple practitioners and that she had apparently forged at least one prescription.

In reviewing the case before binding arbitration, it was the opinion of the orthopedic and psychiatric consultants that, although the initial injury and reported pain were real, the plaintiff consciously elaborated her injuries to obtain the desired narcotic analgesics. (Courtesy of Mark J. Mills, J.D., M.D., and Mark S. Lipian, M.D., Ph.D.)

Child Custody.

Minimizing difficulties or faking good for the sake of obtaining child custody can occur when one party accurately accuses the other of being an unfit parent because of psychological conditions. The accused party may feel compelled to minimize symptoms or to portray himself or herself in a positive light to reduce chances of being deemed unfit and losing custody.

Differential Diagnosis

Malingering must be differentiated from the actual physical or psychiatric illness suspected of being feigned. Furthermore, the possibility of partial malingering, which is an exaggeration of existing symptoms, must be entertained. In addition, the possibility exists of unintentional, dynamically driven misattribution of genuine symptoms (e.g., of depression) to an incorrect environmental cause (e.g., to sexual harassment rather than to narcissistic injury).

It should also be remembered that a real psychiatric disorder and malingering are not mutually exclusive.

Factitious disorder is distinguished from malingering by motivation (sick role vs. tangible pain), whereas the somatoform disorders involve no conscious volition. In conversion disorder, as in malingering, objective signs cannot account for subjective experience, and differentiation between the two disorders can be difficult.

Course and Prognosis

Malingering persists as long as the malingerer believes it will likely produce the desired rewards. In the absence of concurrent diagnoses, once the rewards have been attained, the feigned symptoms disappear. In some structured settings, such as the military or prison units, ignoring the malingered behavior may result in its disappearance, particularly if an expectation of continued productive performance, despite complaints, is made clear. In children, malingering is most likely associated with a predisposing anxiety or conduct disorder; proper attention to this developing problem may alleviate the child's propensity to malinger.

Treatment

The appropriate stance for the psychiatrist is clinical neutrality. If malingering is suspected, a careful differential investigation should ensue. If, at the conclusion of the diagnostic evaluation, malingering seems most likely, the patient should be tactfully but firmly confronted with the apparent outcome. The reasons underlying the ruse need to be elicited, however, and alternative pathways to the desired outcome explored. Coexisting psychiatric disorders should be thoroughly assessed. Only if the patient is utterly unwilling to interact with the physician under any terms other than manipulation should the therapeutic (or evaluative) interaction be abandoned.

BEREAVEMENT

Normal bereavement begins immediately after, or within a few months of, the loss of a loved one. Typical signs and symptoms include feelings of sadness, preoccupation with thoughts about the deceased, tearfulness, irritability, insomnia, and difficulties concentrating and carrying out daily activities. On the basis of the cultural group, bereavement is limited to a varying time, usually 6 months, but it can be longer. Normal bereavement, however, can lead to a full depressive disorder that requires treatment.

The DSM-IV-TR includes the following description of bereavement:

This category can be used when the focus of clinical attention is a reaction to the death of a loved one. As part of their reaction to the loss, some grieving individuals present with symptoms characteristic of a Major Depressive Episode (e.g., feelings of sadness and associated symptoms such as insomnia, poor appetite, and weight loss). The bereaved individual typically regards the depressed mood as "normal," although the person may seek professional help for relief of associated symptoms such as insomnia or anorexia. The duration and expression of "normal" bereavement vary considerably among different cultural groups. The diagnosis of Major Depressive Disorder is generally not given unless the symptoms are still present 2 months after the loss. However, the presence of certain symptoms that are not characteristic of a "normal" grief reaction may be helpful in differentiating bereavement from a Major Depressive Episode. These include (1) guilt about things other than actions taken or not taken by the survivor at the time of the death; (2) thoughts of death other than the survivor feeling that he or she would be better off dead or should have died with the deceased person; (3) morbid preoccupation with worthlessness; (4) marked psychomotor retardation;

(5) prolonged and marked functional impairment; and (6) hallucinatory experiences other than thinking that he or she hears the voice of, or transiently sees the image of, the deceased person.

OCCUPATIONAL PROBLEM

The DSM-IV-TR includes the following statement about occupational problem:

This category can be used when the focus of clinical attention is an occupational problem that is not due to a mental disorder or, if it is due to a mental disorder, is sufficiently severe to warrant independent clinical attention. Examples include job dissatisfaction and uncertainty about career choices.

Occupational problems often arise during stressful changes in work, namely, at initial entry into the workforce or when making job changes within the same organization to a higher position because of good performance or to a parallel position because of corporate need. Distress occurs particularly if these changes are not sought and no preparatory training has taken place, as well as during layoffs and at retirement, especially if retirement is mandatory and the person is unprepared for this event. Work distress can result if initially agreed-to-conditions change to work overload or lack of challenge and opportunity to experience work satisfaction; if an individual feels unable to fulfill conflicting expectations or feels that work conditions prevent accomplishing assignments because of lack of legitimate power; or if an individual believes he or she works in a hierarchy with harsh and unreasonable superiors.

Work Choices and Changes

Young adults without role models or guidance from families, mentors, or others in their communities too often underestimate their lifetime potential abilities to learn a trade or earn a college or postgraduate degree. In addition, women and members of minority groups often feel less prepared to accept work challenges, fear rejection, and do not apply for jobs for which they are qualified. On the other hand, men, in fields in which they are underrepresented, often and confidently move up the career ladder faster ("glass elevator"). As part of initial interviews for evaluation of occupational problems, patients should be encouraged to consider their heretofore unrecognized, unadmitted talents; long-held, yet unexpressed, dreams and goals regarding work; actual successes in work and school; and motivation to risk learning what they would find satisfying.

Minorities and those in low-paying and low-skilled jobs too often have less job security. Business and institutional reorganization and consequent downsizing, factory closings, and moves affect many, often leaving these workers feeling hopeless and helpless about future employment, on welfare, angry, and depressed.

With ongoing and often sudden downsizing of corporations and businesses, men and women continue to struggle with unexpected job loss and premature retirement, even when finances are not an issue. In addition, men, in particular, define themselves by their work roles, and, thus, experience more occupational distress from these changes. Women may adjust faster to retirement, but they often have less financial security than men do (white women earn approximately 80 cents to each dollar for comparable work for men, and African American and Hispanic women earn even less for comparable work); women have generally been in lower-status work positions, find themselves alone after death of a spouse more often than men, and are more likely to be caring for children, grandchildren, and elderly relatives. Women represent more of the single-working-parent group and the working poor.

Stress and the Workplace

More than 30 percent of workers report that they are under stress at work. Workplace distress is implicated in at least 15 percent of occupational disability claims. Expected distress follows recognized and uncontrollable work changes—downsizing, mergers and acquisitions, work overload, and chronic physical strains, including work noise, temperature, bodily injuries, and strain from performing computer work. According to one study, the ten most stressful jobs are (1) president of the United States, (2) firefighter, (3) senior corporate executive, (4) race car driver, (5) taxi driver, (6) surgeon, (7) astronaut, (8) police officer, (9) football player, and (10) air traffic controller. People who work under deadlines, such as bus drivers, are subject to hypertension.

Work frustration can also arise from an individual worker's unrecognized (and therefore unresolved) psychodynamic issues, such as working appropriately with superiors and not relating to one's supervisor as a parent figure. Other developmental issues include unresolved problems with competition, assertiveness, envy, fear of success, and inability to communicate verbally in a constructive manner.

After the September 11, 2001, World Trade Center tragedy, a 32-year-old, married, male firefighter, who had been away on vacation that day with his wife and children, began to exhibit changed behaviors at home and at work. At home, he appeared not to listen to his two latency-aged children and, instead, focused his attention on television sporting events. At work, he also appeared to be more focused on cooking the same dinners for his peers and watching television than on interacting verbally with his remaining peers and the new chief. In the course of several months, a chaplain visited the station several times and talked to the firefighters about survivor guilt and the 9/11 tragedy, and the firefighter began to return somewhat to his former healthier behaviors. (Courtesy of Leah J. Dickstein, M.D.)

Often, work conflicts reflect similar conflicts in the worker's personal life, and referral for treatment, unless there is insight, is in order. Some studies have found that massage therapy, meditation, and yoga at intervals during the work day relieve stress when used on a regular basis. Approaches using cognitive therapy have also helped people reduce work pressure.

Career and Job Problems of Women

Most women work outside of the home out of necessity to support themselves or their dependents (whether children or adults) or as part of a working couple. The divorce rate is 50 percent, and many women find themselves economically poorer after a divorce than when married, although divorced men usually find their economic status improved. Despite more than four decades of increasing knowledge about, and concern for, women's status in the workplace, unique gender issues, bias, and lack of accommodation to their unique needs at certain life stages (i.e., pregnancy and postpartum, major responsibility for young healthy and ill children) continue. Yet, women were the largest group establishing new small businesses in the 1990s. Many have left large corporations where they were not valued for their efforts because of their gender, termed *contra culture*. Women experience problems when they are the sole woman in a man's field. Despite increasing recognition of the need for men in relationships with women to assume home and family responsibilities, less than 25 percent of men do so equitably.

Women of childbearing and child-rearing ages continue to find themselves in conflict with job expectations, opportunities, and personal responsibilities. High-quality, on-site, dependent-care facilities with extended hours are rare and often out of range financially. Major unresolved work issues that are unique to women at certain life stages include flextime and paid and unpaid dependent leave options. Beyond dependent care issues, women in the workforce continue to experience distress after chronic and repeated sexual harassment, despite its illegality and media attention. Increasingly, more women have travel responsibilities, work long hours, work shifts beyond daylight hours, and experience personal workplace violence.

Among dual-career families and partners, the woman is more likely to move when the man chooses to move for a work opportunity than vice versa. Consequently, a woman's career is interrupted more often. Less reluctance is seen, however, to have the two members of a relationship work for the same organization than previously, albeit usually in different departments. Work distress may also stem from continuous miscommunication, especially that based on gender.

Working Teenagers

Many teenagers work part-time while attending high school. Consequently, stress can arise because of less parent–teenager interaction and constructive parental control issues about teens' use of earnings, time spent away from home, and consequent behaviors both in and outside the home. When both parents or a single parent, as well as the teenager, work outside the home, often on different schedules, parent–teen verbal communication must be proactive, clear, and ongoing.

Working within the Home

Although most women with children of all ages must work outside the home, at times they may be home full time or part time or may work at home. When their husbands or significant others work full time outside the home, problems may develop from each partner's perceived expectations of the other. Women who care for children and their home exclusively may be seen by their partners as not only economically dependent and inferior, but also not as competent and not understanding of the man's stressors and needs. Ongoing respectful listening and verbal communication must be encouraged.

People in organizations are increasingly taking work home as their work expectations increase. This work-at-home experience can and does interfere with personal lives and satisfaction, which can then have further repercussions at work.

Chronic Illness

As general and other medical and psychiatric treatments for chronic diseases improve, employers have been increasingly concerned about accommodating patients with acquired immunodeficiency syndrome (AIDS), diabetes mellitus, and other disorders. The issue of mandatory testing for AIDS and substance abuse (alcohol and other illegal substances) continues to be of concern. Employee assistance programs

offering education about general and mental health topics have proved timely and cost-effective.

Domestic Violence

Although occurring in the home, signs and symptoms that interfere with work often trigger identification of those who experience domestic violence. Trained professionals must question all employees experiencing work distress about domestic violence and, when indicated, refer individuals for assistance, which includes safety in the workplace.

Job Loss

Regardless of the reason for job loss, most people experience distress, at least temporarily, including symptoms of normal grief, loss of self-esteem, anger, reactive depressive and anxiety symptoms, as well as somatic symptoms, and, possibly, the onset of, or increase in, substance abuse or domestic violence. Timely education, support programs, and vocational guidance should be instituted and access to treatment made available, if indicated.

ADULT ANTISOCIAL BEHAVIOR

Characterized by activities that are illegal, immoral, or both, antisocial behavior usually begins in childhood and often persists throughout life. DSM-IV-TR includes the following statement about adult antisocial behavior:

This category can be used when the focus of clinical attention is adult antisocial behavior that is not due to a mental disorder (e.g., Conduct Disorder, Antisocial Personality Disorder, or an Impulse-Control Disorder). Examples include the behavior of some professional thieves, racketeers, or dealers in illegal substances.

The term *antisocial behavior* somewhat confusingly applies both to persons' actions that are not due to a mental disorder and to actions by those who never received a neuropsychiatric workup to determine the presence or absence of a mental disorder. As Dorothy Lewis noted, the term can apply to behavior by normal persons who "struggle to make a dishonest living."

Epidemiology

Depending on the criteria and the sampling, estimates of the prevalence of adult antisocial behavior range from 5 to 15 percent of the population. Within prison populations, investigators report prevalence figures between 20 and 80 percent. Men account for more adult antisocial behavior than do women.

Etiology

Antisocial behaviors in adulthood are characteristic of a variety of persons, ranging from those with no demonstrable psychopathology to those who are severely impaired and have psychotic disorders, cognitive disorders, and retardation, among other conditions. A comprehensive neuropsychiatric assessment of antisocial adults is indicated and may reveal potentially treatable psychiatric and neurological impairments that can easily be overlooked. Only in the absence of mental disorders can patients be categorized as displaying adult antisocial behavior. Adult antisocial behavior may be influenced by genetic and social factors.

Genetic Factors.   Data supporting the genetic transmission of antisocial behavior are based on studies that found a 60 percent concordance rate in monozygotic twins and about a 30 percent concordance rate in dizygotic twins. Adoption studies show a high rate of antisocial behavior in the biological relatives of adoptees identified with antisocial behavior and a high incidence of antisocial behavior in the adopted-away offspring of those with antisocial behavior. The prenatal and perinatal periods of those who subsequently display antisocial behavior often are associated with low birthweight, mental retardation, and prenatal exposure to alcohol and other drugs of abuse.

Social Factors.   Studies have shown that in neighborhoods in which families with low socioeconomic status (SES) predominate, the sons of unskilled workers are more likely to commit more offenses and more serious criminal offenses than do the sons of middle-class and skilled workers, at least during adolescence and early adulthood. These data are not as clear for women, but the findings are generally similar in studies from many countries. Areas of family training differ by SES group. Middle-SES parents use love-oriented techniques in discipline. They withdraw affection rather than impose physical punishment as is done in low-SES groups. Negative parental attitudes toward aggressive behavior, attempts to curb aggressive behavior, and the ability to communicate parental values are more characteristic of middle- and high-SES groups than of low ones. Adult antisocial behavior is associated with the use and abuse of alcohol and other substances and with the easy availability of handguns.

Diagnosis and Clinical Features

The diagnosis of adult antisocial behavior is one of exclusion. Substance dependence in such behavior often makes it difficult to separate the antisocial behavior related primarily to substance dependence from disordered behaviors that occurred either before substance use or during episodes unrelated to substance dependence.

During the manic phases of bipolar I disorder, certain aspects of behavior, such as wanderlust, sexual promiscuity, and financial difficulties, can be similar to adult antisocial behavior. Patients with schizophrenia may have episodes of adult antisocial behavior, but the symptom picture is usually clear, especially regarding thought disorder, delusions, and hallucinations on the mental status examination.

Neurological conditions can be associated with adult antisocial behavior, and electroencephalograms (EEGs), computed tomography scans, magnetic resonance imaging, and complete neurological examinations are indicated. Temporal lobe epilepsy should be considered in the differential diagnosis. When a clear-cut diagnosis of temporal lobe epilepsy or encephalitis can be made, the disorder may be considered to contribute to the adult antisocial behavior. Abnormal EEG findings are prevalent among violent offenders: An estimated 50 percent of aggressive criminals have abnormal EEG findings.

Persons with adult antisocial behavior have difficulties in work, marriage, and money matters and conflicts with various authorities. (Antisocial personality disorder is discussed in Chapter 23.)

Treatment

In general, therapists are pessimistic about treating adult antisocial behavior. They have little hope of changing a pattern that has been present almost continuously throughout a person's life. Psychotherapy has not been effective, and no major breakthroughs with biological treatments, including medications, have occurred.

Therapists show more enthusiasm for the use of therapeutic communities and other forms of group treatment, although the data provide little basis for optimism. Many adult criminals who are incarcerated in institutional settings have shown some response to group therapy approaches. The history of violence, criminality, and antisocial behavior has shown that such behaviors seem to decrease after age 40 years. Recidivism in criminals, which can reach 90 percent in some studies, also decreases in middle age.

Prevention.   Because antisocial behavior often begins during childhood, the major focus must be on delinquency prevention. Any measures that improve the physical and mental health of socioeconomically disadvantaged children and their families are likely to reduce delinquency and violent crime. Often, recurrently violent persons have sustained many insults to the central nervous system (CNS), prenatally and throughout childhood and adolescence. Consequently, programs must be developed to educate parents about the dangers to their children of CNS injury from maltreatment, including the effects of psychoactive substances on the brain of the growing fetus. Public education about the releasing effect of alcohol on violent behaviors (not to mention its contribution to vehicular homicide) may also reduce crime.

RELIGIOUS OR SPIRITUAL PROBLEM

According to DSM-IV-TR,

This category can be used when the focus of clinical attention is a religious or spiritual problem. Examples include distressing experiences that involve loss or questioning of faith, problems associated with conversion to a new faith, or questioning other spiritual values which may not necessarily be related to an organized church or religious institution.

Psychiatrists must enable and assist patients to distinguish religious thought or experience from psychopathology and, if this is a problem, encourage patients to work through the issues independently or with assistance. Religious imagery may be recognized in mental illness when persons state they believe they have been commanded by God to take a dangerous or grandiose action.

A midcareer male surgeon, who was very successful but long overcommitted to his private practice and his academic responsibilities, revealed to his often-neglected wife that, at age 9 years, he was approached by his religious leader to get close physically. Believing it was his fault, he never told anyone and decided, then, never to have children. In the weeks after this disclosure, he and his wife began to spend more private time together and even discussed the possibility of starting a family.

Cults

Recently, cults have appeared to be less popular and less attractive to naïve late adolescents and young adults seeking assistance in discovering who they are as they struggle to develop more mature relationships with their parents. Cults are led by charismatic leaders, often out of control themselves, with inappropriate and often unethical values, but purporting to offer acceptance and guidance to troubled followers. Cult members are strongly controlled and forced to dissolve allegiance to family and others to serve the cult leader's directives and personal needs. These young members often come from educated families who then seek professional help in persuading their children to leave the cult and enter deprogramming therapy to restore personal psychological stability to the former cult members. Deprogramming and adjustment back into family, society, and an independent life are time intensive and long term with resultant posttraumatic stress disorder (PTSD), which must be recognized and treated.

ACCULTURATION PROBLEM

The DSM-IV-TR includes the following statement about acculturation problem:

This category can be used when the focus of clinical attention is a problem involving adjustment to a different culture (e.g., following migration).

Culture Shock

Major cultural change can evoke severe distress, termed *culture shock*. This condition arises when individuals suddenly find themselves in a new culture in which they feel completely alien. They may also feel conflict over which lifestyles to maintain, change, or adopt. Children and young adult immigrants often adapt more easily than do middle-aged and elderly immigrants. Younger immigrants often learn the new language more easily and continue to mature in the new culture, whereas those who are more senior, having had more stability and unchanging routines in their former culture, struggle more to adapt. Culture shock from immigration clearly differs from the restless and continuous moving of psychiatric patients secondary to their illness.

Culture shock can occur within a person's own country with geographic, school, and work changes, such as joining the military, experiencing school busing, moving across country, or moving to a vastly different neighborhood or from a rural area to a metropolis. Reactive symptoms, which are understandable, include anxiety, depression, isolation, fear, and a sense of loss of identity as the person adjusts. If the person is part of a family or group making this transition and the move is positive and planned, stress can be lower. Furthermore, if selected cultural mores can be safely maintained as persons integrate into the new culture, stress is also minimized.

Constant geographic moves because of chosen work opportunities or necessity involve a large proportion of workers in the United States. Joining activities in the new community and actively trying to meet neighbors and coworkers can lessen the culture shock.

An 18-year-old, first-year female college student offered an academic scholarship by a small southern college with a major in her field of interest realized on her return home to the Midwest for winter break that she felt like a misfit among her dorm peers. They were friendly, yet generally kept their distance from her after class. At home, she discussed her experiences with high school friends, who replied that they had heard about such cultural dissonance from peers at their midwestern colleges. The student returned to college feeling that it was not her fault or imagination and slowly began to reach out more assertively to her peers so they could get to know her beyond stereotypical beliefs and so she could do the same.

Brainwashing.   First practiced by the Chinese Communists on American prisoners during the Korean War, *brainwashing* is the deliberate creation of culture shock. Individuals are isolated, intimidated, and made to feel different and out of place to break their spirits and destroy their coping skills. Once a person appears mentally weak and helpless, the aggressors impose new ideas on the person that he or she would never have accepted in his or her normal state. As with those involved in cults, on release and return to their homes, brainwashed individuals with PTSD require deprogramming treatment, including reeducation and ongoing supportive psychotherapy, both on an individual and group basis. Treatment is usually long term to rebuild healthy self-esteem and coping skills. (See also Chapter 16, Dissociative Disorders.)

Prisoners of War and Torture Victims.   Prisoners who survive war or torture experiences do so because of personal inner strengths developed in their earlier lives, beginning within their emotionally strong and caring families; if they come from troubled families, they are more likely to commit suicide during imprisonment and torture. Prisoners must constantly cope with ongoing anxiety, fear, isolation from known lives, and complete loss of all control over their lives. Those who appear to cope best believe they must survive for a reason (e.g., to tell others what they experienced or to find and return to loved ones). Prisoners who cope best describe living simultaneously on two levels—coping in the here and now to survive the situation while maintaining constant mental connections to their past values and experiences and those important to them.

Beyond the surviving prisoner's personal difficulties, including PTSD, if and when his or her survival behavior continues, his or her family may be affected by the surviving prisoner's inordinate fear of police and strangers, overprotection and overburdening of children to replace those significant others lost, lack of sharing of the past, continued isolation from current communities, or inappropriate expressed anger. Thus, another generation (i.e., children of survivors) can be affected in their personal development and psychological functioning and may require psychiatric evaluation and treatment. (See also Section 13.5, Posttraumatic Stress Disorder and Acute Stress Disorder.)

A 75-year-old Catholic female survivor of the Pawiak prison in Warsaw, Poland, and then of a concentration camp after her capture as a member of the underground in World War II stated that she had wanted to become a painter. In camp, she carved the Madonna and Child on her toothbrush and sent it home to her mother. She made other clandestine carvings for several women in her barracks to send home to their families, which pleased everyone. After the war, she became a well-known sculptress with exhibits throughout Europe. Many of her art pieces taught people about suffering and respect for others who are of different religions and cultures.

PHASE OF LIFE PROBLEM

The DSM-IV-TR description of phase of life problem includes the following:

This category can be used when the focus of clinical attention is a problem associated with a particular developmental phase or some other life circumstance that is not due to a mental disorder or, if it is due to a mental disorder, is sufficiently severe to warrant independent clinical attention. Examples include: problems associated with entering school, leaving parental control, starting a new job or career, and changes involved in marriage, divorce, relationship loss, illness, and retirement.

Although, on some level, adults recognize that life events will intrude on expected plans in the course of a lifetime, unexpected, multiple, major negative occurrences, especially if they are chronic, overwhelm a person's ability to recover and function constructively. Common phase of life problems include relationship changes, such as a changed significant personal relationship or its loss, job crises, and parenthood.

Because of sex role socialization and consequent cultural expectations, men appear externally better able to handle these phase of life problems, whereas women, the poor, and minority group members appear more vulnerable to negative experiences, perhaps because they feel less empowered psychologically. Major life changes precipitate distress in the form of anxiety and depressive symptoms, inability to express reactive emotions directly, and, often, difficulties in coping with ongoing or changed life responsibilities.

Individuals with positive attitudes, strong family and personal relationships, and mature defense mechanisms and coping styles, including basic trust in self and others, good verbal communication skills, a capacity for creative and positive thinking, and the ability to be flexible, reliable, and energetic, appear to be best able to cope with phase of life problems. Furthermore, a capacity for sublimation, adequate financial and work status, solid values, and healthy feasible goals can enable people to face, accept, and deal realistically with expected and unexpected life problems and changes.

NONCOMPLIANCE WITH TREATMENT

The DSM-IV-TR contains the following statement regarding noncompliance with treatment:

This category can be used when the focus of clinical attention is noncompliance with an important aspect of the treatment for a mental disorder or a general medical condition. The reasons for noncompliance may include discomfort resulting from treatment (e.g., medication side effects), expense of treatment, decisions based on personal value judgments, religious or cultural beliefs about the advantages and disadvantages of the proposed treatment, maladaptive personality traits or coping styles (e.g., denial of illness), or the presence of a mental disorder (e.g., Schizophrenia, Avoidant Personality Disorder). This category should be used only when the problem is sufficiently severe to warrant independent clinical attention.

AGE-RELATED COGNITIVE DECLINE

The DSM-IV-TR includes the following comment regarding age-related cognitive decline:

This category can be used when the focus of clinical attention is an objectively identified decline in cognitive functioning consequent to the aging process that is within normal limits given the person's age. Individuals with this condition may report problems remembering names or appointments or may experience difficulty in solving complex problems. This category should be considered only after it has been determined that the cognitive impairment is not attributable to a specific mental disorder or neurological condition.

Attempts to delay age-related cognitive decline are myriad. They include daily intake of vitamin E (200 to 600 mg), daily intake of nonsteroidal anti-inflammatory drugs, use of the herb ginkgo biloba, and use of male and female sex steroids. Cognitive decline is lower in persons who exercise, do not smoke, drink little or no alcohol, and who challenge their intellect at work or play (e.g., crossword puzzles). The ability to learn new material is maintained through old age; however, it takes longer and requires more practice than in young persons.

30 ▲

Emergency Psychiatric Medicine

▲ 30.1 Suicide

Suicide is derived from the Latin word for "self-murder." It is a fatal act that represents the person's wish to die. There is a range, however, between thinking about suicide and acting it out. Some persons have ideas of suicide that they will never act on; some plan for days, weeks, or even years before acting; and others take their lives seemingly on impulse, without premeditation. Lost in the definition are intentional misclassifications of the cause of death, accidents of undetermined cause, and so-called chronic suicides—for example, death through alcohol and other substance abuse and consciously poor adherence to medical regimens for addiction, obesity, and hypertension.

EPIDEMIOLOGY

Approximately 30,000 deaths are attributed to suicide each year in the United States. This is in contrast to approximately 20,000 deaths annually from homicide. Although significant shifts were seen in the suicide death rates for certain subpopulations during the last century (e.g., increased adolescent and decreased elderly rates), the rate has remained fairly constant, averaging about 12.5 per 100,000 through the 20th century and into the 21st. Whereas the overall suicide rate has remained relatively stable, however, the rate for those 15 to 24 years of age has increased two- to threefold. Suicide is now the eighth-leading overall cause of death in the United States, after heart disease, cancer, cerebrovascular disease, chronic obstructive pulmonary disease, accidents, pneumonia and influenza, and diabetes mellitus.

Suicide rates in the United States are at the midpoint of the rates for industrialized countries as reported to the United Nations. Internationally, suicide rates range from highs of more than 25 per 100,000 persons in Scandinavia, Switzerland, Germany, Austria, the eastern European countries (the so-called suicide belt), and Japan, to fewer than 10 per 100,000 in Spain, Italy, Ireland, Egypt, and the Netherlands.

A state-by-state analysis of suicides in the last decade among persons between the ages of 15 and 44 years revealed that New Jersey had the nation's lowest suicide rates for both sexes. Nevada and New Mexico had the highest rates for men, and Nevada and Wyoming had the highest rates for women. Women in Nevada killed themselves at a higher frequency than did men in New Jersey. The prime suicide site of the world is the Golden Gate Bridge in San Francisco, with more than 800 suicides committed there since the bridge opened in 1937.

Risk Factors

Gender Differences.　　Men commit suicide more than four times as often as women, a rate that is stable over all ages. Women, however, are four times more likely to attempt suicide than men. Men's higher rate of completed suicide is related to the methods they use: firearms, hanging, or jumping from high places. Women more commonly take an overdose of psychoactive substances or a poison, but their use of firearms is increasing. In states with gun control laws, the use of firearms has decreased as a method of suicide. Globally, the most common method of suicide is hanging.

Age.　　Suicide rates increase with age and underscore the significance of the midlife crisis. Among men, suicides peak after age 45 years; among women, the greatest number of completed suicides occurs after age 55 years. Rates of 40 per 100,000 population occur in men age 65 years and older. Older persons attempt suicide less often than younger persons but are more often successful. Although they are only 10 percent of the total population, older persons account for 25 percent of suicides. The rate for those 75 years or older is more than three times the rate among young persons.

The suicide rate, however, is rising most rapidly among young persons, particularly males 15 to 24 years of age. The suicide rate for females in the same age group is increasing more slowly than that for males. Among men 25 to 34 years of age, the suicide rate increased almost 30 percent over the past decade. Suicide is the third-leading cause of death in those 15 to 24 years of age, after accidents and homicides, and attempted suicides in this age group number between 1 million and 2 million annually. Most suicides now occur among those aged 15 to 44 years. Suicide is rare before puberty. (For a thorough discussion of this topic see Chapter 45, Mood Disorders and Suicide in Children and Adolescents.)

Race.　　Two of every three suicides are white males. White male and female rates are approximately two to three times as high as African-American male and female rates across the life cycle. Among young persons who live in inner cities and certain Native American and Inuit groups, suicide rates have greatly exceeded the national rate. Suicide rates among immigrants are higher than those in the native-born population.

Religion.　　Historically, suicide rates among Roman Catholic populations have been lower than rates among Protestants and Jews. The degree of orthodoxy and integration may be a more accurate measure of risk in this category than simple institutional religious affiliation.

Marital Status.　　Marriage lessens the risk of suicide significantly, especially if there are children in the home. Single, never-married persons have an overall rate nearly double that of married persons. Divorce increases suicide risk, with divorced men three times more likely to kill themselves as divorced women. Widows and widowers also have high rates. Suicide occurs more frequently than usual in persons who are socially isolated and have a family history of suicide (attempted or real).

Persons who commit so-called anniversary suicides take their lives on the day a member of their family did.

Occupation.

The higher a person's social status, the greater the risk of suicide, but a fall in social status also increases the risk. Work, in general, protects against suicide. Among occupational rankings, professionals, particularly physicians, have traditionally been considered to be at greatest risk. Other high-risk occupations include law enforcement, dentists, artists, mechanics, lawyers, and insurance agents. Suicide is higher among the unemployed than among employed persons. The suicide rate increases during economic recessions and depressions and decreases during times of high unemployment and during wars.

Climate.

No significant seasonal correlation with suicide has been found. Suicides increase slightly in spring and fall but, contrary to popular belief, not during December and holiday periods.

Physical Health.

The relation of physical health and illness to suicide is significant. Previous medical care appears to be a positively correlated risk indicator of suicide: About one third of all persons who commit suicide have had medical attention within 6 months of death, and a physical illness is estimated to be an important contributing factor in about half of suicides.

Factors associated with illness and contributing to both suicides and suicide attempts are loss of mobility, especially when physical activity is important to occupation or recreation; disfigurement, particularly among women; and chronic, intractable pain. Patients on hemodialysis are at high risk. In addition to the direct effects of illness, the secondary effects—for example, disruption of relationships and loss of occupational status—are prognostic factors.

Certain drugs can produce depression, which may lead to suicide in some cases. Among these drugs are reserpine (Serpasil), corticosteroids, antihypertensives, and some anticancer agents. Alcohol-related illnesses, such as cirrhosis, are associated with higher suicide rates.

Mental Illness.

Almost 95 percent of all persons who commit or attempt suicide have a diagnosed mental disorder. Depressive disorders account for 80 percent of this figure, schizophrenia accounts for 10 percent, and dementia or delirium for 5 percent. Among all persons with mental disorders, 25 percent are also alcohol dependent and have dual diagnoses. Persons with delusional depression are at highest risk of suicide. A history of impulsive behavior or violent acts increases the risk of suicide, as does previous psychiatric hospitalization for any reason. Among adults who commit suicide, significant differences between young and old exist for both psychiatric diagnoses and antecedent stressors. Diagnoses of substance abuse and antisocial personality disorder occurred most often among suicides in persons less than 30 years of age, and diagnoses of mood disorders and cognitive disorders most often among suicides in those age 30 years and older. Stressors associated with suicide in those younger than 30 years were separation, rejection, unemployment, and legal troubles; illness stressors most often occurred among suicide victims older than 30 years.

Psychiatric Patients.

Psychiatric patients' risk for suicide is 3 to 12 times that of nonpatients. The degree of risk varies, depending on age, sex, diagnosis, and inpatient or outpatient status. Male and female psychiatric patients who have at some time been inpatients have 5 and 10 times higher suicide risks, respectively, than their counterparts in the general population. For male and female outpatients who have never been admitted to a hospital for psychiatric treatment, the suicide risks are 3 and 4 times greater, respectively, than those of their counterparts in the general population. The higher suicide risk for psychiatric patients who have been inpatients reflects that patients with severe mental disorders tend to be hospitalized—for example, patients with depressive disorder

who require electroconvulsive therapy (ECT). The psychiatric diagnosis with greatest risk of suicide in both sexes is a mood disorder.

Those in the general population who commit suicide tend to be middle-aged or older, but studies increasingly report that psychiatric patients who commit suicide tend to be relatively young. In one study, the mean age of male suicides was 29.5 years and that of women suicides was 38.4 years. The relative youthfulness of these suicide cases was partly because two early-onset, chronic mental disorders—schizophrenia and recurrent major depressive disorder—accounted for just more than half of these suicides and so reflected an age and diagnostic pattern found in most studies of psychiatric patient suicides.

A small but significant percentage of psychiatric patients who commit suicide do so while they are inpatients. Most of these do not kill themselves in the psychiatric ward itself, but on the hospital grounds, while on a pass or weekend leave, or when absent without leave. For both sexes, the suicide risk is highest in the first week of the psychiatric admission; after 3 to 5 weeks, inpatients have the same risk as the general population. Times of staff rotation, particularly of the psychiatric residents, are periods associated with inpatient suicides. Epidemics of inpatient suicides tend to be associated with periods of ideological change on the ward, staff disorganization, and staff demoralization.

The period after discharge from the hospital is a time of increased suicide risk. A follow-up study of 5,000 patients discharged from an Iowa psychiatric hospital showed that in the first 3 months after discharge, the rate of suicide for female patients was 275 times that of all Iowa women; the rate of suicide for male patients was 70 times that of all Iowa men. Studies show that one third or more of depressed patients who commit suicide do so within 6 months of leaving a hospital; presumably they have relapsed.

The main risk groups are patients with depressive disorders, schizophrenia, and substance abuse and patients who make repeated visits to the emergency room. Patients, especially those with panic disorder, who frequent emergency services also have an increased suicide risk. Thus, mental health professionals working in emergency services must be well trained in assessing suicidal risk and making appropriate dispositions. They must also be aware of the need to contact patients at risk who fail to keep follow-up appointments.

DEPRESSIVE DISORDERS.   Mood disorders are the diagnoses most commonly associated with suicide. The psychopharmacological advances of the past 25 years may have reduced the suicide risk among patients with depressive disorder. Nevertheless, the age-adjusted suicide rates for patients with mood disorders have been estimated to be 400 per 100,000 for male patients and 180 per 100,000 for female patients.

More patients with depressive disorders commit suicide early in the illness than later; more depressed men than women commit suicide; and the chance of depressed persons' killing themselves increases if they are single, separated, divorced, widowed, or recently bereaved. Patients with depressive disorder in the community who commit suicide tend to be middle-aged or older.

Social isolation enhances suicidal tendencies among depressed patients. This finding is in accord with the data from epidemiological studies showing that persons who commit suicide may be poorly integrated into society. Suicide among depressed patients is likely at the onset or the end of a depressive episode. As with other psychiatric patients, the months after discharge from a hospital are a time of high risk.

Regarding outpatient treatment, most depressed suicidal patients had a history of therapy; however, less than half were receiving psychiatric treatment at the time of suicide. Of those who were in treatment, studies have shown that treatment was less than adequate. For example, most patients who received antidepressants were prescribed subtherapeutic doses of the medication.

SCHIZOPHRENIA.   The suicide risk is high among patients with schizophrenia: Up to 10 percent die by committing suicide. In the United States, an estimated 4,000 patients with schizophrenia commit suicide each year. The onset of schizophrenia is typically in adolescence or early adulthood, and most of these patients who commit suicide do so during the first few years of their illness; therefore, those patients with schizophrenia who commit suicide are young.

Thus, the risk factors for suicide among patients with schizophrenia are young age, male gender, single marital status, a previous suicide attempt, a vulnerability to depressive symptoms, and a recent discharge from a hospital. Having three or four hospitalizations during their 20s probably undermines the social, occupational, and sexual adjustment of possibly suicidal patients with schizophrenia. Consequently, potential suicide victims are likely to be male, unmarried, unemployed, socially isolated, and living alone—perhaps in a single room. After discharge from their last hospitalization, they may experience a new adversity or return to ongoing difficulties. As a result, they become dejected, experience feelings of helplessness and hopelessness, reach a depressed state, and have, and eventually act on, suicidal ideas. Only a small percentage committed suicide because of hallucinated instructions or a need to escape persecutory delusions. Up to 50 percent of suicides among patients with schizophrenia occur during the first few weeks and months after discharge from a hospital; only a minority commit suicide while inpatients.

ALCOHOL DEPENDENCE. Up to 15 percent of all alcohol-dependent persons commit suicide. The suicide rate for those who are alcoholic is estimated to be about 270 per 100,000 annually; in the United States, between 7,000 and 13,000 alcohol-dependent persons commit suicide each year.

About 80 percent of all alcohol-dependent suicide victims are male, a percentage that largely reflects the sex ratio for alcohol dependence. Alcohol-dependent suicide victims tend to be white, middle-aged, unmarried, friendless, socially isolated, and currently drinking. Up to 40 percent have made a previous suicide attempt. Up to 40 percent of all suicides by persons who are alcohol dependent occur within a year of the patient's last hospitalization; older alcohol-dependent patients are at particular risk during the postdischarge period.

Studies show that many alcohol-dependent patients who eventually commit suicide are rated depressed during hospitalization and that up to two thirds are assessed as having mood disorder symptoms during the period in which they commit suicide. As many as 50 percent of all alcohol-dependent suicide victims have experienced the loss of a close, affectionate relationship during the previous year. Such interpersonal losses and other types of undesirable life events are probably brought about by the alcohol dependence and contribute to the development of the mood disorder symptoms, which are often present in the weeks and months before the suicide.

The largest group of male alcohol-dependent patients is composed of those with an associated antisocial personality disorder. Studies show that such patients are particularly likely to attempt suicide; to abuse other substances; to exhibit impulsive, aggressive, and criminal behaviors; and to be found among alcohol-dependent suicide victims.

OTHER SUBSTANCE DEPENDENCE. Studies in various countries have found an increased suicide risk among those who abuse substances. The suicide rate for persons who are heroin dependent is about 20 times the rate for the general population. Adolescent girls who use intravenous substances also have a high suicide rate. The availability of a lethal amount of substances, intravenous use, associated antisocial personality disorder, a chaotic lifestyle, and impulsivity are some of the factors that predispose substance-dependent persons to suicidal behavior, particularly when they are dysphoric, depressed, or intoxicated.

PERSONALITY DISORDERS. A high proportion of those who commit suicide have various associated personality difficulties or disorders. Having a personality disorder may be a determinant of suicidal behavior in several ways: by predisposing to major mental disorders such as depressive disorders or alcohol dependence; by leading to difficulties

in relationships and social adjustment; by precipitating undesirable life events; by impairing the ability to cope with a mental or physical disorder; and by drawing persons into conflicts with those around them, including family members, physicians, and hospital staff members.

An estimated 5 percent of patients with antisocial personality disorder commit suicide. Suicide is three times more common among prisoners than among the general population. More than one third of prisoner suicides have had past psychiatric treatment, and half have made a previous suicide threat or attempt, often in the previous 6 months.

ANXIETY DISORDER. Uncompleted suicide attempts are made by almost 20 percent of patients with a panic disorder and social phobia. If depression is an associated feature, however, the risk of completed suicide rises.

Previous Suicidal Behavior.

A past suicide attempt is perhaps the best indicator that a patient is at increased risk of suicide. Studies show that about 40 percent of depressed patients who commit suicide have made a previous attempt. The risk of a second suicide attempt is highest within 3 months of the first attempt.

Depression is associated with both completed suicide and serious attempts at suicide. The clinical feature most often associated with the seriousness of the intent to die is a diagnosis of a depressive disorder. This is shown by studies that relate the clinical characteristics of suicidal patients with various measures of the medical seriousness of the attempt or of the intent to die. In addition, intent-to-die scores correlate significantly with both suicide risk scores and the number and severity of depressive symptoms. Patients having high suicide intent are more often male, older, single or separated, and living alone than those with low intent. In other words, depressed patients who seriously attempt suicide more closely resemble suicide victims than they do suicide attempters.

ETIOLOGY

Sociological Factors

Durkheim's Theory.

The first major contribution to the study of the social and cultural influences on suicide was made at the end of the 19th century by the French sociologist Emile Durkheim. In an attempt to explain statistical patterns, Durkheim divided suicides into three social categories: egoistic, altruistic, and anomic. Egoistic suicide applies to those who are not strongly integrated into any social group. The lack of family integration explains why unmarried persons are more vulnerable to suicide than married ones and why couples with children are the best-protected group. Rural communities have more social integration than urban areas and, thus, fewer suicides. Protestantism is a less cohesive religion than Roman Catholicism, and so Protestants have a higher suicide rate than Catholics.

Altruistic suicide applies to those susceptible to suicide stemming from their excessive integration into a group, with suicide being the outgrowth of the integration—for example, a Japanese soldier who sacrificed his life in battle during World War II. Anomic suicide applies to persons whose integration into society is disturbed so that they cannot follow customary norms of behavior. Anomie explains why a drastic change in economic situation makes persons more vulnerable than they were before their change in fortune. In Durkheim's theory, anomie also refers to social instability and a general breakdown of society's standards and values.

Psychological Factors

Freud's Theory.
Sigmund Freud offered the first important psychological insight into suicide. He described only one patient who made a suicide attempt, but he saw many depressed patients. In his paper "Mourning and Melancholia," Freud stated his belief that suicide represents aggression turned inward against an introjected, ambivalently cathected love object. Freud doubted that there would be a suicide without an earlier repressed desire to kill someone else.

Menninger's Theory.
Building on Freud's ideas, Karl Menninger, in *Man against Himself*, conceived of suicide as inverted homicide because of a patient's anger toward another person. This retroflexed murder is either turned inward or used as an excuse for punishment. He also described a self-directed death instinct (Freud's concept of Thanatos) plus three components of hostility in suicide: the wish to kill, the wish to be killed, and the wish to die.

Recent Theories.
Contemporary suicidologists are not persuaded that a specific psychodynamic or personality structure is associated with suicide. They believe that much can be learned about the psychodynamics of suicidal patients from their fantasies about what would happen and what the consequences would be if they commit suicide. Such fantasies often include wishes for revenge, power, control, or punishment; atonement, sacrifice, or restitution; escape or sleep; rescue, rebirth, reunion with the dead; or a new life. The suicidal patients most likely to act out suicidal fantasies may have lost a love object or received a narcissistic injury, may experience overwhelming affects like rage and guilt, or may identify with a suicide victim. Group dynamics underlie mass suicides such as those at Masada, at Jonestown, and by the Heaven's Gate cult.

Depressed persons may attempt suicide just as they appear to be recovering from their depression. A suicide attempt can cause a long-standing depression to disappear, especially if it fulfills a patient's need for punishment. Of equal relevance, many suicidal patients use a preoccupation with suicide as a way of fighting off intolerable depression and a sense of hopelessness. A study by Aaron Beck showed that hopelessness was one of the most accurate indicators of long-term suicidal risk.

Biological Factors.
Diminished central serotonin plays a role in suicidal behavior. A group at the Karolinska Institute in Sweden first noted that low concentrations of the serotonin metabolite 5-hydroxyindoleacetic acid (5-HIAA) in the lumbar cerebrospinal fluid (CSF) were associated with suicidal behavior. This finding has been replicated many times and in different diagnostic groups. Postmortem neurochemical studies have reported modest decreases in serotonin itself or 5-HIAA in either the brainstem or the frontal cortex of suicide victims. Postmortem receptor studies have reported significant changes in presynaptic and postsynaptic serotonin-binding sites in suicide victims. Together, these CSF, neurochemical, and receptor studies support the hypothesis that reduced central serotonin is associated with suicide. Recent studies also report some changes in the noradrenergic system of suicide victims.

Genetic Factors.
Suicidal behavior, as with other psychiatric disorders, tends to run in families. For example, Margaux Hemingway's 1997 suicide was the fifth suicide among four generations of Ernest Hemingway's family. In psychiatric patients, a family history of suicide increases the risk of attempted suicide and that of completed suicide in most diagnostic groups. In medicine, the strongest evidence for involvement of genetic factors comes from twin and adoption studies and from molecular genetics. Such studies of suicide are reviewed next.

TWIN STUDIES. A landmark study in 1991 investigated 176 twin pairs in which one twin had committed suicide. In 9 of these twin pairs, both twins had committed suicide. Seven of these 9 pairs concordant for suicide were found among the 62 monozygotic pairs, whereas two pairs concordant for suicide were found among the 114 dizygotic twin pairs. This twin group difference for concordance for suicide (11.3 vs. 1.8 percent) is statistically significant ($P < .01$).

Another study collected a group of 35 twin pairs in which one twin had committed suicide, and the living co-twin was interviewed. Ten of the 26 living monozygotic co-twins had themselves attempted suicide, compared with 0 of the 9 living dizygotic co-twins ($P < .04$). Although monozygotic and dizygotic twins may have some differing developmental experiences, these results show that monozygotic twin pairs have significantly higher concordance for both suicide and attempted suicide, which suggests that genetic factors may play a role in suicidal behavior.

MOLECULAR GENETIC STUDIES. Tryptophan hydroxylase (TPH) is an enzyme involved in the biosynthesis of serotonin. A polymorphism in the human TPH gene has been identified, with two alleles—U and L. Because low concentrations of 5-HIAA in CSF are associated with suicidal behavior, it was hypothesized that such individuals may have alterations in genes controlling serotonin synthesis and metabolism. It was found that impulsive alcoholics, who had low CSF 5-HIAA concentrations, had more LL and UL genotypes. Furthermore, a history of suicide attempts was significantly associated with TPH genotype in all of the violent alcoholics; 34 of the 36 violent subjects who attempted suicide had either the UL or LL genotype. Thus, it was concluded that the presence of the L allele was associated with an increased risk of suicide attempts.

Furthermore, a history of multiple suicide attempts was found most often in subjects with the LL genotype and to a lesser extent among those with the UL genotype. This led to the suggestion that the L allele was associated with repetitive suicidal behavior. The presence of one TPH*L allele may indicate a reduced capacity to hydroxylate tryptophan to 5-hydroxytryptophan in the synthesis of serotonin, producing low central serotonin turnover and, thus, a low concentration of 5-HIAA in CSF.

Parasuicidal Behavior
Parasuicide is a term introduced to describe patients who injure themselves by self-mutilation (e.g., cutting the skin) but usually do not wish to die. Studies show that about 4 percent of all patients in psychiatric hospitals have cut themselves; the female-to-male ratio is almost 3:1. The incidence of self-injury in psychiatric patients is estimated to be more than 50 times that in the general population. Psychiatrists note that so-called cutters have cut themselves over several years. Self-injury is found in about 30 percent of all abusers of oral substances and 10 percent of all intravenous users admitted to substance-treatment units.

These patients are usually in their 20s and may be single or married. Most cut delicately, not coarsely, usually in private with a razor blade, knife, broken glass, or mirror. The wrists, arms, thighs, and legs are most commonly cut; the face, breasts, and abdomen are cut infrequently. Most persons who cut themselves claim to experience no pain and give reasons, such as anger at themselves or others, relief of tension, and the wish to die. Most are classified as having personality disorders and are significantly more introverted, neurotic, and hostile than controls. Alcohol abuse and other substance abuse are common, and most cutters have attempted suicide. Self-mutilation has been viewed as localized self-destruction, with mishandling of aggressive impulses caused by a person's unconscious wish to punish himself or herself or an introjected object.

PREDICTION

Clinicians must assess an individual patient's risk for suicide on the basis of a clinical examination. Suicide is grouped into high-risk-related and low-risk-related factors (Table 30.1–1). High-risk characteristics include age greater than 45 years, male gender, alcohol dependence (the suicide rate is 50 times higher in alcohol-dependent persons than in those who are not alcohol dependent), violent behavior, previous suicidal behavior, and previous psychiatric hospitalization.

It is important that questions about suicidal feelings and behaviors be asked, often directly. Asking depressed patients whether they have had thoughts of wanting to kill themselves does not plant the seed of suicide. To the contrary, it may be the first opportunity a patient has had to talk about suicidal ideation that may have been present for some time.

TREATMENT

Most suicides among psychiatric patients are preventable because evidence indicates that inadequate assessment or treatment is often associated with suicide. Some patients experience suffering so great and intense, or so chronic and unresponsive to treatment, that their eventual suicides may be perceived as inevitable. Such patients are relatively uncommon, however. Other patients have severe personality disorders, are highly impulsive, and commit suicide spontaneously, often when dysphoric or intoxicated or both.

The evaluation for suicide potential involves a complete psychiatric history; a thorough examination of the patient's mental state; and an inquiry about depressive symptoms, suicidal thoughts, intents, plans, and attempts. A lack of future plans, giving away personal property, making a will, and having recently experienced a loss all imply increased risk of suicide. The decision to hospitalize a patient depends on diagnosis, depression severity and suicidal ideation, the patient's and the family's coping abilities, the patient's living situation, availability of social support, and the absence or presence of risk factors for suicide.

Inpatient versus Outpatient Treatment

Whether to hospitalize patients with suicidal ideation is the most important clinical decision to be made. Not all such patients require hospitalization; some can be treated on an outpatient basis. However, the absence of a strong social support system, a history

Table 30.1–1
Evaluation of Suicide Risk

Variable	High Risk	Low Risk
Demographic and social profile		
Age	Older than 45 years	Younger than 45 years
Sex	Male	Female
Marital status	Divorced or widowed	Married
Employment	Unemployed	Employed
Interpersonal relationship	Conflictual	Stable
Family background	Chaotic or conflictual	Stable
Health		
Physical	Chronic illness	Good health
	Hypochondriac	Feels healthy
	Excessive substance intake	Low substance use
Mental	Severe depression	Mild depression
	Psychosis	Neurosis
	Severe personality disorder	Normal personality
	Substance abuse	Social drinker
	Hopelessness	Optimism
Suicidal activity		
Suicidal ideation	Frequent, intense, prolonged	Infrequent, low intensity, transient
Suicide attempt	Multiple attempts	First attempt
	Planned	Impulsive
	Rescue unlikely	Rescue inevitable
	Unambiguous wish to die	Primary wish for change
	Communication internalized (self-blame)	Communication externalized (anger)
	Method lethal and available	Method of low lethality or not readily available
Resources		
Personal	Poor achievement	Good achievement
	Poor insight	Insightful
	Affect unavailable or poorly controlled	Affect available and appropriately controlled
Social	Poor rapport	Good rapport
	Socially isolated	Socially integrated
	Unresponsive family	Concerned family

From Adam K. Attempted suicide. *Psychiatr Clin North Am.* 1985;8:183, with permission.

of impulsive behavior, and a suicidal plan of action are indications for hospitalization. To decide whether outpatient treatment is feasible, clinicians should use a straightforward clinical approach: Ask patients who are considered suicidal to agree to call when they become uncertain about their ability to control their suicidal impulses. Patients who can make such an agreement with a doctor with whom they have a relationship reaffirm the belief that they have sufficient strength to control such impulses and to seek help.

In return for a patient's commitment, clinicians should be available to the patient 24 hours a day. If a patient who is considered seriously suicidal cannot make the commitment, immediate emergency hospitalization is indicated; both the patient and the patient's family should be so advised. If, however, the patient is to be treated on an outpatient basis, the therapist should note the patient's home and work telephone numbers for emergency reference; occasionally, a patient hangs up unexpectedly during a late-night call or gives only a name to the answering service. If the patient refuses hospitalization, the family must take the responsibility to be with the patient 24 hours a day.

According to E. S. Shneidman, a clinician has several practical preventive measures for dealing with a suicidal person: reducing the psychological pain by modifying the patient's stressful environment, enlisting the aid of the spouse, the employer, or a friend; building realistic support by recognizing that the patient may have a legitimate complaint; and offering alternatives to suicide.

Many psychiatrists believe that any patient who has attempted suicide, despite its lethality, should be hospitalized. Although most of these patients voluntarily enter a hospital, the danger to self is one of the few clear-cut indications currently acceptable in all states for involuntary hospitalization. In a hospital, patients can receive antidepressant or antipsychotic medications as indicated; individual therapy, group therapy, and family therapy are available, and patients receive the hospital's social support and sense of security. Other therapeutic measures depend on patients' underlying diagnoses. For example, if alcohol dependence is an associated problem, treatment must be directed toward alleviating that condition.

Although patients classified as acutely suicidal may have favorable prognoses, chronically suicidal patients are difficult to treat, and they exhaust the caretakers. Constant observation by special nurses, seclusion, and restraints cannot prevent suicide when a patient is resolute. ECT may be necessary for some severely depressed patients, who may require several treatment courses.

Useful measures for the treatment of depressed suicidal inpatients include searching patients and their belongings on arrival in the ward for objects that could be used for suicide and repeating the search at times of exacerbation of the suicidal ideation. Ideally, suicidally depressed inpatients should be treated on a locked ward where the windows are shatterproof, and the patient's room should be located near the nursing station to maximize observation by the nursing staff. The treatment team must assess how much to restrict the patient and whether to make regular checks or use continuous direct observation.

Vigorous treatment with antidepressant or antipsychotic medication should be initiated, depending on the underlying disorder. Some medications (e.g., risperidone [Risperdal]) have both antipsychotic and antidepressant effects and are useful when the patient has signs and symptoms of both psychosis and depression.

Supportive psychotherapy by a psychiatrist shows concern and may alleviate some of a patient's intense suffering. Some patients may be able to accept the idea that they are suffering from a recognized illness and that they will probably make a complete recovery. Patients should be dissuaded from making major life decisions while they are suicidally depressed because such decisions are often morbidly determined and may be irrevocable. The consequences of such bad decisions can cause further anguish and misery when the patient has recovered.

Patients recovering from a suicidal depression are at particular risk. As the depression lifts, patients become energized and, thus, are able to put their suicidal plans into action (paradoxical suicide). A further complication is the activating effect of serotonergic drugs, such as fluoxetine, which are effective antidepressants, especially with suicidally depressed patients. Such agents may improve psychomotor withdrawal, thus permitting the patient to act on preexisting suicidal impulses because they have more energy. Sometimes, depressed patients, with or without treatment, suddenly appear to be at peace with themselves because they have reached a secret decision to commit suicide. Clinicians should be especially suspicious of such a dramatic clinical change, which may portend a suicide attempt. Although rare, some patients lie to the psychiatrist about their suicidal intent, thus subverting the most careful clinical assessment.

A patient may commit suicide even when in the hospital. According to one survey, about 1 percent of all suicides were committed by patients who were being treated in general medical-surgical or psychiatric hospitals, but the annual suicide rate in psychiatric hospitals is only 0.003 percent.

Legal and Ethical Factors

Liability issues stemming from suicides in psychiatric hospitals frequently involve questions about a patient's rate of deterioration, the presence during hospitalization of clinical signs indicating risk, and psychiatrists' and staff members' awareness of, and response to, these clinical signs.

In about half of cases in which suicides occur while patients are on a psychiatric unit, a lawsuit results. Courts do not require zero suicide rates but do require periodic patient evaluation for suicidal risk, formulation of a treatment plan with a high level of security, and having staff members follow the treatment plan.

Currently, suicide and attempted suicide are variously viewed as a felony and a misdemeanor, respectively; in some states, the acts are considered not crimes but unlawful under common law and statutes. Aiding and abetting a suicide adds another dimension to the legal morass; some court decisions have held that, although neither suicide nor attempted suicide is punishable, anyone who assists in the act may be punished. (Doctor-assisted suicide is discussed in Section 51.2, Euthanasia and Physician-Assisted Suicide.)

National Strategy for Suicide Prevention

In 2001, Surgeon General David Satcher organized the National Strategy for Suicide Prevention, under the auspices of the National Institutes of Health.

The National Strategy for Suicide Prevention creates a framework for suicide prevention for the nation. It is designed to encourage and empower groups and individuals to work together.

The stronger and broader the support and collaboration on suicide prevention, the greater is the chance of success for this public health initiative. Suicide and suicidal behaviors can be reduced as the general public gains more understanding about (1) the extent to which suicide is a problem, (2) the ways in which it can be prevented, and (3) the roles individuals and groups can play in prevention efforts.

SURVIVING SUICIDE

The term *suicide survivor* refers to those who have lost a loved one to suicide, not to someone who has attempted suicide but lived. The toll on suicide survivors appears to be greater than that by other deaths, mainly because the opportunities for guilt are so great. Survivors feel that the loved one intentionally and willfully took his or her life and that if only the survivor had done something differently, the decedent would still be here. Because the decedent cannot tell them otherwise, survivors are at the mercy of their often merciless consciences. What is generally more accurate is that the decedents were not entirely willful but were victims of their genetic or lifetime-experience predispositions to depression and suicide. For children, in particular, the loss of a parent to suicide feels like a shameful abandonment for which the child may blame himself or herself. For parents of children who have killed themselves, their grief is compounded not only by having lost a part of themselves, but also by having failed in what they perceive as their responsibility for the total feelings of their child. To provide mutual support, survivors of suicide groups have appeared throughout the United States, generally led by nonprofessional survivors. Therapists who have lost patients to suicide comprise another survivor group—one too often ignored and unsupported, despite their own considerable suffering and sense of guilt, which is compounded by the specter of litigation potentially being brought to bear.

▲ 30.2 Other Psychiatric Emergencies

A psychiatric emergency is any disturbance in thoughts, feelings, or actions for which immediate therapeutic intervention is necessary. For a variety of reasons—such as the growing incidence of violence, the increased appreciation of the role of medical disease in altered mental status, and the epidemic of alcoholism and other substance use disorders—the number of emergency patients is on the rise. The widening scope of emergency psychiatry goes beyond general psychiatric practice to include such specialized problems as the abuse of substances, children, and spouses; violence in the form of suicide, homicide, and rape; and such social issues as homelessness, aging, competence, and acquired immune deficiency syndrome (AIDS). This subsection provides an overview of psychiatric emergencies in general and in adults in particular. The next subsection covers psychiatric emergencies in children.

PSYCHIATRIC EMERGENCIES IN GENERAL AND IN ADULTS

Epidemiology

Psychiatric emergency rooms are used equally by men and women and more by single than by married persons. About 20 percent of these patients are suicidal, and about 10 percent are violent. The most common diagnoses are mood disorders (including depressive disorders and manic episodes), schizophrenia, and alcohol dependence. About 40 percent of all patients seen in psychiatric emergency rooms require hospitalization. Most visits occur during the night hours, but usage difference is not based on the day of the week or the month of the year. Contrary to popular belief, studies have not found that use of psychiatric emergency rooms increases during the full moon or the Christmas season.

Evaluation

The standard psychiatric interview—consisting of a history, a mental status examination, and, when appropriate and depending on the rules of the emergency room, a full physical examination and ancillary tests—is the cornerstone of the emergency room evaluation. The emergency room psychiatrist, however, must be ready to introduce modifications as needed. For example, the emergency psychiatrist may have to structure the interview with a rambling manic patient, medicate or restrain an agitated patient, or forgo the usual rules of confidentiality to assess an adolescent's risk of suicide. In general, any strategy introduced in the emergency room to accomplish the goal of assessing the patient is considered consistent with good clinical practice as long as the rationale for the strategy is documented in the medical record.

What constitutes a psychiatric emergency is highly subjective. The emergency room has increasingly come to serve as an admitting area, a holding room, a detoxification center, and a private office. Such medical conditions as head traumas, acute intoxications, withdrawal states, and AIDS encephalopathies may present with acute psychiatric manifestations. The emergency psychiatrists must rapidly assess and distinguish the truly emergency psychiatric patients from those who are less acutely ill and from nonpsychiatric emergencies. A triage system using psychiatrists, nurses, and psychiatric social workers is an efficient and effective way to identify emergency, urgent, and nonurgent patients, who can then be prioritized for care.

Patient Safety   Physicians should consider the question of the patient's safety before evaluating every patient. The answer must address the issues of the emergency room's physical layout, staffing patterns and communication, and patient population. Psychiatrists must then take stock of themselves: Are they in the proper frame of mind to conduct an evaluation? Do any issues in the case spark countertransference reactions? The self-assessment should go on throughout the evaluation. The physical and emotional safety of the patient takes priority over all other considerations. If verbal interventions fail or are contraindicated, the use of medication or restraints must be considered and, if necessary, ordered. Careful attention to the possible outbreak of agitation or disruptive behavior beyond acceptable limits is often the best insurance against untoward occurrences.

Medical or Psychiatric?   The most important question for the emergency psychiatrist to address is whether the problem is medical or psychiatric or both. Medical conditions—such as diabetes mellitus, thyroid disease, acute intoxications, withdrawal states, AIDS, and head traumas—can present with prominent mental status changes that mimic common psychiatric illnesses. Such conditions may be life threatening if not treated promptly.

Generally, the treatment of a medical illness is more definitive and the prognosis is better than for a functional psychiatric disorder. The psychiatrist must consider all causal possibilities.

Treatment of Emergencies

Psychotherapy.   In an emergency psychiatric intervention, all attempts are made to help patients' self-esteem. Empathy is critical to healing in a psychiatric emergency. The acquired knowledge of how biogenetic, situational, developmental, and existential forces converge at one point in history to create a psychiatric emergency is tantamount to the maturation of skill in emergency psychiatry. Adjustment disorder in all age groups may result in tantrum-like outbursts of rage. These outbursts are particularly common in marital quarrels, and police are often summoned by neighbors distressed by the sounds of a violent altercation. Such family quarrels should be approached with caution because they may be complicated by alcohol use and the presence of dangerous weapons. The warring couple frequently turn their combined fury on an unwary outsider. Wounded self-esteem is a major issue, and clinicians must avoid patronizing or contemptuous attitudes and try to communicate an attitude of respect and an authentic peacemaking concern.

Pharmacotherapy.   The major indications for the use of psychotropic medication in an emergency room include violent or assaultive behavior, massive anxiety or panic, and extrapyramidal reactions, such as dystonia and akathisia as adverse effects of psychiatric drugs. Laryngospasm is a rare form of dystonia, and psychiatrists should be prepared to maintain an open airway with intubation if necessary.

Persons who are paranoid or in a state of catatonic excitement require tranquilization. Episodic outbursts of violence respond to haloperidol (Haldol), β-adrenergic receptor antagonists (β-blockers), carbamazepine (Tegretol), and lithium. If a history suggests a seizure disorder, use clinical studies to confirm the diagnosis and an evaluation to ascertain the cause. If the findings are positive, anticonvulsant therapy is initiated or appropriate surgery is provided (e.g., in the case of a cerebral mass). Conservative measures may suffice for intoxication from drugs of abuse. Sometimes, drugs such as haloperidol (5 to 10 mg every half-hour to an hour) are needed until a patient is stabilized.

Violent, struggling patients are subdued most effectively with an appropriate sedative or antipsychotic. Diazepam (Valium), 5 to 10 mg, or lorazepam (Ativan), 2 to 4 mg, may be given slowly intravenously (IV) over 2 minutes. Clinicians must give IV medication with great care to avoid respiratory arrest. Patients who require intramuscular (IM) medication can be sedated with haloperidol, 5 to 10 mg IM. If the furor is caused by alcohol or is part of a postseizure psychomotor disturbance, the sleep produced by a relatively small amount of an IV medication may go on for hours. On awakening, patients are often entirely alert and rational and typically have complete amnesia about the violent episode.

If the disturbance is part of an ongoing psychotic process and returns as soon as the IV medication wears off, continuous medication may be given. It is sometimes better to use small IM or oral doses at half-hour to 1-hour intervals (e.g., haloperidol, 2

to 5 mg, or diazepam, 20 mg) until the patient is controlled than to use large doses initially, which can result in an overmedicated patient. As the disturbed behavior is brought under control, successively smaller and less frequent doses should be used. During the preliminary treatment, a patient's blood pressure and other vital signs should be monitored.

Restraints.   Restraints are used when patients are so dangerous to themselves or others that they pose a severe threat that cannot be controlled in any other way. Patients may be restrained temporarily to receive medication or for long periods if medication cannot be used. Usually, patients in restraints quiet down after a time. On a psychodynamic level, such patients may even welcome the control of their impulses provided by restraints.

Documentation.   In the interests of good care, respect for patients' rights, cost control, and medicolegal concerns, documentation has become a central focus for the emergency physician. The medical record should convey a concise picture of the patient, highlighting all pertinent positive and negative findings. Gaps in information and their reason should be mentioned. The names and the telephone numbers of interested parties should be noted. A provisional diagnosis or differential diagnosis must be made. An initial treatment plan or recommendations should clearly follow from the findings of the patient's history, mental status examination and other diagnostic tests, and the medical evaluation. The writing must be legible. The emergency physician has unusual latitude under the law to perform an adequate initial assessment; however, all interventions and decisions must be thought out, discussed, and documented in the patient's record.

PSYCHIATRIC EMERGENCIES IN CHILDREN

Few children or adolescents seek psychiatric intervention on their own, even during crisis; thus, most of their emergency evaluations are initiated by parents, relatives, teachers, therapists, physicians, and child protective service workers. Some referrals are for the evaluation of life-threatening situations for the child or for others, such as suicidal behavior, physical abuse, and violent or homicidal behavior. Other urgent but non–life-threatening referrals pertain to children and adolescents with exacerbations of clear-cut serious psychiatric disorders, such as mania, depression, florid psychosis, and school refusal. Less diagnostically obvious situations occur when a child or adolescent presents with a history of a wide range of disruptive, aberrant behaviors and is accompanied by an overwhelmed, anxious, and distraught adult who perceives the child's actions as an emergency, despite the absence of life-threatening behavior or an obvious psychiatric disorder. In those cases, the spectrum of contributing factors is not immediately clear, and the emergency psychiatrist must assess the entire family or system involved with the child. Familial stressors and parental discord can contribute to the evolution of a crisis for a child. For example, immediate evaluations are sometimes legitimately indicated for a child caught in the crossfire of feuding parents or in a seemingly irreconcilable conflict between a set of parents and a school, therapist, or protective service worker regarding the needs of the child (Table 30.2–1).

Table 30.2–1
Familial Risk Factors

Physical and sexual abuse
Recent family crisis: loss of a parent, divorce, loss of job,
    family move
Severe family dysfunction, including parental mental illness

An emergency setting is often the site of an initial evaluation of a chronic problem behavior. For example, an identified problem—such as severe tantrums, violence, and destructive behavior in a child—may have been present for months or even years. Yet, the initial contact with the mental health system in the emergency room or private office may be the first opportunity for the child or adolescent to disclose underlying stressors, such as physical or sexual abuse.

In view of the integral relation of severe family dysfunction to childhood behavioral disturbance, the emergency psychiatrist must assess familial discord and psychiatric disorder in family members during an urgent evaluation. One way to make the assessment is to interview the child and the individual family members, both alone and together, and to obtain a history from informants outside the family whenever possible. Noncustodial parents, therapists, and teachers may add valuable information regarding the child's daily functioning. Many families, especially those with mental illness and severe dysfunction, may have little or no inclination to seek psychiatric help on a nonurgent basis; therefore, the emergency evaluation becomes the only way to engage them in an extensive psychiatric treatment program.

Life-Threatening Emergencies

Suicidal Behavior

ASSESSMENT. Suicidal behavior is the most common reason for an emergency evaluation in adolescents. Despite the minimal risk for a completed suicide in a child less than 12 years of age, suicidal ideation or behavior in a child of any age must be carefully evaluated, with particular attention to the psychiatric status of the child and the ability of the family or the guardians to provide the appropriate supervision. The assessment must determine the circumstances of the suicidal ideation or behavior, its lethality, and the persistence of the suicidal intention. An evaluation of the family's sensitivity, supportiveness, and competence must be done to assess their ability to monitor the child's suicidal potential. Ultimately, during the course of an emergency evaluation, the psychiatrist must decide whether the child may return home to a safe environment and receive outpatient follow-up care or whether hospitalization is necessary. A psychiatric history, a mental status examination, and an assessment of family functioning help establish the general level of risk.

MANAGEMENT. When self-injurious behavior has occurred, the adolescent likely requires hospitalization on a pediatric unit for treatment of the injury or for the observation of medical sequelae after a toxic ingestion. If the adolescent is medically clear, the psychiatrist must decide whether the adolescent needs psychiatric admission. If the patient persists in suicidal ideation and shows signs of psychosis, severe depression (including hopelessness), or marked ambivalence about suicide, psychiatric admission is indicated. An adolescent who is taking drugs or alcohol should not be released until an assessment can be done when the patient is in a nonintoxicated state. Patients with high-risk profiles—such as late-adolescent males, especially those with substance abuse and aggressive behavior disorders, and those who have severe depression or who have made prior suicide attempts, particularly with lethal weapons—warrant hospitalization. Young children who have made suicide attempts, even when the attempt had a low lethality, need psychiatric admission if the family is so chaotic, dysfunctional, and incompetent that follow-up treatment is unlikely. (For further discussion of suicide in children see Chapter 45, Mood Disorders and Suicide in Children and Adolescents.)

Violent Behavior and Tantrums

ASSESSMENT. The first task in an emergency evaluation of a violent child or adolescent is to make sure that both the child and the staff members are physically protected so that nobody gets hurt. If the child appears to be calming down in the emergency area, the clinician may indicate to the child that it would be helpful if the child recounted what happened and may ask whether the child feels in sufficient control to do so. If the child agrees and the clinician judges the child to be in good control, the clinician may approach the child with the appropriate backup close at hand. If not, the clinician may either give the child several minutes to calm down before reassessing the situation or, with an adolescent, suggest that a medication may help the adolescent relax.

If the adolescent is clearly combative, physical restraint may be necessary before anything else is attempted. Some rageful children and adolescents brought to an emergency setting by overwhelmed families are able to regain control of themselves without the use of physical or pharmacological restraint. Children and adolescents are most likely to calm down if approached calmly in a nonthreatening manner and given a chance to tell their side of the story to a nonjudgmental adult. At this time, the psychiatrist should look for any underlying psychiatric disorder that may be mediating the aggression. The psychiatrist should speak to family members and others who have been witnessing the episode to understand the context in which it occurred and the extent to which the child has been out of control.

MANAGEMENT. Prepubertal children, in the absence of major psychiatric illness, rarely require medication to keep them safe because they are generally small enough to be physically restrained if they begin to hurt themselves or others. It is not immediately necessary to administer medication to a child or an adolescent who was in a rage but is in a calm state when examined. Adolescents and older children who are assaultive, extremely agitated, or overtly self-injurious and who may be difficult to subdue physically may require medication before a dialogue can take place.

Children who have a history of repeated, self-limited, severe tantrums may not require admission to a hospital if they are able to calm down during the course of the evaluation. Yet the pattern, no doubt, will reoccur unless ongoing outpatient treatment for the child and the family is arranged. For adolescents who continue to pose a danger to themselves or others during the evaluation period, admission to a hospital is necessary.

Fire Setting

ASSESSMENT. A sense of emergency and panic often surrounds the parents of a child who has set a fire. Parents or teachers often request an emergency evaluation, even for a very young child who has accidentally lit a fire. Many children, during the course of normal development, become interested in fire, but in most cases, a school-age child who has set a fire has done so accidentally while playing with matches and seeks help to put it out. When a child has a strong interest in playing with matches, the level of supervision by family members must be clarified, so that no further accidental fires occur. The clinician must distinguish between a child who accidentally or even impulsively sets a single fire and a child who engages in repeated fire setting with premeditation and subsequently leaves the fire without making any attempt to extinguish it. In repeated fire setting, the risk is obviously greater than in a single occurrence, and the psychiatrist must determine whether underlying psychopathology exists in the child or in the family members. The psychiatrist should also evaluate family interactions because any factors that interfere with effective supervision and communication—such as high levels of marital discord and harsh, punitive parenting styles—can impede appropriate intervention.

Fire setting is one of a triad of symptoms—enuresis, cruelty to animals, and fire setting—that were believed, some years ago, to be typical of children with conduct disorders; however, no evidence indicates that the three symptoms are truly linked, although conduct disorder is the most frequent psychiatric disorder that occurs with pathological fire setting.

MANAGEMENT.   The critical component of management and treatment for fire setters is to prevent further incidents while treating any underlying psychopathology. In general, fire setting alone is not an indication for hospitalization, unless a continued direct threat exists that the patient will set another fire. The parents of children with a pattern of fire setting must be emphatically counseled that the child must not be left alone at home and should never be left to take care of younger siblings without direct adult supervision. Children who exhibit a pattern of concurrent aggressive behaviors and other forms of destructive behavior are likely to have a poor outcome. Outpatient treatment should be arranged for children who repeatedly set fires. Behavioral techniques that involve both the child and the family are helpful in decreasing the risk for further fire setting, as is positive reinforcement for alternate behaviors.

Child Abuse: Physical and Sexual

ASSESSMENT.   Physical and sexual abuse occurs in girls and boys of all ages, in all ethnic groups, and at all socioeconomic levels. The abuses vary widely with respect to severity and duration, but any form of continued abuse constitutes an emergency situation for a child. No single psychiatric syndrome is a sine qua non of physical or sexual abuse, but fear, guilt, anxiety, depression, and ambivalence regarding disclosure commonly surrounds the child who has been abused.

Young children who are being sexually abused may exhibit precocious sexual behavior with peers and present a detailed sexual knowledge that reflects exposure beyond their developmental level. Children who endure sexual or physical abuse often display sadistic and aggressive behaviors. Children who are abused in any manner are likely to have been threatened with severe and frightening consequences by the perpetrator if they reveal the situation to anyone. Frequently, an abused child who is victimized by a family member is placed in the irreconcilable position of having either to endure continued abuse silently or to defy the abuser by disclosing the experiences and be responsible for destroying the family and risk being disbelieved or abandoned by the family.

In cases of suspected abuse, the child and other family members must be interviewed individually to give each member a chance to speak privately. If possible, the clinician should observe the child with each parent individually to get a sense of the spontaneity, warmth, fear, anxiety, or other prominent features of the relationships. One observation is generally not sufficient to make a final judgment about the family relationship, however; abused children almost always have mixed emotions toward abusive parents.

Physical indicators of sexual abuse in children include sexually transmitted diseases (e.g., gonorrhea); pain, irritation, and itching of the genitalia and the urinary tract; and discomfort while sitting and walking. In many instances of suspected sexual abuse, however, physical evidence is not present. Thus, a careful history is essential. The physician should speak directly about the issues without leading the child in any direction, because already frightened children may be easily influenced to endorse what they think the examiner wants to hear. Furthermore, children who have been abused often retract all or part of what has been disclosed during the course of an interview.

The use of anatomically correct dolls in the assessment of sexual abuse can help the child identify body parts and show what has happened, but no conclusive evidence supports sexual play with dolls as a means of validating abuse. (For a full discussion of child abuse see Chapter 28, Problems Related to Abuse or Neglect.)

Neglect: Failure to Thrive

ASSESSMENT.   In child neglect, a child's physical, mental, or emotional condition has been impaired because of the inability of a parent or caretaker to provide adequate food, shelter, education, or supervision. Similar to abuse, any form of continued neglect is an emergency situation for the child. Parents who neglect their children range widely and may include parents who are very young and ignorant about the emotional and concrete needs of a child, parents with depression and significant passivity, substance-abusing parents, and parents with a variety of incapacitating mental illnesses.

In its extreme form, neglect can contribute to failure to thrive—that is, an infant, usually under 1 year of age, becomes malnourished in the absence of an organic cause. Failure to thrive typically occurs under circumstances in which adequate nourishment is available yet a disturbance within the relationship between the caretaker and the child results in a child who does not eat sufficiently to grow and develop. A negative pattern may exist between the mother and the child in which the child refuses feedings and the mother feels rejected and eventually withdraws. She may then avoid offering food as frequently as the infant needs it. Observation of the mother and the child together may reveal a nonspontaneous, tense interaction, with withdrawal on both sides, resulting in a seeming apathy in the mother. Both the mother and the child may seem depressed.

A rare form of failure to thrive in children who are at least several years old and are not necessarily malnourished is the syndrome of psychosocial dwarfism. In that syndrome, marked growth retardation and delayed epiphyseal malnutrition accompany a disturbed relationship between the caretaker and the child, along with bizarre social and eating behaviors in the child. Those behaviors sometimes include eating from garbage cans, drinking toilet water, binging and vomiting, and diminished outward response to pain. Half of the children with the syndrome have decreased growth hormone. Once the children are removed from the troubled environment and placed in another setting, such as a psychiatric hospital with appropriate supervision and guidance regarding meals, the endocrine abnormalities normalize, and the children begin to grow at a more rapid rate.

MANAGEMENT.   In cases of child neglect, as with physical and sexual abuse, the most important decision to be made during the initial evaluation is whether the child is safe in the home environment. Whenever neglect is suspected, it must be reported to the local child protective service agency. In mild cases, the decision to refer the family for outpatient services, as opposed to hospitalizing the child, depends on the clinician's conviction that the family is cooperative and willing to be educated and to enter into treatment and that the child is not in danger. Before a neglected child is released from an emergency setting, a follow-up appointment must be made.

Education for the family must begin during the evaluation; the family must be told, in a nonthreatening manner, that failure to thrive can become life threatening, that the entire family needs to monitor the child's progress, and that they will receive some help in overcoming the many possible obstacles interfering with the child's emotional and physical well-being.

Anorexia Nervosa.   Anorexia nervosa occurs in females about ten times as often as in males. It is characterized by the refusal to maintain body weight, leading to a weight at least 15 percent below the expected, by a distorted body image, by a persistent fear of becoming fat, and, in females, by the absence of at least three menstrual cycles. The disorder usually begins after puberty, but it has occurred in children of 9 to 10 years of age, in whom the criterion is that expected weight gain does not occur

rather than a loss of 15 percent of body weight. The disorder reaches medical emergency proportions when the weight loss approaches 30 percent of body weight or when metabolic disturbances become severe. Hospitalization then becomes necessary to control the ongoing process of starvation, potential dehydration, and the medical complications of starvation, including electrolyte imbalances, cardiac arrhythmias, and hormonal changes. (For a further discussion of anorexia nervosa and other eating disorders see Chapter 19, Eating Disorders.)

Acquired Immune Deficiency Syndrome

ASSESSMENT. AIDS, which is caused by the human immunodeficiency virus (HIV), occurs in neonate through perinatal transmission from an infected mother, in children and adolescents secondary to sexual abuse by an infected person, and in adolescents through intravenous drug abuse with infected needles and through sexual activities with infected partners. Child and adolescent hemophiliac patients may contract AIDS through tainted blood transfusions.

Children and adolescents may present for emergency evaluations at the urging of a family member or a peer; in some cases, they take the initiative themselves when they are faced with anxiety or panic about high-risk behavior. Early screening of high-risk persons may lead to the treatment of asymptomatic infected patients with such drugs as azidothymidine and possibly other new medications that may slow the course of the disease. During the assessment of the risks for HIV infection, an educational process can be initiated with both the patient and the rest of the family so that an adolescent who is not infected but exhibits high-risk behavior can be counseled about that behavior and about safe-sex practices.

In children, the brain is often a primary site for HIV infection; encephalitis, decreased brain development, and such neuropsychiatric symptoms as impairment in memory, concentration, and attention span may be present before the diagnosis is made. The virus can be present in the cerebrospinal fluid before it shows up in the bloodstream. Changes in cognitive function, frontal lobe disinhibition, social withdrawal, slowed information processing, and apathy constitute some common symptoms of the AIDS dementia complex. Organic mood disorders, organic personality disorder, and frank psychosis can also occur in patients infected with HIV. (HIV infection is discussed in Chapter 8, Neuropsychiatric Aspects of HIV Infection and AIDS.)

Urgent Non–Life-Threatening Situations

School Refusal

ASSESSMENT. Refusal to go to school may occur in a young child who is first entering school or in an older child or adolescent who is making a transition into a new grade or school, or it may emerge in a vulnerable child without an obvious external stressor. In any case, school refusal requires immediate intervention because the longer the dysfunctional pattern continues, the more difficult it is to interrupt.

School refusal is generally associated with separation anxiety, in which the child's distress is related to the consequences of being separated from the parent, so the child resists going to school. School refusal can also occur in children with school phobia, in which the fear and the distress are targeted on the school itself. In either case, a serious disruption of the child's life occurs. Although mild separation anxiety is universal, particularly among very young children who are first facing school, treatment is required when a child actually cannot attend school. Severe psychopathology, including anxiety and depressive disorders, is often present when school refusal occurs for the first time in an adolescent. Children with separation anxiety disorder typically present extreme worries that catastrophic events will befall their mothers or themselves as a result of the separation. Children with separation anxiety disorder may also exhibit many other fears and symptoms of depression, including such somatic complaints such as headaches, stomachaches, and nausea.

Severe tantrums and desperate pleas may ensue when preoccupation that a parent will be harmed during the separation is frequently verbalized; in adolescents, the stated reasons for refusing to go to school are often physical complaints.

As part of an urgent assessment, the psychiatrist must ascertain the duration of the patient's absence from school and must assess the parents' ability to participate in a treatment plan that will undoubtedly involve firm parental guidelines to ensure the child's return to school. The parents of a child with separation anxiety disorder often exhibit excessive separation anxiety or other anxiety disorders themselves, thereby compounding the child's problem. When the parents are unable to participate in a treatment program from home, hospitalization should be considered.

MANAGEMENT. When school refusal caused by separation anxiety is identified during an emergency evaluation, the underlying disorder can be explained to the family, and an intervention can be started immediately. In severe cases, however, a multidimensional, long-term family-oriented treatment plan is necessary. Whenever possible, a separation-anxious child should be brought back to school the next school day, despite the distress, and a contact person within the school (counselor, guidance counselor, or teacher) should be involved to help the child stay in school while praising the child for tolerating the school situation.

When school refusal has been going on for months or years or when the family members are unable to cooperate, a treatment program to move the child back to school from the hospital should be considered. When the child's anxiety is not diminished by behavioral methods alone, tricyclic antidepressants, such as imipramine (Tofranil), are helpful. Medication is generally prescribed not at the initial evaluation but after a behavioral intervention has been tried.

Munchausen's Syndrome by Proxy

ASSESSMENT. Munchausen's syndrome by proxy, essentially, is a form of child abuse in which a parent, usually the mother, or a caretaker repeatedly fabricates or actually inflicts injury or illness in a child for whom medical intervention is then sought, often in an emergency setting. Although it is a rare scenario, mothers who inflict injury often have some prior knowledge of medicine, leading to sophisticated symptoms; the mothers sometimes engage in inappropriate camaraderie with the medical staff regarding the treatment of the child. Careful observation may reveal that the mothers often do not exhibit appropriate signs of distress on hearing the details of the child's medical symptoms. Prototypically, such mothers tend to present themselves as highly accomplished professionals in ways that seem inflated or blatantly untrue.

The illnesses appearing in the child can involve any organ system, but certain symptoms are commonly presented: bleeding from one or may sites, including the gastrointestinal tract, the genitourinary system, and the respiratory system; seizures; and central nervous system depression. At times, the illness is simulated, rather than actually inflicted. This syndrome is covered in Chapter 15.

Other Childhood Disturbances

Posttraumatic Stress Disorder. Children who have been subjected to a severe catastrophic or traumatic event may present for a prompt evaluation because they have extreme fears of the specific trauma occurring again or sudden discomfort with familiar places, people, or situations that previously did not evoke anxiety. Within weeks of a traumatic event, a child may re-create the event in play, in stories, and in dreams that directly replay the terrifying situation. A sense of reliving the experience may occur, including hallucinations and flashback (dissociative) experiences, and intrusive memories of the event come and go. Many traumatized children, over time, go on to reproduce parts of the event through their own victimization behaviors toward others, without being aware that those behaviors reflect their own traumatic experiences.

Table 30.2–2
Common Psychiatric Emergencies

Syndrome	Emergency Manifestations	Treatment Issues
Abuse of child or adult	Signs of physical trauma	Management of medical problems; psychiatric evaluation; report to authorities
Acquired immune deficiency syndrome	Changes in behavior secondary to organic causes; changes in behavior secondary to fear and anxiety; suicidal behavior	Management of neurological illness; management of psychological concomitants; reinforcement of social support
Adolescent crises	Suicidal attempts and ideation; substance abuse, truancy, trouble with the law, pregnancy, running away; eating disorders; psychosis	Evaluation of suicidal potential, extent of substance abuse, family dynamics; crisis-oriented family and individual therapy; hospitalization if necessary; consultation with appropriate extrafamilial authorities
Agoraphobia	Panic; depression	Alprazolam (Xanax), 0.25–2 mg; propranolol (Inderal); antidepressant medication
Agranulocytosis (clozapine [Clozaril] induced)	High fever, pharyngitis, oral and perianal ulcerations	Discontinue medication immediately; administer granulocyte colony–stimulating factor
Akathisia	Agitation, restlessness, muscle discomfort; dysphoria	Reduce antipsychotic dose; propranolol (30–120 mg a day); benzodiazepines; diphenhydramine (Benadryl) orally or IV; benztropine (Cogentin) IM
Alcohol-related emergencies		
Alcohol delirium	Confusion, disorientation, fluctuating consciousness and perception, autonomic hyperactivity; may be fatal	Chlordiazepoxide (Librium); haloperidol (Haldol) for psychotic symptoms may be added if necessary
Alcohol intoxication	Disinhibited behavior, sedation at high doses	With time and protective environment, symptoms abate
Alcohol persisting amnestic disorder	Confusion, loss of memory even for all personal identification data	Hospitalization; hypnosis; amobarbital (Amytal) interview; rule out organic cause
Alcohol persisting dementia	Confusion, agitation, impulsivity	Rule out other causes for dementia; no effective treatment; hospitalization if necessary
Alcohol psychotic disorder with hallucinations	Vivid auditory (at times visual) hallucinations with affect appropriate to content (often fearful); clear sensorium	Haloperidol for psychotic symptoms
Alcohol seizures	Grand mal seizures; rarely status epilepticus	Diazepam (Valium), phenytoin (Dilantin); prevent by using chlordiazepoxide (Librium) during detoxification
Alcohol withdrawal	Irritability, nausea, vomiting, insomnia, malaise, autonomic hyperactivity, shakiness	Fluid and electrolytes maintained; sedation with benzodiazepines; restraints; monitoring of vital signs; 100 mg thiamine IM
Idiosyncratic alcohol intoxication	Marked aggressive or assaultive behavior	Generally no treatment required other than protective environment
Korsakoff's syndrome	Alcohol stigmata, amnesia, confabulation	No effective treatment; institutionalization often needed
Wernicke's encephalopathy	Oculomotor disturbances, cerebellar ataxia; mental confusion	Thiamine, 100 mg IV or IM, with magnesium sulfate given before glucose loading
Amphetamine (or related substance) intoxication	Delusions, paranoia; violence; depression (from withdrawal); anxiety, delirium	Antipsychotics; restraints; hospitalization if necessary; no need for gradual withdrawal; antidepressants may be necessary
Anorexia nervosa	Loss of 15–25% of body weight of the norm for age and sex	Hospitalization; ECG, fluid and electrolytes; neuroendocrine evaluation
Anticholinergic intoxication	Psychotic symptoms, dry skin and mouth, hyperpyrexia, mydriasis, tachycardia, restlessness, visual hallucinations	Discontinue drug, IV physostigmine (Antilirium), 0.5–2 mg, for severe agitation or fever, benzodiazepines; antipsychotics contraindicated
Anticonvulsant intoxication	Psychosis; delirium	Dose of anticonvulsant is reduced
Benzodiazepine intoxication	Sedation, somnolence, and ataxia	Supportive measures; flumazenil (Romazicon), 7.5–45 mg a day, titrated as needed, should be used only by skilled personnel with resuscitative equipment available
Bereavement	Guilt feelings, irritability; insomnia; somatic complaints	Must be differentiated from major depressive disorder; antidepressants not indicated; benzodiazepines for sleep; encouragement of ventilation

(continued)

**Table 30.2–2
(Continued)**

Syndrome	Emergency Manifestations	Treatment Issues
Borderline personality disorder	Suicidal ideation and gestures; homicidal ideations and gestures; substance abuse; micropsychotic episodes; burns, cut marks on body	Suicidal and homicidal evaluation (if great, hospitalization); small doses of antipsychotics; clear follow-up plan
Brief psychotic disorder	Emotional turmoil, extreme lability; acutely impaired reality testing after obvious psychosocial stress	Hospitalization often necessary; low dose of antipsychotics may be necessary but often resolves spontaneously
Bromide intoxication	Delirium; mania; depression; psychosis	Serum levels obtained (>50 mg a day); bromide intake discontinued; large quantities of sodium chloride IV or orally; if agitation, paraldehyde or antipsychotic is used
Caffeine intoxication	Severe anxiety, resembling panic disorder; mania; delirium; agitated depression; sleep disturbance	Cessation of caffeine-containing substances; benzodiazepines
Cannabis intoxication	Delusions; panic; dysphoria; cognitive impairment	Benzodiazepines and antipsychotics as needed; evaluation of suicidal or homicidal risk; symptoms usually abate with time and reassurance
Catatonic schizophrenia	Marked psychomotor disturbance (either excitement or stupor); exhaustion; can be fatal	Rapid tranquilization with antipsychotics; monitor vital signs; amobarbital may release patient from catatonic mutism or stupor but can precipitate violent behavior
Cimetidine psychotic disorder	Delirium; delusions	Reduce dose or discontinue drug
Clonidine withdrawal	Irritability; psychosis; violence; seizures	Symptoms abate with time, but antipsychotics may be necessary; gradual lowering of dose
Cocaine intoxication and withdrawal	Paranoia and violence; severe anxiety; manic state; delirium: schizophreniform psychosis; tachycardia, hypertension, myocardial infarction, cerebrovascular disease; depression and suicidal ideation	Antipsychotics and benzodiazepines; antidepressants or ECT for withdrawal depression if persistent; hospitalization
Delirium	Fluctuating sensorium; suicidal and homicidal risk; cognitive clouding; visual, tactile, and auditory hallucinations; paranoia	Evaluate all potential contributing factors and treat each accordingly; reassurance, structure, clues to orientation; benzodiazepines and low-dose, high-potency antipsychotics must be used with extreme care because of their potential to act paradoxically and increase agitation
Delusional disorder	Most often brought in to emergency room involuntarily; threats directed toward others	Antipsychotics if patient will comply (IM if necessary); intensive family intervention; hospitalization if necessary
Dementia	Unable to care for self; violent outbursts; psychosis; depression and suicidal ideation; confusion	Small doses of high-potency antipsychotics; clues to orientation; organic evaluation, including medication use; family intervention
Depressive disorders	Suicidal ideation and attempts; self-neglect; substance abuse	Assessment of danger to self; hospitalization if necessary, nonpsychiatric causes of depression must be evaluated
L-Dopa intoxication	Mania; depression; schizophreniform disorder, may induce rapid cycling in patients with bipolar I disorder	Lower dose or discontinue drug
Dystonia, acute	Intense involuntary spasm of muscles of neck, tongue, face, jaw, eyes, or trunk	Decrease dose of antipsychotic; benztropine or diphenhydramine IM
Group hysteria	Groups of people exhibit extremes of grief or other disruptive behavior	Group is dispersed with help of other health care workers; ventilation, crisis-oriented therapy; if necessary, small doses of benzodiazepines
Hallucinogen-induced psychotic disorder with hallucinations	Symptom picture is result of interaction of type of substance, dose taken, duration of action, user's premorbid personality, setting; panic; agitation; atropine psychosis	Serum and urine screens; rule out underlying medical or mental disorder; benzodiazepines (2–20 mg) orally; reassurance and orientation; rapid tranquilization; often responds spontaneously
Homicidal and assaultive behavior	Marked agitation with verbal threats	Seclusion, restraints, medication

(continued)

Table 30.2–2
(Continued)

Syndrome	Emergency Manifestations	Treatment Issues
Homosexual panic	Not seen with men or women who are comfortable with their sexual orientation; occurs in those who adamantly deny having any homoerotic impulses; impulses are aroused by talk, a physical overture, or play among same-sex friends, such as wrestling, sleeping together, or touching each other in a shower or hot tub; panicked person sees others as sexually interested in him or her and defends against them	Ventilation, environmental structuring, and, in some instances, medication for acute panic (e.g., alprazolam, 0.25–2 mg) or antipsychotics may be required; opposite-sex clinician should evaluate the patient whenever possible, and the patient should not be touched save for the routine examination; patients have attacked physicians who were examining an abdomen or performing a rectal examination (e.g., on a man who harbors thinly veiled unintegrated homosexual impulses)
Hypertensive crisis	Life-threatening hypertensive reaction secondary to ingestion of tyramine-containing foods in combination with MAOIs; headache, stiff neck, sweating, nausea, vomiting	α-Adrenergic blockers (e.g., phentolamine [Regitinel]); nifedipine (Procardia) 10 mg orally; chlorpromazine (Thorazine); make sure symptoms are not secondary to hypotension (side effect of MAOIs alone)
Hyperthermia	Extreme excitement or catatonic stupor or both; extremely elevated temperature; violent hyperagitation	Hydrate and cool; may be drug reaction, so discontinue any drug; rule out infection
Hyperventilation	Anxiety, terror, clouded consciousness; giddiness, faintness; blurring vision	Shift alkalosis by having patient breathe into paper bag; patient education; antianxiety agents
Hypothermia	Confusion; lethargy; combativeness; low body temperature and shivering; paradoxical feeling of warmth	IV fluids and rewarming, cardiac status must be carefully monitored; avoidance of alcohol
Incest and sexual abuse of child	Suicidal behavior; adolescent crises; substance abuse	Corroboration of charge, protection of victim; contact social services; medical and psychiatric evaluation; crisis intervention
Insomnia	Depression and irritability; early-morning agitation; frightening dreams; fatigue	Hypnotics only in short term; e.g., triazolam (Halcion), 0.25–0.5 mg, at bedtime; treat any underlying mental disorder; rules of sleep hygiene
Intermittent explosive disorder	Brief outbursts of violence; periodic episodes of suicide attempts	Benzodiazepines or antipsychotics for short term; long-term evaluation with computed tomography scan, sleep-deprived EEG, glucose tolerance curve
Jaundice	Uncommon complication of low-potency phenothiazine use (e.g., chlorpromazine)	Change drug to low dose of a low-potency agent in a different class
Leukopenia and agranulocytosis	Side effects within the first 2 months of treatment with antipsychotics	Patient should call immediately for sore throat, fever, etc., and obtain immediate blood count; discontinue drug; hospitalize if necessary
Lithium toxicity	Vomiting; abdominal pain; profuse diarrhea; severe tremor, ataxia; coma; seizures; confusion; dysarthria; focal neurological signs	Lavage with wide-bore tube; osmotic diuresis; medical consultation; may require intensive care unit treatment
Major depressive episode with psychotic features	Major depressive episode symptoms with delusions; agitation, severe guilt; ideas of reference; suicide and homicide risk	Antipsychotics plus antidepressants; evaluation of suicide and homicide risk; hospitalization and ECT if necessary
Manic episode	Violent, impulsive behavior; indiscriminate sexual or spending behavior; psychosis; substance abuse	Hospitalization; restraints if necessary; rapid tranquilization with antipsychotics; restoration of lithium levels
Marital crises	Precipitant may be discovery of an extramarital affair, onset of serious illness, announcement of intent to divorce, or problems with children or work; one or both members of the couple may be in therapy or may be psychiatrically ill; one spouse may be seeking hospitalization for the other	Each partner should be questioned alone regarding extramarital affairs, consultations with lawyers regarding divorce, and willingness to work in crisis-oriented or long-term therapy to resolve the problem; sexual, financial, and psychiatric treatment histories from both, psychiatric evaluation at the time of presentation; may be precipitated by onset of untreated mood disorder or affective symptoms caused by medical illness or insidious-onset dementia; referral for management of the illness reduces

(continued)

Table 30.2–2
(Continued)

Syndrome	Emergency Manifestations	Treatment Issues
		immediate stress and enhances the healthier spouse's coping capacity; children may give insights available only to someone intimately involved in the social system
Migraine	Throbbing, unilateral headache	Sumatriptan (Imitrex), 6 mg IM
Mitral valve prolapse	Associated with panic disorder; dyspnea and palpitations; fear and anxiety	Echocardiogram; alprazolam or propranolol
Neuroleptic malignant syndrome	Hyperthermia; muscle rigidity; autonomic instability; parkinsonian symptoms; catatonic stupor; neurological signs; 10%–30% fatality; elevated creatine phosphokinase	Discontinue antipsychotic; IV dantrolene (Dantrium); bromocriptine (Parlodel) orally; hydration and cooling; monitor creatine phosphokinase levels
Nitrous oxide toxicity	Euphoria and light-headedness	Symptoms abate without treatment within hours of use
Nutmeg intoxication	Agitation; hallucinations; severe headaches; numbness in extremities	Symptoms abate within hours of use without treatment
Opioid intoxication and withdrawal	Intoxication can lead to coma and death; withdrawal is not life threatening	IV naloxone, narcotic antagonist; urine and serum screens; psychiatric and medical illnesses (e.g., AIDS) may complicate picture
Panic disorder	Panic, terror; acute onset	Must differentiate from other anxiety-producing disorders, both medical and psychiatric; ECG to rule out mitral valve prolapse; propranolol (10–30 mg); alprazolam (0.25–2.0 mg); long-term management may include an antidepressant
Paranoid schizophrenia	Command hallucinations; threat to others or themselves	Rapid tranquilization; hospitalization; long-acting depot medication; threatened persons must be notified and protected
Parkinsonism	Stiffness, tremor, bradykinesia, flattened affect, shuffling gait, salivation, secondary to antipsychotic medication	Oral antiparkinsonian drug for 4 wks to 3 mos; decrease dose of the antipsychotic
Perioral (rabbit) tremor	Perioral tumor (rabbit-like facial grimacing) usually appearing after long-term therapy with antipsychotics	Decrease dose or change to a medication in another class
Phencyclidine (or phencyclidine-like intoxication)	Paranoid psychosis; can lead to death; acute danger to self and others	Serum and urine assay; benzodiazepines may interfere with excretion; antipsychotics may worsen symptoms because of anticholinergic side effects; medical monitoring and hospitalization for severe intoxication
Phenelzine-induced psychotic disorder	Psychosis and mania in predisposed people	Reduce dose or discontinue drug
Phenylpropanolamine toxicity	Psychosis; paranoia; insomnia; restlessness; nervousness; headache	Symptoms abate with dose reduction or discontinuation (found in over-the-counter diet aids and oral and nasal decongestants)
Phobias	Panic, anxiety; fear	Treatment same as for panic disorder
Photosensitivity	Easy sunburning secondary to use of antipsychotic medication	Patient should avoid strong sunlight and use high-level sunscreens
Pigmentary retinopathy	Reported with doses of thioridazine (Mellaril) of 800 mg a day or above	Remain <800 mg a day of thioridazine
Postpartum psychosis	Childbirth can precipitate schizophrenia, depression, reactive psychoses, mania, and depression; affective symptoms are most common; suicide risk is reduced during pregnancy but increased in the postpartum period	Danger to self and others (including infant) must be evaluated and proper precautions taken; medical illness presenting with behavioral aberrations is included in the differential diagnosis and must be sought and treated; care must be paid to the effects on father, infant, grandparents, and other children
Posttraumatic stress disorder	Panic, terror; suicidal ideation; flashbacks	Reassurance; encouragement of return to responsibilities; avoid hospitalization if possible to prevent chronic invalidism; monitor suicidal ideation
Priapism (trazodone [Desyrel] induced)	Persistent penile erection accompanied by severe pain	Intracorporeal epinephrine; mechanical or surgical drainage
Propranolol toxicity	Profound depression; confusional states	Reduce dose or discontinue drug; monitor suicidality

(continued)

Table 30.2–2
(Continued)

Syndrome	Emergency Manifestations	Treatment Issues
Rape	Not all sexual violations are reported; silent rape reaction is characterized by loss of appetite, sleep disturbance, anxiety, and, sometimes, agoraphobia; long periods of silence, mounting anxiety, stuttering, blocking, and physical symptoms during the interview when the sexual history is taken; fear of violence and death and of contracting a sexually transmitted disease or being pregnant	Rape is a major psychiatric emergency; victim may have enduring patterns of sexual dysfunction; crisis-oriented therapy, social support, ventilation, reinforcement of healthy traits, and encouragement to return to the previous level of functioning as rapidly as possible; legal counsel; thorough medical examination and tests to identify the assailant (e.g., obtaining samples of pubic hairs with a pubic hair comb, vaginal smear to identify blood antigens in semen); if a woman, methoxyprogesterone or diethylstilbestrol orally for 5 days to prevent pregnancy; if menstruation does not commence within one week of cessation of the estrogen, all alternatives to pregnancy, including abortion, should be offered; if the victim has contracted a venereal disease, appropriate antibiotics; witnessed written permission is required for the physician to examine, photograph, collect specimens, and release information to the authorities; obtain consent, record the history in the patient's own words, obtain required tests, record the results of the examination, save all clothing, defer diagnosis, and provide protection against disease, psychic trauma, and pregnancy; men's and women's responses to rape affectively are reported similarly, although men are more hesitant to talk about homosexual assault for fear they will be assumed to have consented
Reserpine intoxication	Major depressive episodes; suicidal ideation; nightmares	Evaluation of suicidal ideation; lower dose or change drug; antidepressants of ECT may be indicated
Schizoaffective disorder	Severe depression; manic symptoms; paranoia	Evaluation of dangerousness to self or others; rapid tranquilization if necessary; treatment of depression (antidepressants alone can enhance schizophrenic symptoms); use of antimanic agents
Schizophrenia	Extreme self-neglect; severe paranoia; suicidal ideation or assaultiveness; extreme psychotic symptoms	Evaluation of suicidal and homicidal potential; identification of any illness other than schizophrenia; rapid tranquilization
Schizophrenia in exacerbation	Withdrawn; agitation; suicidal and homicidal risk	Suicide and homicide evaluation; screen for medical illness; restraints and rapid tranquilization if necessary; hospitalization if necessary; reevaluation of medication regimen
Sedative, hypnotic, or anxiolytic intoxication and withdrawal	Alterations in mood, behavior, thought—delirium; derealization and depersonalization; can be fatal if untreated; seizures	Naloxone (Narcan) to differentiate from opioid intoxication; slow withdrawal with phenobarbital (Luminal) or sodium thiopental or benzodiazepine; hospitalization
Seizure disorder	Confusion; anxiety; derealization and depersonalization; feelings of impending doom; gustatory or olfactory hallucinations; fugue-like state	Immediate EEG; admission and sleep-deprived and 24-hour EEG; rule out pseudoseizures; anticonvulsants
Substance withdrawal	Abdominal pain; insomnia, drowsiness; delirium; seizures; symptoms of tardive dyskinesia may emerge; eruption of manic or schizophrenic symptoms	Symptoms of psychotropic drug withdrawal disappear with time or disappear with reinstitution of the substance; symptoms of antidepressant withdrawal can be successfully treated with anticholinergic agents, such as atropine; gradual withdrawal of psychotropic substances over 2–4 weeks generally obviates development of symptoms
Suicide attempt	Suicidal ideation; hopelessness	Hospitalization, antidepressants
Sympathomimetic withdrawal	Paranoia; confusional states; depression	Most symptoms abate without treatment; antipsychotics; antidepressants if necessary

(continued)

Table 30.2–2
(Continued)

Syndrome	Emergency Manifestations	Treatment Issues
Tardive dyskinesia	Dyskinesia of mouth, tongue, face, neck, and trunk; choreoathetoid movements of extremities; usually but not always appearing after long-term treatment with antipsychotics, especially after a reduction in dose; incidence highest in the elderly and brain damaged; symptoms are intensified by antiparkinsonian drugs and masked but not cured by increased doses of antipsychotic	No effective treatment reported; may be prevented by prescribing the least amount of drug possible for as little time as is clinically feasible and using drug-free holidays for patients who need to continue taking the drug; decrease or discontinue drug at first sign of dyskinetic movements
Thyrotoxicosis	Tachycardia; gastrointestinal dysfunction; hyperthermia; panic, anxiety, agitation; mania; dementia; psychosis	Thyroid function test (triiodothyronine, thyroxine, thyroid-stimulating hormone); medical consultation
Toluene abuse	Anxiety; confusion; cognitive impairment	Neurological damage is nonprogressive and reversible if toluene use is discontinued early
Vitamin B_{12} deficiency	Confusion; mood and behavior changes; ataxia	Treatment with vitamin B_{12}
Volatile nitrates	Alternations of mood and behavior; light-headedness; pulsating headache	Symptoms abate with cessation of use

AIDS, acquired immune deficiency syndrome; ECG, electrocardiogram; ECT, electroconvulsive therapy; EEG, electroencephalogram; IM, intramuscular; IV, intravenous; MAOIs, monoamine oxidase inhibitors.

Dissociative Disorders.   Dissociative states—including the extreme form, multiple personality disorder—are believed most likely to occur in children who have been subjected to severe and repetitive physical, sexual, or emotional abuse. Children with dissociative symptoms may be referred for evaluation because family members or teachers observe that the children sometimes seem to be spaced out or distracted or act like different persons. Dissociative states are occasionally identified during the evaluation of violent and aggressive behavior, particularly in patients who truly do not remember chunks of their own behavior.

When a child who dissociates is violent or self-destructive or endangers others, hospitalization is necessary. A variety of psychotherapy methods have been used in the complex treatment of children with dissociative disorders, including play techniques and, in some cases, hypnosis. (For a complete discussion of this condition see Chapter 16, Dissociative Disorders.)

SPECIFIC PSYCHIATRIC EMERGENCIES

Table 30.2–2 outlines common psychiatric emergencies in alphabetical order. Readers are referred to the index and to specific chapters of this textbook for a thorough discussion of each disorder.

31

Psychotherapies

▲ 31.1 Psychoanalysis and Psychoanalytic Psychotherapy

Psychoanalysis is virtually synonymous with the renowned name of its founding father, Sigmund Freud. It is also referred to as "classic" or "orthodox" psychoanalysis to distinguish it from more recent variations known as *psychoanalytic psychotherapy* (discussed later). It remains unsurpassed as a method for discovering the meaning and motivation of behavior, especially the unconscious elements informing thoughts and feelings.

As broadly practiced today, psychoanalytic treatment encompasses a wide range of uncovering strategies used in varied degrees and blends. Despite the inevitable blurring of boundaries in actual application, the original modality of classic psychoanalysis and major modes of psychoanalytic psychotherapy (expressive and supportive) are delineated separately here (Table 31.1–1). Analytical practice in all its complexity resides on a continuum. Individual technique is always a matter of emphasis as the therapist titrates the treatment according to the needs and capacities of the patient at every moment.

PSYCHOANALYSIS

Indications and Contraindications

In general, all of the so-called *psychoneuroses* are suitable for psychoanalysis. These include anxiety disorders, obsessional thinking, compulsive behavior, conversion disorder, sexual dysfunction, depressive states, and many other nonpsychotic conditions, such as personality disorders. Significant suffering must be present so that patients are motivated to make the sacrifices of time and financial resources required for psychoanalysis. Patients who enter analysis must have a genuine wish to understand themselves, not a desperate hunger for symptomatic relief. They must be able to withstand frustration, anxiety, and other strong affects that emerge in analysis without fleeing or acting out their feelings in a self-destructive manner. They must also have a reasonable, mature superego that allows them to be honest with the analyst. Intelligence must be at least average, and above all, they must be psychologically minded in the sense that they can think abstractly and symbolically about the unconscious meanings of their behavior.

Psychoanalytic Setting.
As with other forms of psychotherapy, psychoanalysis takes place in a professional setting, apart from the realities of everyday life, in which the patient is offered a temporary sanctuary in which to ease psychic pain and reveal intimate thoughts to an accepting expert. The psychoanalytic environment is designed to promote relaxation and regression. The setting is usually spartan and sensorially neutral, and external stimuli are minimized.

USE OF THE COUCH. The couch has several clinical advantages that are both real and symbolic: (1) the reclining position is relaxing because it is associated with sleep and so eases the patient's conscious control of thoughts; (2) it minimizes the intrusive influence of the analyst, thus curbing unnecessary cues; (3) it permits the analyst to make observations of the patient without interruption; and (4) it holds symbolic value for both parties, a tangible reminder of the Freudian legacy that gives credibility to the analyst's professional identity, allegiance, and expertise. The reclining position of the patient with analyst nearby can also generate threat and discomfort, however, as it recalls anxieties derived from the earlier parent–child configuration that it physically resembles. It may also have personal meanings—for some, a portent of dangerous impulses or of submission to an authority figure; for others, a relief from confrontation by the analyst (e.g., fear of use of the couch and overeagerness to lie down may reflect resistance and, thus, need to be analyzed). Although the use of the couch is requisite to analytical technique, it is not applied automatically; it is introduced gradually and can be suspended whenever additional regression is unnecessary or countertherapeutic.

FUNDAMENTAL RULE. The fundamental rule of *free association* requires patients to tell the analyst everything that comes into their heads—however disagreeable, unimportant, or nonsensical. It differs decidedly from ordinary conversation—instead of connecting personal remarks with a rational thread, the patient is asked to reveal those very thoughts and events that are objectionable precisely because of being averse to doing so.

Aside from its primary purpose of eliciting recall of deeply hidden early memories, the fundamental rule reflects the analytical priority placed on verbalization, which translates the patient's thoughts into words so that they are not channeled physically or behaviorally. As a direct concomitant of the fundamental rule, which prohibits action in favor of verbal expression, patients are expected to postpone making major alterations in their lives, such as marrying or changing careers, until they discuss and analyze them within the context of treatment.

ANALYST AS MIRROR. A second principle is the recommendation that the analyst be impenetrable to the patient and, as a mirror, reflect only what is shown. Analysts are advised to be neutral blank screens and not to bring their own personalities into treatment. This means that they are not to bring their own values or attitudes into the discussion or to share personal reactions or mutual conflicts with their patients, although they may sometimes be tempted to do so. The bringing in of reality and external influences can interrupt or bias the patient's unconscious projections. Neutrality also allows the analyst to accept without censure all forbidden or objectionable responses.

RULE OF ABSTINENCE. The fundamental rule of abstinence does not mean corporal or sexual abstinence, but refers to the frustration of emotional needs and wishes that the patient may have toward the analyst

Table 31.1–1
Scope of Psychoanalytic Practice: A Clinical Continuum[a]

Feature	Psychoanalysis	Psychoanalytic Psychotherapy	
		Expressive Mode	Supportive Mode
Frequency	Regular four to five times/wk; "50-minute hour"	Regular one to three times/wk; $^1/_2$ to full hr	Flexible one time/wk or less; or as needed $^1/_2$ to full hr
Duration	Long-term; usually 3–5+ yrs	Short- or long-term; several sessions to months or years	Short- or intermittent long-term; single session to lifetime
Setting	Patient primarily on couch with analyst out of view	Patient and therapist face-to-face; occasional use of couch	Patient and therapist face-to-face; couch contraindicated
Modus operandi	Systematic analysis of all positive and negative transference and resistance; primary focus on analyst and intrasession events; transference neurosis facilitated; regression encouraged	Partial analysis of dynamics and defenses; focus on current interpersonal events and transference to others outside of sessions; analysis of negative transference; positive transference left unexplored unless impedes progress; limited regression encouraged	Formation of therapeutic alliance and real object relationship; analysis of transference contraindicated with rare exceptions; focus on conscious external events; regression discouraged
Analyst/therapist role	Absolute neutrality; frustration of patient; reflector/mirror role	Modified neutrality; implicit gratification of patient and greater activity	Neutrality suspended; limited explicit gratification, direction, and disclosure
Mutative change agents	Insight predominates within relatively deprived environment	Insight within more empathic environment; identification with benevolent object	Auxiliary or surrogate ego as temporary substitute; holding environment; insight to degree possible
Patient population	Neuroses; mild character psychopathology	Neuroses; mild to moderate character psychopathology, especially narcissistic and borderline disorders	Severe character disorders, latent or manifest psychoses, acute crises, physical illness
Patient requisites	High motivation, psychological mindedness; good previous object relationships; ability to maintain transference neurosis; good frustration tolerance	High to moderate motivation and psychological mindedness; ability to form therapeutic alliance; some frustration tolerance	Some degree of motivation and ability to form therapeutic alliance
Basic goals	Structural reorganization of personality; resolution of unconscious conflicts; insight into intrapsychic events; symptom relief an indirect result	Partial reorganization of personality and defenses; resolution of preconscious and conscious derivatives of conflicts; insight into current interpersonal events; improved object relations; symptom relief a goal or prelude to further exploration	Reintegration of self and ability to cope; stabilization or restoration of preexisting equilibrium; strengthening of defenses; better adjustment or acceptance of pathology; symptom relief and environmental restructuring as primary goals
Major techniques	Free association method predominates; full dynamic interpretation (including confrontation, clarification, and working through), with emphasis on genetic reconstruction	Limited free association; confrontation, clarification, and partial interpretation predominate, with emphasis on here-and-now interpretation and limited genetic interpretation	Free association method contraindicated; suggestion (advise) predominates; abreaction useful; confrontation, clarification, and interpretation in the here-and-now secondary; genetic interpretation contraindicated
Adjunct treatment	Primarily avoided; if applied, all negative and positive meanings and implications are thoroughly analyzed	May be necessary—e.g., psychotropic drugs as temporary measure; if applied, its negative implications explored and diffused	Often necessary—e.g., psychotropic drugs, family rehabilitative therapy, or hospitalization; if applied, its positive implications are emphasized

[a]This division is not categorical; all practice resides on a clinical continuum.

or part of the transference. It allows the patient's longings to persist and serve as driving forces for analytical work and motivation to change. Freud advised that the analyst carry through the analytical treatment in a state of renunciation. The analyst must deny the patient who is longing for love the satisfaction he or she craves.

Limitations.   At present, the predominant treatment constraints are often economic, relating to the high cost in time and money, both for patients and in the training of future practitioners. In addition, because clinical requirements emphasize such requisites as psychological mindedness, verbal and cognitive ability, and stable life situation, psychoanalysis may be unduly restricted to a diagnostically, socioeconomically, or intellectually advantaged patient population. Other intrinsic issues pertain to the use and misuse of its stringent rules, whereby overemphasis on technique may interfere with an authentic human encounter between analyst and patient, and to the major long-term risk of interminability, in which protracted treatment may become a substitute for life. Reification of the classic analytical tradition may interfere with a more open and flexible application of its tenets to meet changing needs. It may also obstruct a comprehensive view of patient care that includes a greater appreciation of other treatment modalities in conjunction with, or as an alternative to, psychoanalysis.

Ms. A, a 25-year-old articulate and introspective medical student, began analysis complaining of mild, chronic anxiety, dysphoria, and a sense of inadequacy, despite above-average intelligence and performance. She also expressed difficulty in long-term relationships with her male peers.

Ms. A began the initial phase of analysis with enthusiastic self-disclosure, frequent reports of dreams and fantasies, and overidealization of the analyst; she tried to please him by being a compliant, good patient, just as she had been a good daughter to her father (a professor of medicine) by going to medical school.

Over the next several months, Ms. A gradually developed a strong attachment to the analyst and settled into a phase of excessive preoccupation with him. Simultaneously, however, she began dating an older psychiatrist and proceeded to complain about the analyst's coldness and unresponsiveness, even considering dropping out of analysis because he did not meet her demands.

In the course of analysis, through dreams and associations, Ms. A recalled early memories of her ongoing competition with her mother for her father's attention and realized that, failing to obtain his exclusive love, she had tried to become like him. She was also able to see how her increasing interest in becoming a psychiatrist (rather than following her original plan to be a pediatrician), as well as her recent choice of a man to date, were recapitulations of the past vis-à-vis the analyst. As this repeated pattern was recognized, the patient began to relinquish her intense erotic and dependent tie to the analyst, viewing him more realistically and beginning to appreciate the ways in which his quiet presence reminded her of her mother. She also became less disturbed by the similarities she shared with her mother and was able to disengage from her father more comfortably. By the fifth year of analysis, she was happily married to a classmate, was pregnant, and was a pediatric chief resident. Her anxiety was now attenuated and situation-specific (that is, she was concerned about motherhood and the termination of analysis). (Courtesy of T. Byram Karasu, M.D.)

PSYCHOANALYTIC PSYCHOTHERAPY

Psychoanalytic psychotherapy, which is based on fundamental dynamic formulations and techniques that derive from psychoanalysis, is designed to broaden its scope. Psychoanalytic psychotherapy, in its narrowest sense, is the use of insight-oriented methods only. As generically applied today to an ever-larger clinical spectrum, it incorporates a blend of uncovering and suppressive measures.

The strategies of psychoanalytic psychotherapy currently range from expressive (insight-oriented, uncovering, evocative, or interpretive) techniques to supportive (relationship-oriented, suggestive, suppressive, or repressive) techniques. Although those two types of methods are sometimes regarded as antithetical, their precise definitions and the distinctions between them are by no means absolute.

The duration of psychoanalytic psychotherapy is generally shorter and more variable than in psychoanalysis. Treatment may be brief, even with an initially agreed-on or fixed time limit, or may extend to a less-definite number of months or years. Brief treatment is chiefly used for selected problems or highly focused conflict, whereas longer treatment may be applied in more chronic conditions or for intermittent episodes that require ongoing attention to deal with pervasive conflict or recurrent decompensation. Unlike psychoanalysis, psychoanalytic psychotherapy rarely uses the couch; instead, patient and therapist sit face to face. This posture helps to prevent regression because it encourages the patient to look on the therapist as a real person from whom to receive direct cues, even though transference and fantasy will continue. The couch is considered unnecessary because the free association method is rarely used, except when the therapist wishes to gain access to fantasy material or dreams to enlighten a particular issue.

Expressive Psychotherapy

Indications and Contraindications. Diagnostically, psychoanalytic psychotherapy in its expressive mode is suited to a range of psychopathology with mild to moderate ego weakening, including neurotic conflicts, symptom complexes, reactive conditions, and the whole realm of nonpsychotic character disorders, including those disorders of the self that are among the more transient and less profound on the severity-of-illness spectrum, such as narcissistic behavior disorders and narcissistic personality disorders. It is also one of the treatments recommended for patients with borderline personality disorders, although special variations may be required to deal with the associated turbulent personality characteristics, primitive defense mechanisms, tendencies toward regressive episodes, and irrational attachments to the analyst.

The persons best suited for the expressive psychotherapy approach have fairly well integrated egos and the capacity to both sustain and detach from a bond of dependency and trust. They are, to some degree, psychologically minded and self-motivated, and they are generally able, at least temporarily, to tolerate doses of frustration without decompensating. They must also have the ability to manage the rearousal of painful feelings outside the therapy hour without additional contact. Patients must have some capacity for introspection and impulse control, and they should be able to recognize the cognitive distinction between fantasy and reality.

Goals. The overall goals of expressive psychotherapy are to increase the patient's self-awareness and to improve object relations through exploration of current interpersonal events and perceptions. In contrast to psychoanalysis, major structural changes in ego function and defenses are modified in light of patient limitations. The aim is to achieve a more limited and, thus, select and focused understanding of one's problems. Rather than uncovering deeply hidden and past motives and tracing them back to their origins in infancy, the major thrust is to deal with preconscious or conscious derivatives of conflicts as they became manifest in present interactions. Although insight is sought, it is less extensive; instead of delving to a genetic level, greater emphasis is on clarifying recent dynamic patterns and maladaptive behaviors in the present.

Major Approach and Techniques.

The major modus operandi involves establishment of a therapeutic alliance and early recognition and interpretation of negative transference. Only limited or controlled regression is encouraged, and positive transference manifestations are generally left unexplored, unless they are impeding therapeutic progress; even here, the emphasis is on shedding light on current dynamic patterns and defenses.

Limitations.

A general limitation of expressive psychotherapy, as of psychoanalysis, is the problem of emotional integration of cognitive awareness. The major danger for patients who are at the more disorganized end of the diagnostic spectrum, however, may have less to do with the overintellectualization that is sometimes seen in neurotic patients than with the threat of decompensation from, or acting out of, deep or frequent interpretations that the patient is unable to integrate properly.

Some therapists fail to accept the limitations of a modified insight-oriented approach and so apply it inappropriately to modulate the techniques and goals of psychoanalysis. Overemphasis on dreams and fantasies, zealous efforts to use the couch, indiscriminate deep interpretations, and continual focus on the analysis of transference may have less to do with the patient's needs than with those of a therapist who is unwilling or unable to be flexible.

Supportive Psychotherapy

Supportive psychotherapy aims at the creation of a therapeutic relationship as a temporary buttress or bridge for the deficient patient. It has roots in virtually every therapy that recognizes the ameliorative effects of emotional support and a stable, caring atmosphere in the management of patients. As a nonspecific attitude toward mental illness, it predates scientific psychiatry, with foundations in 18th-century moral treatment, whereby for the first time patients were treated with understanding and kindness in a humane interpersonal environment free from mechanical restraints.

Supportive psychotherapy has been the chief form used in the general practice of medicine and rehabilitation, frequently to augment extratherapeutic measures, such as prescriptions of medication to suppress symptoms, rest to remove the patient from excessive stimulation, or hospitalization to provide a structured therapeutic environment, protection, and control of the patient. It can be applied as primary or ancillary treatment. The global perspective of supportive psychotherapy (often part of a combined treatment approach) places major etiological emphasis on external rather than intrapsychic events, particularly on stressful environmental and interpersonal influences on a severely damaged self.

Indications and Contraindications.

Supportive psychotherapy is generally indicated for those patients for whom classic psychoanalysis or insight-oriented psychoanalytic psychotherapy is typically contraindicated—those who have poor ego strength and whose potential for decompensation is high. Amenable patients fall into the following major areas: (1) individuals in acute crisis or a temporary state of disorganization and inability to cope (including those who might otherwise be well functioning) whose intolerable life circumstances have produced extreme anxiety or sudden turmoil (e.g., individuals going through grief reactions, illness, divorce, job loss, or who were victims of crime, abuse, natural disaster, or accident); (2) patients with chronic severe pathology with fragile or deficient ego functioning (e.g., those with latent psychosis, impulse disorder, or severe character disturbance); (3) patients whose cognitive deficits and physical symptoms make them particularly vulnerable and, thus, unsuitable for an insight-oriented approach (e.g., certain psychosomatic or medically ill persons); (4) individuals who are psychologically unmotivated, although not necessarily characterologically resistant to a depth approach (e.g., patients who come to treatment in response to family or agency pressure and are interested only in immediate relief or those who need assistance in very specific problem areas of social adjustment as a possible prelude to more exploratory work).

Because support forms a tacit part of every therapeutic modality, it is rarely contraindicated as such. The typical attitude regards better-functioning patients as unsuitable not because they will be harmed by a supportive approach, but because they will not be sufficiently benefited by it. In aiming to maximize the patient's potential for further growth and change, supportive therapy tends to be regarded as relatively restricted and superficial and, thus, is not recommended as the treatment of choice if the patient is available for, and capable of, a more in-depth approach.

Goals.

The general aim of supportive treatment is the amelioration or relief of symptoms through behavioral or environmental restructuring within the existing psychic framework. This often means helping the patient to adapt better to problems and to live more comfortably with his or her psychopathology. To restore the disorganized, fragile, or decompensated patient to a state of relative equilibrium, the major goal is to suppress or control symptomatology and to stabilize the patient in a protective and reassuring benign atmosphere that militates against overwhelming external and internal pressures. The ultimate goal is to maximize the integrative or adaptive capacities so that the patient increases the ability to cope, while decreasing vulnerability by reinforcing assets and strengthening defenses.

Major Approach and Techniques.

Supportive therapy uses several methods, either singly or in combination, including warm, friendly, strong leadership; partial gratification of dependency needs; support in the ultimate development of legitimate independence; help in developing pleasurable activities (e.g., hobbies); adequate rest and diversion; removal of excessive strain, when possible; hospitalization, when indicated; medication to alleviate symptoms; and guidance and advice in dealing with current issues. This therapy uses techniques to help patients feel secure, accepted, protected, encouraged, safe, and not anxious.

Limitations. To the extent that much supportive therapy is spent on practical, everyday realities and on dealing with the external environment of the patient, it may be viewed as more mundane and superficial than depth approaches. Because those patients are seen intermittently and less frequently, the interpersonal commitment may not be as compelling on the part of either the patient or the therapist. Greater severity of illness (and possible psychoses) also makes such treatment potentially more erratic, demanding, and frustrating. The need for the therapist to deal with other family members, caretakers, or agencies (auxiliary treatment, hospitalization) can become an additional complication because the therapist comes to serve as an ombudsman to negotiate with the outside world of the patient and with other professional peers. Finally, the supportive therapist must be able to accept personal limitations and the patient's limited psychological resources and to tolerate the often unrewarded efforts until small gains are made.

CORRECTIVE EMOTIONAL EXPERIENCE. The relationship between therapist and patient gives a therapist an opportunity to display behavior different from the destructive or unproductive behavior of a patient's parent. At times, such experiences seem to neutralize or reverse some effects of the parents' mistakes. If the patient had overly authoritarian parents, the therapist's friendly, flexible, nonjudgmental, nonauthoritarian—but at times firm and limit-setting—attitude gives the patient an opportunity to adjust to, be led by, and identify with a new parent figure. Franz Alexander described this process as a corrective emotional experience. It draws on elements of both psychoanalysis and psychoanalytic psychotherapy.

▲ 31.2 Brief Psychodynamic Psychotherapy

Brief psychodynamic psychotherapy is a time-limited treatment (10 to 12 sessions) that is based on psychoanalysis and psychodynamic theory. It is used to help persons with depression, anxiety, and posttraumatic stress disorder, among others. There are several methods, each having its own treatment technique and specific criteria for selecting patients; however, they are more similar than different. Brief psychodynamic psychotherapy has gained widespread popularity, partly because of the great pressure on health care professionals to contain treatment costs. It is also easier to evaluate treatment efficacy by comparing groups of persons who have had short-term therapy for mental illness with control groups than it is to measure the results of long-term psychotherapy. Thus, short-term therapies have been the subject of much research, especially on outcome measures, which have found them to be effective. Other short-term methods include interpersonal therapy, discussed in Section 31.11, and cognitive therapy, discussed in Section 31.9.

In 1946, Franz Alexander and Thomas French identified the basic characteristics of brief psychodynamic psychotherapy. They described a therapeutic experience designed to put patients at ease, to manipulate the transference, and to use trial interpretations flexibly. Alexander and French conceived psychotherapy as a corrective emotional experience capable of repairing traumatic events of the past and convincing patients that new ways of thinking, feeling, and behaving are possible. At about the same time, Eric Lindemann established a consultation service at the Massachusetts General Hospital in Boston for persons experiencing a crisis. He developed new treatment methods to deal with these situations and eventually applied these techniques to persons who were not in crisis but who were experiencing various kinds of emotional distress. Since then, the field has been influenced by many workers, including David Malan in England, Peter Sifneos in the United States, and Habib Davanloo in Canada.

TYPES

Brief Focal Psychotherapy (Tavistock–Malan)

Brief focal psychotherapy was originally developed in the 1950s by the Balint team at the Tavistock Clinic in London. Malan, a member of the team, reported the results of the therapy. Malan's selection criteria for treatment included eliminating absolute contraindications, rejecting patients for whom certain dangers seemed inevitable, clearly assessing patients' psychopathology, and determining patients' capacities to consider problems in emotional terms, face disturbing material, respond to interpretations, and endure the stress of the treatment. Malan found that high motivation invariably correlated with a successful outcome. Contraindications to treatment were serious suicide attempts, substance dependence, chronic alcohol abuse, incapacitating chronic obsessional symptoms, incapacitating chronic phobic symptoms, and gross destructive or self-destructive acting out.

Requirements and Techniques. In Malan's routine, therapists should identify the transference early and interpret it and the negative transference. They should then link the transferences to patients' relationships to their parents. Both patients and therapists should be willing to become deeply involved and to bear the ensuing tension. Therapists should formulate a circumscribed focus and set a termination date in advance, and patients should work through grief and anger about termination. An experienced therapist should allow about 20 sessions as an average length for the therapy; a trainee should allow about 30 sessions. Malan did not exceed 40 interviews with his patients.

Time-Limited Psychotherapy (Boston University–Mann)

A psychotherapeutic model of exactly 12 interviews focusing on a specified central issue was developed at Boston University by James Mann and his colleagues in the early 1970s. In contrast with Malan's emphasis on clear-cut selection and rejection criteria, Mann was not as explicit about the appropriate candidates for time-limited psychotherapy. Mann considered the major emphases of his theory to be determining a patient's central conflict reasonably correctly and exploring young persons' maturational crises with many psychological and somatic complaints. Mann's exceptions, similar to his rejection criteria, include persons with major depressive disorder that interferes with the treatment agreement, those with acute psychotic states, and desperate patients who need but cannot tolerate object relations.

Requirements and Techniques. Mann's technical requirements included strict limitation to 12 sessions, positive transference predominating early, specification and strict adherence to a central issue involving transference, positive identification, making separation a maturational event for patients, absolute prospect of termination to avoid development of dependence, clarification of present and past experiences and resistances, active therapists who support and encourage patients, and education of patients through direct information, reeducation, and manipulation. The conflicts likely to be encountered include independence versus dependence, activity versus passivity, unresolved or delayed grief, and adequate versus inadequate self-esteem.

Short-Term Dynamic Psychotherapy (McGill University–Davanloo)

As conducted by Davanloo at McGill University, short-term dynamic psychotherapy encompasses nearly all varieties of brief psychotherapy and crisis intervention. Patients treated in Davanloo's series are classified as those whose psychological conflicts are predominantly oedipal, those whose conflicts are not oedipal, and those whose conflicts have more than one focus. Davanloo also devised a specific psychotherapeutic technique for patients with severe, long-standing neurotic problems, specifically those with incapacitating obsessive-compulsive disorders and phobias.

Davanloo's selection criteria emphasize evaluating those ego functions of primary importance to psychotherapeutic work: the establishment of a psychotherapeutic focus; the psychodynamic formulation of the patient's psychological problems; the ability to interact emotionally with evaluators; a history of give-and-take relationships with a significant person in the patient's lives; the patient's ability to experience and tolerate anxiety, guilt, and depression; the patient's motivations for change, psychological mindedness, and ability to respond to interpretation and to link evaluators with persons in the present and past. Both Malan and Davanloo emphasized a patient's responses to interpretation as an important selection and prognostic criterion.

Requirements and Techniques. The highlights of Davanloo's psychotherapeutic approach are flexibility (therapists should adapt the technique to the patient's needs), control, the patient's regressive tendencies, active intervention to avoid having the patient develop overdependence on a therapist, and the patient's intellectual insight and emotional experiences in the transference. These emotional experiences become corrective as a result of the interpretation.

Short-Term Anxiety-Provoking Psychotherapy (Harvard University–Sifneos)

Sifneos developed short-term anxiety-provoking psychotherapy at the Massachusetts General Hospital in Boston during the 1950s. He used the following criteria for selection: a circumscribed chief complaint (implying a patient's ability to select one of a variety of problems to be given top priority and the patient's desire to resolve the problem in treatment), one meaningful or give-and-take relationship during early childhood, the ability to interact flexibly with an evaluator and to express feelings appropriately, above-average psychological sophistication (implying not only above-average intelligence but also an ability to respond to interpretations), a specific psychodynamic formulation (usually a set of psychological conflicts underlying a patient's difficulties and centering on an oedipal focus), a contract between therapist and patient to work on the specified focus and the formulation of minimal expectations of outcome, and good to excellent motivation for change, not just for symptom relief.

Requirements and Techniques. Treatment can be divided into four major phases: patient–therapist encounter, early therapy, height of treatment, and evidence of change and termination. Therapists use the following techniques during the four phases.

PATIENT–THERAPIST ENCOUNTER. A therapist establishes a working alliance by using the patient's quick rapport with, and positive feelings for, the therapist that appear in this phase. Judicious use of open-ended and forced-choice questions enables the therapist to outline and concentrate on a therapeutic focus. The therapist specifies the minimal expectations of outcome to be achieved by the therapy.

EARLY THERAPY. In transference, feelings for the therapist are clarified as soon as they appear, a technique that leads to the establishment of a true therapeutic alliance.

HEIGHT OF THE TREATMENT. Height of treatment emphasizes active concentration on the oedipal conflicts that have been chosen as the therapeutic focus; repeated use of anxiety-provoking questions and confrontations; avoidance of pregenital characterological issues, which the patient uses defensively to avoid dealing with the therapist's anxiety-provoking techniques; avoidance at all costs of a transference neurosis; repetitive demonstration of the patient's neurotic ways or maladaptive patterns of behavior; concentration on the anxiety-laden material, even before the defense mechanisms have been clarified; repeated demonstrations of parent-transference links by the use of properly timed interpretations based on material given by the patient; establishment of a corrective emotional experience; encouragement and support of the patient, who becomes anxious while struggling to understand the conflicts; new learning and problem-solving patterns; and repeated presentations and recapitulations of the patient's psychodynamics until the defense mechanisms used in dealing with oedipal conflicts are understood.

EVIDENCE OF CHANGE AND TERMINATION OF PSYCHOTHERAPY. The final phase of therapy emphasizes the tangible demonstration of change in the patient's behavior outside therapy, evidence that adaptive patterns of behavior are being used, and initiation of talk about terminating the treatment.

Overview and Results. The shared techniques of all the brief psychotherapies described here outdistance their differences. They share the therapeutic alliance or dynamic interaction between therapist and patient, the use of transference, the active interpretation of a therapeutic focus or central issue, the repetitive links between parental and transference issues, and the early termination of therapy. A certain type of patient receiving brief psychotherapy can benefit greatly from a practical working through of his or her nuclear conflict in the transference. Such patients can be recognized in advance through a process of dynamic interaction because they are responsive, motivated, and able to face disturbing feelings and because a circumscribed focus can be formulated for them. The more radical the technique in terms of transference, depth of interpretation, and the link to childhood, the more radical the therapeutic effects will be. For some disturbed patients, a carefully chosen partial focus can be therapeutically effective.

▲ 31.3 Group Psychotherapy, Combined Individual and Group Psychotherapy, and Psychodrama

Group psychotherapy is a treatment in which carefully selected persons who are emotionally ill meet in a group guided by a trained therapist and help one another effect personality change. By using a variety of technical maneuvers and theoretical constructs, the leader directs group members' interactions to bring about changes.

PATIENT SELECTION

To determine a patient's suitability for group psychotherapy, a therapist needs a great deal of information, which is gathered in a screening interview. The psychiatrist should take a psychiatric history and perform a mental status examination to obtain certain dynamic, behavioral, and diagnostic information.

Authority Anxiety

Those patients whose primary problem is their relationship to authority and who are extremely anxious in the presence of authority figures may do well in group therapy because they are more comfortable in a group and more likely will do better in a group than in a dyadic (one-to-one) setting. Patients with a great deal of authority anxiety may be blocked, anxious, resistant, and unwilling to verbalize thoughts and feelings in an individual setting, generally for fear of the therapist's censure or disapproval. Thus, they may welcome the suggestion of group psychotherapy to avoid the scrutiny of the dyadic situation. Conversely, if a patient reacts negatively to the suggestion of group psychotherapy or openly resists the idea, the therapist should consider the possibility that the patient has high peer anxiety.

Peer Anxiety

Patients with conditions such as borderline and schizoid personality disorders who have destructive relationships with their peer groups or who have been extremely isolated from peer group contact generally react negatively or anxiously when placed in a group setting. When such patients can work through their anxiety, however, group therapy can be beneficial.

Robert entered therapy seeking to understand why he was unable to maintain close or lasting relationships. A handsome and successful businessman, he had made a painful and courageous transition away from self-centered, dysfunctional parents early in his life. Although he made good initial impressions in his jobs, he was always puzzled and disappointed when his superiors gradually lost interest in him and his colleagues avoided him. In one-on-one therapy, he was charming and entertaining, but was easily injured by perceived narcissistic slights and would become angry and attacking. Group psychotherapy was suggested when his transference feelings remained intense and therapy was at a seeming impasse. Initially, Robert charmed the group and strove to be the center of attention. Visibly annoyed whenever he felt the group leader was paying more attention to other members, Robert was especially critical and hostile toward older people in the group and displayed little empathy for others. After repeated and forceful confrontations from the group about his antagonistic behavior, he gradually realized that he was repeating childhood patterns in his family of desperately seeking the attention of unloving parents and then entering violent rages when they lost interest. (Courtesy of Normund Wong, M.D.)

Diagnosis

The diagnosis of patients' disorders is important in determining the best therapeutic approach and in evaluating patients' motivations for treatment, capacities for change, and personality structure strengths and weaknesses. Few contraindications exist to group therapy. Antisocial patients generally do poorly in a heterogeneous group setting because they cannot adhere to group standards, but if the group is composed of other antisocial patients, they may respond better to peers than to perceived authority figures. Depressed patients profit from group therapy after they have established a trusting relationship with the therapist. Patients who are actively suicidal or severely depressed should not be treated solely in a group setting. Patients who are manic are disruptive but, once under pharmacological control, do well in the group setting. Patients who are delusional and who may incorporate the group into their delusional system should be excluded, as should patients who pose a physical threat to other members because of uncontrollable aggressive outbursts.

PREPARATION

Patients prepared by a therapist for a group experience tend to continue in treatment longer and report less initial anxiety than those who are not prepared. The preparation consists in having a therapist explain the procedure in as much detail as possible and answer the patient's questions before the first session.

Size

Group therapy has been successful with as few as 3 members and as many as 15, but most therapists consider 8 to 10 members the optimal size. Interaction may be insufficient with fewer members unless they are especially verbal, and with more than 10 members, the interaction may be too great for the members or the therapist to follow.

Frequency and Length of Sessions

Most group psychotherapists conduct group sessions once a week. Maintaining continuity in sessions is important. When there are alternate sessions, the group meets twice a week, once with and once without the therapist. Group sessions generally last anywhere from 1 to 2 hours, but the time limit should be constant.

Marathon groups were most popular in the 1970s but are much less common today. In time-extended therapy (marathon group therapy), the group meets continuously for 12 to 72 hours. Enforced interactional proximity and, during the longest time-extended sessions, sleep deprivation break down certain ego defenses, release affective processes, and theoretically promote open communication. Time-extended sessions, however, can be dangerous for patients with weak ego structures, such as persons with schizophrenia or borderline personality disorder.

Homogeneous versus Heterogeneous Groups

Most therapists believe that groups should be as heterogeneous as possible to ensure maximal interaction. Members with different diagnostic categories and varied behavioral patterns, from all races, social levels, and educational backgrounds, and of varying ages and both sexes should be brought together. Patients between the ages of 20 and 65 years can be included effectively in the same group. Age differences help in developing parent–child and brother–sister models, and patients have the opportunity to relive and rectify interpersonal difficulties that may have appeared insurmountable.

Both children and adolescents are best treated in groups composed mostly of persons in their own age groups. Some adolescent patients are capable of assimilating the material of an adult group, regardless of content, but they should not be deprived of a constructive peer experience that they might otherwise not have.

Open versus Closed Groups

Closed groups have a set number and composition of patients. If members leave, no new members are accepted. In open groups, membership is more fluid, and new members are taken on whenever old members leave.

Therapeutic Factors

Table 31.3–1 outlines 20 significant therapeutic factors that account for change in group psychotherapy.

ROLE OF THE THERAPIST

Although opinions differ about how active or passive a group therapist should be, the consensus is that the therapist's role is primarily facilitative. Ideally, the group members themselves are the primary source of cure and change. The climate produced by the therapist's personality is a potent agent of change. The therapist is more than an expert applying techniques; he or she exerts a personal influence that taps such variables as empathy, warmth, and respect.

INPATIENT GROUP PSYCHOTHERAPY

Group therapy is an important part of hospitalized patients' therapeutic experiences. Groups can be organized in many ways on a ward. In a community meeting, an entire inpatient unit meets with all the staff members (e.g., psychiatrists, psychologists, and nurses). In team meetings, 15 to 20 patients and staff members meet; a regular or small group composed of 8 to 10 patients may meet with 1 or 2 therapists, as in traditional group therapy. Although the goals of each group vary, they all have common purposes: to increase patients' awareness of themselves through their interactions with the other group members, who provide

feedback about their behavior; to provide patients with improved interpersonal and social skills; to help the members adapt to an inpatient setting; and to improve communication between patients and staff. In addition, one type of group meeting is attended only by inpatient hospital staff and is meant to improve communication among the staff members and to provide mutual support and encouragement in their day-to-day work with patients. Community meetings and team meetings are more helpful for dealing with patient treatment problems than they are for providing insight-oriented therapy, which is the province of the small-group therapy meeting.

SELF-HELP GROUPS

Self-help groups are composed of persons who are trying to cope with a specific problem or life crisis and are usually organized with a particular task in mind. Such groups do not attempt to explore individual psychodynamics in great depth or to change personality functioning significantly, but self-help groups have improved the emotional health and well-being of many persons.

A distinguishing characteristic of the self-help groups is their homogeneity. The members have the same disorders and share their experiences—good and bad, successful and unsuccessful—with one another. By so doing, they educate each other, provide mutual support, and alleviate the sense of alienation usually felt by persons drawn to this kind of group.

Self-help groups emphasize cohesion, which is exceptionally strong in these groups. Because the group members have similar problems and symptoms, they develop a strong emotional bond. Each group may have its unique characteristics, to which the members can attribute magical qualities of healing. Examples of self-help groups are Alcoholics Anonymous, Gamblers Anonymous, and Overeaters Anonymous.

The self-help group movement is in ascendancy. These groups meet their members' needs by providing acceptance, mutual support, and help in overcoming maladaptive patterns of behavior or states of feeling that traditional mental health and medical professionals have not generally dealt with successfully. Self-help groups and therapy groups have begun to converge. Self-help groups have enabled their members to give up patterns of unwanted behavior; therapy groups have helped their members understand why and how they got to be the way they were or are.

COMBINED INDIVIDUAL AND GROUP PSYCHOTHERAPY

In combined individual and group psychotherapy, patients see a therapist individually and also take part in group sessions. The therapist for the group and individual sessions is usually the same person. Groups can vary in size from 3 to 15 members, but the most helpful size is 8 to 10. Patients must attend all group sessions. Attendance at individual sessions is also important, and failure to attend either group or individual sessions should be examined as part of the therapeutic process.

Combined therapy is a particular treatment modality, not a system by which individual therapy is augmented by an occasional group session or a group therapy in which a participant meets alone with a therapist from time to time. Rather, it is an

Table 31.3–1
Twenty Therapeutic Factors in Group Psychotherapy

Factor	Definition
Abreaction	A process by which repressed material, particularly a painful experience or conflict, is brought back to consciousness. In the process, the person not only recalls but relives the material, which is accompanied by the appropriate emotional response; insight usually results from the experience.
Acceptance	The feeling of being accepted by other members of the group; differences of opinion are tolerated, and there is an absence of censure.
Altruism	The act of one member helping another; putting another person's need before one's own and learning that there is value in giving to others. The term was originated by Auguste Comte (1798–1857), and Sigmund Freud believed it was a major factor in establishing group cohesion and community feeling.
Catharsis	The expression of ideas, thoughts, and suppressed material that is accompanied by an emotional response that produces a state of relief in the patient.
Cohesion	The sense that the group is working together toward a common goal; also referred to as a sense of "we-ness"; believed to be the most important factor related to positive therapeutic effects.
Consensual validation	Confirmation of reality by comparing one's conceptualizations with those of other group members; interpersonal distortions are thereby corrected. The term was introduced by Harry Stack Sullivan; Trigant Burrow had used the phrase "consensual observation" to refer to the same phenomenon.
Contagion	The process in which the expression of emotion by one member stimulates the awareness of a similar emotion in another member.
Corrective familial experience	The group re-creates the family of origin for some members who can work through original conflicts psychologically through group interaction (e.g., sibling rivalry, anger toward parents).
Empathy	The capacity of a group member to put himself or herself into the psychological frame of reference of another group member and thereby understand his or her thinking, feeling, or behavior.
Identification	An unconscious defense mechanism in which the person incorporates the characteristics and the qualities of another person or object into his or her ego system.
Imitation	The conscious emulation or modeling of one's behavior after that of another (also called *role modeling*); also known as spectator therapy, as one patient learns from another.
Insight	Conscious awareness and understanding of one's own psychodynamics and symptoms of maladaptive behavior. Most therapists distinguish two types: (1) intellectual insight—knowledge and awareness without any changes in maladaptive behavior; (2) emotional insight—awareness and understanding leading to positive changes in personality and behavior.
Inspiration	The process of imparting a sense of optimism to group members; the ability to recognize that one has the capacity to overcome problem; also known as instillation of hope.
Interaction	The free and open exchange of ideas and feelings among group members; effective interaction is emotionally charged.
Interpretation	The process during which the group leader formulates the meaning or significance of a patient's resistance, defenses, and symbols; the result is that the patient has a cognitive framework within which to understand his or her behavior.
Learning	Patients acquire knowledge about new areas, such as social skills and sexual behavior; they receive advice, obtain guidance, and attempt to influence and are influenced by other group members.
Reality testing	Ability of the person to evaluate objectively the world outside the self; includes the capacity to perceive oneself and other group members accurately. *See also* Consensual validation.
Transference	Projection of feelings, thoughts, and wishes onto the therapist, who has come to represent an object from the patient's past. Such reactions, although perhaps appropriate for the condition prevailing in the patient's earlier life, are inappropriate and anachronistic when applied to the therapist in the present. Patients in the group may also direct such feelings toward one another, a process called *multiple transferences*.
Universalization	The awareness of the patient that he or she is not alone in having problems; others share similar complaints or difficulties in learning; the patient is not unique.
Ventilation	The expression of suppressed feelings, ideas, or events to other group members; the sharing of personal secrets that ameliorate a sense of sin or guilt (also referred to as *self-disclosure*).

ongoing plan in which meaningful integration of the group experience with the individual sessions yields reciprocal feedback to help form an integrated therapeutic experience. Although the one-to-one doctor–patient relationship makes a deep examination of the transference reaction possible for some patients, it may not provide other patients with the corrective emotional experiences necessary for therapeutic change. The group gives patients a variety of persons with whom they can have transferential reactions. In the microcosm of the group, patients can relive and work through familial and other important influences.

PSYCHODRAMA

Psychodrama is a method of group psychotherapy originated by the Viennese-born psychiatrist Jacob Moreno in which personality makeup, interpersonal relationships, conflicts, and emotional problems are explored by means of special dramatic methods. Therapeutic dramatization of emotional problems includes the protagonist or patient—the person who acts out problems with the help of auxiliary egos; persons who enact varying aspects of the patient; and the director, psychodramatist, or therapist—the person who guides those in the drama toward the acquisition of insight.

▲ 31.4 Family Therapy and Couples Therapy

FAMILY THERAPY

Family therapy can be defined as any psychotherapeutic endeavor that explicitly focuses on altering the interactions between or among family members and seeks to improve the functioning of the family as a unit, its subsystems, and/or the functioning of individual members of the family. Both family and couple therapy aim at some change in relational functioning. In most cases, they also aim at some other change, typically in the functioning of specific individuals in the family. Family therapy meant to heal a rift between parents and their adult children is an example of the use of family therapy centered on relationship goals. Family therapy aimed at increasing the family's coping with schizophrenia and at reducing the family's expressed emotion is an example of family therapy aimed at individual goals (in this case, the functioning of the person with schizophrenia), as well as family goals. In the early years of family therapy, change in the family system was seen as being sufficient to produce individual change. More recent treatments aimed at change in individuals, as well as in the family system, tend to supplement the interventions that focus on interpersonal relationships with specific strategies that focus on individual behavior.

Techniques

Initial Consultation. Family therapy is familiar enough to the general public for families with a high level of conflict to request it specifically. When the initial complaint is about an individual family member, however, pretreatment work may be needed. Underlying resistance to a family approach typically includes fears by parents that they will be blamed for their child's difficulties, that the entire family will be pronounced sick, that a spouse will object, and that open discussion of one child's misbehavior will have a negative influence on siblings. Refusal by an adolescent or young adult patient to participate in family therapy is frequently a disguised collusion with the fears of one or both parents.

Interview Technique. The special quality of a family interview springs from two important facts. A family comes to treatment with its history and dynamics firmly in place. To a family therapist, the established nature of the group, more than the symptoms, constitutes the clinical problem. Family members usually live together and, at some level, depend on one another for their physical and emotional well-being. Whatever occurs in the therapy session is known to all. Central principles of technique also derive from these facts. For example, the therapist must carefully channel the catharsis of anger by one family member toward another. The person who is the object of the anger will react to the attack, and the anger may escalate into violence and fracture relationships, with one or more member withdrawing from therapy. For another example, free associa-

tion is inappropriate in family therapy because it can encourage one person to dominate a session. Thus, therapists must always control and direct the family interview.

Frequency and Length of Treatment. Unless an emergency arises, sessions are usually held no more than once a week. Each session, however, may require as much as 2 hours. Long sessions can include an intermission to give the therapist time to organize the material and plan a response. A flexible schedule is necessary when geography or personal circumstances make it physically difficult for the family to get together. The length of treatment depends both on the nature of the problem and on the therapeutic model. Therapists who use problem-solving models exclusively may accomplish their goals in a few sessions, whereas therapists who use growth-oriented models may work with a family for years and may schedule sessions at long intervals.

Models of Intervention

Many models of family therapy exist, none of which is superior to the others. The particular model used depends on the training received, the context in which therapy occurs, and the personality of the therapist.

Psychodynamic-Experiential Models. Psychodynamic-experiential models emphasize individual maturation in the context of the family system and are free from unconscious patterns of anxiety and projection rooted in the past. Therapists seek to establish an intimate bond with each family member, and sessions alternate between the therapist's exchanges with the members and the members' exchanges with one another. Clarity of communication and honestly admitted feelings are given high priority. Toward this end, family members may be encouraged to change their seats, to touch each other, and to make direct eye contact. Their use of metaphor, body language, and parapraxes helps reveal the unconscious pattern of family relationships. The therapist may also use family sculpting, in which family members physically arrange one another in tableaus depicting their personal view of relationships, past or present. The therapist both interprets the living sculpture and modifies it in a way to suggest new relationships. In addition, the therapist's subjective responses to the family are given great importance. At appropriate moments, the therapist expresses these responses to the family to form yet another feedback loop of self-observation and change.

Bowen Model. Murray Bowen called his model *family systems*, but in the family therapy field it rightfully carries the name of its originator. The hallmark of the Bowen model is persons' differentiation from their family of origin—their ability to be their true selves in the face of familial or other pressures that threaten the loss of love or social position. Problem families are assessed on two levels: the degree of their enmeshment versus the degree of their ability to differentiate, and the analysis of emotional triangles in the problem for which they seek help.

An emotional triangle is defined as a three-party system (and many of these can exist within a family) arranged so that the closeness of two members expressed as either love or repetitive conflict tends to exclude a third. When the excluded third person attempts to join with one of the other two or when one of the involved parties shifts in the direction of the excluded one, emotional cross-currents are activated. The therapist's role is, first, to stabilize or shift the "hot" triangle—the one producing the presenting symptoms—and, second, to work with the most psychologically available family members, individually if necessary, to achieve sufficient personal differentiation so that the hot triangle does not recur. To preserve his or her neutrality in the family's triangles, the therapist minimizes emotional contact with family members.

Bowen also originated the genogram, a theoretical tool that is a historical survey of the family, going back several generations.

Structural Model.

In a structural model, families are viewed as single, interrelated systems assessed in terms of significant alliances and splits among family members, hierarchy of power (parents in charge of children), clarity and firmness of boundaries between the generations, and family tolerance for each other. The structural model uses concurrent individual and family therapy.

General Systems Model.

Based on general systems theory, a general systems model holds that families are systems and that every action in a family produces a reaction in one or more of its members. Families have external boundaries and internal rules. Every member is presumed to play a role (e.g., spokesperson, persecutor, victim, rescuer, symptom bearer, nurturer), which is relatively stable, but which member fills each role may change. Some families try to scapegoat one member by blaming him or her for the family's problems (the identified patient). If the identified patient improves, another family member may become the scapegoat. The general systems model overlaps with some of the other models presented, particularly the Bowen and structural models.

Goals

Family therapy has several goals: to resolve or reduce pathogenic conflict and anxiety within the matrix of interpersonal relationships; to enhance the perception and fulfillment by family members of one another's emotional needs; to promote appropriate role relationships between the sexes and generations; to strengthen the capacity of individual members and the family as a whole to cope with destructive forces inside and outside the surrounding environment; and to influence family identity and values so that members are oriented toward health and growth. The therapy ultimately aims to integrate families into the large systems of society, extended family, and community groups and social systems, such as schools, medical facilities, and social, recreational, and welfare agencies.

COUPLES (MARITAL) THERAPY

Couples or marital therapy is a form of psychotherapy designed psychologically to modify the interaction of two persons who are in conflict with each other over one parameter or a variety of parameters—social, emotional, sexual, or economic. In couples therapy, a trained person establishes a therapeutic contract with a patient-couple and, through definite types of communication, attempts to alleviate the disturbance, to reverse or change maladaptive patterns of behavior, and to encourage personality growth and development.

Types of Therapies

Individual Therapy.

In individual therapy, the partners may consult different therapists, who do not necessarily communicate with each other and indeed may not even know each other. The goal of treatment is to strengthen each partner's adaptive capacities. At times, only one of the partners is in treatment; in such cases, it is often helpful for the person who is not in treatment to visit the therapist. The visiting partner may give the therapist data about the patient that might otherwise be overlooked; overt or covert anxiety in the visiting partner as a result of change in the

patient can be identified and dealt with; irrational beliefs about treatment events can be corrected; and conscious or unconscious attempts by the partner to sabotage the patient's treatment can be examined.

Individual Couples Therapy.

In individual couples therapy, each partner is in therapy, which is either concurrent—with the same therapist—or collaborative—with each partner seeing a different therapist.

Conjoint Therapy.

In conjoint therapy—the most common treatment method in couples therapy—either one or two therapists treat the partners in joint sessions. Cotherapy with therapists of both sexes prevents a particular patient from feeling ganged up on when confronted by two members of the opposite sex.

Four-Way Session.

In a four-way session, each partner is seen by a different therapist, with regular joint sessions in which all four persons participate. A variation of the four-way session is the roundtable interview, developed by William Masters and Virginia Johnson for the rapid treatment of sexually dysfunctional couples. Two patients and two opposite-sex therapists meet regularly.

Group Psychotherapy.

Group therapy for couples allows a variety of group dynamics to affect the participants. Groups usually consist of three to four couples and one or two therapists. The couples identify with one another and recognize that others have similar problems; each gains support and empathy from fellow group members of the same or opposite sex. They explore sexual attitudes and have an opportunity to gain new information from their peer groups, and each receives specific feedback about his or her behavior, either negative or positive, which may have more meaning and be better assimilated coming from a neutral, nonspouse member, for example, than from the spouse or the therapist.

Combined Therapy.

Combined therapy refers to all or any of the preceding techniques used concurrently or in combination. Thus, a particular patient-couple may begin treatment with one or both partners in individual psychotherapy, continue in conjoint therapy with the partner, and terminate therapy after a course of treatment in a married couples group. The rationale for combined therapy is that no single approach to marital problems has been shown to be superior to another. A familiarity with a variety of approaches thus allows therapists a flexibility that provides maximal benefit for couples in distress.

Indications

Whatever the specific therapeutic technique, initiation of couples therapy is indicated when individual therapy has failed to resolve the relationship difficulties, when the onset of distress in one or both partners is clearly a relational problem, and when couples therapy is requested by a couple in conflict. Problems in communication between partners are a prime indication for couples therapy. In such instances, one spouse may be intimidated by the other, may become anxious when attempting to tell the other about thoughts or feelings, or may project unconscious expectations onto the other. The therapy is geared toward enabling each partner to see the other realistically.

Conflicts in one or several areas, such as the partners' sexual life, are also indications for treatment. Similarly, difficulty in establishing satisfactory social, economic, parental, or emotional roles implies that a couple needs help. Clinicians should evaluate all aspects of the marital relationship before attempting to treat only one problem, which could be a symptom of a pervasive marital disorder.

Contraindications

Contraindications for couples therapy include patients with severe forms of psychosis, particularly patients with paranoid elements and those in whom the marriage's homeostatic mechanism is a protection against psychosis, marriages in which one or both partners really want to divorce, and marriages in which one spouse refuses to participate because of anxiety or fear.

Goals

Nathan Ackerman defined the aims of couples therapy as follows: The goals of therapy for partner relational problems are to alleviate emotional distress and disability and to promote the levels of well-being of both partners together and of each as an individual. Ideally, therapists move toward these goals by strengthening the shared resources for problem solving, by encouraging the substitution of adequate controls and defenses for pathogenic ones, by enhancing both the immunity against the disintegrative effects of emotional upset and the complementarity of the relationship, and by promoting the growth of the relationship and of each partner.

Part of a therapist's task is to persuade each partner in the relationship to take responsibility in understanding the psychodynamic makeup of personality. Each person's accountability for the effects of behavior on his or her own life, the life of the partner, and the lives of others in the environment is emphasized, and the result is often a deep understanding of the problems that created the marital discord.

Couples therapy does not ensure the maintenance of any marriage or relationship. Indeed, in certain instances, it may show the partners that they are in a nonviable union that should be dissolved. In these cases, couples may continue to meet with therapists to work through the difficulties of separating and obtaining a divorce, a process that has been called *divorce therapy*.

▲ 31.5 Dialectical Behavior Therapy

Dialectical behavior therapy (DBT) is a type of psychotherapy that was originally developed for chronically self-injurious patients with borderline personality disorder and parasuicidal behavior. In recent years, its use has extended to other forms of mental illness. The method is eclectic, drawing on concepts derived from supportive, cognitive, and behavioral therapies. Some elements can be traced to Franz Alexander's view of therapy as a corrective emotional experience, and other elements derive from certain Eastern philosophical schools (e.g., Zen).

Patients are seen weekly, with the goal of improving interpersonal skills and decreasing self-destructive behavior using techniques involving advice, metaphor, storytelling, and confrontation, among others. Patients with borderline personality disorder especially are helped to deal with the ambivalent feelings that are characteristic of the disorder. Marsha Linehan, Ph.D., developed the treatment method, based on her theory that such patients cannot identify emotional experiences and cannot tolerate frustration or rejection. As with other behavioral approaches, DBT assumes all behavior (including thoughts and feelings) is learned and that patients with borderline personality disorder behave in ways that reinforce or even reward their behavior, regardless of how maladaptive it is.

FUNCTIONS OF DIALECTICAL BEHAVIOR THERAPY

As described by its originator, there are five essential "functions" in treatment: (1) to enhance and expand the patient's repertoire of skillful behavioral patterns; (2) to improve patient motivation to change by reducing reinforcement of maladaptive behavior, including dysfunctional cognition and emotion; (3) to ensure that new behavioral patterns generalize from the therapeutic to the natural environment; (4) to structure the environment so that effective behaviors, rather than dysfunctional behaviors, are reinforced; and (5) to enhance the motivation and capabilities of the therapist so that effective treatment is rendered.

The four modes of treatment in DBT are as follows: (1) group skills training, (2) individual therapy, (3) phone consultations, and (4) consultation team. Other ancillary treatments used are pharmacotherapy and hospitalization, when needed. These are described in the following.

Group Skills Training

In group format, patients learn specific behavioral, emotional, cognitive, and interpersonal skills. Unlike traditional group therapy, observations about others in the group are discouraged. Rather, a didactic approach, using specific exercises taken from a skills training manual, is used, many of which are geared to control emotional dysregulation and impulsive behavior.

Individual Therapy

Sessions in DBT are held weekly, generally for 50 to 60 minutes, in which skills learned during group training are reviewed and life events in the previous week examined. Particular attention is paid to episodes of pathological behavioral patterns that could have been corrected if learned skills had been put into effect. Patients are encouraged to record their thoughts, feelings, and behavior on diary cards which are analyzed in the session.

Telephone Consultation

Therapists are available for phone consultation 24 hours per day. Patients are encouraged to call when they feel themselves heading toward some crisis that might lead to injurious behavior to themselves or others. Calls are intended to be brief and usually last about 10 minutes.

Consultation Team

Therapists meet in weekly meetings to review their work with their patients. By doing so, they provide support for one another and maintain motivation in their work. The meetings enable them to compare techniques used and to validate those that are most effective.

RESULTS

A study evaluating the effect of DBT for patients with borderline personality disorder found that such therapy was positive. Patients had a low dropout rate from treatment; the incidence of parasuicidal behaviors declined; self-report of angry affect decreased; and social adjustment and work performance improved. The method is now being applied to other disorders, including substance abuse, eating disorders, schizophrenia, and posttraumatic stress disorder.

▲ 31.6 Genetic Counseling

Genetic counseling is a process that provides information (medical, technical, and probabilistic) to the patient (and family) at risk for developing a specific disorder. The provision of information occurs in conjunction with aid to help them to adapt emotionally and psychologically to the diagnosis (or threat of it), thus facilitating informed decision making. The process aims to minimize distress, to increase one's feeling of personal control, and to facilitate informed decision making.

GENETICS AND MENTAL HEALTH

Disorders can recur in families for many reasons, including the functioning of genes (single genes vs. polygenic), shared environmental exposures, a combination of genetic and environmental factors (multifactorial), and cultural transmission. *Single-gene disorders* are caused by defects in one particular gene, and they often have simple and predictable inheritance patterns. By contrast, most psychiatric disorders are *multifactorial* in etiology, influenced by multiple genes as well as environmental factors, making them more difficult to predict.

THE GENETIC COUNSELING PROCESS

The topics that are most often included in counseling sessions are a definition of the disorder and its natural history; explanation of the possible modes of inheritance and their associated recurrence risks; options for medical management, prevention, or treatment; and the availability of genetic testing and the associated risks, benefits, and limitations. The provision of understandable and meaningful information, coupled with empathy, compassion, and sensitivity, moves a simple educational effort to a multifaceted genetic counseling encounter.

The collection and review of the history with the patient might elicit or recall intense feelings of sadness, guilt, anxiety, or anger. Furthermore, the graphic presentation of the family history may bring to light a more concrete realization of an individual's risks; therefore, attention to the patient's affect is important throughout the process.

A couple in their mid 30s contacts a local psychiatrist regarding the woman's diagnosis of bipolar disorder and her use of lithium carbonate during her recently recognized first pregnancy. She has not been able to function well without the medication during her 5-year history with the disorder. They are concerned about the use of medication during the pregnancy. In addition, the husband expressed concern about his partner's family history of other psychiatric disorders, such as schizophrenia. As the family history unfolded, the husband learned of the diagnosis of Huntington's disease in his wife's first cousin.

Patients with Huntington's disease develop significant personality changes (72 percent), affective psychosis (20 to 90 percent), or schizophrenic psychosis (4 to 12 percent). After a description of clinical features associated with Huntington's disease, the couple realized that the woman's symptoms might be presenting signs of Huntington's disease. In this particular case, the woman developed significant anxiety that worsened in response to her husband's anger regarding the discovery.

Issues recognized by the psychiatrist and needing attention in this case include the teratogenic effects of the lithium carbonate, increased risk for chromosomal anomalies because of maternal age, and an assessment of recurrence risks for mental illness and Huntington's disease. Anticipation of a wide variety of emotions may prepare the psychiatrist to assist the couple in their initial adaptation to the various identified risks.

ETHICAL, LEGAL, AND SOCIAL CONSIDERATIONS

Certain individuals and families may experience significant levels of stigma associated with the identification of a genetic disorder, a situation already familiar to individuals and families with mental illness. The added knowledge of a hereditary component may heighten stigmatization. Conversely, having an identified, biological basis may supplant current public perceptions that mental illness is somehow a personal or family failure in moral, spiritual, or attitudinal perspectives.

Questions frequently arise about the privacy of an individual's genetic information, the ability of employers or insurers to access such information and potentially use it against the person by denying insurance, raising rates to unreasonable levels, or denying jobs, and a host of other possible concerns. No overarching federal laws comprehensively protect citizens of the United States from the potential of these abuses, although significant efforts are continuing in this regard. The status of existing and proposed state and federal laws can be reviewed through the Web site of the National Human Genome Research Institute (http://www.genome.gov).

▲ 31.7 Biofeedback

Biofeedback involves the recording and display of small changes in the physiological levels of a feedback parameter. The display can be visual, such as a big meter or a bar of lights, or auditory. Patients are instructed to change the levels of the parameter, using the feedback from the display as a guide. Biofeedback is based on the idea that the autonomic nervous system can come under voluntary control through operant conditioning. Biofeedback can be used by itself or in combination with relaxation. For example, patients with urinary incontinence use biofeedback alone to regain control over the pelvic musculature. Biofeedback is also used in the rehabilitation of neurological disorders. The benefits of biofeedback may be augmented by the relaxation that patients are trained to facilitate.

THEORY

Neal Miller demonstrated the medical potential of biofeedback by showing that the normally involuntary autonomic nervous system can be operantly conditioned by use of appropriate feedback. By means of instruments, patients acquire information about the status of involuntary biological functions, such as skin temperature and electrical conductivity, muscle tension, blood pressure, heart rate, and brain wave activity. Patients then learn to regulate one or more of these biological states that affect symptoms. For example, a person can learn to raise the temperature of his or her hands to reduce the frequency of migraines, palpitations, or angina pectoris. Presumably, patients lower the sympathetic activation and voluntarily self-regulate arterial smooth muscle vasoconstrictive tendencies.

METHODS

Instrumentation

The feedback instrument used depends on the patient and the specific problem. The most effective instruments are the electromyogram (EMG), which measures the electrical potentials of muscle fibers; the electroencephalogram (EEG), which measures alpha waves that occur in relaxed states; the galvanic skin response (GSR) gauge, which shows decreased skin conductivity during a relaxed state; and the thermistor, which measures skin temperature (which drops during tension because of peripheral vasoconstriction). Patients are attached to one of the instruments that measures a physiological function and translates the measurement into an audible or visual signal that patients use to gauge their responses. For example, in the treatment of bruxism, an EMG is attached to the masseter muscle. The EMG emits a high tone when the muscle is contracted and a low tone when it is at rest. Patients can learn to alter the tone to indicate relaxation. Patients receive feedback about the masseter muscle, the tone reinforces the learning, and the condition ameliorates, with all of these events interacting synergistically.

Many less-specific clinical applications (e.g., treating insomnia, dysmenorrhea, and speech problems; improving athletic performance; treating volitional disorders; achieving altered states of consciousness; managing stress; and supplementing psychotherapy for anxiety associated with somatoform disorders) use a model in which frontalis muscle EMG biofeedback is combined with thermal biofeedback and verbal instructions in progressive relaxation.

Relaxation Therapy

Muscle relaxation is used as a component of treatment programs (e.g., systematic desensitization) or as treatment in its own right (relaxation therapy). Relaxation is characterized by (1) immobility of the body, (2) control over the focus of attention, (3) low muscle tone, and (4) cultivation of a specific frame of mind, described as contemplative, nonjudgmental, detached, or mindful. Relaxing breathing exercises are often helpful for patients with panic disorder, especially that considered to be related to

hyperventilation. In the treatment of patients with anxiety disorders, relaxation can serve as an occasion-setting stimulus (i.e., as a context of safety in which other specific intervention can be confidently tried).

Applied Tension

Applied tension is a technique that is the opposite of relaxation; applied tension can be used to counteract the fainting response. The treatment extends over four sessions. In the first session, patients learn to tense the muscles of the arms, legs, and torso for 10 to 15 seconds (as if they were bodybuilders). The tension is maintained long enough for a sensation of warmth to develop in the face. The patients then release the tension but do not progress to a state of relaxation. The maneuver is repeated five times at half-minute intervals. This method can be augmented with feedback of the patient's blood pressure during the muscle contraction; increased blood pressure suggests that appropriate muscle tension was achieved. The patients continue to practice the technique five times a day. An adverse effect of treatment that sometimes develops is headache. In this case, the intensity of the muscle contraction and the frequency of treatment are reduced.

RESULTS

Biofeedback, progressive relaxation, and applied tension have been shown to be effective treatment methods for a broad range of disorders. They form one basis of behavioral medicine in which the patient changes (or learns how to change) behavior that contributes to illness. They form a basis on which many complementary and alternative medical procedures are effective (e.g., yoga and reiki) in which relaxation is an important component. Relaxation also informs more-mainstream treatments, such as hypnosis.

▲ 31.8 Behavior Therapy

The term *behavior* in *behavior therapy* refers to a person's observable actions and responses. Behavior therapy involves changing the behavior of patients to reduce dysfunction and to improve quality of life. Behavior therapy includes a methodology, referred to as *behavior analysis*, for the strategic selection of behaviors to change and a technology to bring about behavior change, such as modifying antecedents or consequences or giving instructions. Behavior therapy has not only influenced mental health care, but, under the rubric of behavioral medicine, it has also made inroads into other medical specialties.

HISTORY

As early as the 1920s, scattered reports about the application of learning principles to the treatment of behavioral disorders began to appear, but they had little effect on the mainstream of psychiatry and clinical psychology. Not until the 1960s did behavior therapy emerge as a systematic and comprehensive approach to psychiatric (behavioral) disorders; at that time, it arose independently on three continents. Joseph Wolpe and his colleagues in Johannesburg, South Africa, used Pavlovian techniques to produce and eliminate experimental neuroses in cats. From this research, Wolpe developed systematic desensitization, the prototype of many current behavioral procedures for the treatment of maladaptive anxiety produced by identifiable stimuli in the environment. At about the same time, a group at the Institute of Psychiatry of the University of London, particularly Hans Jurgen Eysenck and M. B. Shapiro, stressed the importance of an empirical, experimental approach to understanding and treating individual patients, using controlled, single-case experimental paradigms and modern learning theory. The third origin of behavior therapy was work inspired by the research of Harvard psychologist B. F. Skinner. Skinner's students began to apply his operant-conditioning technology, developed in animal-conditioning laboratories, to human beings in clinical settings.

SYSTEMATIC DESENSITIZATION

Developed by Wolpe, systematic desensitization is based on the behavioral principle of counterconditioning, whereby a person overcomes maladaptive anxiety elicited by a situation or an object by approaching the feared situation gradually, in a psychophysiological state that inhibits anxiety. In systematic desensitization, patients attain a state of complete relaxation and are then exposed to the stimulus that elicits the anxiety response. The negative reaction of anxiety is inhibited by the relaxed state, a process called *reciprocal inhibition*. Rather than using actual situations or objects that elicit fear, patients and therapists prepare a graded list or hierarchy of anxiety-provoking scenes associated with a patient's fears. The learned relaxation state and the anxiety-provoking scenes are systematically paired in treatment. Thus, systematic desensitization consists of three steps: relaxation training, hierarchy construction, and desensitization of the stimulus.

Relaxation Training

Relaxation produces physiological effects opposite to those of anxiety: slow heart rate, increased peripheral blood flow, and neuromuscular stability. A variety of relaxation methods have been developed. Some, such as yoga and Zen, have been known for centuries. Most methods use so-called progressive relaxation, developed by the psychiatrist Edmund Jacobson. Patients relax major muscle groups in a fixed order, beginning with the small muscle groups of the feet and working cephalad or vice versa. Some clinicians use hypnosis to facilitate relaxation or use tape-recorded exercise to allow patients to practice relaxation on their own. Mental imagery is a relaxation method in which patients are instructed to imagine themselves in a place associated with pleasant relaxed memories. Such images allow patients to enter a relaxed state or experience (as Herbert Benson termed it) the *relaxation response*.

The physiological changes that take place during relaxation are the opposite of those induced by the adrenergic stress responses that are part of many emotions. Muscle tension, respiration rate, heart rate, blood pressure, and skin conductance decrease. Finger temperature and blood flow to the finger usually increase. Relaxation increases respiratory heart rate variability, an index of parasympathetic tone.

Hierarchy Construction

When constructing a hierarchy, clinicians determine all the conditions that elicit anxiety, and then patients create a hierarchy list of 10 to 12 scenes in order of increasing anxiety. For example, an acrophobic hierarchy may begin with a patient's imagining standing near a window on the second floor and end with being on the roof of a 20-story building, leaning on a guard rail and looking straight down.

Desensitization of the Stimulus

In the final step, called *desensitization*, patients proceed systematically through the list from the least to the most anxiety-provoking scene while in a deeply relaxed state. The rate at which patients progress through the list is determined by their responses to the stimuli. When patients can vividly imagine the most anxiety-provoking scene of the hierarchy with equanimity, they experience little anxiety in the corresponding real-life situation.

Adjunctive Use of Drugs

Clinicians have used various drugs to hasten relaxation, but drugs should be used cautiously and only by clinicians trained and experienced in potential adverse effects. Either the ultrarapidly acting barbiturate sodium methohexital (Brevital) or diazepam (Valium) is given intravenously in subanesthetic doses. If the procedural details are followed carefully, almost all patients find the procedure pleasant, with few unpleasant side effects. The advantages of pharmacological desensitization are that preliminary training in relaxation can be shortened, almost all patients can relax adequately, and the treatment itself seems to proceed more rapidly than without the drugs.

Indications

Systematic desensitization works best in cases of a clearly identifiable anxiety-provoking stimulus. Phobias, obsessions, compulsions, and certain sexual disorders have been treated successfully with this technique.

THERAPEUTIC-GRADED EXPOSURE

Therapeutic-graded exposure is similar to systematic desensitization, except that relaxation training is not involved and treatment is usually carried out in a real-life context. This means that the individual must be brought in contact with (i.e., be exposed to) the warning stimulus to learn firsthand that no dangerous consequences will ensue. Exposure is graded according to a hierarchy. Patients afraid of cats, for example, might progress from looking at a picture of a cat to holding one.

FLOODING

Flooding (sometimes called *implosion*) is similar to graded exposure in that it involves exposing the patient to the feared object in vivo; however, there is no hierarchy. Flooding is based on the premise that escaping from an anxiety-provoking experience reinforces the anxiety through conditioning. Thus, clinicians can extinguish the anxiety and prevent the conditioned avoidance behavior by not allowing patients to escape the situation. Clinicians encourage patients to confront feared situations directly, without a gradual buildup, as in systematic desensitization or graded exposure. No relaxation exercises are used, as in systematic desensitization. Patients experience fear, which gradually subsides after a time. The success of the procedure depends on having patients remain in the fear-generating situation until they are calm and feel a sense of mastery. Prematurely withdrawing from the situation or prematurely terminating the fantasized scene is equivalent to an escape, which then reinforces both the conditioned anxiety and the avoidance behavior and produces the opposite of the desired effect. In a variant called *imaginal flooding*, the feared object or situation is confronted only in the imagination, not in real life. Many patients refuse flooding because of the psychological discomfort involved. It is also contraindicated when intense anxiety would be hazardous to a patient (e.g., those with heart disease or fragile psychological adaptation). The technique works best with specific phobias. An example of in vivo flooding follows.

The patient was a 33-year-old woman with social fears of eating in public. In particular, she was afraid of being observed by others when chewing and swallowing, particularly at dinner parties. A contrived situation was arranged in which the patient came to the session with a prepared meal and drink. She entered a conference room in which five persons in professional attire were already seated along a table. The patient was instructed to eat her meal in front of these individuals. Between bites, she was instructed to look at them often, and they had been instructed to avoid staring contests. She was not to distract herself from her anxiety symptoms. She was to eat her meal slowly, paying attention to the behavior of the observers and to her anxiety symptoms (e.g., dry mouth or difficulty swallowing). No conversation between the patient and observers was permitted. The observers would look at her and observe her chewing and swallowing behaviors, at times writing comments in a notebook. Occasionally, observers would communicate by whispering to each other, exchanging written notes, or giving knowing glances and smiles.

The only other communication occurred between the patient and therapist, and this was limited to the patient providing her subjective units of distress rating. The session lasted 90 minutes. **Note:** this situation may seem quite traumatizing. Because the exposure session is long and continues until ratings decline, the patient becomes desensitized. (Courtesy of Rolf G. Jacob, M.D., and William H. Pelham, M.D.)

PARTICIPANT MODELING

In participant modeling, patients learn a new behavior by imitation, primarily by observation, without having to perform the behavior until they feel ready. Just as irrational fears can be acquired by learning, they can be unlearned by observing a fearless model confront the feared object. The technique has been useful with phobic children who are placed with other children of their own age and sex who approach the feared object or situation. With adults, a therapist may describe the feared activity in a calm manner that a patient can identify. Or, the therapist may act out the process of mastering the feared activity with a patient. Sometimes, a hierarchy of activities is established, with the least anxiety-provoking activity being dealt with first. The participant-modeling technique has been used successfully with agoraphobia by having a therapist accompany a patient into the feared situation. In a variant of the procedure called *behavior rehearsal*, real-life problems are acted out under a therapist's observation or direction.

The following is a self-report by a patient with a contamination phobia, who is afraid to touch objects for fear of being infected or contaminated. She describes her reactions.

[The therapist] started touching everything very slowly. I was told to follow behind and touch everything she touched. It was like we were spreading the contamination. She touched doorknobs, light switches, walls, pictures, and woodwork. She opened drawers in each bedroom and touched the contents. She opened closets and touched clothes hanging on the rods. She touched the towels and sheets in the linen closet. She went through the children's rooms, touching dolls, stuffed animals, models, Star Wars figures, Transformers, and books.

[The therapist] kept talking to me quietly and calmly all the time we went along. I had been anxious when we started, but as we continued, my anxiety level decreased. At one point, when I had begun to think the worst was over, she pointed to the attic door and said we were going inside. I said, "No, that's where the mice were." She told me I didn't want to have a place in my home that was off limits. I agreed but became very anxious. It was very hard for me to go inside. I began touching the boxes too, but I was very upset. Then, she put her hands down on the floor and wanted me to do the same. I said, "I can't. I just can't." Julie said, "Yes you can."

[The therapist] spent several hours with me that day. Before she left, she made a list of things for me to do by myself. Twice a day I was to go through the house touching everything the way she had done with me. I was to invite a friend of mine who had a pet to come and visit and also friends of my children who had pets. (Courtesy of Rolf G. Jacob, M.D., and William H. Pelham, M.D.)

PARADOXICAL THERAPY

With the paradoxical therapy approach, which evolved from the work of Gregory Bateson, a therapist suggests that the patient intentionally engage in the unwanted behavior (called the paradoxical injunction) and, for example, avoid a phobic object or perform a compulsive ritual. Although paradoxical therapy and the use of paradoxical injunctions seem to be counterintuitive, the therapy can create new insights for some patients. It is used in individual therapy as well as in family therapy.

Victor Frankl formulated a related approach called paradoxical intentional therapy in which the patient, in thought, exaggerates his or her symptom. A person with a fear of public speaking for example, imagines collapsing at the podium and becomes desensitized to anxiety as a result.

EXPOSURE TO STIMULI PRESENTED IN VIRTUAL REALITY

Advances in computer technology have made it possible to present environmental cues in virtual reality for exposure treatment. Beneficial effects have been reported with virtual reality exposure of patients with height phobia, fear of flying, spider phobia, and claustrophobia. Much experimental work is being done in the field. One model uses an avatar of the patient walking through a crowded supermarket filled with other avatars (including one of the therapist) as a way of conquering agoraphobia.

ASSERTIVENESS TRAINING

Assertive behavior enables a person to act in his or her best interest, to stand up for himself or herself without undue anxiety, to express honest feelings comfortably, and to exercise personal rights without denying the rights of others.

Two types of situations frequently call for assertive behaviors: (1) setting limits on pushy friends or relatives and (2) commercial situations, such as countering a sales pitch or being persistent when returning defective merchandise. Early assertiveness training programs tended to define specific behaviors as assertive or nonassertive. For example, individuals were encouraged to assert themselves if somebody got in front of them in a supermarket checkout line. Increasing attention is now given to context, that is, what would be assertive behavior in this situation depends on circumstances.

AVERSION THERAPY

When a noxious stimulus (punishment) is presented immediately after a specific behavioral response, theoretically, the response is eventually inhibited and extinguished. Many types of noxious stimuli are used: electric shocks, substances that induce vomiting, corporal punishment, and social disapproval. The negative stimulus is paired with the behavior, which is thereby suppressed. The unwanted behavior may disappear after a series of such sequences. Aversion therapy has been used for alcohol abuse, paraphilias, and other behaviors with impulsive or compulsive qualities, but this therapy is controversial for many reasons. For example, punishment does not always lead to the expected decreased response and can sometimes be positively reinforcing. Aversion therapy has been used with good effect in some cultures in the treatment of opioid addicts.

EYE MOVEMENT DESENSITIZATION AND REPROCESSING

Saccadic eye movements are rapid oscillations of the eyes that occur when a person tracks an object that is moved back and forth across the line of vision. A few studies have demonstrated that inducing saccades while a person is imagining or thinking about an anxiety-producing event can yield a positive thought or image that results in decreased anxiety. Eye movement desensitization and reprocessing has been used in posttraumatic stress disorders and phobias.

POSITIVE REINFORCEMENT

When a behavioral response is followed by a generally rewarding event, such as food, avoidance of pain, or praise, it tends to be strengthened and to occur more frequently than before the reward. This principle has been applied in a variety of situations. On inpatient hospital wards, patients with mental disorder receive a reward for performing a desired behavior, such as tokens that they can use to purchase luxury items or certain privileges.

The process, known as token economy, has successfully altered behavior.

RESULTS

Behavior therapy has been used successfully for a variety of disorders and can be easily taught. It requires less time than other therapies and is less expensive to administer. Although useful for circumscribed behavioral symptoms, the method cannot be used to treat global areas of dysfunction (e.g., neurotic conflicts, personality disorders). Controversy continues between behaviorists and psychoanalysts, which is epitomized by Eysenck's statement: "Learning theory regards neurotic symptoms as simply learned habits; there is no neurosis underlying the symptoms, but merely the symptom itself. Get rid of the symptom and you have eliminated the neurosis." Analytically oriented theorists have criticized behavior therapy by noting that simple symptom removal can lead to symptom substitution: When symptoms are not viewed as consequences of inner conflicts and the core cause of the symptoms is not addressed or altered, the result is the production of new symptoms. Whether this occurs remains open to question, however.

BEHAVIORAL MEDICINE

Behavioral medicine uses the concepts and methods described previously to treat a variety of physical diseases. Emphasis is placed on the role of stress and its influence on the body, particularly on the endocrine system. Attempts to relieve stress are made with the expectation that either the disease state will lessen or the patient's ability to tolerate the disease state will strengthen.

One study measured the effects of a behavioral medicine program on symptoms of acquired immunodeficiency syndrome. The treatment group received training in biofeedback, guided imagery, and hypnosis. Results included significant decreases in fever, fatigue, pain, headache, nausea, and insomnia; and increased vigor and hardiness.

Another study of immunological and psychological outcomes of a stress reduction program was conducted with patients with malignant melanoma. Results included significant increases in large granular lymphocytes and natural killer (NK) cells, along with indications of increased NK cytotoxic activity. Also noted were significantly lower levels of psychological distress and higher levels of positive coping methods in comparison with patients who were not part of the group.

Many other applications of behavior therapy are used in medical care. In general, most patients feel they benefit from such interventions, especially in their ability to cope with chronic illness. For a further discussion of behavioral medicine see Chapter 24, Psychosomatic Medicine.

▲ 31.9 Cognitive Therapy

Cognitive therapy is a short-term, structured therapy that uses active collaboration between patient and therapist to achieve its therapeutic goals, which are oriented toward current problems and their resolution. Cognitive therapy is used with depression, panic disorder, obsessive-compulsive disorder, personality disorders, and somatoform disorders. Therapy is usually conducted on an individual basis, although group methods are sometimes helpful. A therapist may also prescribe drugs in conjunction with therapy.

The treatment of depression can serve as a paradigm of the cognitive approach.

Cognitive therapy assumes that perception and experiencing, in general, are active processes that involve both inspective and introspective data. The patient's cognitions represent a synthesis of internal and external stimuli. The way in which persons appraise a situation is generally evident in their cognitions (thoughts and visual images).

Those cognitions constitute their stream of consciousness or phenomenal field, which reflects their configuration of themselves, their world, their past, and their future.

Alterations in the content of their underlying cognitive structures affect their affective state and behavioral pattern. Through psychological therapy, patients can become aware of their cognitive distortions. Correction of faulty dysfunctional constructs can lead to clinical improvement.

COGNITIVE THEORY OF DEPRESSION

According to the cognitive theory of depression, cognitive dysfunctions are the core of depression, and affective and physical changes and other associated features of depression are consequences of cognitive dysfunctions. For example, apathy and low energy result from a person's expectation of failure in all areas. Similarly, paralysis of will stems from a person's pessimism and feelings of hopelessness. From a cognitive perspective, depression can be explained by the cognitive triad, which explains that negative thoughts are about the self, the world, and the future.

The goal of therapy is to alleviate depression and to prevent its recurrence by helping patients to identify and test negative cognitions, to develop alternative and more flexible schemas, and to rehearse both new cognitive and behavioral responses. Changing the way a person thinks can alleviate the psychiatric disorder.

STRATEGIES AND TECHNIQUES

Therapy is relatively short and lasts about 25 weeks. If a patient does not improve in this time, the diagnosis should be reevaluated. Maintenance therapy can be carried out over years. As with other psychotherapies, therapists' attributes are important to successful therapy. Therapists must exude warmth, understand the life experience of each patient, and be genuine and honest with themselves and with their patients. They must be able to relate skillfully and interactively with their patients. Cognitive therapists set the agenda at the beginning of each session, assign homework to be performed between sessions, and teach new skills. Therapist and patient collaborate actively. The three components of cognitive therapy are didactic aspects, cognitive techniques, and behavioral techniques.

Didactic Aspects

The therapy's didactic aspects include explaining to patients the cognitive triad, schemas, and faulty logic. Therapists must tell patients that they will formulate hypotheses together and test them over the course of the treatment. Cognitive therapy requires a full explanation of the relationship between depression and thinking, affect, and behavior, as well as the rationale for all aspects of treatment. This explanation contrasts with psychoanalytically oriented therapies, which require little explanation.

Cognitive Techniques

The therapy's cognitive approach includes four processes: eliciting automatic thoughts, testing automatic thoughts, identifying maladaptive underlying assumptions, and testing the validity of maladaptive assumptions.

Eliciting Automatic Thoughts.   Automatic thoughts, also called cognitive distortions, are cognitions that intervene between external events and a person's emotional reaction to the event. For example, the belief that "people will laugh at me when they see how badly I bowl" is an automatic thought that occurs to someone who has been asked to go bowling and responds negatively. Another example is the thought, "She doesn't like me," when someone passes in the hall without saying, "Hello." Every psychopathological disorder has its own specific cognitive profile of distorted thought, which, if known, provides a framework for specific cognitive interventions.

Testing Automatic Thoughts.   Acting as a teacher, a therapist helps a patient test the validity of automatic thoughts. The goal is to encourage the patient to reject inaccurate or exaggerated automatic thoughts after careful examination. Patients often blame themselves when things that are outside their control go awry. The therapist reviews the entire situation with the patient and helps reassign the blame or cause of the unpleasant events. Generating alternative explanations for events is another way of undermining inaccurate and distorted automatic thoughts.

Identifying Maladaptive Assumptions.   As the patient and therapist continue to identify automatic thoughts, patterns usually become apparent. The patterns represent rules or maladaptive general assumptions that guide a patient's life. Samples of such rules are "In order to be happy, I must be perfect" and "If anyone doesn't like me, I'm not lovable." Such rules inevitably lead to disappointments and failure and, ultimately, to depression.

Testing the Validity of Maladaptive Assumptions. Testing the accuracy of maladaptive assumptions is similar to testing the validity of automatic thoughts. In a particularly effective test, therapists ask patients to defend the validity of their assumptions. For example, patients may state that they should always work up to their potential, and a therapist may ask, "Why is that so important to you?"

BEHAVIORAL TECHNIQUES

Behavioral and cognitive techniques go hand in hand; behavioral techniques test and change maladaptive and inaccurate cognitions. The overall purposes of such techniques are to help patients understand the inaccuracy of their cognitive assumptions and learn new strategies and ways of dealing with issues.

Among the behavioral techniques in cognitive therapy are scheduling activities, mastery and pleasure, graded task assignments, cognitive rehearsal, self-reliance training, role-playing, and diversion techniques. One of the first things done in therapy is scheduling activities on an hourly basis. Patients keep records of the activities and review them with the therapist. In addition to scheduling activities, patients are asked to rate the amount of mastery and pleasure their activities bring them. Patients are often surprised to learn that they have much more mastery of activities and enjoy them more than they had thought.

To simplify the situation and allow mini accomplishments, therapists often break tasks into subtasks, as in graded task assignments, to show patients that they can succeed. In cognitive rehearsal, patients imagine and rehearse the various steps in meeting and mastering a challenge.

Patients (especially inpatients) are encouraged to become self-reliant by doing such simple things as making their own beds, doing their own shopping, and preparing their own meals. This process is called self-reliance training. Role-playing is a particularly powerful and useful technique for eliciting automatic thoughts and learning new behaviors. Diversion techniques are useful in helping patients get through difficult times and include physical activity, social contact, work, play, and visual imagery.

Imagery or thought stoppage can treat impulsive or obsessive behavior. For instance, patients imagine a stop sign with a police officer nearby or another image that evokes inhibition at the same time that they recognize an impulse or obsession that is alien to the ego. Similarly, obesity can be treated by having patients visualize themselves as thin, athletic, trim, and well muscled and then training them to evoke this image whenever they have an urge to eat. Hypnosis or autogenic training can enhance such imagery. In a technique called guided imagery, therapists encourage patients to have fantasies that can be interpreted as wish fulfillments or attempts to master disturbing affects or impulses.

EFFICACY

Cognitive therapy can be used alone in the treatment of mild to moderate depressive disorders or in conjunction with antidepressant medication for major depressive disorder. Studies have clearly shown that cognitive therapy is effective and in some cases is superior or equal to medication alone. It is one of the most useful psychotherapeutic interventions available for depressive disorders, and it shows promise in the treatment of other disorders.

Cognitive therapy has also been studied as a way of increasing compliance with lithium (Eskalith) prescription by patients with bipolar I disorder and as an adjunct in treating withdrawal from heroin.

▲ 31.10 Hypnosis

Hypnosis is understood as a normal activity of a normal mind through which attention is more focused, critical judgment is partially suspended, and peripheral awareness is diminished. The trance state, being a function of the subject's mind, cannot be forcibly projected by an outside person. The hypnotist, however, may aid in the achievement of the state and use its uncritical, intense focus to facilitate the acceptance of new thoughts and feelings, thereby accelerating therapeutic change. For the subject, hypnosis is typified by a feeling of involuntariness, and movements seem automatic.

TRAIT OF HYPNOTIZABILITY

A person's degree of hypnotizability is a trait that is relatively stable throughout the life cycle and is measurable. The process of hypnosis takes the hypnotizability trait and transforms it into the hypnotized state. Experiencing the hypnotic concentration state requires a convergence of three essential components: absorption, dissociation, and suggestibility.

Absorption is an ability to reduce peripheral awareness that results in a greater focal attention. It can be metaphorically described as a psychological zoom lens that increases attention to the given thought or emotion to the increasing exclusion of all context, even including orientation to time and space.

Dissociation is the separating out from consciousness elements of the patient's identity, perception, memory, or motor response as the hypnotic experience deepens. The result is that components of self-awareness, time, perception, and physical activity can occur without being known to the patient's consciousness and so may seem involuntary.

Suggestibility is the tendency of the hypnotized patient to accept signals and information with a relative suspension of normal critical judgment; it is controversial whether critical judgment can be completely suspended. This trait varies from an almost compulsive response to input in the highly hypnotizable to a sense of automaticity in the less hypnotizable individual.

QUANTIFICATION OF HYPNOTIZABILITY

Quantifying a patient's degree of hypnotizability is useful in a clinical setting because it predicts the effectiveness of hypnosis as a therapeutic modality. Quantification also provides useful information about the way in which patients relate to themselves and the social environment. Highly hypnotizable patients have an increased incidence of spontaneous trance-like states and so may be unduly influenced by ideas and emotions that are not being appropriately self-critiqued.

NEUROPHYSIOLOGICAL CORRELATES OF HYPNOSIS

Neurological testing of individuals in the hypnotized state and those with a high degree of hypnotizability has led to some interesting findings, but no set of changes has been shown to be sensitive or specific for the trance state or hypnotizability trait.

Electroencephalographic (EEG) studies have shown that hypnotized persons exhibit electrical patterns that are similar to those of fully awake and attentive persons and not like those found during sleep. Increased alpha activity and theta power in the left frontal region has been reported in highly hypnotizable patients as compared with those who are less hypnotizable; these differences exist in the trance and nontrance states.

Positron emission tomography (PET) studies that compare regional blood flow in the brain in both hypnotized and nonhypnotized subjects lend further evidence to the hypothesis that hypnosis exerts some of its effects at lower level modalities of the brain. Hypnotic suggestions to add color to a visual image result in increased blood flow to the lingual and fusiform gyri, the color vision processing centers of the brain; suggestions to remove color have the opposite effect. Similarly, the intensity and noxiousness of pain are believed to be processed by different regions of the brain because different areas of reduced blood flow result when each is minimized through hypnosis.

The role of the anterior brain regions, such as the frontal lobes, in hypnosis has been shown physiologically by the positive correlation between homovanillic acid concentrations in the cerebrospinal fluid and degree of hypnotizability. The frontal cortex and basal ganglia have a large number of neurons that use dopamine, of which the metabolite is homovanillic acid. This may explain why pharmacological enhancement of hypnotizability, although difficult, is primarily accomplished with dopaminergic agents, such as amphetamine. The increased activation of the basal ganglia may relate to the increased automaticity of hypnotic motor behavior.

INDICATIONS

A patient's degree of hypnotizability and the technique of hypnosis are clinically useful in diagnosis and in treatment, respectively.

The existence of spontaneous, trance-like states in everyday life and the potential of individuals to uncritically accept emotions and information in these states make a person's degree of hypnotizability a factor in the way in which the world is viewed and processed. A relationship is seen between various Axis I and Axis II conditions and hypnotizability. For example, patients with paranoid personality disorder are low and patients who are histrionic are higher on the hypnotizability spectrum. Patients with dissociative identity disorder are highly hypnotizable. Patients with eating disorders are difficult to hypnotize.

Therapeutically, hypnosis' effectiveness in facilitating acceptance of new thoughts and feelings makes it useful in treating habitual problems and also with symptom management. Smoking, overeating, phobias, anxiety, conversion symptoms, and chronic pain are all indications for hypnosis. They can often be treated in a single session, in which a patient is taught to perform self-hypnosis. Hypnosis can also aid in psychotherapy, notably for posttraumatic stress disorder, and it has been used for memory retrieval.

CONTRAINDICATIONS

No intrinsic dangers to the hypnotic process exist. Because of the increased dependence that the hypnotized patient has on the therapist, a strong transference may occur, however, in which the patient exhibits feelings for the therapist that are inappropriate in regards to their relationship. Strong attachments may occur, and it is important that these are respected and properly interpreted. Negative emotions may also be brought out in the patient, especially those who are emotionally fragile or who have poor reality testing. To minimize the likelihood of this negative transference, caution should be taken when choosing patients who have problems with basic trust, such as those who are paranoid or who require high levels of control. The hypnotized patient also has a reduced ability critically to evaluate hypnotic suggestions and,

thus, the hypnotist must have a strong ethical value system. Controversy exists about whether patients can perform acts during a trance state that they would otherwise find repugnant or that run contrary to their moral system.

▲ 31.11 Interpersonal Therapy

Interpersonal psychotherapy (ITP), a time-limited treatment for major depressive disorder, was developed in the 1970s, defined in a manual, and tested in randomized clinical trials by Gerald L. Klerman and Myrna Weissman. ITP was initially formulated as an attempt to represent the current practice of psychotherapy for depression. It assumes that the development and maintenance of some psychiatric illnesses occur in a social and interpersonal context and that the onset, response to treatment, and outcomes are influenced by the interpersonal relations between the patient and significant others. The overall goal of ITP is to reduce or eliminate psychiatric symptoms by improving the quality of the patient's current interpersonal relations and social functioning.

The typical course of ITP lasts 12 to 20 sessions over a 4- to 5-month period. ITP moves through three defined phases: (1) The initial phase is dedicated to identifying the problem area that will be the target for treatment; (2) the intermediate phase is devoted to working on the target problem area(s); and (3) the termination phase is focused on consolidating gains made during treatment and preparing the patients for future work on their own.

TECHNIQUES

Individual Interpersonal Psychotherapy

Initial Phase.   Sessions 1 through 5 typically constitute the initial phase of ITP. After assessing the patient's current psychiatric symptoms and obtaining a history of these symptoms, the therapist gives the patient a formal diagnosis from the text revision of the fourth edition of the *Diagnostic and Statistical Manual of Mental Disorders* (DSM-IV-TR). Therapist and patient then discuss the diagnosis, as well as what might be expected from treatment. Assignment of the sick role during this phase serves the dual function of granting the patient both the permission to recover and the responsibility to recover. The therapist explains the rationale of ITP, underscoring that therapy will focus on identifying and altering dysfunctional interpersonal patterns related to psychiatric symptomatology. To determine the precise focus of treatment, the therapist conducts an interpersonal inventory with the patient and develops an interpersonal formulation based on this. In the interpersonal formulation, the therapist links the patient's psychiatric symptomatology to one of the four interpersonal problem areas—grief, interpersonal deficits, interpersonal role disputes, or role transitions. The patient's concurrence with the therapist's identification of the problem area and agreement to work on this area are essential before beginning the intermediate treatment phase.

Intermediate Phase.   The intermediate phase—typically sessions 8 to 10—constitutes the "work" of the therapy. An

Table 31.11–1
Interpersonal Problem Areas: Description, Goals, and Strategies

Interpersonal Problem Area	Definition	Goals	Strategies
Grief	Complicated bereavement after the death of a loved one	Facilitate the mourning process Help patient reestablish interest in new activities and relationships to substitute for what has been lost	Reconstruct the patient's relationship with the deceased Explore associated feelings (negative and positive) Consider ways of becoming reinvolved with others
Interpersonal deficits	A history of social impoverishment, inadequate or unsustaining interpersonal relationships	Reduce patient's social isolation Enhance quality of any existing relationships Encourage the formation of new relationships	Review past significant relationships, including negative and positive aspects Explore repetitive patterns in relationships Note problematic interpersonal patterns in the session and relate them to similar patterns in the patient's life
Interpersonal role disputes	Conflicts with a significant other—a partner, other family member, coworker, or close friend	Identify the nature of the dispute Explore options to resolve the dispute Modify expectations and faulty communication to bring about a satisfactory resolution If modification is unworkable, encourage patient to reassess the expectations for the relationship and to generate options to either resolve it or dissolve it and mourn its loss	Determine the stage of the dispute: renegotiation (calm down participants to facilitate resolution); impasse (increase disharmony to reopen negotiation); dissolution (assist mourning and adaptation) Understand how nonreciprocal role expectations relate to the dispute Identify available resources to bring about change in the relationship
Role transitions	Economic or family change—the beginning or end of a relationship or career, a move, promotion, retirement, graduation, diagnosis of a medical illness	Mourn and accept the loss of the old role Recognize the positive and negative aspects of the new role and assets and liabilities of the old role Restore self-esteem by developing a sense of mastery regarding the demands of the new role	Review positive and negative aspects of old and new roles Explore feelings about what is lost Encourage development of social support system and new skills called for in new role

From Treasure J, Schmidt U, van Furth E. *Handbook of Eating Disorders.* 2nd ed. Hoboken, NJ: John Wiley & Sons; 2003:258, with permission.

essential task throughout the intermediate phase is to strengthen the connections the patient makes between the changes he or she is making in his or her interpersonal life and the changes in his or her psychiatric symptoms. During the intermediate phase, the therapist implements the treatment strategies specific to the identified problem area as specified in Table 31.11–1.

Termination Phase.   In the termination phase (usually, sessions 16 through 20), the therapist discusses termination explicitly with the patient and assists him or her in understanding that the end of treatment is a potential time of grief. During this phase, patients are encouraged to describe specific changes in their psychiatric symptoms, especially as they relate to improvements in the identified problem area(s). The therapist also assists the patient in evaluating and consolidating gains, detailing plans for maintaining improvements in the identified interpersonal problem area(s), and outlining remaining work for the patient to continue on his or her own. Patients are also encouraged to identify early warning signs of symptom recurrence and to identify plans of action.

Interpersonal Psychotherapy Delivered in a Group Format

A recent approach in the ongoing development of ITP has been its use in a group format. ITP delivered in a group format has many potential benefits in comparison with individual treatment. For example, a group format in which membership is based on diagnostic similarity (e.g., depression, social phobia, eating disorders) can help alleviate patients' concerns that they are the only one with a particular psychiatric disorder while offering a social environment for patients who have become isolated, withdrawn, or disconnected from others. Given the number and different types of interpersonal interactions in a group setting, the interpersonal skills that are developed may be more readily transferable to the patient's outside social life than are the relationship patterns that are addressed in a one-on-one setting. Moreover, a group modality has therapeutic features not present in individual psychotherapy (e.g., interpersonal learning). The group format also facilitates the identification of problems common to many patients and provides a cost-effective alternative to individual treatment.

▲ 31.12 Psychiatric Rehabilitation

Psychiatric rehabilitation denotes a wide range of interventions designed to help people with disabilities caused by mental illness improve their functioning and quality of life by enabling them to acquire the skills and supports needed to be successful in usual adult roles and in the environments of their choice. Normative adult roles include living independently, attending school, working in competitive jobs, relating to family, having friends, and having intimate relationships. Psychiatric rehabilitation emphasizes independence rather than reliance on professionals, community integration rather than isolation in segregated settings for persons with disabilities, and patient preferences rather than professional goals.

VOCATIONAL REHABILITATION

Impairment of vocational role performance is a common complication related to schizophrenia. Studies across the United States show that less than 15 percent of patients with severe mental illnesses, such as schizophrenia, are employed. Nevertheless, studies also show that competitive employment is a primary goal for 50 to 75 percent of patients with schizophrenia. Because of patient interests and historical factors, vocational rehabilitation has always been a centerpiece of psychiatric rehabilitation.

Antonio is a 45-year-old man who has been a client of a mental health agency for more than 10 years. He attended the rehabilitative day treatment program until it was converted to a supported employment program. His case manager encouraged him to think about the possibility of working part-time. Antonio told his case manager that he could not work because of his schizophrenia and because he was helping to raise his two kids and needed to be home at 3 PM, when they returned from school every day. The case manager explained to Antonio that getting a job does not necessarily mean working 40 hours a week and that lots of people in the agency's supported employment program were working in part-time jobs, even jobs that only require a few hours a week.

Antonio agreed to meet one of the employment specialists to discuss the possibility of work. Over the next couple of weeks, the employment specialist met with Antonio several times, read his clinical record, and talked with his case manager and psychiatrist. The employment specialist learned that Antonio loved to drive his car. He also learned that Antonio had attendance problems in past jobs because he felt unappreciated. The employment specialist found Antonio to be a sociable and likable person.

Antonio told the employment specialist that he was willing to do any job. He did not have one specific job in mind. After discussing options with Antonio and with the team, the employment specialist suggested a job at Meals on Wheels as a driver for the lunch delivery. Antonio was hired and loved it right from the start. Absenteeism was never a problem, because he liked driving around and knew that people were

counting on him for their meals. The hours were perfect (10 AM to 2 PM), so he could be at home when his kids returned from school. He became good friends with the other workers. He told his case manager that it was wonderful to be bringing home a paycheck again. And best of all, he said, was that his kids saw him going to work just like their friends' dads. (Courtesy of Robert E. Drake, M.D., Ph.D., and Alan S. Bellack, Ph.D.)

SOCIAL SKILLS REHABILITATION

Social dysfunction is a defining characteristic of schizophrenia. People with the illness have difficulty fulfilling social roles, such as worker, spouse, and friend, and have difficulty meeting their needs when social interaction is required (e.g., negotiating with merchants, requesting assistance to solve problems). Social dysfunction is semi-independent of symptomatology and plays an important role in the course and outcome of the illness. Social competence is based on three component skills: (1) social perception, or receiving skills; (2) social cognition, or processing skills; and (3) behavioral response, or expressive skills. Social perception is the ability to read or decode social inputs accurately. This includes accurate detection of affect cues, such as facial expressions and nuances of voice, gesture, and body posture, as well as verbal content and contextual information. Social cognition involves effective analysis of the social stimulus, integration of current information with historical information, and planning of an effective response. This domain is also referred to as *social problem solving*.

Methods

The primary modality of social skills training is role play of simulated conversations. The trainer first provides instructions on how to perform the skill and then models the behavior to demonstrate how it is performed. After identifying a relevant social situation in which the skill might be used, the patient engages in role play with the trainer. The trainer next provides feedback and positive reinforcement, which are followed by suggestions for how the response can be improved. The sequence of role play followed by feedback and reinforcement is repeated until the patient can perform the response adequately. Training is typically conducted in small groups (six to eight patients), in which case patients each practice role playing for three to four trials and provide feedback and reinforcement to one another. Teaching is tailored to the individual—for example, a highly impaired group member might simply practice saying "no" to a simple request, whereas a less cognitively impaired peer might learn to negotiate and compromise.

Goals

In a treatment setting, there are four major goals of social skills training: (1) improved social skills in specific situations, (2) moderate generalization of acquired skills to similar situations, (3) acquisition or relearning of social and conversational skills, and (4) decreased social anxiety. Learning, however, is tedious or almost nonexistent when patients are floridly ill with positive symptoms and high levels of distractibility.

Some findings limit the applicability of social skills training. It is more difficult to teach complex conversational skills than to teach briefer, more discrete verbal and nonverbal responses in social situations. Because complex behaviors are more critical for generating social support in the community, methods have been developed to improve the learning and durability of conversational skills. These training methods, focusing on training in social skills and information-processing skills, are discussed in the following paragraphs.

Training in Social Perception Skills.   Recently, efforts have been made to develop strategies for training patients in affect and social cue recognition. Patients with chronic psychotic disorders, such as schizophrenia, often have difficulty perceiving and interpreting the subtle affective and cognitive cues that are critical elements of communication. Social perception abilities are considered the first step in effective interpersonal problem solving; difficulties in this area are likely to lead to a cascade of deficits in social behavior. Training skills in social perception address these deficits and help provide a foundation for developing more specific social and coping skills.

Despite attending several social gatherings, Matt felt apart from the rest of the group. He reported that these events seemed like "a jumble of sights and sounds." His therapist, recognizing Matt's difficulty with social perception, gave him a series of questions designed to help him organize and give meaning to the social stimuli he encountered. For example, when Matt was confused about a conversation someone was having with him, he would ask himself, "What is this person's short-term goal? At what level of disclosure should I be? Should I be talking now or listening?" Identifying the rules and goals of a particular social interaction provided a template for Matt to recognize, and react to, a greater variety of social cues, thus enhancing his behavioral repertoire. (Courtesy of Robert Paul Liberman, M.D., Alex Kopelowicz, M.D., and Thomas E. Smith, M.D.)

Information-Processing Model of Training.   Methods of training that follow a cognitive perspective teach patients to use a set of generative rules that can be adapted for use in various situations. For example, a six-step problem-solving strategy has developed as an outline for helping patients overcome interpersonal dilemmas: (1) adopt a problem-solving attitude, (2) identify the problem, (3) brainstorm alternative solutions, (4) evaluate solutions and pick one to implement, (5) plan the implementation and carry it out, and (6) evaluate the efficacy of the effort and, if it is ineffective, choose another alternative. Although the stepwise, structured, linear process of problem solving occurs intuitively, without conscious awareness in normal persons, it can be a useful interpersonal crutch to help cognitively impaired

psychiatric patients cope with the information needed to fill their social and personal needs.

MILIEU THERAPY

The locus of milieu is a living, learning, or working environment. The defining characteristics of treatment are the use of a team to provide treatment and the time the patient spends in the environment. Recent adaptations of milieu therapy include 24-hour-a-day programs situated in community locales frequented by patients, which provide in vivo support, case management, and training in living skills.

Most milieu therapy programs emphasize group and social interaction; rules and expectations are mediated by peer pressure for normalization of adaptation. When patients are viewed as responsible human beings, the patient role becomes blurred. Milieu therapy stresses a patient's rights to goals and to have freedom of movement and informal relationship with staff; it also emphasizes interdisciplinary participation and goal-oriented, clear communication.

Token Economy

The use of tokens, points, or credits as secondary or generalized reinforcers can be seen as normalizing a mental hospital or day hospital environment with a program mimicking society's use of money to meet instrumental needs. Token economies establish the rules and culture of a hospital inpatient unit or partial hospitalization program, offering coherence and consistency to the interdisciplinary team as it struggles to promote therapeutic progress in difficult patients. These programs are challenging to establish, however, and their widespread dissemination has suffered because of the organizational prerequisites and the additional resources and rewards needed to create a truly positively reinforcing environment.

COGNITIVE REHABILITATION

Increased recognition of the prevalence and importance of neurocognitive deficits over the last decade has stimulated increasing interest in remediation strategies. Much of the work in this area has focused on psychopharmacological approaches, especially on the new-generation antipsychotics. New-generation medications appear to have a positive effect on neurocognitive test performance, but the effect size for any of the medications is small to medium, and little evidence indicates that these medications have a clinically meaningful impact on neurocognitive functioning in the community. As a result, a parallel interest has arisen in the potential for *rehabilitation* or *cognitive remediation*. This body of work is distinguished from cognitive-behavioral therapy and cognitive therapy, which focus on reducing psychotic symptoms.

32

Biological Therapies

▲ 32.1 General Principles of Psychopharmacology

Psychopharmacological advances continue dramatically to expand the parameters of psychiatric treatments. Greater understanding of how the brain functions has led to more effective, less toxic, better-tolerated, and more specifically targeted therapeutic agents. With the ever-increasing sophistication and array of treatment options, clinicians, however, must remain aware of potential adverse effects, drug–drug (and drug–food or drug–supplement) interactions, and how to manage the emergence of unwanted or unintended consequences. Newer drugs may lead ultimately to side effects that are not recognized initially. Keeping up with the latest research findings is increasingly important as these findings proliferate. A thorough understanding of the management of medication-induced side effects (either through treating the effect with another agent or substituting another primary agent) is necessary.

CLASSIFICATION

Medications used to treat psychiatric disorders are referred to as *psychotropic drugs*. These drugs are commonly described by their major clinical application, for example, *antidepressants, antipsychotics, mood stabilizers, anxiolytics, hypnotics, cognitive enhancers,* and *stimulants*. A problem with this approach is that, in many instances, drugs have multiple indications. For example, drugs such as the selective serotonin reuptake inhibitors (SSRIs) are both antidepressants and anxiolytics, and the serotonin-dopamine antagonists (SDAs) are both antipsychotics and mood stabilizers.

Psychotropic drugs have also been organized according to structure (e.g., tricyclic), mechanism (e.g., monoamine oxidase inhibitor), history (e.g., first generation, traditional), uniqueness (e.g., atypical), or indication (e.g., antidepressant). A further problem is that many drugs used to treat medical and neurological conditions are routinely used to treat psychiatric disorders.

In addition, psychotropic drug terminology can be confusing. The first pharmaceutical agents used to treat schizophrenia were termed *tranquilizers*. When newer drugs emerged as therapies for anxiety, a distinction was drawn between *major* and *minor tranquilizers*. More recently, older agents used as treatments for psychosis became known as *typical, conventional,* or *traditional* antipsychotics. Newer ones became *atypical* or *second-generation antipsychotic medication*. To eliminate much of this confusion, in this chapter, drugs are presented according to shared mechanism of action or by similarity of structure. In addition, the terms first- and second-generation antipsychotics are also used.

PHARMACOLOGICAL ACTIONS

Pharmacodynamics

The time course and intensity of a drug's effects are referred to as its *pharmacodynamics*. Major pharmacodynamic considerations include receptor mechanisms, the dose-response curve, the therapeutic index, and the development of tolerance, dependence, and withdrawal phenomena. Drug mechanism of action is subsumed under pharmacodynamics. The clinical response to a drug, including adverse reactions, results from an interaction between that drug and a patient's susceptibility to those actions. Pharmacogenetic studies are beginning to identify genetic polymorphisms linked to individual differences in treatment response and sensitivity to side effects.

Mechanisms

The mechanisms through which most psychotropic drugs produce their therapeutic effects remain poorly understood. Standard explanations focus on ways that drugs alter synaptic concentrations of dopamine, serotonin, norepinephrine, histamine, γ-aminobutyric acid (GABA), or acetylcholine. These changes are said to result from receptor antagonists or agonists, interference with neurotransmitter reuptake, enhancement of neurotransmitter release, or inhibition of enzymes. Specific drugs are associated with permutations or combinations of these actions. For example, a drug can be an agonist for a receptor, thus stimulating the specific biological activity of the receptor, or an antagonist, thus inhibiting the biological activity. Some drugs are partial agonists because they are not capable of fully activating a specific receptor. Some psychotropic drugs also produce clinical effects through mechanisms other than receptor interactions. For example, lithium can act by directly inhibiting the enzyme inositol-1-phosphatase. Some effects are closely linked to a specific synaptic effect. For example, most medications that treat psychosis share the ability to block the dopamine type 2 receptor. Similarly, benzodiazepine agonists bind a receptor complex that contains benzodiazepine and GABA receptors.

Accounts of so-called mechanisms of action should nevertheless be kept in perspective. Explanations of how psychotropic drugs actually work that focus on synaptic elements represent an oversimplification of a complex series of events. If merely raising or lowering levels of neurotransmitter activity is associated with the clinical effects of a drug, then all drugs that cause these changes should produce equivalent benefits. This is not the case. Multiple obscure actions, several steps removed from events at neuronal receptor sites, are probably responsible for the therapeutic effects of psychotropic drugs. These *downstream* elements are postulated to represent the actual reasons that these drugs produce clinical improvement.

Therapeutic Index

Therapeutic index is a relative measure of the toxicity or safety of a drug and is defined as the ratio of the median toxic dose to the median effective dose. The median toxic dose is the dose at which 50 percent of patients experience a specific toxic effect, and the median effective dose is the dose at which 50 percent of patients have a specified therapeutic effect. When the therapeutic index is high, as it is for haloperidol, it is reflected by the wide range of doses in which that drug is prescribed. Conversely, the therapeutic index for lithium is quite low, thus requiring careful monitoring of serum lithium levels in patients for whom the drug is prescribed.

Overdose

Safety in overdose is always a consideration in drug selection. Almost all of the newer agents, however, have a wide margin of safety when taken in overdose. By contrast, a 1-month supply of tricyclic antidepressants could be fatal. The depressed patients they were used to treat were the group most at risk to attempt suicide. Because even the safest drugs can sometimes produce severe medical complications, especially when combined with other agents, clinicians must recognize that the prescribed medication can be used in an attempt to commit suicide. Although it is prudent to write nonrefillable prescriptions for small quantities, this practice passes along increased copay costs to the patient. In fact, many pharmacy benefit management programs encourage the prescribing of a 3-month supply of medication.

In cases in which suicide is a major concern, an attempt should be made to verify that the medication is not being hoarded for a later overdose attempt. Random pill counts or asking a family member to dispense daily doses may be helpful. Some patients attempt suicide just as they are beginning to recover. Large quantities of medications with a low therapeutic index should be prescribed judiciously. Another reason to limit the number of pills prescribed is the possibility of accidental ingestion of medications by children in the household. Psychotherapeutic medications should be kept in a safe place.

Physicians who work in emergency rooms should know which drugs can be hemodialyzed. The issues involved are complex and are not based on any single chemical property of the drug. For example, it is generally presumed that drugs with low protein binding are good candidates for dialysis. Venlafaxine, however, is only 27 percent protein bound and is too large as a molecule dialyzed. Hemodialysis is effective for treating overdose of valproic acid (Depakene).

Pharmacokinetics

Pharmacokinetic drug interactions are the effects of drugs on the plasma concentrations of each other, and pharmacodynamic drug interactions are the effects of drugs on the biological activities of each other. Pharmacokinetic concepts are used to describe and to predict the time course of drug concentrations in different parts of the body, such as plasma, adipose tissue, and the central nervous system (CNS). From a clinical perspective, pharmacokinetic methods help explain or predict the onset and duration of drug activity and interactions between drugs that alter their metabolism or excretion.

Pharmacogenetic research focuses on finding variant alleles that alter drug pharmacokinetics and pharmacodynamics. Researchers are attempting to identify genetic differences in how enzymes metabolize psychotropics, as well as CNS proteins directly involved in drug action. It is likely that identification of patient genotypes will facilitate prediction of clinical response to different types of drugs.

Most clinicians need to consult charts or computer programs to determine when potential interactions may occur and, if so, how clinically relevant they may be. Whenever possible, it is preferable to use a medication that produces minimal risk of drug interactions. In addition, it is recommended that prescribers know the interaction profiles of the drugs that they most commonly prescribe.

Examples of pharmacokinetic interactions include one drug increasing or decreasing the concentrations of a coadministered compound. These types of interactions can also lead to altered concentrations of metabolites. In some cases, there may also be interference with the conversion of a drug to its active metabolite. Enormous variability exists among patients with respect to pharmacokinetic parameters, such as drug absorption and metabolism. Another type of interaction is represented by interactions involving the kidney. Commonly used medications, such as angiotensin-converting enzyme inhibitors, nonsteroidal anti-inflammatory drugs, and thiazides, decrease renal clearance of lithium, increasing the likelihood of severe elevations of lithium. Drug interactions can occur pharmacokinetically or pharmacodynamically.

Pharmacogenetics is being used to study why patients differ in the way that they metabolize drugs. In patients who are ultrarapid or extensive metabolizers, the concentrations of a drug may be lower than expected.

DOSING, DURATION, AND MONITORING

Dosing

The clinically effective dose for treatment depends on the characteristics of the drug and patient factors, such as inherited sensitivity and ability to metabolize a drug, concurrent medical disorders, use of concurrent medications, and history of exposure to previous medications.

Plasma concentrations of many psychotropics can vary up to tenfold. Thus, to some extent, the optimal dose for an individual is ultimately determined by trial and error, guided by the empirical evidence of the usual dose range for that drug. Some drugs demonstrate a clear relationship between increases in dose and clinical response. This dose-response curve plots the drug concentration against the effects of the drug.

The *potency* of a drug refers to the relative dose required to achieve certain effects, not to its efficacy. Haloperidol, for example, is more potent than chlorpromazine because approximately 5 mg of haloperidol is required to achieve the same therapeutic pharmacokinetics and pharmacodynamics. Dosing is another special consideration in drug use with children. Although the small volume of distribution suggests the use of lower doses than those used in adults, a child's higher rate of metabolism suggests that a higher ratio of milligrams of drug to kilograms of body weight should be used. In practice, it is best to begin with a small dose and to increase it until clinical effects are observed. The clinician should not hesitate, however, to use adult doses in children if these doses are effective and the adverse effects are acceptable.

Pregnant and Nursing Women

No definitive assurances exist that any drug is completely without risk during pregnancy and lactation. No psychotropic medication is absolutely contraindicated during pregnancy, although drugs with known risks of birth defects, premature birth, or neonatal complications should be avoided if acceptable alternatives are available.

Women who are pregnant or lactating are excluded from clinical trials, and it is only recently that women of childbearing age have been able to participate in these studies. As a result, there are large gaps in knowledge of the effects of psychotropic agents on the developing fetus and on the neonate. Most of what is known is the result of anecdotal reports or data from registries. The basic rule is to avoid administering any drug to a woman who is pregnant (particularly during the first trimester) or who is breast-feeding a child, unless the mother's psychiatric disorder is severe and it is determined that the therapeutic value of the drug outweighs the theoretical adverse effects on the fetus or newborn. A woman may elect to continue on medication because she does not want to chance a possible recurrence of painful or disabling symptoms.

The administration of psychotherapeutic drugs at or near delivery can cause the baby to be overly sedated at delivery, thus requiring a respirator, or to be physically dependent on the drug, requiring detoxification and the treatment of a withdrawal syndrome. Reports exist of a neonatal withdrawal syndrome associated with third-trimester use of SSRIs in pregnant women. They have also been implicated in producing pulmonary hypertension in newborns.

Virtually all psychiatric drugs are secreted in the milk of a nursing mother; therefore, mothers on those agents should be advised not to breast-feed their infants.

Elderly Patients

The two major concerns when treating geriatric patients with psychotherapeutic drugs are that elderly persons may be more susceptible to adverse effects (particularly cardiac effects) and may metabolize and excrete drugs more slowly, thus requiring lower doses of medication. In practice, clinicians should begin treating geriatric patients with a small dose, usually approximately one half of the usual starting dose. The dose should be raised in small increments, more slowly than for middle-aged adults, until a clinical benefit is achieved or unacceptable adverse effects appear. Although many geriatric patients require a small dose of medication, many others require a full therapeutic dose.

Age-related changes in renal clearance and hepatic metabolism make it more important to be conservative with the starting doses of medication, as well as the rate of dose titration. Within any class of psychotropic agents, those with potentially serious consequences, such as hypotension, cardiac conduction abnormalities, anticholinergic activity, and respiratory depression, are not suitable choices. Drugs that cause cognitive impairment, such as benzodiazepines and anticholinergics, can mimic or exacerbate symptoms of dementia. Similarly, dopamine receptor antagonists can worsen or induce Parkinson's disease, another age-related disorder. Some side effects, such as SSRI-associated syndrome of inappropriate secretion of antidiuretic hormone and oxcarbazepine-associated hyponatremia, occur more commonly in older patients.

Medically Ill Patients

There are special considerations, diagnostic and therapeutic, when administering psychiatric drugs to medically ill patients. The medical disorder should be ruled out as a cause of the psychiatric symptoms. For example, patients with neurological or endocrine disorders or those infected with human immunodeficiency virus may experience disturbances of mood and cognition. Common medications, such as corticosteroids and L-dopa, are associated with induction of mania.

Substance Abuse

Many patients who seek or need treatment for a psychiatric disorder engage in chronic use of illicit substances or drink excessive amounts of alcohol. Marijuana is the most commonly used illicit drug in the United States.

Discontinuation of chronic drug or alcohol use can result not only in craving, but also in clinically significant psychiatric and physiological withdrawal symptoms. For many patients, successful treatment of their underlying psychiatric disorder may not be possible in the presence of ongoing marijuana, cocaine, and alcohol use. If several trials of medications fail, hospitalization for detoxification may be necessary. Little research and no consensus exist about how to use psychotropic agents in patients who are regular users of cocaine, marijuana, or other recreational drugs.

▲ 32.2 Medication-Induced Movement Disorders

The text revision of the fourth edition of the *Diagnostic and Statistical Manual of Mental Disorders* (DSM-IV-TR) includes in the category of "medication-induced movement disorders" both such disorders and any medication-induced adverse effect that becomes a focus of clinical attention. The most common neuroleptic-related movement disorders are Parkinsonism, acute dystonia, and acute akathisia. Neuroleptic malignant syndrome is a life-threatening and often misdiagnosed condition. Neuroleptic-induced tardive dyskinesia is a late-appearing adverse effect of neuroleptic drugs and can be irreversible; recent data, however, indicate that the syndrome, although still serious and potentially disabling, is less pernicious than was previously thought in patients taking dopamine receptor antagonists (DRAs). The newer antipsychotics—the serotonin-dopamine antagonists (SDAs)—block binding to dopamine receptors to a much lesser degree and thereby are less likely to produce such movement disorders.

NEUROLEPTIC-INDUCED PARKINSONISM

Diagnosis, Signs, and Symptoms

Symptoms include muscle stiffness (lead pipe rigidity), cogwheel rigidity, shuffling gait, stooped posture, and drooling. The pill-rolling tremor of idiopathic Parkinsonism is rare, but a regular, coarse tremor similar to essential tremor may be present. The so-called *rabbit syndrome,* a tremor affecting the lips and perioral muscles, is another Parkinsonian effect seen with antipsychotics, although perioral tremor is more likely than other tremors to occur late in the course of treatment.

Epidemiology

Parkinsonian adverse effects occur in about 15 percent of patients who are treated with antipsychotics, usually within 5 to 90 days of the initiation of treatment. Patients who are elderly and female are at the highest risk for neuroleptic-induced Parkinsonism, although the disorder can occur at all ages.

Etiology

Neuroleptic-induced Parkinsonism is caused by the blockade of dopamine type 2 (D_2) receptors in the caudate at the termination of the nigrostriatal dopamine neurons. All antipsychotics can cause the symptoms, especially high-potency drugs with low levels of anticholinergic activity (e.g., trifluoperazine [Stelazine]). Chlorpromazine (Thorazine) and thioridazine (Mellaril) are not likely to be involved. The newer, atypical antipsychotics (e.g., aripiprazole [Abilify], olanzapine [Zyprexa], and quetiapine [Seroquel]) are less likely to cause Parkinsonism.

Differential Diagnosis

Included in the differential diagnosis are idiopathic Parkinsonism, other organic causes of Parkinsonism, and depression, which can also be associated with Parkinsonian symptoms.

Treatment

Parkinsonism can be treated with anticholinergic agents, benztropine (Cogentin), amantadine (Symmetrel), or diphenhydramine (Benadryl). Anticholinergics should be withdrawn after 4 to 6 weeks to assess whether tolerance to the Parkinsonian effects has developed; about half of patients with neuroleptic-induced Parkinsonism require continued treatment. Even after the antipsychotics are withdrawn, Parkinsonian symptoms can last up to 2 weeks and even up to 3 months in elderly patients. With such patients, the clinician may continue the anticholinergic drug after the antipsychotic has been stopped until the Parkinsonian symptoms resolve completely.

NEUROLEPTIC-INDUCED ACUTE DYSTONIA

Diagnosis, Signs, and Symptoms

Dystonias are brief or prolonged contractions of muscles that result in obviously abnormal movements or postures, including oculogyric crises, tongue protrusion, trismus, torticollis, laryngeal–pharyngeal dystonias, and dystonic postures of the limbs and trunk. Other dystonias include blepharospasm and glossopharyngeal dystonia; the latter results in dysarthria, dysphagia, and even difficulty in breathing, which can cause cyanosis. Children are particularly likely to evidence opisthotonos, scoliosis, lordosis, and writhing movements. Dystonia can be painful and frightening and often results in noncompliance with future drug treatment regimens.

Epidemiology

The development of dystonic symptoms is characterized by their early onset during the course of treatment with neuroleptics and their high incidence in men, in patients younger than age 30 years, and in patients given high doses of high-potency medications.

Etiology

Although it is most common with intramuscular doses of high-potency antipsychotics, dystonia can occur with any antipsychotic. The mechanism of action is thought to be dopaminergic hyperactivity in the basal ganglia that occurs when central nervous system levels of the antipsychotic drug begin to fall between doses.

Differential Diagnosis

The differential diagnosis includes seizures and tardive dyskinesia.

Course and Prognosis

Dystonia can fluctuate spontaneously and respond to reassurance, so that the clinician acquires the false impression that the movement is hysterical or completely under conscious control.

Treatment

Prophylaxis with anticholinergics or related drugs usually prevents dystonia, although the risks of prophylactic treatment weigh against that benefit. Treatment with intramuscular anticholinergics or intravenous or intramuscular diphenhydramine (50 mg) almost always relieves the symptoms. Diazepam (Valium) (10 mg intravenously), amobarbital (Amytal), caffeine sodium benzoate, and hypnosis have also been reported to be effective. Although tolerance for the adverse effects usually develops, it is sometimes prudent to change the antipsychotic if the patient is particularly concerned that the reaction may recur.

NEUROLEPTIC-INDUCED ACUTE AKATHISIA

Diagnosis, Signs, and Symptoms

Akathisia is subjective feelings of restlessness, objective signs of restlessness, or both. Examples include a sense of anxiety, inability to relax, jitteriness, pacing, rocking motions while sitting, and rapid alternation of sitting and standing. Akathisia has been associated with the use of a wide range of psychiatric drugs, including antipsychotics, antidepressants, and sympathomimetics. Once akathisia is recognized and diagnosed, the antipsychotic dose should be reduced to the minimal effective level. Akathisia may be associated with a poor treatment outcome.

Epidemiology

Middle-aged women are at increased risk of akathisia, and the time course is similar to that for neuroleptic-induced Parkinsonism.

Treatment

Three basic steps in the treatment of akathisia are reducing medication dose, attempting treatment with appropriate drugs, and considering

Hyperactivity and Aggression in Children

Clonidine and guanfacine can be useful alternatives for the treatment of ADHD. They are used in place of sympathomimetics and antidepressants, which can produce paradoxical worsening of hyperactivity in some children with mental retardation, aggression, or features on the spectrum of autism. Clonidine and guanfacine can improve mood, reduce activity level, and improve social adaptation. Some multiply impaired children may respond favorably to clonidine, whereas others may simply become sedated. The starting dose is 0.05 mg a day; it can be raised to 0.3 mg a day in divided doses. The efficacy of clonidine and guanfacine for control of hyperactivity and aggression often diminishes over several months of use.

Clonidine or guanfacine can be combined with methylphenidate (Ritalin) or amphetamine to treat hyperactivity and inattentiveness, respectively. A few cases have been reported of sudden death of children taking clonidine together with methylphenidate; however, it has not been conclusively demonstrated that these medications contributed to these deaths. The clinician should explain to the family that the efficacy and safety of this combination have not been investigated in controlled trials. Periodic cardiovascular assessments, including vital signs and electrocardiograms, are warranted if this combination is used.

Posttraumatic Stress Disorder

Acute exacerbations of PTSD may be associated with hyperadrenergic symptoms, such as hyperarousal, exaggerated startle response, insomnia, vivid nightmares, tachycardia, agitation, hypertension, and perspiration. These symptoms may respond to the use of clonidine or, especially for overnight benefit, to the use of guanfacine.

Other Disorders

Other potential indications for clonidine include other anxiety disorders (panic disorder, phobias, obsessive-compulsive disorder, and generalized anxiety disorder) and mania, in which it may be synergistic with lithium (Eskalith) or carbamazepine (Tegretol). Anecdotal reports have noted the efficacy of clonidine in schizophrenia and tardive dyskinesia. A clonidine patch can reduce the hypersalivation and dysphagia caused by clozapine (Clozaril).

PRECAUTIONS AND ADVERSE REACTIONS

The most common adverse effects associated with clonidine are dry mouth and eyes, fatigue, sedation, dizziness, nausea, hypotension, and constipation, which result in discontinuation of therapy by about 10 percent of all persons taking the drug. Some persons also experience sexual dysfunction. Tolerance may develop to these adverse effects. A similar but milder adverse effect profile is seen with guanfacine, especially at doses of 3 mg or more per day. Clonidine and guanfacine should not be taken by adults with blood pressure (BP) below 90/60 mm Hg or with cardiac arrhythmias, especially bradycardia. Development of bradycardia warrants gradual, tapered discontinuation of the drug. Clonidine, in particular, is associated with sedation, and tolerance does not usually develop to this adverse effect. Uncommon central nervous system (CNS) adverse effects of clonidine include insomnia, anxiety, and depression; rare CNS adverse effects include vivid dreams, nightmares, and hallucinations. Fluid retention associated with clonidine use can be treated with diuretics.

The transdermal patch formulation of clonidine can cause local skin irritation, which can be minimized by rotating the application sites.

Overdose

Persons who take an overdose of clonidine can present with coma and constricted pupils, symptoms similar to those of an opioid overdose. Other symptoms of overdose are decreased BP, pulse, and respiratory rates. Guanfacine overdose produces a milder version of these symptoms. Clonidine and guanfacine should be used with caution in persons with heart disease, any type of vascular disease, renal disease, Raynaud's syndrome, or a history of depression. Clonidine and guanfacine should be avoided during pregnancy and by nursing mothers. Elderly persons are more sensitive to the drug than are younger adults. Children are susceptible to the same adverse effects as are adults.

Withdrawal

Abrupt discontinuation of clonidine can cause anxiety, restlessness, perspiration, tremor, abdominal pain, palpitations, headache, and a dramatic rise in BP. These symptoms may appear about 20 hours after the last dose of clonidine and, thus, may be seen if one or two doses are skipped. A similar set of symptoms occasionally occurs 2 to 4 days after discontinuation of guanfacine, but the usual course is a gradual return to baseline BP over 2 to 4 days. Because of the possibility of discontinuation symptoms, doses of clonidine and guanfacine should be tapered slowly.

DRUG INTERACTIONS

Coadministration of clonidine and tricyclic drugs can reduce the hypotensive effects of clonidine. Clonidine and guanfacine may enhance the CNS depressive effects of barbiturates, alcohol, other sedative-hypnotics, and trazodone (Desyrel). Clonidine and guanfacine can have an unwanted synergistic hypotensive effect if coadministered with other antihypertensive drugs. The α_2-adrenergic receptor antagonist yohimbine (Yocon) blocks the effects of clonidine and guanfacine. The concomitant use of β-adrenergic receptor antagonists can increase the severity of rebound phenomena when clonidine and guanfacine are discontinued.

LABORATORY INTERFERENCES

No known laboratory interferences are associated with the use of clonidine or guanfacine.

DOSING AND CLINICAL GUIDELINES

Clonidine is available in 0.1-, 0.2-, and 0.3-mg tablets. The usual starting dose is 0.1 mg orally twice a day; the dose can be raised by 0.1 mg a day to an appropriate level (up to 1.2 mg per day).

Clonidine must always be tapered when it is discontinued to avoid rebound hypertension, which may occur about 20 hours after the last clonidine dose. A weekly transdermal formulation of clonidine is available at doses of 0.1, 0.2, and 0.3 mg per day. The usual starting dose is the 0.1-mg-a-day patch, which is changed each week for adults and every 5 days for children; the dose can be increased, as needed, every 1 to 2 weeks. Transition from the oral to the transdermal formulations should be accomplished gradually by overlapping them for 3 to 4 days.

Guanfacine is available in 1- and 2-mg tablets. The usual starting dose is 1 mg before sleep, and this can be increased to 2 mg before sleep after 3 to 4 weeks, if necessary. Regardless of the indication for which clonidine or guanfacine is being used, the drug should be withheld if a person becomes hypotensive (BP below 90/60 mm Hg).

▲ 32.4 β-Adrenergic Receptor Antagonists

The β-adrenergic receptor antagonists, which are variously referred to as *β-blockers* and *β-antagonists,* are commonly used in medical practice for their peripheral effects in the treatment of hypertension, angina, certain cardiac arrhythmias, and migraine. Their effectiveness as peripherally and centrally acting agents has been well demonstrated for social phobia (e.g., performance anxiety), lithium-induced postural tremor, control of aggressive behavior, and neuroleptic-induced akathisia.

The β-receptor antagonists most commonly used in psychiatry are propranolol (Inderal), nadolol (Corgard), pindolol (Visken), labetalol (Normodyne, Trandate), atenolol (Tenormin), metoprolol (Lopressor, Toprol), and acebutolol (Sectral).

PHARMACOLOGICAL ACTIONS

The β-receptor antagonists differ with regard to lipophilicities, metabolic routes, β-receptor selectivity, and half-lives (Table 32.4–1). The absorption of the β-receptor antagonists from the gastrointestinal tract is variable. The agents that are most soluble in lipids (i.e., are lipophilic) are likely to cross the blood–brain barrier and enter the brain; those agents that are least lipophilic are less likely to enter the brain. When central nervous system (CNS) effects are desired, a lipophilic drug may be preferred; when only peripheral effects are desired, a less lipophilic drug may be indicated.

Propranolol, nadolol, pindolol, and labetalol have essentially equal potency at both the β_1- and β_2-receptors, whereas metoprolol, atenolol, and acebutolol have greater affinity for the β_1-receptor than for the β_2-receptor. Relative β_1-selectivity confers few pulmonary and vascular effects on these drugs, although they must be used with caution in asthmatic persons because the drugs retain some activity at the β_2-receptors.

Pindolol has sympathomimetic effects in addition to its β-antagonist effects, which has permitted its use for augmentation of antidepressant drugs. Pindolol, propranolol, and nadolol possess some antagonist activity at the serotonin 5-HT$_{1A}$ receptors.

THERAPEUTIC INDICATIONS

Anxiety Disorders

Propranolol is useful for the treatment of social phobia, primarily of the performance type (e.g., disabling anxiety before a musical performance). Data are also available for its use in treatment of panic disorder, posttraumatic stress disorder, and generalized anxiety disorder. In social phobia, the common treatment approach is to take 10 to 40 mg of propranolol 20 to 30 minutes before the anxiety-provoking situation. A test dose of the β-receptor antagonist can be tried before using it before an anxiety-provoking situation to be sure that the patient does not experience any adverse effects from the drug or the dose. β-Receptor antagonists may blunt cognition in some people. The β-receptor antagonists are less effective for the treatment of panic disorder than are benzodiazepines or selective serotonin reuptake inhibitors (SSRIs).

Lithium-Induced Postural Tremor

The β-receptor antagonists are beneficial for lithium-induced postural tremor and other medication-induced postural tremors—for example, those induced by tricyclic drugs and valproate (Depakene). The initial approach to this movement disorder includes lowering the dose of lithium, eliminating aggravating factors, such as caffeine, and administering lithium at bedtime. If these interventions are inadequate, however, propranolol in the range of 20 to 160 mg a day, given two or three times daily, is generally effective for the treatment of lithium-induced postural tremor.

Neuroleptic-Induced Acute Akathisia

Many studies have shown that β-receptor antagonists can be effective in the treatment of neuroleptic-induced acute akathisia. Most clinicians believe that β-receptor antagonists are more effective for this indication than are anticholinergics and benzodiazepines. The β-receptor

Table 32.4–1
β-Adrenergic Drugs Used in Psychiatry

Generic Name	Trade Name	Lipophilic	Metabolism	Receptor Selectivity	Half-Life (hrs)	Usual Starting Dosage (mg)	Usual Maximum Dosage (mg)
Propranolol	Inderal	Yes	Hepatic	$\beta_1 = \beta_2$	3–6	10–20 two or three times a day	30–40 three times a day
Nadolol	Corgard	No	Renal	$\beta_1 = \beta_2$	14–24	40 once daily	30–240 once daily
Pindolol	Visken	Intermediate	Hepatic	$\beta_1 = \beta_2$	3–4	5 two times a day	30 two times a day
Labetalol	Normodyne, Trandate	Intermediate	Hepatic	$\beta_1 = \beta_2$	4–6	100 two times a day	400–800 three times a day
Metoprolol	Lopressor	Yes	Hepatic	$\beta_1 > \beta_2$	3–4	50 two times a day	75–150 two times a day
Atenolol	Tenormin	No	Renal	$\beta_1 > \beta_2$	5–8	50 once daily	50–100 once daily
Acebutolol	Sectral	No	Hepatic	$\beta_1 > \beta_2$	3–4	400 once daily	600 two times a day

antagonists are not effective in the treatment of such neuroleptic-induced movement disorders as acute dystonia and Parkinsonism.

Aggression and Violent Behavior

The β-receptor antagonists may be effective in reducing the number of aggressive and violent outbursts in persons with impulse disorders, schizophrenia, and aggression associated with brain injuries, such as trauma, tumors, anoxic injury, encephalitis, alcohol dependence, and degenerative disorders (e.g., Huntington's disease). Many studies have added a β-receptor antagonist to the ongoing therapy (e.g., antipsychotics, anticonvulsants, lithium); therefore, it is difficult to distinguish additive effects from independent effects.

Alcohol Withdrawal

Propranolol is reported to be useful as an adjuvant to benzodiazepines but not as a sole agent in the treatment of alcohol withdrawal. The following dose schedule is suggested: no propranolol for a pulse rate below 50 beats per minute (bpm); 50 mg propranolol for a pulse rate between 50 and 79 bpm; and 100 mg propranolol for a pulse rate of 80 bpm or above.

Antidepressant Augmentation

Pindolol has been used to augment and hasten the antidepressant effects of SSRIs, tricyclic drugs, and electroconvulsive therapy. Small studies have shown that pindolol administered at the onset of antidepressant therapy may shorten the usual 2- to 4-week latency of antidepressant response by several days. Because the β-receptor antagonists may possibly induce depression in some persons, augmentation strategies with these drugs need to be further clarified in controlled trials.

Other Disorders

A number of case reports and controlled studies have reported data indicating that β-receptor antagonists may be of modest benefit for persons with schizophrenia and with manic symptoms. They have also been used in some cases of stuttering.

PRECAUTIONS AND ADVERSE REACTIONS

The β-receptor antagonists are contraindicated for use in people with asthma, insulin-dependent diabetes, congestive heart failure, significant vascular disease, persistent angina, and hyperthyroidism. The contraindication in diabetic persons is because the drugs antagonize the normal physiological response to hypoglycemia. The β-receptor antagonists can worsen atrioventricular (AV) conduction defects and lead to complete AV heart block and death. If the clinician decides that the risk-to-benefit ratio warrants a trial of a β-receptor antagonist in a person with one of these coexisting medical conditions, a β_1-selective agent should be the first choice. All available β-receptor antagonists are excreted in breast milk and should be administered with caution to nursing women.

The most common adverse effects of β-receptor antagonists are hypotension and bradycardia. In persons at risk for these adverse effects, a test dose of 20 mg a day of propranolol can be given to assess reaction to the drug. Depression has been associated with lipophilic β-receptor antagonists, such as propranolol,

but it is probably rare. Nausea, vomiting, diarrhea, and constipation can also be caused by treatment with these agents. Serious CNS adverse effects (e.g., agitation, confusion, and hallucinations) are rare.

DRUG INTERACTIONS

Concomitant administration of propranolol results in increases in plasma concentrations of antipsychotics, anticonvulsants, theophylline (Theo-Dur, Slo-bid), and levothyroxine (Synthroid). Other β-receptor antagonists possibly have similar effects. The β-receptor antagonists that are eliminated by the kidneys may have similar effects on drugs that are also eliminated by the renal route. Barbiturates, phenytoin (Dilantin), and cigarette smoking increase the elimination of β-receptor antagonists that are metabolized by the liver. Several reports have associated hypertensive crises and bradycardia with the coadministration of β-receptor antagonists and monoamine oxidase inhibitors. Depressed myocardial contractility and AV nodal conduction can occur from concomitant administration of a β-receptor antagonist and calcium channel inhibitors.

LABORATORY INTERFERENCES

The β-receptor antagonists do not interfere with standard laboratory tests.

DOSING AND CLINICAL GUIDELINES

Propranolol is available in 10-, 20-, 40-, 60-, 80-, and 90-mg tablets; 4-, 8-, and 80-mg/mL solutions; and 60-, 80-, 120-, and 160-mg sustained-release capsules. Nadolol is available in 20-, 40-, 80-, 120-, and 160-mg tablets. Pindolol is available in 5- and 10-mg tablets. Labetalol is available in 100-, 200-, and 300-mg tablets. Metoprolol is available in 50- and 100-mg tablets and 50-, 100-, and 200-mg sustained-release tablets. Atenolol is available in 25-, 50-, and 100-mg tablets. Acebutolol is available in 200- and 400-mg capsules.

For the treatment of chronic disorders, propranolol administration is usually initiated at 10 mg by mouth three times a day or 20 mg by mouth twice daily. The dose can be raised by 20 to 30 mg a day until a therapeutic effect begins to emerge. The dose should be leveled off at the appropriate range for the disorder under treatment. The treatment of aggressive behavior sometimes requires doses up to 800 mg a day, and therapeutic effects may not be seen until the person has been receiving the maximal dose for 4 to 8 weeks. For the treatment of social phobia, primarily the performance type, the patient should take 10 to 40 mg of propranolol 20 to 30 minutes before the performance.

Pulse and blood pressure (BP) readings should be taken regularly, and the drug should be withheld if the pulse rate is below 50 bpm or the systolic BP is below 90 mm Hg. The drug should be temporarily discontinued if it produces severe dizziness, ataxia, or wheezing. Treatment with β-receptor antagonists should never be discontinued abruptly. Propranolol should be tapered by 60 mg a day until a dose of 60 mg a day is reached, after which the drug should be tapered by 10 to 20 mg a day every 3 or 4 days.

▲ 32.5 Anticholinergics and Amantadine

In the clinical practice of psychiatry, the anticholinergic drugs are primarily used to treat medication-induced movement disorders, particularly neuroleptic-induced Parkinsonism, neuroleptic-induced acute dystonia, and medication-induced postural tremor. Amantadine (Symmetrel) is used primarily for the treatment of medication-induced movement disorders, such as neuroleptic-induced Parkinsonism. It is also used as an antiviral agent for the prophylaxis and treatment of influenza A infection.

ANTICHOLINERGICS

Pharmacological Actions

All anticholinergic drugs are well absorbed from the gastrointestinal (GI) tract after oral administration, and all are sufficiently lipophilic to enter the central nervous system (CNS). Trihexyphenidyl (Artane) and benztropine (Cogentin) reach peak plasma concentrations in 2 to 3 hours after oral administration, and their duration of action is 1 to 12 hours. Benztropine is absorbed equally rapidly by intramuscular (IM) and intravenous (IV) administration; IM administration is preferred because of its low risk for adverse effects.

All five anticholinergic drugs listed in this section block muscarinic acetylcholine receptors, and benztropine also has some antihistaminergic effects. None of the available anticholinergic drugs has any effect on the nicotinic acetylcholine receptors. Of the five drugs, trihexyphenidyl is the most stimulating agent, perhaps acting through dopaminergic neurons, and benztropine is the least stimulating and, thus, is least associated with abuse potential.

Therapeutic Indications

The primary indication for the use of anticholinergics in psychiatric practice is for the treatment of *neuroleptic-induced Parkinsonism*, characterized by tremor, rigidity, cogwheeling, bradykinesia, sialorrhea, stooped posture, and festination. All of the available anticholinergics are equally effective in the treatment of Parkinsonian symptoms. Neuroleptic-induced Parkinsonism is most common in the elderly and is most frequently seen with high-potency dopamine receptor antagonists (DRAs), for example, haloperidol (Haldol). The onset of symptoms usually occurs after 2 or 3 weeks of treatment. The incidence of neuroleptic-induced Parkinsonism is lower with the newer antipsychotic drugs of the serotonin-dopamine antagonist (SDA) class.

Another indication is for the treatment of *neuroleptic-induced acute dystonia*, which is most common in young men. The syndrome often occurs early in the course of treatment, is commonly associated with high-potency DRAs (e.g., haloperidol), and most commonly affects the muscles of the neck, the tongue, the face, and the back. Anticholinergic drugs are effective both in the short-term treatment of dystonias and in prophylaxis against neuroleptic-induced acute dystonias.

Akathisia is characterized by a subjective and objective sense of restlessness, anxiety, and agitation. Although a trial of anticholinergics for the treatment of neuroleptic-induced acute akathisia is reasonable, these drugs are not generally considered as effective as the β-adrenergic receptor antagonists, the benzodiazepines, and clonidine (Catapres).

Precautions and Adverse Reactions

The adverse effects of the anticholinergic drugs result from blockade of muscarinic acetylcholine receptors. Anticholinergic drugs should be used cautiously, if at all, by persons with prostatic hypertrophy, urinary retention, and narrow-angle glaucoma. The anticholinergics are occasionally used as drugs of abuse because of their mild mood-elevating properties, most notably, trihexyphenidyl.

The most serious adverse effect associated with anticholinergic toxicity is anticholinergic intoxication, which can be characterized by delirium, coma, seizures, agitation, hallucinations, severe hypotension, supraventricular tachycardia, and peripheral manifestations—flushing, mydriasis, dry skin, hyperthermia, and decreased bowel sounds. Treatment should begin with the immediate discontinuation of all anticholinergic drugs. The syndrome of anticholinergic intoxication can be diagnosed and treated with physostigmine (Antilirium, Eserine), an inhibitor of anticholinesterase, 1 to 2 mg IV (1 mg every 2 minutes) or IM every 30 or 60 minutes. Treatment with physostigmine should be used only in severe cases and only when emergency cardiac monitoring and life-support services are available, because physostigmine can lead to severe hypotension and bronchial constriction.

Drug Interactions

The most common drug–drug interactions with the anticholinergics occur when they are coadministered with psychotropics that also have high anticholinergic activity, such as DRAs, tricyclic and tetracyclic drugs, and monoamine oxidase inhibitors (MAOIs). Many other prescription drugs and over-the-counter cold preparations also induce significant anticholinergic activity. The coadministration of those drugs can result in a life-threatening anticholinergic intoxication syndrome. Anticholinergic drugs can also delay gastric emptying, thereby decreasing the absorption of drugs that are broken down in the stomach and usually absorbed in the duodenum (e.g., levodopa [Larodopa] and DRAs).

Laboratory Interferences

No known laboratory interferences have been associated with anticholinergics.

Dosing and Clinical Guidelines

The five anticholinergic drugs discussed in this section are available in a range of preparations (Table 32.5–1).

Neuroleptic-Induced Parkinsonism.
For the treatment of neuroleptic-induced Parkinsonism, the equivalent of 1 to 3 mg of benztropine should be given one to two times daily. The anticholinergic drug should be administered for 4 to 8 weeks, and then it should be discontinued to assess whether the person

Table 32.5–1
Anticholinergic Drugs

Generic Name	Brand Name	Tablet Size	Injectable	Usual Daily Oral Dose	Short-term IM or IV Dose
Benztropine	Cogentin	0.5, 1, 2 mg	1 mg/mL	1–4 mg one to three times	1–2 mg
Biperiden	Akineton	2 mg	5 mg/mL	2 mg one to three times	2 mg
Ethopropazine	Parsidol	10, 50 mg	—	50–100 mg one to three times	—
Orphenadrine	Norflex, Dispal	100 mg	30 mg/mL	50–100 mg three times	60 mg IV given over 5 min
Procyclidine	Kemadrin	5 mg	—	2–5 mg three times	—
Trihexyphenidyl	Artane, Trihexane, Trihexy-5	2, 5 mg; elixir 2 mg/5 mL	—	2–5 mg two to four times	—

IM, intramuscular; IV, intravenous.

still requires the drug. Anticholinergic drugs should be tapered over a period of 1 to 2 weeks.

Treatment with anticholinergics as prophylaxis against the development of neuroleptic-induced Parkinsonism is usually not indicated because onset of its symptoms is usually sufficiently mild and gradual to allow the clinician to initiate treatment only after it is clearly indicated. In young men, prophylaxis may be indicated, however, especially if a high-potency DRA is being used. The clinician should attempt to discontinue the anti-Parkinsonian agent in 4 to 6 weeks to assess whether its continued use is necessary.

Neuroleptic-Induced Acute Dystonia.   For the short-term treatment and prophylaxis of neuroleptic-induced acute dystonia, 1 to 2 mg of benztropine or its equivalent in another drug should be given IM. The dose can be repeated in 20 to 30 minutes, as needed. If the person still does not improve in another 20 to 30 minutes, a benzodiazepine (e.g., 1 mg IM or IV lorazepam [Ativan]) should be given. Laryngeal dystonia is a medical emergency and should be treated with benztropine, up to 4 mg in a 10-minute period, followed by 1 to 2 mg of lorazepam, administered slowly by the IV route.

Prophylaxis against dystonias is indicated in persons who have had one episode or in persons at high risk (young men taking high-potency DRAs). Prophylactic treatment is given for 4 to 8 weeks and then gradually tapered over 1 to 2 weeks to allow assessment of its continued need. The prophylactic use of anticholinergics in persons requiring antipsychotic drugs has largely become a moot issue because of the availability of SDAs, which are relatively free of Parkinsonian effects.

Akathisia.   As mentioned, anticholinergics are not the drugs of choice for this syndrome. The β-adrenergic receptor antagonists (Section 32.4) and perhaps the benzodiazepines (Section 32.9) and clonidine (Section 32.3) are preferable drugs to try initially.

AMANTADINE

Pharmacological Actions

Amantadine is well absorbed from the GI tract after oral administration, reaches peak plasma concentrations in approximately 2 to 3 hours, has a half-life of about 12 to 18 hours, and attains steady-state concentrations after approximately 4 to 5 days

of therapy. Amantadine is excreted unmetabolized in the urine. Amantadine plasma concentrations can be twice as high in elderly persons as in younger adults. Patients with renal failure accumulate amantadine in their bodies.

Amantadine augments dopaminergic neurotransmission in the CNS; however, the precise mechanism for the effect is unknown. The mechanism may involve dopamine release from presynaptic vesicles, blocking reuptake of dopamine into presynaptic nerve terminals, or an agonist effect on postsynaptic dopamine receptors.

Therapeutic Indications

The primary indication for amantadine use in psychiatry is to treat extrapyramidal signs and symptoms, such as Parkinsonism, akinesia, and so-called rabbit syndrome (focal perioral tremor of the choreoathetoid type) caused by the administration of DRA or SDA drugs. Amantadine is as effective as the anticholinergics (e.g., benztropine [Cogentin]) for these indications and results in improvement in approximately one half of all persons who take it. Amantadine, however, is not generally considered as effective as the anticholinergics for the treatment of acute dystonic reactions and is not effective in treating tardive dyskinesia and akathisia.

Amantadine is a reasonable compromise for persons with extrapyramidal symptoms who would be sensitive to additional anticholinergic effects, particularly those taking a low-potency DRA or the elderly. Elderly persons are susceptible to anticholinergic adverse effects, both in the CNS, such as anticholinergic delirium, and in the peripheral nervous system, such as urinary retention. Amantadine is associated with less memory impairment than are the anticholinergics.

Amantadine has been reported to be of benefit in treating some selective serotonin reuptake inhibitor–associated side effects, such as lethargy, fatigue, anorgasmia, and ejaculatory inhibition.

Amantadine is used in general medical practice for the treatment of Parkinsonism of all causes, including idiopathic Parkinsonism.

Precautions and Adverse Effects

The most common CNS effects of amantadine are mild dizziness, insomnia, and impaired concentration (dose related), which occur in 5 to 10 percent of all persons. Irritability, depression, anxiety, dysarthria, and ataxia occur in 1 to 5 percent of persons. More severe CNS adverse effects, including seizures and psychotic symptoms, have been reported. Nausea is the most common peripheral adverse effect of amantadine. Headache, loss of appetite, and blotchy spots on the skin have also been reported.

Livedo reticularis of the legs (a purple discoloration of the skin, caused by dilation of blood vessels) has been reported in up to 5 percent of persons who take the drug for more than 1 month. It usually diminishes with elevation of the legs and resolves in almost all cases when drug use is terminated.

Amantadine is relatively contraindicated in persons with renal disease or a seizure disorder. Amantadine should be used with caution in persons with edema or cardiovascular disease. Some evidence indicates that amantadine is teratogenic and, therefore, should not be taken by pregnant women. Because amantadine is excreted in milk, women who are breast-feeding should not take the drug.

Suicide attempts with amantadine overdoses are life threatening. Symptoms can include toxic psychoses (confusion, hallucinations, aggressiveness) and cardiopulmonary arrest. Emergency treatment beginning with gastric lavage is indicated.

Drug Interactions

Coadministration of amantadine with phenelzine (Nardil) or other MAOIs can result in a significant increase in resting blood pressure. The coadministration of amantadine with CNS stimulants can result in insomnia, irritability, nervousness, and possibly seizures or irregular heartbeat. Amantadine should not be coadministered with anticholinergics because unwanted side effects—such as confusion, hallucinations, nightmares, dry mouth, and blurred vision—may be exacerbated.

Dosing and Clinical Guidelines

Amantadine is available in 100-mg capsules and as a 50-mg/5 mL syrup. The usual starting dose of amantadine is 100 mg given orally twice a day, although the dose can be cautiously increased up to 200 mg given orally twice a day if indicated. Amantadine should be used in persons with renal impairment *only* in consultation with the physician treating the renal condition. If amantadine is successful in the treatment of the drug-induced extrapyramidal symptoms, it should be continued for 4 to 6 weeks and then discontinued to see whether the person has become tolerant to the neurological adverse effects of the antipsychotic medication. Amantadine should be tapered over 1 to 2 weeks once a decision has been made to discontinue the drug. Persons taking amantadine should not drink alcoholic beverages.

▲ 32.6 Anticonvulsants: Gabapentin, Pregabalin, Tiagabine, Levetiracetam, Topiramate, and Zonisamide

Despite the absence of large placebo-controlled trials proving their efficacy as psychotropics, six anticonvulsant drugs— gabapentin (Neurontin), pregabalin (Lyrica), tiagabine (Gabitril), levetiracetam (Keppra), topiramate (Topamax), and zonisamide (Zonegran)—are occasionally used in psychiatry. Anec-

dotal evidence suggests that some patients benefit from treatment with each of these drugs in certain clinical circumstances; however, their routine use in place of proved treatments is not recommended. These drugs differ in chemical structure.

GABAPENTIN

Gabapentin indirectly increases brain γ-aminobutyric acid (GABA) levels. It is well absorbed, but its bioavailability decreases as doses are increased, because of saturation of the neutral amino acid membrane transporter system in the gut. Because higher amounts are not absorbed, doses should not exceed 1,800 mg per single dose or 5,400 mg a day. Gabapentin absorption is unaffected by food. Steady-state half-life of 5 to 9 hours is reached in 2 days when taken three times a day. Gabapentin does not bind to plasma proteins and is not metabolized. It is excreted unchanged in the urine.

Therapeutic Indications

Gabapentin is used as a hypnotic agent because of its sedating effects. It also has anxiolytic properties, providing benefit to patients with panic attacks and social anxiety disorder. Gabapentin decreases craving for alcohol, helping patients to remain abstinent, and facilitates detoxification. In some cases, patients can be switched to gabapentin following benzodiazepine-facilitated alcohol detoxification. Because gabapentin is renally excreted, it is well suited for use among patients with liver disease. To the extent that gabapentin reduces alcohol use among patients with bipolar disorder, it may prove useful as an adjunct to standard mood stabilizer regimens. Gabapentin is approved by the U.S. Food and Drug Administration (FDA) for the treatment of postherpetic neuralgia. Other pain conditions responsive to gabapentin include trigeminal neuralgia; central pain syndromes; and compression neuropathies, such as carpal tunnel syndrome, radiculopathies, and meralgia paresthetica. Pregabalin, an analog of gabapentin, has been approved for the management of neuropathic pain associated with diabetic peripheral neuropathy and postherpetic neuralgia.

Clinical Guidelines

Gabapentin dose can be escalated to the maintenance range within 2 to 3 days, with sedation being the only dose-related side effect. Other frequent adverse effects of gabapentin are dizziness, ataxia, fatigue, and nystagmus, which are usually transient. Some patients experience peripheral edema, memory impairment, weight gain, and orgasmic dysfunction. Gabapentin has no significant hepatic cytochrome P450 or pharmacodynamic interactions. Antacids containing aluminum hydroxide and magnesium hydroxide (Maalox) decrease gabapentin absorption by 20 percent if administered concurrently but negligibly if administered 2 hours before taking the dose of gabapentin. Gabapentin can cause false-positive readings with the Ames N-Multistix SG dipstick test for urinary protein. The drug should be used cautiously in patients with renal disease or on dialysis.

Gabapentin is available as 100-, 300-, and 400-mg capsules and as 600- and 800-mg tablets. The starting dose of gabapentin is 300 mg three times a day, and the dose can be rapidly titrated up to a maximum of 1,800 mg three times a day over a period of a few days. Most people achieve satisfactory benefit within the range of 600 to 900 mg three times a day. Although abrupt discontinuation of gabapentin does not cause withdrawal effects, use of all anticonvulsant drugs should be gradually tapered.

PREGABALIN

Pregabalin is pharmacologically similar to gabapentin. It is believed to work by inhibiting the release of excess excitatory neurotransmitters, presumably by binding to the α-2-Δ subunit protein of voltage-dependent calcium channels in the brain and spinal cord. It also increases neuronal GABA levels. The binding affinity of pregabalin for the α-2-Δ subunit is six times greater than that of gabapentin, and it has a longer half-life.

Therapeutic Indications

Pregabalin is approved for the management of diabetic peripheral neuropathy and postherpetic neuralgia and for adjunctive treatment of partial onset seizures.

Pregabalin has been found to be of benefit to some patients with generalized anxiety disorder. In studies, no consistent dose-response relationship was found, although 300-mg pregabalin per day was more effective than 150 mg or 450 mg.

Although rejected for that indication by the FDA, the Committee for Medicinal Products for Human Use of the European Medicines Agency issued a positive opinion recommending marketing authorization of pregabalin. Some patients with panic disorder or social anxiety disorder may benefit from pregabalin, but little evidence supports its routine use in treating those disorders.

Clinical Guidelines

Pregabalin exhibits linear pharmacokinetics. It is extremely and rapidly absorbed in proportion to its dose. The time to maximal plasma concentration is about 1 hour, and that to steady state is within 24 to 48 hours. Pregabalin demonstrates high bioavailability, and it has a mean elimination half-life of about 6.5 hours. Food does not affect absorption. Pregabalin does not bind to plasma proteins and is excreted virtually unchanged (<2 percent metabolism) by the kidneys. It is not subject to hepatic metabolism and does not induce or inhibit liver enzymes such as the cytochrome P450 system. Dose adjustment may be necessary in patients with creatinine clearance (CLcr) less than 60 mL per minute. A 50 percent reduction in pregabalin daily dose is recommended for patients with CLcr between 30 and 60 mL per minute compared with those with CLcr greater than 60 mL per minute. Daily doses should be further reduced by approximately 50 percent for each additional 50 percent decrease in CLcr. Pregabalin is highly cleared by hemodialysis, so additional doses may be needed for patients on chronic hemodialysis treatment after each hemodialysis treatment.

The most common adverse events associated with pregabalin use are dizziness, somnolence, blurred vision, peripheral edema, amnesia or loss of memory, and tremors. Pregabalin potentiates sedating effects of alcohol, antihistamines, benzodiazepines, and other central nervous system (CNS) depressants. It remains to be seen if pregabalin is associated with benzodiazepine-type withdrawal symptoms.

The recommended dose for postherpetic neuralgia is 50 or 100 mg orally three times a day. The recommended dose for diabetic peripheral neuropathy is 100 to 200 mg orally three times a day. Pregabalin is available as 25-, 50-, 75-, 100-, 150-, 200-, 225-, and 300-mg capsules.

TOPIRAMATE

Topiramate is a selective inhibitor of glutamate α-amino-3-hydroxy-5-methylisoxazole-4-propionic acid receptors, blocks Na^+ receptors, and has indirect GABAergic activity. It potentiates the action of GABA at a non–benzodiazepine-, non–barbiturate-sensitive $GABA_A$ receptor, is rapidly and completely absorbed, and has a steady-state half-life of 21 hours. Food does not affect its absorption. It is 15 percent protein bound in the plasma, and 70 percent of an oral dose of topiramate is excreted unchanged in the urine, together with small amounts of several inactive metabolites. Topiramate is an inhibitor of state-dependent sodium channels.

Therapeutic Indications

Despite initial reports of mood-stabilizing properties, a series of large, placebo-controlled studies failed to find any evidence of antimanic activity. The fact that some patients lose a substantial amount of weight while taking topiramate is exploited in psychiatry mainly to counteract the weight gain caused by many psychotropic drugs. Topiramate has been shown to benefit patients with primary alcoholism and posttraumatic stress disorder. Topiramate may reduce the frequency of cutting and other forms of self-mutilating behavior in patients with borderline personality disorder. It is effective in treating neuropathic pain and migraine and is also highly effective in treating binge-eating disorder.

The most common non–dose-related adverse effects of topiramate used in combination with other antiepileptic drugs include psychomotor slowing; speech and language problems, especially word-finding difficulties; somnolence; dizziness; ataxia; nystagmus; and paresthesias. The most common dose-related adverse effects are fatigue, nervousness, poor concentration, confusion, taste perversion, depression, anorexia, anxiety, mood problems, weight loss, and tremor. Some 1.5 percent of persons taking topiramate develop renal calculi, a rate ten times that associated with placebo. Patients at risk for calculi should be encouraged to drink plenty of fluids.

Clinical Guidelines

Topiramate has a few well-characterized drug interactions with other anticonvulsant drugs. Topiramate can increase phenytoin concentrations up to 25 percent and valproic acid concentrations 11 percent; it does not affect the concentrations of carbamazepine or its epoxide, phenobarbital (Luminal), or primidone. Topiramate concentrations are decreased by 40 percent to 48 percent with concomitant administration of carbamazepine or phenytoin and by 14 percent with concurrent administration of valproic acid. Topiramate also slightly decreases digoxin (Lanoxin) bioavailability and the efficacy of estrogenic oral contraceptives. Addition of topiramate, a weak inhibitor of carbonic anhydrase, to other inhibitors of carbonic anhydrase, such as acetazolamide (Diamox) or dichlorphenamide (Daranide), may promote development of renal calculi and is to be avoided. Topiramate does not interfere with any laboratory tests.

Topiramate is available as unscored 25-, 100-, and 200-mg tablets. To reduce the risk of adverse cognitive and sedative effects, topiramate dose is titrated gradually over 8 weeks to a maximum of 200 mg twice a day. Higher doses are not associated with increased efficacy. Persons with renal insufficiency should reduce doses by half.

TIAGABINE

Tiagabine is a potent and selective reuptake inhibitor of GABA. It also has mild blocking effects of H_1, serotonin I_B, benzodiazepine, and chloride channel receptors. More than 95 percent of tiagabine is rapidly absorbed. The rate of absorption is slowed by food. Absolute bioavailability of tiagabine is 95 percent, and it is 96 percent protein bound. It has a half-life of 7 to 9 hours and is metabolized by the hepatic cytochrome P450 (CYP450) 3A system. Tiagabine concentrations are about 40 percent lower in the evening than in the morning.

Tiagabine is occasionally used as an anxiolytic or hypnotic agent in patients who have not responded to, or tolerated, standard treatments. It has not been found to be useful in treating manic symptoms, whether used alone or as adjunctive therapy.

Animal studies have found teratogenic effects in rats. Ophthalmic changes can occur with chronic use. CNS side effects include sedation, cognitive impairment, ataxia, dizziness, tremor, paresthesias, confusion, and depression. Other side effects include ecchymosis, nausea, abdominal pain, muscle weakness, and flushing. Cases of serious rash can occur, including Stevens-Johnson syndrome. Lower doses of tiagabine should be used in patients with hepatic impairment. Patients being treated with tiagabine for bipolar disorder have experienced new-onset seizures. Reports of seizures in patients without epilepsy being treated with tiagabine have prompted an FDA warning about its use. Consequently, this drug should not be considered for off-label psychiatric use.

ZONISAMIDE

Zonisamide is sometimes used as an alternative treatment for acute mania and as a weight loss agent for drug-induced weight gain.

Zonisamide blocks sodium channels and may weakly potentiate dopamine and serotonin activity. It also inhibits carbonic anhydrase. Some evidence suggests that it might block calcium channels. Zonisamide is metabolized by the hepatic CYP450 3A system, so enzyme-inducing agents, such as carbamazepine, alcohol, and phenobarbital, increase the clearance and reduce the availability of the drug. Zonisamide does not affect the metabolism of other drugs.

Zonisamide can elevate hepatic alkaline phosphatase and increase blood urea nitrogen and creatinine. Zonisamide is a sulfonamide and, thus, may cause fatal rash and blood dyscrasias, although these events are rare. About 4 percent of patients develop kidney stones. The most common side effects are drowsiness, cognitive impairment, insomnia, ataxia, nystagmus, paresthesia, speech abnormalities, constipation, diarrhea, nausea, and dry mouth. Weight loss is also a common side effect, which has been exploited as a therapy for patients who have gained weight during treatment with psychotropics or who have ongoing difficulty controlling their eating.

Zonisamide is available in 100- and 200-mg capsules. In epilepsy, the dose range is 100 to 400 mg per day, with side effects becoming more pronounced at doses above 300 mg. Because of its long half-life, zonisamide can be given once a day.

LEVETIRACETAM

Levetiracetam has been used to treat acute mania, as add-on therapy to antidepressants to prevent the emergence of mania or cycling, and as an anxiolytic.

The CNS effects of levetiracetam are poorly understood, but it appears to indirectly enhance GABA inhibition. It is rapidly and completely absorbed. Peak concentrations are reached in 1 hour. Food delays the rate of absorption and decreases the amount of absorption. Levetiracetam is not significantly plasma protein bound and is not metabolized through the hepatic CYP system. Its metabolism involves hydrolysis of its acetamide group. No significant drug interactions have been noted. Serum concentrations are not correlated with any therapeutic effect.

The most common side effects of levetiracetam are drowsiness, dizziness, ataxia, diplopia, memory impairment, apathy, and paresthesia. More notably, some patients develop behavioral disturbances during treatment, and hallucinations can occur. Suicidality was noted in a few patients during clinical trials.

Levetiracetam is available as 250-, 500-, and 750-mg tablets. In epilepsy, it is given twice a day, with daily dose ranging from 500 mg to 3,000 mg. The typical daily dose in epilepsy is 1,000 mg.

▲ 32.7 Antihistamines

In clinical psychiatry, certain antihistamines (antagonists of histamine H_1 receptors) are used to treat neuroleptic-induced Parkinsonism and neuroleptic-induced acute dystonia and also as hypnotics and anxiolytics. Diphenhydramine (Benadryl) is used to treat neuroleptic-induced Parkinsonism and neuroleptic-induced acute dystonia and sometimes as a hypnotic. Hydroxyzine hydrochloride (Atarax) and hydroxyzine pamoate (Vistaril) are used as anxiolytics. Promethazine (Phenergan) is used for its sedative and anxiolytic effects. Cyproheptadine (Periactin) has been used for the treatment of anorexia nervosa and inhibited male and female orgasm caused by serotonergic agents. Fexofenadine (Allegra), loratadine (Claritin), and cetirizine (Zyrtec) are less commonly used in psychiatric practice. Terfenadine (Seldane) and astemizole (Hismanal) were withdrawn from commercial availability because they were associated with serious cardiac arrhythmias when coadministered with some drugs (e.g., nefazodone [Serzone], selective serotonin reuptake inhibitors [SSRIs]).

Table 32.7–1 lists antihistaminic drugs not used in psychiatry but which may have psychiatric adverse effects or drug–drug interactions.

PHARMACOLOGICAL ACTIONS

The H_1 antagonists used in psychiatry are well absorbed from the gastrointestinal (GI) tract. The anti-Parkinsonian effects of intramuscular (IM) diphenhydramine have their onset in 15 to 30 minutes, and the sedative effects of diphenhydramine peak in 1 to

Table 32.7–1
Dosing and Administration of Common Histamine Antagonists

Medication	Route	Preparation	Common Dose
Diphenhydramine (Benadryl)	PO	Capsules and tablets: 25 mg, 50 mg Liquid: 12.5 mg/5.0 mL	Adults: 25 to 50 mg three to four times per day Children: 5 mg/kg three to four times per day, not to exceed 300 mg/day
	Deep IM or IV	Solution: 10 or 50 mg/mL	Same as oral
Hydroxyzine Hydrochloride (Atarax)	PO	Tablets: 10, 25, 50, and 100 mg Syrup: 10 mg/5 mL	Adults: 50 to 100 mg three to four times daily Children <6 yrs of age: 2 mg/kg/ day in divided doses Children >6 yrs of age: 12.5 to 25.0 mg, three to four times daily
	IM	Solution: 25 or 50 mg/mL	Same as oral
Pamoate (Vistaril)	PO	Suspension: 25 mg/mL Capsules: 25, 50, and 100 mg	Same as dosages for hydrochloride
Promethazine (Phenergan)	PO	Tablets: 15.2, 25.0, and 50.0 mg Syrup: 3.25 mg/5 mL	Adults: 50–100 mg three to four times daily for sedation Children: 12.5–25.0 mg at night for sedation
	Rectal	Suppositories: 12.5, 25.0, and 50.0 mg	
	IM	Solution: 25 and 50 mg/mL	
Cyproheptadine (Periactin)	PO	Tablets: 4 mg Syrup: 2 mg/5 mL	Adults: 4–20 mg/day Children 2–7 yrs of age: 2 mg two to three times daily (maximum of 12 mg/day) Children 7–14 yrs of age: 4 mg two to three times daily (maximum of 16 mg/day)

IM, intramuscular; IV, intravenous; PO, oral.

3 hours. The sedative effects of hydroxyzine and promethazine begin after 20 to 60 minutes and last for 4 to 6 hours. Because all three drugs are metabolized in the liver, persons with hepatic disease, such as cirrhosis, may attain high plasma concentrations with long-term administration. Cyproheptadine is well absorbed after oral administration, and its metabolites are excreted in the urine.

Activation of H_1 receptors stimulates wakefulness; therefore, receptor antagonism causes sedation. All four agents also possess some antimuscarinic cholinergic activity. Cyproheptadine is unique among the drugs because it has both potent antihistamine and serotonin 5-HT$_2$ receptor antagonist properties.

THERAPEUTIC INDICATIONS

Antihistamines are useful as a treatment for neuroleptic-induced Parkinsonism, neuroleptic-induced acute dystonia, and neuroleptic-induced akathisia. They are an alternative to anticholinergics and amantadine for these purposes. The antihistamines are relatively safe hypnotics but they are not superior to the benzodiazepines, which have been much better studied in terms of efficacy and safety. The antihistamines have not been proved effective for long-term anxiolytic therapy; therefore, either the benzodiazepines, buspirone (BuSpar), or selective serotonin reuptake inhibitors (SSRIs) are preferable for such treatment. Cyproheptadine is sometimes used to treat impaired orgasms, especially delayed orgasm resulting from treatment with serotonergic drugs.

Because it promotes weight gain, cyproheptadine may be of some use in the treatment of eating disorders, such as anorexia nervosa. Cyproheptadine can reduce recurrent nightmares with posttraumatic themes. The antiserotonergic activity of cyproheptadine may counteract the serotonin syndrome caused by concomitant use of multiple serotonin-activating drugs, such as SSRIs and monoamine oxidase inhibitors.

PRECAUTIONS AND ADVERSE REACTIONS

Antihistamines are commonly associated with sedation, dizziness, and hypotension, all of which can be severe in elderly persons, who are also likely to be affected by the anticholinergic effects of those drugs. Paradoxical excitement and agitation are adverse effects seen in a small number of persons. Poor motor coordination can result in accidents; therefore, persons should be warned about driving and operating dangerous machinery. Other common adverse effects include epigastric distress, nausea, vomiting, diarrhea, and constipation. Because of mild anticholinergic activity, some people experience dry mouth, urinary retention, blurred vision, and constipation. For this reason also, antihistamines should be used only at very low doses, if at all, by persons with narrow-angle glaucoma or obstructive GI, prostate, or bladder conditions. A central anticholinergic syndrome with psychosis may be induced by either cyproheptadine or diphenhydramine.

In addition to the above aforementioned effects, antihistamines have some potential for abuse. The coadministration of antihistamines and opioids can increase the euphoria experienced by persons with substance dependence. Overdoses of antihistamines can be fatal. Antihistamines are excreted in breast milk, so their use should be avoided by nursing mothers. Because of some potential for teratogenicity, the use of antihistamines should also be avoided by pregnant women.

Drug Interactions

The sedative property of antihistamines can be additive with other central nervous system depressants, such as alcohol, other sedative-hypnotic drugs, and many psychotropic drugs, including tricyclic drugs and dopamine receptor antagonists. The anticholinergic activity can also be additive with that of other anticholinergic drugs and can sometimes result in severe anticholinergic symptoms or intoxication. The beneficial effects of SSRIs can be antagonized by cyproheptadine.

LABORATORY INTERFERENCES

H_1 antagonists may eliminate the wheal and induration that form the basis of allergy skin tests. Promethazine can interfere with pregnancy tests and can increase blood glucose concentrations. Diphenhydramine may yield a false-positive urine test result for phencyclidine. Hydroxyzine use can falsely elevate the results of certain tests for urinary 17-hydroxycorticosteroids.

DOSING AND CLINICAL GUIDELINES

The antihistamines are available in a variety of preparations. Intramuscular injections should be deep because superficial administration can cause local irritation.

Intravenous (IV) administration of 25 to 50 mg of diphenhydramine is an effective treatment for neuroleptic-induced acute dystonia, which may immediately disappear. Use of 25 mg three times a day—up to 50 mg four times a day, if necessary—can be used to treat neuroleptic-induced Parkinsonism, akinesia, and buccal movements. Diphenhydramine can be used as a hypnotic at a 50-mg dose for mild transient insomnia. Doses of 100 mg have not been shown to be superior to doses of 50 mg, but they produce more anticholinergic effects than do doses of 50 mg.

Hydroxyzine is most commonly used as a short-term anxiolytic. Hydroxyzine should not be given IV because it is irritating to the blood vessels. Doses of 50 to 100 mg given orally four times a day for long-term treatment or 50 to 100 mg IM every 4 to 6 hours for short-term treatment are usually effective.

Anorgasmia induced by SSRIs may sometimes be reversed with 4 to 16 mg a day of cyproheptadine taken by mouth 1 or 2 hours before anticipated sexual activity. A number of case reports and small studies have also reported that cyproheptadine may be of some use in the treatment of eating disorders, such as anorexia nervosa. Cyproheptadine is available in 4-mg tablets and a 2-mg/5 mL solution. Children and elderly patients are more sensitive to the effects of antihistamines than are young adults.

▲ 32.8 Barbiturates and Similarly Acting Drugs

Barbiturates were widely used as sedative-hypnotic agents in the first half of the 20th century. Many problems are associated with these drugs, including high abuse and addiction potential, a narrow therapeutic range with low therapeutic index, and unfavorable side effects. The use of barbiturates and similar compounds such as meprobamate (Miltown) has been practically eliminated by the benzodiazepines, other anxiolytics such as buspirone (BuSpar), and hypnotics such as zolpidem (Ambien) and zaleplon (Sonata), which have a lower abuse potential and a higher therapeutic index than the barbiturates. Nevertheless, the barbiturates and similarly acting drugs still have a role in the treatment of certain mental disorders.

PHARMACOLOGICAL ACTIONS

The barbiturates are well absorbed after oral administration. The binding of barbiturates to plasma proteins is high, but lipid solubility varies. The individual barbiturates are metabolized by the liver and excreted by the kidneys. The half-lives of specific barbiturates range from 1 to 120 hours. Barbiturates may also induce hepatic enzymes (cytochrome P450), thereby reducing the levels of both the barbiturate and any other concurrently administered drugs metabolized by the liver. The mechanism of action of barbiturates involves the γ-aminobutyric acid (GABA) receptor–benzodiazepine receptor–chloride ion channel complex.

THERAPEUTIC INDICATIONS

Electroconvulsive Therapy

Methohexital (Brevital) is commonly used as an anesthetic agent for electroconvulsive therapy (ECT). It has lower cardiac risks than other barbiturate anesthetics. Used intravenously, methohexital produces rapid unconsciousness and, because of its rapid redistribution, it has a brief duration of action (5 to 7 minutes). Typical dosing for ECT is 0.7 to 1.2 mg/kg. Methohexital can also be used to abort prolonged seizures in ECT or to limit postictal agitation.

Seizures

Phenobarbital (Solfoton, Luminal), the most commonly used barbiturate for treatment of seizures, has indications for the treatment of generalized tonic-clonic and simple partial seizures. Parenteral barbiturates are used in the emergency management of seizures independent of cause. Intravenous (IV) phenobarbital should be administered slowly, 10 to 20 mg/kg for status epilepticus.

Narcoanalysis

Amobarbital (Amytal) has been used historically as a diagnostic aid in a number of clinical conditions, including conversion reactions, catatonia, hysterical stupor, and unexplained muteness, and to differentiate stupor of depression, schizophrenia, and structural brain lesions.

The *Amytal interview* is performed by placing the patient in a reclining position and administering amobarbital intravenously, 50 mg a minute. Infusion is continued until lateral nystagmus is sustained or drowsiness is noted, usually at 75 to 150 mg. Following this, 25 to 50 mg can be administered every 5 minutes to maintain narcosis. The patient should be allowed to rest for 15 to 30 minutes after the interview before attempting to walk.

Sleep

The barbiturates reduce sleep latency and the number of awakenings during sleep, although tolerance to these effects generally develops within 2 weeks. Discontinuation of barbiturates often leads to rebound increases on electroencephalogram measures of sleep and a worsening of the insomnia.

Withdrawal from Sedative-Hypnotics

Barbiturates are sometimes used to determine the extent of tolerance to barbiturates or other hypnotics to guide detoxification. Once intoxication has resolved, a test dose of pentobarbital (200 mg) is given orally. One hour later the patient is examined. Tolerance and dose requirements are determined by the degree to which the patient is affected. If the patient is not sedated, another 100 mg of pentobarbital can be administered every 2 hours, up to three times (maximum, 500 mg over 6 hours). The amount needed for mild intoxication corresponds to the approximate daily dose of barbiturate used. Phenobarbital (30 mg) may then be substituted for each 100 mg of pentobarbital. This daily dose requirement can be administered in divided doses and gradually tapered by 10 percent a day, with adjustments made according to withdrawal signs.

PRECAUTIONS AND ADVERSE REACTIONS

Some adverse effects of barbiturates are similar to those of benzodiazepines, including paradoxical dysphoria, hyperactivity, and cognitive disorganization. Rare adverse effects associated with barbiturate use include the development of Stevens-Johnson syndrome, megaloblastic anemia, and neutropenia.

A major difference between the barbiturates and the benzodiazepines is the low therapeutic index of the barbiturates. An overdose of barbiturates can easily prove fatal. In addition to narrow therapeutic indexes, the barbiturates are associated with a significant risk of abuse potential and the development of tolerance and dependence. Barbiturate intoxication is manifested by confusion, drowsiness, irritability, hyporeflexia or areflexia, ataxia, and nystagmus. The symptoms of barbiturate withdrawal are similar to, but more marked than, those of benzodiazepine withdrawal.

Because of some evidence of teratogenicity, barbiturates should not be used by pregnant women or women who are breast-feeding. Barbiturates should be used with caution by patients with a history of substance abuse, depression, diabetes, hepatic impairment, renal disease, severe anemia, pain, hyperthyroidism, or hypoadrenalism. Barbiturates are also contraindicated in patients with acute intermittent porphyria, impaired respiratory drive, or limited respiratory reserve.

DRUG INTERACTIONS

The primary area for concern about drug interactions is the potentially additive effects of respiratory depression. Barbiturates should be used with great caution with other prescribed central nervous system (CNS) drugs (including antipsychotic and antidepressant drugs) and nonprescribed CNS agents (e.g., alcohol). Caution must also be exercised when prescribing barbiturates to patients who are taking other drugs that are metabolized in the liver, especially cardiac drugs and anticonvulsants. Because individual patients have a wide range of sensitivities to barbiturate-induced enzyme induction, it is not possible to predict the degree to which the metabolism of concurrently administered medications is affected. Drugs that may have their metabolism enhanced by barbiturate administration include opioids, antiarrhythmic agents, antibiotics, anticoagulants, anticonvulsants, antidepressants, β-adrenergic receptor antagonists,

dopamine receptor antagonists, contraceptives, and immunosuppressants.

LABORATORY INTERFERENCES

No known laboratory interferences are associated with the administration of barbiturates.

DOSE AND CLINICAL GUIDELINES

Barbiturates and other drugs described later begin to act within 1 to 2 hours of administration. The doses of barbiturates vary (Table 32.8–1), and treatment should begin with low doses that are increased to achieve a clinical effect. Children and older people are more sensitive to the effects of the barbiturates than are young adults. The most commonly used barbiturates are available in a variety of dose forms. Barbiturates with half-lives in the 15- to 40-hour range are preferable because long-acting drugs tend to accumulate in the body. Clinicians should instruct patients clearly about the adverse effects and the potential for dependence associated with barbiturates.

Although determining plasma concentrations of barbiturates is rarely necessary in psychiatry, monitoring of phenobarbital concentrations is standard practice when the drug is used as an anticonvulsant. The therapeutic blood concentrations for phenobarbital in this indication range from 15 to 40 mg/L, although some patients may experience significant adverse effects in that range.

Barbiturates are contained in combination products with which the clinician should be familiar.

OTHER, SIMILARLY ACTING DRUGS

A number of agents that act similarly to the barbiturates are used in the treatment of anxiety and insomnia. Three such available drugs are paraldehyde (Paral), meprobamate, and chloral hydrate. These drugs are rarely used because of their abuse potential and potential toxic effects.

Paraldehyde

Paraldehyde is a cyclic ether, and was first used in 1882 as a hypnotic. It has also been used to treat epilepsy, alcohol withdrawal symptoms, and delirium tremens. Because of its low therapeutic index, it has been supplanted by the benzodiazepines and other anticonvulsants.

Pharmacological Actions. Paraldehyde is rapidly absorbed from the gastrointestinal (GI) tract and from intramuscular (IM) injections. It is primarily metabolized to acetaldehyde by the liver, and unmetabolized drug is expired by the lungs. Reported half-lives range from 3.4 to 9.8 hours. Onset of action is 15 to 30 minutes.

Therapeutic Indications. Paraldehyde is not indicated as an anxiolytic or a hypnotic and has little place in current psychopharmacology.

Precautions and Adverse Reactions. Paraldehyde frequently causes foul breath because of expired unmetabolized drug. It can inflame pulmonary capillaries and cause coughing. It can also cause local thrombophlebitis with IV use. Patients may experience nausea and

Table 32.8–1
Barbiturate Dosages (Adult)

Drug	Trade Name	Available Preparations	Hypnotic Dose Range	Anticonvulsant Dose Range
Amobarbital	Amytal	200 mg	50–300 mg	65–500 mg IV
Aprobarbital	Alurate	40-mg/5-mL elixir	40–120 mg	Not established
Butabarbital	Butisol	15-, 30-, and 50-mg tablets 30-mg/5-mL elixir	45–120 mg	Not established
Mephobarbital	Mebaral	32-, 50-, and 100-mg tablets	100–200 mg	200–600 mg
Methohexital	Brevital	500 mg/50 cc	1 mg/kg for electroconvulsive therapy	Not established
Pentobarbital	Nembutal	50- and 100-mg capsules 50-mg/mL injection or elixir 30-, 60-, 120-, and 200-mg suppository	100–200 mg	100 mg IV, each minute up to 500 mg
Phenobarbital	Luminal	Tablets range from 15–100 mg 20-mg/5-mL elixir 30—130-mg/mL injection	30–150 mg	100–300 mg IV, up to 600 mg/day
Secobarbital	Seconal	100-mg capsule, 50-mg/mL injection	100 mg	5.5 mg/kg IV

IV, intravenous.

vomiting with oral use. Overdose leads to metabolic acidosis and decreased renal output. There is risk of abuse among drug addicts.

Drug Interactions.   Disulfiram (Antabuse) inhibits acetaldehyde dehydrogenase and reduces metabolism of paraldehyde, leading to possible toxic concentration of paraldehyde. Paraldehyde has addictive sedating effects in combination with other CNS depressants such as alcohol or benzodiazepines.

Laboratory Interferences.   Paraldehyde can interfere with the metyrapone, phentolamine, and urinary 17-hydroxycorticosteroid tests.

Dosing and Clinical Guidelines

Paraldehyde is available in 30-mL vials for oral, IV, or rectal use. For seizures in adults, up to 12 mL (diluted to a 10 percent solution) can be administered by gastric tube every 4 hours. For children, the oral dose is 0.3 mg/kg.

Meprobamate

Meprobamate, a carbamate, was introduced shortly before the benzodiazepines, specifically to treat anxiety. It is also used for muscle relaxant effects.

Pharmacological Actions.   Meprobamate is rapidly absorbed from the GI tract and from IM injections. It is primarily metabolized by the liver, and a small portion is excreted unchanged in urine. The plasma half-life is approximately 10 hours.

Therapeutic Indications.   Meprobamate is indicated for short-term treatment of anxiety disorders. It has also been used as a hypnotic and is prescribed as a muscle relaxant.

Precautions and Adverse Reactions.   Meprobamate can cause CNS depression and death in overdose and carries the risk of abuse by patients with drug or alcohol dependence. Abrupt cessation following long-term use can lead to withdrawal syndrome, including seizures and hallucinations. Meprobamate can exacerbate acute intermittent porphyria. Other rare side effects include hypersensitivity reactions,

wheezing, hives, paradoxical excitement, and leukopenia. It should not be used in patients with hepatic compromise.

Drug Interactions.   Meprobamate has additive sedating effects in combination with other CNS depressants, such as alcohol, barbiturates, or benzodiazepines.

Laboratory Interferences.   Meprobamate can interfere with the metyrapone, phentolamine, and urinary 17-hydroxycorticosteroid tests.

Dosing and Clinical Guidelines.   Meprobamate is available in 200-, 400-, and 600-mg tablets; 200- and 400-mg extended-release capsules; and various combinations, for example, aspirin, 325 mg and 200 mg of meprobamate (Equagesic) for oral use. For adults, the usual dose is 400 to 800 mg twice daily. Elderly patients and children ages 6 to 12 years require half the adult dose.

Chloral Hydrate

Chloral hydrate is a hypnotic agent rarely used in psychiatry because numerous safer options, such as benzodiazepines, are available.

Pharmacological Actions.   Chloral hydrate is well absorbed from the GI tract. The parent compound is metabolized within minutes by the liver to the active metabolite trichloroethanol, which has a half-life of 8 to 11 hours. A dose of chloral hydrate induces sleep in about 30 to 60 minutes and maintains sleep for 4 to 8 hours. It probably potentiates GABAergic neurotransmission, which suppresses neuronal excitability.

Therapeutic Indications.   The major indication for chloral hydrate is to induce sleep. It should be used for no more than 2 or 3 days because longer-term treatment is associated with an increased incidence and severity of adverse effects. Tolerance develops to the hypnotic effects of chloral hydrate after 2 weeks of treatment. The benzodiazepines are superior to chloral hydrate for all psychiatric uses.

Precautions and Adverse Reactions.   Chloral hydrate has adverse effects on the CNS, GI system, and skin. High doses (>4 g) may be associated with stupor, confusion, ataxia, falls, or coma. The GI effects include nonspecific irritation, nausea, vomiting, flatulence, and an unpleasant taste. With long-term use and overdose, gastritis and gastric ulceration can develop. In addition to the development of tolerance, dependence on chloral hydrate can occur, with symptoms similar to those of alcohol dependence. The lethal dose of chloral hydrate is between 5,000 and 10,000 mg, thus making it a particularly poor choice for potentially suicidal persons.

Drug Interactions.   It is because of metabolic interference that chloral hydrate should be strictly avoided with alcohol, a notorious concoction known as a *Mickey Finn*. Chloral hydrate may displace warfarin (Coumadin) from plasma proteins and enhance anticoagulant activity; this combination should be avoided.

Laboratory Interferences.   Chloral hydrate administration can lead to false-positive results for urine glucose determinations that use cupric sulfate (e.g., Clinitest) but not in tests that use glucose oxidase (e.g., Clinistix and Tes-Tape). Chloral hydrate can also interfere with the determination of urinary catecholamines in 17-hydroxycorticosteroids.

Dosing and Clinical Guidelines

Chloral hydrate is available in 500-mg capsules, 500-mg/5 mL solution, and 324-, 500-, and 648-mg rectal suppositories. The standard dose of chloral hydrate is 500 to 2,000 mg at bedtime. Because the drug is a GI irritant, it should be administered with excess water, milk, other liquids, or antacids to decrease gastric irritation.

▲ 32.9 Benzodiazepines and Drugs Acting on Benzodiazepine Receptors

The benzodiazepines derive their name from their molecular structure. They share a common effect on receptors that have been termed *benzodiazepine receptors*, which in turn modulate γ-aminobutyric acid (GABA) activity. Nonbenzodiazepine agonists, such as zolpidem (Ambien), zaleplon (Sonata), and eszopiclone (Lunesta)—the so-called "Z drugs"—are discussed in this section because their clinical effects result from interactions with GABA-receptor complexes at binding domains located close to or coupled to benzodiazepine receptors. Flumazenil (Romazicon), a benzodiazepine receptor antagonist used to reverse benzodiazepine-induced sedation and in emergency care of benzodiazepine overdose, is also covered here.

Because benzodiazepines have a rapid anxiolytic sedative effect, they are most commonly used for immediate treatment of insomnia, acute anxiety, and agitation or anxiety associated with any psychiatric disorder. In addition, the benzodiazepines are used as anesthetics, anticonvulsants, and muscle relaxants. Because of the risk of psychological and physical dependence, long-term use of benzodiazepines should be in conjunction with psychotherapy and in cases in which alternative agents have been tried and proved ineffective or poorly tolerated.

PHARMACOLOGICAL ACTIONS

With the exception of clorazepate (Tranxene), all the benzodiazepines are completely absorbed unchanged from the gastrointestinal tract. The absorption, the attainment of peak concentrations, and the onset of action are quickest for diazepam (Valium),

lorazepam (Ativan), alprazolam (Xanax), triazolam (Halcion), and estazolam (ProSom). The rapid onset of effects is important to persons who take a single dose of a benzodiazepine to calm an episodic burst of anxiety or to fall asleep rapidly. Several benzodiazepines are effective following intravenous (IV) injection, whereas only lorazepam and midazolam (Versed) have rapid and reliable absorption following intramuscular (IM) administration.

Diazepam, chlordiazepoxide, clonazepam (Klonopin), clorazepate, flurazepam (Dalmane), prazepam (Centrax), quazepam (Doral), and halazepam (Paxipam) have plasma half-lives of 30 to more than 100 hours and, therefore, are the longest-acting benzodiazepines. The plasma half-lives of these compounds can be as high as 200 hours in persons whose metabolism is genetically slow. Because the attainment of steady-state plasma concentrations of the drugs can take up to 2 weeks, persons may experience symptoms and signs of toxicity after only 7 to 10 days of treatment with a dose that seemed initially to be in the therapeutic range.

The half-lives of lorazepam, oxazepam (Serax), temazepam (Restoril), and estazolam are between 8 and 30 hours. Alprazolam has a half-life of 10 to 15 hours, and triazolam has the shortest half-life (2 to 3 hours) of all the orally administered benzodiazepines.

The advantages of long–half-life drugs over short–half-life drugs include less-frequent dosing, less variation in plasma concentration, and less-severe withdrawal phenomena. The disadvantages include drug accumulation, increased risk of daytime psychomotor impairment, and increased daytime sedation. The advantages of the short–half-life drugs over the long–half-life drugs include no drug accumulation and less daytime sedation. The disadvantages include more-frequent dosing and earlier and more-severe withdrawal syndromes. Rebound insomnia and anterograde amnesia are thought to be more of a problem with the short–half-life drugs than with the long–half-life drugs.

Zaleplon, zolpidem, and eszopiclone are structurally distinct and vary in their binding to the GABA receptor subunits. Benzodiazepines activate all three specific GABA–benzodiazepine (GABA–BZ) binding sites of the GABA type A (GABA$_A$) receptor, which opens chloride channels and reduces the rate of neuronal and muscle firing. Zolpidem, zaleplon, and eszopiclone have selectivity for certain subunits of the GABA receptor. This may account for their selective sedative effects and relative lack of muscle relaxant and anticonvulsant effects.

Zolpidem, zaleplon, and eszopiclone are rapidly and well absorbed after oral administration, although absorption can be delayed by as much as 1 hour if they are taken with food. Zolpidem reaches peak plasma concentrations in 1.6 hours and has a half-life of 2.6 hours. Zaleplon reaches peak plasma concentrations in 1 hour and has a half-life of 1 hour. If taken immediately after a high-fat/heavy meal, the peak is delayed by approximately 1 hour, reducing the effects of eszopiclone on sleep onset. The terminal-phase elimination half-life is approximately 6 hours in healthy adults. Eszopiclone is weakly bound to plasma protein (52 to 59 percent).

The rapid metabolism and lack of active metabolites of zolpidem, zaleplon, and eszopiclone avoid the accumulation of plasma concentrations with long-term use of benzodiazepines.

Gaboxatal.   This is a new hypnotic agent, which works on the α-4 GABA receptor subtype rather than on the α-1 GABA subtype, which the other benzodiazepines affect. α-4 GABA is expressed at high levels in the thalamus.

THERAPEUTIC INDICATIONS

Insomnia

Because insomnia can be a symptom of a physical or psychiatric disorder, hypnotics should not be used for more than 7 to 10 consecutive days without a thorough investigation of the cause of the insomnia. In fact, however, many patients have long-standing sleep difficulties and benefit greatly from chronic use of hypnotic agents. Temazepam, flurazepam, and triazolam are benzodiazepines with a sole indication for insomnia. Zolpidem, zaleplon, and eszopiclone are also indicated only for insomnia. Whereas these "Z-drugs" are not usually associated with rebound insomnia after the discontinuation of their use for short periods, some patients experience increased sleep difficulties the first few nights after discontinuing their use. Use of zolpidem, zaleplon, and eszopiclone for periods longer than 1 month is not associated with the delayed emergence of adverse effects. No development of tolerance to any parameter of sleep measurement was observed over 6 months in clinical trials of eszopiclone.

Flurazepam, temazepam, quazepam, estazolam, and triazolam are the benzodiazepines approved for use as hypnotics. The benzodiazepine hypnotics differ principally in their half-lives; flurazepam has the longest half-life, and triazolam has the shortest. Flurazepam may be associated with minor cognitive impairment on the day after its administration, and triazolam may be associated with mild rebound anxiety and anterograde amnesia. Quazepam may be associated with daytime impairment when used for a long time. Temazepam or estazolam may be a reasonable compromise for most adults. Estazolam produces rapid onset of sleep and a hypnotic effect for 6 to 8 hours.

Anxiety Disorders

Generalized Anxiety Disorder. Benzodiazepines are highly effective for the relief of anxiety associated with generalized anxiety disorder. Most persons should be treated for a predetermined, specific, and relatively brief period. Because generalized anxiety disorder is a chronic disorder with a high rate of recurrence, some persons with generalized anxiety disorder may warrant long-term maintenance treatment with benzodiazepines.

Panic Disorder. Alprazolam and clonazepam, both high-potency benzodiazepines, are commonly used medications for panic disorder, with or without agoraphobia. Although the selective serotonin reuptake inhibitors (SSRIs) are also indicated for treatment of panic disorder, benzodiazepines have the advantage of working quickly and of not causing significant sexual dysfunction and weight gain. SSRIs are still often preferred, however, because they target common comorbid conditions, such as depression or obsessive-compulsive disorder (OCD). Benzodiazepines and SSRIs can be initiated together to treat acute panic symptoms; use of the benzodiazepine can be tapered after 3 to 4 weeks once the therapeutic benefits of the SSRI have emerged.

Social Phobia. Clonazepam has been shown to be an effective treatment for social phobia. In addition, several other benzodiazepines (e.g., diazepam) have been used as adjunctive medications for treatment of social phobia.

Other Anxiety Disorders. Benzodiazepines are used adjunctively for treatment of adjustment disorder with anxiety, pathological anxiety associated with life events (e.g., after an accident), OCD, and posttraumatic stress disorder.

Mixed Anxiety-Depressive Disorder

Alprazolam is indicated for the treatment of anxiety associated with depression. The availability of several antidepressant drugs with more favorable safety profiles makes alprazolam a second-line drug for this indication; however, some patients respond to this medication when other drugs have had minimal effect.

Bipolar I Disorder

Clonazepam, lorazepam, and alprazolam are effective in the management of acute manic episodes and as an adjuvant to maintenance therapy in lieu of antipsychotics. As an adjuvant to lithium (Eskalith) or lamotrigine (Lamictal), clonazepam may result in an increased time between cycles and fewer depressive episodes.

Akathisia

The first-line drug for akathisia is most commonly a β-adrenergic receptor antagonist. Benzodiazepines are also effective in treating some patients with akathisia, however.

Parkinson's Disease

A few persons with idiopathic Parkinson's disease will respond to long-term use of zolpidem with reduced bradykinesia and rigidity. Zolpidem doses of 10 mg four times daily may be tolerated without sedation over a long period of time.

Other Psychiatric Indications

Chlordiazepoxide (Librium) is used to manage the symptoms of alcohol withdrawal. The benzodiazepines (especially IM lorazepam) are used to manage agitation, both substance induced (except amphetamine) and psychotic, in the emergency room. Benzodiazepines have been used instead of amobarbital (Amytal) for drug-assisted interviewing. Benzodiazepines have also been used in the treatment of catatonia. Some patients with delusional disorders with associated anxiety or panic have benefited from the use of benzodiazepines.

Flumazenil for Benzodiazepine Overdose

Flumazenil is used to reverse the adverse psychomotor, amnesic, and sedative effects of benzodiazepine receptor agonists, including benzodiazepines, zolpidem, and zaleplon. Flumazenil is administered IV and has a half-life of 7 to 15 minutes. The most common adverse effects of flumazenil are nausea, vomiting, dizziness, agitation, emotional lability, cutaneous vasodilation, injection-site pain, fatigue, impaired vision, and headache. The most common serious adverse effect associated with use of flumazenil is the precipitation of seizures, which is especially likely to occur in persons with seizure disorders, those who are physically dependent on benzodiazepines, or those who have ingested large quantities of benzodiazepines. Flumazenil alone may impair memory retrieval.

In mixed-drug overdose, the toxic effects (e.g., seizures and cardiac arrhythmias) of other drugs (e.g., tricyclic drugs) may emerge with the reversal of the benzodiazepine effects of flumazenil. For example, seizures caused by an overdose of tricyclic drugs may have been partially treated in a person who had also taken an overdose of benzodiazepines. With flumazenil treatment, the tricyclic-induced seizures or cardiac arrhythmias may appear and result in a fatal outcome. Flumazenil does not reverse the effects of ethanol, barbiturates, or opioids.

For the initial management of a known or suspected benzodiazepine overdose, the recommended initial dose of flumazenil is 0.2 mg (2 mL) administered IV over 30 seconds. If the desired consciousness is not obtained after 30 seconds, a further dose of 0.3 mg (3 mL) can be administered over 30 seconds. Further doses of 0.5 mg (5 mL) can be administered over 30 seconds at 1-minute intervals up to a cumulative dose of 3.0 mg. The clinician should not rush the administration of flumazenil. A secure airway and IV access should be established before the administration of the drug. Persons should be awakened gradually.

Most persons with a benzodiazepine overdose respond to a cumulative dose of 1 to 3 mg of flumazenil; doses greater than 3 mg of flumazenil do not reliably produce additional effects. If a person has not responded 5 minutes after receiving a cumulative dose of 5 mg of flumazenil, the major cause of sedation is probably not benzodiazepine receptor agonists, and additional flumazenil is unlikely to have an effect.

Sedation can return in 1 to 3 percent of persons treated with flumazenil. It can be prevented or treated by giving repeated doses of flumazenil at 20-minute intervals. For repeat treatment, no more than 1 mg (given as 0.5 mg a minute) should be given at any one time, and no more than 3 mg should be given in any 1 hour.

PRECAUTIONS AND ADVERSE REACTIONS

The most common adverse effect of benzodiazepines is drowsiness, which occurs in about 10 percent of all persons. Because of this adverse effect, persons should be advised to be careful while driving or using dangerous machinery when taking the drugs. Drowsiness can be present during the day after the use of a benzodiazepine for insomnia the previous night, so-called *residual daytime sedation*. Some persons also experience ataxia (<2 percent) and dizziness (<1 percent). These symptoms can result in falls and hip fractures, especially in elderly persons. The most serious adverse effects of benzodiazepines occur when other sedative substances, such as alcohol, are taken concurrently. These combinations can result in marked drowsiness, disinhibition, or even respiratory depression. Infrequently, benzodiazepine receptor agonists cause mild cognitive deficits.

High-potency benzodiazepines, especially triazolam, and zolpidem can cause anterograde amnesia. An unusual, paradoxical increase in aggression has been reported in persons given benzodiazepines, although this effect may be most common in persons with preexisting brain damage. Allergic reactions to the drugs are rare, but a few studies report maculopapular rashes and generalized itching. The symptoms of benzodiazepine intoxication include confusion, slurred speech, ataxia, drowsiness, dyspnea, and hyporeflexia.

Triazolam has received significant attention in the media because of an alleged association with serious aggressive behavioral manifestations. The manufacturer, therefore, recommends that the drug be used for no more than 10 days for treatment of insomnia and that physicians carefully evaluate the emergence of any abnormal thinking or behavioral changes in persons treated with triazolam, giving appropriate consideration to all potential causes. Triazolam was banned in Great Britain in 1991.

Persons with hepatic disease and elderly persons are particularly likely to have adverse effects and toxicity from the benzodiazepines, including hepatic coma, especially when the drugs are administered repeatedly or in high doses. Benzodiazepines can produce clinically significant impairment of respiration in persons with chronic obstructive pulmonary disease and sleep apnea. Alprazolam can exert a direct appetite-stimulant effect and may cause weight gain. Benzodiazepines should be used with caution by persons with a history of substance abuse, cognitive disorders, renal disease, hepatic disease, porphyria, central nervous system (CNS) depression, or myasthenia gravis.

Some data indicate that benzodiazepines are teratogenic; therefore, their use during pregnancy is not advised. Moreover, the use of benzodiazepines in the third trimester can precipitate a withdrawal syndrome in the newborn. The drugs are secreted in breast milk in sufficient concentrations to affect the newborn. Benzodiazepines can cause dyspnea, bradycardia, and drowsiness in nursing babies.

Zolpidem and zaleplon are generally well tolerated. At zolpidem doses of 10 mg per day and zaleplon doses above 10 mg per day, a small number of persons will experience dizziness, drowsiness, dyspepsia, or diarrhea. Zolpidem and zaleplon are secreted in breast milk and, therefore, are contraindicated for use by nursing mothers. The dose of zolpidem and zaleplon should be reduced in the elderly and in persons with hepatic impairment.

In rare cases, zolpidem can cause hallucinations and behavioral changes. The coadministration of zolpidem and SSRIs can extend the duration of hallucinations in susceptible patients.

Eszopiclone exhibits a dose-response relationship in elderly adults for the side effects of pain, dry mouth, and unpleasant taste, with this relationship clearest for unpleasant taste.

Tolerance, Dependence, and Withdrawal

When benzodiazepines are used for short periods (1 to 2 weeks) in moderate doses, they usually cause no significant tolerance, dependence, or withdrawal effects. The short-acting benzodiazepines (e.g., triazolam) may be an exception to this rule because some persons have reported increased anxiety the day after taking a single dose of the drug. Some persons also report a tolerance for the anxiolytic effects of benzodiazepines and require increased doses to maintain the clinical remission of symptoms.

The appearance of a withdrawal syndrome, also called a *discontinuation syndrome*, depends on the length of time the person has been taking a benzodiazepine, the dose the person has been taking, the rate at which the drug is tapered, and the half-life of the compound. Benzodiazepine withdrawal syndrome consists of anxiety, nervousness, diaphoresis, restlessness, irritability, fatigue, light-headedness, tremor, insomnia, and weakness. Abrupt discontinuation of benzodiazepines, particularly those with short half-lives, is associated with severe withdrawal symptoms, which can include depression, paranoia, delirium, and seizures. These severe symptoms are more likely to occur if flumazenil is used for rapid reversal of the benzodiazepine receptor agonist effects. Some features of the syndrome can occur in as many as 90 percent of the persons treated with the drugs. The development of a severe withdrawal syndrome is seen only in persons who have taken high doses for long periods. The appearance of the syndrome can be delayed for 1 or 2 weeks in persons who had been taking benzodiazepines with long half-lives. Alprazolam seems to be particularly associated with an immediate and severe withdrawal syndrome and should be tapered gradually.

When the medication is to be discontinued, the drug must be tapered slowly (25 percent a week); otherwise, recurrence or rebound of symptoms is likely. Monitoring of any withdrawal symptoms (possibly with a standardized rating scale) and psychological support of the person are helpful in the successful accomplishment of benzodiazepine discontinuation. Concurrent use of carbamazepine (Tegretol) during benzodiazepine discontinuation has been reported to permit a more rapid and better-tolerated withdrawal than does a gradual taper alone. The dose range of carbamazepine used to facilitate withdrawal is 400 to 500 mg a day. Some clinicians report particular difficulty in tapering and discontinuing alprazolam, especially in persons who have been receiving high doses for long periods. There have been reports of successful discontinuation of alprazolam by switching to clonazepam, which is then gradually withdrawn.

Zolpidem and zaleplon can produce a mild withdrawal syndrome lasting 1 day after prolonged use at higher therapeutic doses. Rarely, a person taking zolpidem has self-titrated up the daily dose to 300 to 400 mg a day. Abrupt discontinuation of such a high dose of zolpidem can cause withdrawal symptoms for 4 or more days. Tolerance does not appear to develop to the sedative effects of zolpidem and zaleplon.

DRUG INTERACTIONS

The most common and potentially serious benzodiazepine receptor agonist interaction results in excessive sedation and respiratory depression occurring when benzodiazepines, zolpidem, or zaleplon are administered concomitantly with other CNS depressants, such as alcohol, barbiturates, tricyclic and tetracyclic drugs, dopamine receptor antagonists, opioids, and antihistamines. Ataxia and dysarthria may likely occur when lithium, antipsychotics, and clonazepam are combined. The combination of benzodiazepines and clozapine (Clozaril) has been reported to cause delirium and should be avoided. Cimetidine (Tagamet), disulfiram (Antabuse), isoniazid, estrogen, and oral contraceptives increase the plasma concentrations of diazepam, chlordiazepoxide, clorazepate, flurazepam, prazepam, and halazepam. Cimetidine increases the plasma concentrations of zaleplon. The plasma concentrations of triazolam and alprazolam are increased to potentially toxic concentrations by nefazodone (Serzone) and fluvoxamine (Luvox). The manufacturer of nefazodone recommends that the dose of triazolam be lowered by 75 percent and the dose of alprazolam lowered by 50 percent when given concomitantly with nefazodone. Over-the-counter preparations of kava plant, advertised as a "natural tranquilizer," can potentiate the action of benzodiazepine receptor agonists through synergistic overactivation of GABA receptors. Carbamazepine can lower the plasma concentration of alprazolam. Antacids and food can decrease the plasma concentrations of benzodiazepines, and smoking can increase the metabolism of benzodiazepines. Rifampin (Rifadin), phenytoin (Dilantin), carbamazepine, and phenobarbital (Solfoton, Luminal) significantly increase the metabolism of zaleplon. The benzodiazepines can increase the plasma concentrations of phenytoin and digoxin (Lanoxin). SSRIs may prolong and exacerbate the severity of zolpidem-induced hallucinations.

LABORATORY INTERFERENCES

No known laboratory interferences are associated with the use of benzodiazepines, zolpidem, and zaleplon.

DOSING AND CLINICAL GUIDELINES

The clinical decision to treat an anxious person with a benzodiazepine should be carefully considered. Medical causes of anxiety (e.g., thyroid dysfunction, caffeinism, and prescription medications) should be ruled out. Benzodiazepine use should be started at a low dose, and the person should be instructed regarding the drug's sedative properties and abuse potential. An estimated length of therapy should be decided at the beginning of treatment, and the need for continued therapy should be reevaluated at least monthly because of the problems associated with long-term use. Certain persons with anxiety disorders, however, are unresponsive to treatments other than benzodiazepines in long-term use.

Benzodiazepines are available in a wide range of formulations. Clonazepam is available in a wafer formulation that facilitates its use in patients who have trouble swallowing pills. Alprazolam is available in an extended-release form, which reduces the frequency of dosing. Some benzodiazepines are more potent than others in that one compound might require a relatively smaller dose than another compound to achieve the same effect. For example, clonazepam requires 0.25 mg to achieve the same effect as 5 mg of diazepam; thus, clonazepam is considered a high-potency benzodiazepine. Conversely, oxazepam has an approximate dose equivalence of 15 mg and is a low-potency drug.

Zaleplon is available in 5- and 10-mg capsules. A single 10-mg dose is the usual adult dose. The dose can be increased to a maximum of 20 mg as tolerated. A single dose of zaleplon can be expected to provide 4 hours of sleep with minimal residual impairment. For persons older than age 65 years or persons with hepatic impairment, an initial dose of 5 mg is advised.

Eszopiclone is available in 1-, 2-, and 3-mg tablets. The starting dose should not exceed 1 mg in patients with severe hepatic impairment or those taking potent cytochrome P450 (CYP) 3A4 inhibitors. The recommended dose to improve sleep onset or maintenance is 2 or 3 mg for adult patients (ages 18 to 64 years) and 2 mg for older adult patients (ages 65 years and older). The 1-mg dose is for sleep onset in older adult patients whose primary complaint is difficulty falling asleep.

RAMELTEON

Ramelteon (Rozerem), a new treatment for insomnia, was approved by the U.S. Food and Drug Administration in 2005. (See also Section 32.21.)

Pharmacological Actions

Unlike the other hypnotic agents discussed in this section, ramelteon does not act on the benzodiazepine or GABA system. It specifically targets the melatonin MT1 and MT2 receptors in the brain's suprachiasmatic nucleus (SCN). The SCN regulates 24-hour, or circadian, rhythms, including the sleep–wake cycle.

Ramelteon is absorbed rapidly, with peak concentrations occurring 30 to 90 minutes after fasting oral administration. The elimination half-life of ramelteon is 1 to 2.6 hours, and that of its active metabolite is 2 to 5 hours.

Therapeutic Indications

Ramelteon is indicated for the treatment of insomnia characterized by difficulty with sleep onset.

Precautions and Adverse Events

The most common adverse events seen with ramelteon were somnolence, dizziness, and fatigue. Ramelteon has been associated with decreased testosterone levels and increased prolactin levels. No evidence suggests abuse or dependence, and the drug is not designated as a controlled substance.

Drug Interactions

CYP 1A2 is the major isozyme involved in the hepatic metabolism of ramelteon.

Laboratory Interferences

Ramelteon is not known to interfere with laboratory tests. Prolactin and testosterone levels should be monitored if patients develop signs and symptoms affecting lactation, menses, libido, or fertility during treatment.

Dosing and Clinical Guidelines

The recommended dose for long-term use in adults is 8 mg taken within 30 minutes before going to bed. Ramelteon should not be combined with fluvoxamine and should not be used by patients with severe hepatic impairment.

▲ 32.10 Bupropion

Unlike other currently used antidepressants, bupropion (Wellbutrin, Wellbutrin SR, Wellbutrin XL) does not act on the serotonin system. It is a norepinephrine and dopamine reuptake inhibitor. This results in a side-effect profile characterized by little risk of sexual dysfunction or sedation and with modest weight loss during acute and long-term treatment. No withdrawal syndrome has been linked to discontinuation of bupropion. Bupropion is approved by the U.S. Food and Drug Administration for the prevention of seasonal depressive episodes of patients with seasonal affective disorder (SAD). Although increasingly used as first-line monotherapy, a significant percentage of bupropion use occurs as add-on therapy to other antidepressants, most commonly selective serotonin reuptake inhibitors (SSRIs). This practice is based on the premise that combining agents with differing mechanisms of action may increase efficacy or mitigate side effects. Bupropion has also been marketed under the name Zyban for use in smoking cessation regimens.

Bupropion is a monocyclic aminoketone that resembles amphetamine and the diet drug diethylpropion (Tenuate) in its molecular structure.

PHARMACOLOGICAL ACTIONS

Three formulations of bupropion are available: immediate release (taken three times daily), sustained release (taken twice daily), and extended release (taken once daily). The different versions of the drug contain the same active ingredient but differ in their pharmacokinetics and dosing.

Immediate-release bupropion is well absorbed from the gastrointestinal (GI) tract. Peak plasma concentrations of bupropion are usually reached within 2 hours of oral administration, and peak levels of the sustained-release version are seen after 3 hours. The mean half-life of the compound is 12 hours, ranging from 8 to 40 hours. Peak levels of extended-release bupropion occur 5 hours after ingestion. This provides a longer time to maximal plasma concentration but comparable peak and trough plasma concentrations. The 24-hour exposure occurring after administration of the extended-release version of 300 mg once daily is equivalent to that provided by sustained release of 150 mg twice daily. Clinically, this permits the drug to be taken once a day in the morning. Plasma levels are also reduced in the evening, making it less likely for some patients to experience treatment-related insomnia.

The mechanism of action for the antidepressant effects of bupropion is poorly understood, although it presumably involves inhibition of dopamine and norepinephrine reuptake. Bupropion binds to the dopamine transporter in the brain. The effects of bupropion on smoking cessation may be related to its effects on dopamine reward pathways or to inhibition of nicotinic acetylcholine receptors.

THERAPEUTIC INDICATIONS

Depression

Although overshadowed by the SSRIs as first-line treatment for major depression, the therapeutic efficacy of bupropion in depression is well established in both outpatient and inpatient settings. Observed rates of response and remission are comparable to those seen with SSRIs.

Seasonal Affective Disorder

Seasonal affective disorder is characterized by recurring fall/winter onset of depressive symptoms that include weight gain, lethargy, and increased sleep. Bupropion has been found to prevent seasonal major depressive episodes in patients with a history of SAD.

Smoking Cessation

Under the brand name Zyban, bupropion is indicated for use in combination with behavioral modification programs for smoking cessation. It is intended to be used in patients who are highly motivated and who receive some form of structured behavioral support. Bupropion is most effective when combined with nicotine substitutes (NicoDerm, Nicotrol).

Bipolar Disorders

Bupropion is less likely than tricyclics to precipitate mania in persons with bipolar I disorder and less likely than other antidepressants to exacerbate or induce rapid-cycling bipolar II disorder; however, the evidence about use of bupropion in the treatment of patients who are bipolar is limited.

Attention-Deficit/Hyperactivity Disorder

Bupropion is used as a second-line agent, after the sympathomimetics, for treatment of attention-deficit/hyperactivity disorder (ADHD). It has not been compared with proved ADHD medications, such as methylphenidate (Ritalin) or atomoxetine (Strattera), for childhood and adult ADHD. Bupropion is an appropriate choice for persons with comorbid ADHD and depression or persons with comorbid ADHD, conduct disorder, or substance abuse. It may also be considered for use in patients who develop tics when treated with psychostimulants.

Cocaine Detoxification

Bupropion may be associated with a euphoric feeling; thus, it may be contraindicated in persons with histories of substance abuse. Because of its dopaminergic effects, however, bupropion has been explored as a treatment to reduce the cravings for cocaine in persons who have withdrawn from the substance. Results have been inconclusive, with some patients showing a reduction in drug craving and others finding their cravings increased.

Hypoactive Sexual Desire Disorder

Bupropion is often added to drugs, such as SSRIs, to counteract sexual side effects and may be helpful as a treatment for nondepressed individuals with hypoactive sexual desire disorder. Bupropion may improve sexual arousal, orgasm completion, and sexual satisfaction.

PRECAUTIONS AND ADVERSE REACTIONS

Headache, insomnia, dry mouth, tremor, and nausea are the most common side effects of bupropion use. Restlessness, agitation, and irritability may also occur. Patients with severe anxiety or panic disorder should not be started on bupropion. Most likely because of its potentiating effects on dopaminergic neurotransmission, bupropion can cause psychotic symptoms, including hallucinations, delusions, and catatonia, as well as delirium. Some bupropion-treated patients experience word-finding difficulties and memory impairment. Most notable about bupropion is the absence of significant drug-induced orthostatic hypotension, weight gain, daytime drowsiness, and anticholinergic effects. Some persons, however, may experience dry mouth or constipation and weight loss. Hypertension can occur in some patients, but bupropion causes no other significant cardiovascular or clinical laboratory changes. Bupropion exerts indirect sympathomimetic activity, producing positive inotropic effects in human myocardium, an effect that may reflect catecholamine release.

Concern about seizure has deterred some physicians from prescribing bupropion. Studies show that at doses of 300 mg a day or less of sustained-release bupropion, the incidence of seizures is 0.05 percent, which is no worse than the incidence of seizures with other antidepressants. The risk of seizures increases to about 0.1 percent with doses of 400 mg a day.

Risk factors for seizures include a history of seizures, use of alcohol, recent benzodiazepine withdrawal, organic brain disease, head trauma, or epileptiform discharges on electroencephalogram.

The use of bupropion by pregnant women is not associated with specific risk of increased rate of birth defects. Bupropion is secreted in breast milk, so the use of bupropion in nursing women should be based on the clinical circumstances of the patient and the judgment of the clinician.

Few deaths have been reported following overdoses of bupropion. Poor outcomes are associated with cases of huge doses and mixed-drug overdoses. Seizures occur in about one third of all overdoses and are dose dependent, with those having seizures ingesting a significantly higher median dose. Fatalities can involve uncontrollable seizures, sinus bradycardia, and cardiac arrest. Symptoms of poisoning most often involve seizures, sinus tachycardia, hypertension, GI symptoms, hallucinations, and agitation. All seizures are typically brief and self-limited. In general, however, bupropion is safer in overdose cases than are other antidepressants, except perhaps SSRIs.

DRUG INTERACTIONS

Given that bupropion is frequently combined with SSRIs or venlafaxine (Effexor), potential interactions are significant. Bupropion has been found to have an effect on the pharmacokinetics of venlafaxine. One study noted a significant increase in venlafaxine levels, and a consequent decrease in its main metabolite O-desmethylvenlafaxine, during combined treatment with sustained-release bupropion. Bupropion hydroxylation is weakly inhibited by venlafaxine. No significant changes in plasma levels of the SSRIs paroxetine and fluoxetine have been reported. A few case reports, however, indicate that the combination of bupropion and fluoxetine (Prozac) may be associated with panic, delirium, or seizures. Bupropion in combination with lithium (Eskalith) may rarely cause central nervous system toxicity, including seizures.

Because of the possibility of inducing a hypertensive crisis, bupropion should not be used concurrently with monoamine oxidase inhibitors (MAOIs). At least 14 days should pass after the discontinuation of an MAOI before initiating treatment with bupropion. In some cases, the addition of bupropion may permit persons taking anti-Parkinsonian medications to lower the doses of their dopaminergic drugs. Delirium, psychotic symptoms, and dyskinetic movements may, however, be associated with the coadministration of bupropion and dopaminergic agents such as levodopa (Larodopa), pergolide (Permax), ropinirole (Requip), pramipexole (Mirapex), amantadine (Symmetrel), and bromocriptine (Parlodel). Sinus bradycardia may occur when bupropion is combined with metoprolol.

Carbamazepine (Tegretol) may decrease plasma concentrations of bupropion, and bupropion may increase plasma concentrations of valproic acid (Depakene).

In vitro biotransformation studies of bupropion have found that formation of a major active metabolite, hydroxybupropion, is mediated by cytochrome P450 (CYP) 2B6. Bupropion has some inhibitory effect on CYP 2D6.

LABORATORY INTERFERENCES

Bupropion may give a false-positive result on urinary amphetamine screens. No other reports have appeared of laboratory interferences clearly associated with bupropion treatment.

Clinically nonsignificant changes in the electrocardiogram (premature beats and nonspecific ST-T changes) and decreases in the white blood cell count (by about 10 percent) have been reported in a small number of persons.

DOSING AND CLINICAL GUIDELINES

Immediate-release bupropion is available in 75-, 100-, and 150-mg tablets. Sustained-release bupropion is available in 100-, 150-, 200-, and 300-mg tablets. Extended-release bupropion comes in 150- and 300-mg strengths, and a 450-mg strength is in development.

Initiation of immediate-release bupropion in the average adult person should be 75 mg orally twice a day. On the fourth day of treatment, the dose can be raised to 100 mg three times a day. Because 300 mg is the recommended dose, the person should be maintained on this dose for several weeks before increasing it further. The maximal dose, 450 mg a day, should be given as 150 mg three times a day. Because of the risk of seizures, increases in dose should never exceed 100 mg in a 3-day period; a single dose of immediate-release bupropion should never exceed 150 mg, and the total daily dose should not exceed 450 mg. The maximum of 400 mg of the sustained-release version should be used as a twice-a-day regimen of either 200 mg twice daily or 300 mg in the morning and 100 mg in the afternoon. A starting dose of the sustained-release version, 100 mg once a day, can be increased to 100 mg twice a day after 4 days. Then, 150 mg twice a day may be used. A single dose of sustained-release bupropion should never exceed 300 mg. The maximal dose is 200 mg twice a day of the immediate-release or extended-release formulations. An advantage of the extended-release preparation is that, after appropriate titration, a total of 450 mg can be given all at once in the morning.

For smoking cessation, the patient should start taking 150 mg a day of sustained-release bupropion 10 to 14 days before quitting smoking. On the fourth day, the dose should be increased to 150 mg twice daily. Treatment generally lasts 7 to 12 weeks.

▲ 32.11 Buspirone

Buspirone (BuSpar) was introduced in 1986 as the first nonsedating drug specifically indicated for the treatment of generalized anxiety disorder. In contrast to existing antianxiety drugs such as the benzodiazepines and barbiturates, it does not cause sedation and is devoid of dependence risk, abuse potential, or a withdrawal syndrome. It also does not have hypnotic, muscle-relaxant, or anticonvulsant properties.

Buspirone is classified as an azaperone and is chemically distinct from other psychotropic agents.

PHARMACOLOGICAL ACTIONS

Buspirone is well absorbed from the gastrointestinal tract, but absorption is delayed by food ingestion. Peak plasma levels are achieved 40 to 90 minutes after oral administration. At doses of 10 to 40 mg, single-dose linear pharmacokinetics is observed. Nonlinear pharmacokinetics is observed after multiple doses. Because of a short half-life (2 to 11 hours), buspirone is dosed three times daily. An active metabolite of buspirone, 1-pyrimidinylpiperazine (1-PP), is about 20 percent less potent than buspirone but up to 30 percent more concentrated in the brain than the parent compound. The elimination half-life of 1-PP is 6 hours.

Buspirone acts as an agonist, partial agonist, or antagonist on serotonin 5-HT$_{1A}$ receptors. Its most pronounced action, as a presynaptic agonist at these receptors, inhibits release of serotonin, with consequent antianxiety effects. Action as an agonist at postsynaptic receptors appears to account for antidepressant activity.

Buspirone has no effect on the γ-aminobutyric acid (GABA)–associated chloride ion channel on that receptor mechanism or the serotonin reuptake transporter, targets of other drugs that are effective in generalized anxiety disorder. Buspirone also has activity at 5-HT$_2$ and dopamine type 2 (D$_2$) receptors, although the significance of the effects at these receptors is unknown. At D$_2$ receptors, it has properties of both an agonist and an antagonist. That buspirone takes 2 to 3 weeks to exert its therapeutic effects implies that, whatever its initial effects, they involve the modulation of several neurotransmitters and intraneuronal mechanisms.

THERAPEUTIC INDICATIONS

Generalized Anxiety Disorder

Buspirone is a narrow-spectrum antianxiety agent, with demonstrated efficacy only in the treatment of generalized anxiety disorder. In contrast to the selective serotonin reuptake inhibitors (SSRIs) or venlafaxine (Effexor), buspirone is not effective in the treatment of panic disorder, obsessive-compulsive disorder (OCD), or social phobia. Buspirone, however, has an advantage over these agents in that it does not typically cause sexual dysfunction or weight gain.

Some evidence suggests that, compared with benzodiazepines, buspirone is generally more effective for symptoms of anger and hostility, equally effective for psychic symptoms of anxiety, and less effective for somatic symptoms of anxiety. The full benefit of buspirone is evident only at doses greater than 30 mg a day. Compared with the benzodiazepines, buspirone has a delayed onset of action and lacks any euphoric effect. Unlike benzodiazepines, buspirone has no immediate effects, and the patient should be told that a full clinical response may take 2 to 4 weeks. If an immediate response is needed, the patient can be started on a benzodiazepine and then withdrawn from the drug after buspirone's effects begin. Sometimes the sedative effects of benzodiazepines, which are not found with buspirone, are desirable; however, these sedative effects can cause impaired motor performance and cognitive deficits.

Other Disorders

Many other clinical uses of buspirone have been reported, but most have not been confirmed in controlled trials. Evidence of the efficacy of high-dose buspirone (30 to 90 mg a day) for depressive disorders is mixed. Buspirone appears to have weak antidepressant activity, which has led to its use as an augmenting agent in patients who have failed standard antidepressant therapy. Buspirone is sometimes used to augment SSRIs in the treatment of OCD. Some reports indicate that buspirone may be beneficial against the increased arousal and flashbacks associated with posttraumatic stress disorder.

Because buspirone does not act on the GABA–chloride ion channel complex, the drug is not recommended for the treatment of withdrawal from benzodiazepines, alcohol, or sedative-hypnotic drugs, except as treatment of comorbid anxiety symptoms.

Scattered trials suggests that buspirone reduces aggression and anxiety in persons with organic brain disease or traumatic brain injury, SSRI-induced bruxism and sexual dysfunction, and nicotine craving, as well as in attention-deficit/hyperactivity disorder.

PRECAUTIONS AND ADVERSE REACTIONS

Buspirone does not cause weight gain, sexual dysfunction, discontinuation symptoms, or significant sleep disturbance. It does not produce sedation or cognitive and psychomotor impairment. The most common adverse effects of buspirone are headache, nausea, dizziness, and, rarely, insomnia. No sedation is associated with buspirone. Some persons may report a minor feeling of restlessness, although that symptom may reflect an incompletely treated anxiety disorder. No deaths have been reported from overdoses of buspirone, and the median lethal dose is estimated to be 160 to 550 times the recommended daily dose. Buspirone should be used with caution by persons with hepatic and renal impairment, pregnant women, and nursing mothers. Buspirone can be used safely by the elderly.

DRUG INTERACTIONS

The coadministration of buspirone and haloperidol (Haldol) results in increased blood concentrations of haloperidol. Buspirone should not be used with monoamine oxidase inhibitors (MAOIs) to avoid hypertensive episodes, and a 2-week washout period should pass between the discontinuation of MAOI use and the initiation of treatment with buspirone. Drugs or foods that inhibit cytochrome 450 3A4—for example, erythromycin (E-mycin), itraconazole (Sporanox), nefazodone (Serzone), and grapefruit juice—increase buspirone plasma concentrations.

LABORATORY INTERFERENCES

Single doses of buspirone can cause transient elevations in growth hormone, prolactin, and cortisol concentrations, although the effects are not clinically significant.

DOSING AND CLINICAL GUIDELINES

Buspirone is available in single-scored 5- and 10-mg tablets and triple-scored 15- and 30-mg tablets; treatment is usually initiated with either 5 mg orally three times daily or 7.5 mg orally twice daily. The dose can be raised 5 mg every 2 to 4 days to the usual dose range of 15 to 60 mg a day.

Switching from a Benzodiazepine to Buspirone

Buspirone is not cross-tolerant with benzodiazepines, barbiturates, or alcohol. A common clinical problem, therefore, is how to initiate buspirone therapy in a person who is taking benzodiazepines. The two alternatives are as follows: First, the clinician can start buspirone treatment gradually while the benzodiazepine

is being withdrawn. Second, the clinician can start buspirone treatment and bring the person up to a therapeutic dose for 2 to 3 weeks, while the person is still receiving the regular dose of the benzodiazepine, and then slowly taper the benzodiazepine dose. Patients who have received benzodiazepines in the past, especially in recent months, may find that buspirone is not as effective as the benzodiazepines in treating their anxiety. This might be explained by the absence of the immediate mildly euphoric and sedative effects of the benzodiazepines. The coadministration of buspirone and benzodiazepines may be effective in the treatment of anxiety disorders that have not responded to treatment with either drug alone.

▲ 32.12 Calcium Channel Inhibitors

Calcium channel inhibitors are used in psychiatry as antimanic agents for persons who are refractory to, or cannot tolerate, treatment with first-line mood-stabilizing agents. Calcium channel inhibitors include nifedipine (Procardia, Adalat), nimodipine (Nimotop), isradipine (DynaCirc), amlodipine (Norvasc, Lotrel), nicardipine (Cardene), nisoldipine (Sular), nitrendipine, and verapamil (Calan). They are used to control mania and ultradian bipolar disorder (mood cycling in <24 hours).

PHARMACOLOGICAL ACTIONS

The calcium channel inhibitors are nearly completely absorbed after oral use, with significant first-pass hepatic metabolism. Considerable intraindividual and interindividual variations are seen in the plasma concentrations of the drugs after a single dose. Peak plasma levels of most of these agents are achieved within 30 minutes. Amlodipine does not reach peak plasma levels for about 6 hours. The half-life of verapamil after the first dose is 2 to 8 hours; the half-life increases to 5 to 12 hours after the first few days of therapy. The half-lives of the other calcium channel blockers range from 1 to 2 hours for nimodipine and isradipine to 30 to 50 hours for amlodipine.

The primary mechanism of action of calcium channel blockers in bipolar illness is not known. The calcium channel inhibitors discussed in this section inhibit the influx of calcium into neurons through L-type (long-acting) voltage-dependent calcium channels.

THERAPEUTIC INDICATIONS

Bipolar Disorder

Nimodipine and verapamil have been demonstrated to be effective as maintenance therapy in bipolar illness. Patients who respond to lithium appear also to respond to treatment with verapamil. Nimodipine may be useful for ultradian cycling and recurrent brief depression. The clinician should begin treatment with a short-acting drug, such as nimodipine or isradipine, beginning with a low dose and increasing the dose every 4 to 5 days until a clinical response is seen or adverse effects appear. Once symptoms are controlled, a longer-acting drug, such as amlodipine, can be substituted as maintenance therapy. Failure to respond to verapamil does not exclude a favorable response to one of the other drugs. Verapamil has been shown to prevent antidepressant-induced mania. Calcium channel blockers can be combined with other agents, such as carbamazepine, in patients who are partial responders to monotherapy.

Depression

None of the calcium channel blockers is effective as treatment for depression, and, in fact, may prevent response to antidepressants.

Other Psychiatric Indications

Nifedipine is used to treat hypertensive crises associated with use of monoamine oxidase inhibitors. Isradipine may reduce the subjective response to methamphetamine. Calcium channel inhibitors may be beneficial in Tourette's disorder, Huntington's disease, panic disorder, intermittent explosive disorder, and tardive dyskinesia.

PRECAUTIONS AND ADVERSE REACTIONS

The most common adverse effects associated with calcium channel inhibitors are those caused by vasodilation: dizziness, headache, tachycardia, nausea, dysesthesias, and peripheral edema. Verapamil and diltiazem (Cardizem), in particular, can cause hypotension, bradycardia, and atrioventricular heart block, all of which necessitate close monitoring and sometimes discontinuation of the drugs. In all patients with cardiovascular disease, the drugs should be used with caution. Other common adverse effects include constipation, fatigue, rash, coughing, and wheezing. Adverse effects noted with diltiazem include hyperactivity, akathisia, and Parkinsonism; with verapamil, delirium, hyperprolactinemia, and galactorrhea; with nimodipine, a subjective sense of chest tightness and skin flushing; and with nifedipine, depression. The drugs have not been evaluated for safety in pregnant women and are best avoided. Because the drugs are secreted in breast milk, nursing mothers should also avoid the drugs.

DRUG INTERACTIONS

Verapamil raises serum levels of carbamazepine, digoxin, and other cytochrome P450 34A substrates. Verapamil and diltiazem, but not nifedipine, have been reported to precipitate carbamazepine-induced neurotoxicity. Calcium channel inhibitors should not be used by persons taking β-adrenergic receptor antagonists, hypotensives (e.g., diuretics, vasodilators, and angiotensin-converting enzyme inhibitors), or antiarrhythmic drugs (e.g., quinidine and digoxin) without consultation with an internist or cardiologist. Cimetidine (Tagamet) has been reported to increase plasma concentrations of nifedipine and diltiazem. Some patients who are treated with lithium and calcium channel inhibitors concurrently may be at increased risk for the signs and symptoms of neurotoxicity, and deaths have occurred.

LABORATORY INTERFERENCES

No known laboratory interferences are associated with the use of calcium channel inhibitors.

DOSING AND CLINICAL GUIDELINES

Verapamil is available in 40-, 80-, and 120-mg tablets; 120-, 180- and 240-mg sustained-release tablets; and 100-, 120-, 180-, 200-, 240-, 300-, and 360-mg sustained-release capsules. The starting dose is 40 mg orally three times a day and can be raised in increments every 4 to 5 days up to 80 to 120 mg three times a day. The patient's blood pressure, pulse, and electrocardiogram (in patients older than 40 years of age or with a history of cardiac illness) should be routinely monitored.

Nifedipine is available in 10- and 20-mg capsules and 30-, 60-, and 90-mg extended-release tablets. Administration should be started at 10 mg orally three or four times a day and can be increased up to a maximal dose of 120 mg a day.

Nimodipine is available in 30-mg capsules. It has been used at 60 mg every 4 hours for ultrarapid-cycling bipolar disorder and sometimes briefly at up to 630 mg per day.

Isradipine is available in 2.5- and 5-mg capsules and 5- or 10-mg controlled-release tablets. Administration should be started at 2.5 mg a day and can be increased up to a maximum of 15 mg a day in divided doses.

Amlodipine is available in 2.5-, 5-, and 10-mg tablets. Administration should start at 5 mg once at night and can be increased to a maximal dose of 10 to 15 mg a day.

Diltiazem is available in 30-, 60-, 90-, and 120-mg tablets; 60-, 90-, 120-, 180-, 240-, 300-, and 360-mg extended-release capsules; and 60-, 90-, 120-, 180-, 240-, 300-, and 360-mg extended-release tablets. Administration should start with 30 mg orally four times a day and can be increased up to a maximum of 360 mg a day.

Elderly persons are more sensitive to the calcium channel inhibitors than are younger adults. No specific information is available regarding the use of these agents for children.

▲ 32.13 Carbamazepine and Oxcarbazepine

Carbamazepine (Equetro, Carbatrol, Tegretol) was first used to treat partial- and generalized-onset epilepsy and trigeminal neuralgia. Outside the United States, carbamazepine has been used for decades as a first-line agent for acute and maintenance treatment for bipolar I disorder. Despite its proved efficacy, carbamazepine was not approved as a treatment for bipolar disorder by the U.S. Food and Drug Administration (FDA) until 2004 and only in the extended-release form. An analog of carbamazepine, oxcarbazepine (Trileptal), was marketed in the United States in 2000, after being used as a treatment for pediatric epilepsy in Europe since 1990. Very small studies and anecdotal reports suggest that oxcarbazepine may possess mood-stabilizing properties, which, however, has not been confirmed in large, placebo-controlled trials.

Both carbamazepine and oxcarbazepine are iminostilbenes, and both drugs are almost structurally identical and are similar to the tricyclic antidepressants. Oxcarbazepine differs structurally from carbamazepine as a result of the replacement of a carbohydrate group with a carboxy moiety. The resulting change in metabolism leads to products that are both safer and better tolerated than carbamazepine. The therapeutic effects of carbamazepine have been linked to blockade of type 2 or batrachotoxin-sensitive sodium channels, action on mitochondrial receptors, and activity at adenosine A_1 receptors. Numerous other receptor effects of carbamazepine have also been described. The primary biochemical effect of oxcarbazepine is potent blockade of sodium channels.

CARBAMAZEPINE

Pharmacological Actions

Absorption of carbamazepine is slow and unpredictable. Food enhances absorption. Peak plasma concentrations are reached 2 to 8 hours after a single dose, and steady-state levels are reached after 2 to 4 days on a steady dose. It is 70 to 80 percent protein bound. The half-life of carbamazepine ranges from 18 to 54 hours, with an average of 26 hours. With chronic administration, however, the half-life of carbamazepine decreases to an average of 12 hours. This results from induction of hepatic cytochrome P450 (CYP) enzymes by carbamazepine, and specifically autoinduction of carbamazepine metabolism. The induction of hepatic enzymes reaches its maximal level after about 3 to 5 weeks of therapy.

The pharmacokinetics of carbamazepine are different for two long-acting preparations of carbamazepine, each of which uses slightly different technology. One formulation, Tegretol XR, requires food to ensure normal gastrointestinal (GI) transit time. The other preparation, Carbatrol, relies on a combination of intermediate, extended-release, and very slow-release beads, making it suitable for bedtime administration.

Carbamazepine is metabolized in the liver, and the 10,11-epoxide metabolite is active as an anticonvulsant. Its activity in the treatment of bipolar disorders is unknown. Long-term use of carbamazepine is associated with an increased ratio of the epoxide to the parent molecule.

The anticonvulsant effects of carbamazepine are thought to be mediated mainly by binding to voltage-dependent sodium channels in the inactive state and prolonging their inactivation. This secondarily reduces voltage-dependent calcium channel activation and, therefore, synaptic transmission. Additional effects include reduction of currents through N-methyl-D-aspartate glutamate-receptor channels, competitive antagonism of adenosine A_1 receptors, and potentiation of central nervous system catecholamine neurotransmission. Whether any or all of these mechanisms also result in mood stabilization is not known.

Therapeutic Indications

Bipolar Disorder

ACUTE MANIA.   The acute antimanic effects of carbamazepine are typically evident within the first several days of treatment. A 50 to 70 percent response is seen within 2 to 3 weeks of initiation. Studies suggest that carbamazepine may be especially effective in persons who are not responsive to lithium, such as persons with dysphoric mania, rapid cycling, or a negative family history of mood disorders. The antimanic effects of carbamazepine can be, and often are, augmented by concomitant administration of lithium, valproic acid, thyroid hormones, dopamine receptor antagonists, or serotonin-dopamine antagonists. Some persons may respond to carbamazepine but not lithium or valproic acid, and vice versa. Comparative data with more recently approved serotonin-dopamine antagonists, also known as the atypical neuroleptics, all of which are also indicated for acute mania, are not available.

PROPHYLAXIS.   Carbamazepine is effective in preventing relapses, particularly among patients with bipolar II illness, schizoaffective disorder, and dysphoric mania.

ACUTE DEPRESSION.   A subgroup of treatment-refractory patients with acute depression responds well to carbamazepine. Patients with more severe episodic and less chronic depression seem to be better responders to carbamazepine. Nevertheless, carbamazepine remains an alternative drug for depressed persons who have not responded to conventional treatments, including electroconvulsive therapy.

Other Disorders.

Carbamazepine helps to control symptoms associated with acute alcohol withdrawal. Although lacking the abuse potential of benzodiazepines in this population, the lack of any advantage of carbamazepine over the benzodiazepines for alcohol withdrawal and the potential risk of adverse effects with carbamazepine limit use in this role. Carbamazepine has been suggested as a treatment for the paroxysmal recurrent component of posttraumatic stress disorder. Uncontrolled studies suggest that carbamazepine is effective in controlling impulsive, aggressive behavior in persons of all ages who are not psychotic, including children and the elderly. Carbamazepine is also effective in controlling nonacute agitation and aggressive behavior in patients with schizophrenia and schizoaffective disorder. Persons with prominent positive symptoms (e.g., hallucinations) may likely respond, as are persons who display impulsive aggressive outbursts.

Precautions and Adverse Reactions

Carbamazepine is relatively well tolerated. Mild GI (nausea, vomiting, gastric distress, constipation, diarrhea, and anorexia) and CNS (ataxia, drowsiness) effects are the most common side effects. The severity of these adverse effects is reduced if the dose of carbamazepine is increased slowly and kept at the minimal effective plasma concentration. In contrast to lithium and valproate—other drugs used to manage bipolar disorder—carbamazepine does not appear to cause weight gain. Because of the phenomenon of autoinduction, with consequent reductions in carbamazepine concentrations, side-effect tolerability may improve over time. Most of the adverse effects of carbamazepine are correlated with plasma concentrations greater than 9 μg/mL. The rarest but most serious adverse effects of carbamazepine are blood dyscrasias, hepatitis, and serious skin reactions.

Blood Dyscrasias.

The drug's hematologic effects are not dose related. Severe blood dyscrasias (aplastic anemia, agranulocytosis) occur in about 1 in 125,000 persons treated with carbamazepine. A correlation does not appear to exist between the degree of benign white blood cell suppression (leukopenia), which is seen in 1 to 2 percent of persons, and the emergence of life-threatening blood dyscrasias. Persons should be warned that the emergence of such symptoms as fever, sore throat, rash, petechiae, bruising, and easy bleeding can potentially herald a serious dyscrasia, and anyone with these symptoms should seek medical evaluation immediately. Routine hematologic monitoring in carbamazepine-treated persons is recommended at 3, 6, 9, and 12 months. With no significant evidence of bone marrow suppression by that time, many experts would reduce the interval of monitoring. Even assiduous monitoring, however, may fail to detect severe blood dyscrasias before they cause symptoms.

Hepatitis.   Within the first few weeks of therapy, carbamazepine can cause both a hepatitis associated with increases in liver enzymes, particularly transaminases, and a cholestasis associated with elevated bilirubin and alkaline phosphatase. Mild transaminase elevations warrant observation only, but persistent elevations more than three times the upper limit of normal indicate the need to discontinue the drug. Hepatitis can recur if the drug is reintroduced to the person and can result in death.

Dermatologic Effects.   About 10 to 15 percent of persons treated with carbamazepine develop a benign maculopapular rash within the first 3 weeks of treatment. Stopping the medication usually leads to resolution of the rash. Some patients may experience life-threatening dermatologic syndromes, including exfoliative dermatitis, erythema multiforme, Stevens-Johnson syndrome, and toxic epidermal necrolysis. The possible emergence of these serious dermatologic problems causes most clinicians to discontinue carbamazepine use in a person who develops any type of rash. The risk of drug rash is about equal between valproic acid and carbamazepine in the first 2 months of use but is subsequently much higher for carbamazepine. If carbamazepine seems to be the only effective drug for a person who has a benign rash with carbamazepine treatment, a retrial of the drug can be undertaken. Many patients can be rechallenged without reemergence of the rash. Pretreatment with prednisone (40 mg a day) may suppress the rash, although other symptoms of an allergic reaction (e.g., fever and pneumonitis) may develop, even with steroid pretreatment.

Renal Effects.   Carbamazepine is occasionally used to treat diabetes insipidus not associated with lithium use. This activity results from direct or indirect effects at the vasopressin receptor. It also can lead to the development of hyponatremia and water intoxication in some patients, particularly the elderly or when used in high doses.

Other Adverse Effects.   Carbamazepine decreases cardiac conduction (although less than the tricyclic drugs do) and, thus, can exacerbate preexisting cardiac disease. Carbamazepine should be used with caution in persons with glaucoma, prostatic hypertrophy, diabetes, or a history of alcohol abuse. Carbamazepine occasionally activates vasopressin receptor function, which results in a condition resembling the syndrome of secretion of inappropriate antidiuretic hormone, characterized by hyponatremia and, rarely, water intoxication. This is the opposite of the renal effects of lithium (i.e., nephrogenic diabetes insipidus). Augmentation of lithium with carbamazepine does not reverse the lithium effect, however. Emergence of confusion, severe weakness, or headache in a person taking carbamazepine should prompt measurement of serum electrolytes.

Carbamazepine use rarely elicits an immune hypersensitivity response consisting of fever, rash, eosinophilia, and possibly fatal myocarditis.

Minor cranial facial abnormalities, fingernail hypoplasia, and spina bifida in infants may be associated with the maternal use of carbamazepine during pregnancy. Pregnant women should not use carbamazepine unless absolutely necessary. All women with childbearing potential should take 1 to 4 mg of folic acid daily, even if they are not trying to conceive. Carbamazepine is secreted in breast milk.

Drug Interactions

Carbamazepine decreases serum concentrations of numerous drugs as a result of prominent induction of hepatic CYP 3A4. Monitoring for a decrease in clinical effects is frequently indicated. Carbamazepine can decrease the blood concentrations of oral contraceptives, resulting in breakthrough bleeding and uncertain prophylaxis against pregnancy. Carbamazepine should not be administered with monoamine oxidase inhibitors, which

should be discontinued at least 2 weeks before initiating treatment with carbamazepine. Grapefruit juice inhibits the hepatic metabolism of carbamazepine. When carbamazepine and valproate are used in combination, the dose of carbamazepine should be decreased because valproate displaces carbamazepine binding on proteins, and the dose of valproate may need to be increased.

Laboratory Interferences

Circulating increased levels of thyroxine and triiodothyronine without an associated increase in thyroid-stimulating hormone may be associated with carbamazepine treatment. Carbamazepine is also associated with an increase in total serum cholesterol, primarily by increasing high-density lipoproteins. The thyroid and cholesterol effects are not clinically significant. Carbamazepine can interfere with the dexamethasone-suppression test and may also cause false-positive pregnancy test results.

Dosing and Administration

The target dose for antimanic activity is 1,200 mg a day, although this varies considerably. Immediate-release carbamazepine needs to be taken three or four times a day, which leads to lapses in compliance. Extended-release formulations are thus preferred because they can be taken just once or twice a day. One form of extended-release carbamazepine, Carbatrol, comes as 100-, 200-, and 300-mg capsules. Another form, called Equetro, is identical to Carbatrol and marketed as a treatment for bipolar disorder. These capsules contain tiny beads with three different types of coatings so that they dissolve at different times. Capsules should not be crushed or chewed. The contents can be sprinkled over food, however, without affecting the extended-release qualities. This formulation can be taken either with or without meals. The entire daily dose can be given at bedtime. The rate of absorption is faster when it is given with a high-fat meal. Another extended-release form of carbamazepine, Tegretol XR, uses a different drug-delivery system than Carbatrol. It is available in 100-, 200-, and 300-mg tablets.

Preexisting hematologic, hepatic, and cardiac diseases can be relative contraindications for carbamazepine treatment. Persons with hepatic disease require only one third to one half of the usual dose; the clinician should be cautious about raising the dose in such persons and should do so only slowly and gradually. The laboratory examination should include a complete blood count with platelet count, liver function tests, serum electrolytes, and an electrocardiogram in persons older than 40 years of age or those with a preexisting cardiac disease. An electroencephalogram is not necessary before the initiation of treatment, but it may be helpful in some cases for the documentation of objective changes correlated with clinical improvement.

Routine Laboratory Monitoring.   Serum levels for antimanic efficacy have not been established. The anticonvulsant blood concentration range for carbamazepine is 4 to 12 μg/mL, and this range should be reached before determining that carbamazepine is not effective in the treatment of a mood disorder. A clinically insignificant suppression of the white blood count commonly occurs during carbamazepine treatment. This benign decrease can be reversed by adding lithium, which enhances colony-stimulating factor. Potential serious hematologic effects of carbamazepine, such as pancytopenia, agranulocytosis, and aplastic anemia, occur in about 1 of 125,000 patients. Complete laboratory blood assessments may be performed every 2 weeks for the first 2 months of treatment and quarterly thereafter, but the FDA has revised the package insert for carbamazepine to suggest that blood monitoring be performed at the discretion of the physician. Patients should be informed that fever, sore throat, rash, petechiae, bruising, or unusual bleeding may indicate a hematologic problem and should prompt immediate notification of a physician. This approach is probably more effective than is frequent blood monitoring during long-term treatment. It has also been suggested that liver and renal function tests be conducted quarterly, although the benefit of conducting tests this frequently has been questioned. It seems reasonable, however, to assess hematologic status, along with liver and renal functions, whenever a routine examination of the person is being conducted.

Carbamazepine treatment should be discontinued, and a consult with a hematologist be obtained, if the following laboratory values are found: total white blood cell count less than 3,000/mm^3, erythrocytes less than 4.0×10^6/mm^3, neutrophils less than 1,500/mm^3, hematocrit less than 32 percent, hemoglobin less than 11 g/100 mL, platelet count less than 100,000/mm^3, reticulocyte count less than 0.3 percent, and a serum iron concentration less than 150 mg/100 mL.

OXCARBAZEPINE

Although structurally related to carbamazepine, the usefulness of oxcarbazepine as a treatment for mania or other psychiatric disorders has not been established in controlled trials.

Pharmacokinetics

Absorption is rapid and unaffected by food. Peak concentrations occur after about 45 minutes. The elimination half-life of the parent compound is 2 hours, which remains stable over long-term treatment. The monohydroxide has a half-life of 9 hours. Most of the drug's anticonvulsant activity is presumed to result from this monohydroxy derivative.

Side Effects

The most common side effects are sedation and nausea. Less frequent side effects are cognitive impairment, ataxia, diplopia, nystagmus, dizziness, and tremor. In contrast to carbamazepine, oxcarbazepine does not have an increased risk of serious blood dyscrasias, so hematologic monitoring is not necessary. The frequency of benign rash is lower than observed with carbamazepine, and serious rashes are extremely rare. About 25 to 30 percent of patients who develop an allergic rash on carbamazepine, however, also develop a rash with oxcarbazepine. Oxcarbazepine is more likely to cause hyponatremia than carbamazepine. Approximately 3 to 5 percent of patients taking oxcarbazepine develop this side effect. It is advisable to obtain serum sodium concentrations early in the course of treatment because hyponatremia may be clinically silent. In severe cases, confusion and seizure may occur.

Dosing and Administration

Oxcarbazepine dosing for psychiatric disorders has not been established. It is available in 150-, 300-, and 600-mg tablets. The dose range may vary from 150 to 2,400 mg per day, given in divided doses twice a day. In clinical trials for mania, the doses typically used were from 900 to 1,200 mg per day, with a starting dose of 150 or 300 mg at night.

Drug Interactions

Drugs such as phenobarbital and alcohol, which induce CYP 3A4, increase the clearance and reduce oxcarbazepine concentrations. Oxcarbazepine induces CYP 3A4/5 and inhibits CYP 2C19, which may affect the metabolism of drugs that utilize that pathway. Women taking oral contraceptives should be told to consult with their gynecologist because oxcarbazepine may reduce concentrations of their contraceptive and, thus, decrease its efficacy.

▲ 32.14 Cholinesterase Inhibitors and Memantine

Donepezil (Aricept), rivastigmine (Exelon), galantamine (Reminyl), and tacrine (Cognex) are cholinesterase inhibitors used to treat mild to moderate cognitive impairment in dementia of the Alzheimer's type. They reduce the inactivation of the neurotransmitter acetylcholine and, thus, potentiate cholinergic neurotransmission, which in turn produces a modest improvement in memory and goal-directed thought. Memantine (Namenda) is not a cholinesterase inhibitor, and produces its effects through blockade of N-methyl-D-aspartate (NMDA) receptors. Unlike the cholinesterase inhibitors, which are indicated for the mild to moderate stages of Alzheimer's disease, memantine is indicated for the moderate to severe stages of the disease. Tacrine, the first cholinesterase inhibitor to be introduced, is rarely used because of its multiple-daily-dosing regimens, its potential for hepatotoxicity, and the consequent need for frequent laboratory monitoring.

PHARMACOLOGICAL ACTIONS

Donepezil is absorbed completely from the gastrointestinal (GI) tract. Peak plasma concentrations are reached about 3 to 4 hours after oral dosing. The half-life of donepezil is 70 hours in the elderly, and it is taken only once daily. Steady-state levels are achieved within about 2 weeks. Presence of stable alcoholic cirrhosis reduces clearance of donepezil by 20 percent. Rivastigmine is rapidly and completely absorbed from the GI tract and reaches peak plasma concentrations in 1 hour, but this is delayed by up to 90 minutes if rivastigmine is taken with food. The half-life of rivastigmine is 1 hour, but because it remains bound to cholinesterases, a single dose is therapeutically active for 10 hours, and it is taken twice daily. Galantamine is an alkaloid similar to codeine and is extracted from bulbs and flowers of the plant *Galanthus nivalis* and related species. It is readily absorbed, with maximal concentrations reached after 30 minutes to 2 hours. Food decreases the maximal concentration by 25 percent. The elimination half-life of galantamine is approximately 6 hours.

Tacrine is absorbed rapidly from the GI tract. Peak plasma concentrations are reached about 90 minutes after oral dosing.

The half-life of tacrine is about 2 to 4 hours, thereby necessitating four–times-daily dosing.

The primary mechanism of action of cholinesterase inhibitors is reversible, nonacylating inhibition of acetylcholinesterase and butyrylcholinesterase, the enzymes that catabolize acetylcholine in the central nervous system (CNS). The enzyme inhibition increases synaptic concentrations of acetylcholine, especially in the hippocampus and cerebral cortex. Unlike tacrine, which is nonselective for all forms of acetylcholinesterase, donepezil appears to be selectively active within the CNS and to have little activity in the periphery. Donepezil's favorable side-effect profile appears to correlate with its lack of inhibition of cholinesterases in the GI tract. Rivastigmine appears to have somewhat more peripheral activity than donepezil and, thus, is more likely to cause GI adverse effects than is donepezil.

THERAPEUTIC INDICATIONS

Cholinesterase inhibitors are effective for the treatment of mild to moderate cognitive impairment in dementia of the Alzheimer's type. In long-term use, they slow the progression of memory loss and diminish apathy, depression, hallucinations, anxiety, euphoria, and purposeless motor behaviors. Functional autonomy is less well preserved. Some persons note immediate improvement in memory, mood, psychotic symptoms, and interpersonal skills. Others note little initial benefit but are able to retain their cognitive and adaptive faculties at a relatively stable level for many months. A practical benefit of cholinesterase inhibitor use is a delay or reduction of the need for nursing home placement.

Donepezil and rivastigmine may be beneficial for patients with Parkinson's disease and Lewy body disease and for the treatment of cognitive deficits caused by traumatic brain injury. Donepezil is under study for treatment of mild cognitive impairment less severe than that caused by Alzheimer's disease. People with vascular dementia may respond to acetylcholinesterase inhibitors. Occasionally, cholinesterase inhibitors elicit an idiosyncratic catastrophic reaction, with signs of grief and agitation, which is self-limited once the drug is discontinued. Use of cholinesterase inhibitors to improve cognition by nondemented individuals should be discouraged.

PRECAUTIONS AND ADVERSE REACTIONS

Donepezil

Donepezil is generally well tolerated at recommended doses. Less than 3 percent of persons taking donepezil experience nausea, diarrhea, and vomiting. These mild symptoms are more common with a 10-mg dose than with a 5-mg dose and, when present, they tend to resolve after 3 weeks of continued use. Donepezil can cause weight loss. Donepezil treatment has been infrequently associated with bradyarrhythmias, especially in persons with underlying cardiac disease. A few persons experience syncope.

Rivastigmine

Rivastigmine is generally well tolerated, but recommended doses may need to be scaled back in the initial period of treatment to limit GI and CNS adverse effects. These mild symptoms are more common at doses above 6 mg a day and, when present, they tend to resolve once the dose is lowered. The most common adverse effects associated with rivastigmine are nausea, vomiting, dizziness, headache, diarrhea, abdominal pain, anorexia, fatigue, and somnolence. Rivastigmine can cause weight loss, but it does not appear to cause hepatic, renal, hematologic, or electrolyte abnormalities.

Galantamine

The most common side effects of galantamine are dizziness, headache, nausea, vomiting, diarrhea, and anorexia. These side effects tend to be mild and transient.

Tacrine

Tacrine is the least used of the cholinesterase inhibitors, but its use requires more discussion with the patient than the others because it is cumbersome to titrate and use, and it poses the risk of potentially significant elevations in hepatic transaminase levels. These increases occur in 25 to 30 percent of persons. Aside from elevated transaminase levels, the most common specific adverse effects associated with tacrine treatment are nausea, vomiting, myalgia, anorexia, and rash, but only nausea, vomiting, and anorexia have been found to have a clear relation to the dose. Transaminase elevations characteristically develop during the first 6 to 12 weeks of treatment, and cholinergically mediated events are dose related.

Hepatotoxicity.   Tacrine is associated with increases in the plasma activities of alanine aminotransferase (ALT) and aspartate aminotransferase (AST). The ALT measurement is the more sensitive indicator of the hepatic effects of tacrine. About 95 percent of patients who develop elevated ALT serum levels do so in the first 18 weeks of treatment. Four weeks is the average length of time for elevated ALT concentrations to return to normal after stopping tacrine treatment.

For routine monitoring of hepatic enzymes, AST and ALT activities should be measured weekly for the first 18 weeks, every month for the second 4 months, and every 3 months thereafter. Weekly assessments of AST and ALT should be performed for at least 6 weeks after any increase in dose. Patients with mildly elevated ALT activity should be monitored weekly and not be rechallenged with tacrine until the ALT activity returns to the normal range. For any patient with elevated ALT activity and jaundice, tacrine treatment should be stopped, and the patient should not be given the drug again.

DRUG INTERACTIONS

All cholinesterase inhibitors should be used cautiously with drugs that also possess cholinomimetic activity, such as succinylcholine (Anectine) or bethanechol (Urecholine). The coadministration of cholinesterase inhibitors and drugs that have cholinergic antagonist activity (e.g., tricyclic drugs) is probably counterproductive. Paroxetine has the most marked anticholinergic effects of any of the newer antidepressant and anxiolytic drugs and should be avoided for that reason, as well as for its inhibiting effect on the metabolism of some of the cholinesterase inhibitors.

Donepezil undergoes extensive metabolism via both cytochrome P450 (CYP) 2D6 and 3A4 isozymes. The metabolism of donepezil may be increased by phenytoin (Dilantin), carbamazepine (Tegretol), dexamethasone (Decadron), rifampin

(Rifadin), or phenobarbital (Solfoton). Commonly used agents, such as paroxetine, ketoconazole, and erythromycin, can significantly increase donepezil concentrations. Donepezil is highly protein bound, but it does not displace other protein-bound drugs, such as furosemide (Lasix), digoxin (Lanoxin), or warfarin (Coumadin). Rivastigmine circulates mostly unbound to serum proteins and has no significant drug interactions.

As with donepezil, galantamine is metabolized by both CYP 2D6 and 3A4 isozymes and, thus, may interact with drugs that inhibit these pathways. Paroxetine and ketoconazole should be used with great caution.

LABORATORY INTERFERENCES

No laboratory interferences have been associated with use of cholinesterase inhibitors.

DOSING AND CLINICAL GUIDELINES

Before initiating cholinesterase inhibitor therapy, potentially treatable causes of dementia should be ruled out and the diagnosis of dementia of the Alzheimer's type established.

Donepezil is available in 5- and 10-mg tablets. Treatment should be initiated at 5 mg each night. If well tolerated and of some discernible benefit after 4 weeks, the dose should be increased to a maintenance dose of 10-mg each night. Donepezil absorption is unaffected by meals.

Rivastigmine is available in 1.5-, 3-, 4.5-, and 6-mg capsules. The recommended initial dose is 1.5 mg twice daily for a minimum of 2 weeks, after which increases of 1.5 mg a day can be made at intervals of at least 2 weeks to a target dose of 6 mg a day, taken in two equal doses. If tolerated, the dose can be further titrated upward to a maximum of 6 mg twice daily. The risk of adverse GI events can be reduced by administration of rivastigmine with food.

Galantamine is available in 4-, 8-, and 16-mg tablets. The suggested dose range is 16 to 32 mg per day given twice a day. The higher dose is actually better tolerated than the lower dose. The initial dose is 8 mg per day and, after a minimum of 4 weeks, the dose can be raised. All subsequent dose increases should occur at 4-week intervals and should be based on tolerability.

Tacrine is available in 10-, 20-, 30-, and 40-mg capsules. Before the initiation of tacrine treatment, a complete physical and laboratory examination should be conducted, with special attention to liver function tests and baseline hematological indexes. Treatment should be initiated at 10 mg four times a day and then raised by increments of 10 mg a dose every 6 weeks up to 160 mg a day; the person's tolerance of each dose is indicated by the absence of unacceptable side effects and lack of elevation of ALT activity. Tacrine should be given four times daily—ideally 1 hour before meals because tacrine absorption is reduced by about 25 percent when it is taken during the first 2 hours after meals. If tacrine is used, the specific guidelines for tacrine-induced ALT listed previously should be followed.

MEMANTINE

Pharmacological Actions

Memantine is well absorbed after oral administration, with peak concentrations reached in about 3 to 7 hours. Food has no effect on the absorption of memantine. Memantine has linear pharmacokinetics over the therapeutic dose range and has a terminal elimination half-life of about 60 to 80 hours. Plasma protein binding is 45 percent.

Memantine undergoes little metabolism, with most (57 to 82 percent) of an administered dose excreted unchanged in urine; the remainder is converted primarily to three polar metabolites: the N-gludantan conjugate, 6-hydroxy memantine, and 1-nitroso-deaminated memantine. These metabolites possess minimal NMDA receptor antagonist activity. Memantine is a low- to moderate-affinity NMDA receptor antagonist. It is thought that overexcitation of NMDA receptors by the neurotransmitter glutamate may play a role in Alzheimer's disease because glutamate plays an integral role in the neural pathways associated with learning and memory. Excess glutamate overstimulates NMDA receptors to allow too much calcium into nerve cells, leading to the eventual cell death observed in Alzheimer's disease. Memantine may protect cells against excess glutamate by partially blocking NMDA receptors associated with abnormal transmission of glutamate while allowing for physiological transmission associated with normal cell functioning.

Therapeutic Indications

Memantine is the only approved therapy in the United States for moderate to severe Alzheimer's disease.

Precautions and Adverse Reactions

Memantine is safe and well tolerated. The most common adverse effects are dizziness, headache, constipation, and confusion. The use of memantine in patients with severe renal impairment is not recommended. In a documented case of an overdose with up to 400 mg of memantine, the patient experienced restlessness, psychosis, visual hallucinations, somnolence, stupor, and loss of consciousness. The patient recovered without permanent sequelae.

Drug Interactions

In vitro studies conducted with marker substrates of CYP enzymes (CYP 1A2, 2A6, 2C9, 2D6, 2E1, and 3A4) showed minimal inhibition of these enzymes by memantine. No pharmacokinetic interactions with drugs metabolized by these enzymes are expected.

Because memantine is eliminated in part by tubular secretion, coadministration of drugs that use the same renal cationic system, including hydrochlorothiazide triamterene, cimetidine, ranitidine, quinidine, and nicotine, could potentially result in altered plasma levels of both agents. Coadministration of memantine and a combination of hydrochlorothiazide and triamterene did not affect the bioavailability of either memantine or triamterene, and the bioavailability of hydrochlorothiazide decreased by 20 percent.

Urine pH is altered by diet, drugs (e.g., carbonic anhydrase inhibitors, topiramate, sodium bicarbonate), and the clinical state of the patient (e.g., renal tubular acidosis or severe infections of the urinary tract). Memantine clearance is reduced by about 80 percent under alkaline urine conditions at pH 8. Therefore, alterations of urine pH toward the alkaline condition may lead to an accumulation of the drug with a possible increase in adverse

Indications

Acamprosate is used for treating alcohol-dependent individuals seeking to continue to remain alcohol-free after they have stopped drinking. Its efficacy in promoting abstinence has not been demonstrated in persons who have not undergone detoxification and who have not achieved alcohol abstinence before beginning treatment.

Precautions and Adverse Effects

Side effects, which are mostly seen early in treatment, are usually mild and transient in nature. The most common side effects are headache, diarrhea, flatulence, abdominal pain, paresthesias, and various skin reactions. No adverse events occur following abrupt withdrawal of acamprosate, even after long-term use. No evidence indicates addiction to the drug. Patients with severe renal impairment (creatinine clearance of <30 mL/min) should not be given acamprosate.

Drug Interactions

The concomitant intake of alcohol and acamprosate does not affect the pharmacokinetics of either alcohol or acamprosate. Administration of disulfiram or diazepam does not affect the pharmacokinetics of acamprosate. Coadministration of naltrexone with acamprosate produces an increase in concentrations of acamprosate. No adjustment of dose is recommended in such patients. The pharmacokinetics of naltrexone and its major metabolite 6-β-naltrexol were unaffected following coadministration with acamprosate. During clinical trials, patients taking acamprosate concomitantly with antidepressants more commonly reported both weight gain and weight loss compared with patients taking either medication alone.

Laboratory Interferences

Acamprosate has not been shown to interfere with commonly done laboratory tests.

Dosing and Clinical Guidelines

It is important to remember that acamprosate should not be used to treat alcohol withdrawal symptoms. It should only be started after the individual has been successfully weaned off the alcohol. Patients should show a commitment to remaining abstinent, and treatment should be part of a comprehensive management program that includes counseling or support group attendance.

Each tablet contains acamprosate calcium 333 mg, which is equivalent to 300 mg of acamprosate. The dose of acamprosate is different for different patients. The recommended dose is two 333-mg tablets (each dose should total 666 mg) taken three times daily. Although dosing may be done without regard to meals, dosing with meals was used during clinical trials and is suggested as an aid to compliance in those patients who regularly eat three meals daily. A lower dose may be effective in some patients. A missed dose should be taken as soon as possible. If it is almost time for the next dose, however, the missed dose should be skipped, and then the regular dosing schedule should be resumed. Doses should not be doubled up. For patients with moderate re-

nal impairment (creatinine clearance of 30 to 50 mL/min), a starting dose of one 333-mg tablet taken three times daily is recommended.

▲ 32.17 Dopamine Receptor Agonists and Precursors: Apomorphine, Bromocriptine, Levodopa, Pergolide, Pramipexole, and Ropinirole

Dopamine receptor agonists and precursors were developed to treat idiopathic Parkinson's disease. On occasion, they are used by psychiatrists to treat such adverse effects of antipsychotic drugs as (1) Parkinsonism, (2) extrapyramidal symptoms, (3) akinesia, (4) focal perioral tremors, (5) hyperprolactinemia, (6) galactorrhea, and (7) neuroleptic malignant syndrome. The drugs in this class most commonly prescribed are bromocriptine (Parlodel); levodopa, also called L-Dopa, (Larodopa); and carbidopa-levodopa (Sinemet). New dopamine receptor agonists include ropinirole (Requip), pramipexole (Mirapex), pergolide (Permax), and apomorphine (Apokyn).

Levodopa is the natural precursor of dopamine. The formulation of levodopa combined with carbidopa reduces the incidence of non–central nervous system (non-CNS) adverse effects experienced with use of levodopa alone. Bromocriptine and pergolide are ergotamine derivatives. Pramipexole is a nonergot dopamine agonist. Apomorphine, also a nonergot dopamine agonist, has been used in medicine for more than a century. It has been available since the 1970s in Europe and Canada but was only approved for use in the United States in 2004. It is indicated for the treatment of motor symptoms associated with late-stage Parkinson's disease. Apomorphine is structurally related to morphine and other opioids.

PHARMACOLOGICAL ACTIONS

L-Dopa is rapidly absorbed after oral administration, and peak plasma levels are reached after 30 to 120 minutes. The half-life of L-Dopa is 90 minutes. Absorption of L-Dopa can be significantly reduced by changes in gastric pH and by ingestion with meals. Bromocriptine, pergolide, and ropinirole are rapidly absorbed but undergo first-pass metabolism such that only about 30 to 55 percent of the dose is bioavailable. Peak concentrations are achieved 1.5 to 3 hours after oral administration. Pergolide has a half-life of about 27 hours, and a single dose has 5 to 6 hours of clinical activity. The half-life of ropinirole is 6 hours. Pramipexole is rapidly absorbed with little first-pass metabolism and reaches peak concentrations in 2 hours. Its half-life is 8 hours. Oral forms of apomorphine have been studied, although they are not available in the United States. Subcutaneous apomorphine injection results in rapid and controlled systemic delivery, with linear pharmacokinetics over a dose ranging from 2 to 8 mg.

Once L-Dopa enters the dopaminergic neurons of the CNS, it is converted into the neurotransmitter dopamine. Apomorphine, bromocriptine, pergolide, ropinirole, and pramipexole act directly on dopamine receptors. Dopamine, pramipexole, and ropinirole bind about 20 times more selectively to dopamine D_3 than D_2 receptors; the corresponding ratio for pergolide is 5:1 and for bromocriptine is less than 2:1. Apomorphine binds selectively to D_1 and D_2 receptors, with little affinity for D_3 and D_4 receptors. L-Dopa, pramipexole, and ropinirole have no significant activity at nondopaminergic receptors, but pergolide and bromocriptine bind to serotonin 5-HT$_1$ and 5-HT$_2$ and α_1-, α_2-, and β-adrenergic receptors.

THERAPEUTIC INDICATIONS

Medication-Induced Movement Disorders

In present-day clinical psychiatry, dopamine receptor agonists are used to treat medication-induced Parkinsonism, extrapyramidal symptoms, akinesia, and focal perioral tremors. Their use has diminished, however, because the incidence of medication-induced movement disorders is much lower with the use of the newer, atypical antipsychotics (serotonin–dopamine antagonists). Dopamine receptor agonists are effective in treating idiopathic restless leg syndrome and may also be helpful when this is a medication side effect.

For the treatment of medication-induced movement disorders, most clinicians rely on anticholinergics, amantadine (Symmetrel), and antihistamines because they are equally effective and have few adverse effects. Bromocriptine remains in use in the treatment of neuroleptic malignant syndrome; however, the incidence of this disorder is diminishing with the decreasing use of dopamine receptor antagonists.

Dopamine receptor agonists are also used to counteract the hyperprolactinemic effects of dopamine receptor antagonists, which result in the side effects of amenorrhea and galactorrhea.

Mood Disorders

Bromocriptine has long been used to enhance response to antidepressant drugs in refractory patients. Ropinirole and pergolide have been reported to be useful as augmentation to antidepressant therapy and for the treatment of medication-resistant bipolar II depression. Ropinirole may also be helpful in the treatment of antidepressant-induced sexual dysfunction.

Sexual Dysfunction

All dopamine receptor agonists can improve erectile dysfunction. They are rarely used, however, because, at therapeutic doses, they frequently cause adverse effects. Recently introduced phosphodiesterase-5 inhibitors agents are better tolerated and more effective.

PRECAUTIONS AND ADVERSE REACTIONS

Adverse effects are common with dopamine receptor agonists, thus limiting the usefulness of these drugs. Adverse effects, which are dose dependent, include nausea, vomiting, orthostatic hypotension, headache, dizziness, and cardiac arrhythmias. To reduce the risk of orthostatic hypotension, the initial dose of all dopamine receptor agonists should be quite low, with incremental increases in dose at intervals of at least 1 week. These

drugs should be used with caution in persons with hypertension, cardiovascular disease, and hepatic disease. After long-term use, persons, particularly elderly persons, may experience choreiform and dystonic movements and psychiatric disturbances—including hallucinations, delusions, confusion, depression, and mania—and other behavioral changes.

Long-term use of bromocriptine and pergolide can produce retroperitoneal and pulmonary fibrosis, pleural effusions, and pleural thickening.

In general, ropinirole and pramipexole have a similar but much milder adverse effect profile than L-Dopa, bromocriptine, and pergolide. Pramipexole and ropinirole can cause irresistible sleep attacks that occur suddenly without warning and have caused motor vehicle accidents.

The most common adverse effects of apomorphine are yawning, dizziness, nausea, vomiting, drowsiness, bradycardia, syncope, and perspiration. Hallucinations have also been reported. Apomorphine's sedative effects are exacerbated with concurrent use of alcohol or other CNS depressants.

Dopamine receptor agonists are contraindicated during pregnancy and for nursing mothers especially, because they inhibit lactation.

DRUG INTERACTIONS

Dopamine receptor antagonists are capable of reversing the effects of dopamine receptor agonists, but this is not usually clinically significant. The concurrent use of tricyclic drugs and dopamine receptor agonists has been reported to cause symptoms of neurotoxicity, such as rigidity, agitation, and tremor. They may also potentiate the hypotensive effects of diuretics and other antihypertensive medications. Dopamine receptor agonists should not be used in conjunction with monoamine oxidase inhibitors (MAOIs), including selegiline (Eldepryl), and MAOIs should be discontinued at least 2 weeks before the initiation of dopamine receptor agonist therapy.

Benzodiazepines, phenytoin (Dilantin), and pyridoxine may interfere with the therapeutic effects of dopamine receptor agonists. Ergot alkaloids and bromocriptine should not be used concurrently because they can cause hypertension and myocardial infarction. Progestins, estrogens, and oral contraceptives may interfere with the effects of bromocriptine and may raise plasma concentrations of ropinirole. Ciprofloxacin (Cipro) can raise plasma concentrations of ropinirole, and cimetidine (Tagamet) can raise plasma concentrations of pramipexole.

LABORATORY INTERFERENCES

L-Dopa administration has been associated with false reports of elevated serum and urinary uric acid concentrations, urinary glucose test results, urinary ketone test results, and urinary catecholamine concentrations. No laboratory interferences have been associated with the administration of the other dopamine receptor agonists.

DOSING AND CLINICAL GUIDELINES

Table 32.17–1 lists the various dopamine receptor agonists and their formulations. For the treatment of antipsychotic-induced Parkinsonism, the clinician should start with a 100-mg dose of levodopa three times a day, which may be increased until the person is functionally improved. The maximum dose of L-Dopa is 2,000 mg a day, but most persons respond to doses below

The most common side effects of DRAs are neurological. Medication-induced movement disorders, such as Parkinsonism, dystonia, akathisia, and tardive dyskinesia, are discussed in Section 32.2. As a rule, low-potency drugs cause most nonneurological adverse effects, whereas the high-potency drugs cause most neurological adverse effects.

PRECAUTIONS AND ADVERSE REACTIONS

Neuroleptic Malignant Syndrome

A potentially fatal side effect of DRA treatment, neuroleptic malignant syndrome, can occur at any time during the course of DRA treatment. Symptoms include extreme hyperthermia, severe muscular rigidity and dystonia, akinesia, mutism, confusion, agitation, and increased pulse rate and blood pressure (BP) leading to cardiovascular collapse. Laboratory findings include increased white blood cell (WBC) count, creatinine phosphokinase, liver enzymes, plasma myoglobin, and myoglobinuria, occasionally associated with renal failure. The symptoms usually evolve over 24 to 72 hours, and the untreated syndrome lasts 10 to 14 days. The diagnosis is often missed in the early stages, and the withdrawal or agitation may mistakenly be considered to reflect increased psychosis. Men are affected more frequently than are women, and young persons are affected more commonly than are elderly persons. The mortality rate can reach 20 to 30 percent or even higher when depot medications are involved. Rates are also increased when high doses of high-potency agents are used.

If neuroleptic malignant syndrome is suspected, the DRA should be stopped immediately and the following done: medical support to cool the person; monitoring of vital signs, electrolytes, fluid balance, and renal output; and symptomatic treatment of fever. Anti-Parkinsonian medications may reduce some of the muscle rigidity. Dantrolene (Dantrium), a skeletal muscle relaxant (0.8 to 2.5 mg/kg every 6 hours, up to a total dose of 10 mg a day) may be useful in the treatment of this disorder. Once the person can take oral medications, dantrolene can be given in doses of 100 to 200 mg a day. Bromocriptine (20 to 30 mg a day in four divided doses) or amantadine can be added to the regimen. Treatment should usually be continued for 5 to 10 days. When drug treatment is restarted, the clinician should consider switching to a low-potency drug or an SDA, although these agents—including clozapine—can also cause neuroleptic malignant syndrome.

Seizure Threshold

The DRAs may lower the seizure threshold. Chlorpromazine, thioridazine, and other low-potency drugs are thought to be more epileptogenic than are high-potency drugs. Molindone may be the least epileptogenic of the DRA drugs. The risk of inducing a seizure by drug administration warrants consideration when the person already has a seizure disorder or brain lesion.

Sedation

Blockade of histamine H_1 receptors is the usual cause of sedation associated with DRAs. Giving the entire daily dose at bedtime usually eliminates any problems from sedation, and tolerance for this adverse effect often develops.

Central Anticholinergic Effects

The symptoms of central anticholinergic activity include severe agitation; disorientation to time, person, and place; hallucina-

tions; seizures; high fever; and dilated pupils. Stupor and coma may ensue. The treatment of anticholinergic toxicity consists of discontinuing the causal agent or agents, close medical supervision, and physostigmine (Antilirium, Eserine), 2 mg by slow intravenous (IV) infusion, repeated within 1 hour as necessary. Too much physostigmine is dangerous, and symptoms of physostigmine toxicity include hypersalivation and sweating. Atropine sulfate (0.5 mg) can reverse the effects of physostigmine toxicity.

Cardiac Effects

The DRAs decrease cardiac contractility, disrupt enzyme contractility in cardiac cells, increase circulating levels of catecholamines, and prolong atrial and ventricular conduction time and refractory periods. Low-potency DRAs are more cardiotoxic than are high-potency drugs. Chlorpromazine causes prolongation of the QT and PR intervals, blunting of the T waves, and depression of the ST segment. Thioridazine and mesoridazine, in particular, are associated with substantial QT prolongation and risk of *torsade de pointes*. These drugs, thus, are indicated only when other agents have been ineffective.

Sudden Death

Occasional reports of sudden cardiac death during treatment with DRAs may be the result of cardiac arrhythmias. Other causes may include seizure, asphyxiation, malignant hyperthermia, heat stroke, and neuroleptic malignant syndrome. There is a slight increase in the incidence of sudden death linked to the use of antipsychotics in patients with dementia.

Orthostatic (Postural) Hypotension

Orthostatic (postural) hypotension is most common with low-potency drugs, particularly chlorpromazine, thioridazine, and chlorprothixene. When using intramuscular (IM) low-potency DRAs, the clinician should measure the person's BP (lying and standing) before and after the first dose and during the first few days of treatment.

Orthostatic hypotension is mediated by adrenergic blockade and occurs most frequently during the first few days of treatment. Tolerance often develops for this side effect, which is why initial dosing of these drugs is lower than the usual therapeutic dose. Fainting or falls, although uncommon, can lead to injury. Patients should be warned of this side effect and instructed to rise slowly after sitting or reclining. Patients should avoid all caffeine and alcohol; they should drink at least 2 L of fluid a day and, if not under treatment for hypertension, should add liberal amounts of salt to their diet. Support hose may help some persons.

Hypotension can usually be managed by having patients lie down with their feet higher than their heads and pump their legs as if bicycling. Volume expansion or vasopressor agents, such as norepinephrine (Levophed), may be indicated in severe cases. Because hypotension is produced by α-adrenergic blockade, the drugs also block the α-adrenergic stimulating properties of epinephrine, leaving the β-adrenergic stimulating effects untouched. Therefore, the administration of epinephrine results in a paradoxical worsening of hypotension and is contraindicated in cases of antipsychotic-induced hypotension. Pure α-adrenergic pressor agents, such as metaraminol (Aramine) and norepinephrine, are the drugs of choice in the treatment of the disorder.

Hematological Effects

A temporary leukopenia with a WBC count of about 3,500 is a common but not serious problem. Agranulocytosis, a life-threatening hematological problem, occurs in about 1 of 10,000 persons treated with DRAs. Thrombocytopenic or nonthrombocytopenic purpura, hemolytic anemias, and pancytopenia may occur rarely in persons treated with DRAs. Although routine complete blood counts (CBCs) are not indicated, if a person reports a sore throat and fever, a CBC should be done immediately to check for the possibility. If the blood indexes are low, administration of DRAs should be stopped, and the person should be transferred to a medical facility. The mortality rate for the complication may be as high as 30 percent.

Peripheral Anticholinergic Effects

Peripheral anticholinergic effects, consisting of dry mouth and nose, blurred vision, constipation, urinary retention, and mydriasis, are common, especially with low-potency DRAs, for example, chlorpromazine, thioridazine, mesoridazine (Serentil). Some persons also have nausea and vomiting.

Constipation should be treated with the usual laxative preparations, but severe constipation can progress to paralytic ileus. A decrease in the DRA dose or a change to a less anticholinergic drug is warranted in such cases. Pilocarpine (Salagen) can be used to treat paralytic ileus, although the relief is only transitory. Bethanechol (Urecholine) (20 to 40 mg a day) may be useful in some persons with urinary retention.

Weight gain is associated with increased mortality and morbidity and with medication noncompliance. Low-potency DRAs can cause significant weight gain but not as much as is seen with the SDAs olanzapine (Zyprexa) and clozapine (Clozaril). Molindone (Moban) and, perhaps, loxapine (Loxitane) appear to be least likely to cause weight gain.

Endocrine Effects

Blockade of the dopamine receptors in the tuberoinfundibular tract results in the increased secretion of prolactin, which can result in breast enlargement, galactorrhea, amenorrhea, and inhibited orgasm in women and impotence in men. The SDAs, with the exception of risperidone, are not particularly associated with an increase in prolactin levels and may be the drugs of choice for persons experiencing disturbing side effects from increased prolactin release.

Sexual Adverse Effects

Both men and women taking DRAs can experience anorgasmia and decreased libido. As many as 50 percent of men taking antipsychotics report ejaculatory and erectile disturbances. Sildenafil (Viagra), vardenafil (Levitra), and tadalafil (Cialis) are often used to treat psychotropic-induced orgasmic dysfunction, but they have not been studied in combination with DRAs. Thioridazine is particularly associated with decreased libido and retrograde ejaculation in men. Priapism and reports of painful orgasms have also been described, both possibly resulting from α$_1$-adrenergic antagonist activity.

Skin and Eye Effects

Allergic dermatitis and photosensitivity can occur, especially with low-potency agents. Urticarial, maculopapular, petechial, and edematous eruptions can occur early in treatment, generally in the first few weeks, and remit spontaneously. A photosensitivity reaction that resembles a severe sunburn also occurs in some persons taking chlorpromazine. Persons should be warned of this adverse effect, spend no more than 30 to 60 minutes in the sun, and use sunscreens. Long-term chlorpromazine use is associated with blue-gray discoloration of skin areas exposed to sunlight. The skin changes often begin with a tan or golden brown color and progress to such colors as slate gray, metallic blue, and purple. These discolorations resolve when the patient is switched to another medication.

Irreversible retinal pigmentation is associated with use of thioridazine at doses above 1,000 mg a day. An early symptom of the side effect can sometimes be nocturnal confusion related to difficulty with night vision. The pigmentation can progress even after thioridazine administration is stopped, finally resulting in blindness. It is for this reason that the maximal recommended dose of thioridazine is 800 mg per day.

Patients taking chlorpromazine can develop a relatively benign pigmentation of the eyes, characterized by whitish brown granular deposits concentrated in the anterior lens and posterior cornea and visible only by slit-lens examination. The deposits can progress to opaque white and yellow-brown granules, often stellate. Occasionally, the conjunctiva is discolored by a brown pigment. No retinal damage is seen, and vision is almost never impaired. This condition gradually resolves when the chlorpromazine is discontinued.

Jaundice

Elevations of liver enzymes during treatment with a DRA tend to be transient and not clinically significant. When chlorpromazine first came into use, cases of obstructive or cholestatic jaundice were reported. It usually occurred in the first month of treatment and was heralded by symptoms of upper abdominal pain, nausea, and vomiting. This was followed by fever, rash, eosinophilia, bilirubin in the urine, and increases in serum bilirubin, alkaline phosphatase, and hepatic transaminases. Reported cases are now extremely rare, but if jaundice occurs, the medication should be discontinued.

Overdoses

Overdoses typically consist of exaggerated DRA side effects. Symptoms and signs include central nervous system (CNS) depression, extrapyramidal symptoms, mydriasis, rigidity, restlessness, decreased deep tendon reflexes, tachycardia, and hypotension. The severe symptoms of overdose include delirium, coma, respiratory depression, and seizures. Haloperidol may be among the safest typical antipsychotics in overdose. After an overdose, the electroencephalogram shows diffuse slowing and low voltage. Extreme overdose can lead to delirium and coma, with respiratory depression and hypotension. Life-threatening overdose usually involves ingestion of other CNS depressants, such as alcohol or benzodiazepines.

Activated charcoal, if possible, and gastric lavage should be administered if the overdose is recent. Emetics are not indicated, because the antiemetic actions of DRAs inhibit their efficacy.

Seizures can be treated with IV diazepam (Valium) or phenytoin (Dilantin). Hypotension can be treated with either norepinephrine or dopamine, but not epinephrine.

Pregnancy and Lactation

A low correlation exists between the use of antipsychotics during pregnancy and congenital malformations. Nevertheless, antipsychotics should be avoided during pregnancy, particularly in the first trimester, unless the benefit outweighs the risk. High-potency drugs, particularly fluphenazine (Prolixon), are preferable to low-potency drugs because the low-potency drugs are associated with hypotension.

The DRAs are secreted in the breast milk, although concentrations are low. Women taking these agents should be advised against breast-feeding.

DRUG INTERACTIONS

Many pharmacokinetic and pharmacodynamic drug interactions are associated with these drugs. Cytochrome P450 (CYP) 2D6 is the most common hepatic isozyme involved in DRA pharmacokinetic interactions. Other common drug interactions affect the absorption of the DRAs.

Antacids, activated charcoal, cholestyramine, kaolin, pectin, and cimetidine (Tagamet) taken within 2 hours of antipsychotic administration can reduce the absorption of these drugs. Anticholinergics can decrease the absorption of DRAs. The additive anticholinergic activity of DRAs, anticholinergics, and tricyclic drugs can result in anticholinergic toxicity. Digoxin and steroids, both of which decrease gastric motility, can increase DRA absorption.

Phenothiazines, especially thioridazine, can decrease the metabolism of, and cause toxic concentrations of, phenytoin. Barbiturates can increase the metabolism of DRAs, and these drugs may lower the person's seizure threshold.

Tricyclic drugs and selective serotonin reuptake inhibitors (SSRIs) that inhibit CYP 2D6—paroxetine, fluoxetine, and fluvoxamine—interact with DRAs, resulting in increased plasma concentrations of both drugs. The anticholinergic, sedative, and hypotensive effects of the drugs may also be additive.

Typical antipsychotics may inhibit the hypotensive effects of α-methyldopa (Aldomet). Conversely, typical antipsychotics may have an additive effect on some hypotensive drugs. Antipsychotic drugs have a variable effect on the hypotensive effects of clonidine. Propranolol coadministration increases the blood concentrations of both drugs.

The DRAs potentiate the CNS-depressant effects of sedatives, antihistamines, opiates, opioids, and alcohol, particularly in persons with impaired respiratory status. When these agents are taken with alcohol, the risk for heat stroke may be increased.

Cigarette smoking may decrease the plasma levels of typical antipsychotic drugs. Epinephrine has a paradoxical hypotensive effect in persons taking typical antipsychotics. These drugs may decrease the blood concentration of warfarin (Coumadin), resulting in decreased bleeding time. Phenothiazines, thioridazine, and pimozide should not be coadministered with other agents that prolong the QT interval. Thioridazine is contraindicated in

patients taking drugs that inhibit the CYP 2D6 isozyme or in patients with reduced levels of CYP 2D6.

LABORATORY INTERFERENCES

Chlorpromazine and perphenazine (Trilafon) may cause both false-positive and false-negative results in immunological pregnancy tests and falsely elevated bilirubin (with reagent test strips) and urobilinogen (with Ehrlich's reagent test) values. These drugs have also been associated with an abnormal shift in results of the glucose tolerance test, although that shift may reflect the effects of the drugs on the glucose-regulating system. Phenothiazines have been reported to interfere with the measurement of 17-ketosteroids and 17-hydroxycorticosteroids and produce false-positive results in tests for phenylketonuria.

DOSING AND CLINICAL GUIDELINES

Contraindications to the use of DRAs include (1) a history of a serious allergic response, (2) the possible ingestion of a substance that will interact with the antipsychotic to induce CNS depression (e.g., alcohol, opioids, barbiturates, and benzodiazepines) or anticholinergic delirium (e.g., scopolamine and possibly phencyclidine), (3) the presence of a severe cardiac abnormality, (4) a high risk for seizures, (5) the presence of narrow-angle glaucoma or prostatic hypertrophy if a drug with high anticholinergic activity is to be used, and (6) the presence or a history of tardive dyskinesia. Antipsychotics should be administered with caution in persons with hepatic disease because impaired hepatic metabolism can result in high plasma concentrations. The usual assessment should include a CBC with WBC indexes, liver function tests, and an electrocardiogram, especially in women older than 40 years of age and men older than 30 years of age. The elderly and children are more sensitive to side effects than are young adults, so the dose of the drug should be adjusted accordingly.

Various patients may respond to widely different doses of antipsychotics; therefore, no set dose exists for any given antipsychotic drug. Because tolerance develops to many side effects, it is reasonable clinical practice to begin at a low dose and increase it as necessary. It is important to remember that the maximal effects of a particular dose may not be evident for 4 to 6 weeks. Available preparations and doses of DRAs are given in Table 32.18–1.

Short-Term Treatment

The equivalent of 5 to 20 mg of haloperidol is a reasonable dose for an adult person in an acute state. A geriatric person may benefit from as little as 1 mg of haloperidol. The administration of more than 25 mg of chlorpromazine in one injection can result in serious hypotension. Administration of the antipsychotic IM results in peak plasma levels in about 30 minutes versus 90 minutes using the oral route. Doses of drugs for IM administration are about half those given by the oral route. In a short-term treatment setting, the person should be observed for 1 hour after the first dose of medication. After that time, most clinicians administer a second dose or a sedative agent (e.g., a benzodiazepine) to achieve effective behavioral control. Possible sedatives include lorazepam (Ativan) (2 mg IM) and amobarbital (Amytal) (50 to 250 mg IM).

Table 32.18–1
Dopamine Receptor Antagonists

Generic or Chemical	Trade	Tablets (mg)	Capsules (mg)	Solution	Parenteral	Rectal Suppositories (mg)	Adult Dose Range (mg/day) Acute	Maintenance
Chlorpromazine	Thorazine	10, 25, 50, 100, 200	30, 75, 150, 200, 300	10 mg/5 mL, 30 mg/mL, 100 mg/mL	25 mg/mL	25, 100	100 to 1,600 p.o. 25 to 400 IM	50 to 400 p.o.
Prochlorperazine	Compazine	5, 10, 25	10, 15, 30	5 mg/5 mL	5 mg/mL	2.5, 5, 25	15 to 200 p.o. 40 to 80 IM	15 to 60 p.o.
Perphenazine	Trilafon	2, 4, 8, 16	—	16 mg/5 mL	5 mg/mL	—	12 to 64 p.o. 15 to 30 IM	8 to 24 p.o.
Trifluoperazine	Stelazine	1, 2, 5, 10	—	10 mg/mL	2 mg/mL	—	4 to 40 p.o. 4 to 10 IM	5 to 20 p.o.
Fluphenazine	Prolixin	1, 2.5, 5, 10	—	2.5 mg/5 mL, 5 mg/mL	2.5 mg/mL (IM only)	—	2.5 to 40.0 p.o. 5 to 20 IM	1.0 to 15.0 p.o. 12.5 to 50.0 IM (decanoate or enanthate, weekly or biweekly)
Fluphenazine decanoate	—	—	—	—	2.5 mg/mL	—		
Fluphenazine enanthate	—	—	—	2.5 mg/mL	—	—		
Thioridazine	Mellaril	10, 15, 25, 50, 100, 150, 200	—	25 mg/5 mL, 100 mg/5 mL, 30 mg/mL, 100 mg/mL	—	—	200 to 800 p.o.	100 to 300 p.o.
Mesoridazine	Serentil	10, 25, 50, 100	—	25 mg/mL	25 mg/mL	—	100 to 400 p.o. 25 to 200 IM	30 to 150 p.o.
Haloperidol	Haldol	0.5, 1, 2, 5, 10, 20	—	2 mg/5 mL	5 mg/mL (IM only)	—	5 to 20 p.o.	1 to 10 p.o.
Haloperidol decanoate	—	—	—	—	50 mg/mL, 100 mg/mL (IM only)	—	12.5 to 25 IM	25 to 200 IM (decanoate, monthly)
Chlorprothixene	Taractan	10, 25, 50, 100	—	100 mg/5 mL (suspension)	12.5 mg/mL	—	75 to 600 p.o. 75 to 200 IM	50 to 400
Thiothixene	Navane	—	1, 2, 5, 10, 20	5 mg/mL	5 mg/mL (IM only), 20 mg/mL (IM only)	—	6 to 100 p.o. 8 to 30 IM	6 to 30
Loxapine	Loxitane	—	5, 10, 25, 50	25 mg/5 mL	50 mg/mL	—	20 to 250, 20 to 75 IM	20 to 100
Molindone	Moban	5, 10, 25, 50, 100	—	20 mg/mL	—	—	50 to 225	5 to 150
Pimozide	Orap	2	—	—	—	—	0.5 to 20	0.5 to 5.0

p.o., oral; IM, intramuscular.

Rapid Neuroleptization

Rapid neuroleptization (also called *psychotolysis*) is the practice of administering hourly IM doses of antipsychotic medications until marked sedation of the person is achieved. Several research studies have shown, however, that merely waiting several more hours after one dose yields the same clinical improvement as is seen with repeated doses. Nevertheless, clinicians must be careful to keep persons from becoming violent while they are psychotic. Clinicians can help prevent violent episodes by using adjuvant sedatives or by temporarily using physical restraints until such persons can control their behavior.

Early Treatment

A full 6 weeks may be necessary to evaluate the extent of the improvement in psychotic symptoms. Agitation and excitement usually improve quickly with antipsychotic treatment, however. About 75 percent of persons with a short history of illness show significant improvement in their psychosis. Psychotic symptoms, both positive and negative, usually continue to improve 3 to 12 months after the initiation of treatment.

About 5 mg of haloperidol or 300 mg of chlorpromazine is the usual effective daily dose. In the past, much higher doses were used, but evidence suggests that this resulted in more side effects without additional benefits. A single daily dose is usually given at bedtime to help induce sleep and to reduce the incidence of adverse effects. Bedtime dosing for elderly persons may increase their risk of falling, however, if they get out of bed during the night. The sedative effects of typical antipsychotics last only a few hours, in contrast to the antipsychotic effects, which last for 1 to 3 days.

Intermittent Medications

It is common clinical practice to order medications to be given intermittently as needed (p.r.n.). Although this practice may be reasonable during the first few days that a person is hospitalized, the amount of time the person takes antipsychotic drugs, rather than an increase in dose, is what produces therapeutic improvement. Clinicians on in-patient services may feel pressured by staff members to write p.r.n. antipsychotic orders; such orders should include specific symptoms, how often the drugs should be given, and how many doses can be given each day. Clinicians may choose to use small doses for the p.r.n. doses (e.g., 2 mg of haloperidol) or use a benzodiazepine instead (e.g., 2 mg of lorazepam IM). If p.r.n. doses of an antipsychotic are necessary after the first week of treatment, the clinician may want to consider increasing the standing daily dose of the drug.

Maintenance Treatment

The first 3 to 6 months after a psychotic episode is usually considered a period of stabilization. After that time, the dose of the antipsychotic can be decreased about 20 percent every 6 months until the minimal effective dose is found. A person is usually maintained on antipsychotic medications for 1 to 2 years after the first psychotic episode. Antipsychotic treatment is often continued for 5 years after a second psychotic episode, and lifetime maintenance is considered after the third psychotic episode, although attempts to reduce the daily dose can be made every 6 to 12 months.

Antipsychotic drugs are effective in controlling psychotic symptoms, but persons may report that they prefer being off the drugs because they feel better without them. This problem is less common with the newer antipsychotic SDAs. The clinician must discuss maintenance medication with patients and take into account their wishes, the severity of their illnesses, and the quality of their support systems. It is essential for the clinician to know enough about the patient's life to try to predict upcoming stressors that might require increasing the dose or closely monitoring compliance.

Long-Acting Depot Medications

Long-acting depot preparations may be needed to overcome problems with compliance. IM preparations are typically given once every 1 to 4 weeks.

Two depot preparations, a decanoate and an enanthate, of fluphenazine and a decanoate preparation of haloperidol are available in the United States. The preparations are injected IM into an area of large muscle tissue, from which they are absorbed slowly into the blood. Decanoate preparations can be given less frequently than enanthate preparations because they are absorbed more slowly. Although stabilizing a person on the oral preparation of the specific drugs is not necessary before initiating the depot form, it is good practice to give at least one oral dose of the drug to assess the possibility of an adverse effect, such as severe extrapyramidal symptoms or an allergic reaction.

It is reasonable to begin with either 12.5 mg (0.5 mL) of fluphenazine preparation or 25 mg (0.5 mL) of haloperidol decanoate. If symptoms emerge in the next 2 to 4 weeks, the person can be treated temporarily with additional oral medications or with additional small depot injections. After 3 to 4 weeks, the depot injection can be increased to a single dose equal to the total of the doses given during the initial period.

A good reason to initiate depot treatment with low doses is that the absorption of the preparations may be faster than usual at the onset of treatment, resulting in frightening episodes of dystonia that eventually discourage compliance with the medication. Some clinicians keep persons drug free for 3 to 7 days before initiating depot treatment and give small doses of the depot preparations (3.125 mg of fluphenazine or 6.25 mg of haloperidol) every few days to avoid those initial problems.

Plasma Concentrations

Genetic differences among persons and pharmacokinetic interactions with other drugs influence the metabolism of the antipsychotics. If a person has not improved after 4 to 6 weeks of treatment, the plasma concentration of the drug should be determined, if feasible. After a patient has been on a particular dose for at least five times the half-life of the drug and, thus, approaches steady-state concentrations, blood levels may be helpful. It is standard practice to obtain plasma samples at trough levels—just before the daily dose is given, usually at least 12 hours after the previous dose and most commonly 20 to 24 hours after the previous dose. In fact, most antipsychotics have no well-defined dose-response curve. The best-studied drug is haloperidol, which may have a therapeutic window ranging from 2 to 15 ng/mL. Other therapeutic ranges that have been reasonably well documented are

30 to 100 ng/mL for chlorpromazine and 0.8 to 2.4 ng/mL for perphenazine.

Treatment-Resistant Persons

Approximately 10 to 35 percent of persons with schizophrenia do not obtain significant benefit from the antipsychotic drugs. Treatment resistance is failure on at least two adequate trials of antipsychotics from two pharmacological classes. It is useful to determine plasma concentrations for such persons because they may be slow or rapid metabolizers or may not be taking their medication. Clozapine has been conclusively shown to be effective when given to patients who have failed multiple trials of DRAs.

Adjunctive Medications

It is common practice to use DRAs in conjunction with other psychotropic agents, either to treat side effects or further improve symptoms. Most commonly, this involves the use of lithium or other mood-stabilizing agents, SSRIs, or benzodiazepines. It was once held that antidepressant drugs exacerbated psychosis in patients with schizophrenia. In all likelihood, this observation involved patients with bipolar disorder who were misdiagnosed as being schizophrenic. Abundant evidence suggests that antidepressants, in fact, lessen symptoms of depression in patients with schizophrenia. In some cases, amphetamines can be added to DRAs if patients remain withdrawn and apathetic.

Choice of Drug

Given their proved efficacy in managing acute psychotic symptoms and that prophylactic administration of anti-Parkinsonian medication prevents or minimizes acute motor abnormalities, DRAs are still valuable—especially for short-term therapy. Considerable cost advantage exists to a DRA anti-Parkinsonian regimen as compared with monotherapy with a newer antipsychotic agent. Concern about the development of DRA-induced tardive dyskinesia is the major deterrent to long-term use of these drugs, yet it is not clear that SDAs are completely risk free of this complication. Side effects, such as extreme weight gain, are more common with SDAs than with DRAs, which can contribute to the risk of diabetes mellitus. Thus, DRAs still occupy an important role in psychiatric treatment. DRAs are not predictably interchangeable. For reasons that cannot be explained, some patients do better on one drug than another. Choice of a particular DRA should be based on the known adverse-effect profile of the drugs. Other than a significant advantage in terms of medication cost, the choice is an SDA. If a DRA is felt to be preferable, a high-potency antipsychotic is favored, even though it may be associated with more neurological adverse effects, mainly because a higher incidence exists of other adverse effects (e.g., cardiac, hypotensive, epileptogenic, sexual, and allergic) with the low-potency drugs. If sedation is a desired goal, either a low-potency antipsychotic can be given in divided doses or a benzodiazepine can be coadministered.

An unpleasant or dysphoric reaction (a subjective sense of restlessness, oversedation, and acute dystonia) to the first dose of an antipsychotic predicts future poor response and noncompliance. Prophylactic use of anti-Parkinsonian medications may prevent this reaction.

▲ 32.19 Lamotrigine

Lamotrigine (Lamictal) was originally developed as an antiepileptic drug used as adjunctive therapy for general and partial seizures in adults and pediatric patients. It was approved by the U.S. Food and Drug Administration for maintenance treatment of bipolar I disorder in 2003. In clinical trials, it was shown to keep patients euthymic longer and was particularly effective in preventing depressive episodes. As a maintenance treatment, lamotrigine can be used in situations in which lithium has traditionally been prescribed.

Although comparatively new as compared with lithium, the gold standard of bipolar maintenance therapy, lamotrigine has very real advantages compared with that agent in terms of tolerability, safety, and convenience. For example, lamotrigine treatment is associated with no significant metabolic or neurological effects, and it does not require laboratory testing of plasma concentrations. In contrast to lithium, however, lamotrigine does not have any acute antimanic effects.

Lamotrigine is a novel three-ringed (phenyltriazine) compound. It has antiglutamatergic and sodium channel blocking effects, as well as other properties.

PHARMACOLOGICAL ACTIONS

Lamotrigine is completely absorbed, has a bioavailability of 98 percent, and has a steady-state plasma half-life of 25 hours. The rate of lamotrigine's metabolism varies, however, over a six-fold range, depending on which other drugs are administered concomitantly. Dosing is escalated slowly to twice-a-day maintenance dosing. Food does not affect its absorption, and it is 55 percent protein bound in the plasma; 94 percent of lamotrigine and its inactive metabolites are excreted in the urine. Among the better-delineated biochemical actions of lamotrigine are blockade of voltage-sensitive sodium channels, which in turn modulate release of glutamate and aspartate, and a slight effect on calcium channels. Lamotrigine modestly increases plasma serotonin concentrations, possibly through inhibition of serotonin reuptake, and is a weak inhibitor of serotonin 5-HT$_3$ receptors.

THERAPEUTIC INDICATIONS

Bipolar Disorder

Lamotrigine is indicated in the maintenance treatment of bipolar disorder and may prolong the time between episodes of depression and mania. It is more effective in lengthening the intervals between depressive episodes than manic episodes. It is also effective as treatment for rapid-cycling bipolar disorder.

Other Indications

Therapeutic benefit has been reported in the treatment of borderline personality disorder and in the treatment for various pain syndromes.

PRECAUTIONS AND ADVERSE REACTIONS

Lamotrigine is remarkably well tolerated. The absence of sedation, weight gain, or other metabolic effects is noteworthy. The most common adverse effects—dizziness, ataxia, somnolence, headache, diplopia, blurred vision, and nausea—are typically mild. Cognitive impairment and joint or back pain may occur.

The appearance of a rash, which is common and occasionally very severe, is a source of concern. About 8 percent of patients started on lamotrigine develop a benign maculopapular rash during the first 4 months of treatment, and the drug should be discontinued if a rash develops. Although these rashes are benign, concern is that in some cases, they may represent early manifestations of Stevens-Johnson syndrome or toxic epidermal necrolysis. Nevertheless, even if lamotrigine is discontinued immediately on development of rash or other signs of hypersensitivity reaction, such as fever and lymphadenopathy, this may not prevent subsequent development of a life-threatening rash or permanent disfiguration.

Estimates of the rate of serious rash vary, depending on the source of the data. In some studies, the incidence of serious rashes was 0.08 percent in adult patients receiving lamotrigine as initial monotherapy and 0.13 percent in adult patients receiving lamotrigine as adjunctive therapy. German registry data, based on clinical practice, suggest that the risk of rash may be as low as 1 in 5,000 patients. The appearance of any type of rash necessitates immediate discontinuation of drug administration.

It is known that the likelihood of a rash increases if the recommended starting dose and speed of dose increase exceed what is recommended. Concomitant administration of valproic acid also increases risk and should be avoided if possible. If valproate is used, a more conservative dosing regimen is followed. Children and adolescents younger than 16 years of age appear to be more susceptible to rash with lamotrigine. If patients miss more than four consecutive days of lamotrigine treatment, they need to restart therapy at the initial starting dose and titrate upward as if they had not already been on the medication.

Pregnancy registry data suggest a possible association between lamotrigine and an increased risk of nonsyndromic oral clefts in infants exposed to lamotrigine during the first trimester of pregnancy.

LABORATORY TESTING

No proven correlation exists between lamotrigine blood concentrations and either antiseizure effects or efficacy in bipolar disorders. Laboratory tests are not useful in predicting the occurrence of adverse events.

DRUG INTERACTIONS

Lamotrigine has significant, well-characterized drug interactions involving other anticonvulsants. The most potentially serious lamotrigine drug interaction involves concurrent use of valproic acid, which doubles serum lamotrigine concentrations conversely. Lamotrigine decreases the plasma concentration of valproic acid by 25 percent. Sertraline (Zoloft) also increases plasma lamotrigine concentrations but to a lesser extent than does valproic acid. Lamotrigine concentrations are decreased by 40 to 50 percent with concomitant administration of carbamazepine, phenytoin, or phenobarbital. Combinations of lamotrigine and other anticonvulsants have complex effects on the time of peak plasma concentration and the plasma half-life of lamotrigine.

LABORATORY INTERFERENCES

Lamotrigine and topiramate do not interfere with any laboratory tests.

DOSING AND ADMINISTRATION

In the clinical trials leading to the approval of lamotrigine as a treatment for bipolar disorder, no consistent increase in efficacy was associated with doses greater than 200 mg per day. Most patients should take between 100 and 200 mg a day. In epilepsy, the drug is administered twice daily; in bipolar disorder, however, the total dose can be taken once a day, either in the morning or at night, depending on whether the patient finds the drug activating or sedating.

Lamotrigine is available as unscored 25-, 100-, 150-, and 200-mg tablets. The major determinant of lamotrigine dosing is minimization of the risk of rash. Lamotrigine should not be taken by anyone younger than the age of 16 years. Because valproic acid markedly slows the elimination of lamotrigine, concomitant administration of these two drugs necessitates a much slower titration. People with renal insufficiency should aim for a lower maintenance dose. Appearance of any type of rash necessitates immediate discontinuation of lamotrigine administration. Lamotrigine should usually be discontinued gradually over 2 weeks unless a rash emerges, in which case it should be discontinued over 1 to 2 days.

Chewable dispersible tablets of 2, 5, and 25 mg are also available.

▲ 32.20 Lithium

Lithium (Eskalith, Lithobid, Lithonate) was approved by the U.S. Food and Drug Administration for the treatment of mania in 1970, more than 20 years after the first favorable reports by John F. J. Cade, an Australian psychiatrist. It is used for short-term, long-term, and prophylactic treatment of bipolar I disorder. Until recently, it was the only drug approved for both acute and maintenance treatment. It is also used as an adjunctive medication in the treatment of major depressive disorder.

Lithium (Li), a monovalent ion, is a member of the group IA alkaline metals on the periodic table, a group that also includes sodium, potassium, rubidium, cesium, and francium. Lithium exists in nature as both ^{6}Li (7.42 percent) and ^{7}Li (92.58 percent). The latter isotope allows the imaging of lithium by magnetic resonance spectroscopy. Some 300 mg of lithium is contained in 1,597 mg of lithium carbonate. Most lithium used in the United States is obtained from dry lake mining in Chile and Argentina.

PHARMACOLOGICAL ACTIONS

Lithium is rapidly and completely absorbed after oral administration, with peak serum concentrations occurring in 1 to 1.5 hours with standard preparations and in 4 to 4.5 hours with slow- and controlled-released preparations. Lithium does not bind to plasma proteins, is not metabolized, and is excreted through the kidneys. The plasma half-life is initially 1.3 days and is 2.4 days after administration for more than 1 year. The blood–brain barrier permits only slow passage of lithium, which is why a single overdose does not necessarily cause toxicity and why long-term lithium intoxication is slow to resolve. The elimination half-life of lithium is 18 to 24 hours in young adults but is shorter in children and longer in the elderly. Renal clearance of lithium is decreased with renal insufficiency. Equilibrium is reached after 5 to 7 days of regular intake. Obesity is associated with higher rates of lithium clearance. The excretion of lithium is complex during pregnancy; excretion increases during pregnancy but decreases after delivery. Lithium is excreted in breast milk and in insignificant amounts in the feces and sweat. Thyroid and renal concentrations of lithium are higher than serum levels.

An explanation for the mood-stabilizing effects of lithium remains elusive. Theories include alterations of ion transport and effects on neurotransmitters and neuropeptides, signal transduction pathways, and second messenger systems.

THERAPEUTIC INDICATIONS

Bipolar I Disorder

Manic Episodes. Lithium controls acute mania and prevents relapse in about 80 percent of persons with bipolar I disorder and in a somewhat smaller percentage of persons with mixed (mania and depression) episodes, rapid-cycling bipolar disorder, or mood changes in encephalopathy. Lithium has a relatively slow onset of action and exerts its antimanic effects over 1 to 3 weeks. Thus, a benzodiazepine, dopamine receptor antagonist (DRA), serotonin–dopamine antagonist (SDAs), or valproic acid is usually administered for the first few weeks. Patients with mixed or dysphoric mania, rapid cycling, comorbid substance abuse, or organicity respond less well to lithium than do those with classic mania.

Bipolar Depression. Lithium has been shown to be effective in the treatment of depression associated with bipolar I disorder, as well as in add-on therapy for patients with severe major depressive disorder. Augmentation of lithium therapy with valproate (Depakene) or carbamazepine (Tegretol) is usually well tolerated, with little risk of mania precipitation.

When a depressive episode occurs in a person taking maintenance lithium, the differential diagnosis should include lithium-induced hypothyroidism, substance abuse, and lack of compliance with the lithium therapy. Possible treatment approaches include increasing the lithium concentration (up to 1 to 1.2 mEq/L), adding supplemental thyroid hormone (e.g., 25 μg a day of liothyronine [Cytomel]) even in the presence of normal findings on thyroid function tests, augmentation with valproate or carbamazepine, the judicious use of antidepressants, or electroconvulsive therapy (ECT). Once the acute depressive episode resolves, other therapies should be tapered off in favor of lithium monotherapy, if clinically tolerated.

Maintenance. Maintenance treatment with lithium markedly decreases the frequency, the severity, and the duration of manic and depressive episodes in persons with bipolar I disorder. Lithium provides relatively more effective prophylaxis for mania than for depression, and supplemental antidepressant strategies may be necessary, either intermittently or continuously. Lithium maintenance is almost always indicated after the second episode of bipolar I disorder depression or mania and should be considered after the first episode for adolescents or for persons who have a family history of bipolar I disorder. Others who benefit from lithium maintenance are those who have poor support systems, had no precipitating factors for the first episode, have a high suicide risk, had a sudden onset of the first episode, or had a first episode of mania. Clinical studies have shown that lithium reduces the incidence of suicide in patients with bipolar I disorder sixfold or sevenfold. Lithium is also effective treatment for persons with severe cyclothymic disorder.

Initiating maintenance therapy after the first manic episode is considered a wise approach based on several observations. First, each episode of mania increases the risk of subsequent episodes. Second, among people responsive to lithium, relapses are 28 times more likely after lithium use is discontinued. Third, case reports describe persons who initially responded to lithium, discontinued taking it, and then had a relapse but no longer responded to lithium in subsequent episodes. Continued maintenance treatment with lithium is often associated with increasing efficacy and reduced mortality. An episode of depression or mania that occurs after a relatively short time of lithium maintenance, therefore, does not necessarily represent treatment failure. Lithium treatment alone may begin to lose its effectiveness, however, after several years of successful use. If this occurs, then supplemental treatment with carbamazepine or valproate may be useful.

Maintenance lithium doses often can be adjusted to achieve plasma concentration somewhat lower than that needed for treatment of acute mania. If lithium use is to be discontinued, then the dose should be slowly tapered. Abrupt discontinuation of lithium therapy is associated with increased risk of recurrence of manic and depressive episodes.

Major Depressive Disorder

Lithium is effective in the long-term treatment of major depression but is not more effective than antidepressant drugs. The most common role for lithium in major depressive disorder is as an adjuvant to antidepressant use in persons who have failed to respond to the antidepressants alone. About 50 to 60 percent of antidepressant nonresponders do respond when lithium, 300 mg three times daily, is added to the antidepressant regimen. In some cases, a response may be seen within days, but most often, several weeks are required to see the efficacy of the regimen. Lithium alone may effectively treat depressed persons who have bipolar I disorder but have not yet had their first manic episode. Lithium has been reported to be effective in persons with major depressive disorder whose disorder has a particularly marked cyclicity.

Schizoaffective Disorder and Schizophrenia

Persons with prominent mood symptoms—either bipolar type or depressive type—with schizoaffective disorder are more likely to respond to lithium than are those with predominant psychotic symptoms. Whereas SDAs and DRAs are the treatments of choice for persons with schizoaffective disorder, lithium is a useful augmentation agent. This is particularly true for persons whose symptoms are resistant to treatment with SDAs and DRAs. Lithium augmentation of an SDA or DRA treatment may be effective for persons with schizoaffective disorder even in the absence of a prominent mood disorder component. Some persons with schizophrenia who cannot take antipsychotic drugs may benefit from lithium treatment alone.

Other Indications

Over the years, reports have appeared about the use of lithium to treat a wide range of other psychiatric and nonpsychiatric conditions. The effectiveness and safety of lithium for most of these disorders has not been confirmed. Lithium has antiaggressive activity that is separate from its effects on mood. Aggressive outbursts in persons with schizophrenia, violent prison inmates, and children with conduct disorder and aggression or self-mutilation in persons with mental retardation can sometimes be controlled with lithium.

PRECAUTIONS AND ADVERSE EFFECTS

More than 80 percent of patients taking lithium experience side effects. It is important to minimize the risk of adverse events through monitoring of lithium blood levels and to use appropriate pharmacological interventions to counteract unwanted effects when they occur. Patient education can play an important role in reducing the incidence and severity of side effects. Patients taking lithium should be advised that changes in the body's water and salt content can affect the amount of lithium excreted, resulting in either increases or decreases in lithium concentrations. Excessive sodium intake (e.g., a dramatic dietary change) lowers lithium concentrations. Conversely, too little sodium (e.g., fad diets) can lead to potentially toxic concentrations of lithium. Decreases in body fluid (e.g., excessive perspiration) can lead to dehydration and lithium intoxication. Patients should report whenever medications are prescribed by another clinician because many commonly used agents can affect lithium concentrations.

Gastrointestinal Effects

Gastrointestinal (GI) symptoms—which include nausea, decreased appetite, vomiting, and diarrhea—can be diminished by dividing the dose, administering the lithium with food, or switching to another lithium preparation. The lithium preparation least likely to cause diarrhea is lithium citrate. Some lithium preparations contain lactose, which can cause diarrhea in lactose-intolerant persons. Persons taking slow-release formulations of lithium who experience diarrhea because of unabsorbed medication in the lower part of the GI tract may experience less diarrhea than with standard-release preparations. Diarrhea may also respond to antidiarrheal preparations such as loperamide (Imodium, Kaopectate), bismuth subsalicylate (Pepto-Bismol), and diphenoxylate with atropine (Lomotil).

Weight Gain

Weight gain results from a poorly understood effect of lithium on carbohydrate metabolism. Weight gain can also result from lithium-induced hypothyroidism, lithium-induced edema, or excessive consumption of soft drinks and juices to quench lithium-induced thirst.

Neurological Effects

Tremor.   A lithium-induced postural tremor can occur that is usually 8 to 12 Hz and is most notable in outstretched hands, especially in the fingers, and during tasks involving fine manipulations. The tremor can be reduced by dividing the daily dose, using a sustained-release formulation, reducing caffeine intake, reassessing the concomitant use of other medicines, and treating comorbid anxiety. β-Adrenergic receptor antagonists, such as propranolol, 30 to 120 mg a day in divided doses, and primidone (Mysoline), 50 to 250 mg a day, are usually effective in reducing the tremor. In persons with hypokalemia, potassium supplementation may improve the tremor. When a person taking lithium has a severe tremor, the possibility of lithium toxicity should be suspected and evaluated.

Cognitive Effects.   Lithium use has been associated with dysphoria, lack of spontaneity, slowed reaction times, and impaired memory. The presence of these symptoms should be noted carefully because they are a frequent cause of noncompliance. The differential diagnosis for such symptoms should include depressive disorders, hypothyroidism, hypercalcemia, other illnesses, and other drugs. Some, but not all, persons have reported that fatigue and mild cognitive impairment decrease with time.

Other Neurological Effects.   Uncommon neurological adverse effects include symptoms of mild Parkinsonism, ataxia, and dysarthria, although the latter two symptoms may also be caused by lithium intoxication. Lithium is rarely associated with development of peripheral neuropathy, benign intracranial hypertension (pseudotumor cerebri), findings resembling myasthenia gravis, and increased risk of seizures.

Renal Effects

The most common adverse renal effect of lithium is polyuria with secondary polydipsia. The symptom is particularly a problem in 25 to 35 percent of persons taking lithium who may have a urine output of more than 3 L a day (normal, 1 to 2 L a day). The polyuria primarily results from lithium antagonism to the effects of antidiuretic hormone, which thus causes diuresis. When polyuria is a significant problem, the person's renal function should be evaluated and followed up with 24-hour urine collections for creatinine clearance determinations. Treatment consists in fluid replacement, the use of the lowest effective dose of lithium, and single daily dosing of lithium. Treatment can also involve the use of a thiazide or potassium-sparing diuretic—for example, amiloride (Midamor), spironolactone (Aldactone), triamterene (Dyrenium), or amiloride-hydrochlorothiazide (Moduretic). If treatment with a diuretic is initiated, the lithium dose should be halved, and the diuretic should not be started for 5 days because the diuretic is likely to increase lithium retention.

The most serious renal adverse effects, which are rare and associated with continuous lithium administration for 10 years or more, involve appearance of nonspecific interstitial fibrosis, associated with gradual decreases in glomerular filtration rate and increases in serum creatinine concentrations, and rarely with renal failure. Lithium occasionally is associated with nephrotic syndrome and features of distal renal tubular acidosis. It is prudent for persons taking lithium to check their serum creatinine concentration, urine chemistries, and 24-hour urine volume at 6-month intervals.

Thyroid Effects

Lithium causes a generally benign and often transient diminution in the concentrations of circulating thyroid hormones. Reports have attributed goiter (5 percent of persons), benign reversible exophthalmos, hyperthyroidism, and hypothyroidism (7 to 10 percent of persons) to lithium treatment. Lithium-induced hypothyroidism is more common in women (14 percent) than in men (4.5 percent). Women are at highest risk during the first 2 years of treatment. Persons taking lithium to treat bipolar disorder are twice as likely to develop hypothyroidism if they develop rapid cycling. About 50 percent of persons receiving long-term lithium treatment have laboratory abnormalities, such as an abnormal thyrotropin-releasing hormone response, and about 30 percent have elevated concentrations of thyroid-stimulating hormone (TSH). If symptoms of hypothyroidism are present, replacement with levothyroxine (Synthroid) is indicated. Even in the absence of hypothyroid symptoms, some clinicians treat persons with significantly elevated TSH concentrations with levothyroxine. In lithium-treated persons, TSH concentrations should be measured every 6 to 12 months. Lithium-induced hypothyroidism should be considered when evaluating depressive episodes that emerge during lithium therapy.

Cardiac Effects

The cardiac effects of lithium resemble those of hypokalemia on the electrocardiogram (ECG). They are caused by the displacement of intracellular potassium by the lithium ion. The most common changes on the ECG are T-wave flattening or inversion. The changes are benign and disappear after the lithium is excreted from the body.

Lithium depresses the pacemaking activity of the sinus node, sometimes resulting in sinus dysrhythmias, heart block, and episodes of syncope. Lithium treatment, therefore, is contraindicated in persons with sick sinus syndrome. In rare cases, ventricular arrhythmias and congestive heart failure have been associated with lithium therapy. Lithium cardiotoxicity is more prevalent in persons on a low-salt diet, those taking certain diuretics or angiotensin-converting enzyme (ACE) inhibitors, and those with fluid-electrolyte imbalances or any renal insufficiency.

Dermatological Effects

Dermatological effects may be dose dependent. They include acneiform, follicular and maculopapular eruptions; pretibial ulcerations; and worsening of psoriasis. Occasionally, aggravated psoriasis or acneiform eruptions may force the discontinuation of lithium treatment. Alopecia has also been reported. Many of those conditions respond favorably to changing to another lithium preparation and the usual dermatological measures. Lithium concentrations should be monitored if tetracycline is used for the treatment of acne because it can increase lithium retention.

Lithium Toxicity and Overdoses

The early signs and symptoms of lithium toxicity include neurological symptoms, such as coarse tremor, dysarthria, and ataxia; GI symptoms; cardiovascular changes; and renal dysfunction.

The later signs and symptoms include impaired consciousness, muscular fasciculations, myoclonus, seizures, and coma. Risk factors include exceeding the recommended dose, renal impairment, low-sodium diet, drug interaction, and dehydration. Elderly persons are more vulnerable to the effects of increased serum lithium concentrations. The greater the degree and duration of elevated lithium concentrations, the worse are the symptoms of lithium toxicity.

Lithium toxicity is a medical emergency, potentially causing permanent neuronal damage and death. In cases of toxicity, lithium should be stopped and dehydration treated. Unabsorbed lithium can be removed from the GI tract by ingestion of polystyrene sulfonate (Kayexalate) or polyethylene glycol solution (GoLYTELY) but not activated charcoal. Ingestion of a single large dose may create clumps of medication in the stomach, which can be removed by gastric lavage with a widebore tube. The value of forced diuresis is debated. In severe cases, hemodialysis rapidly removes excessive amounts of serum lithium. Postdialysis serum lithium concentrations may rise as lithium is redistributed from tissues to blood, so repeat dialysis may be needed. Neurological improvement may lag behind clearance of serum lithium by several days because lithium crosses the blood–brain barrier slowly.

Adolescents

The serum lithium concentrations for adolescents are similar to those for adults. Weight gain and acne associated with lithium use can be particularly troublesome to an adolescent.

Elderly Persons

Lithium is a safe and effective drug for the elderly. Treatment of elderly persons taking lithium may be complicated, however, by the presence of other medical illnesses, decreased renal function, special diets that affect lithium clearance, and generally increased sensitivity to lithium. Elderly persons should initially be given low doses, their doses should be switched less frequently than those of younger persons, and a longer time must be allowed for renal excretion to equilibrate with absorption before lithium can be assumed to have reached its steady-state concentrations.

Pregnant Women

Lithium should not be administered to pregnant women in the first trimester because of the risk of birth defects. The most common malformations involve the cardiovascular system, most commonly Ebstein's anomaly of the tricuspid valves. The risk of Ebstein's malformation in lithium-exposed fetuses is 1 of 1,000, which is 20 times the risk in the general population. The possibility of fetal cardiac anomalies can be evaluated with fetal echocardiography. The teratogenic risk of lithium (4 to 12 percent) is higher than that for the general population (2 to 3 percent) but appears to be lower than that associated with use of valproate or carbamazepine. A woman who continues to take lithium during pregnancy should use the lowest effective dose. The maternal lithium concentration must be monitored closely during pregnancy and especially after pregnancy because of the significant decrease in renal lithium excretion as renal function returns to normal in the first few days after delivery. Adequate hydration can reduce the risk of lithium toxicity during labor. Lithium prophylaxis is recommended for all women with bipolar disorder as they enter the postpartum period. Lithium is excreted into breast milk and should be taken by a nursing mother only after careful evaluation of potential risks and benefits. Signs of lithium toxicity in infants include lethargy, cyanosis, abnormal reflexes, and sometimes hepatomegaly.

Miscellaneous Effects

Lithium should be used with caution in diabetic persons, who should monitor their blood glucose concentrations carefully to avoid diabetic ketoacidosis. Benign, reversible leukocytosis is commonly associated with lithium treatment. Dehydrated, debilitated, and medically ill persons are most susceptible to adverse effects and toxicity.

DRUG INTERACTIONS

Lithium is commonly used in conjunction with DRAs. This combination is typically effective and safe. Coadministration of higher doses of a DRA and lithium, however, may result in a synergistic increase in the symptoms of lithium-induced neurological side effects and neuroleptic extrapyramidal symptoms. In rare instances, encephalopathy has been reported with this combination.

The coadministration of lithium and carbamazepine, lamotrigine, valproate, and clonazepam may increase lithium concentrations and aggravate lithium-induced neurological adverse effects. Treatment with the combination should be initiated at slightly lower doses than usual, and the doses should be increased gradually. Changes from one to another treatment for mania should be made carefully, with as little temporal overlap between the drugs as possible.

Most diuretics (e.g., thiazide and potassium sparing) can increase lithium concentrations; when treatment with such a diuretic is stopped, the clinician may need to increase the person's daily lithium dose. Osmotic and loop diuretics, carbonic anhydrase inhibitors, and xanthines (including caffeine) can reduce lithium concentrations to below therapeutic concentrations. ACE inhibitors can cause an increase in lithium concentrations, whereas the AT_1 angiotensin II receptor inhibitors losartan (Cozaar) and irbesartan (Avapro) do not alter lithium concentrations. A wide range of nonsteroidal antiinflammatory drugs (NSAIDs) can decrease lithium clearance, thereby increasing lithium concentrations. These drugs include indomethacin (Indocin), phenylbutazone (Azolid), diclofenac (Voltaren), ketoprofen (Orudis), oxyphenbutazone (Oxalid), ibuprofen (Motrin, Advil), piroxicam (Feldene), and naproxen (Naprosyn). Aspirin and sulindac (Clinoril) do not affect lithium concentrations.

The coadministration of lithium and quetiapine (Seroquel) can cause somnolence but is otherwise well tolerated. The coadministration of lithium and ziprasidone (Geodon) may modestly increase the incidence of tremor. The coadministration of lithium and calcium channel inhibitors should be avoided because of potentially fatal neurotoxicity.

A person taking lithium who is about to undergo ECT should discontinue taking lithium 2 days before beginning ECT to reduce the risk of delirium.

LABORATORY INTERFERENCES

Lithium does not interfere with any laboratory tests, but lithium-induced alterations include increased white blood cell count, decreased serum thyroxine, and increased serum calcium. Blood collected in a lithium–heparin anticoagulant tube will produce falsely elevated lithium concentrations.

DOSING AND CLINICAL GUIDELINES

Initial Medical Workup

All patients should have a routine laboratory workup and physical examination before being started on lithium. The laboratory tests should include serum creatinine concentration (or a 24-hour urine creatinine if the clinician has any reason to be concerned about renal function), electrolytes, thyroid function (TSH, triiodothyronine, and thyroxine), a complete blood count, ECG, and a pregnancy test in women of childbearing age.

Dosing Recommendations

Lithium formulations include immediate-release 150-, 300-, and 600-mg lithium carbonate capsules (Eskalith and generic), 300-mg lithium carbonate tablets (Lithotabs), 450-mg controlled-release lithium carbonate capsules (Eskalith CR and Lithonate), and 8 mEq/5 mL of lithium citrate syrup.

The starting dose for most adults is 300 mg of the regular-release formulation three times daily. The starting dose for elderly persons or persons with renal impairment should be 300 mg once or twice daily. After stabilization, doses between 900 and 1,200 mg a day usually produce a therapeutic plasma concentration of 0.6 to 1 mEq/L, and a daily dose of 1,200 to 1,800 mg usually produces a therapeutic concentration of 0.8 to 1.2 mEq/L. Maintenance dosing can be given either in two or three divided doses of the regular-release formulation or in a single dose of the sustained-release formulation equivalent to the combined daily dose of the regular-release formulation. The use of divided doses reduces gastric upset and avoids single high-peak lithium concentrations. Discontinuation of lithium should be gradual to minimize the risk of early recurrence of mania and also to permit recognition of early signs of recurrence.

Laboratory Monitoring

Regular monitoring of serum lithium concentrations is essential. Lithium levels should be obtained every 2 to 6 months, except when signs of toxicity are seen, during dose adjustments, and in persons suspected to be noncompliant with the prescribed doses. Baseline ECGs are essential and should be repeated annually.

When obtaining blood for lithium levels, patients should be at steady-state lithium dosing (usually after 5 days of constant dosing), preferably using a twice- or three-times daily dosing regimen, and the blood sample must be drawn 12 hours (±30 minutes) after a given dose. Lithium concentrations 12 hours postdose in persons treated with sustained-release preparations are generally about 30 percent higher than the corresponding concentrations obtained from those taking the regular-release preparations. Because data are based on a sample population following a multiple-dose regimen, regular-release formulations given at least twice daily should be used for initial determination of the appropriate doses. Factors that can cause fluctuations in lithium measurements include dietary sodium intake, mood state, activity level, body position, and use of an improper blood sample tube.

Laboratory values that do not seem to correspond to clinical status may result from the collection of blood in a tube with a lithium–heparin anticoagulant (which can give results falsely elevated by as much as 1 mEq/L) or aging of the lithium ion-selective electrode (which can cause inaccuracies of up to 0.5 mEq/L). Once the daily dose has been set, it is reasonable to change to the sustained-release formulation given once daily.

Effective serum concentrations for mania are 1.0 to 1.5 mEq/L, a level associated with 1,800 mg a day. The recommended range for maintenance treatment is 0.4 to 0.8 mEq/L, which is usually achieved with a daily dose of 900 to 1,200 mg. A few persons will not achieve therapeutic benefit with a lithium concentration of 1.5 mEq/L yet will have no signs of toxicity. For such persons, titration of the lithium dose to achieve a concentration above 1.5 mEq/L may be warranted. Some patients can be maintained at concentrations below 0.4 mEq/L. Considerable variation is seen from patient to patient, so it is best to follow the maxim "treat the patient, not the laboratory results." The only way to establish an optimal dose for a patient may be through trial and error.

If no response occurs after 2 weeks at a concentration that is beginning to cause adverse effects, then the person should taper off lithium use over 1 to 2 weeks and should try other mood-stabilizing drugs.

Patient Education

Lithium has a narrow therapeutic index, and many factors can upset the balance between lithium concentrations that are well tolerated and produce therapeutic benefit and those that produce side effects or toxicity. Thus, it is imperative that persons taking lithium be educated about signs and symptoms of toxicity, factors that affect lithium levels, how and when to obtain laboratory testing, and the importance of regular communication with the prescribing physician. Common factors, such as excessive sweating caused by ambient heat or exercise or use of widely prescribed agents, such as ACE inhibitors or NSAIDs, can seriously disrupt lithium concentrations. Patients may stop taking their lithium because they are feeling well or because they are experiencing side effects. They should be advised against discontinuing or modifying their lithium regimen.

▲ 32.21 Melatonin Agonists: Ramelteon and Melatonin

RAMELTEON

Ramelteon (Rozerem) is a melatonin receptor agonist used to treat sleep onset insomnia. Unlike benzodiazepines, ramelteon has no appreciable affinity for the γ-aminobutyric acid receptor complex.

Pharmacological Actions

Ramelteon essentially mimics melatonin's sleep-promoting properties. It has high affinity for melatonin MT_1 and MT_2 receptors in the brain. These receptors are believed to be critical in the regulation of the body's sleep–wake cycle. Melatonin (N-acetyl-5 methoxytryptamine) is a hormone mainly produced at night in the pineal gland. Its secretion is stimulated by the dark and inhibited by light. It is naturally synthesized from the amino acid tryptophan. Tryptophan is converted to serotonin and finally converted to melatonin. The suprachiasmatic nuclei (SCN) of the hypothalamus have melatonin receptors, and melatonin may have a direct action on SCN to influence "circadian" rhythms. These include jet lag and sleep disturbances. Melatonin is also produced in the retina and gastrointestinal tract.

Peak absorption occurs between 30 and 90 minutes after ingestion. The half-life of ramelteon is between 1 and 2.6 hours.

Therapeutic Indications

Ramelteon mainly shortens latency to sleep onset and, to a lesser extent, increases total duration of sleep.

Clinical trials and animal studies failed to find evidence of rebound insomnia or withdrawal effects.

Precautions and Adverse Events

Headache is the most common side effect. Other adverse effects of ramelteon may include somnolence, fatigue, dizziness, worsening insomnia, depression, nausea, and diarrhea. This drug should not be used in patients with severe hepatic impairment. It is also not recommended in patients with severe sleep apnea or severe chronic obstructive pulmonary disease.

Ramelteon has been found to sometimes decrease blood cortisol and testosterone and to raise prolactin. Female patients should be monitored for cessation of menses or galactorrhea, decreased libido, or fertility problems. Safety and effectiveness of ramelteon in children has not been established. Its use is not recommended during lactation.

Drug Interactions

Cytochrome P450 (CYP) 1A2 is the major isozyme involved in the hepatic metabolism of ramelteon. Accordingly, fluvoxamine (Luvox) and other CYP 1A2 inhibitors may increase side effects of ramelteon.

Efficacy of ramelteon may be reduced when it is used in combination with potent CYP enzyme inducers, such as rifampin.

Rozerem should be administered with caution in patients taking other CYP 1A2 inhibitors, strong CYP 3A4 inhibitors such as ketoconazole, and strong CYP 2C9 inhibitors such as fluconazole (Diflucan). No clinically meaningful interactions were found when ramelteon was coadministered with omeprazole, theophylline, dextromethorphan, midazolam, digoxin, and warfarin.

Dosing and Clinical Guidelines

The usual dose of ramelteon is 8 mg within 30 minutes of going to bed. It should not be taken with or immediately after high-fat meals.

MELATONIN

Ingested melatonin has been shown to be capable of reaching and binding to melatonin-binding sites in the brains of mammals and to produce somnolence when used at higher doses. Accordingly, melatonin has become available as a dietary supplement. It is not a medication, however, and few well-controlled clinical trials have been conducted to determine its effectiveness in treating such conditions as insomnia, jet lag, and sleep disturbances related to shift work.

Melatonin can cause severe headaches, mental impairment, and mood changes. Melatonin concentrations are increased when taken in combination with monoamine oxidase inhibitors (MAOIs) because MAOIs inhibit the breakdown of melatonin by the body. Melatonin can suppress libido by inhibiting secretion of luteinizing hormone and follicle-stimulating hormone from the anterior pituitary gland. β-Blockers may decrease nocturnal melatonin release. The elimination half-life of melatonin is 32 to 40 minutes.

Over-the-counter melatonin is available in the following formulations: 1-, 2.5-, 3-, and 5-mg capsules; 1-mg/mL and 1-mg/4 mL liquid; 0.5- and 3-mg lozenges; 2.5-mg sublingual tablets; and 1-, 2-, and 3-mg timed-release tablets.

AGOMELATINE (VALDOXAN)

Agomelatine (Valdoxan) is structurally related to melatonin and is being investigated as a treatment of major depressive disorder. It acts as an agonist at melatonin (MT_1 and MT_2) receptors. It is also an antagonist at serotonin-2C ($5-HT_{2C}$) receptors. It is hypothesized that the antidepressant-like activity of agomelatine most probably involves a combination of its melatonin agonist and $5-HT_{2C}$ receptor antagonist properties. The effective dose in clinical trials is 25 mg/day. If found to be effective and safe, this compound could be very useful because sleep complaints are a feature of depression.

▲ 32.22 Mirtazapine

Mirtazapine (Remeron) is unique among drugs used to treat major depression in that it increases both norepinephrine and serotonin through a mechanism other than reuptake blockade (as in the case of tricyclic agents or selective serotonin reuptake inhibitors [SSRIs]) or monoamine oxidase inhibition (as in the case of phenelzine or tranylcypromine). Mirtazapine is also more likely to reduce rather than cause nausea and diarrhea, the result of its effects on serotonin $5-HT_3$ receptors. Characteristic side effects include increased appetite and sedation.

PHARMACOLOGICAL ACTIONS

Mirtazapine is administered orally and is rapidly and completely absorbed. It has a half-life of about 30 hours. Peak concentration is achieved within 2 hours of ingestion, and steady-state is reached after 6 days. Plasma clearance may be slowed up to 30 percent in persons with impaired hepatic function, up to 50 percent in those with impaired renal function, up to 40 percent in elderly males, and up to 10 percent in elderly females.

The mechanism of action of mirtazapine is antagonism of central presynaptic α_2-adrenergic receptors and blockade of postsynaptic serotonin $5-HT_2$ and $5-HT_3$ receptors. The α_2-adrenergic receptor antagonism causes increased firing of norepinephrine and serotonin neurons. The potent antagonist of serotonin $5-HT_2$ and $5-HT_3$ receptors serves to decrease anxiety, relieve insomnia, and stimulate appetite. Mirtazapine is a potent antagonist of histamine H_1 receptors and is a moderately potent antagonist at α_1-adrenergic and muscarinic-cholinergic receptors.

THERAPEUTIC INDICATIONS

Mirtazapine is effective for the treatment of depression. It is highly sedating, making it a reasonable choice for use in depressed patients with severe or long-standing insomnia. Some patients find the residual daytime sedation associated with initiation of treatment to be quite pronounced. The more extreme sedating properties of the drug generally lessen over the first week of treatment. Combined with the tendency to cause a sometimes ravenous appetite, mirtazapine is well suited for depressed patients with melancholic features such as insomnia, weight loss, and agitation. Elderly depressed patients, in particular, are good candidates for mirtazapine, whereas young adults are more likely to object to this side-effect profile.

Mirtazapine's blockade of $5-HT_3$ receptors, a mechanism associated with medications used to combat the severe gastrointestinal side effects of cancer chemotherapy agents, has led to use of the drug in a similar role. In this population, sedation and stimulation of appetite clearly could be seen as being beneficial instead of unwelcome side effects.

Mirtazapine is often combined with SSRIs or venlafaxine (Effexor) to augment antidepressant response or counteract serotonergic side effects of those drugs, particularly nausea, agitation, and insomnia. Mirtazapine has no significant pharmacokinetic interactions with other antidepressants.

PRECAUTIONS AND ADVERSE REACTIONS

Somnolence, the most common adverse effect of mirtazapine, occurs in greater than 50 percent of persons. Persons starting mirtazapine, thus, should exercise caution when driving or operating dangerous machinery, or even when getting out of bed at night. This adverse effect is why mirtazapine is almost always given before sleep. Mirtazapine potentiates the sedative effects of other central nervous system depressants, so potentially sedating prescription or over-the-counter drugs and alcohol should be avoided during use of mirtazapine. Mirtazapine also causes dizziness in 7 percent of persons. It does not appear to increase the risk for seizures. Mania or hypomania occurred in clinical trials at a rate similar to that with other antidepressant drugs.

Mirtazapine increases appetite in about one third of patients. Mirtazapine may also increase serum cholesterol concentration to 20 percent or more above the upper limit of normal in 15 percent of persons and increase triglycerides to 500 mg/dL or more in 6 percent of persons. Elevations of alanine transaminase levels to more than three times the upper limit of normal were seen in 2 percent of mirtazapine-treated persons, as opposed to 0.3 percent of placebo controls.

In limited premarketing experience, the absolute neutrophil count dropped to 500/mm^3 or less within 2 months of onset of use in 0.3 percent of persons, some of whom developed symptomatic infections. This hematological condition, which was reversible in all cases, was more likely to occur when other risk factors for neutropenia were present. Increases in the frequency of neutropenia, however, have not been reported during the extensive postmarketing period. Persons who develop fever, chills, sore throat, mucous membrane ulceration, or other signs of infection should nevertheless be evaluated medically. If a low white blood cell count is found, mirtazapine should be immediately discontinued, and the infectious disease status should be followed closely.

A few persons experience orthostatic hypotension while taking mirtazapine. Although no data exist regarding effects on fetal development, mirtazapine should be used with caution during pregnancy.

Mirtazapine use by pregnant women has not been studied; because the drug may be excreted in breast milk, it should not be taken by nursing mothers. Because of the risk of agranulocytosis associated with mirtazapine use, persons should be attuned to signs of infection, as discussed previously. Because of the sedating effects of mirtazapine, persons should determine the degree to which they are affected before engaging in driving or other potentially dangerous activities.

DRUG INTERACTIONS

Mirtazapine can potentiate the sedation of alcohol and benzodiazepines. Mirtazapine should not be used within 14 days of use of a monoamine oxidase inhibitor.

LABORATORY INTERFERENCES

No laboratory interferences have been described for mirtazapine.

DOSING AND ADMINISTRATION

Mirtazapine is available in 15-, 30-, and 45-mg scored tablets. Mirtazapine is also available in 15-, 30- and 45-mg orally disintegrating tablets for persons who have difficulty swallowing pills. If persons fail to respond to the initial dose of 15 mg of mirtazapine before sleep, the dose may be increased in 15-mg increments every 5 days to a maximum of 45 mg before sleep. Lower doses may be necessary in elderly persons or persons with renal or hepatic insufficiency.

▲ 32.23 Monoamine Oxidase Inhibitors

The monoamine oxidase inhibitors (MAOIs), which were introduced as antidepressants in 1957, are effective in treating both depression and panic disorder. The first of these drugs were hydrazine derivatives developed as treatments for tuberculosis. Their antidepressant properties were discovered by chance when some of the patients were observed to experience elevation of mood during treatment. Despite their effectiveness, prescription of MAOIs as first-line agents has always been limited by concern about the development of potentially lethal hypertension and the consequent need for a restrictive diet. Use of MAOIs declined further after the introduction of the selective serotonin reuptake

inhibitors (SSRIs) and other new agents. They are now mainly relegated to use in treatment-resistant cases. Thus, the second-line status of MAOIs has less to do with considerations of efficacy than with concerns for safety. The available MAOIs include phenelzine (Nardil), isocarboxazid (Marplan), tranylcypromine (Parnate), and selegiline (Eldepryl). Oral selegiline is a selective inhibitor of MAO_B used for the treatment of Parkinsonism. A transdermal delivery system to administer selegiline has been developed for use as an antidepressant. Reversible inhibitors of MAO_A (RIMAs), which are not available in the United States (e.g., moclobemide [Manerix] and befloxatone), require few dietary restrictions.

Isocarboxazid and phenelzine are derivatives of hydrazine, whereas tranylcypromine is structurally similar to amphetamine.

PHARMACOLOGICAL ACTIONS

Phenelzine, tranylcypromine, and isocarboxazid are readily absorbed after oral administration and reach peak plasma concentrations within 2 hours. Their plasma half-lives are in the range of 2 to 3 hours, whereas their tissue half-lives are considerably longer. Because they irreversibly inactivate MAOs, the therapeutic effect of a single dose of irreversible MAOIs may persist for as long as 2 weeks. The RIMA moclobemide is rapidly absorbed and has a half-life of 0.5 to 3.5 hours. Because it is a reversible inhibitor, moclobemide has a much briefer clinical effect following a single dose than do irreversible MAOIs.

The MAO enzymes are found on the outer membranes of mitochondria, where they degrade cytoplasmic and extraneuronal monoamine neurotransmitters, such as norepinephrine, serotonin, dopamine, epinephrine, and tyramine. MAOIs act in the central nervous system (CNS), the sympathetic nervous system, the liver, and the gastrointestinal (GI) tract. The two types of MAOs are MAO_A and MAO_B. MAO_A primarily metabolizes norepinephrine, serotonin, and epinephrine; dopamine and tyramine are metabolized by both MAO_A and MAO_B.

THERAPEUTIC INDICATIONS

The MAOIs are used to treat depression. Some research indicates that phenelzine is more effective than tricyclic antidepressants (TCAs) in depressed patients with mood reactivity, extreme sensitivity to interpersonal loss or rejection, prominent anergia, hyperphagia, and hypersomnia—a constellation of symptoms conceptualized as atypical depression. Evidence also indicates that MAOIs are more effective than TCAs as a treatment for bipolar depression.

A 38-year-old divorced mother of two teenage daughters presented at the Mood Disorders Clinic with a history of failed antidepressant treatment trials. Two years earlier, she had become increasingly irritable, exhausted, and tearful after the breakup of her marriage. She could not tolerate fluoxetine (Prozac) or sertraline (Zoloft) and discontinued each of these SSRIs after only a few days because of GI symptoms. Although she could tolerate desipramine (Norpramin) up to 300 mg daily, she felt no benefit after 4 months and was reluctant to continue this tricyclic antidepressant medication because of adverse effects (weight gain and sweating, in particular). Because of her increasing fatigue and sleep needs, and generally atypical profile, she was offered a trial of phenelzine. After 4 weeks, at a dosage of 60 mg daily, she reported significant improvement in her energy level, mood, and sleep pattern. Two years later, she continues to take 45 mg of phenelzine daily with some adverse effects (occasional insomnia and anorgasmia). (Courtesy of Sidney H. Kennedy, M.D., Andrew Holt, Ph.D., and Glen B. Baker, Ph.D., D.Sc.)

Patients with panic disorder and social phobia respond well to MAOIs. MAOIs have also been used to treat bulimia nervosa, posttraumatic stress disorder, anginal pain, atypical facial pain, migraine, attention-deficit hyperactivity disorder, idiopathic orthostatic hypotension, and depression associated with traumatic brain injury.

PRECAUTIONS AND ADVERSE REACTIONS

The most frequent adverse effects of MAOIs are orthostatic hypotension, insomnia, weight gain, edema, and sexual dysfunction. Orthostatic hypotension can lead to dizziness and falls. Thus, cautious upward tapering of the dose should be used to determine the maximal tolerable dose. Treatment for orthostatic hypotension includes avoidance of caffeine, intake of 2 L of fluid per day, addition of dietary salt or adjustment of antihypertensive drugs (if applicable), support stockings, and, in severe cases, treatment with fludrocortisone (Florinef), a mineralocorticoid, 0.1 to 0.2 mg a day. Orthostatic hypotension associated with tranylcypromine use can usually be relieved by dividing the daily dose.

Insomnia can be treated by dividing the dose, not giving the medication after dinner, and using trazodone (Desyrel) or a benzodiazepine hypnotic, if necessary. Weight gain, edema, and sexual dysfunction often do not respond to any treatment and may warrant switching to another agent. When switching from one MAOI to another, the clinician should taper and stop use of the first drug for 10 to 14 days before beginning use of the second drug.

Paresthesias, myoclonus, and muscle pains are occasionally seen in persons treated with MAOIs. Paresthesias may be secondary to MAOI-induced pyridoxine deficiency, which may respond to supplementation with pyridoxine, 50 to 150 mg orally each day. Occasionally, persons complain of feeling drunk or confused, perhaps indicating that the dose should be reduced and then increased gradually. Reports that the hydrazine MAOIs are associated with hepatotoxic effects are relatively uncommon. MAOIs are less cardiotoxic and less epileptogenic than are the tricyclic and tetracyclic drugs.

The most common adverse effects of the RIMA moclobemide are dizziness, nausea, and insomnia or sleep disturbance. RIMAs cause fewer GI adverse effects than do SSRIs. Moclobemide does not have adverse anticholinergic or cardiovascular effects, and it has not been reported to interfere with sexual function.

Persons with renal disease, cardiovascular disease, or hyperthyroidism should use the MAOIs with caution. MAOIs may alter the dose of a hypoglycemic agent required by diabetic persons. MAOIs have been particularly associated with induction of mania in persons in the depressed phase of bipolar I disorder

and triggering of a psychotic decompensation in persons with schizophrenia. MAOIs are contraindicated during pregnancy, although data on their teratogenic risk are minimal. MAOIs should not be taken by nursing women because the drugs can pass into the breast milk.

Tyramine-Induced Hypertensive Crisis

The most worrisome side effect of MAOIs is the tyramine-induced hypertensive crisis. The amino acid tyramine is normally transformed via GI metabolism. MAOIs, however, inactivate GI metabolism of dietary tyramine, thus allowing intact tyramine to enter the circulation. A hypertensive crisis may subsequently occur as a result of a powerful pressor effect of the amino acid. It is to allow resynthesis of adequate concentrations of MAOs that tyramine-containing foods be avoided until 2 weeks after the last dose of an irreversible MAOI.

Accordingly, foods rich in tyramine (Table 32.23–1) or other sympathomimetic amines, such as ephedrine, pseudoephedrine (Sudafed), or dextromethorphan (Trocal), should be avoided by persons who are taking irreversible MAOIs. Patients should be advised to continue the dietary restrictions for 2 weeks after they stop MAOI treatment to allow the body to resynthesize the enzyme. Bee stings may cause a hypertensive crisis. In addition to severe hypertension, other symptoms may include headache,

Table 32.23–1
Tyramine-Rich Foods to Be Avoided in Planning MAOI Diets

High tyramine content[a] (≥2 mg of tyramine a serving)
  Cheese: English Stilton, blue cheese, white (3 years old), extra old, old cheddar, Danish blue, mozzarella, cheese snack spreads
  Fish, cured meats, sausage, pâtés and organs, salami, mortadella, air-dried sausage
  Alcoholic beverages:[b] liqueurs and concentrated after-dinner drinks
  Marmite (concentrated yeast extract)
  Sauerkraut

Moderate tyramine content[a] (0.5 to 1.99 mg of tyramine a serving)
  Cheese: Swiss Gruyere, muenster, feta; parmesan; gorgonzola, blue cheese dressing: Black Diamond
  Fish, cured meats, sausage, pâtés and organs: chicken liver (5 days old), bologna; aged sausage, smoked meat, salmon mousse
  Alcoholic beverages: Beer and ale (12 oz per bottle)—Amstel, Export Draft, Blue Light, Guinness Extra Stout, Old Vienna, Canadian, Miller Light, Export, Heineken; Blue Wines (per 4-oz glass)—Rioja (red wine)

Low tyramine content[a] (0.01 to >0.49 mg of tyramine a serving)
  Cheese: Brie, Camembert, Cambozola with or without rind
  Fish, cured meat, sausage, organs, and pâtés, pickled herring, smoked fish, kielbasa sausage, chicken livers, liverwurst (<2 days old)
  Alcoholic beverages: red wines, sherry, scotch[c]
  Others: banana or avocado (ripe or not), banana peel

MAOI, monoamine oxidase inhibitor.
[a]Any food left out to age or spoil can spontaneously develop tyramine through fermentation.
[b]Alcohol can produce profound orthostasis interacting with MAOIs, but cannot produce direct hypotensive reactions.
[c]White wines, gin, and vodka have no tyramine content.
Table by Jonathan M. Himmelhoch, M.D.

stiff neck, diaphoresis, nausea, and vomiting. A patient with these symptoms should seek immediate medical treatment.

An MAOI-induced hypertensive crisis should be treated with α-adrenergic antagonists—for example, phentolamine (Regitine) or chlorpromazine (Thorazine). These drugs lower blood pressure within 5 minutes. Intravenous furosemide (Lasix) can be used to reduce fluid load, and a β-adrenergic receptor antagonist can control tachycardia. A sublingual 10-mg dose of nifedipine (Procardia) can be given and repeated after 20 minutes. MAOIs should not be used by persons with thyrotoxicosis or pheochromocytoma.

The risk of tyramine-induced hypertensive crises is relatively low for persons who are taking RIMAs, such as moclobemide and befloxatone. These drugs have relatively little inhibitory activity for MAO_B and, because they are reversible, normal activity of existing MAO_A returns within 16 to 48 hours of the last dose of a RIMA. Therefore, the dietary restrictions are less stringent for RIMAs, and apply only to foods containing high concentrations of tyramine, which need be avoided for only 3 days after the last dose of a RIMA. A reasonable dietary recommendation for persons taking RIMAs is not to eat tyramine-containing foods for a period from 1 hour before to 2 hours after taking a RIMA.

Spontaneous, non–tyramine-induced hypertensive crisis is a rare occurrence, usually shortly after the first exposure to an MAOI. Persons experiencing such a crisis should avoid MAOIs altogether.

A 57-year-old man had been successfully treated with tranylcypromine for 10 years after failing to respond to previous antidepressants. At his follow-up appointments, he admitted to being somewhat complacent about following a low-tyramine diet, because there appeared to be no hazardous sequelae. A confirmed hypertensive crisis occurred some time later and was successfully treated with sublingual nifedipine (Procardia; 10 mg). The cause of this reaction was ultimately traced to a change in his beer-drinking habit. For years, he had consumed one or two standard domestic beers every week. Just before the reaction, he sampled a microbrewery bottled draft beer that, on subsequent analysis, turned out to have a high tyramine content. (Courtesy of Sidney H. Kennedy, M.D., Andrew Holt, Ph.D., and Glen B. Baker, Ph.D., D.Sc.)

WITHDRAWAL

Abrupt cessation of regular doses of MAOIs can cause a self-limited discontinuation syndrome consisting of arousal, mood disturbances, and somatic symptoms. To avoid these symptoms when discontinuing use of an MAOI, doses should be gradually tapered over several weeks.

OVERDOSE

Often, an asymptomatic period of 1 to 6 hours occurs after an MAOI overdose before the occurrence of the symptoms of toxicity. MAOI overdose is characterized by agitation that progresses to coma with hyperthermia, hypertension, tachypnea, tachycardia, dilated pupils, and hyperactive deep tendon reflexes. Involuntary movements may be present, particularly in the face and

the jaw. Acidification of the urine markedly hastens the excretion of MAOIs, and dialysis can be of some use. Phentolamine or chlorpromazine may be useful if hypertension is a problem. Moclobemide alone in overdose causes relatively mild and reversible symptoms.

DRUG INTERACTIONS

Most antidepressants, as well as precursor agents, should be avoided. Persons should be instructed to tell any other physicians or dentists who are treating them that they are taking an MAOI. MAOIs may potentiate the action of CNS depressants, including alcohol and barbiturates. MAOIs should not be coadministered with serotonergic drugs, such as SSRIs and clomipramine (Anafranil), because this combination can trigger a serotonin syndrome. Use of lithium or tryptophan with an irreversible MAOI may also induce a serotonin syndrome. Initial symptoms of a serotonin syndrome can include tremor, hypertonicity, myoclonus, and autonomic signs, which can then progress to hallucinosis, hyperthermia, and even death. Fatal reactions have occurred when MAOIs were combined with meperidine (Demerol) or fentanyl (Sublimaze).

When switching from an irreversible MAOI to any other type of antidepressant drug, persons should wait at least 14 days after the last dose of the MAOI before beginning use of the next drug to allow replenishment of the body's MAOs. When switching from an antidepressant to an irreversible MAOI, persons should wait 10 to 14 days (or 5 weeks for fluoxetine [Prozac]) before starting use of the MAOI to avoid drug–drug interactions. In contrast, MAO activity recovers completely 24 to 48 hours after the last dose of a RIMA.

The effects of the MAOIs on hepatic enzymes are poorly studied. Tranylcypromine inhibits cytochrome P450 (CYP) 2C19. Moclobemide inhibits CYP 2D6, CYP 2C19, and CYP 1A2 and is a substrate for 2C19.

Cimetidine (Tagamet) and fluoxetine significantly reduce the elimination of moclobemide. Modest doses of fluoxetine and moclobemide administered concurrently may be well tolerated, with no significant pharmacodynamic or pharmacokinetic interactions.

LABORATORY INTERFERENCES

The MAOIs may lower blood glucose concentrations. MAOIs artificially raise urinary metanephrine concentrations and may cause a false-positive test result for pheochromocytoma or neuroblastoma. MAOIs have been reported to be associated with a minimal false elevation in thyroid function test results.

DOSING AND CLINICAL GUIDELINES

No definitive rationale exists for choosing one irreversible MAOI over another. Table 32.23–2 lists MAOI preparations and typical doses. Phenelzine use should begin with a test dose of 15 mg on the first day. The dose can be increased to 15 mg three times daily during the first week and increased by 15 mg a day each week thereafter until the dose of 90 mg a day, in divided doses, is reached by the end of the fourth week. Tranylcypromine and isocarboxazid use should begin with a test dose of 10 mg and may be increased to 10 mg three times daily by the end of the

Table 32.23–2
Available Preparations and Typical Doses of MAOIs

Generic Name	Trade Name	Preparations	Usual Daily Dose (mg)	Usual Maximal Daily Dose (mg)
Isocarboxazid[a]	Marplan	10-mg tablets	20–40	60
Moclobemide[b]	Manerix	100-, 150-mg tablets	300–600	600
Phenelzine	Nardil	15-mg tablets	30–60	90
Selegiline[c]	Eldepryl, Atapryl	5-mg capsules, 5-mg tablets	10	30
Tranylcypromine	Parnate	10-mg tablets	20–60	60

MAOIs, monoamine oxidase inhibitors.
[a] Available directly from the manufacturer.
[b] Not available in the United States.
[c] Also available as Emsam, 6-, 9-, 12-mg patch, used once daily.

first week. Many clinicians and researchers have recommended upper limits of 50 mg a day for isocarboxazid and 40 mg a day for tranylcypromine. Administration of tranylcypromine in multiple, small daily doses may reduce its hypotensive effects.

Although coadministration of MAOIs with TCAs, SSRIs, or lithium is generally contraindicated, these combinations have been used successfully and safely to treat patients with refractory depression, but they should be used with extreme caution.

Hepatic transaminase serum concentrations should be monitored periodically because of the potential for hepatotoxicity, especially with phenelzine and isocarboxazid. Elderly persons may be more sensitive to MAOI adverse effects than are younger adults. MAO activity increases with age, so that MAOI doses for elderly persons are the same as those required for younger adults. The use of MAOIs for children has had minimal study.

Moclobemide use is initiated at 300 to 450 mg a day, divided three times a day, and may be increased to a maximum of 600 mg a day after several weeks. Dietary restrictions consist of avoidance of only large quantities of tyramine-containing foods and the administration of moclobemide after, rather than before, tyramine-containing meals. RIMAs can be used in combination with other antidepressants with somewhat less concern for hypertensive crises but still with caution.

TRANSDERMAL SELEGILINE (EMSAM)

Oral selegiline is approved only as an adjunct to levodopa or carbidopa for patients with Parkinson's disease, but some studies have found it to be effective for treating depression. Antidepressant doses are greater than 30 mg per day, a level that results in loss of selective inhibition of MAO_B and consequent risk of the same tyramine reactions seen with the older MAOIs. For this reason, oral selegiline is rarely used off-label as an antidepressant.

A transdermal formulation of selegiline was approved in 2006 for treating major depressive disorder. The fact that it is absorbed through the skin eliminates first-pass hepatic metabolism and, thus, alters the mix of available medication. At the lowest (6 mg) strength, transdermal selegiline delivers more selegiline to the bloodstream than does low-dose oral selegiline but without inhibiting gut MAO_A. By selectively inhibiting MAO_B, it appears to have a lower risk of potentially fatal hypertensive reaction than that seen with other MAOIs. The 6-mg patch provides the brain MAO_A and MAO_B inhibition necessary for an antidepressant effect while eliminating the need for dietary restrictions at this lowest dose. At higher doses, 9 and 12 mg per day, transder-

mal selegiline may inhibit too much gastrointestinal MAO_A to clear tyramine from foods. The same food restrictions that apply to the older MAOIs, therefore, are necessary when prescribing transdermal selegiline at 9 or 12 mg per day.

Transdermal selegiline achieves therapeutic blood levels and reaches sustained concentration within 4 to 8 hours of administration. Compared with oral selegiline, transdermal delivery results in higher plasma selegiline concentrations (1,500 pg/mL with the 6-mg patch) with much lower exposure to metabolites.

As with oral selegiline, the transdermal patch should not be used concurrently with SSRIs, serotonin-norepinephrine reuptake inhibitors, tricyclic antidepressants, mirtazapine, or bupropion. Other contraindicated drugs include carbamazepine or oxcarbazepine, meperidine, tramadol, methadone, propoxyphene, St. John's wort, cough syrups containing dextromethorphan, amphetamines, cyclobenzaprine, and drugs containing pseudoephedrine, phenylephrine, phenylpropanolamine, or ephedrine.

Because MAO inhibition persists for 2 weeks after the last dose of selegiline, a 2-week "wash out" is required before starting a new antidepressant or stopping food restrictions in patients taking the 9-mg and 12-mg patches.

Inflammation at the application site is the most common side effect. Fair-skinned females are most at risk for this reaction. Insomnia can also occur. In clinical trials, transdermal selegiline did not impair sexual function, alter appetite, or change body weight or blood pressure compared with placebo. Transdermal selegiline was not tapered in clinical trials, yet no withdrawal symptoms were reported even after 1 year of continuous treatment.

Transdermal selegiline is started at 6 mg per day. The patch is applied to the upper torso (chest, back, or stomach), where vascularity is richer than in the buttocks and legs. The patch is changed daily and is applied to a different spot each day to prevent inflammation. The dose can be increased after 2 or 3 months if response is inadequate. Transdermal selegiline patches contain 1 mg/cm^2 of selegiline and deliver approximately 0.3 mg/cm^2 of selegiline over 24 hours. Available dosing forms are 6-, 9-, and 12-mg patches. Patches should not be cut.

▲ 32.24 Nefazodone

Nefazodone (Serzone) is indicated for the treatment of major depression. It is an analog of trazodone (Desyrel). It was found to produce problematic sedation, nausea, dizziness, and visual disturbances, and there are also reports of sometimes fatal hepatotoxicity. Consequently, nefazodone was never extensively adopted, and the manufacturer discontinued production of branded nefazodone in 2004. Generic nefazodone remains available in the United States.

Nefazodone is structurally related to trazodone and unrelated to the classic tricyclic and tetracyclic drugs, the monoamine oxidase inhibitors (MAOIs), selective serotonin reuptake inhibitors (SSRIs), and other available antidepressant drugs.

PHARMACOLOGICAL ACTIONS

Nefazodone is rapidly and completely absorbed but is then extensively metabolized, so that the bioavailability of active compounds is about 20 percent of the oral dose. Its half-life is 2 to 4 hours. Steady-state concentrations of nefazodone and its principal active metabolite hydroxynefazodone are achieved within 4 to 5 days. Metabolism of nefazodone in the elderly, especially women, is about half that seen in younger persons, so lowered doses are recommended for elderly persons. An important metabolite of nefazodone is *meta*-chlorophenylpiperazine (mCPP), which has some serotonergic effects and can cause migraine, anxiety, and weight loss.

Although nefazodone is an inhibitor of serotonin uptake and, more weakly, of norepinephrine reuptake, its antagonism of serotonin 5-HT$_{2A}$ receptors is thought to produce its antianxiety and antidepressant effects. Nefazodone is also a mild antagonist of the α_1-adrenergic receptors, which predisposes some persons to orthostatic hypotension, but is not sufficiently potent to produce priapism.

THERAPEUTIC INDICATIONS

Nefazodone is effective for the treatment of major depression. The usual effective dose is 300 to 600 mg a day. In direct comparison with SSRIs, nefazodone is less likely to cause inhibition of orgasm or decreased sexual desire. Nefazodone is also effective for treatment of panic disorder, panic with comorbid depression or depressive symptoms, of generalized anxiety disorder, and of premenstrual dysphoric disorder and for the management of chronic pain. It is not effective for the treatment of obsessive-compulsive disorder. Nefazodone increases rapid eye movement sleep and increases sleep continuity. Nefazodone is also of use in patients with posttraumatic stress disorder and chronic fatigue syndrome. It may also be effective in patients who have been treatment resistant to other antidepressant drugs.

PRECAUTIONS AND ADVERSE REACTIONS

The most common reasons for discontinuing nefazodone use are sedation, nausea, dizziness, insomnia, weakness, and agitation. Many patients report no specific side effect but describe a vague sense of feeling medicated. Nefazodone also causes visual trails, in which patients see an afterimage when looking at moving objects or when moving their heads quickly.

Some patients taking nefazodone may experience a drop in blood pressure that can cause episodes of postural hypotension. Nefazodone, therefore, should be used with caution by persons with underlying cardiac conditions, history of stroke or heart attack, dehydration, or hypovolemia or by persons being treated with antihypertensive medications. Patients switched from SSRIs to nefazodone may experience an increase in side effects, possibly because nefazodone does not protect against SSRI withdrawal symptoms. One of its metabolites, mCPP, may actually intensify these discontinuation symptoms.

The effects of nefazodone on the fetus are not yet as well understood as those of the SSRIs. Nefazodone, therefore, should be used during pregnancy only if the potential benefit to the mother outweighs the potential risks to the fetus. It is not known whether nefazodone is excreted in human breast milk. Therefore, it should be used with caution by lactating mothers. The nefazodone dose should be lowered in persons with severe hepatic disease, but no adjustment is necessary for persons with renal disease.

DRUG INTERACTIONS AND LABORATORY INTERFERENCES

Nefazodone should not be given concomitantly with MAOIs. In addition, nefazodone has particular drug–drug interactions with the triazolobenzodiazepines triazolam (Halcion) and alprazolam (Xanax) because of the inhibition of cytochrome P450 3A4 by nefazodone. Potentially elevated levels of each of these drugs can develop after administration of nefazodone, whereas the levels of nefazodone are generally not affected. The dose of triazolam should be lowered by 75 percent and the dose of alprazolam by 50 percent when given concomitantly with nefazodone.

Nefazodone may slow the metabolism of digoxin; therefore, digoxin levels should be monitored carefully in persons taking both medications. Nefazodone also slows the metabolism of haloperidol (Haldol), so the dose of haloperidol should be reduced in persons taking both medications. Addition of nefazodone may also exacerbate the adverse effects of lithium (Eskalith).

No known laboratory interferences are associated with nefazodone use.

DOSING AND CLINICAL GUIDELINES

Nefazodone is available in 50-, 200-, and 250-mg unscored tablets and 100- and 150-mg scored tablets. The recommended starting dose of nefazodone is 100 mg twice a day, but 50 mg twice a day may be better tolerated, especially by elderly persons. To limit the development of adverse effects, the dose should be slowly raised in increments of 100 to 200 mg a day at intervals of no less than 1 week per increase. The optimal dose is 300 to 600 mg daily in two divided doses. Some studies, however, report that nefazodone is effective when taken once a day, especially at bedtime. Geriatric persons should receive doses about two thirds of the usual nongeriatric doses, with a maximum of 400 mg a day. Similar to other antidepressants, clinical benefit of nefazodone usually appears after 2 to 4 weeks of treatment. Patients with premenstrual syndrome are treated with a flexible dose that averages about 250 mg a day.

▲ 32.25 Opioid Receptor Agonists: Methadone, Buprenorphine, and Levomethadyl

The drugs discussed in this section are used to deal with opioid addiction, commonly referred to as psychological dependence, physical dependence, or tolerance that develops after long-term abuse. Commonly abused opioids include heroin, hydromorphone (Dilaudid), codeine, meperidine (Demerol), butorphanol (Stadol), and hydrocodone (Robidone). Annually, approximately 2.6 million Americans use prescription pain relievers for nonmedical reasons and more than 3 million Americans use heroin.

The drugs discussed in this section include methadone (Dolophine), buprenorphine (Buprenex), and levomethadyl acetate, also called L-α-acetylmethadol (LAAM). Because of severe adverse reactions (described in the following text), LAAM was removed from the European market in 2001 and from the United States in 2003.

PHARMACOLOGICAL ACTIONS

Methadone, levomethadyl, and buprenorphine are absorbed rapidly from the gastrointestinal (GI) tract. Hepatic first-pass metabolism significantly affects the bioavailability of each of the drugs, but in markedly different ways. For methadone, hepatic enzymes reduce the bioavailability of an oral dose by about half, an effect that is easily managed with dose adjustments.

For levomethadyl, hepatic enzymes metabolize an oral dose into normethyl-LAAM and dinormethyl-LAAM, which are several times more potent as μ-opioid receptor agonists than is levomethadyl itself.

For buprenorphine, in contrast, first-pass intestinal and hepatic metabolism eliminates oral bioavailability almost completely. When used in opioid detoxification, buprenorphine is given sublingually, in either a liquid or a tablet formulation.

The peak plasma concentrations of oral methadone are reached within 2 to 6 hours, and the plasma half-life initially is 4 to 6 hours in opioid-naïve persons and 24 to 36 hours after steady dosing of any type of opioid. Methadone is highly protein bound and equilibrates widely throughout the body, which ensures little postdose variation in steady-state plasma concentrations.

The peak plasma concentrations of oral levomethadyl are reached within 1.5 to 2 hours, and the plasma half-lives of levomethadyl and its active metabolites range from 2 to 4 days.

Elimination of a sublingual dose of buprenorphine occurs in two phases: an initial phase with a half-life of 3 to 5 hours and a terminal phase with a half-life of more than 24 hours. Buprenorphine dissociates from its receptor binding site slowly, which permits an every-other-day dosing schedule.

Methadone and levomethadyl act as pure agonists at μ-opioid receptors and have negligible agonist or antagonist activity at κ- or δ-opioid receptors. Buprenorphine is a partial agonist at μ-receptors, a potent antagonist at κ-receptors, and neither an agonist nor an antagonist at δ-receptors.

THERAPEUTIC INDICATIONS

Methadone

Methadone is used for short-term detoxification (7 to 30 days), long-term detoxification (up to 180 days), and maintenance (treatment beyond 180 days) of opioid-dependent individuals. For these purposes, it is available only through designated clinics called methadone maintenance treatment programs and in hospitals and prisons. Methadone is a schedule II drug, which means that its administration is tightly governed by specific federal laws and regulations.

Enrollment in a methadone program reduces the risk of death by 70 percent and reduces (1) illicit use of opioids and other substances of abuse, (2) criminal activity, (3) the risk of infectious diseases of all types, most importantly human immunodeficiency virus and hepatitis B and C infection, and (4) in pregnant women, the risk of fetal and neonatal morbidity and mortality. The use of methadone maintenance frequently requires lifelong treatment.

Some opioid-dependence treatment programs use a stepwise detoxification protocol in which a person addicted to heroin switches first to the strong agonist methadone, then to the weaker agonist buprenorphine, and finally to maintenance on an opioid receptor antagonist, such as naltrexone (ReVia). This approach minimizes the appearance of opioid withdrawal effects, which, if they occur, are mitigated with clonidine (Catapres). Compliance with opioid receptor antagonist treatment is poor, however, outside of settings using intensive cognitive-behavioral techniques. In contrast, noncompliance with methadone maintenance precipitates opioid withdrawal symptoms, which serve to reinforce use of methadone and make cognitive-behavioral therapy less than essential. Thus, some well-motivated, socially integrated former heroin addicts are able to use methadone for years without participation in a psychosocial support program.

Data pooled from many reports indicate that methadone is more effective when taken at doses in excess of 60 mg a day. The analgesic effects of methadone are sometimes used in the management of chronic pain when less addictive agents are ineffective.

Pregnancy.   Methadone maintenance, combined with effective psychosocial services and regular obstetric monitoring, significantly improves obstetric and neonatal outcomes for women addicted to heroin. Enrollment of a heroin-addicted pregnant woman in such a maintenance program reduces the risk of malnutrition, infection, preterm labor, spontaneous abortion, preeclampsia, eclampsia, abruptio placenta, and septic thrombophlebitis.

The dose of methadone during pregnancy should be the lowest effective dose, and no withdrawal to abstinence should be attempted during pregnancy. Methadone is metabolized more rapidly in the third trimester, which may necessitate higher doses. To avoid potentially sedating postdose peak plasma concentrations, the daily dose can be administered in two divided doses during the third trimester. Methadone treatment has no known teratogenic effects.

Neonatal Methadone Withdrawal Symptoms.   Withdrawal symptoms in newborns frequently include tremor, high-pitched cry, increased muscle tone and activity, poor sleep and eating, mottling, yawning, perspiration, and skin excoriation. Convulsions that require aggressive anticonvulsant therapy may also occur. Withdrawal symptoms can be delayed in onset and prolonged in neonates because of their immature hepatic metabolism. Women taking methadone are sometimes counseled to initiate breast-feeding as a means of gently weaning their infants from methadone dependence, but they should not breast-feed their babies while still taking methadone.

Levomethadyl

Levomethadyl is no longer used. It had been used only for maintenance treatment of opioid-dependent patients. It was not used for detoxification treatment or for analgesia.

Buprenorphine

Buprenorphine at a dose of 8 to 16 mg a day appears to reduce heroin use. Buprenorphine also is effective in thrice-weekly dosing because of its slow dissociation from opioid receptors. The analgesic effects of buprenorphine are sometimes used in the management of chronic pain when less addictive agents are ineffective.

PRECAUTIONS AND ADVERSE REACTIONS

The most common adverse effects of opioid receptor agonists are lightheadedness, dizziness, sedation, nausea, constipation, vomiting, perspiration, weight gain, decreased libido, inhibition of orgasm, and insomnia or sleep irregularities. Opioid receptor agonists can induce tolerance as well as produce physiological and psychological dependence. Other central nervous system (CNS) adverse effects include depression, sedation, euphoria, dysphoria, agitation, and seizures. Delirium has been reported in rare cases. Occasional non-CNS adverse effects include peripheral edema, urinary retention, rash, arthralgia, dry mouth, anorexia, biliary tract spasm, bradycardia, hypotension, hypoventilation, syncope, antidiuretic hormone–like activity, pruritus, urticaria, and visual disturbances. Menstrual irregularities are common in women, especially in the first 6 months of use. Various abnormal endocrine laboratory indexes of little clinical significance may also be seen.

Most persons develop tolerance to the pharmacological adverse effects of opioid agonists during long-term maintenance, and relatively few adverse effects are experienced after the induction period.

Levomethadyl is associated with prolonged QT intervals and torsades de pointes, which may be fatal. As mentioned, for these reasons, this drug is no longer in use.

Overdose

The acute effects of opioid receptor agonist overdose include sedation, hypotension, bradycardia, hypothermia, respiratory suppression, miosis, and decreased GI motility. Severe effects include coma, cardiac arrest, shock, and death. The risk of overdose is greatest in the induction stage of treatment and in persons with slow drug metabolism because of preexisting hepatic insufficiency. Deaths have been caused during the first week of induction by methadone doses of only 50 to 60 mg a day.

The risk of overdose with buprenorphine appears to be lower than with methadone. Deaths have been caused, however, by use of buprenorphine in combination with benzodiazepines.

Withdrawal Symptoms

Abrupt cessation of methadone use triggers withdrawal symptoms within 3 to 4 days, which usually reach peak intensity on the sixth day. Withdrawal symptoms include weakness, anxiety, anorexia, insomnia, gastric distress, headache, sweating, and hot and cold flashes. The withdrawal symptoms usually resolve after 2 weeks. A protracted methadone abstinence syndrome is possible, however, which may include restlessness and insomnia.

The withdrawal symptoms associated with buprenorphine are similar to, but less marked than, those caused by methadone. In particular, buprenorphine is sometimes used to ease the transition from methadone to opioid receptor antagonists or abstinence because of the relatively mild withdrawal reaction associated with discontinuation of buprenorphine.

DRUG–DRUG INTERACTIONS

Opioid receptor agonists can potentiate the CNS depressant effects of alcohol, barbiturates, benzodiazepines, other opioids, low-potency dopamine receptor antagonists, tricyclic and tetracyclic drugs, and monoamine oxidase inhibitors (MAOIs). Carbamazepine (Tegretol), phenytoin (Dilantin), barbiturates, and rifampin (Rimactane, Rifadin), and heavy long-term consumption of alcohol can induce hepatic enzymes, which can lower the plasma concentration of methadone or buprenorphine and thereby precipitate withdrawal symptoms. In contrast, however, hepatic enzyme induction can raise the plasma concentration of active levomethadyl metabolites and cause toxicity.

Acute opioid withdrawal symptoms can be precipitated in persons on methadone maintenance therapy who take pure opioid receptor antagonists, such as naltrexone, nalmefene (Revex), and naloxone (Narcan); partial agonists, such as buprenorphine; or mixed agonist-antagonists, such as pentazocine (Talwin). These symptoms may be mitigated by use of clonidine, a benzodiazepine, or both.

Competitive inhibition of methadone or buprenorphine metabolism following short-term use of alcohol or administration of cimetidine (Tagamet), erythromycin, ketoconazole (Nizoral), fluoxetine (Prozac), fluvoxamine (Luvox), loratadine (Claritin), quinidine (Quinidex), and alprazolam (Xanax) can lead to higher plasma concentrations or prolonged duration of action of methadone or buprenorphine. Medications that alkalinize the urine can reduce methadone excretion.

Methadone maintenance can also increase plasma concentrations of desipramine (Norpramin, Pertofrane) and fluvoxamine. Use of methadone can increase zidovudine (Retrovir) concentrations, which increases the possibility of zidovudine toxicity at otherwise standard doses. In vitro human liver microsome studies, moreover, demonstrate competitive inhibition of methadone demethylation by several protease inhibitors, including ritonavir (Norvir), indinavir (Crixivan), and saquinavir (Invirase). The clinical relevance of this finding is unknown.

Fatal drug–drug interactions with the MAOIs are associated with use of the opioids fentanyl (Sublimaze) and meperidine

(Demerol) but not with use of methadone, levomethadyl, or buprenorphine.

LABORATORY INTERFERENCES

Methadone, levomethadyl, and buprenorphine can be tested for separately in urine toxicology to distinguish them from other opioids. No known laboratory interferences are associated with use of methadone, levomethadyl, or buprenorphine.

DOSING AND CLINICAL GUIDELINES

Methadone

Methadone is supplied in 5-, 10-, and 40-mg dispersible scored tablets; 40-mg scored wafers; 5-mg/5 mL, 10-mg/5 mL, and 10-mg/mL solutions; and a 10-mg/mL parenteral form. In maintenance programs, methadone is usually dissolved in water or juice, and dose administration is directly observed to ensure compliance. For induction of opioid detoxification, an initial methadone dose of 15 to 20 mg will usually suppress craving and withdrawal symptoms. Some individuals, however, may require up to 40 mg a day in single or divided doses. Higher doses should be avoided during induction of treatment to reduce the risk of acute toxicity from overdose.

Over several weeks, the dose should be raised to at least 70 mg a day. The maximal dose is usually 120 mg a day, and higher doses require prior approval from regulatory agencies. Doses above 60 mg a day are associated with much more complete abstinence from use of illicit opioids than are doses of less than 60 mg a day.

Treatment duration should not be predetermined but should be based on response to treatment and assessment of psychosocial factors. All studies of methadone maintenance programs endorse long-term treatment (i.e., several years) as more effective than short-term programs (i.e., <1 year) for prevention of relapse into opioid abuse. In practice, however, a few programs are permitted by policy or approved by insurers to provide even 6 months of continuous maintenance treatment. Moreover, some programs encourage withdrawal from methadone in less than 6 months after induction. This is quite ill conceived because more than 80 percent of persons who terminate methadone maintenance treatment eventually return to illicit drug use within 2 years. In those programs that offer both maintenance and withdrawal treatments, the overwhelming majority of participants enroll in the maintenance treatment.

Levomethadyl

Levomethadyl is no longer marketed. Because of the tendency of levomethadyl to accumulate toxic concentrations if taken daily, it was prescribed thrice weekly in doses of 60 to 90 mg.

Buprenorphine

Buprenorphine is supplied as a 0.3-mg/mL solution in 1-mL ampules. Sublingual tablet formulations of buprenorphine containing buprenorphine only or buprenorphine combined with naloxone in a 4:1 ratio are used for opioid maintenance treatment. Buprenorphine is not used for short-term opioid detoxification.

Maintenance doses of 8 to 16 mg three times a week have effectively reduced heroin use. Physicians must be trained and certified to carry out this therapy in their private offices. A number of approved training programs are available in the United States.

▲ 32.26 Opioid Receptor Antagonists: Naltrexone, Nalmefene, and Naloxone

The three opioid receptor antagonists are naltrexone (ReVia), Naloxone (Narcan), and nalmefene (Revex). Opioid receptor antagonists appear to reduce or eliminate the subjective "high" associated with consumption of opioids or alcohol, thus interrupting their reinforcing effects. Opioid receptor antagonists also reduce or eliminate the craving associated with withdrawal from chronic opioid or alcohol abuse.

Of the three opioid receptor antagonists, only oral naltrexone is approved by the U.S. Food and Drug Administration for treatment of alcohol dependence and for blockade of the effects of exogenously administered opioids. The only available formulation of nalmefene and naltrexone is for intravenous administration, and both of these drugs are used to treat respiratory depression induced by opioids and to manage known or suspected overdose of synthetic or natural opioid preparations.

PHARMACOLOGICAL ACTIONS

Oral opioid receptor antagonists are rapidly absorbed from the gastrointestinal (GI) tract, but because of first-pass hepatic metabolism, only 60 percent of a dose of naltrexone and 40 to 50 percent of a dose of nalmefene reach the systemic circulation unchanged. Peak concentrations of naltrexone and its active metabolite, $6\text{-}\beta\text{-naltrexol}$, are achieved within 1 hour of ingestion. The half-life of naltrexone is 1 to 3 hours, and the half-life of $6\text{-}\beta\text{-naltrexol}$ is 13 hours. Peak concentrations of nalmefene are achieved in about 1 to 2 hours, and the half-life is 8 to 10 hours. Clinically, a single dose of naltrexone effectively blocks the rewarding effects of opioids for 72 hours. Traces of $6\text{-}\beta\text{-naltrexol}$ can linger for up to 125 hours after a single dose.

Naltrexone and nalmefene are competitive antagonists of opioid receptors. Understanding the pharmacology of opioid receptors can explain the difference in adverse effects caused by naltrexone and nalmefene. Opioid receptors in the body are typed pharmacologically as either μ-, κ-, or δ. Activation of the κ- and δ-receptors is thought to reinforce opioid and alcohol consumption centrally, whereas activation of μ-receptors is more closely associated with central and peripheral antiemetic effects. Because naltrexone is a relatively weak antagonist of κ- and δ-receptors and a potent μ-receptor antagonist, doses of naltrexone that effectively reduce opioid and alcohol consumption also strongly block μ-receptors and, therefore, may cause nausea. Nalmefene, in contrast, is an equally potent antagonist of all three opioid receptor types, and doses of nalmefene that effectively reduce opioid and alcohol consumption have no particularly increased effect on μ-receptors. Thus, nalmefene is associated clinically with few GI adverse effects.

Naloxone has the highest affinity for the μ-receptor, but is a competitive antagonist at the μ-, κ-, and δ-receptors.

Whereas the effects of opioid receptor antagonists on opioid use are easily understood in terms of competitive inhibition of opioid receptors, the effects of opioid receptor antagonists on alcohol dependence are less straightforward and probably relate to the fact that the desire for, and effects of, alcohol consumption appear to be regulated by several neurotransmitter systems, both opioid and nonopioid.

THERAPEUTIC INDICATIONS

The combination of a cognitive-behavioral program plus use of opioid receptor antagonists is more successful than either the cognitive-behavioral program or use of opioid receptor antagonists alone. Naltrexone is used as a screening test to ensure that the patient is opioid free before the induction of therapy with naltrexone (see later discussion of the naloxone challenge test).

Opioid Dependence

Patients in detoxification programs are usually weaned from potent opioid agonists such as heroin over a period of days to weeks, during which emergent adrenergic withdrawal effects are treated as needed with clonidine (Catapres). A serial protocol is sometimes used in which potent agonists are gradually replaced by weaker agonists, followed by mixed agonist–antagonists, and then finally by pure antagonists. For example, an abuser of the potent agonist heroin would switch first to the weaker agonist methadone (Dolophine), then to the partial agonist buprenorphine (Buprenex) or levomethadyl acetate (ORLAAM)—commonly called LAAM—and finally, following a 7- to 10-day washout period, to a pure antagonist, such as naltrexone or nalmefene. Even with gradual detoxification, some persons, however, continue to experience mild adverse effects or opioid withdrawal symptoms for the first several weeks of treatment with naltrexone.

As the opioid receptor agonist potency diminishes, so do the adverse consequences of discontinuing the drug. Thus, because no pharmacological barriers exist to discontinuation of pure opioid receptor antagonists, the social environment and frequent cognitive-behavioral intervention become extremely important factors supporting continued opioid abstinence. Because of poorly tolerated adverse symptoms, most persons not simultaneously enrolled in a cognitive-behavioral program stop taking opioid receptor antagonists within 3 months. Compliance with administration of an opioid receptor antagonist regimen can also be increased with participation in a well-conceived voucher program.

Issues of medication compliance should be a central focus of treatment. If a person with a history of opioid addiction stops taking a pure opioid receptor antagonist, the person's risk of relapse into opioid abuse is exceedingly high because reintroduction of a potent opioid agonist would yield a very rewarding subjective "high." In contrast, compliant persons do not develop tolerance to the therapeutic benefits of naltrexone, even if it is administered continuously for 1 year or longer. Individuals may undergo several relapses and remissions before achieving long-term abstinence.

Persons taking opioid receptor antagonists should also be warned that sufficiently high doses of opioid agonists can over-come the receptor antagonism of naltrexone or nalmefene, which can lead to hazardous and unpredictable levels of receptor activation (see Precautions and Adverse Reactions).

Rapid Detoxification.   To avoid the 7- to 10-day period of opioid abstinence generally recommended before use of opioid receptor antagonists, rapid detoxification protocols have been developed. Continuous administration of adjunct clonidine—to reduce the adrenergic withdrawal symptoms—and adjunct benzodiazepines, such as oxazepam (Serax)—to reduce muscle spasms and insomnia—can permit use of oral opioid receptor antagonists on the first day of opioid cessation. Detoxification, thus, can be completed within 48 to 72 hours, at which point opioid receptor antagonist maintenance is initiated. Moderately severe withdrawal symptoms may be experienced on the first day, but they tail off rapidly thereafter.

Because of the potential hypotensive effects of clonidine, the blood pressure (BP) of persons undergoing rapid detoxification must be closely monitored for the first 8 hours. Outpatient rapid detoxification settings, therefore, must be adequately prepared to administer emergency care.

The main advantage of rapid detoxification is that the transition from opioid abuse to maintenance treatment occurs over just 2 or 3 days. The completion of detoxification in as little time as possible minimizes the risk that the person will relapse into opioid abuse during the detoxification protocol.

Alcohol Dependence

Opioid receptor antagonists are also used as adjuncts to cognitive-behavioral programs for treatment of alcohol dependence. Opioid receptor antagonists reduce alcohol craving and alcohol consumption, and they ameliorate the severity of relapses. The risk of relapse into heavy consumption of alcohol attributable to an effective cognitive-behavioral program alone may be halved with concomitant use of opioid receptor antagonists.

The newer agent nalmefene has a number of potential pharmacological and clinical advantages over its predecessor naltrexone for treatment of alcohol dependence. Whereas naltrexone may cause reversible transaminase elevations in persons who take doses of 300 mg a day (which is six times the recommended dose for treatment of alcohol and opioid dependence [50 mg a day]), nalmefene has not been associated with any hepatotoxicity. Clinically effective doses of naltrexone are discontinued by 10 to 15 percent of persons because of adverse effects, most commonly nausea. In contrast, discontinuation of nalmefene because of an adverse event is rare at the clinically effective dose of 20 mg a day and in the range of 10 percent at excessive doses—that is, 80 mg a day. Because of its pharmacokinetic profile, a given dose of nalmefene can also produce a more sustained opioid antagonist effect than does naltrexone.

The efficacy of opioid receptor antagonists in reducing alcohol craving can be augmented with a selective serotonin reuptake inhibitor, although data from large trials are needed to assess this potential synergistic effect more fully.

PRECAUTIONS AND ADVERSE REACTIONS

Because opioid receptor antagonists are used to maintain a drug-free state after opioid detoxification, great care must be taken to ensure that an adequate washout period elapses after the last dose of opioids and before the first dose of an opioid receptor antagonist is taken: at least 5 days for a short-acting opioid such as heroin and at least 10 days for longer-acting opioids such as methadone. The opioid-free state should be determined by self-report and urine toxicology screens. If any question persists of whether opioids are in the body despite a negative urine screen result, then a *naloxone challenge test* should be performed. Naloxone challenge is used because its opioid antagonism lasts less than 1 hour, whereas those of naltrexone and nalmefene can persist for more than 24 hours. Thus, any withdrawal effects elicited by naloxone will be relatively short-lived (see Dosing and Clinical Guidelines). Symptoms of acute opioid withdrawal include drug craving, feeling of temperature change, musculoskeletal pain, and GI distress. Signs of opioid withdrawal include confusion, drowsiness, vomiting, and diarrhea. Naltrexone and nalmefene should not be taken if naloxone infusion causes any signs of opioid withdrawal, except as part of a supervised rapid detoxification protocol.

A set of adverse effects, resembling a vestigial withdrawal syndrome, tends to affect up to 10 percent of persons who take opioid receptor antagonists. Up to 15 percent of persons taking naltrexone may experience abdominal pain, cramps, nausea, and vomiting, which may be limited by transiently halving the dose or altering the time of administration. Adverse central nervous system effects of naltrexone, experienced by up to 10 percent of persons, include headache, low energy, insomnia, anxiety, and nervousness. Joint and muscle pains may occur in up to 10 percent of persons taking naltrexone, as may rash.

Naltrexone can cause dose-related hepatic toxicity at doses well in excess of 50 mg a day; 20 percent of persons taking 300 mg a day of naltrexone may experience serum aminotransferase concentrations 3 to 19 times the upper limit of normal. The hepatocellular injury of naltrexone appears to be a dose-related toxic effect rather than an idiosyncratic reaction. At the lowest doses of naltrexone required for effective opioid antagonism, hepatocellular injury is not typically observed. Naltrexone doses as low as 50 mg a day may be hepatotoxic, however, in persons with underlying liver disease, such as persons with cirrhosis of the liver caused by chronic alcohol abuse. Serum aminotransferase concentrations should be monitored monthly for the first 6 months of naltrexone therapy and thereafter on the basis of clinical suspicion. Hepatic enzyme concentrations usually return to normal after discontinuation of naltrexone therapy.

If analgesia is required while a dose of an opioid receptor antagonist is pharmacologically active, opioid agonists should be avoided in favor of benzodiazepines or other nonopioid analgesics. Persons taking opioid receptor antagonists should be instructed that low doses of opioids will have no effect, but larger doses could overcome the receptor blockade and suddenly produce symptoms of profound opioid overdose, with sedation possibly progressing to coma or death. Use of opioid receptor antagonists is contraindicated in persons who are taking opioid agonists, small amounts of which may be present in over-the-counter antiemetic and antitussive preparations; in persons with acute hepatitis or hepatic failure; and in persons who are hypersensitive to the drugs.

Because naltrexone is transported across the placenta, opioid receptor antagonists should only be taken by pregnant women if a compelling need outweighs the potential risks to the fetus. It is not known whether opioid receptor antagonists are distributed into maternal milk.

Opioid receptor antagonists are relatively safe drugs, and ingestion of high doses of them should be treated with supportive measures combined with efforts to decrease GI absorption.

DRUG INTERACTIONS

Because of its extensive hepatic metabolism, naltrexone can affect, or be affected by, other drugs that influence hepatic enzyme levels. The clinical importance of these potential interactions, however, is not known.

One potentially hepatotoxic drug that has been used in some cases with opioid receptor antagonists is disulfiram (Antabuse). Although no adverse effects were observed, frequent laboratory monitoring is indicated when such combination therapy is contemplated. Opioid receptor antagonists have been reported to potentiate the sedation associated with use of thioridazine (Mellaril), an interaction that probably applies equally to all low-potency dopamine receptor antagonists.

LABORATORY INTERFERENCES

No laboratory interferences have been described for opioid receptor antagonists, although relatively nonspecific immune-based toxicology screens for opioids could potentially yield positive results in persons taking only opioid receptor antagonists, because of their structural similarities to other opioids.

DOSING AND CLINICAL GUIDELINES

To avoid the possibility of precipitating an acute opioid withdrawal syndrome, several steps should be taken to ensure that the person is opioid free. Within a supervised detoxification setting, at least 5 days should elapse following the last dose of short-acting opioids, such as heroin, hydromorphone (Dilaudid), meperidine (Demerol), or morphine, and at least 10 days should elapse after the last dose of longer-acting opioids, such as methadone, before opioid antagonists are initiated. Briefer periods off opioids have been used in rapid detoxification protocols. To confirm that opioid detoxification is complete, urine toxicological screens should demonstrate no opioid metabolites. An individual may, however, have a negative urine opioid screen result and yet still be physically dependent on opioids and, thus, susceptible to antagonist-induced withdrawal effects. Therefore, once the urine screen result is negative, a naloxone challenge test is recommended, unless an adequate period of opioid abstinence can be reliably confirmed by observers.

The initial dose of naltrexone for treatment of opioid or alcohol dependence is 50 mg a day, which should be achieved through gradual introduction, even when the naloxone challenge test result is negative. Various authorities begin with 5, 10, 12.5, or 25 mg and titrate up to the 50-mg dose over a period ranging from 1 hour to 2 weeks while constantly monitoring for evidence of opioid withdrawal. Once a daily dose of 50 mg is well tolerated, it may be averaged over a week by giving 100 mg on alternate days or 150 mg every third day. Such schedules may increase compliance. The corresponding therapeutic dose of nalmefene is 20 mg a day, divided into two equal doses. Gradual titration of nalmefene to this daily dose is probably a wise strategy, although clinical data on dosing strategies for nalmefene are not available.

To maximize compliance, it is recommended that ingestion of each dose be directly observed, either in a facility or by family members, and that random urine tests be taken for opioid receptor antagonists and their metabolites and for ethanol or opioid metabolites. Opioid receptor antagonists should be continued until the person is no longer considered psychologically at risk for relapse into opioid or alcohol abuse. This generally requires at least 6 months, but may take longer, particularly if there are external stresses.

Rapid Detoxification

Rapid detoxification has been standardized using naltrexone, although nalmefene would be expected to be equally effective with fewer adverse effects. In rapid detoxification protocols, the addicted person stops opioid use abruptly and begins the first opioid-free day by taking clonidine, 0.2 mg, orally every 2 hours for nine doses, to a maximal dose of 1.8 mg, during which time BP is monitored every 30 to 60 minutes for the first 8 hours. Naltrexone, 12.5 mg, is administered 1 to 3 hours after the first dose of clonidine. To reduce muscle cramps and later insomnia, a short-acting benzodiazepine, such as oxazepam, 30 to 60 mg, is administered simultaneously with the first dose of clonidine, and half of the initial dose is readministered every 4 to 6 hours as needed. The maximal daily dose of oxazepam should not exceed 180 mg. The person undergoing rapid detoxification should be accompanied home by a reliable escort. On the second day, similar doses of clonidine and the benzodiazepine are administered but with a single dose of naltrexone, 25 mg, taken in the morning. Relatively asymptomatic persons may return home after 3 to 4 hours. Administration of the daily maintenance dose of naltrexone, 50 mg, is begun on the third day, and the doses of clonidine and the benzodiazepine are gradually tapered off over 5 to 10 days.

▲ 32.27 Phosphodiesterase-5 Inhibitors

The introduction of the first phosphodiesterase (PDE)-5 inhibitor, sildenafil (Viagra), in 1998 revolutionized the treatment of the major sexual dysfunction affecting men—erectile disorder. Two congeners have since come on the market—vardenafil (Levitra) and tadalafil (Cialis). All have a similar method of action and have changed people's expectations of sexual functioning. Although indicated only for the treatment of male erectile dysfunction, anecdotal evidence suggests their being effective in women. They are also being misused as recreational drugs that are believed to enhance sexual performance. These drugs have been used by more than 20 million men, if not more, around the world.

The development of sildenafil provided important information about the physiology of erection. Sexual stimulation causes the release of the neurotransmitter nitric oxide (NO), which increases the synthesis of cyclic guanosine monophosphate (cGMP), causing smooth muscle relaxation in the corpus cavernosum that allows blood to flow into the penis and that results in turgidity and tumescence. The concentration of cGMP is regulated by the enzyme PDE-5, which, when inhibited, allows cGMP to increase and enhance erectile function. Because sexual stimulation is required to cause the release of NO, PDE-5 inhibitors have no effect in the absence of such stimulation, an important point to understand when providing information to patients about their use. The congeners vardenafil and tadalafil work in the same way, by inhibiting PDE-5, thus allowing an increase in cGMP and enhancing the vasodilatory effects of NO. For this reason, these drugs are sometimes referred to as NO enhancers.

PHARMACOLOGICAL ACTIONS

All three substances are fairly rapidly absorbed from the gastrointestinal tract, with maximal plasma concentrations reached in 30 to 120 minutes (median, 60 minutes) in the fasting state. Because it is lipophilic, concomitant ingestion of a high-fat meal delays the rate of absorption by up to 60 minutes and reduces the peak concentration by one fourth. These drugs are principally metabolized by the cytochrome 450 (CYP) 3A4 system, which can lead to clinically significant drug–drug interactions, not all of which have been documented. Excretion of 80 percent of the dose is via feces, and another 13 percent is eliminated in the urine. Elimination is reduced in persons older than age 65 years, which results in plasma concentrations 40 percent higher than in persons aged 18 to 45 years. Elimination is also reduced in the presence of severe renal or hepatic insufficiency.

The mean half-lives of sildenafil and vardenafil are 3 to 4 hours, and that of tadalafil is about 18 hours. Tadalafil can be detected in the bloodstream 5 days after ingestion, and because of its long half-life, it has been marketed as effective for up to 36 hours—the so-called weekend pill; however, the effects of inhibiting PDE for long periods of time may require further investigation. The onset of sildenafil occurs about 30 minutes after ingestion on an empty stomach; tadalafil and vardenafil act somewhat more quickly. More than once-a-day use can cause excessive accumulation of the drug.

The clinician needs to be aware of the important clinical observation that these drugs do not by themselves create an erection. Rather, the mental state of sexual arousal brought on by erotic stimulation must first lead to activity in the penile nerves, which then release NO into the cavernosum, triggering the erectile cascade, the resulting erection being prolonged by the NO enhancers. Then, full advantage may be taken of a sexually exciting stimulus, but the drug is not a substitute for foreplay and emotional arousal. By contrast, the penile injection of alprostadil (Caverject) causes an erection to occur in the absence of or with minimal erotic stimulation.

THERAPEUTIC INDICATIONS

Erectile dysfunctions have traditionally been classified as organic, psychogenic, or mixed. Over the last 20 years, the prevailing view of the cause of erectile dysfunction has shifted away from psychological causes toward organic causes. The latter include diabetes mellitus, hypertension, hypercholesterolemia, cigarette smoking, peripheral vascular disease, pelvic or spinal cord injury, pelvic or abdominal surgery (especially, prostate surgery), multiple sclerosis, peripheral neuropathy, and Parkinson's disease. Erectile dysfunction is often induced by alcohol, nicotine, and other substances of abuse and by prescription drugs.

These drugs are effective regardless of the baseline severity of erectile dysfunction, race, or age. Among those responding to sildenafil are men with coronary artery disease, hypertension, other cardiac disease, peripheral vascular disease, diabetes mellitus, depression, coronary artery bypass graft, radical prostatectomy, transurethral resection of the prostate, spina bifida, and spinal cord injury, as well as persons taking antidepressants, antipsychotics, antihypertensives, and diuretics. The response rate, however, is variable.

Sildenafil has been reported to reverse selective serotonin reuptake inhibitor–induced anorgasmia in men. Anecdotal reports indicate that sildenafil has an effect in women as well, causing clitoral erectile tissue to become engorged.

PRECAUTIONS AND ADVERSE REACTIONS

The most important potential adverse effect associated with use of these drugs is myocardial infarction (MI). The U.S. Food and Drug Administration (FDA) distinguished the risk of MI caused directly by these drugs from that caused by underlying conditions, such as hypertension, atherosclerotic heart disease, diabetes mellitus, and other atherogenic conditions. The FDA concluded that, when used according to the approved labeling, the drugs do not by themselves confer an increased risk of death. Increased oxygen demand and stress is placed on the cardiac muscle by sexual intercourse, however. Thus, coronary perfusion may be severely compromised, and cardiac failure may occur as a result. For that reason, any person with a history of MI, stroke, renal failure, hypertension, or diabetes mellitus and any person older than the age of 70 years should discuss plans to use these drugs with an internist or a cardiologist. The cardiac evaluation should specifically address exercise tolerance and the use of nitrates.

Use of PDE-5 inhibitors is contraindicated in persons who are taking organic nitrates in any form. In addition, amyl nitrate (poppers), a popular substance of abuse sometimes used by gay men and others to enhance the intensity of orgasm, should not be used with any of the erection-enhancing drugs. The combination of organic nitrates and PDE inhibitors can cause a precipitous lowering of blood pressure and can reduce coronary perfusion to the point of causing MI and death.

Adverse effects are dose dependent, occurring at higher rates with higher doses. The most common adverse effects are headache, flushing, and stomach pain. Other, less common adverse effects include nasal congestion, urinary tract infection, abnormal vision (colored tinge [usually blue], increased sensitivity to light, or blurred vision), diarrhea, dizziness, and rash. No cases of priapism were reported in premarketing trials. Supportive management is indicated in cases of overdose. Tadalafil has been associated with back and muscle pain in about 10 percent of patients.

Recently there have been 50 reports and 14 verified cases of a serious condition in men taking sildenafil called nonarteritic anterior ischemic optic neuropathy. This is an eye ailment that causes restriction of blood flow to the optic nerve and can result in permanent vision loss. The first symptoms appear within 24 hours after use of sildenafil and include blurred vision and some degree of vision loss. The incidence of this effect is very rare—1 in 1 million. In the reported cases, many patients had preexisting eye problems that may have increased their risk, and many had a history of heart disease and diabetes, which may indicate a vulnerability in these men to endothelial damage.

No data are available on the effects on human fetal growth and development or testicular morphological or functional changes.

Because these drugs are not considered an essential treatment, they should not be used during pregnancy.

DRUG INTERACTIONS

The major route of PDE-5 metabolism is through CYP 3A4, and the minor route is through CYP 2C9. Inducers or inhibitors of these enzymes, therefore, will affect the plasma concentration and half-life of sildenafil. For example, 800 mg of cimetidine (Tagamet), a nonspecific CYP inhibitor, increases plasma sildenafil concentrations by 56 percent, and erythromycin (E-mycin) increases plasma sildenafil concentrations by 182 percent. Other, stronger inhibitors of CYP 3A4 include ketoconazole (Nizoral), itraconazole (Sporanox), and mibefradil (Posicor). In contrast, rifampicin (Rifadin), a CYP 3A4 inducer, decreases plasma concentrations of sildenafil.

LABORATORY INTERFERENCES

No laboratory interferences have been described.

DOSING AND CLINICAL GUIDELINES

Sildenafil is available as 25-, 50-, and 100-mg tablets. The recommended dose of sildenafil is 50 mg taken by mouth 1 hour prior to intercourse. Sildenafil, however, may take effect within 30 minutes. The duration of the effect is usually 4 hours, but in healthy young men, the effect may persist for 8 to 12 hours. Based on effectiveness and adverse effects, the dose should be titrated between 25 and 100 mg. Sildenafil is recommended for use no more than once a day. The dosing guidelines for use by women, an off-label use, are the same as those for men.

Increased plasma concentrations of sildenafil can occur in persons older than 65 years of age and those with cirrhosis or severe renal impairment or using CYP 3A4 inhibitors. A starting dose of 25 mg should be used in these circumstances.

An investigational nasal spray formulation of sildenafil has been developed that acts within 5 to 15 minutes of administration. This formulation is highly water soluble, and it is rapidly absorbed directly into the bloodstream. Such a formulation would permit more ease of use.

Vardenafil is supplied in 2.5-, 5-, 10-, and 20-mg tablets. The initial dose is usually 10 mg taken with or without food about 1 hour before sexual activity. The dose can be increased to a maximum of 20 mg or decreased to 5 mg based on efficacy and side effects. The maximal dosing frequency is once per day. As with sildenafil, doses may have to be adjusted in patients with hepatic impairment or in patients using certain CYP 3A4 inhibitors.

The recommended dose of tadalafil is 10 mg before sexual activity, which may be increased to 20 mg or decreased to 5 mg, depending on efficacy and side effects. Because of its long half-life, it should probably not be used more than once every 36 hours, although the manufacturer states that once-a-day use is acceptable for most patients. Similar cautions apply as mentioned earlier in patients with hepatic impairment and in those taking concomitant potent inhibitors of CYP 3A4. As with other PDE-5 inhibitors, concomitant use of nitrates in any form is contraindicated.

▲ 32.28 Selective Serotonin–Norepinephrine Reuptake Inhibitors

Venlafaxine (Effexor) and duloxetine (Cymbalta) are selective serotonin–norepinephrine reuptake inhibitors (SNRIs). Originally marketed as an antidepressant, venlafaxine is now also indicated for the treatment of generalized anxiety and social anxiety disorders. Duloxetine is indicated for the treatment of depression, generalized anxiety disorder, and painful diabetic neuropathy and is awaiting the indication for stress urinary incontinence.

Venlafaxine and duloxetine are not unique with respect to their dual action. Tricyclic and tetracyclic antidepressants (TCAs) also inhibit reuptake of norepinephrine and serotonin. TCAs, however, also possess numerous other receptor properties, such as muscarinic, adrenergic, and histaminergic effects, and thus are not considered selective.

VENLAFAXINE

Pharmacological Actions

Venlafaxine is well absorbed from the gastrointestinal tract. The extended-release formulation of venlafaxine (Effexor XR) and the metabolite O-desmethylvenlafaxine (ODV) reach peak plasma concentrations in 5.5 and 9 hours, respectively. Venlafaxine has a half-life of about 3.5 hours, and ODV has a half-life of 9 hours. It is metabolized by hepatic cytochrome P450 (CYP) 2D6. Thus, inhibitors of this isozyme, such as quinidine or paroxetine, reduce the formation of ODV. Venlafaxine is not highly bound to plasma proteins.

Venlafaxine is a potent inhibitor of serotonin and norepinephrine reuptake and a weak inhibitor of dopamine reuptake. It does not have activity at muscarinic, nicotinic, histaminergic, opioid, or adrenergic receptors, and it is not active as a monoamine oxidase inhibitor.

Therapeutic Indications

Depression.   The U.S. Food and Drug Administration (FDA) does not recognize any class of antidepressant as being more effective than any other. This does not mean that differences do not exist, but no study has sufficiently demonstrated such superiority. There is some evidence to suggest that venlafaxine has a potential to induce higher rates of remission in depressed patients than do the selective serotonin reuptake inhibitors (SSRIs). This difference of the venlafaxine advantage is about 6 percent.

Generalized Anxiety Disorder.   The extended-release formulation of venlafaxine is approved for treatment of generalized anxiety disorder. In clinical trials lasting 6 months, doses of 75 to 225 mg a day were effective against insomnia, poor concentration, restlessness, irritability, and excessive muscle tension related to generalized anxiety disorder.

Social Anxiety Disorder.   The extended-release formulation of venlafaxine is approved for treatment of social anxiety disorder. Its efficacy was established in 12-week studies.

Panic Disorder.   The extended-release formulation of venlafaxine is also approved for treatment of panic disorder.

Other Indications.   Case reports and uncontrolled studies have indicated that venlafaxine may be beneficial in the treatment of obsessive-compulsive disorder, agoraphobia, attention-deficit/hyperactivity disorder, and in patients with a dual diagnosis of depression and cocaine dependence. It has also been used in chronic pain syndromes with good effect.

Precautions and Adverse Reactions

The frequency of specific side effects varied in studies involving different disorders. Overall, the most common adverse reactions are nausea, somnolence, dry mouth, dizziness, nervousness, constipation, asthenia, anxiety, anorexia, blurred vision, abnormal ejaculation or orgasm, erectile disturbances, and impotence. Sweating is also more common with venlafaxine than with the SSRIs (and is frequently treated with terazosin). The incidence of nausea can be considerably reduced by initiating treatment using 37.5-mg per day capsules.

Abrupt discontinuation of venlafaxine use can produce a discontinuation syndrome consisting of dizziness, anxiety, nausea, somnolence, paresthesias, and insomnia. Therefore, venlafaxine use should be tapered gradually over 2 to 4 weeks.

Venlafaxine can cause an increase in blood pressure (BP) in some persons. Diastolic hypertension was seen more often in patients treated with doses of venlafaxine greater than 300 mg per day, a dose higher than needed in most patients.

A common misconception is that risk of venlafaxine-induced hypertension is greater among persons with preexisting hypertension. It is wise periodically to monitor the BP of any patient taking venlafaxine. If a patient develops significant rise in BP but otherwise shows a good therapeutic response, it is reasonable to consider either lowering the dose, adding antihypertensive therapy, or both.

Venlafaxine can cause mydriasis, so patients with raised intraocular pressure or those at risk for acute narrow-angle glaucoma should be monitored during venlafaxine treatment. As in the case of SSRIs, abnormal bleeding or ecchymosis may be associated with venlafaxine use, the result of serotonin-related impairment of platelet aggregation.

The pharmacokinetic dispositions of both venlafaxine and ODV are altered in patients with hepatic cirrhosis. Venlafaxine elimination half-life is prolonged by about 30 percent, and its clearance is decreased by about 50 percent. ODV elimination half-life is also prolonged (by about 60 percent), and its clearance decreased by about 30 percent. In patients with more severe cirrhosis, there may be a 90 percent decrease in venlafaxine clearance. Dose adjustment, thus, is necessary in patients with liver disease.

Information concerning use of venlafaxine by pregnant and nursing women is not available. Venlafaxine and ODV are excreted in human milk. Clinicians should carefully weigh the risks and benefits of venlafaxine use by pregnant and nursing women.

Drug Interactions

Cimetidine (Tagamet) appears to inhibit the first-pass hepatic metabolism of venlafaxine and to raise the levels of the unmetabolized drug. Because the metabolite is mainly responsible for the therapeutic effect, this interaction is of concern only in persons with preexisting hypertension or hepatic disease, in whom this combination should be avoided. Combined use of sustained-release bupropion (Wellbutrin SR) has been shown to increase plasma concentrations of venlafaxine. Venlafaxine may raise plasma concentrations of concurrently administered haloperidol (Haldol). As with all antidepressant medications, venlafaxine should not be used within 14 days of the use of monoamine oxidase inhibitors, and it may potentiate the sedative effects of other drugs that act on the central nervous system.

Laboratory Interferences

No data are available on laboratory interferences with venlafaxine.

Dosing and Administration

Venlafaxine is available in 25-, 37.5-, 50-, 75-, and 100-mg tablets and 37.5-, 75-, and 150-mg extended-release capsules. The tablets and the extended-release capsules are equally potent, and persons stabilized with one can switch to an equivalent dose of the other. The immediate-release tablets are rarely used because of their tendency to cause nausea and need for multiple daily doses, and so the dosing recommendations that follow refer to use of the extended-release capsules.

In depressed persons, venlafaxine demonstrates a dose-response curve. The initial therapeutic dose is 75 mg a day, given once a day. Most persons, however, are started at a dose of 37.5 mg for 4 to 7 days to minimize adverse effects, particularly nausea. A convenient starter kit for the drug contains a 1-week supply of both the 37.5- and 75-mg strengths. Should a rapid titration be preferred, the dose can be raised to 150 mg per day after day 4. As a rule, the dose can be raised in increments of 75 mg a day every 4 or more days. Although the recommended upper dose of the extended-release preparation (Effexor XR) is 225 mg per day, it is approved by the FDA for use at doses up to 375 mg a day. The dose of venlafaxine should be halved in persons with significantly diminished hepatic or renal function. If discontinued, venlafaxine use should be gradually tapered over 2 to 4 weeks to avoid withdrawal symptoms.

Minor differences exist in the doses used for major depression, generalized anxiety disorder, and social anxiety disorder. In the treatment of these disorders, for example, a dose-response effect has not been found. In addition, lower mean doses are typically used, with most patients taking 75 to 150 mg per day.

DULOXETINE

Pharmacological Actions

Duloxetine is formulated as a delayed-release capsule to reduce the risk of severe nausea associated with the drug. It is well absorbed, but a 2-hour delay occurs before absorption begins. Peak plasma concentrations occur 6 hours after ingestion. Food delays the time to achieve maximal concentrations from 6 to 10 hours and reduces the extent of absorption by about 10 percent. Duloxetine has an elimination half-life of about 12 hours (range 8 to 17 hours). Steady-state plasma concentrations occur after 3 days. Elimination is mainly through the isozymes CYP 2D6 and CYP 1A2. Duloxetine undergoes extensive hepatic metabolism to numerous metabolites. About 70 percent of the drug appears in the urine as metabolites, and about 20 percent is excreted in the feces. Duloxetine is 90 percent protein bound.

Therapeutic Indications

Depression and Generalized Anxiety Disorder (GAD).   In contrast to venlafaxine, a small number of studies have compared duloxetine with SSRIs in depression. These studies are suggestive of some advantage in efficacy with duloxetine. In GAD, higher doses are also used with good results.

Neuropathic Pain Associated with Diabetes and Stress Urinary Incontinence.   Duloxetine is the first drug to be approved by the FDA as a treatment for neuropathic pain associated with diabetes. The drug has been studied for its effects on physical symptoms, including pain, in depressed patients, but these effects have not been compared with those seen with other widely used agents such as venlafaxine and the tricyclic antidepressants. Duloxetine is awaiting approval as a treatment for stress urinary incontinence—the inability to voluntarily control bladder voiding—which is the most frequent type of incontinence in women. The action of duloxetine in the treatment of stress urinary incontinence is associated with its effects in the sacral spinal cord, which in turn increase the activity of the striated urethral sphincter. Duloxetine will be marketed under the name Yantreve for this indication.

Although duloxetine is approved for the treatment of diabetic peripheral neuropathic pain, it may worsen control of blood sugar levels. Pooled data from clinical trials show that short-term treatment with duloxetine causes an increase in fasting glucose and hemoglobin A1c levels. Body weight decreased with short-term duloxetine treatment but increased during long-term treatment. Modest increases in cholesterol may occur during duloxetine therapy.

Precautions and Adverse Reactions

The most common adverse reactions are nausea, dry mouth, dizziness, constipation, fatigue, decreased appetite, anorexia, somnolence, and increased sweating. Nausea was the most common side effect leading to treatment discontinuation in clinical trials. The true incidence of sexual dysfunction is not known, nor are the long-term effects on body weight. In clinical trials, treatment with duloxetine was associated with mean increases in BP averaging 2 mm Hg systolic and 0.5 mm Hg diastolic versus placebo. No studies have compared BP effects of venlafaxine and duloxetine at equivalent therapeutic doses.

Patients with substantial alcohol use should not be treated with duloxetine because of possible hepatic effects. It also should not be prescribed for patients with hepatic insufficiency and end-stage renal disease or for patients with uncontrolled narrow-angle glaucoma.

Abrupt discontinuation of duloxetine should be avoided because it can produce a discontinuation syndrome similar to that of venlafaxine. A gradual dose reduction is recommended.

Because of limited clinical experience with duloxetine, risks associated with its use by pregnant and nursing women are not available. Clinicians should avoid the use of duloxetine by pregnant and nursing women unless the potential benefits justify the potential risks.

Drug Interactions

Duloxetine is a moderate inhibitor of CYP 450 enzymes.

Laboratory Interferences

No data are available on laboratory interferences with duloxetine.

Dosing and Administration

Duloxetine is available in 20-, 30-, and 60-mg tablets. The recommended therapeutic, and maximal, dose is 60 mg per day. The 20- and 30-mg doses are useful for either initial therapy or for twice-daily use as strategies to reduce side effects. In clinical trials, doses of up to 120 mg per day were studied, but no consistent advantage in efficacy was noted at doses higher than 60 mg per day. Duloxetine, thus, does not appear to demonstrate a dose-response curve. Difficulties in tolerability were seen, however, with single doses above 60 mg. Accordingly, when doses of 80 and 120 mg per day were used, they were administered as 40 or 60 mg twice daily. Because of limited clinical experience with duloxetine, it remains to be seen to what extent doses above 60 mg per day will be necessary and whether, in fact, this will require divided doses to make the drug tolerable.

Other SNRIs

Desvenlafaxine Succinate (DVS) (Pristiq).
DVS is the salt form of the isolated major active metabolite of venlafaxine, developed as separated drug. Like venlafaxine, DVS is mechanistically an SNRI. It has been developed for the treatment of depression and for the alleviation of vasomotor symptoms (VMS) associated with menopause. Symptoms of VMS include hot flashes and night sweats. There are also plans to pursue DVS indications for fibromyalgia and diabetic neuropathic pain.

As is typical of the SNRI class, most common side effects of DVS are abdominal pain, asthenia, anorexia, constipation, dry mouth, nausea, vomiting, dizziness, insomnia, nervousness, somnolence, sweating, tremor, vertigo, increased blood pressure, and abnormal ejaculation. The optimal dosing of DVS has not been established, but in clinical trials, doses of 200- to 300-mg were effective in treating depression, whereas doses up to 600 mg were needed to alleviate VMS. At these doses, no effect on the QT interval was observed.

Milnacipran.
This is another SNRI that has been available in many countries as an antidepressant. It has not been studied in the United States solely as a treatment for fibromyalgia. No drugs are FDA-approved for use in the treatment of fibromyalgia.

Sibutramine (Meridia).
This is an SNRI marketed as a short-term antiobesity treatment. The effectiveness and safety of the drug beyond 1 year have not been studied. Sibutramine has not been shown to act as an antidepressant. Side effects are similar to those of other SNRIs and include dose-related increase in blood pressure, heart rate, and arrhythmias.

▲ 32.29 Selective Serotonin Reuptake Inhibitors

The first selective serotonin reuptake inhibitor (SSRI), fluoxetine (Prozac), which was introduced in 1987, altered attitudes about pharmacological treatment of depression. The reasons for this included the fact that initial side effects of fluoxetine were generally better tolerated than those of existing treatments, such as the tricyclic antidepressants (TCAs) and monoamine oxidase inhibitors (MAOIs), and the simplicity of dosing of fluoxetine.

Subsequently, other SSRIs have been introduced, all of which share the same basic properties of fluoxetine. Since 1990, the list of approved indications for drugs in the class has expanded to include not only depression, but also obsessive-compulsive disorder (OCD), panic disorder, generalized anxiety disorder, premenstrual dysphoric disorder, social anxiety disorder, and eating disorders (Table 32.29–1). All SSRIs appear to be equally effective in the treatment of these disorders.

The SSRIs are each structurally and chemically distinct. Escitalopram (Lexapro), an isomer of citalopram (Celexa), is the only exception. This molecular diversity explains why individual responses to and tolerability of SSRIs are so varied. The SSRIs possess significantly different pharmacokinetic profiles, as suggested by their diverse chemical structures.

Table 32.29–1
Approved Indications of the Selective Serotonin Reuptake Inhibitors in the United States for Adult and Pediatric Populations

	Citalopram (Celexa)	Escitalopram (Lexapro)	Fluoxetine (Prozac)	Fluvoxamine (Luvox)	Paroxetine (Paxil)	Sertraline (Zoloft)
Major depressive disorder	Adult	Adult	Adult[a] and pediatric	—	Adult[c]	Adult
Generalized anxiety disorder	—	Adult	—	—	Adult	—
OCD	—	—	Adult and pediatric	Adult and pediatric	Adult	Adult and pediatric
Panic disorder	—	—	Adult	—	Adult[c]	Adult
PTSD	—	—	—	—	Adult	Adult
Social anxiety disorder	—	—	—	—	Adult[c]	Adult
Bulimia nervosa	—	—	Adult	—	—	—
Premenstrual dysphoric disorder	—	—	Adult[b]	—	Adult[d]	Adult

OCD, obsessive-compulsive disorder; PTSD, posttraumatic stress disorder.
[a] Weekly fluoxetine is approved for continuation and maintenance therapy in adults.
[b] Marketed as Sarafem.
[c] Paroxetine and paroxetine controlled release.
[d] Paroxetine controlled release is approved for premenstrual dysphoric disorder.

PHARMACOLOGICAL ACTIONS

Pharmacokinetics

The most significant difference among the SSRIs is their broad range of serum half-lives. Fluoxetine has the longest half-life: 4 to 6 days; its active metabolite has a half-life of 7 to 9 days. The half-life of sertraline is 26 hours, and its less active metabolite has a half-life of 3 to 5 days. The half-lives of the other three, which do not have metabolites with significant pharmacological activity, are 35 hours for citalopram, 27 to 32 hours for escitalopram, 21 hours for paroxetine, and 15 hours for fluvoxamine. As a rule, SSRIs are well absorbed after oral administration and have their peak effects in the range of 3 to 8 hours. Absorption of sertraline may be slightly enhanced by food.

Differences in plasma protein binding percentages are also found among the SSRIs, with sertraline, fluoxetine, and paroxetine being the most highly bound and escitalopram being the least bound.

All SSRIs are metabolized in the liver by the cytochrome P450 (CYP) enzymes. Because SSRIs have such a wide therapeutic index, it is rare that other drugs produce problematic increases in SSRI concentrations. The most important drug–drug interactions involving the SSRIs occur as a result of the SSRIs inhibiting the metabolism of a coadministered medication. Each of the SSRIs possesses a potential for slowing or blocking the metabolism of many drugs (Table 32.29–2). Fluvoxamine is the most problematic of the drugs in this respect. It has a marked effect on several of the CYP enzymes. Examples of clinically significant interactions include fluvoxamine and theophylline (Theo-Dur) through CYP 1A2 interaction; fluvoxamine and clozapine (Clozaril) through CYP 1A2 inhibition; and fluvoxamine with alprazolam (Xanax) or clonazepam (Klonopin) through CYP 3A4 inhibition. Fluoxetine and paroxetine also possess significant effects on the CYP 2D6 isozyme, which may interfere with the efficacy of opiate analogs, such as codeine and hydrocodone, by blocking the conversion of these agents to their active form. Thus, coadministration of fluoxetine and paroxetine with an opiate interferes with its analgesic effects. Sertraline, citalopram, and escitalopram are least likely to complicate treatment because of interactions.

Pharmacodynamics

The SSRIs are believed to exert their therapeutic effects through 5-HT reuptake inhibition. They derive their name from the fact that they have little effect on reuptake of norepinephrine or dopamine. Often, adequate clinical activity and saturation of the 5-HT transporters are achieved at starting doses. As a rule, higher doses do not increase antidepressant efficacy, but they may increase the risk of adverse effects.

Citalopram and escitalopram are the most selective inhibitors of serotonin reuptake, with very little inhibition of norepinephrine or dopamine reuptake and very low affinities for histamine H_1, γ-aminobutyric acid, or benzodiazepine receptors. The other SSRIs have a similar profile, except that fluoxetine weakly inhibits norepinephrine reuptake and binds to 5-HT_{2C} receptors; sertraline weakly inhibits norepinephrine and dopamine reuptake; and paroxetine has significant anticholinergic activity at higher doses and binds to nitric oxide synthase.

A pharmacodynamic interaction appears to underlie the antidepressant effects of combined fluoxetine–olanzapine. When taken together, these drugs increase brain concentrations of norepinephrine. Concomitant use of SSRIs and drugs in the triptan class (sumatriptan [Imitrex], naratriptan [Amerge], rizatriptan [Maxalt], and zolmitriptan [Zomig]) may result in a serious pharmacodynamic interaction, the development of a serotonin syndrome (see Precautions and Adverse Reactions). Many people, however, use triptans while taking a low dose of an SSRI for headache prophylaxis without adverse reaction. A similar reaction may occur when SSRIs are combined with tramadol (Ultram).

THERAPEUTIC INDICATIONS

Depression

In the United States, all SSRIs other than fluvoxamine have been approved by the U.S. Food and Drug Administration (FDA) for treatment of depression. Several studies have found that antidepressants with serotonin–norepinephrine activity, drugs such as the MAOIs, TCAs, venlafaxine, and mirtazapine, produce higher rates of remission than SSRIs in head-to-head studies. The continued role of SSRIs as first-line treatments, thus, reflects their simplicity of use, safety, and broad spectrum of action.

Table 32.29–2
Cytochrome P450 Inhibitory Potential of Commonly Prescribed Antidepressants

Relative Rank	CYP 1A2	CYP 2C	CYP 2D6	CYP 3A
Higher	Fluvoxamine (Luvox)	Fluoxetine Fluvoxamine	Bupropion Fluoxetine Paroxetine	Fluvoxamine Nefazodone Tricyclics
Moderate	Tertiary amine tricyclics Fluoxetine (Prozac)	Sertraline	Secondary amine tricyclics Citalopram (Celexa) Escitalopram (Lexapro) Sertraline	Fluoxetine Sertraline
Low or minimal	Bupropion (Wellbutrin) Mirtazapine (Remeron) Nefazodone (Serzone) Paroxetine (Paxil) Sertraline (Zoloft) Venlafaxine (Effexor)	Paroxetine Venlafaxine (Effexor)	Fluvoxamine Mirtazapine Nefazodone Venlafaxine	Citalopram Escitalopram Mirtazapine Paroxetine Venlafaxine

CYP, cytochrome P450.

Direct comparisons of individual SSRIs have not revealed any to be consistently superior to another. Nevertheless, considerable diversity is seen in response to the various SSRIs among individuals. For example, more than 50 percent of people who respond poorly to one SSRI will respond favorably to another. Thus, before shifting to non-SSRI antidepressants, it is most reasonable to try other agents in the SSRI class for persons who did not respond to the first SSRI.

Some clinicians have attempted to select a particular SSRI for a specific person on the basis of the drug's unique adverse effect profile. For example, thinking that fluoxetine is an activating and stimulating SSRI, some may assume that it is a better choice for an abulic person than paroxetine, which is presumed to be a sedating SSRI. These differences, however, usually vary from person to person.

Suicide. In the late 1980s, a widely publicized report suggested an association between fluoxetine use and violent acts, including suicide, but many subsequent reviews have failed to confirm this association. A few patients, however, become especially anxious and agitated when started on an SSRI. Thus, all suicidally depressed patients should be closely monitored during the period of maximal risk—the first few days and weeks they are taking SSRIs. It is important to keep in mind that SSRIs, as with all antidepressants, prevent potential suicides as a result of their primary action—the shortening and prevention of depressive episodes.

Depression during Pregnancy and Postpartum. Rates of relapse of major depression during pregnancy among women who discontinue, attempt to discontinue, or modify their antidepressant regimen are extremely high. Rates range from 68 to 100 percent of patients. Thus, many women need to continue taking their medication during pregnancy and postpartum. The impact of maternal depression on infant development is unknown. No increased risk is seen for major congenital malformations following exposure to SSRIs during pregnancy. Thus, the risk of relapse into depression when a newly pregnant mother is taken off SSRIs is several times higher than the risk to the fetus of exposure to SSRIs.

Some evidence suggests increased rates of special care nursery admissions after delivery for children of mothers taking SSRIs. In addition, a potential exists for a discontinuation syndrome with paroxetine. No clinically significant neonatal complications are associated with SSRI use.

Studies that have followed children into their early school years have failed to find any perinatal complications, congenital fetal anomalies, decreases in global intelligence quotient, language delays, or specific behavioral problems attributable to the use of fluoxetine during pregnancy.

Postpartum depression (with or without psychotic features) affects a small percentage of mothers. Some clinicians start administering SSRIs if the postpartum blues extend beyond a few weeks or if a woman becomes depressed during pregnancy. The head start afforded by starting SSRI administration during pregnancy if a woman is at risk for postpartum depression also protects the newborn, toward whom the woman may have harmful thoughts after parturition.

The SSRIs are secreted in breast milk, but the plasma of babies breast-feeding from mothers who are taking SSRIs is typically very low. In some cases, however, concentrations have been reported that are higher than average. No decision regarding the use of an SSRI is risk free. It is important to document that communication of potential risks to the patient has taken place.

Depression in the Elderly and Medically Ill. SSRIs are safe and well tolerated when used to treat the elderly and medically ill. As a class, they have little or no cardiotoxic, anticholinergic, antihistaminergic, or α-adrenergic adverse effects. Paroxetine does have some anticholinergic activity, which may lead to constipation and worsening of cognition. SSRIs can produce subtle cognitive deficits, prolonged bleeding time, and hyponatremia, all of which may have an impact on the health of this population. SSRIs are effective in poststroke depression and dramatically reduce the symptom of crying.

Depression in Children. SSRIs are widely accepted as useful antidepressants in the treatment of child and adolescent depressions. In 2004, the FDA accumulated data that found an increase in suicidal thoughts and behavior in children taking these drugs. As a result, they placed a "black box" warning on the label cautioning against their use. Subsequently, the use of this class of drug in children dropped markedly. Reviews since then have shown that accompanying this decrease in prescribing SSRIs was an increase in the rate of suicide. This correlation prompted experts in the field to suggest that the "black box" warning be removed and that psychiatrists be encouraged to use these drugs in their depressed patients. Careful monitoring of suicidal patients should always be practiced, regardless of the type of medication employed.

Anxiety Disorders

Obsessive-Compulsive Disorder. Fluvoxamine, paroxetine, sertraline, and fluoxetine are indicated for treatment of OCD in persons older than the age of 18 years. Fluvoxamine and sertraline have also been approved for treatment of pediatric OCD (ages 6 to 17 years). About 50 percent of persons with OCD begin to show symptoms in childhood or adolescence, and more than half of these respond favorably to medication. Beneficial responses can be dramatic. Long-term data support the model of OCD as a genetically determined, lifelong condition that is best treated continuously with drugs and cognitive-behavioral therapy from the onset of symptoms in childhood throughout the lifespan.

The SSRI doses for OCD may need to be higher than those required to treat depression. Although some response can be seen in the first few weeks of treatment, it may take several months for the maximal effects to become evident. Patients who fail to obtain adequate relief of their OCD symptoms with an SSRI often benefit from the addition of a small dose of risperidone (Risperdal). Apart from the extrapyramidal side effects of Risperdal, patients should be monitored for increases in prolactin levels when this combination is used. Clinically, hyperprolactinemia may manifest as gynecomastia and galactorrhea (in both men and women) and loss of menses.

A number of disorders are now considered to be within the OCD spectrum. This includes a number of conditions and symptoms characterized by nonsuicidal self-mutilation, such as trichotillomania, eyebrow-picking, nose-picking, nail-biting, compulsive picking of skin blemishes, and cutting. Patients with these behaviors benefit from treatment with SSRIs. Other spectrum disorders include compulsive gambling, compulsive shopping, hypochondriasis, and body dysmorphic disorder.

Panic Disorder.   Paroxetine and sertraline are indicated for treatment of panic disorder, with or without agoraphobia. These agents work less rapidly than do the benzodiazepines alprazolam and clonazepam but are far superior to benzodiazepines for treatment of panic disorder with comorbid depression. Citalopram, fluvoxamine, and fluoxetine also can reduce spontaneous or induced panic attacks. Because fluoxetine can initially heighten anxiety symptoms, persons with panic disorder must begin by taking small doses (5 mg a day) and have the dose raised slowly. Low doses of benzodiazepines may be given to manage this side effect.

Social Anxiety Disorder.   SSRIs are effective agents in the treatment of social phobia. They reduce both symptoms and disability. The response rate is comparable to that seen with the MAOI phenelzine (Nardil), the previous standard treatment. SSRIs are safer to use than MAOIs or benzodiazepines.

Posttraumatic Stress Disorder.   Pharmacotherapy for posttraumatic stress disorder (PTSD) must target specific symptoms in three clusters: reexperiencing, avoidance, and hyperarousal. For long-term treatment, SSRIs appear to have a broader spectrum of therapeutic effects on specific PTSD symptom clusters than do TCAs and MAOIs. Benzodiazepine augmentation is useful in the acute symptomatic state. SSRIs are associated with marked improvement of both intrusive and avoidant symptoms.

Generalized Anxiety Disorder.   SSRIs may be useful for the treatment of specific phobias, generalized anxiety disorder, and separation anxiety disorder. A thorough, individualized evaluation is the first approach, with particular attention to identifying conditions amenable to drug therapy. In addition, cognitive-behavioral or other psychotherapies can be added for greater efficacy.

Bulimia Nervosa and Other Eating Disorders

Fluoxetine is indicated for treatment of bulimia, which is best done in the context of psychotherapy. Doses of 60 mg a day are significantly more effective than 20 mg a day. In several well-controlled studies, fluoxetine in a dose of 60 mg a day was superior to placebo in reducing binge eating and induced vomiting. Some experts recommend an initial course of cognitive-behavioral therapy alone. If no response occurs in 3 to 6 weeks, then fluoxetine administration is added. The appropriate duration of treatment with fluoxetine and psychotherapy has not been determined.

Fluvoxamine was not effective at a statistically significant level in one double-blind, placebo-controlled trial for inpatients with bulimia.

Anorexia Nervosa.   Fluoxetine has been used in inpatient treatment of anorexia nervosa to attempt to control comorbid mood disturbances and obsessive-compulsive symptoms. At least two careful studies, one of 7 months and one of 24 months, however, failed to find that fluoxetine affected the overall outcome and the maintenance of weight. Effective treatments for

anorexia include cognitive-behavioral, interpersonal, psychodynamic, and family therapies in addition to a trial with SSRIs.

Obesity.   Fluoxetine, in combination with a behavioral program, has been shown to be only modestly beneficial for weight loss. A significant percentage of all persons who take SSRIs, including fluoxetine, lose weight initially, but later they may gain weight. All SSRIs may cause initial weight gain, however.

Premenstrual Dysphoric Disorder

Premenstrual dysphoric disorder is characterized by debilitating mood and behavioral changes in the week preceding menstruation that interfere with normal functioning. Sertraline, paroxetine, fluoxetine, and fluvoxamine have been reported to reduce the symptoms of premenstrual dysphoric disorder. Controlled trials of fluoxetine and sertraline administered either throughout the cycle or only during the luteal phase (the 2-week period between ovulation and menstruation) showed both schedules to be equally effective.

An additional observation of unclear significance was that fluoxetine was associated with changing the duration of the menstrual period by more than 4 days, either lengthening or shortening it. The effects of SSRIs on menstrual cycle length are mostly unknown and may warrant careful monitoring in women of reproductive age.

Off-Label Uses

Premature Ejaculation.   The antiorgasmic effects of SSRIs make them useful as a treatment for men with premature ejaculation. SSRIs permit intercourse for a significantly longer period and are reported to improve sexual satisfaction in couples in which the man has premature ejaculation. Fluoxetine and sertraline have been shown to be effective for this purpose.

Paraphilias.   SSRIs may reduce obsessive-compulsive behavior in people with paraphilias. SSRIs diminish the average time per day spent in unconventional sexual fantasies, urges, and activities. Evidence suggests a greater response for sexual obsessions than for paraphilic behavior.

Autism.   Obsessive-compulsive behavior, poor social relatedness, and aggression are prominent autistic features that may respond to serotonergic agents such as SSRIs and clomipramine. Sertraline and fluvoxamine have been shown in controlled and open-label trials to mitigate aggressiveness, self-injurious behavior, repetitive behaviors, some degree of language delay, and, rarely, lack of social relatedness in adults with autistic spectrum disorders. Fluoxetine has been reported to be effective for features of autism in children, adolescents, and adults.

PRECAUTIONS AND ADVERSE REACTIONS

The side effects of SSRIs need to be considered in terms of their onset, duration, and severity. For example, nausea and jitteriness are early, generally mild, and time-limited side effects.

Sexual Dysfunction

All SSRIs cause sexual dysfunction, and it is the most common adverse effect of SSRIs associated with long-term treatment. It has an estimated incidence of between 50 and 80 percent. The most common complaints are anorgasmia, inhibited orgasm, and decreased libido. Some studies suggest that sexual dysfunction is dose related, but this has not been clearly established. Unlike most of the other adverse effects of SSRIs, sexual inhibition rarely resolves in the first few weeks of use, but it usually continues as long as the drug is taken. In some cases, there may be improvement over time.

Strategies to counteract SSRI-induced sexual dysfunction are too numerous to mention, and none has been proved to be very effective. Some reports suggest decreasing the dose or adding bupropion. Reports have described successful treatment of SSRI-induced sexual dysfunction with agents such as sildenafil (Viagra), which are used to treat erectile dysfunction. Ultimately, patients may need to be switched to antidepressants that do not interfere with sexual functioning—drugs such as mirtazapine or bupropion.

Gastrointestinal Adverse Effects

Gastrointestinal (GI) side effects, which are very common, are mediated largely through effects on the serotonin $5HT_3$ receptor. The most frequent GI complaints are nausea, diarrhea, anorexia, vomiting, flatulence, and dyspepsia. Sertraline and fluvoxamine produce the most intense GI symptoms. Delayed-release paroxetine, when compared with the immediate-release preparation of paroxetine, has less intense GI side effects during the first week of treatment. Paroxetine, because of its anticholinergic activity, frequently causes constipation, however. Nausea and loose stools are usually dose related and transient, resolving within a few weeks. Sometimes, flatulence and diarrhea persist, especially during sertraline treatment. Initial anorexia can also occur and is most common with fluoxetine. SSRI-induced appetite and weight loss begin as soon as the drug is taken and peak at 20 weeks, after which weight often returns to baseline. Up to one third of persons taking SSRIs gain weight, sometimes more than 20 pounds. This effect is mediated through a metabolic mechanism, increase in appetite, or both. It happens gradually and is usually resistant to diet and exercise regimens. Paroxetine is associated with more frequent and more pronounced weight gain than the other SSRIs, especially among young women.

Headaches

The incidence of headache in SSRI trials was 18 to 20 percent, only 1 percentage point higher than the placebo rate. Fluoxetine is the SSRI most likely to cause headache. On the other hand, all SSRIs are effective prophylaxis against both migraine and tension-type headaches in many persons.

Central Nervous System Adverse Effects

Anxiety.   Fluoxetine can cause anxiety, particularly in the first few weeks. These initial effects, however, usually give way to an overall reduction in anxiety after a few weeks. Increased anxiety is caused considerably less frequently by paroxetine or escitalopram, which may be a better choice if sedation is desired, as in mixed anxiety and depressive disorders.

Insomnia and Sedation.   The major effect SSRIs exert in the area of insomnia and sedation is improved sleep resulting from treatment of depression and anxiety. As many as one

fourth of persons taking SSRIs, however, note either trouble sleeping or excessive somnolence or overwhelming fatigue. Fluoxetine is the most SSRI likely to cause insomnia, for which reason it is often taken in the morning. Sertraline and fluvoxamine are about equally likely to cause insomnia as somnolence, and citalopram and, especially, paroxetine often cause somnolence. Escitalopram is more likely to interfere with sleep than its isomer, citalopram. Some persons benefit from taking their SSRI dose before going to bed, whereas others prefer to take it the morning. SSRI-induced insomnia can be treated with benzodiazepines, trazodone (Desyrel) (clinicians must explain the risk of priapism), or other sedating medicines. Significant SSRI-induced somnolence often requires switching to use of another SSRI or bupropion.

Other Sleep Effects.   Many persons taking SSRIs report recalling extremely vivid dreams or nightmares. They describe sleep as "busy." Other sleep effects of the SSRIs include bruxism, restless legs, nocturnal myoclonus, and sweating.

Emotional Blunting.   Emotional blunting is a largely overlooked but frequent side effect associated with chronic SSRI use. Patients report an inability to cry in response to emotional situations, a feeling of apathy or indifference, or a restriction in the intensity of emotional experiences. This side effect often leads to treatment discontinuation even when the drugs are providing relief from depression or anxiety.

Yawning.   Close clinical observation of patients taking SSRIs reveals an increase in yawning. This side effect is not a reflection of fatigue or of poor nocturnal sleep but is the result of SSRI effects on the hypothalamus.

Seizures.   Seizures have been reported in 0.1 to 0.2 percent of all patients treated with SSRIs, an incidence comparable to that reported with other antidepressants and not significantly different from that with placebo. Seizures are more frequent at the highest doses of SSRIs (e.g., fluoxetine 100 mg a day or higher).

Extrapyramidal Symptoms.   SSRIs may rarely cause akathisia, dystonia, tremor, cogwheel rigidity, torticollis, opisthotonos, gait disorders, and bradykinesia. Rare cases of tardive dyskinesia have been reported. People with well-controlled Parkinson's disease may experience acute worsening of their motor symptoms when they take SSRIs.

Anticholinergic Effects

Paroxetine has mild anticholinergic activity that causes dry mouth, constipation, and sedation in a dose-dependent fashion. Nevertheless, most persons taking paroxetine do not experience cholinergic adverse effects. Other SSRIs are associated with dry mouth, but this effect is not mediated by muscarinic activity.

Hematological Adverse Effects

The SSRIs can cause functional impairment of platelet aggregation but not a reduction in platelet number. This is manifested by easy bruising and excessive or prolonged bleeding. When patients exhibit these signs, a test for bleeding time should be performed. Special monitoring is suggested when patients use SSRIs in conjunction with anticoagulants or aspirin.

Electrolyte and Glucose Disturbances

The SSRIs can acutely decrease glucose concentrations; therefore, diabetic patients should be carefully monitored. Rare cases of SSRI-associated hyponatremia and the secretion of inappropriate antidiuretic hormone have been seen in patients treated with diuretics who are also water deprived.

Endocrine and Allergic Reactions

The SSRIs can decrease prolactin levels and cause mammoplasia and galactorrhea in both men and women. Breast changes are reversible on discontinuation of the drug, but this can take several months to occur.

Various types of rashes appear in about 4 percent of patients; in a small subset of these patients, the allergic reaction may generalize and involve the pulmonary system, resulting rarely in fibrotic damage and dyspnea. SSRI treatment may have to be discontinued in patients with drug-related rashes.

Serotonin Syndrome

Concurrent administration of an SSRI with an MAOI, L-tryptophan, or lithium can raise plasma serotonin concentrations to toxic levels, producing a constellation of symptoms called the *serotonin syndrome*. This serious and possibly fatal syndrome of serotonin overstimulation is composed, in order of appearance as the condition worsens, of (1) diarrhea; (2) restlessness; (3) extreme agitation, hyperreflexia, and autonomic instability with possible rapid fluctuations in vital signs; (4) myoclonus, seizures, hyperthermia, uncontrollable shivering, and rigidity; and (5) delirium, coma, status epilepticus, cardiovascular collapse, and death.

Treatment of the serotonin syndrome consists in removing the offending agents and promptly instituting comprehensive supportive care with nitroglycerine, cyproheptadine, methysergide (Sansert), cooling blankets, chlorpromazine (Thorazine), dantrolene (Dantrium), benzodiazepines, anticonvulsants, mechanical ventilation, and paralyzing agents.

Sweating

Some patients experience sweating while being treated with SSRIs. The sweating is unrelated to ambient temperature. Nocturnal sweating may drench bed sheets and require a change of night clothes. Terazosin, 1 or 2 mg per day, is often dramatically effective in counteracting sweating.

SSRI Withdrawal

The abrupt discontinuance of SSRI use, especially one with a shorter half-life (e.g., paroxetine or fluvoxamine), has been associated with a withdrawal syndrome that can include dizziness, weakness, nausea, headache, rebound depression, anxiety, insomnia, poor concentration, upper respiratory symptoms, paresthesias, and migraine-like symptoms. It usually does not appear

until after at least 6 weeks of treatment and usually resolves spontaneously in 3 weeks. Persons who experienced transient adverse effects in the first weeks of taking an SSRI were more likely to experience discontinuation symptoms.

Fluoxetine is the SSRI least likely to be associated with this syndrome because the half-life of its metabolite is more than 1 week and it effectively tapers itself. Fluoxetine, therefore, has been used in some cases to treat the discontinuation syndrome caused by termination of other SSRIs. Nevertheless, a delayed and attenuated withdrawal syndrome occurs with fluoxetine as well.

DRUG INTERACTIONS

The SSRIs do not interfere with most other drugs. A serotonin syndrome (Table 36.29–3) can develop with concurrent administration of MAOIs, tryptophan, lithium (Eskalith), or other antidepressants that inhibit reuptake of serotonin. Fluoxetine, sertraline, and paroxetine can raise plasma concentrations of tricyclic antidepressants, which can cause clinical toxicity. A number of potential pharmacokinetic interactions have been described based on in vitro analyses of the CYP enzymes, but clinically relevant interactions are rare.

The combination of lithium and any serotonergic drug should be used with caution because of the possibility of precipitating seizures. SSRIs, particularly fluvoxamine, should not be used with clozapine because it raises clozapine concentrations, and seizures may result. SSRIs may increase the duration and severity of zolpidem (Ambien)-induced hallucinations.

Fluoxetine

Fluoxetine can be administered with tricyclic drugs, but the clinician should use low doses of the tricyclic drug. Because it is metabolized by the hepatic enzyme CYP 2D6, fluoxetine can interfere with the metabolism of other drugs in the 7 percent of the population that has an inefficient isoform of this enzyme, the so-called *poor metabolizers*. Fluoxetine may slow the metabolism of carbamazepine (Tegretol), antineoplastic agents, diazepam (Valium), and phenytoin (Dilantin). Drug interactions have been described for fluoxetine that may affect the plasma levels of benzodiazepines, antipsychotics, and lithium. Fluoxetine has no interactions with warfarin (Coumadin), tolbutamide (Orinase), or chlorothiazide (Diuril).

Sertraline

Sertraline may displace warfarin from plasma proteins and may increase the prothrombin time. The drug interaction data on sertraline support a generally similar profile to that of fluoxetine, although sertraline does not interact as strongly with the CYP 2D6 enzyme.

Table 32.29–3
Serotonin Syndrome

Diarrhea	Myoclonus
Diaphoresis	Hyperactive reflexes
Tremor	Disorientation
Ataxia	Lability of mood

Paroxetine

Paroxetine has a higher risk for drug interactions than does either fluoxetine or sertraline because it is a more potent inhibitor of the CYP 2D6 enzyme. Cimetidine (Tagamet) can increase the concentration of sertraline and paroxetine, and phenobarbital (Luminal) and phenytoin can decrease the concentration of paroxetine. Because of the potential for interference with the CYP 2D6 enzyme, the coadministration of paroxetine with other antidepressants, phenothiazines, and antiarrhythmic drugs should be undertaken with caution. Paroxetine can increase the anticoagulant effect of warfarin. Coadministration of paroxetine and tramadol (Ultram) may precipitate a serotonin syndrome in elderly persons.

Fluvoxamine

Among the SSRIs, fluvoxamine appears to present the most risk for drug–drug interactions. Fluvoxamine is metabolized by the enzyme CYP 3A4, which may be inhibited by ketoconazole (Nizoral). Fluvoxamine can increase the half-life of alprazolam, triazolam (Halcion), and diazepam, and it should not be coadministered with these agents. Fluvoxamine can increase theophylline (Slo-bid, Theo-Dur) levels threefold and warfarin levels twofold, with important clinical consequences; thus, the serum levels of the latter drugs should be closely monitored and the doses adjusted accordingly. Fluvoxamine raises concentrations and may increase the activity of clozapine, carbamazepine, methadone (Dolophine, Methadose), propranolol (Inderal), and diltiazem (Cardizem). Fluvoxamine has no significant interactions with lorazepam (Ativan) or digoxin (Lanoxin).

Citalopram

Citalopram is not a potent inhibitor of any CYP enzymes. Concurrent administration of cimetidine increases concentrations of citalopram by about 40 percent. Citalopram does not significantly affect the metabolism of, nor is its metabolism significantly affected by, digoxin, lithium, warfarin, carbamazepine, or imipramine (Tofranil). Citalopram increases the plasma concentrations of metoprolol twofold, but this usually has no effect on blood pressure or heart rate. Data on coadministration of citalopram and potent inhibitors of CYP 3A4 or CYP 2D6 are not available.

Escitalopram

Escitalopram is a moderate inhibitor of CYP 2D6 and has been shown to significantly raise desipramine and metoprolol concentrations.

LABORATORY INTERFERENCES

The SSRIs do not interfere with any laboratory tests.

DOSING AND CLINICAL GUIDELINES

Fluoxetine

Fluoxetine is available in 10- and 20-mg capsules, in a scored 10-mg tablet, as a 90-mg enteric-coated capsule for once-weekly administration, and as an oral concentrate (20 mg/5 mL). Fluoxetine is also marketed as Sarafem for premenstrual dysphoric disorder. For depression, the initial dose is usually 10 or 20 mg orally each day, usually given in the morning, because insomnia is a potential adverse effect of the drug. Fluoxetine should be taken with food to minimize the possible nausea. The long half-lives of the drug and its metabolite contribute to a 4-week period to reach steady-state concentrations. A 20-mg dose is often as effective as higher doses for treating depression. The maximal dose recommended by the manufacturer is 80 mg a day. To minimize the early side effects of anxiety and restlessness, some clinicians initiate fluoxetine use at 5 to 10 mg a day, either with the scored 10-mg tablet or by using the liquid preparation. Alternatively, because of the long half-life of fluoxetine, its use can be initiated with an every-other-day administration schedule. The dose of fluoxetine and other SSRIs that is effective in other indications may differ from the dose generally used for depression.

Sertraline

Sertraline is available in scored 25-, 50-, and 100-mg tablets. For the initial treatment of depression, sertraline use should be initiated with a dose of 50 mg once daily. To limit the GI effects, some clinicians begin at 25 mg a day and increase to 50 mg a day after 3 weeks. Patients who do not respond after 1 to 3 weeks may benefit from dose increases of 50 mg every week up to a maximum of 200 mg, given once daily. Sertraline can be administered in the morning or the evening. Administration after eating may reduce the GI adverse effects. Sertraline oral concentrate (1 mL = 20 mg) has 12 percent alcohol content and must be diluted before use. When used to treat panic disorder, sertraline should be initiated at 25 mg to reduce the risk of provoking a panic attack.

Paroxetine

Immediate-release paroxetine is available in scored 20-mg tablets; in unscored 10-, 30-, and 40-mg tablets; and as an orange-flavored, 10–mg/5 mL oral suspension. Paroxetine use for the treatment of depression is usually initiated at a dose of 10 or 20 mg a day. An increase in the dose should be considered when an adequate response is not seen in 1 to 3 weeks. At that point, the clinician can initiate upward dose titration in 10-mg increments at weekly intervals to a maximum of 50 mg a day. Persons who experience GI upset may benefit by taking the drug with food. Paroxetine can be taken initially as a single daily dose in the evening; higher doses can be divided into two doses per day.

A delayed-release formulation of paroxetine (Paxil CR) is available in 12.5-, 25-, and 37.5-mg tablets. The starting dose for depression is 25 mg per day, and that for panic disorder is 12.5 mg per day.

Paroxetine is the SSRI most likely to produce a discontinuation syndrome because plasma concentrations drop rapidly in the absence of continuous dosing. To limit the development of symptoms of abrupt discontinuation, paroxetine use should be tapered gradually, with dose reductions every 2 to 3 weeks.

Fluvoxamine

Fluvoxamine is available in unscored 25-mg tablets and scored 50- and 100-mg tablets. The effective daily dose range is 50 to

300 mg. A usual starting dose is 50 mg once a day at bedtime for the first week, after which the dose can be adjusted according to the adverse effects and clinical response. Doses above 100 mg a day can be divided into twice-daily dosing. A temporary dose reduction or slower upward titration may be necessary if nausea develops over the first 2 weeks of therapy. Fluvoxamine can also be administered as a single evening dose to minimize its adverse effects. Tablets should be swallowed with food without chewing the tablet. Abrupt discontinuation of fluvoxamine can cause a discontinuation syndrome.

Citalopram

Citalopram is available in 20- and 40-mg scored tablets and as a liquid (10 mg/5 mL). The usual starting dose is 20 mg a day for the first week, after which it usually is increased to 40 mg a day. For elderly persons or persons with hepatic impairment, 20 mg a day is recommended, with an increase to 40 mg a day only with no response at 20 mg a day. Tablets should be taken once daily, in either the morning or the evening, with or without food.

Escitalopram

Escitalopram is available as 10- and 20-mg scored tablets, as well as an oral solution at a concentration of 5 mg/5 mL. The recommended dose of escitalopram is 10 mg per day. In clinical trials, no additional benefit was noted when 20 mg per day was used.

Loss of Efficacy

Some patients report a lessened response to SSRIs with recurrence of depressive symptoms after a period of time (e.g., 4 to 6 months). The exact mechanism is unknown. Potential remedies for the attenuation of response to SSRIs include increasing or decreasing the dose; tapering drug use and then rechallenging with the same medication; switching to another SSRI or non-SSRI antidepressant; and augmenting with bupropion or another augmentation agent.

▲ 32.30 Serotonin–Dopamine Antagonists: Second-Generation Antipsychotics

The serotonin–dopamine antagonists (SDAs) are also known as second-generation or atypical antipsychotic drugs. These drugs include risperidone (Risperdal), olanzapine (Zyprexa), quetiapine (Seroquel), clozapine (Clozaril), and ziprasidone (Geodon). They are called SDAs because they have a higher ratio of serotonin type 2 (5-HT$_2$)- to D$_2$-dopamine receptor blockades than the typical, or conventional, dopamine receptor antagonists (DRAs) that previously were the mainstay of treatment. The SDAs also appear to be more specific for the mesolimbic than striatal dopamine system and, in some cases, are associated with rapid dissociation from the D$_2$ receptor. It is hypothesized that these properties account for the improved tolerability associated with the SDAs.

All of the SDAs share the following characteristics: (1) low D$_2$-receptor blocking effects when compared with DRAs, which have high D$_2$-receptor blockades; (2) a reduced risk of extrapyramidal side effects compared with older agents, a reduced risk that probably extends to the occurrence of tardive dyskinesia as well; (3) proven efficacy as treatments for schizophrenia; and (4) proven efficacy as treatments for acute mania. In all other respects, these agents differ markedly. All have different chemical structures, receptor affinities, and side-effect profiles. No SDA is identical to another in its combination of receptor affinities, and the relative contribution of each receptor interaction to the clinical effects is unknown.

Aripiprazole (Abilify), which exhibits a novel mechanism as a partial dopamine antagonist, is discussed separately later in this section. It represents a further advance, beyond second-generation antipsychotics, in the treatment of psychotic disorders.

Although associated with a lowered but not absent risk of extrapyramidal side effects, some of the drugs in this group often produce substantial weight gain, which, in turn, increases the potential for development of diabetes mellitus. The U.S. Food and Drug Administration (FDA) has requested that all SDAs carry a warning label that patients on the drugs be monitored closely for the development of glucose abnormalities.

Among these drugs, clozapine sits apart. It is not considered a first-line agent because of side effects and need for weekly blood tests. Although highly effective in treating both mania and depression, clozapine does not have an FDA indication for those conditions. Olanzapine is indicated for the treatment of acute and chronic manic episodes associated with bipolar I disorders; however, it is frequently used in patients who fail to respond to other interventions.

THERAPEUTIC INDICATIONS

Although approved for the treatment of acute mania, these drugs also are useful as adjunctive therapy in treatment-resistant depression, posttraumatic stress disorder, and behavioral disturbances associated with dementia. All of these agents are considered first-line drugs, except clozapine, which causes adverse hematological effects that require weekly blood sampling.

Schizophrenia and Schizoaffective Disorder

The SDAs are effective for treating acute and chronic psychoses, such as schizophrenia and schizoaffective disorder, in both adults and adolescents. SDAs are as good as, or better than, typical antipsychotics (DRAs) for the treatment of positive symptoms in schizophrenia and clearly superior to DRAs for the treatment of negative symptoms. Compared with persons treated with DRAs, persons treated with SDAs have fewer relapses and require less frequent hospitalization, fewer emergency room visits, less phone contact with mental health professionals, and less treatment in day programs.

Because clozapine has potentially life-threatening adverse effects, it is appropriate only for patients with schizophrenia that is resistant to all other antipsychotics. Other indications for clozapine include treatment of persons with severe tardive dyskinesias—which can be reversed with high doses in some cases—and those with a low threshold for extrapyramidal symptoms. Persons who tolerate clozapine have done well on long-term therapy. The effectiveness of clozapine can be increased by augmentation with risperidone and aripiprazole, which raise clozapine concentrations, and sometimes this results in dramatic clinical improvement.

Mood Disorders

All of the SDAs are FDA approved for treatment of acute mania. Olanzapine is also approved for maintenance treatment of bipolar disorder. In general, however, typical antipsychotics and benzodiazepines exert calming effects in mania more rapidly than do SDAs. The SDAs improve depressive symptoms in schizophrenia, and both clinical experience and clinical trials show that all of the SDAs augment antidepressants in the acute management of major depression. A combination of SDAs and antidepressants is frequently used in treatment-resistant depression, and a fixed combination of olanzapine and fluoxetine (Symbyax) is approved by the FDA as a treatment for acute bipolar depression.

Other Indications

About 10 percent of patients with schizophrenia exhibit outwardly aggressive or violent behavior. SDAs are effective for treatment of such aggression. Other indications include acquired immunodeficiency syndrome, autistic spectrum disorders, Tourette's disorder, Huntington's disease, and Lesch-Nyhan syndrome. Risperidone and olanzapine have been used to control aggression and self-injury in children. These drugs have also been coadministered with sympathomimetics, such as methylphenidate (Ritalin) and dextroamphetamine (Dexedrine, Dextrostat), to children with attention-deficit/hyperactivity disorder who are comorbid for either opposition-defiant disorder or conduct disorder. SDAs—especially olanzapine, quetiapine, and clozapine—are useful in persons who have severe tardive dyskinesia. SDA treatment suppresses the abnormal movements of tardive dyskinesia but does not appear to worsen the movement disorder. SDAs are also effective for treating psychotic depression and for psychosis secondary to head trauma, dementia, or treatment drugs. When used for dementia, low doses should be used because of reports of increased mortality in dementia patients treated with SDAs. Extended-release preparations should be avoided.

Treatment with SDAs decreases the risk of suicide and water intoxication in patients with schizophrenia. Patients with treatment-resistant obsessive-compulsive disorder (OCD) have responded to SDAs; however, a few persons treated with SDAs have noted treatment-emergent symptoms of OCD. Some patients with borderline personality disorder may improve with SDAs.

ADVERSE EFFECTS

The SDAs share a similar spectrum of adverse reactions but differ considerably in terms of frequency or severity of their occurrence. Specific side effects that are more common with an individual SDA are emphasized in the discussion of each drug.

PHARMACOLOGY, SIDE EFFECTS, DOSAGES, AND INTERACTIONS

Risperidone

Pharmacology.   Risperidone is a benzisoxazole. It undergoes extensive first-pass hepatic metabolism to 9-hydroxyrisperidone, a metabolite with equivalent antipsychotic activity. Peak plasma levels of the parent compound occur within 1 hour for the parent compound and 3 hours for the metabolite. Risperidone has a bioactivity of 70 percent. The combined half-life of risperidone and 9-hydroxyrisperidone averages 20 hours, so it is effective in once-daily dosing. Risperidone is an antagonist of the serotonin $5\text{-}HT_{2A}$, dopamine D_2, $\alpha_1\text{-}$ and α_2-adrenergic, and histamine H_1 receptors. It has a low affinity for α-adrenergic and muscarinic cholinergic receptors. Although it is as potent an antagonist of D_2 receptors as haloperidol (Haldol), risperidone is much less likely (except in high doses) than haloperidol to cause extrapyramidal symptoms in humans.

Side Effects.   Extrapyramidal effects of risperidone are largely dose dependent, and a trend is seen to using lower doses than initially recommended. Weight gain, anxiety, nausea and vomiting, rhinitis, erectile dysfunction, orgasmic dysfunction, and increased pigmentation are associated with risperidone use. The most common drug-related reasons for discontinuation of risperidone use are extrapyramidal symptoms, dizziness, hyperkinesias, somnolence, and nausea. Marked elevation of prolactin can occur. Weight gain occurs more commonly with risperidone use in children than in adults.

Dosage.   The recommended dose range and frequency of risperidone dosing has changed since the drug first came into clinical use. Risperidone is available in 1-, 2-, 3-, and 4-mg tablets, as a 1-mg/mL oral solution, and in M-tab form (rapidly dissolving). The initial dose is usually 1 to 2 mg at night, which can then be raised to 4 mg per day. Positron emission tomography (PET) studies have shown that doses of 1 to 4 mg per day provide the required D_2 blockade needed for a therapeutic effect. At first it was believed that because of its short elimination half-life, risperidone should be given twice a day, but studies have shown equal efficacy with once-a-day dosing. Doses above 6 mg a day are associated with a higher incidence of adverse effects, particularly extrapyramidal symptoms. No correlation has been found between plasma concentrations and therapeutic effect.

Risperidone (Risperdal Consta) is the only SDA available in a depot formulation. It is given as an intramuscular injection formulation every 2 weeks. The dose may be 25, 50, or 75 mg. Oral risperidone should be coadministered with Risperdal Consta for the first 3 weeks before being discontinued.

Drug Interactions.   Inhibition of cytochrome P450 (CYP 2D6) by drugs such as paroxetine and fluoxetine can block the formation of risperidone's active metabolite. Risperidone is a weak inhibitor of CYP 2D6 and has little effect on other drugs. Combined use of risperidone and selective serotonin reuptake inhibitors (SSRIs) can result in significant elevation of prolactin, with associated galactorrhea and breast enlargement.

Olanzapine

Pharmacology.   Approximately 85 percent of olanzapine is absorbed from the gastrointestinal (GI) tract, and about 40 percent of the dose is inactivated by first-pass hepatic metabolism. Peak concentrations are reached in 5 hours, and the half-life averages 31 hours (range 21 to 54 hours). It is given in once-daily dosing. In addition to $5\text{-}HT_{2A}$ and D_2 antagonism, olanzapine is an antagonist of the D_1, D_4, α_1, $5\text{-}HT_{1A}$, muscarinic M_1 through M_5, and H_1 receptors.

Side Effects.   Other than clozapine, olanzapine consistently causes a greater amount and more frequent weight gain than other atypical antipsychotics, which plateaus after about 10 months. This effect is not dose related. Somnolence, dry mouth, dizziness, constipation, dyspepsia, increased appetite, akathisia, and tremor are associated with olanzapine use. A few patients (2 percent) may need to discontinue use of the drug because of transaminase elevation. A dose-related risk exists of extrapyramidal side effects. The manufacturer recommends "periodic" assessment of blood sugar and transaminases during treatment with olanzapine. An FDA mandate warns about an increased risk of stroke among patients with dementia treated with olanzapine and other SDAs, but this risk is small and is outweighed by improved behavioral control that treatment may produce.

Dosage.   Olanzapine is available in 2.5-, 5-, 7.5-, 10-, 15-, and 20-mg tablets. The initial dose for treatment of psychosis is usually 5 or 10 mg and for treatment of acute mania is usually 10 or 15 mg, given once daily. It is also available as 5-, 10-, 15-, and 20-mg orally disintegrating tablets that might be useful for patients who have difficulty swallowing pills or who "cheek" their medication. A 10-mg injection form is available for treatment of acute agitation in schizophrenia and bipolar disorder.

A starting daily dose of 5 to 10 mg is recommended. After 1 week, the dose can be raised to 10 mg a day. Given the long half-life, 1 week must be allowed to achieve each new steady-state blood level. Doses in clinical use ranges vary, with 5 to 20 mg a day being most commonly used, but 30 to 40 mg a day is needed in treatment-resistant patients. A word of caution, however, is that the higher doses are associated with increased extrapyramidal and other adverse effects, and doses greater than 20 mg a day were not studied in the pivotal trials that led to the approval of olanzapine.

Drug Interactions.   Fluvoxamine (Luvox) and cimetidine (Tagamet) increase, whereas carbamazepine (Tegretol) and phenytoin decrease, serum concentrations of olanzapine. Ethanol increases olanzapine absorption by more than 25 percent, leading to increased sedation. Olanzapine has little effect on the metabolism of other drugs.

Quetiapine

Pharmacology.   Quetiapine is a dibenzothiazepine structurally related to clozapine, but it differs markedly from that agent in biochemical effects. It is rapidly absorbed from the GI tract, with peak plasma concentrations reached in 1 to 2 hours. Steady-state half-life is about 7 hours, and optimal dosing is two or three times per day. Quetiapine, in addition to being an antagonist of D_2 and 5-HT_2, also blocks 5-HT_6, D_1 and H_1, and α_1 and α_2 receptors. It does not block muscarinic or benzodiazepine receptors. The receptor antagonism for quetiapine is generally lower than that for other antipsychotic drugs, and it is not associated with extrapyramidal symptoms.

Side Effects.   Somnolence, postural hypotension, and dizziness are the most common adverse effects of quetiapine. These are usually transient and are best managed with initial gradual upward titration of the dose. Quetiapine is the SDA least likely to cause extrapyramidal side effects, regardless of dose. This makes it particularly useful in treating patients with Parkinson's disease who develop dopamine agonist-induced psychosis. Prolactin elevation is rare and both transient and mild when it occurs. Quetiapine is associated with modest weight gain in some persons, but some patients occasionally gain a considerable amount of weight. Small increases in heart rate and constipation and a transient rise in liver transaminases can also occur. Initial concerns about cataract formation, based on animal studies, have not been borne out since the drug has been in clinical use. Nevertheless, it might be prudent to test for lens abnormalities early in treatment and periodically thereafter.

Dosage.   Quetiapine is available in 25-, 100-, and 200-mg tablets. In schizophrenia a target of 400 mg a day is desired, and in mania and bipolar depression 800 and 300 mg, respectively, are desired. It has become evident that the target dose can be achieved rapidly and that some patients benefit from doses of as much as 1,200 to 1,600 mg a day. Despite its short elimination half-life, quetiapine can be given once a day to many patients. This is consistent with the observation that quetiapine receptor occupancy remains even when concentrations in the blood have markedly declined. Quetiapine in doses of 25 to 300 mg at night has been used for insomnia.

Drug Interactions.   The potential interactions between quetiapine and other drugs have been well studied. Other than a finding that phenytoin increases quetiapine clearance fivefold, no major pharmacokinetic interactions have been noted.

Ziprasidone

Pharmacology.   Ziprasidone is a benzothiazolyl piperazine. Peak plasma concentrations of ziprasidone are reached in 2 to 6 hours. Steady-state levels ranging from 5 to 10 hours are reached between the first and third days of treatment. The mean terminal half-life at steady state ranges from 5 to 10 hours, which accounts for the recommendation that twice-daily dosing is necessary. Bioavailability doubles when ziprasidone is taken with food.

Peak serum concentrations of IM ziprasidone occur after approximately 1 hour, with a half-life of 2 to 5 hours.

Ziprasidone, as with the other SDAs, blocks 5-HT_{2A} and D_2 receptors. It is also an antagonist of 5-HT_{1D}, 5-HT_{2C}, D_3, D_4, α_1, and H_1 receptors. It has very low affinity for D_1, M_1, and α_2 receptors. Ziprasidone also has agonist activity at the serotonin 5-HT_{1A} receptors and is a serotonin reuptake inhibitor and a norepinephrine reuptake inhibitor. This is consistent with clinical reports that ziprasidone has antidepressant-like effects in nonschizophrenic patients.

Side Effects.   Somnolence, headache, dizziness, nausea, and lightheadedness are the most common adverse effects in patients taking ziprasidone. It has almost no significant effects outside the central nervous system and is associated with almost no weight gain and does not cause sustained prolactin elevation. Concerns about prolongation of the QT_c complex have deterred some clinicians from using ziprasidone as a first choice. The QT_c interval has been shown to increase by an average of 4.7 to 1.4 ms in patients treated with 40 and 120 mg per day, respectively. Ziprasidone is contraindicated in combination with other drugs known to prolong the QT_c interval. These include, but are not limited to, dofetilide, sotalol, quinidine, other class

Ia and III antiarrhythmics, mesoridazine, thioridazine, chlorpromazine, droperidol, pimozide, sparfloxacin, gatifloxacin, moxifloxacin, halofantrine, mefloquine, pentamidine, arsenic trioxide, levomethadyl acetate, dolasetron mesylate, probucol, and tacrolimus. Ziprasidone should be avoided in patients with congenital long-QT syndrome and in patients with a history of cardiac arrhythmias.

Dosage.   Ziprasidone is available in 20-, 40-, 60-, and 80-mg capsules. Ziprasidone for IM use comes as a single-use 20-mg/mL vial. Oral ziprasidone dosing should be initiated at 40 mg a day, divided into two daily doses. Studies have shown efficacy in the range of 80 to 160 mg a day, divided twice daily. In clinical practice, doses as high as 240 mg a day are being used. The recommended IM dosage is 10 to 20 mg every 2 hours for the 10-mg dose and every 4 hours for the 20-mg dose. The maximal total daily dose of IM ziprasidone is 40 mg.

Drug Interactions.   Other than interactions with other drugs that prolong the QT_c complex, ziprasidone appears to have low potential for clinically significant drug interactions.

Clozapine

Pharmacology.   Clozapine is a dibenzodiazepine. It is rapidly absorbed, with peak plasma levels reached in about 2 hours. Steady state is achieved in less than 1 week if twice-daily dosing is used. The elimination half-life is about 12 hours. Clozapine has two major metabolites, one of which, N-dimethyl clozapine, may have some pharmacological activity. Clozapine is an antagonist of 5-HT$_{2A}$, D_1, D_3, D_4, and α (especially α_1) receptors. It has relatively low potency as a D_2-receptor antagonist. Data from PET scanning show that 10 mg of haloperidol produces 80 percent occupancy of striatal D_2 receptors, whereas clinically effective doses of clozapine occupy only 40 to 50 percent of striatal D_2 receptors. This difference in D_2-receptor occupancy is probably why clozapine does not cause extrapyramidal adverse effects. It has also been postulated that clozapine, as well as other SDAs, bind more loosely to the D_2 receptor, and as a result of this "fast dissociation," more normal dopamine neurotransmission is possible.

Special Indications.   In addition to being the most effective drug treatment for patients who have failed on standard therapies, clozapine has been shown to benefit patients with severe tardive dyskinesia. Clozapine suppresses these dyskinesias, but the abnormal movements return when clozapine is discontinued. This is true despite the fact that clozapine, on rare occasions, can cause tardive dyskinesia. Other clinical situations in which clozapine can be used include the treatment of psychotic patients who are intolerant of extrapyramidal side effects caused by other agents, treatment-resistant mania, severe psychotic depression, idiopathic Parkinson's disease, Huntington's disease, and suicidal patients with schizophrenia or schizoaffective disorder. Other treatment-resistant disorders that have demonstrated response to clozapine include pervasive developmental disorder, autism of childhood, and OCD (either alone or in combination with an SSRI). Used by itself, clozapine, very rarely, induces obsessive-compulsive symptoms.

Side Effects.   The most common drug-related adverse effects are sedation, dizziness, syncope, tachycardia, hypotension,

electrocardiogram (ECG) changes, nausea, and vomiting. Other common adverse effects include fatigue, weight gain, various GI symptoms (most commonly, constipation), anticholinergic effects, and subjective muscle weakness. Sialorrhea, or hypersalivation, is a side effect that begins early in treatment and is most evident at night. Patients report that their pillows are drenched with saliva. This side effect is most likely the result of impairment of swallowing. Although reports suggest that clonidine or amitriptyline may help reduce hypersalivation, the most practical solution is to put a towel over the pillow.

The risk of seizures is about 4 percent in patients taking doses greater than 600 mg a day. Leukopenia, granulocytopenia, agranulocytosis, and fever occur in about 1 percent of patients. During the first year of treatment, a 0.73 percent risk is seen of clozapine-induced agranulocytosis. The risk during the second year is 0.07 percent. For neutropenia, the risk is 2.32 and 0.69 percent during the first and second years of treatment, respectively. The only contraindications to the use of clozapine are a white blood cell (WBC) count less than 3,500/mm^3 cells, a previous bone marrow disorder, a history of agranulocytosis during clozapine treatment, or the use of another drug that is known to suppress the bone marrow, for example, carbamazepine.

During the first 6 months of treatment, weekly WBC counts are indicated to monitor the patient for the development of agranulocytosis. If the WBC count remains normal, the frequency of testing can be decreased to every 2 weeks. Although monitoring is expensive, early indication of agranulocytosis can prevent a fatal outcome. Clozapine should be discontinued if the WBC count is less than 3,000/mm^3 cells or the granulocyte count is less than 1,500/mm^3. In addition, a hematological consultation should be obtained, and obtaining a bone marrow sample should be considered. Persons with agranulocytosis should not be reexposed to the drug. To avoid situations in which a physician or patient fails to comply with the required blood tests, clozapine cannot be dispensed without proof of monitoring.

Myocarditis is also a serious risk in the use of clozapine.

Dosage.   Clozapine is available in 25- and 100-mg tablets. The initial dose is usually 25 mg one or two times daily, although a conservative initial dose is 12.5 mg twice daily. The dose can then be raised gradually (25 mg a day every 2 or 3 days) to 300 mg a day in divided doses, usually two or three times daily. Doses up to 900 mg a day can be used. Testing for blood concentrations of clozapine may be helpful in patients who fail to respond. Studies have found that plasma concentrations greater than 350 mg/mL are associated with a better likelihood of response.

Drug Interactions.   Clozapine should not be used with any other drug that is associated with the development of agranulocytosis or bone marrow suppression. Such drugs include carbamazepine, phenytoin, propylthiouracil, sulfonamides, and captopril (Capoten). Lithium combined with clozapine can increase the risk of seizures, confusion, and movement disorders. Lithium should not be used in combination with clozapine by persons who have experienced an episode of neuroleptic malignant syndrome. Clomipramine (Anafranil) can increase the risk of seizure by lowering the seizure threshold and by increasing clozapine plasma concentrations. Risperidone, fluoxetine, paroxetine, and fluvoxamine increase serum concentrations of clozapine. Addition of paroxetine may precipitate clozapine-associated neutropenia.

PARTIAL DOPAMINE D$_2$ AGONISTS

A new type of atypical antipsychotic is characterized by a partial D$_2$ agonism, in contrast to the effect of SDAs on D$_2$-receptor antagonism. The main drugs in this class are apiprazole (Abilify) and paliperidone (Invega), which is the metabolite of risperidone. Both are discussed later. Partial D$_2$ agonism is believed to decrease dopamine activity in an overactive dopamine system while simultaneously increasing dopamine activity in regions of the brain where dopaminergic activity is too low. By blocking overstimulated receptors and stimulating underactive ones, partial D$_2$ agonists act as dopamine stabilizers.

Paliperidone (Invega)

Pharmacological Action.   Paliperidone is the major active metabolite of risperidone. The mechanism of action is mediated through a combination of central D$_2$ and 5-HT$_{2A}$ receptor antagonism. Paliperidone is also active as an antagonist at α_1- and α_2-adrenergic receptors and H$_1$ histaminergic receptors, which may explain some of the other effects of the drug. Paliperidone has no affinity for cholinergic muscarinic or β_1- and β_2-adrenergic receptors.

Following a single dose, the plasma concentrations of paliperidone gradually rise to reach peak plasma concentration approximately 24 hours after dosing. The pharmacokinetics of paliperidone administration are dose proportional within the dose range of 3 to 12 mg. Steady-state concentrations are attained within 4 to 5 days. The drug does not substantially inhibit the metabolism of drugs metabolized by CYP isozymes.

Dosages.   Paliperidone is available only in extended-release tablets of 3, 6, and 9 mg. Initial dose titration is not required. Although it has not been systematically established that doses greater than 6 mg have additional benefit, there may be a general trend for greater effects with higher doses. This should be weighed against the dose-related increase in adverse effects. Thus, some patients may benefit from higher doses, up to 12 mg per day, and for some patients, a lower dose of 3 mg per day may be sufficient. Dose increases above 6 mg per day should be made only after clinical reassessment and generally should occur at intervals of more than 5 days. When dose increases are indicated, small increments of 3 mg per day are recommended. The maximum recommended dose is 12 mg per day. Concomitant use of paliperidone with risperidone has not been studied.

Paliperidone is contained within a nonabsorbable shell designed to release the drug at a controlled rate. The tablet shell, along with insoluble core components, is eliminated from the body; patients should not be concerned if they occasionally notice in their stool something that looks like a tablet.

Side Effects.   Common side effects include anxiety, somnolence, dizziness, dyspepsia, and constipation. Akathisia and extrapyramidal symptoms may occur as with risperidone. A modest increase in the QT$_c$ interval can occur, and the drug should be avoided in persons with congenital long-QT syndrome or a history of chronic arrhythmias. In general, paliperidone has a similar side-effect profile to its precursor, risperidone. The dose should be reduced in patients with renal impairment.

Drug Interactions.   Inhibition of CYP 2D6 by drugs such as paroxetine, fluoxetine, and other SSRIs can block the action of paliperidone. Combined use of SSRIs and paliperidone can result in significant elevation of prolactin and possible gynecomastia in men. Galactorrhea may occur in women.

ARIPIPRAZOLE

Unlike the SDAs, aripiprazole is not a D$_2$ antagonist, but is a partial D$_2$ agonist. Partial D$_2$ agonists compete at D$_2$ receptors for endogenous dopamine, thereby producing a functional reduction of dopamine activity. Because schizophrenia and mania are disorders associated with increased dopamine activity, this reduction may account for its therapeutic effects.

Aripiprazole is usually nonsedating and has not been found to pose an increased risk of weight gain and diabetes. Aripiprazole is particularly effective in sparing, and possibly enhancing, neurocognitive functions. Use of aripiprazole is relatively new, and, thus, little off-label use has been described. Aripiprazole is a quinoline derivative.

Pharmacological Actions

Aripiprazole is well absorbed, reaching peak plasma concentrations after 3 to 5 hours. Absorption is not affected by food. The mean elimination half-life of aripiprazole is about 75 hours. It has a weakly active metabolite with a half-life of 96 hours. These relatively long half-lives make aripiprazole suitable for once-daily dosing. Clearance is reduced in the elderly. Aripiprazole exhibits linear pharmacokinetics and is primarily metabolized by CYP 3A4 and CYP 2D6 enzymes. It is 99 percent protein bound. Aripiprazole is excreted in breast milk in lactating rats.

Mechanistically, aripiprazole acts as a modulator rather than a blocker, and it acts on both postsynaptic D$_2$ receptors and presynaptic autoreceptors. In theory, this mechanism addresses excessive limbic dopamine (hyperdopaminergic) activity and decreased dopamine (hypodopaminergic) activity in frontal and prefrontal areas—abnormalities that are thought to be present in schizophrenia. The absence of complete D$_2$ blockade in the striatal areas would be expected to minimize extrapyramidal side effects. Aripiprazole is an α_1-adrenergic receptor antagonist, which can cause some patients to experience orthostatic hypotension. As with the so-called atypical antipsychotic agents, aripiprazole is a 5-HT$_{2A}$ antagonist.

Therapeutic Indications

Schizophrenia.   Short-term, 4- to 6-week studies comparing aripiprazole with haloperidol and risperidone in patients with schizophrenia and schizoaffective disorder have shown comparable efficacy. Doses of 15, 20, and 30 mg a day were found to be effective. Long-term studies suggest that aripiprazole is effective as a maintenance treatment at a daily dose of 15 to 30 mg.

Acute Mania.   Aripiprazole is useful for the initial control of agitation during a manic episode. Despite being largely devoid of sedation as a side effect, the antimanic effects of aripiprazole were evident in clinical trials as early as day 4. No studies have compared aripiprazole with lithium, divalproex, or olanzapine, other drugs that are used to treat acute mania.

Other Uses. Aripiprazole has been reported to be successful as an add-on to SSRIs in treatment-resistant patients with mood or anxiety disorders. Doses of 15 to 30 mg per day were used. A small study of aripiprazole as a treatment for psychotic symptoms associated with Alzheimer's disease found no clinical benefit from aripiprazole. A study of aggressive children and adolescents with oppositional defiant disorder or conduct disorder found a positive response in about 60 percent of the patients. In this study, vomiting and somnolence led to a reduction in initial aripiprazole dosage.

Adverse Effects

The most commonly reported adverse effects of aripiprazole are headache, somnolence, agitation, dyspepsia, anxiety, and nausea. Although it is not a frequent cause of extrapyramidal side effects, aripiprazole does cause akathisia-like activation. Described as restlessness or agitation, it can be highly distressing and often leads to discontinuation of medication. Insomnia is another common complaint. Data do not indicate that weight gain or diabetes mellitus has an increased incidence with aripiprazole use. Prolactin elevation does not typically occur. Aripiprazole does not cause significant QT_c-interval changes. Seizures have been reported.

Drug Interactions

Carbamazepine and valproate reduce, whereas ketoconazole, fluoxetine, paroxetine, and quinidine increase, aripiprazole serum concentrations. Lithium and valproic acid, two drugs likely to be combined with aripiprazole when treating bipolar disorder, do not affect the steady-state concentrations of aripiprazole. Combined use with antihypertensives can cause hypotension. Drugs that inhibit CYP 2D6 activity reduce aripiprazole elimination.

Dosing and Clinical Guidelines

Aripiprazole is available as 5-, 10-, 15-, 20-, and 30-mg tablets. The effective dose range is 10 to 30 mg per day. Although the starting dose is 10 to 15 mg per day, problems with nausea, insomnia, and akathisia have led to use of lower-than-recommended starting doses of aripiprazole. Many clinicians find that an initial dose of 5 mg increases tolerability. It is too early to predict optimal dosing strategy for aripiprazole in clinical practice.

Bifeprunox. Bifeprunox, a dopamine partial agonist, is an investigational atypical antipsychotic for the treatment of schizophrenia. Although bifeprunox has been shown to have a smaller mean effect in acute psychosis compared to other atypical antipsychotics, it may be an alternative in terms of side effects. In studies, gastrointestinal side effects were the most common adverse events. These included nausea, vomiting, constipation, and abdominal discomfort. In some studies, bifeprunox was associated with a decrease in weight and improvement in the lipid profile compared to placebo.

CLINICAL GUIDELINES

All SDAs are appropriate for the management of an initial psychotic episode, whereas clozapine is reserved for persons refractory to all other antipsychotic drugs. If a person does not respond to the first SDA, other SDAs should be tried. Drug choice should be based on the patient's clinical status and history of response to medication. SDAs usually require 4 to 6 weeks to reach full effectiveness, and it may take up to 8 weeks for the full clinical effects of an SDA to become apparent. Much of the observed initial clinical improvement, thus, may reflect nonspecific sedation. At first glance, this would suggest that highly sedating SDAs, such as olanzapine or quetiapine, would be preferred agents for acute treatment of agitated, violent, or highly anxious patients. Of interest, head-to-head studies do not show differences between SDAs with respect to acute effects. Nevertheless, it is acceptable practice to augment an SDA with a high-potency DRA or benzodiazepine in the first few weeks of use. Lorazepam 1 to 2 mg orally or IM can be used as needed for acute agitation. Once effective, doses can be lowered as tolerated. Clinical improvement may take 6 months of treatment with SDAs in some particularly treatment-refractory persons.

Use of all SDAs must be initiated at low doses and gradually tapered upward to therapeutic doses. The gradual increase in dose is necessitated by the potential development of adverse effects. If a person stops taking an SDA for more than 36 hours, drug use should be resumed at the initial titration schedule. After the decision to terminate olanzapine or clozapine use, doses should be tapered whenever possible to avoid cholinergic rebound symptoms, such as diaphoresis, flushing, diarrhea, and hyperactivity.

Once a clinician has determined that a trial of an SDA is warranted for a particular person, the risks and the benefits of SDA treatment must be explained to the person and the family. In the case of clozapine, an informed-consent procedure should be documented in the person's chart. The patient's history should include information about blood disorders, epilepsy, cardiovascular disease, hepatic and renal diseases, and drug abuse. The presence of a hepatic or renal disease necessitates using low starting doses of the drug. Physical examination should include supine and standing blood pressure measurements to screen for orthostatic hypotension. The laboratory examination should include an ECG; several complete blood counts with WBC counts, which can then be averaged; and liver and renal function tests. Periodic monitoring of blood glucose, lipids, and body weight is recommended.

Although the transition from a DRA to an SDA may be made abruptly, it is wise to taper off the DRA slowly while titrating up the SDA. Clozapine and olanzapine both have anticholinergic effects, and the transition from one to the other can usually be accomplished with little risk of cholinergic rebound. The transition from risperidone to olanzapine is best accomplished by tapering the risperidone off over 3 weeks and simultaneously beginning olanzapine at 10 mg a day. Risperidone, quetiapine, and ziprasidone lack anticholinergic effects, and the abrupt transition from a DRA, olanzapine, or clozapine to one of these agents can cause cholinergic rebound, which consists in excessive salivation, nausea, vomiting, and diarrhea. The risk of cholinergic rebound can be mitigated by initially augmenting risperidone, quetiapine, or ziprasidone with an anticholinergic drug, which is then tapered off slowly. Any initiation and termination of SDA use should be accomplished gradually.

It is wise to overlap administration of the new drug with the old drug. Of interest, some people have a more robust clinical response while taking the two agents during the transition and then regressing on monotherapy with the newer drug. Little is known about the effectiveness and safety of a strategy of combining one SDA with another SDA or with a DRA.

Persons receiving regular injections of depot formulations of a DRA who are to switch to SDA use are given the first dose of the SDA on the day the next injection is due.

Persons who develop agranulocytosis while taking clozapine can safely switch to olanzapine use, although initiation of olanzapine use in the midst of clozapine-induced agranulocytosis can prolong the time of recovery from the usual 3 to 4 days up to 11 to 12 days. It is prudent to wait for resolution of agranulocytosis before initiating olanzapine use. Emergence or recurrence of agranulocytosis has not been reported with olanzapine, even in persons who developed it while taking clozapine.

Use of an SDA by pregnant women has not been studied, but consideration should be given to the potential of risperidone to raise prolactin concentrations, sometimes up to three to four times the upper limit of the normal range. Because the drugs can be excreted in breast milk, they should not be taken by nursing mothers.

▲ 32.31 Sympathomimetics and Related Drugs

Stimulant drugs, also referred to as *psychostimulants*, mimic the effects of naturally occurring sympathomimetic amines. They increase motivation, mood, energy, and wakefulness. Psychostimulants used in psychiatry include methylphenidate (Ritalin), dexmethylphenidate (Focalin), dextroamphetamine (Dexedrine), a combination of amphetamine and dextroamphetamine (Adderall), and pemoline (Cylert), now considered a second-line agent because of rare but potentially fatal hepatic toxicity. A prodrug of amphetamine, lisdexamfetamine (Vyvanse), was recently approved. The drugs are indicated for the treatment of attention-deficit/hyperactivity disorder (ADHD) and narcolepsy and are also effective in the treatment of depression in some patients. Both amphetamine and nonamphetamine sympathomimetics have been used as appetite suppressants. Other sympathomimetics used for appetite suppression include methamphetamine (Desoxyn), phentermine (Adipex-P, Ionamin), diethylpropion (Tenuate), and phendimetrazine (Bontril). A novel stimulant approved for treatment of narcolepsy in the United States, modafinil (Provigil), has been used as an antidepressant and a treatment for ADHD. Atomoxetine (Strattera), although not a stimulant, is indicated for use in ADHD and is included in this section.

PHARMACOLOGICAL ACTIONS

All of these drugs are well absorbed from the gastrointestinal tract. Amphetamine and dextroamphetamine reach peak plasma concentrations in 2 to 3 hours and have a half-life of about 6 hours, thereby necessitating once- or twice-daily dosing.

Lisdexamfetamine is an extended-release preparation that lasts for 12 hours. Methylphenidate is available in immediate-release (Ritalin), sustained-release (Ritalin SR), and extended-release (Concerta) formulations. Immediate-release methylphenidate reaches peak plasma concentrations in 1 to 2 hours and has a short half-life of 2 to 3 hours, thereby necessitating multiple daily dosing. The sustained-release formulation reaches peak plasma concentrations in 4 to 5 hours and doubles the effective half-life of methylphenidate. The extended-release formulation reaches peak plasma concentrations in 6 to 8 hours and is designed to be effective for 12 hours in once-daily dosing. Dexmethylphenidate reaches peak plasma concentration in about 3 hours and is prescribed twice daily. Pemoline reaches peak plasma concentrations in 2 to 4 hours and has a half-life of about 12 hours, and modafinil reaches peak plasma concentrations in 2 to 4 hours and has a half-life of 15 hours, thereby allowing once-daily dosing of these two agents.

Methylphenidate, dextroamphetamine, and amphetamine are indirectly acting sympathomimetics, with the primary effect of causing the release of catecholamines from presynaptic neurons. Clinical effectiveness is associated with increased release of both dopamine and norepinephrine. Dextroamphetamine and methylphenidate are also weak inhibitors of catecholamine reuptake and inhibitors of monoamine oxidase. Pemoline may indirectly stimulate dopaminergic activity by a poorly understood mechanism, but it has little actual sympathomimetic activity.

The specific mechanism of action of modafinil is unknown. Narcolepsy–cataplexy results from deficiency of hypocretin, a hypothalamic neuropeptide. Hypocretin-producing neurons are activated after modafinil administration. Modafinil does not appear to work through a dopaminergic mechanism. It does have α_1-adrenergic agonist properties, which may account for its alerting effects, because the wakefulness induced by modafinil can be attenuated by prazosin, an α_1-adrenergic antagonist. Some evidence suggests that modafinil has some norepinephrine reuptake blocking effects.

THERAPEUTIC INDICATIONS

Attention-Deficit/Hyperactivity Disorder

Sympathomimetics are the first-line drugs for treatment of ADHD in children and are effective about 75 percent of the time. Methylphenidate and dextroamphetamine are equally effective and work within 15 to 30 minutes. Pemoline requires 3 to 4 weeks to reach its full efficacy; however, it is rarely used because of toxicity. Sympathomimetic drugs decrease hyperactivity, increase attentiveness, and reduce impulsivity. They may also reduce comorbid oppositional behaviors associated with ADHD. Many persons take these drugs throughout their schooling and beyond. In responsive persons, use of a sympathomimetic may be a critical determinant of scholastic success.

Sympathomimetics improve the core ADHD symptoms of hyperactivity, impulsivity, and inattentiveness and permit improved social interactions with teachers, family, other adults, and peers. The success of long-term treatment of ADHD with sympathomimetics, which are efficacious for most of the various constellations of ADHD symptoms present from childhood to adulthood, supports a model in which ADHD results from a genetically determined neurochemical imbalance that requires lifelong pharmacological management.

Methylphenidate is the most commonly used initial agent, at a dose of 5 to 10 mg every 3 to 4 hours. Doses may be increased to a maximum of 20 mg four times daily or 1 mg/kg a day. Use of the 20-mg sustained-release formulation to achieve 6 hours of benefit and eliminate the need for dosing at school is supported by many experts, although other authorities feel that it is less effective than the immediate-release formulation. Dextroamphetamine is about twice as potent as methylphenidate on a per-milligram basis and provides 6 to 8 hours of benefit. Some 70 percent of nonresponders to one sympathomimetic may benefit from another. All of the sympathomimetic drugs should be tried before switching to drugs of a different class. The previous dictum that sympathomimetics worsen tics and, therefore, should be avoided by persons with comorbid ADHD and tic disorders has been questioned. Small doses of sympathomimetics do not appear to cause an increase in the frequency and severity of tics. Alternatives to sympathomimetics for ADHD include bupropion (Wellbutrin), venlafaxine (Effexor), guanfacine (Tenex), clonidine (Catapres), and tricyclic drugs. Further studies are needed to determine whether modafinil decreases the symptoms of ADHD.

Short-term use of the sympathomimetics induces a euphoric feeling; however, tolerance develops for both the euphoric feeling and the sympathomimetic activity. Of note, tolerance does not develop for the therapeutic effects in ADHD.

Narcolepsy and Hypersomnolence

Narcolepsy consists of sudden sleep attacks (*narcolepsy*), sudden loss of postural tone (*cataplexy*), loss of voluntary motor control going into (hypnagogic) or coming out of (hypnopompic) sleep (*sleep paralysis*), and hypnagogic or hypnopompic *hallucinations*. Sympathomimetics reduce narcoleptic sleep attacks and also improve wakefulness in other types of hypersomnolent states. Modafinil is approved as an antisomnolence agent for treatment of narcolepsy, for people who cannot adjust to night shift work, and for those who do not sleep well because of obstructive sleep apnea.

Other sympathomimetics are also used to maintain wakefulness and accuracy of motor performance in persons subject to sleep deprivation, such as pilots and military personnel. Persons with narcolepsy, unlike persons with ADHD, may develop tolerance for the therapeutic effects of the sympathomimetics.

In direct comparison with amphetamine-like drugs, modafinil is equally effective at maintaining wakefulness, with a lower risk of excessive activation.

Depressive Disorders

Sympathomimetics can be used for treatment-resistant depressive disorders, usually as augmentation of standard antidepressant drug therapy. Possible indications for use of sympathomimetics as monotherapy include depression in the elderly, who are at increased risk for adverse effects from standard antidepressant drugs; depression in medically ill persons, especially persons with acquired immunodeficiency syndrome; obtundation because of chronic use of opioids; and clinical situations in which a rapid response is important but for which electroconvulsive therapy is contraindicated. Depressed patients with abulia and anergia may also benefit.

Dextroamphetamine may be useful in differentiating pseudodementia of depression from dementia. A depressed person generally responds to a 5-mg dose with increased alertness and improved cognition. Sympathomimetics are thought to provide only short-term benefit (2 to 4 weeks) for depression because most persons rapidly develop tolerance for the antidepressant effects of the drugs. Some clinicians, however, report that long-term treatment with sympathomimetics can benefit some persons.

Encephalopathy Caused by Brain Injury

Sympathomimetics increase alertness, cognition, motivation, and motor performance in persons with neurological deficits caused by strokes, trauma, tumors, or chronic infections. Treatment with sympathomimetics may permit earlier and more robust participation in rehabilitative programs. Poststroke lethargy and apathy may respond to long-term use of sympathomimetics.

Obesity

Sympathomimetics are used in the treatment of obesity because of their anorexia-inducing effects. Because tolerance develops for the anorectic effects and because of the drugs' high abuse potential, their use for this indication is limited. Of the sympathomimetic drugs, phentermine is the most widely used for appetite suppression. Phentermine was the second half of "fen-phen," an off-label combination of fenfluramine and phentermine that was widely used to promote weight loss until fenfluramine and dexfenfluramine were withdrawn from commercial availability because of an association with cardiac valvular insufficiency, primary pulmonary hypertension, and irreversible loss of cerebral serotoninergic nerve fibers. The toxicity of fenfluramine is attributed to its stimulating release of massive amounts of serotonin from nerve endings, a mechanism of action not shared by phentermine. Use of phentermine alone has not been reported to cause the same adverse effects as those caused by fenfluramine or dexfenfluramine.

Careful limitation of caloric intake and judicious exercise are at the core of any successful weight loss program. Sympathomimetic drugs facilitate loss of, at most, an additional fraction of a pound per week. Sympathomimetic drugs are effective appetite suppressants only for the first few weeks of use; then the anorexigenic effects tend to decrease.

Fatigue

Between 70 and 90 percent of individuals with multiple sclerosis experience fatigue. Modafinil, amphetamines, methylphenidate, and the dopamine receptor agonist amantadine (Symmetrel) are sometimes effective in combating this symptom. Other causes of fatigue, such as chronic fatigue syndrome, respond to stimulants in many cases.

PRECAUTIONS AND ADVERSE REACTIONS

The most common adverse effects associated with amphetamine-like drugs are stomach pain, anxiety, irritability, insomnia, tachycardia, cardiac arrhythmias, and dysphoria. Sympathomimetics cause decreased appetite, although tolerance usually develops for this effect. The drugs can also cause increases in heart rate and blood pressure (BP) and may cause palpitations. Less common adverse effects include the possible induction of movement disorders, such as tics, Tourette's disorder–like symptoms, and dyskinesias, which are often self-limited over 7 to 10 days. If a person taking a sympathomimetic develops one of these movement disorders, a correlation between the dose of the medication and the severity of the disorder must be firmly established before adjustments are made in the medication dose. In severe cases, augmentation with risperidone (Risperdal), clonidine, or guanfacine is necessary. Methylphenidate may worsen tics in one third of persons; these persons fall into two groups: those whose methylphenidate-induced tics resolve immediately on metabolism of the dose and a smaller group in whom methylphenidate appears to trigger tics that persist for several months but eventually resolve spontaneously.

Longitudinal studies do not indicate that sympathomimetics cause growth suppression. Sympathomimetics can exacerbate glaucoma, hypertension, cardiovascular disorders, hyperthyroidism, anxiety disorders, psychotic disorders, and seizure disorders.

High doses of sympathomimetics can cause dry mouth, pupillary dilation, bruxism, formication, excessive ebullience, restlessness, and emotional lability. Long-term use of high doses can cause a delusional disorder that resembles paranoid schizophrenia. Overdoses of sympathomimetics result in hypertension, tachycardia, hyperthermia, toxic psychosis, delirium, and occasionally seizures. Overdoses of sympathomimetics can also result in death, often caused by cardiac arrhythmias. Seizures can be treated with benzodiazepines, cardiac effects with β-adrenergic receptor antagonists, fever with cooling blankets, and delirium with dopamine receptor antagonists.

The most limiting adverse effect of sympathomimetics is their association with psychological and physical dependence. At the doses used for treatment of ADHD, psychological dependence virtually never develops. A greater concern is the presence of adolescent or adult cohabitants who might confiscate the supply of sympathomimetics for abuse or sale.

Sympathomimetic use should be avoided during pregnancy, especially during the first trimester. Dextroamphetamine and methylphenidate pass into the breast milk, and it is not known whether pemoline or modafinil do.

A review of postmarketing experience with pemoline found several cases of acute hepatic failure, some of which were in children. This prompted the U.S. Food and Drug Administration (FDA) to change the package insert to recommend that pemoline no longer be considered first-line therapy for ADHD. It is now rarely used.

DRUG INTERACTIONS

The coadministration of sympathomimetics and tricyclic or tetracyclic antidepressants, warfarin (Coumadin), primidone (Mysoline), phenobarbital (Luminal), phenytoin (Dilantin), or phenylbutazone (Butazolidin) decreases the metabolism of these compounds, resulting in increased plasma levels. Sympathomimetics decrease the therapeutic efficacy of many antihypertensive drugs, especially guanethidine (Esimil, Ismelin). The sympathomimetics should be used with extreme caution with monoamine oxidase inhibitors (MAOIs).

LABORATORY INTERFERENCES

Dextroamphetamine can elevate plasma corticosteroid levels and interfere with some assay methods for urinary corticosteroids.

DOSING AND ADMINISTRATION

Many psychiatrists believe that amphetamine use has been overly regulated by governmental authorities. Amphetamines are listed as schedule II drugs by the Drug Enforcement Agency. In some states, physicians must use triplicate prescriptions for such drugs; one copy is filed with a state government agency. Such mandates worry both patients and physicians about breaches in confidentiality, and physicians are concerned that their prescribing practices may be misinterpreted by official agencies. Consequently, some physicians may withhold prescription of sympathomimetics, even from persons who may benefit from the medications.

The dose ranges and the available preparations for sympathomimetics are presented in Table 32.31–1. Dextroamphetamine, methylphenidate, amphetamine, lisdexamfetamines, benzphetamine, and methamphetamine are schedule II drugs; in some states, they require triplicate prescriptions. Phendimetrazine and phenmetrazine are schedule III drugs, and modafinil, phentermine, diethylpropion, and mazindol are schedule IV drugs.

Pretreatment evaluation should include an evaluation of the person's cardiac function, with particular attention to the presence of hypertension or tachyarrhythmias. The clinician should also examine the person for the presence of movement disorders, such as tics and dyskinesia, because these conditions can be exacerbated by the administration of sympathomimetics. If tics are present, many experts will not use sympathomimetics but will instead choose clonidine or antidepressants. Recent data, however, indicate that sympathomimetics may cause only a mild increase in motor tics and may actually suppress vocal tics. Liver function and renal function should be assessed, and doses of sympathomimetics should be reduced for persons with impaired metabolism. In the case of pemoline, any elevation of liver enzymes is a compelling reason to discontinue the medication.

Persons with ADHD can take immediate-release methylphenidate at 8 AM, 12 noon, and 4 PM. Dextroamphetamine, sustained-release methylphenidate, or 18 mg of extended-release methylphenidate may be taken once at 8 AM. Pemoline is taken at 8 AM. The starting dose of methylphenidate ranges from 2.5 mg of regular to 20 mg of sustained-release drug in children and 90 mg daily in adults. If this is inadequate, the dose may be increased to a maximal dose of 80 mg. The dose of dextroamphetamine is 2.5 to 40 mg a day up to 0.5 mg/kg a day. Pemoline is given in doses of 18.75 to 112.5 mg a day. Liver function tests should be monitored when using pemoline. Although it is not clear that the routine liver screening can predict acute liver failure caused by pemoline, it is certainly necessary to stop pemoline use if screening tests give any hint of hepatic dysfunction. Children are generally more sensitive to adverse effects than are adults. Dosing for treatment of narcolepsy and depression is comparable to that for treatment of ADHD. Lifdexamfetamine is given once daily in the morning in an oral dose of 30-, 50-, or 70-mg extended-release capsule. The average therapeutic dose is 70 mg.

Table 32.31–1
Sympathomimetics Commonly Used in Psychiatry

Generic Name	Trade Name	Preparations	Initial Daily Dose	Usual Daily Dose for ADHD[a]	Usual Daily Dose for Narcolepsy	Maximal Daily Dose
Atomoxetine	Strattera	10-, 18-, 25-, 40-, 60-mg tablets	20 mg	40–80 mg	Not used	Children 80 mg, adults 100 mg
Amphetamine-dextroamphetamine	Adderall	5-, 10-, 20-, 30-mg tablets	5 to 10 mg	20–30 mg	5–60 mg	Children 40 mg, adults 60 mg
Dexmethylphenidate	Focalin	2.5-, 5-, 10-mg capsules	5 mg	5–20 mg	Not used	20 mg
Dextroamphetamine	Dexedrine, Dextrostat	5-, 10-, 15-mg ER capsules; 5-, 10-mg tablets	5 to 10 mg	20–30 mg	5–60 mg	Children 40 mg, adults 60 mg
Lisdexamfetamine	Vyvanse	30-, 50-, 70-mg ER tablets	30 mg	30–70 mg	Not used	70 mg
Modafinil	Provigil	100-, 200-mg tablets	100 mg	Not used	400 mg	400 mg
Methamphetamine	Desoxyn	5-mg tablets; 5-, 10-, 15-mg ER tablets	5–10 mg	20–25 mg	Not generally used	45 mg
Methylphenidate	Ritalin, Methidate, Methylin, Attenade	5-, 10-, 20-mg tablets; 10-, 20-mg SR tablets	5–10 mg	5–60 mg	20–30 mg	Children 80 mg, adults 90 mg
	Concerta	18-, 36-mg ER tablets	18 mg	18–54 mg	Not yet established	54 mg
Pemoline	Cylert	18.75-, 37.5-, 75-mg tablets; 37.5-mg chewable tablets	37.5 mg	56.25–75 mg	Not used	112.5 mg

ADHD, attention-deficit/hyperactivity disorder; ER, extended release; SR, sustained released.
[a]For children 6 years of age or older.

The starting dose of modafinil is 200 mg in the morning in medically healthy individuals and 100 mg in the morning in persons with hepatic impairment. Some persons take a second 100- or 200-mg dose in the afternoon. The maximal recommended daily dose is 400 mg, although doses of 600 to 1,200 mg a day have been used safely. Adverse effects become prominent at doses greater than 400 mg a day. Compared with amphetamine-like drugs, modafinil promotes wakefulness but produces less attentiveness and less irritability. Some persons with excessive daytime sleepiness extend the activity of the morning modafinil dose with an afternoon dose of methylphenidate.

ATOMOXETINE (STRATTERA)

Atomoxetine is the first nonstimulant drug to be approved by the FDA as a treatment of ADHD in children, adolescents, and adults. It is included in this section because it shares this indication with the stimulants described previously.

Pharmacological Actions

Atomoxetine is believed to produce a therapeutic effect through selective inhibition of the presynaptic norepinephrine transporter. It is well absorbed after oral administration and is minimally affected by food. High-fat meals may decrease the rate but not the extent of absorption. Maximal plasma concentrations are reached after approximately 1 to 2 hours. At therapeutic concentrations, 98 percent of atomoxetine in plasma is bound to protein, mainly albumin. Atomoxetine has a half-life of approximately 5 hours and is metabolized principally by the cytochrome P450 (CYP) 2D6 pathway. Poor metabolizers of this compound have a fivefold-higher area under the curve and a fivefold-higher peak plasma concentration than do normal or extensive metabolizers. This is important to consider in patients receiving medications that inhibit the CYP 2D6 enzyme. For example, the antidepressant-like pharmacology of atomoxetine has led to its use as an add-on to selective serotonin reuptake inhibitors or other antidepressants. Drugs such as fluoxetine (Prozac), paroxetine (Paxil), or bupropion are CYP 2D6 inhibitors and may raise atomoxetine levels.

Therapeutic Indications

Atomoxetine is used for the treatment of ADHD. It should be considered for use in patients who find stimulants too activating or who experience other intolerable side effects. Because atomoxetine has no abuse potential, it a reasonable choice in the treatment of patients with both ADHD and substance abuse, patients who complain of ADHD symptoms but are suspected of seeking stimulant drugs, or patients who are in recovery.

Atomoxetine may enhance cognition when used to treat patients with schizophrenia. It also can be used as an alternative or add-on to antidepressants in patients who fail to respond to standard therapies.

Precautions and Adverse Reactions

Common side effects of atomoxetine include abdominal discomfort, decreased appetite with resulting weight loss, sexual dysfunction, dizziness, vertigo, irritability, and mood swings. Minor increases in BP and heart rate have also been observed. Cases have been seen of severe liver injury in a few patients taking atomoxetine. The drug should be discontinued in patients with jaundice (yellowing of the skin or whites of the eyes, itching) or laboratory evidence of liver injury. Atomoxetine should not be taken at the same time as, or within 2 weeks of taking, an MAOI or by patients with narrow-angle glaucoma.

The effects of overdose greater than twice the maximal recommended daily dose in humans are unknown. No specific information is available on the treatment of overdose with atomoxetine.

Dosing and Clinical Guidelines

Atomoxetine is available as 10-, 18-, 25-, 40-, and 60-mg capsules. In children and adolescents up to 70 kg in body weight, atomoxetine should be initiated at a total daily dose of approximately 0.5 mg/kg and increased after a minimum of 3 days to a target total daily dose of approximately 1.2 mg/kg administered either as a single daily dose in the morning or as evenly divided doses in the morning and late afternoon or early evening. The total daily dose in smaller children and adolescents should not exceed 1.4 mg/kg or 100 mg, whichever is less. Dosing of children and adolescents greater than 70 kg in body weight and adults should start at a total daily dose of 40 mg and then be increased after a minimum of 3 days to a target total daily dose of approximately 80 mg. The doses can be administered either as a single daily dose in the morning or as evenly divided doses in the morning and late afternoon or early evening. After 2 to 4 additional weeks, the dose may be increased to a maximum of 100 mg in patients who have not achieved an optimal response. The maximal recommended total daily dose in children and adolescents greater than 70 kg and adults is 100 mg.

▲ 32.32 Thyroid Hormones

Thyroid hormones—levothyroxine (Synthroid, Levothroid, Levoxine) and liothyronine (Cytomel)—are used in psychiatry either alone or as augmentation to treat persons with depression or rapid-cycling bipolar I disorder. They can convert an antidepressant-nonresponsive person into an antidepressant-responsive person. Thyroid hormones are also used as replacement therapy for persons treated with lithium (Eskalith) who develop a hypothyroid state.

Liothyronine and levothyroxine are the levorotatory forms of the endogenous hormones triiodothyronine (T_3) and thyroxine (T_4), respectively.

PHARMACOLOGICAL ACTIONS

Thyroid hormones are administered orally, and their absorption from the gastrointestinal tract is variable. Absorption is increased if the drug is administered on an empty stomach. In the brain, T_4 crosses the blood–brain barrier and diffuses into neurons, where it is converted into T_3, which is the physiologically active form. The half-life of T_4 is 6 to 7 days, and that of T_3 is 1 to 2 days.

The mechanism of action for thyroid hormone effects on antidepressant efficacy is unknown. Thyroid hormone binds to intracellular receptors that regulate the transcription of a wide range of genes, including several receptors for neurotransmitters.

THERAPEUTIC INDICATIONS

The major indication for thyroid hormones in psychiatry is as an adjuvant to antidepressants. No clear correlation has been found between the laboratory measures of thyroid function and the response to thyroid hormone supplementation of antidepressants. If a patient has not responded to a 6-week course of antidepressants at appropriate doses, adjuvant therapy with either lithium or a thyroid hormone is an alternative. Most clinicians use adjuvant lithium before trying a thyroid hormone. Several controlled trials have indicated that liothyronine use converts about 50 percent of antidepressant nonresponders to responders.

The dose of liothyronine is 25 or 50 μg a day added to the patient's antidepressant regimen. Liothyronine has been used primarily as an adjuvant for tricyclic drugs; however, evidence suggests that liothyronine augments the effects of all the antidepressant drugs.

Thyroid hormones have not been shown to cause particular problems in pediatric or geriatric patients; however, the hormones should be used with caution in the elderly, who may have occult heart disease.

PRECAUTIONS AND ADVERSE REACTIONS

At the doses usually used for augmentation—25 to 50 μg a day—adverse effects occur infrequently. The most common adverse effects associated with thyroid hormones are transient headache, weight loss, palpitations, nervousness, diarrhea, abdominal cramps, sweating, tachycardia, increased blood pressure, tremors, and insomnia. Osteoporosis can also occur with long-term treatment, but this has not been found in studies involving liothyronine augmentation. Overdoses of thyroid hormones can lead to cardiac failure and death.

Thyroid hormones should not be taken by persons with cardiac disease, angina, or hypertension. The hormones are contraindicated in thyrotoxicosis and uncorrected adrenal insufficiency and in persons with acute myocardial infarctions. Thyroid hormones can be administered safely to pregnant women, provided that laboratory thyroid indexes are monitored. Thyroid hormones are minimally excreted in the breast milk and have not been shown to cause problems in nursing babies.

DRUG INTERACTIONS

Thyroid hormones can potentiate the effects of warfarin (Coumadin) and other anticoagulants by increasing the catabolism of clotting factors. They may increase the insulin requirement for diabetic persons and the digitalis requirement for persons with cardiac disease. Thyroid hormones should not be coadministered with sympathomimetics, ketamine (Ketalar), or maprotiline (Ludiomil) because of the risk of cardiac decompensation. Administration of selective serotonin reuptake inhibitors, tricyclic and tetracyclic drugs, lithium, or carbamazepine (Tegre-

tol) can mildly lower serum thyroxine and raise serum thyrotropin concentrations in euthyroid persons or persons taking thyroid replacements. This interaction warrants close serum monitoring and may require an increase in the dose or initiation of thyroid hormone supplementation.

LABORATORY INTERFERENCES

Levothyroxine has not been reported to interfere with any laboratory test other than thyroid function indexes. Liothyronine, however, suppresses the release of endogenous T_4, thereby lowering the result of any thyroid function test that depends on the measure of T_4.

THYROID FUNCTION TESTS

Several thyroid function tests are available, including tests for T_4 by competitive protein binding and by radioimmunoassay involving a specific antigen–antibody reaction. More than 90 percent of T_4 is bound to serum protein and is responsible for thyroid-stimulating hormone (TSH) secretion and cellular metabolism. Other thyroid measures include the free T_4 index, T_3 uptake, and total serum T_3 measured by radioimmunoassay. Those tests are used to rule out hypothyroidism, which can be associated with symptoms of depression. In some studies, up to 10 percent of patients complaining of depression and associated fatigue had incipient hypothyroid disease. Lithium can cause hypothyroidism and, more rarely, hyperthyroidism. Neonatal hypothyroidism results in mental retardation and is preventable if the diagnosis is made at birth.

Thyrotropin-Releasing Hormone Stimulation Test

The thyrotropin-releasing hormone (TRH) stimulation test is indicated for patients who have marginally abnormal thyroid test results with suspected subclinical hypothyroidism, which may account for clinical depression. It is also used in patients with possible lithium-induced hypothyroidism. The procedure entails an intravenous injection of 500 mg of protirelin (TRH), which produces a sharp rise in serum TSH levels, which are measured at 15, 30, 60, and 90 minutes. An increase in serum TSH of 5 to 25 mIU/mL above the baseline is normal. An increase of less than 7 mIU/mL is considered a blunted response, which may correlate with a diagnosis of depression. Of all patients with depression, 8 percent have some thyroid illness.

DOSING AND CLINICAL GUIDELINES

Liothyronine is available in 5-, 25-, and 50-μg tablets. Levothyroxine is available in 12.5-, 25-, 50-, 75-, 88-, 100-, 112-, 125-, 150-, 175-, 200-, and 300-μg tablets; it is also available in a 200- and 500-μg parenteral form. The dose of liothyronine is 25 or 50 μg a day added to the person's antidepressant regimen. Liothyronine has been used as an adjuvant for all the available antidepressant drugs. An adequate trial of liothyronine supplementation should last 2 to 3 weeks. If liothyronine supplementation is successful, it should be continued for 2 months and then tapered off at the rate of 12.5 μg a day every 3 to 7 days.

▲ 32.33 Trazodone

Trazodone (Desyrel) was introduced as a treatment of major depression in 1998 but never achieved widespread use in that role because many patients found it to be too sedating at therapeutic doses. It has become extensively used, however, at low doses as an alternative to hypnotic agents, particularly to counteract the frequent sleep disturbances associated with selective serotonin reuptake inhibitors. Trazodone is structurally related to nefazodone (Serzone) and structurally unrelated to other available antidepressant drugs.

PHARMACOLOGICAL ACTIONS

Trazodone is readily absorbed from the gastrointestinal tract and reaches peak plasma levels in about 1 hour. It has a half-life of 5 to 9 hours. Trazodone is metabolized in the liver, and 75 percent of its metabolites are excreted in the urine.

Trazodone is a weak inhibitor of serotonin reuptake and a potent antagonist of serotonin 5-HT_{2A} and 5-HT_{2C} receptors. The active metabolite of trazodone is m-chlorophenylpiperazine (mCPP), which is an agonist at 5-HT_{2C} receptors and has a half-life of 14 hours. mCPP has been associated with migraine, anxiety, and weight loss. The adverse effects of trazodone are partially mediated by α_1-adrenergic receptor antagonism.

THERAPEUTIC INDICATIONS

Depressive Disorders

The main indication for the use of trazodone is major depressive disorder. A clear dose–response relationship is seen, with doses of 250 to 600 mg a day being necessary for trazodone to have therapeutic benefit. Trazodone increases total sleep time, decreases the number and the duration of nighttime awakenings, and decreases the amount of rapid eye movement sleep. Unlike tricyclic drugs, trazodone does not decrease stage 4 sleep. Trazodone, thus, is useful for depressed persons with anxiety and insomnia.

Insomnia

Trazodone is a first-line agent for the treatment of insomnia because of its marked sedative qualities and favorable effects on sleep architecture (see preceding comments), combined with its lack of anticholinergic effects. Trazodone is effective for insomnia caused both by depression and by use of drugs. When used as a hypnotic, the usual initial dose is 25 to 100 mg at bedtime.

Erectile Disorder

Trazodone is associated with an increased risk of priapism. Trazodone can potentiate erections resulting from sexual stimulation, and thus it has been used to prolong erectile time and turgidity in some men with erectile disorder. The dose for this indication is 150 to 200 mg a day. Trazodone-triggered priapism (an erection lasting more than 3 hours with pain) is a medical emergency. The use of trazodone for treatment of male erectile dysfunction has diminished considerably since the introduction of phosphodiesterase-5 agents.

Other Indications

Trazodone may be useful in low doses (50 mg a day) to control severe agitation in children with developmental disabilities and elderly persons with dementia. At doses above 250 mg a day, trazodone reduces the tension and apprehension associated with generalized anxiety disorder. It has been used to treat depression in patients with schizophrenia. Trazodone may have a beneficial effect on insomnia and nightmares in posttraumatic stress disorder.

PRECAUTIONS AND ADVERSE REACTIONS

The most common adverse effects associated with trazodone are sedation, orthostatic hypotension, dizziness, headache, and nausea. Some persons experience dry mouth or gastric irritation. The drug is not associated with anticholinergic adverse effects, such as urinary retention, weight gain, and constipation. A few case reports have noted an association between trazodone and arrhythmias in persons with preexisting, premature ventricular contractions or mitral valve prolapse. Neutropenia, usually not of clinical significance, can develop, which should be considered if persons have fever or sore throat.

Trazodone can cause significant orthostatic hypotension 4 to 6 hours after a dose is taken, especially if it is taken concurrently with antihypertensive agents or if a large dose is taken without food. Administration of trazodone with food slows absorption and reduces the peak plasma concentration, thus reducing the risk of orthostatic hypotension.

Trazodone causes priapism—prolonged erection in the absence of sexual stimuli—in 1 of every 10,000 men. Trazodone-induced priapism usually appears in the first 4 weeks of treatment but can occur as late as 18 months into treatment. It can appear at any dose. In such cases, trazodone use should be discontinued and another antidepressant should be used. Painful erections or erections lasting more than 1 hour are warning signs that warrant immediate discontinuation of the drug and medical evaluation. The first step in the emergency management of priapism is intracavernosal injection of an α_1-adrenergic agonist pressor agent, such as metaraminol (Aramine) or epinephrine. Trazodone is less likely to precipitate mania in vulnerable persons than are other antidepressant drugs.

Trazodone use is contraindicated in pregnant and nursing women. Trazodone should be used with caution in persons with hepatic and renal diseases.

DRUG INTERACTIONS

Trazodone potentiates the central nervous system–depressant effects of other centrally acting drugs and alcohol. Concurrent use of trazodone and antihypertensives can cause hypotension. No cases of hypertensive crisis have been reported when trazodone has been used to treat monoamine oxidase inhibitor–associated insomnia. Trazodone can increase levels of digoxin and phenytoin. Trazodone should be used with caution in combination with warfarin. Drugs that inhibit cytochrome P450 3A4 can increase levels of trazodone's major metabolite, mCPP, leading to an increase in side effects.

LABORATORY INTERFERENCES

No known laboratory interferences are associated with the administration of trazodone.

DOSING AND CLINICAL GUIDELINES

Trazodone is available in 50-, 100-, 150-, and 300-mg tablets. Once-a-day dosing is as effective as divided dosing and reduces daytime sedation. The usual starting dose is 50 mg before sleep. The dose can be increased in increments of 50 mg every 3 days if sedation or orthostatic hypotension does not become a problem. The therapeutic range for trazodone is 200 to 600 mg a day in divided doses. Some reports indicate that doses of 400 to 600 mg a day are required for maximal therapeutic effects; other reports indicate that 250 to 400 mg a day is sufficient. The dose can be titrated up to 300 mg a day; then, the person can be evaluated for the need for further dose increases on the basis of the presence or the absence of signs of clinical improvement.

▲ 32.34 Tricyclics and Tetracyclics

The tricyclic antidepressants and tetracyclic antidepressants (TCAs) have a long history of use in psychiatry, having become available in the mid-1950s. Introduced as antidepressants, their therapeutic indications now also include panic disorder, generalized anxiety disorder, posttraumatic stress disorder (PTSD), obsessive-compulsive disorder (OCD), and pain syndromes. The introduction of newer agents, such as the selective serotonin reuptake inhibitors (SSRIs), bupropion (Wellbutrin), venlafaxine (Effexor), and mirtazapine (Remeron), has sharply decreased prescriptions of the TCAs; nevertheless, they remain extremely useful.

PHARMACOLOGICAL ACTIONS

Absorption of most TCAs is complete after oral administration, and significant metabolism occurs from the first-pass effect. Peak plasma concentrations occur within 2 to 8 hours, and the half-lives of the TCAs vary from 10 to 70 hours; nortriptyline (Aventyl, Pamelor), maprotiline (Ludiomil), and, particularly, protriptyline (Vivactil) can have longer half-lives. The long half-lives allow all of the compounds to be given once daily; 5 to 7 days are needed to reach steady-state plasma concentrations. Imipramine pamoate (Tofranil) is a depot form of the drug for intramuscular (IM) administration; indications for the use of this preparation are limited.

The TCAs undergo hepatic metabolism by the cytochrome P450 (CYP) enzyme system. Clinically relevant drug interactions can result from competition for enzyme CYP 2D6 between TCAs and quinidine, cimetidine (Tagamet), fluoxetine (Prozac), sertraline (Zoloft), paroxetine (Paxil), phenothiazines, carbamazepine (Tegretol), and the type IC antiarrhythmics propafenone (Rythmol) and flecainide (Tambocor). Concomitant administration of TCAs and these inhibitors may slow the metabolism and raise the plasma concentrations of TCAs. In addition, genetic variations in the activity of CYP 2D6 may account for up to a 40-times difference in plasma TCA concentrations in different persons. The dosage of the TCA may need to be adjusted to correct changes in the rate of hepatic TCA metabolism.

The TCAs block the transporter site for norepinephrine and serotonin, thus increasing synaptic concentrations of these neurotransmitters. Each drug differs in its affinity for each of these transporters, with clomipramine (Anafranil) being the most serotonin selective and desipramine (Norpramin, Pertofrane) the most norepinephrine selective of the TCAs. Secondary effects of the TCAs include antagonism at the muscarinic acetylcholine, histamine H_1, and α_1- and α_2-adrenergic receptors. It is the potency of these effects on other receptors that largely determines the side-effect profile of each drug. Amoxapine (Asendin), nortriptyline, desipramine, and maprotiline have the least anticholinergic activity; doxepin (Adapin, Sinequan) has the most antihistaminergic activity. Although they are more likely to cause constipation, sedation, dry mouth, or lightheadedness than the SSRIs, the TCAs are less likely to cause sexual dysfunction, significant long-term weight gain, and sleep disturbances than the SSRIs. The half-life and plasma clearance for most TCAs are very similar.

THERAPEUTIC INDICATIONS

Each of the following indications is also an indication for SSRIs, which have widely replaced the TCAs in clinical practice. TCAs, however, represent a reasonable alternative for persons who cannot tolerate the adverse effects of the SSRIs.

Major Depressive Disorder

The treatment of a major depressive episode and the prophylactic treatment of major depressive disorder are the principal indications for using TCAs. Whereas the TCAs are effective in the treatment of depression in persons with bipolar I disorder, they are more likely to induce mania, hypomania, or cycling than newer antidepressants, most notably the SSRIs and bupropion. Thus, it is not advised that TCAs be routinely used to treat depression associated with bipolar I or bipolar II disorder.

Melancholic features, prior major depressive episodes, and a family history of depressive disorders increase the likelihood of a therapeutic response. All available TCAs are equally effective in the treatment of depressive disorders. In the case of an individual person, however, one tricyclic or tetracyclic may be effective, whereas another one may be ineffective. The treatment of a major depressive episode with psychotic features almost always requires the coadministration of an antipsychotic drug and an antidepressant.

Although it is used worldwide as an antidepressant, clomipramine is only approved in the United States for the treatment of OCD.

Panic Disorder with Agoraphobia

Imipramine is the TCA most studied for panic disorder with agoraphobia, but other TCAs are also effective when taken at the usual antidepressant doses. Because of the potential initial anxiogenic effects of the TCAs, starting doses should be small, and the dose should be titrated upward slowly. Small doses of benzodiazepines can be used initially to deal with this side effect.

Generalized Anxiety Disorder

The use of doxepin for the treatment of anxiety disorders is approved by the U.S. Food and Drug Administration. Some research data show that imipramine may also be useful. Although rarely used anymore, a chlordiazepoxide–amitriptyline combination (Limbitrol) is available for mixed anxiety and depressive disorders.

Obsessive-Compulsive Disorder

Obsessive-compulsive disorder appears to respond specifically to clomipramine, as well as the SSRIs. Some improvement is usually seen in 2 to 4 weeks, but a further reduction in symptoms may continue for the first 4 to 5 months of treatment. None of the other TCAs appears to be nearly as effective as clomipramine for treatment of this disorder. Clomipramine may also be a drug of choice for depressed persons with marked obsessive features.

Pain

The TCAs are widely used to treat chronic neuropathic pain and in prophylaxis of migraine headache. Amitriptyline is the TCA most often used in this role. During treatment of pain, doses are generally lower than those used in depression; for example, 75 mg of amitriptyline may be effective. These effects also appear more rapidly.

Other Disorders

Childhood enuresis is often treated with imipramine. Peptic ulcer disease can be treated with doxepin, which has marked antihistaminergic effects. Other indications for TCAs are narcolepsy, nightmare disorder, and PTSD. The drugs are sometimes used for treatment of children and adolescents with attention-deficit/hyperactivity disorder, sleepwalking disorder, separation anxiety disorder, and sleep terror disorder. Clomipramine has also been used to treat premature ejaculation, movement disorders, and compulsive behavior in children with autistic disorders; however, because TCAs have caused sudden death in several children and adolescents, their use is best avoided in this population.

PRECAUTIONS AND ADVERSE REACTIONS

The TCAs are associated with a wide range of problematic side effects and can be lethal when taken in overdose.

Psychiatric Effects

The TCAs can induce a switch to mania or hypomania in susceptible individuals. TCAs can also exacerbate psychotic disorders in susceptible persons. At high plasma concentrations (levels >300 ng/mL), the anticholinergic effects of the TCAs can cause confusion or delirium. Patients with dementia are particularly vulnerable to this development.

Anticholinergic Effects

Anticholinergic effects often limit the tolerable dose to relatively low ranges. Some persons may develop a tolerance for the anticholinergic effects with continued treatment. Anticholinergic effects include dry mouth, constipation, blurred vision, delirium, and urinary retention. Sugarless gum, candy, or fluoride lozenges can alleviate the dry mouth. Bethanechol (Urecholine), 25 to 50 mg three or four times a day, may reduce urinary hesitancy and

may be helpful in erectile dysfunction when the drug is taken 30 minutes before sexual intercourse. Narrow-angle glaucoma can also be aggravated by anticholinergic drugs, and the precipitation of glaucoma requires emergency treatment with a miotic agent. TCAs should be avoided in persons with narrow-angle glaucoma, and an SSRI should be substituted. Severe anticholinergic effects can lead to a central nervous system (CNS) anticholinergic syndrome with confusion and delirium, especially if TCAs are administered with dopamine receptor antagonists (DRAs) or anticholinergic drugs. IM or intravenous physostigmine (Antilirium, Eserine) is used to diagnose and treat anticholinergic delirium.

Cardiac Effects

When administered in their usual therapeutic doses, the TCAs can cause tachycardia, flattened T waves, prolonged QT intervals, and depressed ST segments in the electrocardiographic (ECG) recording. Imipramine has a quinidine-like effect at therapeutic plasma concentrations and may reduce the number of premature ventricular contractions. Because the drugs prolong conduction time, their use is contraindicated in persons with preexisting conduction defects. In persons with a history of any type of heart disease, TCAs should be used only after SSRIs or other newer antidepressants have been found ineffective, and, if used, they should be introduced at low doses, with gradual increases in dose and monitoring of cardiac functions. All TCAs can cause tachycardia, which may persist for months and is one of the most common reasons for drug discontinuation, especially in younger persons. At high plasma concentrations, as seen in overdoses, the drugs become arrhythmogenic.

Other Autonomic Effects

Orthostatic hypotension is the most common cardiovascular autonomic adverse effect and the most common reason TCAs are discontinued. It can result in falls and injuries in affected persons. Nortriptyline may be the drug least likely to cause this problem. Orthostatic hypotension is treated with avoidance of caffeine, intake of at least 2 L of fluid per day, and addition of salt to the diet unless the person is being treated for hypertension. In persons taking antihypertensive agents, a dose reduction may reduce the risk of orthostatic hypotension. Other possible autonomic effects are profuse sweating, palpitations, and increased blood pressure (BP). Although some persons respond to fludrocortisone (Florinef), 0.02 to 0.05 mg twice a day, substitution of an SSRI is preferable to addition of a potentially toxic mineralocorticoid such as fludrocortisone. TCA use should be discontinued several days before elective surgery because of the occurrence of hypertensive episodes during surgery in persons receiving TCAs.

Sedation

Sedation is a common effect of TCAs and may be welcomed if sleeplessness has been a problem. The sedative effect of TCAs is a result of anticholinergic and antihistaminergic activities. Amitriptyline, trimipramine, and doxepin are the most-sedating agents; imipramine, amoxapine, nortriptyline, and maprotiline are less sedating; and desipramine and protriptyline are the least-sedating agents.

Neurological Effects

A fine rapid tremor may occur. Myoclonic twitches and tremors of the tongue and the upper extremities are common. Rare effects include speech blockage, paresthesia, peroneal palsies, and ataxia.

Amoxapine is unique in causing Parkinsonian symptoms, akathisia, and even dyskinesia because of the dopaminergic blocking activity of one of its metabolites. Amoxapine can also cause neuroleptic malignant syndrome in rare cases. Maprotiline can cause seizures when the dose is increased too quickly or is kept at high levels for too long. Clomipramine and amoxapine may lower the seizure threshold more than other drugs in the class. As a class, however, the TCAs have a relatively low risk for inducing seizures, except in persons who are at risk for seizures (e.g., persons with epilepsy and those with brain lesions). Although TCAs can still be used by such persons, the initial doses should be lower than usual, and subsequent dose increases should be gradual.

Allergic and Hematological Effects

Exanthematous rashes are seen in 4 to 5 percent of all persons treated with maprotiline. Jaundice is rare. Agranulocytosis, leukocytosis, leukopenia, and eosinophilia are rare complications of TCA treatment. A person who has a sore throat or a fever during the first few months of TCA treatment, however, should have a complete blood count done immediately.

Hepatic Effects

Mild and self-limited rise in serum transaminase concentrations can occur and should be monitored. TCAs can also produce a fulminant acute hepatitis in 0.1 to 1 percent of persons. This can be life threatening, and the antidepressant should be discontinued.

Other Adverse Effects

Modest weight gain is common. Amoxapine exerts a DRA effect and can cause hyperprolactinemia, impotence, galactorrhea, anorgasmia, and ejaculatory disturbances. Other TCAs have also been associated with gynecomastia and amenorrhea. Inappropriate secretion of antidiuretic hormone has also been reported with TCAs. Other effects include nausea, vomiting, and hepatitis.

Precautions

The TCAs can cause a withdrawal syndrome in newborns, consisting of tachypnea, cyanosis, irritability, and poor sucking reflex. The drugs do pass into breast milk, but at concentrations that are usually undetectable in the infant's plasma. The drugs should be used with caution in persons with hepatic and renal diseases. TCAs should not be administered during a course of electroconvulsive therapy, primarily because of the risk of serious adverse cardiac effects.

DRUG INTERACTIONS

Monoamine Oxidase Inhibitors

The TCAs should not be taken within 14 days of administration of a monoamine oxidase inhibitor.

Antihypertensives

The TCAs block the neuronal reuptake of guanethidine (Esimil, Ismelin), which is required for antihypertensive activity. The antihypertensive effects of β-adrenergic receptor antagonists (e.g., propranolol [Inderal] and clonidine [Catapres]) can also be blocked by TCAs. The coadministration of a TCA and α-methyldopa (Aldomet) can cause behavioral agitation.

Antiarrhythmic Drugs

The antiarrhythmic properties of TCAs can be additive to those of quinidine, an effect that is further exacerbated by the inhibition of TCA metabolism by quinidine.

Dopamine Receptor Antagonists

Concurrent administration of TCAs and DRAs increases the plasma concentrations of both drugs. Desipramine plasma concentrations can rise twofold during concurrent administration with perphenazine (Trilafon). DRAs also add to the anticholinergic and sedative effects of the TCAs.

Central Nervous System Depressants

Opioids, alcohol, anxiolytics, hypnotics, and over-the-counter cold medications have additive effects by causing CNS depression when coadministered with TCAs. Persons should be advised to avoid driving or using dangerous equipment if they are sedated by TCAs.

Sympathomimetics

Tricyclic drug use with sympathomimetic drugs can cause serious cardiovascular effects.

Oral Contraceptives

Birth control pills can decrease TCA plasma concentrations through the induction of hepatic enzymes.

Other Drug Interactions

Nicotine can reduce TCA concentrations. Plasma concentrations can also be lowered by ascorbic acid, ammonium chloride, barbiturates, cigarette smoking, carbamazepine, chloral hydrate, lithium (Eskalith), and primidone (Mysoline). TCA plasma concentrations can be increased by concurrent use of acetazolamide (Diamox), sodium bicarbonate, acetylsalicylic acid, cimetidine, thiazide diuretics, fluoxetine, paroxetine, and fluvoxamine (Luvox). Plasma concentrations of TCAs can rise three- to fourfold when administered concurrently with fluoxetine, fluvoxamine, and paroxetine.

LABORATORY INTERFERENCES

Laboratory interferences with the TCAs have not been reported.

DOSING AND CLINICAL GUIDELINES

Persons who intend to take TCAs should have a routine physical and laboratory examination, including a complete blood count, a white blood cell count with differential, and serum electrolytes with liver function tests. An ECG should be obtained for all persons, especially women older than 40 years of age and men older than 30 years of age. TCAs are contraindicated in persons with a QT_c greater than 450 ms. The initial dose should be small and should be raised gradually. Because of the availability of highly effective alternatives to TCAs, a newer agent should be used in the presence of any medical condition that could interact adversely with the TCAs.

The elderly and children are more sensitive to TCA adverse effects than are young adults. In children, the ECG should be regularly monitored during use of a TCA.

The available preparations of TCAs are presented in Table 32.34–1. The doses and therapeutic blood levels for the TCAs vary among the drugs. With the exception of protriptyline, all TCAs can be started at 25 mg a day and increased as tolerated. Divided doses at first reduce the severity of the adverse effects, although most of the dose should be given at night to help induce sleep if a sedating drug, such as amitriptyline, is used. Eventually, the entire daily dose can be given at bedtime. A common clinical mistake is to stop increasing the dose when the person is tolerating the drug but taking less than the maximal therapeutic dose and does not show clinical improvement. The clinician should routinely assess the person's pulse and orthostatic changes in BP while the dose is being increased.

Nortriptyline use should be started at 25 mg a day. Most patients need only 75 mg a day to achieve a blood level of 100 mg/nL. The dose, however, can be raised to 150 mg a day, if needed. Amoxapine can be started at 150 mg a day and raised to 400 mg a day. Protriptyline use should be started at 15 mg a day and raised to 60 mg a day. Maprotiline has been associated with an increased incidence of seizures if the dose is raised too quickly or is maintained at too high a level. Maprotiline use should be started at 25 mg a day and increased over 4 weeks to 225 mg a day. It should be kept at that level for only 6 weeks and then be reduced to 175 to 200 mg a day.

Persons with chronic pain can be particularly sensitive to adverse effects when TCA use is started. Therefore, treatment should begin with low doses that are raised in small increments.

Persons with chronic pain may experience relief, however, on long-term low-dose therapy, such as amitriptyline or nortriptyline at 10 to 75 mg a day.

The TCAs should be avoided in children, except as a last resort. Dosing guidelines in children for imipramine include initiation at 1.5 mg/kg a day. The dose can be titrated to no more than 5 mg/kg a day. In enuresis, the dose is usually 50 to 100 mg a day taken at bedtime. Clomipramine use can be initiated at 50 mg a day and increased to no more than 3 mg/kg a day or 200 mg a day.

When TCA treatment is discontinued, the dose should first be decreased to three fourths of the maximal dose for a month. At that time, if no symptoms are present, drug use can be tapered by 25 mg (5 mg for protriptyline) every 4 to 7 days. Slow tapering avoids a cholinergic rebound syndrome consisting of nausea, upset stomach, sweating, headache, neck pain, and vomiting. This syndrome can be treated by reinstituting a small dose of the drug and tapering more slowly than before. Several case reports note the appearance of rebound mania or hypomania after the abrupt discontinuation of TCA use.

Plasma Concentrations and Therapeutic Drug Monitoring

Clinical determinations of plasma concentrations should be conducted after 5 to 7 days on the same dose of medication and 8 to 12 hours after the last dose. Because of variations in absorption and metabolism, a 30 to 50 times difference may be noted in the plasma concentrations in persons given the same dose of a TCA. Nortriptyline is unique in its association with a therapeutic window; that is, plasma concentrations less than 50 ng/mL or greater than 150 ng/mL may reduce its efficacy.

Plasma concentrations can be useful in confirming compliance, assessing reasons for drug failures, and documenting effective plasma concentrations for future treatment. Clinicians should always treat the person's condition and not the plasma concentration. Some persons have adequate clinical responses with seemingly subtherapeutic plasma concentrations, and other persons only respond at supratherapeutic plasma concentrations, without experiencing adverse effects. The latter situation, however, should alert the clinician to monitor the person's condition with, for example, serial ECG recordings.

Table 32.34–1
Tricyclic and Tetracyclic Drug Preparations

Drug	Tablets	Capsules	Parenteral	Solution
Imipramine (Tofranil)	10, 25, and 50 mg	75, 100, 125, and 150 mg	12.5 mg/mL	—
Desipramine (Norpramin, Pertofrane)	10, 25, 50, 75, 100, and 150 mg	—	—	—
Trimipramine (Surmontil)	—	25, 50, and 100 mg	—	—
Amitriptyline (Elavil)	10, 25, 50, 75, 100, and 150 mg	—	10 mg/mL	—
Nortriptyline (Aventyl, Pamelor)	—	10, 25, 50, and 75 mg	—	10 mg/5 mL
Protriptyline (Vivactil)	5 and 10 mg	—	—	—
Amoxapine (Asendin)	25, 50, 100, and 150 mg	—	—	—
Doxepin (Sinequan)	—	10, 25, 50, 75, 100, and 150 mg	—	10 mg/mL
Maprotiline (Ludiomil)	25, 50, and 75 mg	—	—	—
Clomipramine (Anafranil)	—	25, 50, and 75 mg	—	—

Overdose Attempts

Overdose attempts with TCAs are serious and can often be fatal. Prescriptions for these drugs should be nonrefillable and for no longer than a week at a time for patients at risk for suicide. Amoxapine may be more likely than the other TCAs to result in death when taken in overdose. The newer antidepressants are safer in overdose.

Symptoms of overdose include agitation, delirium, convulsions, hyperactive deep tendon reflexes, bowel and bladder paralysis, dysregulation of BP and temperature, and mydriasis. The patient then progresses to coma and perhaps respiratory depression. Cardiac arrhythmias may not respond to treatment. Because of the long half-lives of TCAs, patients are at risk of cardiac arrhythmias for 3 to 4 days after the overdose, so they should be monitored in an intensive care medical setting.

▲ 32.35 Valproate

Valproate (Depakene, Depakote), or valproic acid, is used for the treatment of acute manic or mixed episodes associated with bipolar I disorder. Other indications include seizure disorder and migraine prophylaxis.

Valproate is a simple-chain branch carboxylic acid. It is called valproic acid because it is rapidly converted to the acid form in the stomach. Multiple formulations of valproic acid are marketed. These include valproic acid (Depakene); divalproex sodium (Depakote), an enteric-coated delayed release 1:1 mixture of valproic acid and sodium valproate; and sodium valproate injection (Depacon). An extended-release preparation is also available. Each of these is therapeutically equivalent because at physiological pH, valproic acid dissociates into valproate ion.

PHARMACOLOGICAL ACTIONS

Regardless of how it is formulated, valproate is rapidly and completely absorbed 1 to 2 hours after oral administration, with peak concentrations occurring 4 to 5 hours after oral administration. The plasma half-life of valproate is 10 to 16 hours. Valproate is highly protein bound. Protein binding becomes saturated, and concentrations of therapeutically effective free valproate increase at serum concentrations above 50 to 100 μg/mL. The extended-release preparation produces lower peak concentrations and higher minimal concentrations and can be given once a day. Valproate is metabolized primarily by hepatic glucuronidation and mitochondrial β oxidation.

The biochemical basis of valproate's therapeutic effects is poorly understood. Postulated mechanisms include enhancement of γ-aminobutyric acid activity, modulation of voltage-sensitive sodium channels, and action on extrahypothalamic neuropeptides.

THERAPEUTIC INDICATIONS

Bipolar I Disorder

Acute Mania.   About two thirds of persons with acute mania respond to valproate. Most patients with mania usually respond within 1 to 4 days after achieving valproate serum concentrations above 50 μg/mL. Antimanic response is generally associated with levels greater than

50 μg/mL, in a range of 50 to 150 μg/mL. Using gradual-dosing strategies, this serum concentration can be achieved within 1 week of initiation of dosing, but newer, rapid oral loading strategies achieve therapeutic serum concentrations in 1 day and can control manic symptoms within 5 days. The short-term antimanic effects of valproate can be augmented with addition of lithium (Eskalith), carbamazepine (Tegretol), or dopamine receptor antagonists (DRAs). Because of its more favorable profile of cognitive, dermatological, thyroid, and renal adverse effects, valproate is preferred to lithium for treatment of acute mania in children and elderly persons.

Mixed Episodes.   Divalproex sodium extended-release tablets are approved for the treatment of acute manic or mixed episodes associated with bipolar disorder, with or without psychotic features. Mixed mania is a state of mind characterized by symptoms of both mania and depression. Patients often simultaneously feel agitated, angry, depressed, and irritable.

Acute Bipolar Depression.   Valproate possesses some activity as a short-term treatment of depressive episodes in bipolar I disorder, but this effect is far less pronounced than for treatment of manic episodes. Among depressive symptoms, valproate is more effective for treatment of agitation than dysphoria. In clinical practice, valproate is most often used as add-on therapy to an antidepressant to prevent the development of mania or rapid cycling.

Prophylaxis.   Studies suggest that valproate is effective in the prophylactic treatment of bipolar I disorder, resulting in fewer, less severe, and shorter manic episodes. In direct comparison, valproate is at least as effective as, and better tolerated than, lithium. It may be particularly effective in persons with rapid-cycling and ultrarapid-cycling bipolar disorders, dysphoric or mixed mania, and mania due to a general medical condition as well as in persons who have comorbid substance abuse or panic attacks and in persons who have not had complete favorable responses to lithium treatment.

Schizophrenia and Schizoaffective Disorder

Valproate may accelerate response to antipsychotic therapy in patients with schizophrenia or schizoaffective disorder. Valproate alone is generally less effective in schizoaffective disorder than in bipolar I disorder. Valproate alone is ineffective for treatment of psychotic symptoms and is typically used in combination with other drugs in patients with these symptoms.

Other Mental Disorders

Valproate has been studied for possible efficacy in a broad range of psychiatric disorders. These include alcohol withdrawal and relapse prevention, panic disorder, posttraumatic stress disorder, impulse control disorder, borderline personality disorder, and behavioral agitation and dementia. Evidence supporting use in these cases is weak, and any observed therapeutic effects may be related to treatment of comorbid bipolar disorder.

PRECAUTIONS AND ADVERSE REACTIONS

The two most serious adverse effects of valproate treatment affect the pancreas and the liver. Risk factors for potentially fatal hepatotoxicity include young age (<3 years), concurrent use of phenobarbital, and the presence of neurological disorders, especially inborn errors of metabolism. The rate of fatal hepatotoxicity in persons who have been treated with only valproate is 0.85 per 100,000 persons; no person older than the age of 10 years is reported to have died from hepatotoxicity. Therefore, the risk of this adverse reaction in adult psychiatric patients seems low. Nevertheless, if symptoms of lethargy, malaise, anorexia, nausea and vomiting, edema, and abdominal pain occur in a person treated with valproate, the clinician must consider the possibility of severe hepatotoxicity. A modest increase in liver function test results does not correlate with the development of serious hepatotoxicity. Rare cases of pancreatitis have been reported; they occur most often in the first 6 months of treatment, and the condition occasionally results in death. Pancreatic function can be assessed and followed with serum amylase concentrations. Other potentially serious consequences of treatment include hyperammonemia-induced encephalopathy and thrombocytopenia. Thrombocytopenia and platelet dysfunction occur most commonly at high doses and result in the prolongation of bleeding times.

If at all possible, valproate should not be used by pregnant women. Women who require valproate therapy, therefore, should inform their physicians if they intend to become pregnant. The drug is associated with neural tube defects (e.g., spina bifida) in about 1 to 4 percent of all women who take valproate during the first trimester of the pregnancy. The risk of valproate-induced neural tube defects can be reduced with daily folic acid supplements (1 to 4 mg a day). All women on the drug with childbearing potential should be given folic acid supplements. Infants breast-fed by mothers taking valproate develop serum valproate concentrations 1 to 10 percent of maternal serum concentrations, and no data suggest that this poses a risk to the infant. Valproate is not contraindicated in nursing mothers. Clinicians should not administer the drug to persons with hepatic diseases. Valproate may be especially problematic for adolescent and young adult females. Cases of polycystic ovary disease have been reported in women using valproate. Even when the full syndromal criteria for this syndrome are not met, many of these women develop menstrual irregularities, hair loss, and hirsutism. These effects are thought to result from a metabolic syndrome that is driven by insulin resistance and hyperinsulinemia.

The common adverse effects associated with valproate are those affecting the gastrointestinal (GI) system, such as nausea, vomiting, dyspepsia, and diarrhea. The GI effects are generally most common in the first month of treatment, particularly if the dose is increased rapidly. Unbuffered valproic acid (Depakene) is more likely to cause GI symptoms than are the enteric-coated "sprinkle" or the delayed-release divalproex sodium formulations. Other common adverse effects involve the nervous system, such as sedation, ataxia, dysarthria, and tremor. Valproate-induced tremor may respond well to treatment with β-adrenergic receptor antagonists or gabapentin. Treatment of the other neurological adverse effects usually requires lowering the valproate dose.

Weight gain is a common adverse effect, especially in long-term treatment, and can best be treated by strict limitation of caloric intake. Hair loss can occur in 5 to 10 percent of all persons treated, and rare cases of complete loss of body hair have been reported. Some clinicians have recommended treatment of valproate-associated hair loss with vitamin supplements that contain zinc and selenium. Of persons taking valproate, 5 to 40 percent experience a persistent but clinically insignificant elevation in liver transaminases up to three times the upper limit of

normal, which is usually asymptomatic and resolves after discontinuation of the drug. High doses of valproate (>1,000 mg a day) may rarely produce mild to moderate hyponatremia, most likely because of some degree of the syndrome of secretion of inappropriate antidiuretic hormone, which is reversible on lowering of the dose. Overdoses of valproate can lead to coma and death.

DRUG INTERACTIONS

Valproate is commonly prescribed as part of a regimen involving other psychotropic agents. The only consistent drug interaction with lithium, if both drugs are maintained in their respective therapeutic ranges, is the exacerbation of drug-induced tremors, which can usually be treated with β-receptor antagonists. The combination of valproate and DRAs can result in increased sedation, as can be seen when valproate is added to any central nervous system depressant (e.g., alcohol), and increased severity of extrapyramidal symptoms, which usually respond to treatment with anti-Parkinsonian drugs. Valproate can usually be safely combined with carbamazepine or serotonin–dopamine antagonists. Perhaps the most worrisome interaction of valproate and a psychotropic drug involves lamotrigine. Since the approval of lamotrigine for the treatment of bipolar disorder, the likelihood that patients will be treated with both agents has increased. Valproate more than doubles lamotrigine concentrations, increasing the risk of a serious rash.

The plasma concentrations of carbamazepine, diazepam (Valium), amitriptyline (Elavil), nortriptyline (Pamelor), and phenobarbital (Luminal) can also be increased when these drugs are coadministered with valproate, and the plasma concentrations of phenytoin (Dilantin) and desipramine (Norpramin) can be decreased when they are combined with valproate. The plasma concentrations of valproate may be decreased when the drug is coadministered with carbamazepine and may be increased when coadministered with guanfacine (Tenex), amitriptyline, or fluoxetine (Prozac). Valproate can be displaced from plasma proteins by carbamazepine, diazepam, and aspirin. Persons who are treated with anticoagulants (e.g., aspirin and warfarin [Coumadin]) should also be monitored when valproate use is initiated to assess the development of any undesired augmentation of the anticoagulation effects.

LABORATORY INTERFERENCES

Valproate can cause laboratory increase of serum free fatty acids. Valproate metabolites can produce a false-positive test result for urinary ketones as well as falsely abnormal thyroid function test results.

DOSING AND CLINICAL GUIDELINES

When starting valproate therapy, a baseline hepatic panel, complete blood cell and platelet counts, and pregnancy testing should be ordered. Additional testing should include amylase and coagulation studies, if baseline pancreatic disease or coagulopathy is suspected. In addition to baseline laboratory tests, white blood cell and platelet counts and hepatic transaminase concentrations should be obtained 1 month after initiation of therapy and every 6 to 24 months thereafter. Because even frequent monitoring may not predict serious organ toxicity, it is more prudent, however, to reinforce the need for prompt evaluation of any illnesses when

Table 32.35–1
Valproate Preparations Available in the United States

Generic Name	Trade Name, Form (Dose)	Time to Peak
Valproate sodium injection	Depacon injection (100 mg valproic acid/mL)	1 hr
Valproic acid	Depakene, syrup (250 mg/5 mL)	1–2 hrs
	Depakene, capsules (250 mg)	1–2 hrs
Divalproex sodium	Depakote, delayed-released tablets (125, 250, 500 mg)	3–8 hrs
Divalproex sodium coated particles in capsules	Depakote, sprinkle capsules (125 mg)	Compared with divalproex tablets, divalproex sprinkle has earlier onset and slower absorption, with slightly lower peak plasma concentration

reviewing the instructions with patients. Asymptomatic elevation of transaminase concentrations up to three times the upper limit of normal are common and do not require any change in dose.

Valproate is available in a number of formulations (Table 32.35–1). For treatment of acute mania, an oral loading strategy of initiation with 20 to 30 mg/kg a day can be used to accelerate control of symptoms. This is usually well tolerated but can cause excessive sedation and tremor in elderly persons. Agitated behavior can be rapidly stabilized with intravenous infusion of valproate. If acute mania is absent, it is best to initiate drug treatment gradually to minimize the common adverse effects of nausea, vomiting, and sedation. The dose on the first day should be 250 mg administered with a meal. The dose can be raised up to 250 mg orally three times daily over the course of 3 to 6 days. The plasma concentrations can be assessed in the morning before the first daily dose is administered. Therapeutic plasma concentrations for the control of seizures range between 50 and 150 μg/mL, but concentrations up to 200 μg/mL are usually well tolerated. It is reasonable to use the same range for the treatment of mental disorders; most of the controlled studies have used 50 to 125 μg/mL. Most persons attain therapeutic plasma concentrations on a dose between 1,200 and 1,500 mg a day in divided doses. Once a person's symptoms are well controlled, the full daily dose can be taken all at once before sleep.

▲ 32.36 Yohimbine

Yohimbine (Yocon) is an α_2-adrenergic receptor antagonist that is sometimes used as a treatment for both idiopathic and medication-induced erectile disorder. Sildenafil (Viagra) and its congeners (see Section 32.27) and alprostadil (Impulse, Caverject) are considered more efficacious for this indication than yohimbine. Yohimbine hydrochloride is derived from an alkaloid found in *rubaceae* and related trees and in the *rauwolfia serpentina* plant.

PHARMACOLOGICAL ACTIONS

Yohimbine is erratically absorbed following oral administration, with bioavailability ranging from 7 to 87 percent. There is extensive hepatic first-pass metabolism. Yohimbine affects the sym-

pathomimetic autonomic nervous system by increasing plasma concentrations of norepinephrine. The half-life of yohimbine is 0.5 to 2 hours.

Yohimbine is an antagonist of α_2-receptors located both presynaptically and postsynaptically on noradrenergic neurons. The α_2-receptors are also located on synaptic terminals of some serotonergic neurons. Stimulation of presynaptic α_2-receptors results in a decrease in the release of neurotransmitters from the neuron; therefore, blockade of the receptors results in an increase in the release of neurotransmitters. Both norepinephrine and serotonin are involved in the physiology of male sexual response. Clinically, yohimbine produces increased parasympathetic (cholinergic) tone.

THERAPEUTIC INDICATIONS

Yohimbine has been used to treat erectile dysfunction. Penile erection has been linked to cholinergic activity and to α_2-adrenergic blockade, which theoretically results in increased penile inflow of blood, decreased penile outflow of blood, or both.

Yohimbine is reported to help counteract the loss of sexual desire and the orgasmic inhibition caused by some serotonergic antidepressants (e.g., selective serotonin reuptake inhibitors). It has not been found useful in women for these indications.

PRECAUTIONS AND ADVERSE EFFECTS

The side effects of yohimbine include anxiety, elevated blood pressure (BP) and heart rate, increased psychomotor activity, irritability, tremor, headache, skin flushing, dizziness, urinary frequency, nausea, vomiting, and sweating. Patients with panic disorder show heightened sensitivity to yohimbine and experience increased anxiety, increased BP, and increased plasma 3-methoxy-4-hydroxyphenylglycol.

Yohimbine should be used with caution in female patients and should not be used in patients with renal disease, cardiac disease, glaucoma, or a history of gastric or duodenal ulcer.

DRUG INTERACTIONS

Yohimbine blocks the effects of clonidine (Catapres), guanfacine (Tenex), and other α_2-receptor agonists.

LABORATORY INTERFERENCES

No known laboratory interferences are associated with yohimbine use.

DOSING AND CLINICAL GUIDELINES

Yohimbine is available in 5.4-mg tablets. The dosage of yohimbine in the treatment of erectile disorder is approximately 18 mg a day given in doses that range from 2.7 to 5.4 mg three times a day. In the event of significant adverse effects, dose should first be reduced and then gradually increased again. Yohimbine should be used judiciously in psychiatric patients because it may have an adverse effect on their mental status. Because yohimbine has no consistent effect on erectile dysfunction, its use remains controversial. Phosphodiesterase-5 inhibitors are the preferred medication for this disorder.

▲ 32.37 Electroconvulsive Therapy

Use of electroconvulsive therapy (ECT) has diminished since the middle of the 20th century. However, because ECT remains the most effective treatment for major depression and a rapidly effective treatment for life-threatening psychiatric conditions, unlike its contemporaneous somatic therapies, ECT remains in the active treatment portfolio of modern therapeutics. Its use has shifted from public to private institutions, and it is estimated that approximately 100,000 patients receive ECT annually in the United States. A limiting factor in its use has been the adverse effect of confusion and memory loss associated with the course of treatment; however, both are reversible, and most of the major innovations in ECT technique over the past 20 years have sought to diminish cognitive effects while maintaining benefits. New developments in ECT technique offer the hope that this form of treatment will find better acceptance among psychiatrists and patients.

INDICATIONS

Major Depressive Disorder

The most common indication for ECT is major depressive disorder, for which ECT is the fastest and most effective therapy. ECT should be considered for use in patients who have failed medication trials, have not tolerated medications, have severe or psychotic symptoms, are acutely suicidal or homicidal, or have marked symptoms of agitation or stupor. Controlled studies have shown that up to 70 percent of patients who fail to respond to antidepressant medications may respond positively to ECT.

Electroconvulsive therapy is effective for depression in both major depressive disorder and bipolar I disorder. Delusional or psychotic depression has long been considered particularly responsive to ECT; recent studies, however, have indicated that major depressive episodes with psychotic features are no more responsive to ECT than are nonpsychotic depressive disorders. Nevertheless, because major depressive episodes with psychotic features respond poorly to antidepressant pharmacotherapy alone, ECT should be considered much more often as the first-line treatment for patients with the disorder. Major depressive disorder with melancholic features (e.g., markedly severe symptoms, psychomotor retardation, early-morning awakening, diurnal variation, decreased appetite and weight, and agitation) is considered likely to respond to ECT. ECT is particularly indicated for persons who are severely depressed, who have psychotic symptoms, who show suicidal intent, or who refuse to eat. Depressed patients less likely to respond to ECT include those with somatization disorder. Elderly patients tend to respond to ECT more slowly than do young patients. ECT is a treatment for major depressive episode and does not provide prophylaxis unless it is administered on a long-term maintenance basis.

Manic Episodes

Electroconvulsive therapy is at least equal to lithium (Eskalith) in the treatment of acute manic episodes. The pharmacological treatment of manic episodes, however, is so effective in the short term and for prophylaxis that the use of ECT to treat manic episodes is generally limited to situations with specific contraindications to all available pharmacological approaches. The relative rapidity of the ECT response indicates its usefulness for patients whose manic behavior has produced dangerous levels of exhaustion. ECT should not be used for a patient who is receiving lithium, because lithium can lower the seizure threshold and cause a prolonged seizure.

Schizophrenia

Although an effective treatment for the symptoms of acute schizophrenia, ECT is not for those of chronic schizophrenia. Patients with schizophrenia who have marked positive symptoms, catatonia, or affective symptoms are considered most likely to respond to ECT. In such patients, the efficacy of ECT is about equal to that of antipsychotics, but improvement may occur faster.

Other Indications

Small studies have found ECT effective in the treatment of catatonia, a symptom associated with mood disorders, schizophrenia, and medical and neurological disorders. ECT is also reportedly useful in treating episodic psychoses, atypical psychoses, obsessive-compulsive disorder, and delirium and such medical conditions as neuroleptic malignant syndrome, hypopituitarism, intractable seizure disorders, and the on-off phenomenon of Parkinson's disease. ECT may also be the treatment of choice for depressed suicidal pregnant women who require treatment and cannot take medication; for geriatric and medically ill patients who cannot take antidepressant drugs safely; and perhaps even for severely depressed and suicidal children and adolescents who may be less likely to respond to antidepressant drugs than are adults. ECT is not effective in somatization disorder (unless accompanied by depression), personality disorders, and anxiety disorders.

CLINICAL GUIDELINES

Patients and their families are often apprehensive about ECT; therefore, clinicians must explain both beneficial and adverse effects and alternative treatment approaches. The informed-consent process should be documented in the patients' medical records and should include a discussion of the disorder, its natural course, and the option of receiving no treatment. Printed literature and videotapes about ECT may be useful in attempting to obtain a truly informed consent. The use of involuntary ECT is rare today and should be reserved for patients who urgently need treatment and who have a legally appointed guardian who has agreed to its use. Clinicians must know local, state, and federal laws about the use of ECT.

Pretreatment Evaluation

Pretreatment evaluation should include standard physical, neurological, and preanesthesia examinations and a complete medical history. Laboratory evaluations should include blood and urine chemistries, a chest X-ray, and an electrocardiogram. A dental examination to assess the state of patients' dentition is advisable for elderly patients and patients who have had inadequate dental care. An X-ray of the spine is needed if other evidence of a spinal disorder is seen. Computed tomography or magnetic resonance imaging should be performed if a clinician suspects the presence of a seizure disorder or a space-occupying lesion. Practitioners of ECT no longer consider even a space-occupying lesion to be an absolute contraindication to ECT, but with such patients the procedure should be performed only by experts.

Concomitant Medications.
Patients' ongoing medications should be assessed for possible interactions with the induction of a seizure, for effects (both positive and negative) on the seizure threshold, and for drug interactions with the medications used during ECT. The use of tricyclic and tetracyclic drugs, monoamine oxidase inhibitors, and antipsychotics is generally considered acceptable. Benzodiazepines used for anxiety should be withdrawn because of their anticonvulsant activity; lithium (Eskalith) should be withdrawn because it can result in increased postictal delirium and can prolong seizure activity; clozapine (Clozaril) and bupropion (Wellbutrin) should be withdrawn because they are associated with the development of late-appearing seizures. Lidocaine (Xylocaine) should not be administered during ECT because it markedly increases the seizure threshold; theophylline (Theo-Dur) is contraindicated because it increases the duration of seizures. Reserpine (Serpasil) is also contraindicated because it is associated with further compromise of the respiratory and cardiovascular systems during ECT.

Premedications, Anesthetics, and Muscle Relaxants

Patients should not be given anything orally for 6 hours before treatment. Just before the procedure, the patient's mouth should be checked for dentures and other foreign objects, and an intravenous (IV) line should be established. A bite block is inserted in the mouth just before the treatment is administered to protect the patient's teeth and tongue during the seizure. Except for the brief interval of electrical stimulation, 100 percent oxygen is administered at a rate of 5 L a minute during the procedure until spontaneous respiration returns. Emergency equipment for establishing an airway should be immediately available in case it is needed.

Muscarinic Anticholinergic Drugs.
Muscarinic anticholinergic drugs are administered before ECT to minimize oral and respiratory secretions and to block bradycardias and asystoles, unless the resting heart rate is above 90 beats a minute. Some ECT centers have stopped the routine use of anticholinergics as premedications, although their use is still indicated for patients taking β-adrenergic receptor antagonists and those with ventricular ectopic beats. The most commonly used drug is atropine, which can be administered 0.3 to 0.6 mg intramuscularly (IM) or subcutaneously (SC) 30 to 60 minutes before the anesthetic or 0.4 to 1.0 mg IV 2 or 3 minutes before the anesthetic. An option is to use glycopyrrolate (Robinul) (0.2 to 0.4 mg IM, IV, or SC), which is less likely to cross the blood–brain barrier and less likely to cause cognitive dysfunction and nausea, although it is thought to have less cardiovascular protective activity than does atropine.

Anesthesia.
Administration of ECT requires general anesthesia and oxygenation. The depth of anesthesia should be as light as possible, not only to minimize adverse effects, but also to avoid elevating the seizure threshold associated with many anesthetics. Methohexital (Brevital) (0.75- to 1.0-mg/kg IV bolus) is the most commonly used anesthetic because of its shorter duration of action and lower association with postictal arrhythmias than thiopental (Pentothal) (usual dose 2 to 3 mg/kg IV), although this difference in cardiac effects is not universally accepted. Four other anesthetic alternatives are etomidate (Amidate), ketamine (Ketalar), alfentanil (Alfenta), and propofol (Diprivan). Etomidate (0.15 to 0.3 mg/kg IV) is sometimes used because it does not increase the seizure threshold; this effect is particularly useful for elderly patients because the seizure threshold increases with age. Ketamine (6 to 10 mg/kg IM) is sometimes used because it does not increase the seizure threshold, although its use is limited by the frequent association of psychotic symptoms with emergence from anesthesia with this drug. Alfentanil (2 to 9 mg/kg IV) is sometimes coadministered with barbiturates to allow the use of low doses of the barbiturate anesthetics and, thus, reduce the seizure threshold less than usual, although its use can be associated with an increased incidence of nausea. Propofol (0.5 to 3.5 mg/kg IV) is less useful because of its strong anticonvulsant properties.

Muscle Relaxants.
After the onset of the anesthetic effect, usually within 1 minute, a muscle relaxant is administered to minimize the risk of bone fractures and other injuries resulting from motor activity during the seizure. The goal is to produce profound relaxation of the muscles, not necessarily to paralyze them, unless the patient has a history of osteoporosis or spinal injury or has a pacemaker and, therefore, is at risk for injury related to motor activity during the seizure. Succinylcholine, an ultrafast-acting depolarizing blocking agent, has gained virtually universal acceptance for the purpose. Succinylcholine is usually administered in a dose of 0.5 to 1 mg/kg as an IV bolus or drip. Because succinylcholine is a depolarizing agent, its action is marked by the presence of muscle fasciculations, which move in a rostrocaudal progression. The disappearance of these movements in the feet or the absence of muscle contractions after peripheral nerve stimulation indicates maximal muscle relaxation. In some patients, tubocurarine (3 mg IV) is administered to prevent myoclonus and increases in potassium and muscle enzymes; these reactions can be a problem in patients with musculoskeletal or cardiac disease. To monitor the duration of the convulsion, a blood pressure cuff may be inflated at the ankle to a pressure in excess of the systolic pressure before infusion of the muscle relaxant, to allow observation of relatively innocuous seizure activity in the foot muscles.

If a patient has a known history of pseudocholinesterase deficiency, atracurium (Tracrium) (0.5 to 1 mg/kg IV) or curare can be used instead of succinylcholine. In such a patient, the metabolism of succinylcholine is disrupted, and prolonged apnea may necessitate emergency airway management. In general, however, because of the short half-life of succinylcholine, the duration of apnea after its administration is generally shorter than the delay in regaining consciousness caused by the anesthetic and the postictal state.

Electrode Placement

Electroconvulsive therapy can be conducted with either bilaterally or unilaterally placed electrodes. Bilateral placement usually yields a more rapid therapeutic response, and unilateral placement results in less marked cognitive adverse effects in the first week or weeks after treatment, although this difference between placements is absent 2 months after treatment. In bilateral placement, which was introduced first, one stimulating electrode is placed several centimeters apart over each hemisphere of the brain. In unilateral ECT, both electrodes are placed several centimeters apart over the nondominant hemisphere, almost always the right hemisphere. Some attempts have been made to vary the location of the electrodes in unilateral ECT, but these attempts have not obtained the rapidity of response seen with bilateral ECT or have further reduced the cognitive adverse effects. The most common approach is to initiate treatment with unilateral ECT because of its more favorable adverse effect profile. If a patient does not improve after four to six unilateral treatments, bilateral placement is used. Initial bilateral placement of the electrodes may be indicated in the following situations: severe depressive symptoms, marked agitation, immediate suicide risk, manic symptoms, catatonic stupor, and treatment-resistant schizophrenia. Some patients are particularly at risk for anesthetic-related adverse effects, and these patients may also be treated with bilateral placement from the beginning to minimize the number of treatments and exposure to anesthetics.

In traditional bilateral ECT, the electrodes are placed bifrontotemporally with the center of each electrode about 1 inch above the midpoint of an imaginary line drawn from the tragus to the external canthus. With unilateral ECT, one stimulus electrode typically is placed over the nondominant frontotemporal area. Although several locations for the second stimulus electrode have been proposed, placement on the nondominant centroparietal scalp, just lateral to the midline vertex, appears to provide the most effective configuration.

Which cerebral hemisphere is dominant can generally be determined by a simple series of performance tasks (e.g., for handedness and footedness) and stated preference. Right-body responses correlate highly with left-brain dominance. If the responses are mixed or if they clearly indicate left-body dominance, clinicians should alternate the polarity of unilateral stimulation during successive treatments. Clinicians should also monitor the time that it takes for patients to recover consciousness and to answer simple orientation and naming questions. The side of stimulation associated with less rapid recovery and return of function is considered dominant. The left hemisphere is dominant in most persons; therefore, unilateral electrode placement is almost always over the right hemisphere.

Electrical Stimulus

The electrical stimulus must be sufficiently strong to reach the seizure threshold (the level of intensity needed to produce a seizure). The electrical stimulus is given in cycles, and each cycle contains a positive and a negative wave. Old machines use a sine wave; however, this type of machine is now considered obsolete because of the inefficiency of that wave shape. When a sine wave is delivered, the electrical stimulus in the sine wave before the seizure threshold is reached and after the seizure is activated is unnecessary and excessive. Modern ECT machines use a brief pulse waveform that administers the electrical stimulus usually in 1 to 2 ms at a rate of 30 to 100 pulses a second. Machines that use an ultrabrief pulse (0.5 ms) are not as effective as brief-pulse machines.

Induced Seizures

A brief muscular contraction, usually strongest in a patient's jaw and facial muscles, is seen concurrently with the flow of stimulus current, regardless of whether a seizure occurs. The first behavioral sign of the seizure is often a plantar extension, which lasts 10 to 20 seconds and marks the tonic phase. This phase is followed by rhythmic (i.e., clonic) contractions that decrease in frequency and finally disappear. The tonic phase is marked by high-frequency, sharp EEG activity on which a higher-frequency muscle artifact may be superimposed. During the clonic phase, bursts of polyspike activity occur simultaneously with the muscular contractions, but these usually persist for at least a few seconds after the clonic movements stop.

Monitoring Seizures.   A physician must have an objective measure that a bilateral generalized seizure has occurred after the stimulation. The physician should be able to observe either some evidence of tonic-clonic movements or electrophysiological evidence of seizure activity from the EEG or electromyogram. Seizures with unilateral ECT are asymmetrical, with higher ictal EEG amplitudes over the stimulated hemisphere than over the nonstimulated hemisphere. Occasionally, unilateral seizures are induced; for this reason, at least a single pair of EEG electrodes should be placed over the contralateral hemisphere when using unilateral ECT. For a seizure to be effective in the course of ECT, it should last at least 25 seconds.

Failure to Induce Seizures.   If a particular stimulus fails to cause a seizure of sufficient duration, up to four attempts at seizure induction can be tried during a course of treatment. The onset of seizure activity is sometimes delayed as long as 20 to 40 seconds after the stimulus administration. If a stimulus fails to result in a seizure, the contact between the electrodes and the skin should be checked, and the intensity of the stimulus should be increased by 25 to 100 percent. The clinician can also change the anesthetic agent to minimize increases in the seizure threshold caused by the anesthetic. Additional procedures to lower the seizure threshold include hyperventilation and administration of 500 to 2,000 mg IV of caffeine sodium benzoate 5 to 10 minutes before the stimulus.

Prolonged and Tardive Seizures.   Prolonged seizures (seizures lasting >180 seconds) and status epilepticus can be terminated either with additional doses of the barbiturate anesthetic agent or with IV diazepam (Valium) (5 to 10 mg). Management of such complications should be accompanied by intubation because the oral airway is insufficient to maintain adequate ventilation over an extended apneic period. Tardive seizures—that is, additional seizures appearing some time after the ECT treatment—may develop in patients with preexisting seizure disorders. Rarely, ECT precipitates the development of an epileptic disorder in patients. Such situations should be managed clinically as if they were pure epileptic disorders.

Number and Spacing of Treatments

Electroconvulsive therapy treatments are usually administered two to three times a week; twice-weekly treatments are associated with less memory impairment than thrice-weekly treatments. In general, the course of treatment of major depressive disorder can take 6 to 12 treatments (although up to 20 sessions are possible); the treatment of manic episodes can take 8 to 20 treatments; the treatment of schizophrenia can take more than 15 treatments; and the treatment of catatonia and delirium can take as few as 1 to 4 treatments. Treatment should continue until the patient achieves what is considered the maximal therapeutic response. Further treatment does not yield any therapeutic benefit but increases the severity and duration of the adverse effects. The point of maximal improvement is usually thought to occur when a patient fails to continue to improve after 2 consecutive treatments. If a patient is not improving after 6 to 10 sessions, bilateral placement and high-density treatment (three times the seizure threshold) should be attempted before ECT is abandoned.

Multiple Monitored Electroconvulsive Therapy. Multiple monitored ECT (MMECT) involves giving multiple ECT stimuli during a single session, most commonly two bilateral stimuli within 2 minutes. This approach may be warranted in severely ill patients and in those at especially high risk from the anesthetic procedures. MMECT is associated with the most frequent occurrences of serious cognitive adverse effects.

Maintenance Treatment

A short-term course of ECT induces a remission in symptoms but does not, of itself, prevent a relapse. Post-ECT maintenance treatment should always be considered. Maintenance therapy is generally pharmacological, but maintenance ECT treatments (weekly, biweekly, or monthly) have been reported to be effective relapse prevention measures, although data from large studies are lacking. Indications for maintenance ECT treatments can include rapid relapse after initial ECT, severe symptoms, psychotic symptoms, and the inability to tolerate medications. If ECT was used because a patient was unresponsive to a specific medication, then, following ECT, the patient should be given a trial of a different medication.

Failure of Electroconvulsive Therapy Trial

Patients who fail to improve after a trial of ECT should again be treated with the pharmacological agents that failed in the past. Although the data are primarily anecdotal, many reports indicate that patients who had previously failed to improve while taking an antidepressant drug do improve while taking the same drug after receiving a course of ECT treatments, even if the ECT seemed to be a therapeutic failure. Nonetheless, with the increased availability of drugs that act at diverse receptor sites, it is less often necessary to return to a drug that has failed than it was formerly.

ADVERSE EFFECTS

Contraindications

Electroconvulsive therapy has no absolute contraindications, only situations in which a patient is at increased risk and has an increased need for close monitoring. Pregnancy is not a contraindication for ECT, and fetal monitoring is generally considered unnecessary unless the pregnancy is high risk or complicated. Patients with space-occupying central nervous system lesions are at increased risk for edema and brain herniation after ECT. If the lesion is small, however, pretreatment with dexamethasone (Decadron) is given and hypertension is controlled during the seizure; the risk of serious complications can be minimized for these patients.

Patients who have increased intracerebral pressure or are at risk for cerebral bleeding (e.g., those with cerebrovascular diseases and aneurysms) are at risk during ECT because of the increased cerebral blood flow during the seizure. This risk can be lessened, although not eliminated, by control of the patient's blood pressure during the treatment. Patients with recent myocardial infarctions are another high-risk group, although the risk is greatly diminished 2 weeks after the myocardial infarction and is even further reduced 3 months after the infarction. Patients with hypertension should be stabilized on their antihypertensive medications before ECT is administered. Propranolol (Inderal) and sublingual nitroglycerin can also be used to protect such patients during treatment.

Mortality

The mortality rate with ECT is about 0.002 percent per treatment and 0.01 percent for each patient. These numbers compare favorably with the risks associated with general anesthesia and childbirth. ECT death is usually from cardiovascular complications and is most likely to occur in patients whose cardiac status is already compromised.

Central Nervous System Effects

Common adverse effects associated with ECT are headache, confusion, and delirium shortly after the seizure while the patient is coming out of anesthesia. Marked confusion may occur in up to 10 percent of patients within 30 minutes of the seizure and can be treated with barbiturates and benzodiazepines. Delirium is usually most pronounced after the first few treatments and in patients who receive bilateral ECT or who have coexisting neurological disorders. The delirium characteristically clears within days or a few weeks at the longest.

Memory. The greatest concern about ECT is the association between ECT and memory loss. About 75 percent of all patients given ECT say that the memory impairment is the worst adverse effect. Although memory impairment during a course of treatment is almost the rule, follow-up data indicate that almost all patients are back to their cognitive baselines after 6 months. Some patients, however, complain of persistent memory difficulties. For example, a patient may not remember the events leading up to the hospitalization and ECT, and such autobiographical memories may never be recalled. The degree of cognitive impairment during treatment and the time it takes to return to baseline are related, in part, to the amount of electrical stimulation used during treatment. Memory impairment is most often reported by patients who have experienced little improvement with ECT. Despite the memory impairment, which usually resolves, no evidence indicates brain damage caused by ECT. This subject has been the focus of several brain-imaging studies, using a variety of modalities; virtually all concluded that permanent brain damage is not an adverse effect of ECT. Neurologists and epileptologists generally agree that seizures that last less than 30 minutes do not cause permanent neuronal damage.

Other Adverse Effects of Electroconvulsive Therapy

Fractures often accompanied treatments in the early days of ECT. With routine use of muscle relaxants, fractures of long bones or vertebrae should not occur. Some patients, however, may break teeth or experience back pain because of contractions during the procedure. Muscle soreness can occur in some individuals, but it often results from the effects of muscle depolarization by succinylcholine and is most likely to be particularly troublesome after the first session in a series. This soreness can be treated with mild analgesics, including nonsteroidal antiinflammatory drugs (NSAIDs). A significant minority of patients experience nausea, vomiting, and headaches following an ECT treatment. Nausea and vomiting can be prevented by treatment with antiemetics at the time of ECT (e.g., metoclopramide [Reglan], 10 mg IV, or prochlorperazine [Compazine], 10 mg IV; ondansetron [Zofran] is an acceptable alternative if adverse effects preclude use of dopamine receptor antagonists).

Electroconvulsive therapy can be associated with headaches, although this effect is usually readily manageable. Headaches often respond to NSAIDs given in the ECT recovery period. In patients with severe headaches, pretreatment with ketorolac (Toradol) (30 to 60 mg IV), an NSAID approved for brief parenteral use, can be helpful. Acetaminophen (Tylenol), tramadol (Ultram), propoxyphene (Darvon), and more potent analgesia provided by opioids can be used individually or in various combinations (e.g., pretreatment with ketorolac and postseizure management with acetaminophen-propoxyphene) to manage more intractable headache. ECT can induce migrainous headache and related symptoms; sumatriptan (Imitrex) (6 mg SC or 25 mg orally) may be a useful addition to the agents just described. Ergot compounds can exacerbate cardiovascular changes observed during ECT and probably should not be a component of ECT pretreatment.

▲ 32.38 Other Brain Stimulation Methods

In addition to electroconvulsive therapy, described in Section 32.37, a variety of other techniques have been developed to modify the brain anatomically and functionally in an effort to cure mental illness. These techniques were developed to treat patients who had not responded to repeated exposures to conventional treatments and whose illnesses were extraordinarily severe and incapacitating. Some of these methods are described in this section.

REPEATED TRANSCRANIAL MAGNETIC STIMULATION

Repeated transcranial magnetic stimulation (rTMS) is a noninvasive technique for stimulating cells of the cerebral cortex. It creates a time-varying magnetic field in which a localized pulse magnetic field over the surface of the head depolarizes the superficial neurons. TMS uses a hand-held magnet to allow focused electrical stimulation across the scalp and cranium without the pain associated with percutaneous electrical stimulation. If TMS pulses are delivered repetitively and rhythmically, the technique is called rTMS. rTMS was originally used to map cortical motor control and hemisphere dominance. Stimulating the motor cortex with rTMS results in a contralateral motor response. Likewise, stimulating Broca's area with rTMS has resulted in speech blockage. The potential use of rTMS for the treatment of neurological and psychiatric disorders is actively being explored.

Some psychiatric conditions, such as major depression, may be characterized by hypoactive cortical areas. Functional imaging, including positron emission tomography (PET) has revealed a relative hypofrontality in some patients with major depression. It has been proposed that rTMS stimulation of these frontal areas would relieve symptoms of depression.

The application of rTMS to psychiatric conditions has lagged behind its neurological applications. rTMS has been used to map the motor cortex, to help determine hemispheric dominance, and to probe short-term memory. In some symptoms of Parkinson's disease, including bradykinesia, diminished reaction time has improved transiently with rTMS. Finally, rTMS has been used to help elucidate the pathophysiology of migraine headache, and some patients have had temporary symptom relief with rTMS.

Studies are underway by the National Institute of Mental Health to fully evaluate this method. The neurobiological mechanisms of action require further study, as does determining which patients are most likely to respond. Further work is needed.

VAGAL NERVE STIMULATION

Since 1985, a tremendous amount of work has been done on how the sensory afferent fibers from the vagal nerve cause brain changes. The vagal nerve (cranial nerve X) is a parasympathetic efferent nerve that relays information from the nucleus tractus solitarius to many areas of the brain, including the locus ceruleus. Vagal nerve stimulation (VNS) refers to stimulation of the left vagus nerve using commercially available devices. The VNS is delivered through a bipolar pulse generator, which is multiprogrammable and implanted in the left chest wall through a bipolar lead.

Vagal nerve stimulation is an alternative treatment for patients with refractory epilepsy who cannot tolerate surgery for the epileptic seizures. With increasing use and knowledge of safety (minimal gastrointestinal and cardiac side effects despite VNS), it is used in the less severely ill patient. It has been estimated that VNS leads to a 50 percent reduction of seizures in approximately 30 percent of patients with seizure who are treated, with approximately 10 percent of patients becoming seizure free over long periods of time.

Observations of mood effects of VNS in patients with epilepsy have led to a possible indication for the use of VNS in depression. It has been shown through brain-imaging studies that VNS affects the metabolism of limbic structures that are involved in mood stabilization, and neurochemical effects on brain monoamines are known to be involved in regulation of depressed mood.

Vagal nerve stimulation was recently approved by the U.S. Food and Drug Administration as an adjunctive long-term treatment for patients with recurrent or chronic major depressive disorders who have failed at least four antidepressant medication trials.

DEEP BRAIN STIMULATION

Deep brain stimulation (DBS) involves creating a small hole in the skull and passing a fine wire into selected brain regions. This wire can be excited on its terminal end by a pacemaker-like device connected subdermally and implanted in the chest wall. When the DBS is implanted, the wire stimulates at high frequencies and temporarily stops the function at that region.

Deep brain stimulation in the thalamus is approved for the treatment of Parkinson's disease. The technique involves implanting DBS at the subthalamic nucleus and the internal globus pallidus. This allows determination of motor regions that impair movements, and, thus, the ability to counteract this with high-frequency DBS gives more fluid movement.

Deep brain stimulation of the internal capsule has shown some positive effects for obsessive-compulsive disorder (OCD). The mood effects are sometimes worsened, as a case report noted that a patient became depressed with DBS at the subthalamic nucleus. It is possible that, with respect to the improvement in Parkinson's disease, mood-enhancing effects with DBS may exist at other locations. The technique has been of use in reducing abnormal movements in patients with Tourette's disorder.

Deep brain stimulation is less invasive than ablative surgery. The device can be turned off, and wires can be removed without significant sequelae. Whether it will be approved for general use is under review.

PSYCHOSURGERY

Psychosurgery involves surgical modification of the brain with the goal of reducing the symptoms of the most severely ill psychiatric patients who have not responded adequately to less radical treatments. Psychosurgical procedures focus on lesion-specific brain regions (e.g., lobotomies and cingulotomies) or their connecting tracts (e.g., tractotomies and leukotomies). Psychosurgical techniques are also used in the treatment of neurological disorders, such as epilepsy and chronic pain disorder.

The interest in psychosurgical approaches to mental disorders has only recently been rekindled. The renewed interest is based on several factors, including much-improved techniques that allow neurosurgeons to make exact stereotactically placed lesions, improved preoperative diagnoses, and comprehensive preoperative and postoperative psychological assessments. New techniques also facilitate gathering complete follow-up data and enable a growing understanding of the neuroanatomical basis of some mental disorders.

Stereotactic neurosurgical equipment now allows neurosurgeons to place discrete lesions in the brain. Radioactive implants, cryoprobes, electrical coagulation, proton beams, and ultrasonic waves are used to make the actual lesions.

The major indication for psychosurgery is the presence of a debilitating, chronic mental disorder that has not responded to any other treatment. A reasonable guideline is that the disorder should have been present for 5 years, during which a wide variety of alternative treatment approaches was attempted. Chronic intractable major depressive disorder and OCD are the two disorders reportedly most responsive to psychosurgery. The presence of vegetative symptoms and marked anxiety further increases the likelihood of a successful therapeutic outcome. Whether psychosurgery is a reasonable treatment for intractable and extreme aggression is still controversial. Psychosurgery is not indicated for the treatment of schizophrenia, and data about manic episodes are controversial.

When patients are carefully selected, between 50 and 70 percent have significant therapeutic improvement with psychosurgery. Fewer than 3 percent become worse. Continued improvement is often noted from 1 to 2 years after surgery, and patients often respond better to traditional pharmacological and behavioral treatment approaches than they did before psychosurgery. Postoperative seizures are present in fewer than 1 percent of patients, and these seizures are usually controlled with phenytoin (Dilantin). As measured by intelligence quotient scores, cognitive abilities improve after surgery, probably because of patients' increased ability to attend to cognitive tasks. No undesired changes in personality have been noted with modern limited procedures.

33

Child Psychiatry: Assessment, Examination, and Psychological Testing

Psychiatric assessment of a child or adolescent includes identifying the reasons for referral; assessing the nature and extent of the child's psychological and behavioral difficulties; and determining family, school, social, and developmental factors that may be influencing the child's emotional well-being.

CLINICAL INTERVIEWS

To conduct a useful interview with a child of any age, clinicians must be familiar with normal development to place the child's responses in the proper perspective. For example, a young child's discomfort on separation from a parent and a school-age child's lack of clarity about the purpose of the interview are both perfectly normal and should not be misconstrued as psychiatric symptoms. Furthermore, behavior that is normal in a child at one age, such as temper tantrums in a 2-year-old, takes on a different meaning, for example, in a 17-year-old.

The interviewer's first task is to engage the child and develop a rapport so that the child is comfortable. The interviewer should inquire about the child's concept of the purpose of the interview and should ask what the parents have told the child. If the child appears to be confused about the reason for the interview, the examiner may opt to summarize the parents' concerns in a developmentally appropriate and supportive manner. During the interview with the child, the clinician seeks to learn about the child's relationships with family members and peers, academic achievement and peer relationships in school, and the child's pleasurable activities. An estimate of the child's cognitive functioning is a part of the mental status examination.

The extent of confidentiality in child assessment is correlated with the age of the child. In most cases, almost all specific information can appropriately be shared with the parents of a very young child, whereas privacy and permission of an older child or adolescent are mandated before sharing information with parents. School-age and older children are informed that if the clinician becomes concerned that any child is dangerous to himself or herself or to others, this information must be shared with parents and, at times, additional adults. As part of a psychiatric assessment of a child of any age, the clinician must determine whether that child is safe in his or her environment and must develop an index of suspicion about whether the child is a victim of abuse or neglect. Whenever there is a suspicion of child maltreatment, the local child protective service agency must be notified.

Toward the end of the interview, the child may be asked in an open-ended manner whether he or she would like to bring up anything else. Each child should be complimented for his or her cooperation and thanked for participating in the interview, and the interview should end on a positive note.

Infants and Young Children

Assessments of infants usually begin with the parents present because very young children may be frightened by the interview situation; the interview with the parents present also allows the clinician to assess the parent–infant interaction. Infants may be referred for a variety of reasons, including high levels of irritability, difficulty being consoled, eating disturbances, poor weight gain, sleep disturbances, withdrawn behavior, lack of engagement in play, and developmental delay. The clinician assesses areas of functioning that include motor development, activity level, verbal communication, ability to engage in play, problem-solving skills, adaptation to daily routines, relationships, and social responsiveness.

The child's developmental level of functioning is determined by combining observations made during the interview with standardized developmental measures. Observations of play reveal a child's developmental level and reflect the child's emotional state and preoccupations. The examiner can interact with an infant age 18 months or younger in a playful manner by using such games as peek-a-boo. Children between the ages of 18 months and 3 years can be observed in a playroom. Children ages 2 years or older may exhibit symbolic play with toys, revealing more in this mode than through conversation. The use of puppets and dolls with children younger than 6 years of age is often an effective way to elicit information, especially if questions are directed to the dolls rather than to the child.

School-Age Children

Some school-age children are at ease when conversing with an adult; others are hampered by fear, anxiety, poor verbal skills, or oppositional behavior. School-age children can usually tolerate a 45-minute session. The room should be sufficiently spacious for

568

the child to move around but not so large as to reduce intimate contact between the examiner and the child. Part of the interview can be reserved for unstructured play, and various toys can be made available to capture the child's interest and to elicit themes and feelings. Children in lower grades may be more interested in the toys in the room, whereas by the sixth grade, children may be more comfortable with the interview process and less likely to show spontaneous play.

The initial part of the interview explores the child's understanding of the reasons for the meeting. The clinician should confirm that the interview was not set up because the child is "in trouble" or as a punishment for "bad" behavior. Techniques that can facilitate disclosure of feelings include asking the child to draw peers, family members, a house, or anything else that comes to mind. The child can then be questioned about the drawings. Children may be asked to reveal three wishes, to describe the best and worst events of their lives, and to name a favorite person to be stranded with on a desert island. Games such as Donald W. Winnicott's "squiggle," in which the examiner draws a curved line and then the child and the examiner take turns continuing the drawing, may facilitate conversation.

Questions that are partially open-ended with some multiple choices may elicit the most complete answers from school-age children. Simple, closed (yes or no) questions may not elicit sufficient information, and completely open-ended questions can overwhelm a school-age child who cannot construct a chronological narrative. These techniques often result in a shoulder shrug from the child. The use of indirect commentary—such as, "I once knew a child who felt very sad when he moved away from all his friends"—is helpful, although the clinician must be careful not to lead the child into confirming what the child thinks the clinician wants to hear. School-age children respond well to clinicians who help them compare moods or feelings by asking them to rate feelings on a scale of 1 to 10.

Adolescents

Adolescents usually have distinct ideas about why the evaluation was initiated and can usually give a chronological account of the recent events leading to the evaluation, although some may disagree with the need for the evaluation. The clinician should clearly communicate the value of hearing the story from an adolescent's point of view and must be careful to reserve judgment and not assign blame. Adolescents may be concerned about confidentiality, and clinicians can assure them that permission will be requested from them before any specific information is shared with parents, except situations involving danger to the adolescent or others, in which case confidentiality must be sacrificed. Adolescents can be approached in an open-ended manner; however, when silences occur during the interview, the clinician should attempt to reengage the patient. Clinicians can explore what the adolescent believes the outcome of the evaluation will be (change of school, hospitalization, removal from home, removal of privileges).

Some adolescents approach the interview with apprehension or hostility but open up when it becomes evident that the clinician is neither punitive nor judgmental. Clinicians must be aware of their responses to adolescents' behavior (countertransference) and stay focused on the therapeutic process even in the face of defiant, angry, or difficult teenagers. Clinicians should set appropriate limits and should postpone or discontinue an interview if they feel threatened or if patients become destructive to property or engage in self-injurious behavior. Every interview should include an exploration of suicidal thoughts, assaultive behavior, psychotic symptoms, substance use, and knowledge of safe sexual practices along with a sexual history. Once rapport has been established, many adolescents appreciate the opportunity to tell their side of the story and may reveal things that they have not disclosed to anyone else.

Family Interview

An interview with parents and the patient may take place first or may occur later in the evaluation. Sometimes, an interview with the entire family, including siblings, can be enlightening. The purpose is to observe the attitudes and behavior of the parents toward the patient and the responses of the children to their parents. The clinician's job is to maintain a nonthreatening atmosphere in which each member of the family can speak freely without feeling that the clinician is taking sides with any particular member. Although child psychiatrists generally function as advocates for the child, the clinician must validate each family member's feelings in this setting because lack of communication often contributes to the patient's problems.

Parents

The interview with the patient's parents or caretakers is necessary to get a chronological picture of the child's growth and development. A thorough developmental history and details of any stressors or important events that have influenced the child's development must be elicited. The parents' view of the family dynamics, their marital history, and their own emotional adjustment are also elicited. The family's psychiatric history and the upbringing of the parents are pertinent. Parents are usually the best informants about the child's early development and previous psychiatric and medical illnesses. They may be better able to provide an accurate chronology of past evaluations and treatment. In some cases, especially with older children and adolescents, the parents may be unaware of significant current symptoms or social difficulties of the child. Clinicians elicit the parents' formulation of the causes and nature of their child's problems and ask about expectations about the current assessment.

DIAGNOSTIC INSTRUMENTS

The two main types of diagnostic instruments used by clinicians and researchers are diagnostic interviews and questionnaires. Diagnostic interviews are administered to either children or their parents and are often designed to elicit sufficient information on numerous aspects of functioning to determine whether criteria are met from the text revision of the fourth edition of the *Diagnostic and Statistical Manual of Mental Disorders* (DSM-IV-TR).

Diagnostic instruments aid the collection of information in a systematic way. Diagnostic instruments, even the most comprehensive, however, cannot replace clinical interviews because clinical interviews are superior in understanding the chronology of symptoms, the interplay between environmental stressors and emotional responses, and developmental issues. Clinicians often

Table 33–1
Child Psychiatric Evaluation

Identifying data
    Identified patient and family members
    Source of referral
    Informants
History
    Chief complaint
    History of present illness
    Developmental history and milestones
    Psychiatric history
    Medical history, including immunizations
    Family social history and parents' marital status
    Educational history and current school functioning
    Peer relationship history
    Current family functioning
    Family psychiatric and medical histories
    Current physical examination
Mental status examination
Neuropsychiatric examination (when applicable)
Developmental, psychological, and educational testing
Formulation and summary
DSM-IV-TR diagnosis
Recommendations and treatment plan

DSM-IV-TR, text revision of the fourth edition of the *Diagnostic and Statistical Manual of Mental Disorders.*

find it helpful to combine the data from diagnostic instruments with clinical material gathered in a comprehensive evaluation.

Questionnaires can cover a broad range of symptom areas, such as the *Achenbach Child Behavior Checklist*, or they can be focused on a particular type of symptomatology and are often called rating scales, such as the *Connors Parent Rating Scale for ADHD.*

COMPONENTS OF THE CHILD PSYCHIATRIC EVALUATION

Psychiatric evaluation of a child includes a description of the reason for the referral, the child's past and present functioning, and any test results. An outline of the evaluation is given in Table 33–1.

Identifying Data

To understand the clinical problems to be evaluated, the clinician must first identify the patient and keep in mind the family constellation surrounding the child. The clinician must also pay attention to the source of the referral—that is, whether it is the child's family, school, or another agency—because this influences the family's attitude toward the evaluation. Finally, many informants contribute to the child's evaluation, and each must be identified to gain insight into the child's functioning in different settings.

History

A comprehensive history contains information about the child's current and past functioning from the child's report, from clinical and structured interviews with the parents, and from in-

Table 33–2
Mental Status Examination for Children

1. Physical appearance
2. Parent–child interaction
3. Separation and reunion
4. Orientation to time, place, and person
5. Speech and language
6. Mood
7. Affect
8. Thought process and content
9. Social relatedness
10. Motor behavior
11. Cognition
12. Memory
13. Judgment and insight

formation from teachers and previous treating clinicians. The chief complaint and the history of the present illness are generally obtained from both the child and the parents. Naturally, the child will articulate the situation according to his or her developmental level. The developmental history is more accurately obtained from the parents. Psychiatric and medical histories, current physical examination findings, and immunization histories can be augmented with reports from psychiatrists and pediatricians who have treated the child. The child's report is critical in understanding the current situation regarding peer relationships and adjustment to school. Adolescents are the best informants regarding their knowledge of safe sexual practices, drug or alcohol use, and suicidal ideation. The family's psychiatric and social histories and family function are best obtained from the parents.

Mental Status Examination

A detailed description of the child's current mental functioning can be obtained through observation and specific questioning. An outline of the mental status examination is presented in Table 33–2. Table 33–3 lists components of a comprehensive neuropsychiatry mental status.

Physical Appearances. The examiner should document the child's size, grooming, nutritional state, any bruising present, head circumference, physical signs of anxiety, facial expressions, and mannerisms.

Parent–Child Interaction. The examiner can observe the interactions between parents and child in the waiting area before the interview and in the family session. The manner in which parents and child converse and the emotional overtones are pertinent.

Separation and Reunion. The examiner should note both the manner in which the child responds to the separation from a parent for an individual interview and the reunion behavior. Either lack of affect at separation and reunion or severe distress on separation or reunion can indicate problems in the parent–child relationship or other psychiatric disturbances.

Orientation to Time, Place, and Persons. Impairments in orientation can reflect organic damage, low intelligence, or a thought disorder. The age of the child must be kept in mind, however, because very young children are not expected to know the date, other chronological information, or the name of the interview site.

Speech and Language. The examiner should evaluate the child's speech and language acquisition. Is it appropriate for the child's

Table 33–3
Neuropsychiatric Mental Status Examination

A. General Description
1. General appearance and dress
2. Level of consciousness and arousal
3. Attention to environment
4. Posture (standing and seated)
5. Gait
6. Movements of limbs, trunk, and face (spontaneous, resting, and after instruction)
7. General demeanor (including evidence of responses to internal stimuli)
8. Response to examiner (eye contact, cooperation, ability to focus on interview process)
9. Native or primary language

B. Language and Speech
1. Comprehension (words, sentences, simple and complex commands, and concepts)
2. Output (spontaneity, rate, fluency, melody or prosody, volume, coherence, vocabulary, paraphasic errors, complexity of usage)
3. Repetition
4. Other aspects
   a. Object naming
   b. Color naming
   c. Body part identification
   d. Ideomotor praxis to command

C. Thought
1. Form (coherence and connectedness)
2. Content
   a. Ideational (preoccupations, overvalued ideas, delusions)
   b. Perceptual (hallucinations)

D. Mood and Affect
1. Internal mood state (spontaneous and elicited; sense of humor)
2. Future outlook
3. Suicidal ideas and plans
4. Demonstrated emotional status (congruence with mood)

E. Insight and Judgment
1. Insight
   a. Self-appraisal and self-esteem
   b. Understanding of current circumstances
   c. Ability to describe personal psychological and physical status
2. Judgment
   a. Appraisal of major social relationships
   b. Understanding of personal roles and responsibilities

F. Cognition
1. Memory
   a. Spontaneous (as evidenced during interview)
   b. Tested (incidental, immediate repetition, delayed recall, cued recall, recognition; verbal, nonverbal; explicit, implicit)
2. Visuospatial skills
3. Constructional ability
4. Mathematics
5. Reading
6. Writing
7. Fine sensory function (stereognosis, graphesthesia, two-point discrimination)
8. Finger gnosis
9. Right-left orientation
10. "Executive functions"
11. Abstraction

Note: Questions should be adapted to the age of the child.
Courtesy of Eric D. Caine, M.D., and Jeffrey M. Lyness, M.D.

age? A disparity between expressive language usage and receptive language is notable. The examiner should also note the child's rate of speech, rhythm, latency to answer, spontaneity of speech, intonation, articulation of words, and prosody. Echolalia, repetitive stereotypical phrases, and unusual syntax are important psychiatric findings. Children who do not use words by age 18 months or who do not use phrases by age 2.5 to 3 years but who have a history of normal babbling and responding appropriately to nonverbal cues are probably developing normally. The examiner should consider the possibility that a hearing loss is contributing to a speech and language deficit.

Mood. A child's sad expression, lack of appropriate smiling, tearfulness, anxiety, euphoria, and anger are valid indicators of mood, as are verbal admissions of feelings. Persistent themes in play and fantasy also reflect the child's mood.

Affect. The examiner should note the child's range of emotional expressivity, appropriateness of affect to thought content, ability to move smoothly from one affect to another, and sudden labile emotional shifts.

Thought Process and Content.
In evaluating a thought disorder in a child, the clinician must always consider what is developmentally expected for the child's age and what is deviant for any age group. The evaluation of thought form considers loosening of associations, excessive magical thinking, perseveration, echolalia, the ability to distinguish fantasy from reality, sentence coherence, and the ability to reason logically. The evaluation of thought content considers delusions, obsessions, themes, fears, wishes, preoccupations, and interests.

Suicidal ideation is always a part of the mental status examination for children who are sufficiently verbal to understand the questions and old enough to understand the concept. Children of average intelligence older than 4 years of age usually have some understanding of what is real and what is make-believe and may be asked about suicidal ideation, although a firm concept of the permanence of death may not be present until several years later.

Aggressive thoughts and homicidal ideation are assessed here. Perceptual disturbances, such as hallucinations, are also assessed. Very young children are expected to have short attention spans and may change the topic and conversation abruptly without exhibiting a symptomatic flight of ideas. Transient visual and auditory hallucinations in very young children do not necessarily represent major psychotic illnesses, but they do deserve further investigation.

Social Relatedness. The examiner assesses the appropriateness of the child's response to the interviewer, general level of social skills, eye contact, and degree of familiarity or withdrawal in the interview process. Overly friendly or familiar behavior may be as troublesome, as are extremely retiring and withdrawn responses. The examiner assesses the child's self-esteem, general and specific areas of confidence, and success with family and peer relationships.

Motor Behavior. The motor behavior part of the mental status examination includes observations of the child's coordination and activity level and ability to pay attention and carry out developmentally appropriate tasks. It also involves involuntary movements, tremors, motor hyperactivity, and any unusual focal asymmetries of muscle movement.

Cognition. The examiner assesses the child's intellectual functioning and problem-solving abilities. An approximate level of intelligence can be estimated by the child's general information, vocabulary, and comprehension. For a specific assessment of the child's cognitive abilities, the examiner can use a standardized test.

Memory. School-age children should be able to remember three objects after 5 minutes and to repeat five digits forward and three digits backward. Anxiety can interfere with the child's performance, but an obvious inability to repeat digits or to add simple numbers may reflect brain damage, mental retardation, or learning disabilities.

Judgment and Insight.   The child's view of the problems, reactions to them, and suggested solutions may give the clinician a good idea of the child's judgment and insight. In addition, the child's understanding of what he or she can realistically do to help and what the clinician can do adds to the assessment of the child's judgment.

Neuropsychiatric Assessment

A neuropsychiatric assessment is appropriate for children who are suspected of having a neurological disorder, a psychiatric impairment that coexists with neurological signs, or psychiatric symptoms that may be caused by neuropathology. The neuropsychiatric evaluation combines information from neurological, physical, and mental status examinations. The neurological examination can identify asymmetrical abnormal signs (hard signs) that may indicate lesions in the brain. A physical examination can evaluate the presence of physical stigmata of particular syndromes in which neuropsychiatric symptoms or developmental aberrations play a role (e.g., fetal alcohol syndrome, Down syndrome).

An important part of the neuropsychiatric examination is the assessment of neurological soft signs and minor physical anomalies. The term *neurological soft signs* was first noted by Loretta Bender in the 1940s in reference to nondiagnostic abnormalities in the neurological examinations of children with schizophrenia. Soft signs do not indicate focal neurological disorders, but they are associated with a wide variety of developmental disabilities and occur frequently in children with low intelligence, learning disabilities, and behavioral disturbances. Soft signs may refer to both behavioral symptoms (which are sometimes associated with brain damage, such as severe impulsivity and hyperactivity), physical findings (including contralateral overflow movements), and a variety of nonfocal signs (e.g., mild choreiform movements, poor balance, mild incoordination, asymmetry of gait, nystagmus, and the persistence of infantile reflexes). Soft signs can be divided into those that are normal in a young child but become abnormal when they persist in an older child, and those that are abnormal at any age. The *Physical and Neurological Examination for Soft Signs* is an instrument used with children up to the age of 15 years. It consists of 15 questions about general physical status and medical history and 43 physical tasks (e.g., touch your finger to your nose, hop on one foot to the end of the line, tap quickly with your finger). Neurological soft signs are important to note, but they are not useful in making a specific psychiatric diagnosis.

Minor physical anomalies or dysmorphic features occur with a higher than usual frequency in children with developmental disabilities, learning disabilities, speech and language disorders, and hyperactivity. As with soft signs, the documentation of minor physical anomalies is part of the neuropsychiatric assessment, but it is rarely helpful in the diagnostic process and does not imply a good or bad prognosis. Minor physical anomalies include a high-arched palate, epicanthal folds, hypertelorism, low-set ears, transverse palmar creases, multiple hair whorls, a large head, a furrowed tongue, and partial syndactyly of several toes.

When a seizure disorder is being considered in the differential diagnosis or a structural abnormality in the brain is suspected, an electroencephalogram, computed tomography, or magnetic resonance imaging may be indicated.

Developmental, Psychological, and Educational Testing

Psychological tests are not always required to assess psychiatric symptoms, but they are valuable in determining a child's developmental level, intellectual functioning, and academic difficulties. A measure of adaptive functioning (including the child's competence in communication, daily living skills, socialization, and motor skills) is a prerequisite when a diagnosis of mental retardation is being considered.

Development Tests for Infants and Preschoolers.

The *Gesell Infant Scale*, the *Cattell Infant Intelligence Scale*, *Bayley Scales of Infant Development*, and the *Denver Developmental Screening Test* include developmental assessments of infants as young as 2 months of age. When used with very young infants, the tests focus on sensorimotor and social responses to a variety of objects and interactions. When these instruments are used with older infants and preschoolers, emphasis is placed on language acquisition. The *Gesell Infant Scale* measures development in four areas: motor, adaptive functioning, language, and social.

An infant's score on one of these developmental assessments is not a reliable way to predict a child's future intelligence quotient (IQ) in most cases. Infant assessments are valuable, however, in detecting developmental deviation and mental retardation and in raising suspicions of a developmental disorder. Whereas infant assessments rely heavily on sensorimotor functions, intelligence testing in older children and adolescents includes later-developing functions, including verbal, social, and abstract cognitive abilities.

Intelligence Tests for School-Age Children and Adolescents.

The most widely used test of intelligence for school-age children and adolescents is the third edition of the *Wechsler Intelligence Scale for Children* (WISC-III-R). It can be given to children from 6 to 17 years of age and yields a verbal IQ, a performance IQ, and a combined full-scale IQ. The verbal subtests consist of vocabulary, information, arithmetic, similarities, comprehension, and digit span (supplemental) categories. The performance subtests include block design, picture completion, picture arrangement, object assembly, coding, mazes (supplemental), and symbol search (supplemental). The scores of the supplemental subtests are not included in the computation of IQ.

Each subcategory is scored from 1 to 19, with 10 being the average score. An average full-scale IQ is 100; 70 to 80 represents borderline intellectual function; 80 to 90 is in the low average range; 90 to 109 is average; 110 to 119 is high average; and above 120 is in the superior or very superior range. The multiple breakdowns of the performance and verbal subscales allow great flexibility in identifying specific areas of deficit and scatter in intellectual abilities. Because a large part of intelligence testing measures abilities used in academic settings, the breakdown of the WISC-III-R can also be helpful in pointing out skills in which a child is weak and may benefit from remedial education.

The *Stanford-Binet Intelligence Scale* covers an age range from 2 to 24 years. It relies on pictures, drawings, and objects for very young children and on verbal performance for older children and adolescents. This intelligence scale, the earliest version of an intelligence test of its kind, leads to a mental age score as well as an intelligence quotient.

The *McCarthy Scales of Children's Abilities* and the *Kaufman Assessment Battery for Children* are two other intelligence tests that are available for preschool and school-age children. They do not cover the adolescent age group.

LONG-TERM STABILITY OF INTELLIGENCE.   Although a child's intelligence is relatively stable throughout the school-age years and adolescence, some factors can influence intelligence and a child's score on an intelligence test. The intellectual functions of children with severe mental illnesses and of those from low socioeconomic levels may decrease over time, whereas the IQs of children whose environments have been enriched may increase over time. Factors that influence a child's score on a given test of intellectual functioning and, thus, affect the accuracy of the test are motivation, emotional state, anxiety, and cultural milieu.

Perceptual and Perceptual Motor Tests.

The *Bender Visual Motor Gestalt Test* can be given to children between the ages of 4 and 12 years. The test consists of a set of spatially related figures that the child is asked to copy. The scores are based on the number of errors. Although not a diagnostic test, it is useful in identifying developmentally age-inappropriate perceptual performances.

Personality Tests.

Personality tests are not of much use in making diagnoses, and they are less satisfactory than intelligence tests in regard to norms, reliability, and validity, but they can be helpful in eliciting themes and fantasies.

The Rorschach test is a projective technique in which ambiguous stimuli—a set of bilaterally symmetrical inkblots—are shown to a child, who is then asked to describe what he or she sees in each. The hypothesis is that the child's interpretation of the vague stimuli reflects basic characteristics of personality. The examiner notes the themes and patterns. Two sets of norms have been established for the Rorschach test, one for children between 2 and 10 years of age and one for adolescents between 10 and 17 years of age.

A more structured projective test is the *Children's Apperception Test* (CAT), which is an adaptation of the *Thematic Apperception Test*. The CAT consists of cards with pictures of animals in scenes that are somewhat ambiguous but are related to parent–child and sibling issues, caretaking, and other relationships. The child is asked to describe what is happening and to tell a story about the scene. Animals are used because it was hypothesized that children might respond more readily to animal images than to human figures.

Drawings, toys, and play are also applications of projective techniques that can be used during the evaluation of children. Dollhouses, dolls, and puppets have been especially helpful in allowing a child to use a nonconversational mode in which to express a variety of attitudes and feelings. Play materials that reflect household situations are likely to elicit a child's fears, hopes, and conflicts about the family.

Projective techniques have not fared well as standardized instruments. Rather than being considered tests, projective techniques are best considered as additional clinical modalities.

Educational Tests.

Achievement tests measure the attainment of knowledge and skills in a particular academic curriculum. The *Wide-Range Achievement Test-Revised* consists of tests of knowledge and skills and timed performances of reading, spelling, and mathematics. It is used with children from 5 years of age to adulthood. The test yields a score that is compared with the average expected score for the child's chronological age and grade level.

The *Peabody Individual Achievement Test* includes word identification, spelling, mathematics, and reading comprehension.

The *Kaufman Test of Educational Achievement*, the *Gray Oral Reading Test-Revised*, and the *Sequential Tests of Educational Progress* are achievement tests that determine whether a child has achieved the educa-

tional level expected for his or her grade level. Children with an average IQ whose achievement is significantly lower than expected for their grade level in one or more subjects are considered to be learning disabled. Thus, achievement testing, combined with a measure of intellectual function, can identify specific learning disabilities for which remediation is recommended. Children who do not reach their grade level according to their chronological age but who function intellectually in the borderline range or lower are not necessarily learning disabled unless a disparity exists between their IQs and their levels of achievement.

Biopsychosocial Formulation.

The clinician's task is to integrate all of the information obtained into a formulation that takes into account the biological predisposition, psychodynamic factors, environmental stressors, and life events that have led to the child's current level of functioning. Psychiatric disorders and any specific physical, neuromotor, or developmental abnormalities must be considered in the formulation of etiologic factors for current impairment. The clinician's conclusions are an integration of clinical information along with data from standardized psychological and developmental assessments. The psychiatric formulation includes an assessment of family function as well as the appropriateness of the child's educational setting. A determination of the child's overall safety in his or her current situation is made. Any suspected maltreatment must be reported to the local child protective service agency. The child's overall well-being regarding growth, development, and academic and play activities is considered.

Diagnosis

Evidence suggests that the use of structured and semistructured (evidence-based) assessment tools enhance a clinician's ability to make the most accurate diagnoses. These instruments, described earlier, include the *Kiddie-Schedule for Affected Disorders and Schizophrenia* (K-SADS), the *Child and Adolescent Psychiatric Assessment* (CAPA), and the *National Institute of Mental Health Diagnostic Interview for Children Version IV* (NIMH DISC-IV) interviews. The advantages of including an evidence-based instrument in the diagnostic process include decreasing potential clinician bias to make a diagnosis without all of the necessary symptoms information and serving as guides for the clinician to consider each symptom that could contribute to a given diagnosis. These data can enable the clinician to optimize his or her expertise to make challenging judgments regarding child and adolescent disorders that may possess overlapping symptoms. The clinician's ultimate task includes making all appropriate diagnoses according to DSM-IV-TR. Some clinical situations do not fulfill criteria for DSM-IV-TR diagnoses but cause impairment and require psychiatric attention and intervention. Clinicians who evaluate children are frequently in the position of determining the impact of behavior of family members on the child's well-being. In many cases, a child's level of impairment is related to factors extending beyond a psychiatric diagnosis, such as the child's adjustment to his or her family life, peer relationships, and educational placement.

RECOMMENDATIONS AND TREATMENT PLAN

The recommendations for treatment are derived by a clinician who integrates the data gathered during the evaluation into a coherent formulation of the factors that are contributing to the child's problems, the consequences of the problems, and strategies that may ameliorate the difficulties. The recommendations can be broken down into their biological, psychological, and social components. That is, identification of a biological predisposition to a particular psychiatric disorder may be clinically relevant to inform a psychopharmacologic recommendation. As part of the formulation, an understanding of the psychodynamic interactions among family members may lead a clinician to recommend treatment that includes a family component. Educational and academic problems are addressed in the formulation and may lead to a recommendation to seek a more effective academic placement. The overall social situation of the child or adolescent is taken into account when recommendations for treatment are developed. Of course, the physical and emotional safety of a child or adolescent is of the utmost importance and always at the top of the list of recommendations.

The child or adolescent's family, school life, peer interactions, and social activities often have a direct impact on the child's success in overcoming his or her difficulties. The psychological education and cooperation of a child or adolescent's family are essential ingredients in successful application of treatment recommendations. Communications from clinicians to parents and family members that balance the observed positive qualities of the child and family with the weak areas are often perceived as more helpful than a focus only on the problem areas. Finally, the most successful treatment plans are those developed cooperatively among the clinician, child, and family members during which each member of the team perceives that he or she has been given credit for positive contributions.

34 ▲

Mental Retardation

The conceptualization of mental retardation includes deficits in cognitive abilities, as well as in behaviors required for social and personal sufficiency, known as *adaptive functioning*. Wide acceptance of this definition has led to the consensus that an assessment of both social adaptation and intelligence quotient (IQ) is necessary to determine the level of mental retardation. Measures of adaptive function assess competency in performance of everyday tasks, whereas measures of intellectual function focus on cognitive abilities. Evidence shows that individuals with a given intellectual level do not all have the same adaptive function, yet it is likely that IQ contributes an upper limit or ceiling to adaptive accomplishments.

CLASSIFICATION

According to the text revision of the fourth edition of the *Diagnostic and Statistical Manual of Mental Disorders* (DSM-IV-TR), mental retardation is defined as significantly subaverage general intellectual functioning resulting in, or associated with, concurrent impairment in adaptive behavior and manifested during the developmental period, before the age of 18 years. The diagnosis is made regardless of whether the person has a co-existing physical disorder or other mental disorder. Table 34–1 presents an overview of developmental levels in communication, academic functioning, and vocational skills expected of persons with various degrees of mental retardation.

General intellectual functioning is determined by the use of standardized tests of intelligence, and the term *significantly subaverage* is defined as an IQ of approximately 70 or below or two standard deviations below the mean for the particular test. Adaptive functioning can be measured by using a standardized scale, such as the *Vineland Adaptive Behavior Scale*. This scale scores communications, daily living skills, socialization, and motor skills (up to 4 years, 11 months) and generates an adaptive behavior composite that is correlated with the expected skills at a given age.

Approximately 85 percent of persons with mental retardation fall within the mild mental retardation category (IQ between 50 and 70). The adaptive functions of persons with mild mental retardation are effective in several areas, such as communications, self-care, social skills, work, leisure, and safety. Mental retardation is influenced by genetic, environmental, and psychosocial factors; previously, the development of mild retardation was often attributed to severe psychosocial deprivation. More recently, however, researchers have increasingly recognized the likely contribution of a host of subtle biological factors, including chromosomal abnormalities, subclinical lead intoxication, and prenatal exposure to drugs, alcohol, and other toxins. Furthermore, evidence is increasing that subgroups of persons with mental retardation, such as

those with fragile X syndrome, Down syndrome, and Prader-Willi syndrome, have characteristic patterns of social, linguistic, and cognitive development and typical behavioral manifestations.

The DSM-IV-TR includes in its text on mental retardation additional information regarding the etiological factors and their association with mental retardation syndromes (e.g., fragile X syndrome).

EPIDEMIOLOGY

The prevalence of mental retardation at any one time is estimated to range from 1 to 3 percent of the population. The incidence of mental retardation is difficult to calculate because mild mental retardation sometimes goes unrecognized until middle childhood. In some cases, even when intellectual function is limited, good adaptive skills are not challenged until late childhood or early adolescence, and the diagnosis is not made until that time. The highest incidence is in school-age children, with the peak at ages 10 to 14 years. Mental retardation is about 1.5 times more common among men than among women. In older persons, prevalence is lower; those with severe or profound mental retardation have high mortality rates because of the complications of associated physical disorders.

COMORBIDITY

Prevalence

Epidemiological surveys indicate that up to two thirds of children and adults with mental retardation have comorbid mental disorders; this rate is several times higher than that in the community samples of those without mental retardation. The prevalence of psychopathology seems to be correlated with the severity of mental retardation; the more severe the mental retardation, the higher the risk for other mental disorders. A recent epidemiological study found that 40.7 percent of intellectually disabled children between 4 and 18 years of age met criteria for at least one psychiatric disorder. The severity of retardation affected the type of psychiatric disorder. Disruptive and conduct-disorder behaviors occurred more commonly in the group with mild retardation; the group with more severe retardation exhibited psychiatric problems more often associated with autistic disorder, such as self-stimulation and self-mutilation. In contrast to the epidemiology of psychopathology in children in general, age and sex did not affect the prevalence of psychiatric disorders in this study. Those with profound mental retardation were less likely to exhibit psychiatric symptoms.

The mental disorders that occur among persons with mental retardation appear to run the gamut of those seen in persons without mental retardation, including mood disorders, schizophrenia, attention-deficit/hyperactivity disorder (ADHD), and conduct disorder. Those with

Table 34–1
Developmental Characteristics of Persons with Mental Retardation

Degree of Mental Retardation	Preschool Age (0–5 yrs): Maturation and Development	School Age (6–20 yrs): Training and Education	Adult (≥21 yrs): Social and Vocational Adequacy
Profound	Gross retardation; minimal capacity for functioning in sensorimotor areas; need nursing care; constant aid and supervision required	Some motor development present; may respond to minimal or limited training in self-help	Some motor and speech development; may achieve very limited self-care; need nursing care
Severe	Poor motor development; speech minimal; generally unable to profit from training in self-help; little or no communication skills	Can talk or learn to communicate; can be trained in elemental health habits; profit from systematic habit training; unable to profit from vocational training	May contribute partially to self-maintenance under complete supervision; can develop self-protection skills to a minimal useful level in controlled environment
Moderate	Can talk or learn to communicate; poor social awareness; fair motor development; profit from training in self-help; can be managed with moderate supervision	Can profit from training in social and occupational skills; unlikely to progress beyond second-grade level in academic subjects; may learn to travel alone in familiar places	May achieve self-maintenance in unskilled or semiskilled work under sheltered conditions; need supervision and guidance when under mild social or economic stress
Mild	Can develop social and communication skills; minimal retardation in sensorimotor areas; often not distinguished from normal until later age	Can learn academic skills up to approximately sixth-grade level by late teens; can be guided toward social conformity	Can usually achieve social and vocational skills adequate to minimal self-support, but may need guidance and assistance when under unusual social or economic stress

DSM-IV criteria are adapted essentially from this chart.
Adapted from *Mental Retardation: Activities of the U.S. Department of Health, Education and Welfare*. Washington, DC: U.S. Government Printing Office; 1989:2, with permission.

severe mental retardation have a particularly high rate of autistic disorder and pervasive developmental disorders. About 2 to 3 percent of persons with mental retardation meet the criteria for schizophrenia; this percentage is several times higher than the rate for the general population. Up to 50 percent of children and adults with mental retardation had a mood disorder when such instruments as the *Kiddie Schedule for Affective Disorders and Schizophrenia*, the *Beck Depression Inventory*, and the *Children's Depression Inventory* were used in pilot studies, but because these instruments have not been standardized within this population, these findings must be considered preliminary.

Highly prevalent psychiatric symptoms that can occur in persons with mental retardation outside the context of a mental disorder include hyperactivity and short attention span, self-injurious behaviors (e.g., head-banging and self-biting), and repetitive stereotypical behaviors (hand-flapping and toe-walking). Personality styles and traits in persons with mental retardation are not unique to them, but negative self-image, low self-esteem, poor frustration tolerance, interpersonal dependence, and a rigid problem-solving style are overrepresented. Specific causal syndromes seen in mental retardation can also predispose affected persons to various types of psychopathologies.

Neurological Disorders

Comorbid psychiatric disorders are increased in individuals with mental retardation who also have known neurological conditions, such as seizure disorders. Rates of psychopathology increase with the severity of mental retardation; thus, neurological impairment increases as intellectual impairment increases. In a recent review of psychiatric disorders in children and adolescents with mental retardation and epilepsy, approximately one third also had autistic disorder or an autistic-like condition. The combination of mental retardation, active epilepsy, and autism or an autistic-like condition occurs at a rate of 0.07 percent in the general population.

Psychosocial Features

A negative self-image and poor self-esteem are common features of persons with mild and moderate mental retardation, who are well aware of being different from others. They experience repeated failure and disappointment in not meeting their parents' and society's expectations and in falling progressively behind their peers and even their younger siblings. Communication difficulties further increase their vulnerability to feelings of ineptness and frustration. Inappropriate behaviors, such as withdrawal, are common. The perpetual sense of isolation and inadequacy has been linked to feelings of anxiety, anger, dysphoria, and depression.

ETIOLOGY

Etiological factors in mental retardation can be primarily genetic, developmental, acquired, or a combination of these. Genetic causes include chromosomal and inherited conditions; developmental factors include prenatal exposure to infections and toxins; and acquired syndromes include perinatal trauma (e.g., prematurity) and sociocultural factors. The severity of the resulting mental retardation is related to the timing and duration of the trauma as well as to the degree of exposure to the central nervous system (CNS). The more severe the mental retardation, the more likely it is that the cause is evident. In about three fourths of persons with severe mental retardation, the cause is known, whereas the cause is apparent in only half of those with mild mental retardation. A recent study of 100 consecutive children with mental retardation admitted to a clinical genetics unit of a university pediatric hospital reported that in 41 percent of cases, a causative diagnosis was made. In general, etiological classifications used included genetic, multifactorial, environmental, and unknown etiology. No cause is known for three fourths of persons with borderline intellectual functioning. Overall, in up to two thirds of all persons with mental retardation, the probable cause can be identified. Among chromosomal and metabolic disorders, Down syndrome, fragile X syndrome, and phenylketonuria (PKU) are the most common disorders that usually produce at least moderate mental retardation. Those with mild mental retardation sometimes have a familial pattern apparent in parents and siblings. Deprivation of nutrition, nurturance, and social stimulation can contribute to the development of mental retardation. Current knowledge suggests that genetic, environmental, biological, and psychosocial factors work additively in mental retardation.

Genetic Etiological Factors in Mental Retardation

Abnormalities in autosomal chromosomes are frequently associated with mental retardation, whereas aberrations in sex chromosomes can result in characteristic physical syndromes that do not include mental retardation (e.g., Turner's syndrome with XO and Klinefelter's syndrome with XXY, XXXY, and XXYY variations). Some children with Turner's syndrome have normal to superior intelligence. Agreement exists on a few predisposing factors for chromosomal disorders—among them, advanced maternal age, increased age of the father, and X-ray radiation.

Down Syndrome. The description of Down syndrome, first made by the English physician Langdon Down in 1866, was based on the physical characteristics associated with subnormal mental functioning. Since then, Down syndrome has been the most investigated, and most discussed, syndrome in mental retardation. Children with this syndrome were originally called *mongoloid* because of their physical characteristics of slanted eyes, epicanthal folds, and flat nose. Despite a plethora of theories and hypotheses advanced in the last 100 years, the cause of Down syndrome is still unknown.

The problem of cause is complicated even further by the recent recognition of three types of chromosomal aberration in Down syndrome:

1. Patients with trisomy 21 (three chromosome 21 instead of the usual two) represent the overwhelming majority; they have 47 chromosomes, with an extra chromosome 21. The mothers' karyotypes are normal. A nondisjunction during meiosis, occurring for unknown reasons, is held to be responsible for the disorder.
2. Nondisjunction occurring after fertilization in any cell division results in mosaicism, a condition in which both normal and trisomic cells are found in various tissues.
3. In translocation, a fusion occurs of two chromosomes, usually 21 and 15, resulting in a total of 46 chromosomes, despite the presence of an extra chromosome 21. The disorder, unlike trisomy 21, is usually inherited, and the translocated chromosome may be found in unaffected parents and siblings. The asymptomatic carriers have only 45 chromosomes.

The incidence of Down syndrome in the United States is about 1 in every 700 births. In his original description, Down mentioned the frequency of 10 percent among all patients with mental retardation. For a middle-aged mother (>32 years of age), the risk of having a child with Down syndrome with trisomy 21 is about 1 in 100 births, but when translocation is present, the risk is about 1 in 3. These facts assume special importance in genetic counseling.

Mental retardation is the overriding feature of Down syndrome. Most persons with the syndrome have moderate or severe retardation, with only a minority having an IQ greater than 50. Mental development seems to progress normally from birth to 6 months of age; IQ scores gradually decrease from near normal at 1 year of age to about 30 at older ages. The decline in intelligence may not be readily apparent. Infantile tests may not reveal the full extent of the defect, which may become manifest when sophisticated tests are used in early childhood. According to many sources, children with Down syndrome are placid, cheerful, and cooperative and adapt easily at home. With adolescence, the picture changes: Youngsters may experience various emotional difficulties, behavior disorders, and (rarely) psychotic disorders.

In Down syndrome, language function is a relative weakness, whereas sociability and social skills, such as interpersonal cooperation and conformity with social conventions, are relative strengths. Most studies have noted muted affect in children with Down syndrome relative to children of the same mental age who do not have retardation. Those with Down syndrome also manifest deficiencies in scanning the environment; they are likely to focus on a single stimulus and have difficulty noticing environmental changes. A variety of mental disorders occurs in persons with Down syndrome, but the rates appear to be lower than those in other mental retardation syndromes, especially autistic disorder.

The diagnosis of Down syndrome is made with relative ease in an older child but is often difficult in newborn infants. The most important signs in a newborn include general hypotonia; oblique palpebral fissures; abundant neck skin; a small, flattened skull; high cheekbones; and a protruding tongue. The hands are broad and thick, with a single palmar transversal crease, and the little fingers are short and curved inward. Moro reflex is weak or absent. More than 100 signs or stigmata are described in Down syndrome, but rarely are all found in one person. Life expectancy was once about 12 years; with the advent of antibiotics, few young patients die from Down syndrome, but many do not live beyond the age of 40 years. Life expectancy is increasing, however.

Persons with Down syndrome tend to exhibit marked deterioration in language, memory, self-care skills, and problem solving in their 30s. Postmortem studies of those with Down syndrome older than the age of 40 years have shown a high incidence of senile plaques and neurofibrillary tangles, as seen in Alzheimer's disease. Neurofibrillary tangles are known to occur in a variety of degenerative diseases, whereas senile plaques seem to be found most often in Alzheimer's disease and in Down syndrome. Thus, the two disorders may share some pathophysiology.

Fragile X Syndrome. Fragile X syndrome is the second-most-common cause of mental retardation. The syndrome results from a mutation on the X chromosome at what is known as the fragile site (Xq27.3). The fragile site is expressed in only some cells, and it may be absent in asymptomatic males and female carriers. Much variability is present in both genetic and phenotypic expression. Fragile X syndrome is believed to occur in about 1 of every 1,000 males and 1 of every 2,000 females. The typical phenotype includes a large, long head and ears, short stature, hyperextensible joints, and postpubertal macroorchidism. The mental retardation ranges from mild to severe. The behavioral profile of persons with the syndrome includes a high rate of ADHD, learning disorders, and pervasive developmental disorders, such as autism. Deficits in language function include rapid perseverative speech with abnormalities in combining words into phrases and sentences. Persons with fragile X syndrome seem to have relatively strong skills in communication and socialization; their intellectual functions seem to decline in the pubertal period. Female carriers are often less impaired than males with fragile X syndrome, but females can also manifest the typical physical characteristics and can have mild retardation.

Prader-Willi Syndrome. Prader-Willi syndrome is postulated to result from a small deletion involving chromosome 15, usually occurring sporadically. Its prevalence is less than 1 in 10,000. Persons with the syndrome exhibit compulsive eating behavior and often obesity, mental retardation, hypogonadism, small stature, hypotonia, and small hands and feet. Children with the syndrome often have oppositional and defiant behavior.

Cat's Cry (Cri-du-Chat) Syndrome.

Children with cat's cry syndrome lack part of chromosome 5. They have severe retardation and show many signs often associated with chromosomal aberrations, such as microcephaly, low-set ears, oblique palpebral fissures, hypertelorism, and micrognathia. The characteristic cat-like cry caused by laryngeal abnormalities that gave the syndrome its name gradually changes and disappears with increasing age.

Phenylketonuria.

PKU was first described by Ivar Asbjörn Fölling in 1934 as the paradigmatic inborn error of metabolism. PKU is transmitted as a simple recessive autosomal Mendelian trait and occurs in about 1 of every 10,000 to 15,000 live births. For parents who have already had a child with PKU, the chance of having another child with PKU is 1 in every 4 to 5 successive pregnancies. Although the disease is reported predominantly in persons of North European origin, a few cases have been described in blacks, Yemenite Jews, and Asians. The frequency among institutionalized patients with retardation is about 1 percent. The basic metabolic defect in PKU is an inability to convert phenylalanine, an essential amino acid, to paratyrosine because of the absence or inactivity of the liver enzyme phenylalanine hydroxylase, which catalyzes the conversion. Two other types of hyperphenylalaninemia have recently been described. One is caused by a deficiency of the enzyme dihydropteridine reductase and the other by a deficiency of a cofactor, biopterin. The first defect can be detected in fibroblasts, and biopterin can be measured in body fluids. Both of these rare disorders carry a high risk of fatality.

Most patients with PKU have severe retardation, but some are reported to have borderline or normal intelligence. Eczema, vomiting, and convulsions occur in about one third of all patients. Although the clinical picture varies, typical children with PKU are hyperactive; they exhibit erratic, unpredictable behavior and are difficult to manage. They frequently have temper tantrums and often display bizarre movements of their bodies and upper extremities, including twisting hand mannerisms; their behavior sometimes resembles that of children with autism or schizophrenia. Verbal and nonverbal communication is usually severely impaired or nonexistent. The children's coordination is poor, and they have many perceptual difficulties.

In the United States, newborn infants are now routinely screened for PKU. Early diagnosis is important because a low-phenylalanine diet, in use since 1955, significantly improves both behavior and developmental progress. The best results seem to be obtained with early diagnosis and the start of dietary treatment before the child is 6 months of age. Dietary treatment, however, is not without risk. Phenylalanine is an essential amino acid, and its omission from the diet can lead to such severe complications as anemia, hypoglycemia, edema, and even death. Dietary treatment of PKU should be continued indefinitely. Children who receive a diagnosis before the age of 3 months and are placed on an optimal dietary regimen may have normal intelligence. A low-phenylalanine diet does not influence the level of mental retardation in untreated older children and adolescents with PKU, but the diet does decrease irritability and abnormal electroencephalogram (EEG) changes and does increase social responsiveness and attention span. The parents of children with PKU and some of the children's normal siblings are heterozygous carriers. The disease can be detected by a phenylalanine tolerance test, which may be important in genetic counseling of the family members.

Rett's Disorder.

Rett's disorder is hypothesized to be an X-linked dominant mental retardation syndrome that is degenerative and affects only females. In 1966, Andreas Rett reported on 22 girls with a serious progressive neurological disability. Deterioration in communica-

tions skills, motor behavior, and social functioning starts at about 1 year of age. Autistic-like symptoms are common, as are ataxia, facial grimacing, teeth-grinding, and loss of speech. Intermittent hyperventilation and a disorganized breathing pattern are characteristic while the child is awake. Stereotypical hand movements, including hand-wringing, are typical. Progressive gait disturbance, scoliosis, and seizures occur. Severe spasticity is usually present by middle childhood. Cerebral atrophy occurs with decreased pigmentation of the substantia nigra, which suggests abnormalities of the dopaminergic nigrostriatal system.

Neurofibromatosis.

Also called *von Recklinghausen's* disease, neurofibromatosis is the most common of the neurocutaneous syndromes caused by a single dominant gene, which may be inherited or be a new mutation. The disorder occurs in about 1 of 5,000 births and is characterized by café au lait spots on the skin and by neurofibromas, including optic gliomas and acoustic neuromas, caused by abnormal cell migration. Mild mental retardation occurs in up to one third of those with the disease.

Tuberous Sclerosis.

Tuberous sclerosis is the second-most common of the neurocutaneous syndromes; a progressive mental retardation occurs in up to two thirds of all affected persons. It occurs in about 1 of 15,000 persons and is inherited by autosomal dominant transmission. Seizures are present in all of those with mental retardation and in two thirds of those without it. Infantile spasms may occur as early as 6 months of age. The phenotypic presentation includes adenoma sebaceum and ash-leaf spots that can be identified with a slit lamp.

Lesch-Nyhan Syndrome.

Lesch-Nyhan syndrome is a rare disorder caused by a deficiency of an enzyme involved in purine metabolism. The disorder is X-linked; patients have mental retardation, microcephaly, seizures, choreoathetosis, and spasticity. The syndrome is also associated with severe compulsive self-mutilation by biting the mouth and fingers. Lesch-Nyhan syndrome is another example of a genetically determined syndrome with a specific, predictable behavioral pattern.

Adrenoleukodystrophy.

The most common of several disorders of sudanophilic cerebral sclerosis, adrenoleukodystrophy is characterized by diffuse demyelination of the cerebral white matter resulting in visual and intellectual impairment, seizures, spasticity, and progression to death. The cerebral degeneration in adrenoleukodystrophy is accompanied by adrenocortical insufficiency. The disorder is transmitted by a sex-linked gene located on the distal end of the long arm of the X chromosome. The clinical onset is generally between 5 and 8 years of age, with early seizures, disturbances in gait, and mild intellectual impairment. Abnormal pigmentation reflecting adrenal insufficiency sometimes precedes the neurological symptoms, and attacks of crying are common. Spastic contractures, ataxia, and swallowing disturbances are also frequent. Although the course is often rapidly progressive, some patients may have a relapsing and remitting course. The story of a child with the disorder was presented in the 1992 film *Lorenzo's Oil*.

Maple Syrup Urine Disease.

The clinical symptoms of maple syrup urine disease appear during the first week of life. The infant deteriorates rapidly and has decerebrate rigidity, seizures, respiratory irregularity, and hypoglycemia. If untreated, most patients die in the first months of life, and the survivors have severe retardation. Some variants have been reported with transient ataxia and only mild retardation. Treatment follows the general principles established for PKU and consists in a diet very low in the three involved amino acids—leucine, isoleucine, and valine.

Other Enzyme Deficiency Disorders.

Several enzyme deficiency disorders associated with mental retardation have been identified, and still more diseases are being added as new discoveries are made, including Hartnup's disease, galactosemia, and glycogen-storage disease.

Acquired and Developmental Factors

Prenatal Period.   Important prerequisites for the overall development of the fetus include the mother's physical, psychological, and nutritional health during pregnancy. Maternal chronic illnesses and conditions affecting the normal development of the fetus's CNS include uncontrolled diabetes, anemia, emphysema, hypertension, and long-term use of alcohol and narcotic substances. Maternal infections during pregnancy, especially viral infections, have been known to cause fetal damage and mental retardation. The extent of fetal damage depends on such variables as the type of viral infection, the gestational age of the fetus, and the severity of the illness. Although numerous infectious diseases have been reported to affect the fetus's CNS, the following medical disorders have been definitely identified as high-risk conditions for mental retardation.

Rubella (German Measles).   Rubella has replaced syphilis as the major cause of congenital malformations and mental retardation caused by maternal infection. The children of affected mothers may show several abnormalities, including congenital heart disease, mental retardation, cataracts, deafness, microcephaly, and microphthalmia. Timing is crucial because the extent and frequency of the complications are inversely related to the duration of the pregnancy at the time of maternal infection. When mothers are infected in the first trimester of pregnancy, 10 to 15 percent of the children are affected, but the incidence rises to almost 50 percent when the infection occurs in the first month of pregnancy. The situation is often complicated by subclinical forms of maternal infection that often go undetected. Maternal rubella can be prevented by immunization.

Cytomegalic Inclusion Disease.   In many cases, cytomegalic inclusion disease remains dormant in the mother. Some children are stillborn, and others have jaundice, microcephaly, hepatosplenomegaly, and radiographic findings of intracerebral calcification. Children with mental retardation from the disease frequently have cerebral calcification, microcephaly, or hydrocephalus. The diagnosis is confirmed by positive findings of the virus in throat and urine cultures and the recovery of inclusion-bearing cells in the urine.

Syphilis.   Syphilis in pregnant women was once the main cause of various neuropathological changes in their offspring, including mental retardation. Today, the incidence of syphilitic complications of pregnancy fluctuates with the incidence of syphilis in the general population. Some recent alarming statistics from several major cities in the United States indicate that there is still no room for complacency.

Toxoplasmosis.   Toxoplasmosis can be transmitted by the mother to the fetus. It causes mild or severe mental retardation and, in severe cases, hydrocephalus, seizures, microcephaly, and chorioretinitis.

Herpes Simplex.   The herpes simplex virus can be transmitted transplacentally, although the most common mode of infection is during birth. Microcephaly, mental retardation, intracranial calcification, and ocular abnormalities may result.

Acquired Immune Deficiency Syndrome (AIDS).
Many fetuses of mothers with AIDS never come to term because of stillbirth or spontaneous abortion. Of infants born infected with the human

immunodeficiency virus (HIV), up to half have progressive encephalopathy, mental retardation, and seizures within the first year of life. Children born with HIV infection often live only a few years; however, most babies born to HIV-infected mothers are not infected with the virus.

Fetal Alcohol Syndrome.   Fetal alcohol syndrome results in mental retardation and a typical phenotypic picture of facial dysmorphism that includes hypertelorism, microcephaly, short palpebral fissures, inner epicanthal folds, and a short, turned-up nose. Often, the affected children have learning disorders and ADHD. Cardiac defects are also frequent. The entire syndrome occurs in up to 15 percent of babies born to women who regularly ingest large amounts of alcohol. Babies born to women who consume alcohol regularly during pregnancy have a high incidence of ADHD, learning disorders, and mental retardation without the facial dysmorphism.

Prenatal Drug Exposure.   Prenatal exposure to opioids, such as heroin, often results in infants who are small for their gestational age, with a head circumference below the tenth percentile and withdrawal symptoms that appear within the first 2 days of life. The withdrawal symptoms of infants include irritability, hypertonia, tremor, vomiting, a high-pitched cry, and an abnormal sleep pattern. Seizures are unusual, but the withdrawal syndrome can be life threatening to infants if it is untreated. Diazepam (Valium), phenobarbital (Luminal), chlorpromazine (Thorazine), and paregoric have been used to treat neonatal opioid withdrawal. The long-term sequelae of prenatal opioid exposure are not fully known; the children's developmental milestones and intellectual functions may be within the normal range, but they have an increased risk for impulsivity and behavioral problems. Infants prenatally exposed to cocaine are at high risk for low birthweight and premature delivery. In the early neonatal period, they may have transient neurological and behavioral abnormalities, including abnormal results on EEGs, tachycardia, poor feeding patterns, irritability, and excessive drowsiness. Rather than a withdrawal reaction, the physiological and behavioral abnormalities are a response to the cocaine, which may be excreted for up to 1 week postnatally.

Complications of Pregnancy.   Toxemia of pregnancy and uncontrolled maternal diabetes present hazards to the fetus and sometimes result in mental retardation. Maternal malnutrition during pregnancy often results in prematurity and other obstetrical complications. Vaginal hemorrhage, placenta previa, premature separation of the placenta, and prolapse of the cord can damage the fetal brain by causing anoxia. The potential teratogenic effect of pharmacological agents administered during pregnancy was widely publicized after the thalidomide tragedy (the drug produced a high percentage of deformed babies when given to pregnant women). So far, with the exception of metabolites used in cancer chemotherapy, no usual doses of medications are known to damage the fetus's CNS, but caution and restraint in prescribing drugs to pregnant women are certainly indicated. The use of lithium during pregnancy was recently implicated in some congenital malformations, especially of the cardiovascular system (e.g., Ebstein's anomaly).

Perinatal Period.   Some evidence indicates that premature infants and infants with low birthweight are at high risk for neurological and intellectual impairments that appear during their school years. Infants who sustain intracranial hemorrhages or show evidence of cerebral ischemia are especially vulnerable to cognitive abnormalities. The degree of neurodevelopmental impairment generally correlates with the severity of the intracranial hemorrhage. Recent studies have documented that, among children with very low birthweight (<1,000 g), 20 percent had significant disabilities, including cerebral palsy, mental retardation, autism, and low intelligence with severe learning problems. Very premature children and those who suffered intrauterine growth retardation were found to be at high risk for developing both social problems and academic difficulties. Socioeconomic deprivation can also affect the adaptive function of these vulnerable infants. Early intervention may improve their cognitive, language, and perceptual abilities.

Acquired Childhood Disorders.   Occasionally, a child's developmental status changes dramatically as a result of a specific disease or physical trauma. In retrospect, it is sometimes difficult to ascertain the full picture of the child's developmental progress before the insult, but the adverse effects on the child's development or skills are apparent afterward.

Infection.   The most serious infections affecting cerebral integrity are encephalitis and meningitis. Measles encephalitis has been virtually eliminated by the universal use of measles vaccine, and the incidence of other bacterial infections of the CNS has been markedly reduced with antibacterial agents. Most episodes of encephalitis are caused by viruses. Sometimes a clinician must retrospectively consider a probable encephalitic component in a previous obscure illness with high fever. Meningitis that was diagnosed late, even when followed by antibiotic treatment, can seriously affect a child's cognitive development. Thrombotic and purulent intracranial phenomena secondary to septicemia are rarely seen today except in small infants.

Head Trauma.   The best-known causes of head injury in children that produces developmental handicaps, including seizures, are motor vehicle accidents, but more head injuries are caused by household accidents, such as falls from tables, from open windows, and on stairways. Child abuse is also a cause of head injury.

Other Issues.   Brain damage from cardiac arrest during anesthesia is rare. One cause of complete or partial brain damage is asphyxia associated with near drowning. Long-term exposure to lead is a well-established cause of compromised intelligence and learning skills. Intracranial tumors of various types and origins, surgery, and chemotherapy can also adversely affect brain function.

Environmental and Sociocultural Factors

Mild retardation can result from significant deprivation of nutrition and nurturance. Children who have endured these conditions are subject to long-lasting damage to their physical and emotional development. Prenatal environment compromised by poor medical care and poor maternal nutrition can be contributing factors in the development of mild mental retardation. Teenage pregnancies are risk factors, and they are associated with obstetrical complications, prematurity, and low birthweight. Poor postnatal medical care, malnutrition, exposure to such toxic substances as lead, and physical trauma are risk factors for mild mental retardation. Family instability, frequent moves, and multiple but inadequate caretakers may deprive an infant of necessary emotional relationships, leading to failure to thrive and potential risk to the developing brain.

An incapacitating mental disorder in a parent may interfere with appropriate child care and stimulation and cause developmental risk. Children of parents with mood disorders and schizophrenia are known to be at risk for these and related disorders. Some studies indicate a higher-than-expected prevalence of motor skills disorder and developmental disorders, but not necessarily mental retardation, among the children of parents with chronic mental disorders.

DIAGNOSIS

The diagnosis of mental retardation can be made after the history, a standardized intellectual assessment, and a measure of adaptive function indicate that a child's current behavior is significantly below the expected level (Table 34–2). The diagnosis itself does not specify either the cause or the prognosis. A history and psychiatric interview are useful in obtaining a longitudinal picture of the child's development and functioning, and examination of physical signs, neurological abnormalities, and laboratory tests can be used to ascertain the cause and prognosis.

History

The history is most often obtained from the parents or the caretaker, with particular attention to the mother's pregnancy, labor, and delivery; the presence of a family history of mental retardation; consanguinity of the parents; and hereditary disorders. As part of the history, the clinician assesses the overall level of functioning and intellectual capacity of the parents and the emotional climate of the home.

Table 34–2
DSM-IV-TR Diagnostic Criteria for Mental Retardation

A. Significantly subaverage intellectual functioning: an IQ of approximately 70 or below on an individually administered IQ test (for infants, a clinical judgment of significantly subaverage intellectual functioning).

B. Concurrent deficits or impairments in present adaptive functioning (i.e., the person's effectiveness in meeting the standards expected for his or her age by his or her cultural group) in at least two of the following areas: communication, self-care, home living, social/interpersonal skills, use of community resources, self-direction, functional academic skills, work, leisure, health, and safety.

C. The onset is before age 18 years.

Code based on degree of severity reflecting level of intellectual impairment:

Mild mental retardation:	IQ level 50–55 to approximately 70
Moderate mental retardation:	IQ level 35–40 to 50–55
Severe mental retardation:	IQ level 20–25 to 35–40
Profound mental retardation:	IQ level below 20 or 25
Mental retardation, severity unspecified:	When there is strong presumption of mental retardation but the person's intelligence is untestable by standard tests

(From American Psychiatric Association. *Diagnostic and Statistical Manual of Mental Disorders.* 4th ed. Text rev. Washington, DC: American Psychiatric Association; copyright 2000, with permission.)

Psychiatric Interview

Two factors are of paramount importance when interviewing the patient: the interviewer's attitude and manner of communicating. The interviewer should not be guided by the patient's mental age, which cannot fully characterize the person. An adult with mild mental retardation with a mental age of 10 years is not a 10-year-old child. When addressed as if they were children, some persons with mental retardation become justifiably insulted, angry, and uncooperative. Passive and dependent persons, alternatively, may assume the child's role that they think is expected of them. In neither case can valid diagnostic data be obtained.

The patient's verbal abilities, including receptive and expressive language, should be assessed as soon as possible by observing the communication between the caretakers and the patient and by taking the history. The clinician often finds it helpful to see the patient and the caretakers together. If the patient uses sign language, the caretaker may have to stay during the interview as an interpreter. Persons with retardation often have the lifelong experience of failing in many areas, and they may be anxious about seeing an interviewer. The interviewer and the caretaker should attempt to give such patients a clear, supportive, concrete explanation of the diagnostic process, particularly patients with sufficiently receptive language. Giving patients the impression that their bad behavior is the cause of the referral should be avoided. Support and praise should be offered in language appropriate to the patient's age and understanding. Leading questions should be avoided because persons with retardation may be suggestible and wish to please others. Subtle direction, structure, and reinforcement may be necessary to keep them focused on the task or topic.

The patient's control over motility patterns should be ascertained, and clinical evidence of distractibility and distortions in perception and memory may be evaluated. The use of speech, reality testing, and the ability to generalize from experiences should be noted. The nature and maturity of the patient's defenses—particularly exaggerated or self-defeating uses of avoidance, repression, denial, introjection, and isolation—should be observed. Frustration, tolerance, and impulse control—especially over motor, aggressive, and sexual drives—should be assessed. Also important are self-image and its role in the development of self-confidence, as well as an assessment of tenacity, persistence, curiosity, and willingness to explore the unknown. In general, the psychiatric examination of a person with retardation should reveal how the patient has coped with the stages of development.

Physical Examination

Various parts of the body may have certain characteristics that have prenatal causes and are commonly found in persons with mental retardation. For example, the configuration and the size of the head offer clues to a variety of conditions, such as microcephaly, hydrocephalus, and Down syndrome. The patient's face may have some signs of mental retardation that greatly facilitate the diagnosis, such as hypertelorism, a flat nasal bridge, prominent eyebrows, epicanthal folds, corneal opacities, retinal changes, low-set and small or misshapen ears, a protruding tongue, and a disturbance in dentition. Facial expression, such as a dull appearance, can be misleading and should not be relied on without other supporting evidence. The color and texture of the skin and hair, a high-arched palate, the size of the thyroid gland, and the size of the child and his or her trunk and extremities should also be explored. The circumference of the head should be measured as part of the clinical investigation. Dermatoglyphics may offer another diagnostic tool because uncommon ridge patterns and flexion creases on the hand are often found in persons with mental retardation. Abnormal dermatoglyphics occur in chromosomal disorders and in persons who were prenatally infected with rubella. The clinician should bear in mind during the examination that children with mental retardation, particularly those with associated behavioral problems, are at increased risk for child abuse.

Neurological Examination

Sensory impairments occur frequently among persons with mental retardation; for example, up to 10 percent are hearing impaired, a rate that is four times that of the general population. Sensory disturbances can include hearing difficulties, ranging from cortical deafness to mild hearing deficits. Visual disturbances can range from blindness to disturbances of spatial concepts, design recognition, and concepts of body image. Various other neurological impairments also occur frequently in persons with mental retardation; seizure disorders occur in about 10 percent of all persons with mental retardation and in one third of those with severe retardation. When neurological abnormalities are present, their incidence and severity generally rise in direct proportion to the degree of retardation. Many children with severe retardation, however, have no neurological abnormalities; conversely, about 25 percent of all children with cerebral palsy have normal intelligence. Disturbances in motor areas are manifested in abnormalities of muscle tone (spasticity or hypotonia), reflexes (hyperreflexia), and involuntary movements (choreoathetosis). Less disability is revealed in clumsiness and poor coordination.

The infants with the poorest prognoses are those who manifest a combination of inactivity, general hypotonia, and exaggerated response to stimuli. In older children, hyperactivity, short attention span, distractibility, and a low frustration tolerance are often signs of brain damage. In general, the younger the child at the time of investigation, the more caution is indicated in predicting future ability, because the recovery potential of the infantile brain is very good. Observing the child's development at regular intervals is probably the most reliable approach.

Skull X-rays are usually taken routinely but are illuminating in only a relatively few conditions, such as craniosynostosis, hydrocephalus, and other disorders that result in intracranial calcifications (e.g., toxoplasmosis, tuberous sclerosis, cerebral angiomatosis, and hypoparathyroidism). Computed tomography scans and magnetic resonance imaging (MRI) have become important tools for uncovering CNS pathology associated with mental retardation. Occasionally, findings are of internal hydrocephalus, cortical atrophy, or porencephaly in brain-damaged children with severe retardation. An EEG is best interpreted with caution in cases of mental retardation. The exceptions are patients with hypsarrhythmia and grand mal seizures, in whom the EEG may help establish the diagnosis and suggest treatment. In most other conditions, a diffuse cerebral disorder produces nonspecific EEG changes, characterized by slow frequencies with bursts of spikes and sharp or blunt wave complexes. The confusion over the significance of the EEG in the diagnosis of mental retardation is best illustrated by the reports of frequent EEG abnormalities in Down syndrome, which are in the range of 25 percent in most patients examined.

CLINICAL FEATURES

Mild mental retardation may not be diagnosed until the affected children enter school; their social skills and communication may be adequate in the preschool years. As they get older, however, such cognitive deficits as poor ability to abstract and egocentric thinking may distinguish them from others of their age. Although persons with mild retardation can function academically at the high elementary level and their vocational skills suffice to support themselves in some cases, social assimilation can be difficult. Communication deficits, poor self-esteem, and dependence can contribute to their relative lack of social spontaneity. Some persons with mild retardation may fall into relationships with peers who exploit their shortcomings. In most cases, persons with mild mental retardation can achieve some social and vocational success in a supportive environment.

Moderate mental retardation is likely to be diagnosed at a younger age than mild mental retardation; communication skills develop more slowly in persons with moderate retardation, and their social isolation may begin in the elementary school years. Although academic achievement is usually limited to the middle-elementary level, children with moderate retardation benefit from individual attention focused on the development of self-help skills. Children with moderate mental retardation are aware of their deficits and often feel alienated from their peers and frustrated by their limitations. They continue to require a relatively high level of supervision but can become competent at occupational tasks in supportive settings.

Severe mental retardation is generally obvious in the preschool years; affected children's speech is minimal, and their motor development is poor. Some language development may occur in the school-age years. By adolescence, if language is poor, nonverbal forms of communication may have evolved; the inability to articulate needs fully may reinforce the physical means of communicating. Behavioral approaches can help promote some self-care, although those with severe mental retardation generally need extensive supervision.

Children with profound mental retardation require constant supervision and are severely limited in communication and motor skills. By adulthood, some speech development may be present, and simple self-help skills may be acquired. Even in adulthood, nursing care is needed.

Surveys have identified several clinical features that occur with greater frequency in persons with mental retardation than in the general population. These features, which can occur in isolation or as part of a mental disorder, include hyperactivity, low frustration tolerance, aggression, affective instability, repetitive and stereotypic motor behaviors, and various self-injurious behaviors. Self-injurious behaviors seem to be more frequent and more intense with increasingly severe mental retardation. It is often difficult to decide whether these clinical features are comorbid mental disorders or direct sequelae of the developmental limitations imposed by mental retardation.

LABORATORY EXAMINATION

Laboratory tests used to elucidate the causes of mental retardation include chromosomal analysis, urine and blood testing for metabolic disorders, and neuroimaging. Chromosomal abnormalities are the most common cause of mental retardation found in individuals for whom a cause can be identified.

Chromosome Studies

The determination of the karyotype in a genetic laboratory is considered whenever a chromosomal disorder is suspected or when the cause of the mental retardation is unknown. Amniocentesis, in which a small amount of amniotic fluid is removed from the amniotic cavity transabdominally at about the 15th week of gestation, has been useful in diagnosing prenatal chromosomal abnormalities. It is often considered when an increased fetal risk exists, such as with increased maternal age. Amniotic fluid cells, mostly fetal in origin, are cultured for cytogenetic and biochemical studies. Many serious hereditary disorders can be predicted with amniocentesis, and it should be considered by pregnant women older than the age of 35 years.

Chronic villi sampling is a screening technique to determine fetal chromosomal abnormalities. It is done at 8 to 10 weeks of gestation, 6 weeks earlier than amniocentesis is done. The results are available in a short time (hours or days), and, if the result is abnormal, the decision to terminate the pregnancy can be made within the first trimester. The procedure has a miscarriage risk between 2 and 5 percent; the risk in amniocentesis is lower (1 in 200).

Urine and Blood Analysis

Lesch-Nyhan syndrome, galactosemia, PKU, Hurler's syndrome, and Hunter's syndrome are examples of disorders that include mental retardation that can be identified through assays of the appropriate enzyme or organic or amino acids. Enzymatic abnormalities in chromosomal disorders, particularly Down syndrome, promise to become useful diagnostic tools. Unexplained growth abnormality, seizure disorder, poor muscle tone, ataxia, bone or skin abnormalities, and eye abnormalities are some indications for testing metabolic function.

Electroencephalography

Electroencephalography is indicated whenever a seizure disorder is considered.

Neuroimaging

Neuroimaging studies are being utilized to gather data that may uncover biological mechanisms contributing to mental retardation syndromes. MRI, including structural MRI, functional MRI, and other forms of neuroimaging, are being used by researchers seeking to identify specific etiologies of mental retardation syndromes. For example, data suggest that individuals with fragile X syndrome who exhibit attentional deficits are also more likely to show aberrant frontal-striatal pathways seen on MRI. MRI can show abnormalities in the brain such as myelination patterns. MRI studies can also provide a baseline for comparison of a later, potentially degenerative process in the brain.

Hearing and Speech Evaluations

Hearing and speech should be evaluated routinely. Speech development may be the most reliable criterion in investigating mental retardation. Various hearing impairments often occur in persons with mental retardation, but in some instances impairments can simulate mental retardation. The commonly used methods of hearing and speech evaluation, however, require the patient's cooperation and, thus, are often unreliable in persons with severe retardation.

Psychological Assessment

Examining clinicians can use several screening instruments for infants and toddlers. As in many areas of mental retardation, the controversy over the predictive value of infant psychological tests is heated. Some report that the correlation of abnormalities during infancy with later abnormal functioning is very low, and others report that it is very high. The correlation rises in direct proportion to the age of the child at the time of the developmental examination; however, copying geometric figures, the *Goodenough Draw-a-Person Test*, the *Kohs Block Test*, and geometric puzzles all may be used as quick screening tests of visual-motor coordination. Psychological testing, performed by an experienced psychologist, is a standard part of an evaluation for mental retardation. The Gesell and Bayley scales and the *Cattell Infant Intelligence Scale* are most commonly used with infants. For children, the *Stanford-Binet Intelligence Scale* and the third edition of the *Wechsler Intelligence Scale for Children* are those most widely used in the United States. Both tests have been criticized for penalizing culturally deprived children, for being culturally biased, for testing mainly the potential for academic achievement and not for adequate social functioning, and for their unreliability in children with IQs less than 50. Some researchers have tried to overcome the language barrier of persons with mental retardation by devising picture vocabulary tests, of which the *Peabody Vocabulary Test* is the most widely used. The tests often found to be useful in detecting brain damage are the *Bender Gestalt Test* and the *Benton Visual Retention Test*. These tests are also useful for children with mild retardation. In addition, a psychological evaluation should assess perceptual, motor, linguistic, and cognitive abilities. Information about motivational, emotional, and interpersonal factors is also important.

COURSE AND PROGNOSIS

In most cases of mental retardation, the underlying intellectual impairment does not improve, yet the affected person's level of adaptation can be influenced positively by an enriched and supportive environment. In general, persons with mild and moderate mental retardation have the most flexibility in adapting to various environmental conditions. As in those without mental retardation, the more comorbid mental disorders there are, the more guarded is the overall prognosis. When clear-cut mental disorders are superimposed on mental retardation, standard treatments for the comorbid mental disorders are often beneficial. However, clarity about the classification of such aberrant behaviors as hyperactivity, emotional lability, and social dysfunction is lacking.

DIFFERENTIAL DIAGNOSIS

By definition, mental retardation must begin before the age of 18 years. A child with mental retardation has to cope with so many difficult social and academic situations that maladaptive patterns often complicate the diagnostic process. Children whose family life provides inadequate stimulation may manifest motor and mental retardation that can be reversed if an enriched, stimulating environment is provided in early childhood. Several sensory disabilities, especially deafness and blindness, can be mistaken for mental retardation if no compensation is allowed during testing. Speech deficits and cerebral palsy often make a child seem to have retardation, even in the presence of borderline or normal intelligence. Chronic, debilitating diseases of any kind can depress a child's functioning in all areas. Convulsive disorders can give an impression of mental retardation, especially in the

presence of uncontrolled seizures. Chronic brain syndromes can result in isolated handicaps—failure to read (alexia), failure to write (agraphia), failure to communicate (aphasia), and several others—that can exist in a person of normal and even superior intelligence. Children with learning disorders (which can coexist with mental retardation) experience a delay or failure of development in a specific area, such as reading or mathematics, but they develop normally in other areas. In contrast, children with mental retardation show general delays in most areas of development.

Mental retardation and pervasive developmental disorders often coexist; 70 to 75 percent of those with pervasive developmental disorders have an IQ of less than 70. A pervasive developmental disorder results in distortion of the timing, rate, and sequence of many basic psychological functions necessary for social development. Because of their general level of functioning, children with pervasive developmental disorders have more problems with social relatedness and more deviant language than those with mental retardation. In mental retardation, generalized delays in development are present, and children with mental retardation behave in some ways as though they were passing through an earlier normal developmental stage rather than one with completely aberrant behavior.

A most difficult differential diagnostic problem concerns children with severe mental retardation, brain damage, autistic disorder, schizophrenia with childhood onset, or, according to some, Heller's disease. The confusion stems from details of the child's early history that are often unavailable or unreliable. In addition, when the children are evaluated, many with these conditions display similar bizarre and stereotyped behavior—mutism, echolalia, or functioning on a level of retardation. By the time the children are usually seen, it does not matter from a practical point of view whether their retardation is secondary to a primary early infantile autistic disorder or schizophrenia or whether the personality and behavioral distortions are secondary to brain damage or mental retardation. In a recent epidemiological study, pervasive developmental disorders (such as autistic disorder) were found in 19.8 percent of children with mental retardation.

Children younger than the age of 18 years who meet the diagnostic criteria for dementia and who have an IQ of less than 70 are given the diagnoses of dementia and mental retardation. Those whose IQs drop to less than 70 after the age of 18 years and who have new onsets of cognitive disorders are not given the diagnosis of mental retardation but only the diagnosis of dementia.

TREATMENT

The treatment of individuals with mental retardation is based on an assessment of social, educational, psychiatric, and environmental need. Mental retardation is associated with a variety of comorbid psychiatric disorders that often require specific treatment in addition to psychosocial support. Of course, when preventative measures are available, optimal treatment of conditions that could lead to mental retardation include primary, secondary, and tertiary prevention.

Primary Prevention

Primary prevention concerns actions taken to eliminate or reduce the conditions that lead to development of the disorders associated with mental retardation. Such measures include education to increase the general public's knowledge and awareness of mental retardation; continuing efforts of health professionals to ensure and upgrade public health policies; legislation to provide optimal maternal and child health care; and eradication of the known disorders associated with CNS damage. Family and genetic counseling helps reduce the incidence of mental retardation in a family with a history of a genetic disorder associated with mental retardation. For children and mothers of low socioeconomic status, proper prenatal and postnatal medical care and various supplementary enrichment programs and social service assistance may help minimize medical and psychosocial complications.

Secondary and Tertiary Prevention

Once a disorder associated with mental retardation has been identified, the disorder should be treated to shorten the course of the illness (secondary prevention) and to minimize the sequelae or consequent disabilities (tertiary prevention). Hereditary metabolic and endocrine disorders, such as PKU and hypothyroidism, can be treated effectively in an early stage by dietary control or hormone replacement therapy. Children with mental retardation frequently have emotional and behavioral difficulties requiring psychiatric treatment. Their limited cognitive and social capabilities require modified psychiatric treatment modalities based on their level of intelligence.

Education for the Child.   Educational settings for children with mental retardation should include a comprehensive program that addresses training in adaptive skills, social skills, and vocation. Particular attention should focus on communication and efforts to improve the quality of life. Group therapy has often been a successful format in which children with mental retardation can learn and practice hypothetical real-life situations and receive supportive feedback.

Behavioral, Cognitive, and Psychodynamic Therapies.   The difficulties in adaptation among persons with mental retardation are widespread and so varied that several interventions alone or in combination may be beneficial. Behavior therapy has been used for many years to shape and enhance social behaviors and to control and minimize aggressive and destructive behaviors. Positive reinforcement for desired behaviors and benign punishment (e.g., loss of privileges) for objectionable behaviors have been helpful. Cognitive therapy, such as dispelling false beliefs and relaxation exercises with self-instruction, has

also been recommended for persons with mental retardation who can follow the instructions. Psychodynamic therapy has been used with patients and their families to decrease conflicts about expectations that result in persistent anxiety, rage, and depression.

Family Education.   One of the most important areas that a clinician can address is educating the family of a patient with mental retardation about ways to enhance competence and self-esteem while maintaining realistic expectations for the patient. The family often finds it difficult to balance the fostering of independence and the providing of a nurturing and supportive environment for a child with mental retardation, who is likely to experience some rejection and failure outside the family context. The parents may benefit from continuous counseling or family therapy and should be allowed opportunities to express their feelings of guilt, despair, anguish, recurring denial, and anger about their child's disorder and future. The psychiatrist should be prepared to give the parents all the basic and current medical information regarding causes, treatment, and other pertinent areas (e.g., special training and the correction of sensory defects).

Social Intervention.   One of the most prevalent problems among persons with mental retardation is a sense of social isolation and social skills deficits. Thus, improving the quantity and quality of social competence is a critical part of their care. Special Olympics International is the largest recreational sports program geared for this population. In addition to providing a forum to develop physical fitness, Special Olympics also enhances social interactions, friendships, and (it is hoped) general self-esteem. A recent study confirmed positive effects of the Special Olympics on the social competence of the adults with mental retardation who participated.

Pharmacology.   Pharmacological approaches to the treatment of behavioral and psychological symptoms in patients with mental retardation are much the same as for those patients without retardation. Increasing data support the use of a variety of medications for patients with mental disorders who do not have mental retardation, and some studies have focused on the use of medications for behavioral syndromes that are frequent among persons with mental retardation.

35

Learning Disorders

Learning disorders in a child or adolescent are characterized by academic underachievement in reading, written expression, or mathematics in comparison with the overall intellectual ability of the child. Children with learning disorders often find it difficult to keep up with their peers in certain academic subjects, whereas they excel in others. Learning disorders affect at least 5 percent of school-age children. This represents approximately half of all public school children who receive special education services in the United States. In 1975, Public Law 94-142 (the Education for All Handicapped Children Act) mandated all states to provide free and appropriate educational services to all children. Since that time, the number of children identified with learning disorders has increased, and a variety of definitions of learning disabilities has arisen. The term *learning disorders*, formally referred to as *academic skills disorders*, was introduced by the fourth edition of the *Diagnostic and Statistical Manual of Mental Disorders* (DSM-IV). To meet the criteria for a diagnosis of learning disorder, a child's achievement in that particular learning area must be significantly lower than expected and the learning problems must interfere with academic achievement or activities of daily living.

The most recent revised version of the DSM-IV (DSM-IV-TR) includes four diagnostic categories of learning disorders: reading disorder, mathematics disorder, disorder of written expression, and learning disorder not otherwise specified. Children with a learning disorder, such as reading disorder, for example, can be identified in two different ways: children who read poorly compared with most other children of the same age and children whose achievement in reading is significantly lower than their overall intelligence quotient (IQ) would predict. DSM-IV-TR criteria for learning disorders require a substantial IQ–achievement discrepancy and significantly poor achievement in reading compared with that of most children of the same age. Research studies have led to questions regarding inclusion of an IQ–achievement discrepancy component in the definition of a learning disorder because current data suggest that most children with reading disorders, for example, have similar deficits in phonological processing skills, regardless of their IQ. That is, most children with reading disorders have trouble with word recognition and "sounding out" words because they cannot understand and use phonemes, the smaller bits of words that are associated with particular sounds.

READING DISORDER

Reading disorders are present in approximately 75 percent of children and adolescents with learning disorders. Students who have learning problems in other academic areas most commonly experience difficulties with reading as well.

Reading disorder is defined as reading achievement below the expected level for a child's age, education, and intelligence, with the impairment interfering significantly with academic success or the daily activities that involve reading. According to DSM-IV-TR, if a neurological condition or sensory disturbance is present, the reading disability exhibited exceeds that usually associated with the other condition.

Reading disorder is characterized by an impaired ability to recognize words, slow and inaccurate reading, and poor comprehension. In addition, children with attention-deficit/hyperactivity disorder (ADHD) are at high risk for reading disorder. Historically, many different labels have been used to describe reading disabilities, including word blindness, reading backward, learning disability, alexia, and developmental word blindness. The term *developmental alexia* was accepted and defined as a developmental deficit in the recognition of printed symbols. This term was simplified by adopting the term *dyslexia* in the 1960s. Dyslexia was used extensively for many years to describe a reading disability syndrome that often included speech and language deficits and right-left confusion.

Epidemiology

An estimated 4 percent of school-age children in the United States have reading disorder; prevalence studies find rates ranging between 2 and 8 percent. Three to four times as many boys as girls are reported to have reading disability in clinically referred samples. No clear gender differential is seen among adults who report reading difficulties.

Comorbidity

Children with reading disorder are at higher-than-average risk for attentional problems, disruptive behavior disorders, and depressive disorders, particularly older children and adolescents. Data suggest that up to 25 percent of children with reading disorder also have ADHD. Conversely, it is estimated that between 15 and 30 percent of children diagnosed with ADHD have a learning disorder. Children with reading disorders experience higher levels of anxiety symptoms than children without learning disorders. Furthermore, children with reading disorders tend to be at increased risk for problematic peer relationships and have less skills responding to subtle social cues.

Etiology

Data from cognitive, neuroimaging, and genetic studies indicate that reading disorder is most accurately described as a

585

neurobiological disorder with a genetic origin. It is believed to reflect a deficiency in processing sounds of spoken language. That is, children who struggle with reading have a deficit in phonological processing skills. These children cannot identify effectively the parts of words that denote specific sounds, which leads to grave difficulty in recognizing and sounding out words. Children with reading disorders are slower than average in naming letters and numbers, even when controlling for IQ. Thus, the core deficit for children with reading disorders lies within the domain of language use.

Complications during pregnancy and prenatal and perinatal difficulties are common in the histories of children with reading disorder. Extremely low birthweight and severely premature children are at higher risk for reading disorder and other learning disorders than children who are born full term and have normal birthweight. A recent study reviewed the relationship between critical periods for brain growth and babies born significantly preterm. Children who are born very preterm who attend mainstream schools have been noted to be at increased risk of minor motor, behavioral, and learning disorders. These appear to be associated with postnatal growth, particularly of the head. Although intrauterine growth retardation may play a role in compromised intellectual capacity, interventions that aim to improve motor ability and potentially learning disorders should focus on optimal nutrition and care postnatally.

Diagnosis

Reading disorder is diagnosed when a child's reading achievement is significantly below that expected of a child of the same age and intellectual capacity (Table 35–1). Characteristic diagnostic features include difficulty recalling, evoking, and sequencing printed letters and words; processing sophisticated grammatical constructions; and making inferences. Clinically, a child may be first identified with a reading disorder after becoming demoralized or exhibiting symptoms of depression related to being unable to succeed in school. School failure and ensuing poor self-esteem can exacerbate the problems as the child becomes more consumed with a sense of failure and spends less time focusing on academic work. Students suspected of having reading disorders are entitled to an educational evaluation through the school district to determine eligibility for special education services. Special education classification, however, is not uniform across states or regions, and students with identical reading difficulties may be eligible for services in one region but ineligible in another. In some cases, an evaluation is requested on the basis of disruptive behavioral problems that occur in conjunction with the reading disorder.

Clinical Features

Children who have reading disorder can usually be identified by the age of 7 years (second grade). Reading difficulty may be apparent among students in classrooms where reading skills are expected as early as the first grade. Children can sometimes compensate for reading disorder in the early elementary grades by the use of memory and inference, particularly when the disorder is associated with high intelligence. In such instances, the disorder may not be apparent until age 9 years (fourth grade) or later. Children with reading disorder make many errors in their oral reading. The errors are characterized by omissions, additions, and distortions of words. Such children have difficulty in distinguishing between printed letter characters and sizes, especially those that differ only in spatial orientation and length of line. The problems in managing printed or written language can pertain to individual letters, sentences, and even a page. The child's reading speed is slow, often with minimal comprehension. Most children with reading disorder have an age-appropriate ability to copy from a written or printed text, but nearly all spell poorly.

Associated problems include language difficulties, exhibited often as impaired sound discrimination and difficulty in sequencing words properly. A child with disorders may start a word either in the middle or at the end of a printed or written sentence. At times, because of a poorly established left-right tracking sequence, such children transpose letters to be read. Failures in both memory recall and sustained elicitation result in poor recall of letter names and sounds.

Most children with reading disorder dislike and avoid reading and writing. Their anxiety is heightened when they are confronted with demands that involve printed language. Many children with the disorder who do not receive remedial education have a sense of shame and humiliation because of their continuing failure and subsequent frustration. These feelings grow more intense with time. Older children tend to be angry and depressed and exhibit poor self-esteem.

Pathology and Laboratory Examination

No specific physical signs or laboratory measures are helpful in the diagnosis of reading disorder. Psychoeducational testing, however, is critical in determining this diagnosis. The diagnosis of reading disorder is made after collecting data from a standardized intelligence test and an educational assessment of achievement. The diagnostic battery generally includes a standardized spelling test, written composition, processing and use of oral language, design copying, and judgment of the adequacy of pencil use. The reading subtests of the *Woodcock-Johnson Psycho-Educational Battery-Revised* and the *Peabody Individual Achievement Test-Revised* are useful in identifying reading disability. A screening projective battery may include human-figure drawings, picture-story tests, and sentence completion. The evaluation should also include systematic observation of behavioral variables.

Table 35–1
DSM-IV-TR Diagnostic Criteria for Reading Disorder

A. Reading achievement, as measured by individually administered standardized tests of reading accuracy or comprehension, is substantially below that expected given the person's chronological age, measured intelligence, and age-appropriate education.

B. The disturbance in Criterion A significantly interferes with academic achievement or activities of daily living that require reading skills.

C. If a sensory deficit is present, the reading difficulties are in excess of those usually associated with it.

Coding note: If a general medical (e.g., neurological) condition or sensory deficit is present, code the condition on Axis III.

From American Psychiatric Association. *Diagnostic and Statistical Manual of Mental Disorders.* 4th ed. Text rev. Washington, DC: American Psychiatric Association; copyright 2000, with permission.

Course and Prognosis

Many children with reading disorder gain some knowledge of printed language during their first 2 years in grade school, even without any remedial assistance. By the end of the first grade, many children with reading disorder, in fact, have learned how to read a few words; however, by the time a child with a reading disorder reaches the third grade, keeping up with classmates is exceedingly difficult without remedial educational intervention. In the best circumstances, a child is recognized as being at risk for a reading disorder during the kindergarten year or early in the first grade. When remediation is instituted early, in milder cases, it is no longer necessary by the end of the first or second grade. In severe cases and depending on the pattern of deficits and strengths, remediation may be continued into the middle and high school years.

Differential Diagnosis

Reading disorder is often accompanied by comorbid disorders, such as expressive language disorder, disorder of written expression, and ADHD. A recent study indicates that children with reading disorder consistently present difficulties with linguistic abilities, whereas children with ADHD do not. Children with reading disorder who do not qualify for a diagnosis of ADHD, however, were shown to have some overlapping deficits in the area of cognitive inhibition such that they perform impulsively on continuous performance tasks. Deficits in expressive language and speech discrimination in reading disorder can be sufficiently severe to warrant the additional diagnosis of expressive language disorder or mixed receptive-expressive language disorder. Some children exhibit a discrepancy between scores on verbal and performance intelligence. Visual perceptual deficits occur in only about 10 percent of cases. Reading disorder must be differentiated from mental retardation syndromes in which reading, along with other skills, is below the achievement expected for a child's chronological age. Intellectual testing helps to differentiate global deficits from more specific reading difficulties.

Poor reading skills resulting from inadequate schooling can be detected by finding out whether other children in the same school have similarly poor reading performances on standardized reading tests. Hearing and visual impairments should be ruled out with screening tests.

Treatment

Most current remediation strategies for children with reading disorder are characterized by direct instruction of the various components of reading that focus a child's attention to the connections between speech sounds and spelling. A recent survey of the efficacy of specific word study with text reading practice or word study tutoring in first graders who scored within the lowest quartile for reading skills indicated that students exposed to either of the foregoing instructions outperformed those who received only classroom instruction. Improvements were noted on measures of reading accuracy, reading comprehension, reading efficiency, passage reading fluency, and spelling. Many effective remediation programs begin by teaching the child to make accurate associations between letters and sounds. This approach is based on the current consensus that, in most cases, the core deficits in reading disorders are related to difficulty recognizing and remembering the associations between letters and sounds. After individual letter–sound associations have been mastered, remediation can target larger components of reading such as syllables and words. The exact focus of any reading program can be determined only after accurate assessment of a child's specific deficits and weaknesses. Positive coping strategies include small, structured reading groups that offer individual attention and make it easier for a child to ask for help.

As in psychotherapy, the therapist–patient relationship is important to a successful treatment outcome in remedial educational therapy. Children should be placed in a grade as close as possible to their social functional level and given special remedial work in reading. Coexisting emotional and behavioral problems should be treated by appropriate psychotherapeutic means. Parental counseling may also be helpful. Approximately 75 percent of children with learning disorders can be differentiated from comparison samples by lower measures of social competence. It is important, therefore, to include social skills improvement as a therapeutic component of a treatment program for children with reading disorders.

MATHEMATICS DISORDER

Children with mathematics disorder have difficulty learning and remembering numerals, cannot remember basic facts about numbers, and are slow and inaccurate in computation. Poor achievement in four groups of skills have been identified in mathematics disorder: linguistic skills (those related to understanding mathematical terms and converting written problems into mathematical symbols), perceptual skills (the ability to recognize and understand symbols and order clusters of numbers), mathematical skills (basic addition, subtraction, multiplication, division, and following sequencing of basic operations), and attentional skills (copying figures correctly and observing operational symbols correctly). A variety of terms over the years, including *dyscalculia, congenital arithmetic disorder, acalculia, Gerstmann's syndrome,* and *developmental arithmetic disorder* have been used to denote the difficulties present in mathematics disorder.

Epidemiology

Mathematics disorder alone is estimated to occur in about 1 percent of school-age children, that is, approximately 1 of every 5 children with learning disorder. Epidemiological studies have indicated that up to 6 percent of school-age children have some difficulty with mathematics. Mathematics disorder may occur with greater frequency in girls. Many studies of learning disorders in children have grouped several disorders together rather than separating them into individual disorders, which makes it more difficult to ascertain the precise prevalence of mathematics disorder.

Comorbidity

Mathematics disorder is commonly found comorbid with reading disorder and disorder of written expression. Children with mathematics disorder may also be at higher risk for expressive language disorder, mixed receptive-expressive language disorder, and developmental coordination disorder.

Etiology

Mathematics disorder, as with other learning disorders, is probably at least partly caused by genetic factors. An early theory proposed a neurological deficit in the right cerebral hemisphere, particularly in the occipital lobe areas. These regions are responsible for processing visual-spatial stimuli that, in turn, are responsible for mathematical skills. This theory, however, has received little support in subsequent neuropsychiatric studies.

Currently, the cause is thought to be multifactorial, so that maturational, cognitive, emotional, educational, and socioeconomic factors account in varying degrees and combinations for mathematics disorder. Compared with reading, arithmetic abilities seem to depend more on the amount and quality of instruction.

Diagnosis

The diagnosis of mathematics disorder is made when a child's skills in mathematics fall significantly below what is expected for that child's age, intellectual ability, and education. Many different skills are needed for mathematics proficiency. These include linguistic skills, conceptual skills, and computational skills. Linguistic skills involve being able to understand mathematical terms, understand word problems, and translate them into the proper mathematical process. Conceptual skills involve recognition of mathematical symbols and being able to use mathematical signs correctly. Computational skills include the ability to line up numbers correctly and to follow the "rules" of the mathematical operation. A definitive diagnosis can be made only after a child takes an individually administered standardized arithmetic test and scores markedly below the level expected in view of the child's schooling and intellectual capacity as measured by a standardized intelligence test. A pervasive developmental disorder and mental retardation should also be ruled out before confirming the diagnosis of mathematics disorder. The DSM-IV-TR diagnostic criteria for mathematics disorder are given in Table 35–2.

Table 35–2
DSM-IV-TR Diagnostic Criteria
for Mathematics Disorder

A. Mathematical ability, as measured by individually administered standardized tests, is substantially below that expected given the person's chronological age, measured intelligence, and age-appropriate education.

B. The disturbance in Criterion A significantly interferes with academic achievement or activities of daily living that require mathematical ability.

C. If a sensory deficit is present, the difficulties in mathematical ability are in excess of those usually associated with it.

Coding note: If a general medical (e.g., neurological) condition or sensory deficit is present, code the condition on Axis III.

From American Psychiatric Association. *Diagnostic and Statistical Manual of Mental Disorders.* 4th ed. Text rev. Washington, DC: American Psychiatric Association; copyright 2000, with permission.

Clinical Features

Common features of mathematics disorder include difficulty with various components of mathematics, such as learning number names, remembering the signs for addition and subtraction, learning multiplication tables, translating word problems into computations, and doing calculations at the expected pace. Most children with mathematics disorder can be detected during the second and third grades in elementary school. A child with mathematics disorder generally has significant problems with concepts, such as counting and adding even one-digit numbers, compared with classmates of the same age. During the first 2 or 3 years of elementary school, a child with mathematics disorder may just get by in mathematics by relying on rote memory. Soon, however, as mathematics problems require discrimination and manipulation of spatial and numerical relations, a child with mathematics disorder is overwhelmed.

Mathematics disorder often coexists with other disorders affecting reading, expressive writing, coordination, and expressive and receptive language. Spelling problems, deficits in memory or attention, and emotional or behavioral problems may be present. Young grade-school children often first show other learning disorders and should be checked for mathematics disorder. Children with cerebral palsy may have mathematics disorder with normal overall intelligence.

The relation between mathematics disorder and other communication and learning disorders is not clear. Although children with mixed receptive-expressive language disorder and expressive language disorder are not necessarily affected by mathematics disorder, the conditions often coexist because they are associated with impairments in both decoding and encoding processes.

Pathology and Laboratory Examination

No physical signs or symptoms indicate mathematics disorder, but educational testing and standardized measurement of intellectual function are necessary to make this diagnosis. The *Keymath Diagnostic Arithmetic Test* measures several areas of mathematics including knowledge of mathematical content, function, and computation. It is used to assess ability in mathematics of children in grades 1 to 6.

Course and Prognosis

A child with a mathematics disorder can usually be identified by the age of 8 years (third grade). In some children, the disorder is apparent as early as age 6 years (first grade); in others, it may not be apparent until age 10 years (fifth grade) or later. Too few data are available from longitudinal studies to predict clear patterns of developmental and academic progress of children classified as having mathematics disorder in early school grades. On the other hand, children with a moderate mathematics disorder who do not receive intervention may have complications, including continuing academic difficulties, shame, poor self-concept, frustration, and depression. These complications can lead to reluctance to attend school, truancy, and eventual hopelessness about academic success.

Differential Diagnosis

Mathematics disorder must be differentiated from global causes of impaired functioning such as mental retardation syndromes.

Arithmetic difficulties in mental retardation are accompanied by generalized impairment in overall intellectual functioning. In unusual cases of mild mental retardation, arithmetic skills may be significantly below the level expected on the basis of a person's schooling and level of mental retardation. In such cases, an additional diagnosis of mathematics disorder should be made. Treatment of the arithmetic difficulties can particularly help a child's chances for employment in adulthood. Inadequate schooling can often affect a child's poor arithmetic performance on a standardized arithmetic test. Conduct disorder or ADHD can occur with mathematics disorder, and, in these cases, both diagnoses should be made.

Treatment

The presence of mathematics difficulties for children has not been shown to be a stable disorder over time; thus, early intervention may lead to improved skills in basic computation. The presence of reading disorder along with mathematics difficulties can impede progress, yet children are responsive to remediation in early grade school. For children as early as in kindergarten, indications of mathematics disorder and the need for intervention include lack of mastery in knowledge of which digit in a pair is larger, counting abilities, identification of numbers, and poor working memory for numbers, such as difficulty with reverse digit span. The most effective treatments for mathematics disorder combine teaching mathematics concepts with continuous practice in solving math problems. Flash cards, workbooks, and computer games can be a viable part of this treatment. A recent report indicates that mathematics instruction is most helpful when the focus is on problem-solving activities, including word problems, rather than only computation. Project MATH, a multimedia self-instructional or group-instructional in-service training program, has been successful for some children with mathematics disorder. Computer programs can be helpful and can increase compliance with remediation efforts.

Social skills deficits can contribute to a child's hesitation in asking for help, so a child identified with a mathematics disorder may benefit from gaining positive problem-solving skills in a social arena as well as in mathematics.

DISORDER OF WRITTEN EXPRESSION

Written expression is the most complex skill acquired to convey an understanding of language and to express thoughts and ideas. Writing skills are highly correlated with reading for most children; for some children, however, reading comprehension may far surpass their ability to express complex thoughts. Written expression in some cases is a sensitive index of more subtle, although impairing, deficits in language usage that typically are not detected by standardized reading and language tests.

Disorder of written expression is characterized by writing skills that are significantly below the expected level for a child's age and intellectual capacity. These difficulties impair the child's academic performance and writing in everyday life. The many components of writing disorder include poor spelling, errors in grammar and punctuation, and poor handwriting. Spelling errors are among the most common difficulties for a child with a writing disorder. Spelling mistakes are most often phonetic errors; that is, an erroneous spelling that sounds like the correct spelling.

Examples of common types of spelling errors are *fone* for *phone* and *beleeve* for *believe*.

Historically, dysgraphia (i.e., poor writing skills) was considered to be a form of reading disorder; however, evidence indicates that disorder of written expression can occur on its own. Terms once used to describe writing disability include *spelling disorder* and *spelling dyslexia*. Writing disabilities are often associated with other learning disorders, but they may be diagnosed later because expressive writing is acquired later than language and reading.

Epidemiology

The prevalence of disorder of written expression alone has not been studied, but, as with reading disorder, it is estimated to occur in approximately 4 percent of school-age children. The gender ratio in writing disorder is believed to be similar that of reading disorder, occurring in about three times as many boys. Disorder of written expression often occurs along with reading disorder, but not always.

Comorbidity

Children with writing disorder are at higher risk for a variety of other learning and language disorders, including reading disorder, mathematics disorder, and expressive and receptive language disorders. ADHD occurs with greater frequency in children with writing disorders than in the general population. Finally, children with writing disorders are believed to be at higher risk for social skills difficulties, and some go on to develop poor self-esteem and depressive symptoms.

Etiology

Causes of writing disorders are believed to be similar to those of reading disorder, that is, a deficit in the use of the components of language related to letter sounds. It is likely that genetic factors are significant in the development of writing disorder. Writing difficulties often accompany language disorders in which a given child may have trouble understanding grammatical rules, finding words, and expressing ideas clearly. According to one hypothesis, a disorder of written expression may result from the combined effects of one or more of the following: expressive language disorder, mixed receptive-expressive language disorder, and reading disorder. Hereditary predisposition to the disorder is supported by findings that most children with disorder of written expression have first-degree relatives with the disorder. Children with limited attention spans and high levels of distractibility may find writing an arduous task.

Diagnosis

A diagnosis of disorder of written expression is based on a child's poor performance on composing written text, including handwriting and impaired ability to spell and to place words sequentially in coherent sentences, compared with most other children of the same age and intellectual ability. In addition to spelling mistakes, a child with writing disorder may make serious grammatical mistakes, such as using incorrect tenses, forgetting words in sentences, and placing words in the wrong order. Punctuation may be incorrect, and the child may have poor ability to remember which words begin with capital letters. Poor handwriting may also contribute to writing disorder, including letters that are not legible, inverted letters, and mixtures of uppercase and lowercase letters in a given word. Other features of writing disorders include poor organization of written stories, which lack critical elements such as "where," "when," and "who" or clear expression of the plot.

Clinical Features

Children with disorder of written expression have difficulties early in grade school in spelling words and expressing their thoughts according to age-appropriate grammatical norms. Their spoken and written sentences contain an unusually large number of grammatical errors and poor paragraph organization. During and after the second grade, these children commonly make simple grammatical errors in writing a short sentence. For example, despite constant reminders, they frequently fail to capitalize the first letter of the first word in a sentence and to end the sentence with a period. Common features of the disorder of written expression are spelling errors, grammatical errors, punctuation errors, poor paragraph organization, and poor handwriting.

As they grow older and progress into higher grades in school, such children's spoken and written sentences become more conspicuously primitive, odd, and inferior to what is expected of students at their grade level. Their word choices are erroneous and inappropriate; their paragraphs are disorganized and are not in proper sequence; and spelling correctly becomes increasingly difficult as their vocabulary becomes larger and more abstract. Associated features of disorder of written expression include refusal or reluctance to go to school and to do assigned written homework, poor academic performance in other areas (e.g., mathematics), general avoidance of school work, truancy, attention deficit, and conduct disturbance.

Many children with disorder of written expression become frustrated and angry because of feelings of inadequacy and failure in their academic performance. In severe cases, depressive disorders can result from a growing sense of isolation, estrangement, and despair. Young adults with disorder of written expression who do not receive remedial intervention continue to have difficulties in social adaptation involving writing skills and a continuing sense of incompetence, inferiority, isolation, and estrangement. Some even try to avoid writing a response letter or a simple greeting card for fear of exposing their writing incompetence.

Pathology and Laboratory Examination

Whereas no physical stigmata of a writing disorder exist, educational testing is used in making a diagnosis of writing disorder. Diagnosis is based on a child's writing performance being markedly below his or her intellectual capacity, as confirmed by an individually administered standardized expressive writing test (Table 35–3). The presence of a major disorder, such as a pervasive developmental disorder, or mental retardation may obviate the diagnosis of disorder of written expression. Other disorders to be differentiated from disorder of written expression are communication disorders, reading disorder, and impaired vision and hearing.

A child suspected of having disorder of written expression should first be given a standardized intelligence test, such as the third edition of the *Wechsler Intelligence Scale for Children* or

Table 35–3
DSM-IV-TR Diagnostic Criteria for Disorder of Written Expression

A. Writing skills, as measured by individually administered standardized tests (or functional assessments of writing skills), are substantially below those expected given the person's chronological age, measured intelligence, and age-appropriate education.

B. The disturbance in Criterion A significantly interferes with academic achievement or activities of daily living that require the composition of written texts (e.g., writing grammatically correct sentences and organized paragraphs).

C. If a sensory deficit is present, the difficulties in writing skills are in excess of those usually associated with it.

Coding note: If a general medical (e.g., neurological) condition or sensory deficit is present, code the condition on Axis III.

From American Psychiatric Association. *Diagnostic and Statistical Manual of Mental Disorders.* 4th ed. Text rev. Washington, DC: American Psychiatric Association; copyright 2000, with permission.

the revised Wechsler Adult Intelligence Scale, to determine the child's overall intellectual capacity.

Course and Prognosis

Because writing, language, and reading disorders often coexist and because a child normally speaks well before learning to read and learns to read well before writing well, a child with all these disorders has expressive language disorder diagnosed first and disorder of written expression diagnosed last. In severe cases, a disorder of written expression is apparent by age 7 years (second grade); in less severe cases, the disorder may not be apparent until age 10 years (fifth grade) or later. Most persons with mild and moderate disorder of written expression fare well if they receive timely remedial education early in grade school. Severe disorder of written expression requires continual, extensive remedial treatment through the late part of high school and even into college.

The prognosis depends on the severity of the disorder, the age or grade when the remedial intervention is started, the length and continuity of treatment, and presence or absence of associated or secondary emotional or behavioral problems. Those who later become well compensated or who recover from disorder of written expression are often from families with high socioeconomic backgrounds.

Differential Diagnosis

It is important to determine whether another disorder, such as ADHD or a depressive disorder, is preventing a child from being able to concentrate on writing tasks in the absence of writing disorder itself. If this is the case, treatment for the other disorder should improve a child's writing performance. Disorder of written expression can also occur with a variety of other language and learning disorders. Common associated disorders are reading disorder, mixed receptive-expressive language disorder, expressive language disorder, mathematics disorder, developmental coordination disorder, and disruptive behavior disorder and ADHD.

Table 35–4
DSM-IV-TR Diagnostic Criteria for Learning Disorder Not Otherwise Specified

This category is for disorders in learning that do not meet criteria for any specific learning disorder. This category might include problems in all three areas (reading, mathematics, written expression) that together significantly interfere with academic achievement even though performance on tests measuring each individual skill is not substantially below that expected given the person's chronological age, measured intelligence, and age-appropriate education.

From American Psychiatric Association. *Diagnostic and Statistical Manual of Mental Disorders*. 4th ed. Text rev. Washington, DC: American Psychiatric Association; copyright 2000, with permission.

Treatment

Remedial treatment for writing disorder includes direct practice in spelling and sentence writing as well as a review of grammatical rules. Intensive and continuous administration of individually tailored, one-on-one expressive and creative writing therapy appears to effect favorable outcome. Teachers in some special schools devote as much as 2 hours a day to such writing instruction. The effectiveness of a writing intervention largely depends on an optimal relationship between the child and the writing specialist. Success or failure in sustaining the patient's motivation greatly affects the treatment's long-term efficacy. Associated secondary emotional and behavioral problems should be given prompt attention, with appropriate psychiatric treatment and parental counseling.

LEARNING DISORDER NOT OTHERWISE SPECIFIED

Learning disorder not otherwise specified is a new category in DSM-IV-TR for disorders that do not meet the criteria for any specific learning disorder but cause impairment and reflect learning abilities below those expected for a person's intelligence, education, and age (Table 35–4). An example of a disability that could be placed in this category is a spelling skills deficit.

36

Motor Skills Disorder: Developmental Coordination Disorder

Children with developmental motor coordination struggle to perform accurately the motor activities of daily life, such as jumping, hopping, running, or catching a ball. Children with coordination problems may also agonize over using utensils correctly, tying their shoelaces, or writing. A child with developmental coordination disorder may exhibit delays in achieving motor milestones, such as sitting, crawling, and walking, because of clumsiness, and yet excel at verbal skills.

Children with developmental coordination disorder may resemble younger children because of their inability to master motor activities typical for their age group. For example, children with developmental coordination disorder in elementary school may not be adept at bicycle riding, skateboarding, running, skipping, or hopping. In the middle school years, children with this disorder may have trouble in team sports, such as soccer, baseball, or basketball. Fine motor skill manifestations of developmental coordination disorder typically include clumsiness using utensils and difficulty with buttons and zippers in the preschool age group. In older children, using scissors and more complex grooming skills, such as styling hair or putting on makeup, is difficult. Children with developmental coordination disorder are often ostracized by peers because of their poor skills in many sports, and they often have long-standing difficulties with peer relationships. Developmental coordination disorder is the sole disorder in the text revision of the fourth edition of the *Diagnostic and Statistical Manual of Mental Disorders* (DSM-IV-TR) category motor skills disorder. Gross and fine motor impairment in this disorder cannot be explained on the basis of a medical condition, such as cerebral palsy, muscular dystrophy, or any other neuromuscular disorder.

EPIDEMIOLOGY

The prevalence of developmental coordination disorder has been estimated at about 5 percent of school-age children. The male-to-female ratio in referred populations tends to show increased rates of the disorder in males, but schools refer boys more often for testing and special education evaluations. Reports in the literature of the male-to-female ratio have ranged from 2:1 to as much as 4:1. These rates may also be inflated because motor behaviors in boys are scrutinized more closely than those in girls.

COMORBIDITY

Developmental coordination disorder is strongly associated with speech and language disorders. Children with coordination difficulties have higher-than-expected rates of speech and language disorders, and studies of children with speech disorders report very high rates of "clumsiness." Some studies have found associations between fine motor skills in the upper arms and expressive and receptive language disorders, whereas gross motor problems and visual motor coordination problems were not associated with language disturbance. Developmental coordination disorder is also associated with reading disorders, mathematics disorder, and disorder of written expression. Higher-than-expected rates of attention-deficit/hyperactivity disorders (ADHD) are also associated with developmental coordination disorder.

ETIOLOGY

The causes of developmental coordination disorder are believed to include both "organic" and "developmental" factors. Risk factors postulated to contribute to this disorder include prematurity, hypoxia, perinatal malnutrition, and low birthweight. Prenatal exposure to alcohol, cocaine, and nicotine has also been hypothesized to contribute to both low birthweight and cognitive and behavioral abnormalities. Neurochemical abnormalities and parietal lobe lesions have also been suggested to contribute to coordination deficits. Developmental coordination disorder and communication disorders have strong associations, although the specific causative agents are unknown for both. Coordination problems are also more frequently found in children with hyperactivity syndromes and learning disorders. Recent studies of postural control, that is, the ability to regain balance after being in motion, indicate that children with developmental coordination disorder who do not have significant difficulties with balance when standing still are unable accurately to correct for movement, resulting in impaired balance compared with other children. A recent study concluded that, in children with developmental coordination disorder, signals from the brain to particular muscles (including the tibialis anterior and peroneus muscles) involved in balance are not being optimally sent or received. These findings have implicated the cerebellum as a contributing origin of dysfunction for developmental coordination disorder.

DIAGNOSIS

The diagnosis of developmental coordination disorder depends on poor performance, for a child's age and intellectual level, in

Table 36–1
DSM-IV-TR Diagnostic Criteria for Developmental Coordination Disorder

A. Performance in daily activities that require motor coordination is substantially below that expected given the person's chronological age and measured intelligence. This may be manifested by marked delays in achieving motor milestones (e.g., walking, crawling, sitting), dropping things, "clumsiness," poor performance in sports, or poor handwriting.

B. The disturbance in Criterion A significantly interferes with academic achievement or activities of daily living.

C. The disturbance is not due to a general medical condition (e.g., cerebral palsy, hemiplegia, or muscular dystrophy) and does not meet criteria for a pervasive developmental disorder.

D. If mental retardation is present, the motor difficulties are in excess of those usually associated with it.

Coding note: If a general medical (e.g., neurological) condition or sensory deficit is present, code the condition on Axis III.

From American Psychiatric Association. *Diagnostic and Statistical Manual of Mental Disorders.* 4th ed. Text rev. Washington, DC: American Psychiatric Association; copyright 2000, with permission.

activities requiring coordination. Diagnosis is based on a history of the child's delay in achieving early motor milestones, as well as on direct observation of current deficits in coordination. An informal screen for developmental coordination disorder involves asking the child to perform tasks involving gross motor coordination (e.g., hopping, jumping, and standing on one foot); fine motor coordination (e.g., finger-tapping and shoelace tying); and hand–eye coordination (e.g., catching a ball and copying letters). Judgments regarding poor performance must be based on what is expected for a child's age. A child who is mildly clumsy but whose functioning is not impaired does not qualify for a diagnosis of developmental coordination disorder.

The diagnosis may be associated with below-normal scores on performance subtests of standardized intelligence tests and by normal or above-normal scores on verbal subtests. Specialized tests of motor coordination can be useful, such as the *Bender Visual Motor Gestalt Test*, the *Frostig Movement Skills Test Battery*, and the *Bruininks-Oseretsky Test of Motor Development*. The child's chronological age and intellectual capacity must be taken into account, and the disorder cannot be caused by a neurological or neuromuscular condition. Examination, however, may occasionally reveal slight reflex abnormalities and other soft neurological signs. The DSM-IV-TR diagnostic criteria are given in Table 36–1.

CLINICAL FEATURES

The clinical signs suggesting the existence of developmental coordination disorder are evident as early as infancy in some cases, when a child begins to attempt tasks requiring motor coordination. The essential clinical feature is significantly impaired performance in motor coordination. The difficulties in motor coordination may vary with a child's age and developmental stage.

In infancy and early childhood, the disorder may be manifested by delays in developmental motor milestones, such as turning over, crawling, sitting, standing, walking, buttoning shirts, and zipping up pants. Between the ages of 2 and 4 years, clumsiness appears in almost all activities requiring motor coordination. Affected children cannot hold objects and drop them

easily, their gait may be unsteady, they often trip over their own feet, and they may bump into other children while attempting to go around them. Older children may display impaired motor coordination in table games, such as putting together puzzles or building blocks, and in any type of ball game. Although no specific features are pathognomonic of developmental coordination disorder, developmental milestones are frequently delayed. Many children with the disorder also have speech and language difficulties. Older children may have secondary problems, including academic difficulties, as well as poor peer relationships based on social rejection. It has been reported widely that children with motor coordination problems are more likely to have problems understanding subtle social cues and are often rejected by peers. A recent study indicated that children with motor difficulties were found to perform more poorly on scales that measure recognition of static and changing facial expressions of emotion. This finding is likely to be correlated with the clinical observations that children with motor coordination have difficulties in social behavior and peer relationships.

DIFFERENTIAL DIAGNOSIS

The differential diagnosis includes medical conditions that produce coordination difficulties (e.g., cerebral palsy and muscular dystrophy), pervasive developmental disorders, and mental retardation. In mental retardation and in the pervasive developmental disorders, coordination usually does not stand out as a significant deficit compared with other skills. Children with neuromuscular disorders may exhibit more global muscle impairment rather than clumsiness and delayed motor milestones. Neurological examination and workups usually reveal more extensive deficits in neurological conditions than in developmental coordination disorder. Extremely hyperactive and impulsive children may be physically careless because of their high levels of motor activity. Clumsy gross and fine motor behavior and ADHD seem to be associated.

COURSE AND PROGNOSIS

Few data are available on the prospective longitudinal outcomes of both treated and untreated children with developmental coordination disorder. For the most part, although clumsiness may continue, some children can compensate by developing interests in other skills. Some studies suggest a favorable outcome for children who have an average or above-average intellectual capacity, in that they come up with strategies to develop friendships that do not depend on physical activities. Clumsiness generally persists into adolescence and adult life. One study following a group of children with developmental coordination problems over a decade found that the clumsy children remained less dexterous, showed poor balance, and continued to be physically awkward. The affected children were also more likely to have both academic problems and poor self-esteem. Commonly associated features include delays in nonmotor milestones, expressive language disorder, and mixed receptive-expressive language disorder.

TREATMENT

Interventions for children with developmental coordination disorder utilize multiple modalities, including visual, auditory, and tactile materials targeting perceptual motor training for specific motor tasks. More recently, motor imagery training has been incorporated into treatment. These approaches are visual imagery exercises using CD-ROM; they have a broad range of foci, including predictive timing for motor tasks, relaxation and mental preparation, visual modeling of fundamental motor skills, and mental rehearsal of various tasks. This type of intervention is based on the notion that improved internal representation of a movement task will improve a child's motor behavior. The treatment of developmental coordination disorder generally includes versions of sensory-integration programs and modified physical education. Sensory integration programs, usually administered by occupational therapists, consist in physical activities that increase awareness of motor and sensory function. For example, a child who bumps into objects often might be given the task of trying to balance on a scooter, under supervision, to improve balance and body awareness. Children who have difficulty writing letters are often given tasks to increase awareness of hand movements. School-based occupational therapies for motor coordination problems in writing include utilizing mechanisms that provide resistance or vibration during writing exercises to improve grip and practicing vertical writing on a chalk board to increase arm strength and stability while writing. These programs have been shown to improve legibility of student's writing but not necessarily speed because students learn to write with greater accuracy and deliberate letter formation. Many schools also allow and may even encourage children with coordination difficulties that affect writing to use computers to aid in writing reports and long papers.

Adaptive physical education programs are designed to help children enjoy exercise and physical activities without the pressures of team sports. These programs generally incorporate certain sports actions, such as kicking a soccer ball or throwing a basketball. Children with coordination disorder may also benefit from social skills groups and other prosocial interventions. The Montessori technique (developed by Maria Montessori) may promote motor skill development, especially with preschool children, because this educational program emphasizes the development of motor skills. Small studies have suggested that exercise in rhythmic coordination, practicing motor movements, and learning to use word processing keyboards may be beneficial. Parental counseling may help reduce parents' anxiety and guilt about their child's impairment, increase their awareness, and facilitate their confidence to cope with the child.

A recent investigation of children with developmental coordination disorder showed positive results using a computer game designed to improve ability to catch a ball. These children were able to improve their game score by practicing virtual catching without specific instructions on how to utilize the visual cues. This has implications for treatment in that certain types of motor task coordination can be positively influenced through the practice of specific motor tasks, even without overt instructions.

37 ▲

Communication Disorders

Communication disorders are among the most common disorders in childhood. To communicate effectively, children must have a mastery of language—that is, the ability to understand and express ideas—using words and speech—the manner in which words are spoken. Language disorders include expressive and mixed receptive-expressive language disorder, whereas speech disorders include phonological disorder and stuttering. Children with expressive language disorders have difficulties expressing their thoughts with words and sentences at a level of sophistication expected for their age and developmental level in other areas. These children may struggle with limited vocabularies, speak in sentences that are short or ungrammatical, and often present descriptions of situations that are disorganized, confusing, and infantile. They may be delayed in developing an understanding and a memory of words compared with others their age.

EXPRESSIVE LANGUAGE DISORDER

Expressive language disorder is diagnosed when a child demonstrates a selective deficit in expressive language development relative to receptive language skills and nonverbal intelligence. Thus, a child with expressive language disorder may be identified using the *Wechsler Intelligence Scale for Children III*, in that verbal intellectual level may appear to be depressed compared with the child's overall intelligence quotient. A child with expressive language disorder is likely to function below the expected levels of acquired vocabulary, correct tense usage, complex sentence constructions, and word recall. Children with expressive language disorder often present verbally as younger than their age. Language disability can be acquired at any time during childhood (e.g., secondary to a trauma or a neurological disorder) or it can be developmental; it is usually congenital, without an obvious cause. Most childhood language disorders fall in the developmental category. In either case, deficits in receptive skills (language comprehension) or expressive skills (ability to use language) can occur. Expressive language disturbance often appears in the absence of comprehension difficulties, whereas receptive dysfunction generally diminishes proficiency in the expression of language. Children with expressive language disorder alone have courses and prognoses that differ from those of children with mixed receptive-expressive language disorder.

Epidemiology

The prevalence of expressive language disorder is estimated to be as high as 6 percent in children between the ages of 5 and 11 years of age. Surveys have indicated rates of expressive language

disorder as high as 15 percent in children younger than age 3 years. In school-age children older than the age of 11 years, the estimates are lower, ranging from 3 percent to 5 percent. The disorder is two to three times more common in boys than in girls and is most prevalent among children whose relatives have a family history of phonological disorder or other communication disorders.

Comorbidity

Children with developmental language disorders, such as expressive language disorder, have above-average rates of comorbid psychiatric disorders. In one large study of children with speech and language disorders by Lorian Baker and Dennis Cantwell, the most common comorbid disorders were attention-deficit/hyperactivity disorder (ADHD) (19 percent), anxiety disorders (10 percent), and oppositional defiant disorder and conduct disorder (7 percent combined). Children with expressive language disorder are also at higher risk for a speech disorder, receptive difficulties, and other learning disorders.

Many disorders—such as reading disorder, developmental coordination disorder, and other communication disorders—are associated with expressive language disorder. Children with expressive language disorder often have some receptive impairment, although not always sufficiently significant for the diagnosis of mixed receptive-expressive language disorder. Delayed motor milestones and a history of enuresis are common in children with expressive language disorder. Phonological disorder is commonly found in young children with the disorder, and neurological abnormalities have been reported in a number of children, including soft neurological signs, depressed vestibular responses, and electroencephalogram (EEG) abnormalities. On the other hand, a recent study found that boys with serious behavior problems also had high levels of unidentified expressive language disorders; thus, it may be important to screen for language dysfunction in children who are extremely behaviorally disordered.

Etiology

The specific cause of developmental expressive language disorder is likely to be multifactorial. Subtle cerebral damage and maturational lags in cerebral development have been postulated as underlying causes. Some children with language disorders have difficulty processing information in a time-limited manner. Scant data are available on the specific brain structure of children with language disorder, but limited magnetic resonance imaging (MRI) studies suggest that language disorders are associated with a loss of the normal left–right brain asymmetry in the perisylvian and planum temporale regions. Results of one small MRI study suggested possible inversion of brain asymmetry (right > left). Left-handedness or ambilaterality appears to be associated with expressive language problems. Evidence shows that language disorders occur with higher frequency in certain families. Genetic factors have been suspected to play a role, and several studies of twins show significant concordance for monozygotic twins for developmental language disorders. Some studies have found that some individuals with Williams-Beuren syndrome are at an increased risk of expressive language disorder. Environmental and educational factors are also postulated to contribute to developmental language disorders. Data suggest that prenatal exposure to substances such as alcohol and cocaine, for example, are likely to be associated with both delays in language acquisition and expressive language ability.

Diagnosis

Expressive language disorder is present when a child has a selective deficit in language skills and is functioning well in nonverbal areas and in receptive skills. Markedly below-age-level verbal or sign language, accompanied by a low score on standardized expressive verbal tests, is diagnostic of expressive language disorder (Table 37–1). The disorder is not caused by a pervasive developmental disorder, and a child with an expressive language disorder usually develops some nonverbal strategies to aid in socialization. A child with an expressive language disorder exhibits the following features: limited vocabulary, simple grammar, and variable articulation. "Inner language" or the appropriate use of toys and household objects is present. To confirm the diagnosis, a child is given standardized expressive language and nonverbal intelligence tests. Observations of children's verbal and sign language patterns in various settings (e.g., schoolyard, classroom, home, and playroom) and during interactions with other children help ascertain the severity and specific areas of a child's impairment and aid in early detection of behavioral and emotional complications. Family history should include the presence or absence of expressive language disorder among relatives.

Clinical Features

The essential feature of expressive language disorder is marked impairment in the development of age-appropriate expressive language, which results in the use of verbal or sign language markedly below the expected level in view of a child's nonverbal intellectual capacity. Language understanding (decoding) skills remain relatively intact. When severe, the disorder becomes recognizable by about the age of 18 months, when a child fails to utter spontaneously or even echo single words or sounds. Even simple words, such as "Mama" and "Dada," are absent from the child's active vocabulary, and the child points or uses gestures to indicate desires. The child seems to want to communicate, maintains eye contact, relates well to the mother, and enjoys games such as pat-a-cake and peek-a-boo. The child's vocabulary is severely limited. At 18 months, the child may be limited to pointing to common objects when they are named.

When a child with expressive language disorder begins to speak, the language impairment gradually becomes apparent. Articulation is often immature; numerous articulation errors occur but are inconsistent, particularly with such sounds as *th, r, s, z, y,* and *l,* which are either omitted or are substituted for other sounds.

By the age of 4 years, most children with expressive language disorder can speak in short phrases but may have difficulty retaining new words. After beginning to speak, they acquire language more slowly than do most children. Their use of various grammatical structures is also markedly below the age-expected level, and their developmental milestones may be slightly delayed. Emotional problems involving poor self-image, frustration, and depression may develop in school-age children.

Table 37–1
DSM-IV-TR Diagnostic Criteria for Expressive Language Disorder

A. The scores obtained from standardized individually administered measures of expressive language development are substantially below those obtained from standardized measures of both nonverbal intellectual capacity and receptive language development. The disturbance may be manifest clinically by symptoms that include having a markedly limited vocabulary, making errors in tense, or having difficulty recalling words or producing sentences with developmentally appropriate length or complexity.

B. The difficulties with expressive language interfere with academic or occupational achievement or with social communication.

C. Criteria are not met for mixed receptive-expressive language disorder or a pervasive developmental disorder.

D. If mental retardation, a speech-motor or sensory deficit, or environmental deprivation is present, the language difficulties are in excess of those usually associated with these problems.

Coding note: If a speech-motor or sensory deficit or a neurological condition is present, code the condition on Axis III.

From American Psychiatric Association. *Diagnostic and Statistical Manual of Mental Disorders.* 4th ed. Text rev. Washington, DC: American Psychiatric Association; copyright 2000, with permission.

Josh was an alert, energetic 2-year-old whose expressive vocabulary was limited to only four words (*mama, daddy, hi,* and *more*). He used these words one at a time in appropriate situations. He supplemented his infrequent verbal communications with pointing and other simple gestures to request desired objects or actions. He rarely communicated, however, for other purposes (e.g., commenting or protesting). Josh appeared to be developing normally in all other areas, except for expressive language. He sat, stood, and walked at the expected times. He played happily with other children, enjoying activities and toys that were appropriate for 2-year-olds. Although he had a history of frequent ear infections, a recent hearing test revealed normal hearing. Of importance, he showed age-appropriate comprehension for the names of familiar objects and actions and for simple verbal instructions (e.g., "Put that down." "Get your shirt." "Clap your hands."). Of course, at his age, comprehension testing had to be carefully conducted to ensure his attention and motivation.

Despite Josh's slow start in language development, most specialists would be reluctant to diagnose an expressive language disorder at his young age. Prospective research on the development of late talkers such Josh has demonstrated that most of them spontaneously overcome their initial slow start in language development. A parental report measure of vocabulary comprehension has shown promise as a prognostic indicator that can be used as early as 10 months of age. (Courtesy of Carla J. Johnson, Ph.D. and Joseph H. Beitchman, M.D.)

Differential Diagnosis

Language disorders are associated with many other psychiatric disorders, and, thus, the language disorder itself may be difficult to separate from other difficulties. In mental retardation, patients have an overall impairment in intellectual functioning, as shown by below-normal intelligence test scores in all areas, but the nonverbal intellectual capacity and functioning of children with expressive language disorder are within normal limits. In mixed receptive-expressive language disorder, language comprehension (decoding) is markedly below the expected age-appropriate level, whereas in expressive language disorder, language comprehension remains within normal limits.

In pervasive developmental disorders, in addition to the cardinal cognitive characteristics, affected children have no inner language, symbolic or imagery play, appropriate use of gesture, or capacity to form warm and meaningful social relationships. Moreover, children show little or no frustration with the inability to communicate verbally. In contrast, all these characteristics are present in children with expressive language disorder.

Children with acquired aphasia or dysphasia have a history of early normal language development; the disordered language had its onset after a head trauma or other neurological disorder (e.g., a seizure disorder). Children with selective mutism have a history of normal language development. Often these children will speak only in front of family members (e.g., mother, father, and siblings). Children affected by selective mutism are socially anxious and withdrawn outside of the family.

Pathology and Laboratory Examination

Children with speech and language disorders should have an audiogram to rule out hearing loss.

Course and Prognosis

The prognosis for expressive language disorder is related to the severity of the disorder. Studies of "late talkers" concur that 50 to 80 percent of these children master language skills that are within the expected level during the preschool years. Most children who begin to talk later than average but catch up during preschool years are not at high risk to develop further language or learning disorders. Outcome of expressive language disorder is influenced by other comorbid disorders. If children do not develop mood disorders or disruptive behavior problems, the prognosis is better. The rapidity and extent of recovery depend on the severity of the disorder, the child's motivation to participate in therapy, and the timely institution of speech and other therapeutic interventions. The presence or absence of other factors—such as moderate to severe hearing loss, mild mental retardation, and severe emotional problems—also affects the prognosis for recovery. As many as 50 percent of children with mild expressive

language disorder recover spontaneously without any sign of language impairment, but children with severe expressive language disorder may later display features of mild to moderate language impairment.

Treatment

Controversy exists among experts whether intervention for young children with expressive language difficulties should be initiated as soon as it is noted or whether waiting until age 4 or 5 years is the optimal time to begin treatment. Treatment for expressive language disorder is generally not initiated unless it persists after the preschool years. Various techniques have been used to help a child improve use of such parts of speech as pronouns, correct tenses, and question forms. Direct interventions use a speech and language pathologist who works directly with the child. Mediated interventions, in which a speech and language professional teaches a child's teacher or parent how to promote therapeutic language techniques, have also been efficacious. Language therapy is often aimed at using words to improve communication strategies and social interactions as well. Such therapy consists in behaviorally reinforced exercises and practice with phonemes (sound units), vocabulary, and sentence construction. The goal is to increase the number of phrases by using block-building methods and conventional speech therapies.

Psychotherapy may be useful for children whose language impairment has affected their self-esteem, insofar as it can be used as a positive model for more effective communication and broadening social skills. Supportive parental counseling may be indicated in some cases. Parents may need help to reduce intrafamilial tensions arising from difficulties in rearing language-disordered children and to increase their awareness and understanding of the disorder.

More research is needed to establish whether early intervention for preschoolers with language deficits has long-term benefits and to develop comprehensive treatment programs that may address the direct language interventions along with interventions for common comorbid communication and learning disorders.

MIXED RECEPTIVE-EXPRESSIVE LANGUAGE DISORDER

Children with mixed receptive-expressive learning disorders exhibit impaired skills in the expression and reception (understanding and comprehension) of spoken language. The expressive difficulties in these children may be similar to those of children with only expressive language disorder, which is characterized by limited vocabulary, use of simplistic sentences, and short sentence usage. Children with receptive language difficulties may be experiencing additional deficits in basic auditory processing skills, such as discriminating between sounds, rapid sound changes, association of sounds and symbols, and the memory of sound sequences. These deficits may lead to a whole host of communication barriers for a child, including a lack of understanding of questions or directives from others and inability to follow the conversations of peers or family members. Recognition of the disorder in children with mixed expressive-receptive language disorders may be delayed because of early misattribution of their communication by teachers and parents as a behavioral problem rather than a deficit in understanding.

Epidemiology

Mixed receptive-expressive language disorder is believed to occur in about 5 percent of preschoolers and to persist in approximately 3 percent of school-age children. It is less common than expressive language disorder alone. Mixed receptive-expressive language disorder is believed to be at least twice as prevalent in boys as in girls.

Comorbidity

Children with mixed receptive-expressive disorder are at high risk for additional speech and language disorders, learning disorders, and additional psychiatric disorders. About half of children with this disorder also have pronunciation difficulties leading to phonological disorder, and about half also have reading disorder. These rates are significantly higher than the comorbidity found in children with expressive language disorder alone. ADHD is present in at least one third of children with mixed receptive-expressive language disorder.

Etiology

Language disorders most likely have multiple determinants, including genetic factors, developmental brain abnormalities, environmental influences, neurodevelopmental immaturity, and auditory processing features in the brain. As with expressive language disorder alone, evidence is found of familial aggregation of mixed receptive-expressive language disorder. Genetic contribution to this disorder is implicated by twin studies, but no mode of genetic transmission has been proved. Some studies of children with various speech and language disorders have also shown cognitive deficits, particularly slower processing of tasks involving naming objects, as well as fine motor tasks. Slower myelinization of neural pathways has been hypothesized to account for the slow processing found in children with developmental language disorders. Several studies suggest an underlying impairment of auditory discrimination because most children with the disorder are more responsive to environmental sounds than to speech sounds.

Diagnosis

Children with mixed receptive-expressive language disorder develop language more slowly than their peers and have trouble understanding conversations that peers can follow. In mixed receptive-expressive language disorder, receptive dysfunction coexists with expressive dysfunction. Therefore, standardized tests for both receptive and expressive language abilities must be given to anyone suspected of having mixed receptive-expressive language disorder.

A markedly below-expected level of comprehension of verbal or sign language with intact age-appropriate nonverbal intellectual capacity, confirmation of language difficulties by standardized receptive language tests, and the absence of pervasive developmental disorders confirm the diagnosis of mixed receptive-expressive language disorder (Table 37–2).

**Table 37–2
DSM-IV-TR Diagnostic Criteria for Mixed Receptive-Expressive Language Disorder**

A. The scores obtained from a battery of standardized individually administered measures of both receptive and expressive language development are substantially below those obtained from standardized measures of nonverbal intellectual capacity. Symptoms include those for expressive language disorder as well as difficulty understanding words, sentences, or specific types of words, such as spatial terms.

B. The difficulties with receptive and expressive language significantly interfere with academic or occupational achievement or with social communication.

C. Criteria are not met for a pervasive developmental disorder.

D. If mental retardation, a speech-motor or sensory deficit, or environmental deprivation is present, the language difficulties are in excess of those usually associated with these problems.

Coding note: If a speech-motor or sensory deficit or a neurological condition is present, code the condition on Axis III.

From American Psychiatric Association. *Diagnostic and Statistical Manual of Mental Disorders.* 4th ed. Text rev. Washington, DC: American Psychiatric Association; copyright 2000, with permission.

Clinical Features

The essential clinical feature of the disorder is significant impairment in both language comprehension and language expression. In the mixed disorder, the expressive impairments are similar to those of expressive language disorder, but they can be more severe. The clinical features of the receptive component of the disorder typically appear before the age of 4 years. Severe forms are apparent by the age of 2 years; mild forms may not become evident until age 7 years (second grade) or older, when language becomes complex. Children with mixed receptive-expressive language disorder show markedly delayed and below-normal ability to comprehend (decode) verbal or sign language, although they have age-appropriate nonverbal intellectual capacity. In most cases of receptive dysfunction, verbal or sign expression (encoding) of language is also impaired. The clinical features of mixed receptive-expressive language disorder in children between the ages of 18 and 24 months result from a child's failure to utter a single phoneme spontaneously or to mimic another person's words.

Many children with mixed receptive-expressive language disorder have auditory sensory difficulties or cannot process visual symbols, such as explaining the meaning of a picture. They have deficits in integrating both auditory and visual symbols—for example, recognizing the basic common attributes of a toy truck and a toy passenger car. Whereas at 18 months, a child with expressive language disorder only can comprehend simple commands and can point to familiar household objects when told to do so, a child of the same age with mixed receptive-expressive language disorder cannot either point to common objects or obey simple commands. A child with mixed receptive-expressive language disorder usually appears to be deaf, but the child can hear. He or she responds normally to nonlanguage sounds from the environment but not to spoken language. If the child later starts to speak, the speech contains numerous articulation errors, such as omissions, distortions, and substitutions of phonemes. Language acquisition is much slower for children with mixed receptive-expressive language disorder than for children without this disorder.

Children with mixed receptive-expressive language disorder have difficulty recalling early visual and auditory memories and recognizing and reproducing symbols in proper sequence. In some cases, bilateral EEG abnormalities are seen. Some children with mixed receptive-expressive language disorder have a partial hearing defect for true tones, an increased threshold of auditory arousal, and an inability to localize sound sources. Seizure disorders and reading disorder are more common among the relatives of children with mixed receptive-expressive language disorder than they are in the general population.

Pathology and Laboratory Examination

An audiogram is indicated for all children thought to have mixed receptive-expressive language disorder to rule out or confirm the presence of deafness and to determine the types of auditory deficits. A history of the child and family and observation of the child in various settings help to clarify the diagnosis.

> Susan was a pleasant 2-year-old who did not yet use any spoken words. She made her needs known with vocalizations and simple gestures (e.g., showing or pointing) such as those typically used by younger children. She seemed to understand the names for a few familiar people and objects (e.g., *mommy*, *daddy*, *cat*, *bottle*, and *cookie*). Compared with other children her age, she had a small comprehension vocabulary and showed limited understanding of simple verbal directions (e.g., "Get your doll"; "Close your eyes"). Nonetheless, her hearing was normal, and her motor and play skills were developing as expected for her age. She showed interest in her environment and in the activities of the other children at her day care. (Courtesy of Carla J. Johnson, Ph.D., and Joseph H. Beitchman, M.D.)

Differential Diagnosis

Children with significant mixed receptive-expressive language disorder have a deficit in language comprehension. This deficit may be overlooked at first because the expressive language deficit may be more obvious. In expressive language disorder alone, comprehension of spoken language (decoding) remains within age norms. Children with phonological disorder or stuttering have normal expressive and receptive language competence, despite the speech impairments. Hearing impairment should be ruled out.

Course and Prognosis

The overall prognosis for mixed receptive-expressive language disorder is less favorable than that for expressive language disorder alone. When the mixed disorder is identified in a young child, it is usually severe, and the short-term prognosis is poor. Language develops at a rapid rate in early childhood, and young children with the disorder may appear to be falling behind. In view of the likelihood of comorbid learning disorders and other mental disorders, the prognosis is guarded. Young children with

severe mixed receptive-expressive language disorder are likely to have learning disorders in the future. In children with mild versions, mixed disorder may not be identified for several years, and the disruption in everyday life may be less overwhelming than that in severe forms of the disorder. Over the long run, some children with mixed receptive-expressive language disorder achieve close-to-normal language functions. The prognosis for children who have mixed receptive-expressive language disorder varies widely and depends on the nature and severity of the damage.

Treatment

A comprehensive speech and language evaluation is recommended for children with mixed receptive-expressive language disorder before embarking on a speech and language remediation program. Preschoolers with mixed receptive-expressive language disorder optimally receive interventions designed to promote social communication and literacy as well as oral language. For children at the kindergarten level, optimal intervention includes direct teaching of key prereading skills as well as social skills training. An important early goal of interventions for young children with mixed receptive-expressive language disorder is the achievement of rudimentary reading skills, in that these skills are protective against the academic and psychosocial ramifications of falling behind early on in reading skills. Some language therapists favor a low-stimuli setting in which children are given individual linguistic instruction. Others recommend that speech and language instruction be integrated into a varied setting with several children who are taught several language structures simultaneously. Often, a child with mixed receptive-expressive language disorder will benefit from a small, special-educational setting that allows more individualized learning.

Psychotherapy may be helpful for children with mixed receptive-expressive language disorder who have associated emotional and behavioral problems. Particular attention should be paid to evaluating the child's self-image and social skills. Family counseling in which parents and children can develop more effective, less frustrating means of communicating may be beneficial.

PHONOLOGICAL DISORDER

Children with phonological disorder are unable to produce speech sounds correctly because of omissions of sounds, distortions of sounds, or atypical pronunciation. Typical speech disturbances in this disorder include omitting the last sounds of the word (e.g., saying *mou* for *mouse* or *drin* for *drink*) or substituting one sound for another (saying *bwu* instead of *blue* or *tup* for *cup*). Distortions in sounds can occur when children allow too much air to escape from the side of their mouths while saying sounds like *sh* or producing sounds like *s* or *z* with their tongue protruded. Speech sound errors can also occur in patterns because a child has an interrupted air flow instead of a steady airflow, preventing the entire word to be pronounced (e.g., *pat* for *pass* or *bacuum* for *vacuum*).

Children with a phonological disorder can be mistaken for younger children because of their difficulties in producing speech sounds correctly. The diagnosis of a phonological disorder is made by comparing the skills of a given child with the expected skill level of others of the same age. The disorder results in errors in whole words because of incorrect pronunciation of consonants, substitution of one sound for another, omission of entire phonemes, and, in some cases, dysarthria (slurred speech because of incoordination of speech muscles) or dyspraxia (difficulty planning and executing speech). Speech sound development is believed to be based on both linguistic and motor development that must be integrated to produce sounds. According to the text revision of the 4th edition of the *Diagnostic and Statistical Manual of Mental Disorders* (DSM-IV-TR), if mental retardation, a speech-motor or sensory deficit, or environmental deprivation is present, the language dysfunction must exceed that associated with those problems.

Epidemiology

Surveys indicate that the prevalence of phonological disorder is at least 3 percent in preschoolers, 2 percent in children 6 to 7 years of age, and 0.5 percent in 17-year-old adolescents. Approximately 7 to 8 percent of 5-year-old children in one large community sample had speech sound production problems of developmental, structural, or neurological origins. Another study found that up to 7.5 percent of children between the ages of 7 and 11 years had phonological disorders. Of those, 2.5 percent had speech delay (deletion and substitution errors past the age of 4 years), and 5 percent had residual articulation errors beyond the age of 8 years. Developmental phonological disorders occur much more frequently than disorders with known structural or neurological origin. The disorder is approximately two to three times more common in boys than in girls. It is also more common among first-degree relatives of patients with the disorder than in the general population. According to DSM-IV-TR, the prevalence falls to 0.5 percent by mid to late adolescence.

Comorbidity

More than half of children with developmental phonological disorder have some difficulty with expressive language. Disorders that commonly present with phonological disorder are expressive language disorder, mixed receptive-expressive language disorder, reading disorder, and developmental coordination disorder. Enuresis may also accompany the disorder. A delay in reaching speech milestones (e.g., first word and first sentence) has been reported in some children with phonological disorder, but most children with the disorder begin speaking at the appropriate age. Children with phonological disorder who also have language disorders are at greatest risk for attentional problems and learning disorders. Children with phonological disorder who do not have language dysfunction have lower risk of comorbid psychiatric or behavioral problems.

Etiology

The likely causes of phonological disturbance include multiple variables—perinatal problems, genetic factors, auditory processing problems, hearing impairment, and structural abnormalities related to speech. A developmental lag or maturational delay in the neurological process underlying speech has been postulated in some cases. The likelihood of a subtle brain abnormality is supported by the observation that children with phonological disorder are also more likely to manifest "soft neurological signs" as well as additional disorders, including receptive and expressive language difficulties and a higher-than-expected rate of reading disorder. Genetic factors are implicated by data from twin studies that show concordance rates for monozygotic twins that are higher than chance.

Environmental factors may play a role in developmental phonological disorder, but constitutional factors seem to make the most significant contribution. The high proportion of phonological disorder in certain families implies a genetic component in the development of this disorder. Poor motor coordination, laterality, and handedness are not associated with phonological disorder.

Diagnosis

The essential feature of phonological disorder is a child's delay or failure to produce developmentally expected speech sounds, especially consonants, resulting in sound omissions, substitutions, and distortions of phonemes. A rough guideline for clinical assessment of children's articulation is that normal 3-year-olds correctly articulate *m, n, ng, b, p, h, t, k, q,* and *d*; normal 4-year-olds correctly articulate *f, y, ch, sh,* and *z*; and normal 5-year-olds correctly articulate *th, s,* and *r*.

Phonological disorder cannot be attributed to structural or neurological abnormalities, and it is accompanied by normal language development. The DSM-IV-TR diagnostic criteria for phonological disorder are given in Table 37–3.

Clinical Features

Children with phonological disorder are delayed in, or incapable of, producing speech sounds that are expected for their age, intelligence, and dialect. The sounds are often substitutions—for example, the use of *t* instead of *k*—and omissions, such as leaving off the final consonants of words. Phonological disorder can be recognized in early childhood. In severe cases, the disorder is first recognized at about 3 years of age. In less severe cases, the

Table 37–3
DSM-IV-TR Diagnostic Criteria for Phonological Disorder

A. Failure to use developmentally expected speech sounds that are appropriate for age and dialect (e.g., errors in sound production, use, representation, or organization such as, but not limited to, substitutions of one sound for another [use of /t/ for target /k/ sound] or omissions of sounds such as final consonants).

B. The difficulties in speech sound production interfere with academic or occupational achievement or with social communication.

C. If mental retardation, a speech-motor or sensory deficit, or environmental deprivation is present, the speech difficulties are in excess of those usually associated with these problems.

Coding note: If a speech-motor or sensory deficit or a neurological condition is present, code the condition on Axis III.

From American Psychiatric Association. *Diagnostic and Statistical Manual of Mental Disorders.* 4th ed. Text rev. Washington, DC: American Psychiatric Association; copyright 2000, with permission.

disorder may not be apparent until the age of 6 years. A child's articulation is judged disordered when it is significantly behind that of most children at the same age level, intellectual level, and educational level.

In very mild cases, a single speech sound (i.e., phoneme) may be affected. When a single phoneme is affected, it is usually one that is acquired late in normal language acquisition. The speech sounds most frequently misarticulated are also those acquired late in the developmental sequence, including *r, sh, th, f, z, l,* and *ch.* In severe cases and in young children, sounds such as *b, m, t, d, n,* and *h* may be mispronounced. One or many speech sounds may be affected, but vowel sounds are not among them.

Children with phonological disorder cannot articulate certain phonemes correctly and may distort, substitute, or even omit the affected phonemes. With omissions, the phonemes are absent entirely— for example, *bu* for *blue, ca* for *car,* or *whaa?* for *what's that?* With substitutions, difficult phonemes are replaced with incorrect ones— for example, *wabbit* for *rabbit, fum* for *thumb,* or *whath dat?* for *what's that?* With distortions, the correct phoneme is approximated but is articulated incorrectly. Rarely, additions (usually of the vowel *uh*) occur—for example, *puhretty* for *pretty, what's uh that uh?* for *what's that?*

Omissions are thought to be the most serious type of misarticulation, with substitutions the next most serious, and distortions the least serious type. Omissions, which are most frequent in the speech of young children, usually occur at the ends of words or in clusters of consonants (*ka* for *car, scisso* for *scissors*). Distortions, which are found mainly in the speech of older children, result in a sound that is not part of the speaker's dialect. Distortions may be the last type of misarticulation remaining in the speech of children whose articulation problems have mostly remitted. The most common types of distortions are the lateral slip—in which a child pronounces *s* sounds with the airstream going across the tongue, producing a whistling effect—and the palatal or lisp—in which the *s* sound, formed with the tongue too close to the palate, produces a *ssh* sound effect.

The misarticulations of children with phonological disorder are often inconsistent and random. A phoneme may be pronounced correctly one time and incorrectly another time. Misarticulations are most common at the ends of words, in long and syntactically complex sentences, and during rapid speech.

Omissions, distortions, and substitutions also occur normally in the speech of young children learning to talk. Whereas young, normally speaking children soon replace these misarticulations, however, children with phonological disorder do not. Even as children with phonological disorder grow and finally acquire the correct phoneme, they may use it only in newly acquired words and may not correct the words learned earlier that they have been mispronouncing for some time.

Most children eventually outgrow phonological disorder, usually by the third grade. After the fourth grade, however, spontaneous recovery is unlikely, and so it is important to try to remediate the disorder before the development of complications. Often, beginning kindergarten or school precipitates the improvement when recovery from phonological disorder is spontaneous. Speech therapy is clearly indicated for children who have not shown spontaneous improvement by the third or fourth grade. Speech therapy should be initiated at an early age for children whose articulation is significantly unintelligible and who are clearly troubled by their inability to speak clearly.

Natasha was a shy, reserved 8-year-old with a history of significant speech delay. During her preschool and early school years, she had overcome many of her earlier speech errors. A few late-developing sounds ($/r/$, $/l/$, and */th/*), however, continued to pose a challenge for her. Natasha often substituted $/f/$ or $/d/$ for */th/* and produced $/w/$ for $/r/$ and $/l/$. Overall, her speech was easily understood, despite these minor errors. Nonetheless, she was often reluctant to speak in front of others because of the teasing she received from her classmates about her speech. (Courtesy of Carla J. Johnson, Ph.D., and Joseph H. Beitchman, M.D.)

Differential Diagnosis

The differential diagnosis of phonological disorder includes a careful determination of symptoms severity and possible medical conditions that might be producing the symptoms. First, the clinician must determine that the misarticulations are sufficiently severe to be considered impairing rather than a normative developmental process of learning to speak. Second, the clinician must determine that no physical abnormalities account for the articulation errors and must rule out neurological disorders that may cause dysarthria, hearing impairment, mental retardation, and pervasive developmental disorders. Third, the clinician must obtain an evaluation of receptive and expressive language to determine that the speech difficulty is not solely attributable to the foregoing disorders.

Neurological, oral structural, and audiometric examinations may be necessary to rule out physical factors that cause certain types of articulation abnormalities. Children with dysarthria—a disorder caused by structural or neurological abnormalities— differ from children with developmental phonological disorder in that dysarthria is less likely to remit spontaneously and may be more difficult to remediate. Drooling, slow, or uncoordinated motor behavior, abnormal chewing or swallowing, and awkward or slow protrusion and retraction of the tongue indicate dysarthria. A slow rate of speech also indicates dysarthria.

Course and Prognosis

Spontaneous remission of symptoms is common in children whose misarticulations involve only a few phonemes. Children who persist in exhibiting articulation problems after the age of 5 years may be experiencing a myriad of other speech and language impairments, so that a comprehensive evaluation may be indicated at this time. Children older than the age of 5 years with articulation problems are at higher risk for auditory perceptual problems. Spontaneous recovery is rare after the age of 8 years.

Treatment

Treatment is typically recommended for children with moderate to severe developmental phonological disorders. Two main approaches have been used successfully to improve phonological difficulties. The first one, the *phonological approach,* is usually chosen for children with extensive patterns of multiple speech sound errors that may include final consonant deletion or consonant cluster reduction. Exercises in this approach to treatment focus on guided practice of specific sounds, such as final consonants, and when that skill is mastered, practice is extended to use in meaningful words and sentences. The other approach, the *traditional approach*, is used for children who produce substitution or distortion errors in just a few sounds. In this approach, the child practices the production of the problem sound while the clinician provides immediate feedback and cues concerning the correct placement of the tongue and mouth for improved articulation. Children who have errors in articulation because of abnormal swallowing resulting in tongue thrust and lisps are treated with exercises that improve swallowing patterns and, in turn, improve speech. Speech therapy is typically provided by a speech-language pathologist, yet parents can be taught to provide adjunctive help by practicing techniques used in the treatment. Early intervention can be helpful because, for many children with mild articulation difficulties, even several months of intervention may be helpful in early elementary school. In general, when a child's articulation and intelligibility is noticeably different than peers by the age of 8 years, speech deficits often lead to problems with peers, learning, and self-image, especially when the disorder is so severe that many consonants are misarticulated and when errors involve omissions and substitutions of phonemes rather than distortions.

STUTTERING

Stuttering is a condition in which the normal flow of speech is disrupted by involuntary speech motor events. Stuttering can include a variety of specific disruptions of fluency, including sound or syllable repetitions, sound prolongations, dysrhythmic phonations, and complete blocking or unusual pauses between sounds and syllables of words. In severe cases, the stuttering may be accompanied by accessory or secondary attempts to compensate, such as respiratory, abnormal voice phonations, or tongue clicks. Associated behaviors, such as eye blinks, facial grimacing, head jerks, and abnormal body movements, may be observed before or during the disrupted speech. The disorder usually originates in childhood.

Controversy is found among speech and language experts as to whether stuttering should be considered an independent entity or part of a broader speech and language disorder. Some question whether stuttering should be considered a psychiatric condition at all. Many children who stutter do endure significant psychological distress, and stuttering does cause impairment in everyday life for many children with this condition.

Epidemiology

Surveys conducted mainly in the United States and Europe indicate that the prevalence of stuttering is about 1 percent in the general population. Stuttering tends to be most common in young children and has often resolved spontaneously by the time the child is older. The typical age of onset is 2 to 7 years of age, with a peak at age 5 years. Estimates are that up to 3 to 4 percent of individuals may have stuttered at some time in their lives. Approximately 80 percent of young children who stutter are likely to have a spontaneous remission over time. According to DSM-IV-TR, it dips to 0.8 percent by adolescence. Stuttering affects about three to four males for every female. The disorder is significantly more common among family members of affected children than in the general population. According to DSM-IV-TR, for male

persons who stutter, 20 percent of their male children and 10 percent of their female children will also stutter.

Comorbidity

Very young children who stutter typically show some delay in the development of language and articulation without additional disorders of speech and language. Preschoolers and school-age children who stutter exhibit an increased incidence of social anxiety, school refusal, and other anxiety symptoms. Older children who stutter also do not necessarily have comorbid speech and language disorders but often manifest anxiety symptoms and disorders. When stuttering persists into adolescence, social isolation occurs at higher rates than in the general adolescent population. Stuttering is also associated with a variety of abnormal motor movements, upper body tics, and facial grimaces. Other disorders that coexist with stuttering include phonological disorder, expressive language disorder, mixed receptive-expressive language disorder, and ADHD.

Etiology

Converging evidence indicates that cause of stuttering is multifactorial, including genetic, neurophysiological, and psychological factors that predispose a child to have poor speech fluency. Although research evidence does not indicate that anxiety or conflicts cause stuttering or that persons who stutter have more psychiatric disturbances than those with other forms of speech and language disorders, stuttering can be exacerbated by certain stressful situations.

Other theories about the cause of stuttering include organic models and learning models. Organic models include those that focus on incomplete lateralization or abnormal cerebral dominance. Several studies using EEG found that stuttering males had right-hemispheric alpha suppression across stimulus words and tasks; nonstutterers had left-hemispheric suppression. Some studies of stutterers have noted an overrepresentation of left-handedness and ambidexterity. Twin studies and striking gender differences in stuttering indicate that stuttering has some genetic basis.

Learning theories about the cause of stuttering include the semantogenic theory, in which stuttering is basically a learned response to normative early childhood dysfluencies. Another learning model focuses on classic conditioning, in which the stuttering becomes conditioned to environmental factors. In the cybernetic model, speech is viewed as a process that depends on appropriate feedback for regulation; stuttering is hypothesized to occur because of a breakdown in the feedback loop. The observations that stuttering is reduced by white noise and that delayed auditory feedback produces stuttering in normal speakers lend support to the feedback theory.

The motor functioning of some children who stutter appears to be delayed or slightly abnormal. The observation of difficulties in speech planning exhibited by some children who stutter suggests that higher-level cognitive dysfunction may contribute to stuttering. Although children who stutter do not routinely exhibit other speech and language disorders, family members of these children often exhibit an increased incidence of a variety of speech and language disorders. Stuttering is

Table 37–4
DSM-IV-TR Diagnostic Criteria for Stuttering

A. Disturbance in the normal fluency and time patterning of speech (inappropriate for the individual's age), characterized by frequent occurrences of one or more of the following:
  (1) sound and syllable repetitions
  (2) sound prolongations
  (3) interjections
  (4) broken words (e.g., pauses within a word)
  (5) audible or silent blocking (filled or unfilled pauses in speech)
  (6) circumlocutions (word substitutions to avoid problematic words)
  (7) words produced with an excess of physical tension
  (8) monosyllabic whole-word repetitions (e.g., "I-I-I-I see him")

B. The disturbance in fluency interferes with academic or occupational achievement or with social communication.

C. If a speech-motor or sensory deficit is present, the speech difficulties are in excess of those usually associated with these problems.

Coding note: If a speech-motor or sensory deficit or a neurological condition is present, code the condition on Axis III.

From American Psychiatric Association. *Diagnostic and Statistical Manual of Mental Disorders.* 4th ed. Text rev. Washington, DC: American Psychiatric Association; copyright 2000, with permission.

most likely to be caused by a set of interacting variables that include both genetic and environmental factors.

Diagnosis

The diagnosis of stuttering is not difficult when the clinical features are apparent and well developed and each of the four phases (described in the next section) can be readily recognized. Diagnostic difficulties can arise when trying to determine the existence of stuttering in young children because some preschool children experience transient dysfluency. It may not be clear whether the nonfluent pattern is part of normal speech and language development or represents the initial stage in the development of stuttering. If incipient stuttering is suspected, referral to a speech pathologist is indicated. Table 37–4 presents the DSM-IV-TR diagnostic criteria for stuttering.

Clinical Features

Stuttering usually appears between the ages of 18 months and 9 years, with two sharp peaks of onset between the ages of 2 to 3.5 years and 5 to 7 years. Some, but not all, stutterers have other speech and language problems, such as phonological disorder and expressive language disorder. Stuttering does not begin suddenly; it typically develops over weeks or months with a repetition of initial consonants, whole words that are usually the first words of a phrase, or long words. As the disorder progresses, the repetitions become more frequent, with consistent stuttering on the most important words or phrases. Even after it develops, stuttering may be absent during oral readings, singing, and talking to pets or inanimate objects.

Stutterers show a vivid, fearful anticipation of stuttering. They fear words, sounds, and situations. Word substitutions and circumlocutions are common. Stutterers avoid situations requiring speech and show other evidence of fear and embarrassment.

Stutterers may have associated clinical features: vivid, fearful anticipation of stuttering, with avoidance of particular words, sounds, or situations in which stuttering is anticipated; and eye blinks, tics, and tremors of the lips or jaw. Frustration, anxiety, and depression are common among those with chronic stuttering.

Differential Diagnosis

Normal speech dysfluency in preschool years is difficult to differentiate from incipient stuttering. In stuttering, more nonfluencies, part-word repetitions, sound prolongations, and disruptions in voice airflow through the vocal track occur. Children who stutter appear to be tense and uncomfortable with their speech pattern, in contrast to young children who are nonfluent in their speech but seem to be at ease. Spastic dysphonia is a stuttering-like speech disorder distinguished from stuttering by the presence of an abnormal breathing pattern.

Cluttering is a speech disorder characterized by erratic and dysrhythmic speech patterns of rapid and jerky spurts of words and phrases. In cluttering, those affected are usually unaware of the disturbance, whereas, after the initial phase of the disorder, stutterers are aware of their speech difficulties. Cluttering is often an associated feature of expressive language disorder.

Course and Prognosis

The course of stuttering is usually long term, with some periods of partial remission lasting for weeks or months and exacerbations occurring most frequently when a stutterer is under pressure to communicate. Of all children who stutter, mostly those with mild cases, 50 to 80 percent recover spontaneously. School-age children who stutter chronically may have impaired peer relationships as a result of testing and social ostracism. The children may face academic difficulties if they avoid speaking in class. Later major complications include an affected person's limitations in occupational choice and advancement.

Treatment

Two distinct forms of intervention have been used in the treatment of stuttering. Direct speech therapy typically targets modification of the stuttering response to fluent-sounding speech by systematic steps and rules of speech mechanics that the person can practice. Another form of therapy for stuttering targets diminishing tension and anxiety during speech. These treatments use breathing exercises and relaxation techniques to help children slow the rate of speaking and modulate speech volume. Until the end of the 19th century, the most common treatments for stuttering were distraction, suggestion, and relaxation. Recent approaches using distraction include teaching stutterers to talk in time to rhythmic movements of the arm, hand, or fingers. Stutterers are also advised to speak slowly in a sing-song or monotone manner. These approaches, however, remove stuttering only temporarily. Suggestion techniques, such as hypnosis, also stop stuttering but, again, only temporarily. Relaxation techniques are based on the premise that it is nearly impossible to be relaxed and stutter in the usual manner at the same time. Current interventions for stuttering use individualized combinations of behavioral distraction, relaxation techniques, and directed speech modification.

Stutterers who have poor self-image, comorbid anxiety disorders, or depressive disorders are likely to require additional treatments. Most modern treatments of stuttering include components that target stuttering as, in part, a learned behavior that can be modified through behavioral techniques regardless of the complexity of how they emerged. These approaches work directly with the speech difficulty to minimize stuttering responses, to modify or decrease the severity of stuttering by eliminating the secondary symptoms, and to encourage stutterers to speak, even when stuttering, in a relatively easy and effortless fashion that aims to eliminate fear and blocks.

One example of this approach is the self-therapy proposed by the Speech Foundation of America. Self-therapy is based on the premise that stuttering is not a symptom, but a behavior that can be modified. Stutterers are told that they can learn to control their difficulty partly by modifying their feelings about stuttering and attitudes toward it and partly by modifying the deviant behaviors associated with their stuttering blocks. The approach includes desensitizing; reducing the emotional reaction to, and fears of, stuttering; and substituting positive action to control the moment of stuttering.

Recently developed therapies focus on restructuring fluency. The entire speech production pattern is reshaped, with emphasis on a variety of target behaviors, including rate reduction, easy or gentle onset of voicing, and smooth transitions between sounds, syllables, and words. The approaches have met with substantial success in establishing perceptually fluent speech in adults, but fluency maintenance over long periods and relapses remain problems for all involved in adult-stuttering treatment.

Psychopharmacological intervention, such as treatment with benzodiazepines (e.g., clonazepam [Klonopin]), have been used to promote relaxation; no data exist to assess the efficacy of this approach. Whichever therapeutic approach is used, individual and family assessments and supportive interventions may be helpful. A team assessment of a child or adolescent and his or

Table 37–5
DSM-IV-TR Diagnostic Criteria for Communication Disorder Not Otherwise Specified

This category is for disorders in communication that do not meet criteria for any specific communication disorder; for example, a voice disorder (i.e., an abnormality of vocal pitch, loudness, quality, tone, or resonance).

From American Psychiatric Association. *Diagnostic and Statistical Manual of Mental Disorders.* 4th ed. Text rev. Washington, DC: American Psychiatric Association; copyright 2000, with permission.

her family should be made before any approaches to treatment are begun.

COMMUNICATION DISORDER NOT OTHERWISE SPECIFIED

Disorders that do not meet the diagnostic criteria for any specific communication disorder fall into the category of communication disorder not otherwise specified. An example is voice disorder, in which the patient has an abnormality in pitch, loudness, quality, tone, or resonance. To be coded as a disorder, the voice abnormality must be sufficiently severe to impair academic achievement or social communication (Table 37–5). Operationally, speech production can be broken down into five interacting subsystems, including respiration (airflow from the lungs), phonation (sound generation in the larynx), resonance (shaping of the sound quality in the pharynx and nasal cavity), articulation (modulation of the sound stream into consonant and vowel sounds with the tongue, jaw, and lips), and suprasegmentalia (speech rhythm, loudness, and intonation). Together, these systems work to convey information, and, as important, voice quality conveys information about the speaker's emotional, psychological, and physical status. Thus, voice abnormalities can cover a broad area of communication as well as indicate many different types of abnormalities.

Cluttering is not listed as a disorder in DSM-IV-TR, but it is an associated speech abnormality in which the disturbed rate and rhythm of speech impair intelligibility. Speech is erratic and dysrhythmic and consists of rapid, jerky spurts that are inconsistent with normal phrasing patterns. The disorder usually occurs in children between 2 and 8 years of age; in two thirds of cases, the patient recovers spontaneously by early adolescence. Cluttering is associated with learning disorders and other communication disorders.

Pervasive Developmental Disorders

Pervasive developmental disorders include several disorders that are characterized by impaired reciprocal social interactions, aberrant language development, and restricted behavioral repertoire. Pervasive developmental disorders typically emerge in young children before the age of 3 years, and parents often become concerned about a child by 18 months as language development does not occur as expected. In about 25 percent of cases, some language develops and is subsequently lost. Some children with pervasive developmental disorders are not identified with problems until school age because they make relatively few demands and have minimal conflicts with others owing to their infrequent social engagement. Children with pervasive developmental disorders often exhibit idiosyncratic intense interest in a narrow range of activities, resist change, and are not appropriately responsive to the social environment. These disorders affect multiple areas of development, are manifested early in life, and cause persistent dysfunction.

The text revision of the fourth edition of the *Diagnostic and Statistical Manual of Mental Disorders* (DSM-IV-TR) includes five pervasive developmental disorders: autistic disorder, Rett's disorder, childhood disintegrative disorder, Asperger's disorder, and pervasive developmental disorder not otherwise specified. These are discussed in this chapter.

AUTISTIC DISORDER

Autistic disorder (historically called *early infantile autism*, *childhood autism*, or *Kanner's autism*) is characterized by symptoms from each of the following three categories: qualitative impairment in social interaction, impairment in communication, and restricted repetitive and stereotyped patterns of behavior or interests.

In 1943 Leo Kanner, in his classic paper "Autistic Disturbances of Affective Contact," coined the term *infantile autism* and provided a clear, comprehensive account of the early childhood syndrome. He described children who exhibited extreme autistic aloneness; failure to assume an anticipatory posture; delayed or deviant language development with echolalia and pronominal reversal (using you for I); monotonous repetitions of noises or verbal utterances; excellent rote memory; limited range of spontaneous activities, stereotypies, and mannerisms; anxiously obsessive desire for the maintenance of sameness and dread of change; poor eye contact; abnormal relationships with persons; and a preference for pictures and inanimate objects. Kanner suspected that the syndrome was more frequent than it seemed and suggested that some children with this disorder had been misclassified as mentally retarded or schizophrenic. Before 1980, children with pervasive developmental disorders were generally diagnosed with childhood schizophrenia. Over time, it became evident that autistic disorder and schizophrenia were two distinct psychiatric entities. In some cases, however, a child with autistic disorder may develop a comorbid schizophrenic disorder later in childhood.

Epidemiology

Prevalence. Autistic disorder is believed to occur at a rate of about 8 cases per 10,000 children (0.08 percent). Multiple epidemiological surveys mainly in Europe have resulted in variable rates of autistic disorder ranging from 2 to 30 cases per 10,000. By definition, the onset of autistic disorder is before the age of 3 years, although in some cases, it is not recognized until a child is much older.

Some recent studies have shown an apparent increase in the prevalence of autistic disorder. One study reported a prevalence of 19.5 per 10,000 in California, which was also accompanied by a decreased prevalence of mental retardation. Other studies reported rates of up to 60 per 10,000 for autism. The evidence suggests that the majority, if not all, of the reported rise in incidence and prevalence is due to changes in diagnostic criteria; whether there has been a true increase in incidence is under investigation.

Sex Distribution. Autistic disorder is four to five times more frequent in boys than in girls. Girls with autistic disorder are more likely to have more-severe mental retardation.

Socioeconomic Status. Early studies suggested that a high socioeconomic status was more common in families with autistic children; however, these findings were probably based on referral bias. Over the last 25 years, no epidemiological studies have demonstrated an association between autistic disorder and any socioeconomic status.

Etiology and Pathogenesis

Genetic Factors. Evidence supports a genetic basis for the development of autistic disorder in most cases, with a contribution of up to four or five genes. Family studies have demonstrated a 50 to 200 times increase in the rate of autism in siblings of an index child with autistic disorder. In addition, even when not affected with autism, siblings are at increased risk for a variety of developmental disorders often related to communication and social skills. These difficulties in the nonautistic relatives of persons with autistic disorder are also known by researchers as the "broad phenotype." The specific modes of inheritance are not clear. Hypotheses include genetic inheritance of a more general predisposition to developmental difficulties and specific genetic etiology of autistic disorder.

verbal autistic children may say more than they understand. Words and even entire sentences may drop in and out of a child's vocabulary. It is not atypical for a child with autistic disorder to use a word once and then not use it again for a week, a month, or years. Children with autistic disorder typically exhibit speech that contains echolalia, both immediate and delayed, or stereotyped phrases that seem out of context. These language patterns are frequently associated with pronoun reversals. A child with autistic disorder might say, "You want the toy" when she means that she wants it. Difficulties in articulation are also common. Many children with autistic disorder use peculiar voice quality and rhythm. About 50 percent of autistic children never develop useful speech. Some of the brightest children show a particular fascination with letters and numbers. Children with autistic disorder sometimes excel in certain tasks or have special abilities; for example, a child may learn to read fluently at preschool age (hyperlexia), often astonishingly well. Very young autistic children who can read many words, however, have little comprehension of the words read.

STEREOTYPED BEHAVIOR.   In the first years of an autistic child's life, much of the expected spontaneous exploratory play is absent. Toys and objects are often manipulated in a ritualistic manner, with few symbolic features. Autistic children generally do not show imitative play or use abstract pantomime. The activities and play of these children are often rigid, repetitive, and monotonous. Ritualistic and compulsive phenomena are common in early and middle childhood. Children often spin, bang, and line up objects and may exhibit an attachment to a particular inanimate object. Many autistic children, especially those with severe mental retardation, exhibit movement abnormalities. Stereotypies, mannerisms, and grimacing are most frequent when a child is left alone and may decrease in a structured situation. Autistic children are generally resistant to transition and change. Moving to a new house, seeing that furniture in a room has been moved, or encountering a change, such as having breakfast before a bath when the reverse was the routine, may evoke panic, fear, or temper tantrums.

INSTABILITY OF MOOD AND AFFECT.   Some children with autistic disorder exhibit sudden mood changes, with bursts of laughing or crying without an obvious reason. It is difficult to learn more about these episodes if the child cannot express the thoughts related to the affect.

RESPONSE TO SENSORY STIMULI.   Autistic children have been observed to overrespond to some stimuli and underrespond to other sensory stimuli (e.g., to sound and pain). It is not uncommon for a child with autistic disorder to appear deaf, at times showing little response to a normal speaking voice; on the other hand, the same child may show intent interest in the sound of a wristwatch. Some children with autistic disorder have a heightened pain threshold or an altered response to pain. Indeed, some autistic children do not respond to an injury by crying or seeking comfort. Many autistic children reportedly enjoy music. They frequently hum a tune or sing a song or commercial jingle before saying words or using speech. Some particularly enjoy vestibular stimulation—spinning, swinging, and up-and-down movements.

ASSOCIATED BEHAVIORAL SYMPTOMS.   Hyperkinesis is a common behavior problem in young autistic children. Hypokinesis is less frequent; when present, it often alternates with hyperactivity. Aggression and temper tantrums are observed, often prompted by change or demands. Self-injurious behavior includes head banging, biting, scratching, and hair pulling. Short

attention span, poor ability to focus on a task, insomnia, feeding and eating problems, and enuresis are also common among children with autism.

ASSOCIATED PHYSICAL ILLNESS.   Young children with autistic disorder have been reported to have a higher-than-expected incidence of upper respiratory infections and other minor infections. Gastrointestinal symptoms commonly found among children with autistic disorder include excessive burping, constipation, and loose bowel movements. Also seen is an increased incidence of febrile seizures in children with autistic disorder. Some autistic children do not show temperature elevations with minor infectious illnesses and may not show the typical malaise of ill children. In some children, behavior problems and relatedness seem to improve noticeably during a minor illness, and in some, such changes are a clue to physical illness.

A standardized instrument that can be very helpful in eliciting comprehensive information regarding developmental disorders is the *Autism Diagnostic Observation Schedule-Generic*.

John was the second of two children born to middle-class parents after normal pregnancy, labor, and delivery. As an infant, John appeared undemanding and relatively placid; motor development proceeded appropriately, but language development was delayed. Although his parents indicated that they were first concerned about his development when he was 18 months of age and still not speaking, in retrospect, they noted that, in comparison to their previous child, he had seemed relatively uninterested in social interaction and the social games of infancy. Stranger anxiety had never really developed, and John did not exhibit differential attachment behaviors toward his parents. Their pediatrician initially reassured John's parents that he was a "late talker," but they continued to be concerned. Although John seemed to respond to some unusual sounds, the pediatrician obtained a hearing test when John was 24 months old. Levels of hearing appeared adequate for development of speech, and John was referred for developmental evaluation. At 24 months, motor skills were age appropriate, and John exhibited some nonverbal problem-solving skills close to age level. His language and social development, however, were severely delayed, and he was noted to be resistant to changes in routine and unusually sensitive to aspects of the inanimate environment. His play skills were quite limited, and he used play materials in unusual and idiosyncratic ways. His older sister had a history of some learning difficulties, but the family history was otherwise negative. A comprehensive medical evaluation revealed a normal EEG and CT scan; genetic screening and chromosome analysis were normal as well.

John was enrolled in a special education program, in which he gradually began to speak. His speech was characterized by echolalia, extreme literalness, a monotonic voice quality, and pronoun reversal. He rarely used language in interaction and remained quite isolated. By school age, John had developed some evidence of differential attachments to family members; he also had developed a number of self-stimulatory behaviors and engaged in occasional periods of head banging. Extreme sensitivity to change continued.

Intelligence testing revealed marked scatter, with a full-scale intelligence quotient (IQ) in the moderately retarded range. As an adolescent, John's behavioral functioning deteriorated, and he developed a seizure disorder. Now an adult, he lives in a group home and attends a sheltered workshop. He has a rather passive interactional style but exhibits occasional outbursts of aggression and self-abuse. (Courtesy of Fred Volkmar, M.D.)

Intellectual Functioning. About 70 to 75 percent of children with autistic disorder function in the mentally retardation range of intellectual function. About 30 percent of children function in the mild to moderate range, and about 45 to 50 percent have severe to profound mental retardation. Epidemiological and clinical studies show that the risk for autistic disorder increases as the IQ decreases. About one fifth of all autistic children have a normal, nonverbal intelligence. The IQ scores of autistic children tend to reflect most severe problems with verbal sequencing and abstraction skills, with relative strengths in visuospatial or rote memory skills. This finding suggests the importance of defects in language-related functions.

Unusual or precocious cognitive or visuomotor abilities occur in some autistic children. The abilities, which may exist even in the overall retarded functioning, are referred to as *splinter functions* or *islets of precocity*. Perhaps the most striking examples are so-called idiot or autistic savants, who have prodigious rote memories or calculating abilities, usually beyond the capabilities of their normal peers. Other precocious abilities in young autistic children include hyperlexia—an early ability to read well (although they cannot understand what they read)—facility at memorizing and reciting, and high musical abilities (singing or playing tunes or recognizing musical pieces).

Differential Diagnosis

Autism must first be differentiated from one of the other pervasive developmental disorders such as Asperger's disorder and pervasive developmental disorder not otherwise specified. Furthermore, it must be differentiated from other developmental disorders, including mental retardation syndromes and developmental language disorders. Other disorders in the differential diagnosis are schizophrenia with childhood onset, congenital deafness or severe hearing disorder, psychosocial deprivation, and disintegrative (regressive) psychoses. It is sometimes difficult to make the diagnosis of autism because of its overlapping symptoms with childhood schizophrenia, mental retardation syndromes with behavioral symptoms, mixed receptive-expressive language disorder, and hearing disorders. Because children with a pervasive developmental disorder usually have many concurrent problems, Michael Rutter and Lionel Hersov suggested a stepwise approach to the differential diagnosis (Table 38–2).

Schizophrenia with Childhood Onset.
Although a wealth of literature on autistic disorder is available, few data exist on children younger than the age of 12 years who meet the diagnostic criteria for schizophrenia. Schizophrenia is rare in children younger than the age of 5 years. It is accompanied by hallucinations or delusions, with a lower incidence of seizures and mental retardation and a more even IQ than autistic children

Table 38–2
Procedure for Differential Diagnosis on a Multiaxial System

1. Determine intellectual level
2. Determine level of language development
3. Consider whether child's behavior is appropriate for
   (a) chronological age
   (b) mental age
   (c) language age
4. If not appropriate, consider differential diagnosis of psychiatric disorder according to
   (a) pattern of social interaction
   (b) pattern of language
   (c) pattern of play
   (d) other behaviors
5. Identify any relevant medical conditions
6. Consider whether there are any relevant psychosocial factors

From Rutter M, Hersov I. *Child and Adolescent Psychiatry: Modern Approaches.* 2nd ed. Oxford: Blackwell; 1985:73, with permission.

exhibit. Table 38–3 compares autistic disorder and schizophrenia with childhood onset.

Mental Retardation with Behavioral Symptoms.
About 40 percent of autistic children have moderate, severe, or profound retardation, and children with retardation may have behavioral symptoms that include autistic features. When both disorders are present, both should be diagnosed. The main differentiating features between autistic disorder and mental retardation are that children with mental retardation usually relate to adults and other children in accordance with their mental age, use the language they do have to communicate with others, and exhibit a relatively even profile of impairments without splinter functions.

Mixed Receptive-Expressive Language Disorder.
Some children with mixed receptive-expressive language disorder have mild autistic-like features and may present a diagnostic problem. Table 38–4 summarizes the major differences between autistic disorder and mixed receptive-expressive language disorder.

Acquired Aphasia with Convulsion.
Acquired aphasia with convulsion is a rare condition that is sometimes difficult to differentiate from autistic disorder and childhood disintegrative disorder. Children with the condition are normal for several years before losing both their receptive and their expressive language over a period of weeks or months. Most have a few seizures and generalized EEG abnormalities at the onset, but these signs usually do not persist. A profound language comprehension disorder then follows, characterized by deviant speech pattern and speech impairment. Some children recover, but with considerable residual language impairment.

Congenital Deafness or Severe Hearing Impairment.
Because autistic children are often mute or show a selective disinterest in spoken language, they are often thought to be deaf. Differentiating factors include the following: Autistic infants may babble only infrequently, whereas deaf infants have a history of relatively normal babbling that then gradually tapers off and may

Table 38–5
DSM-IV-TR Diagnostic Criteria for Rett's Disorder

A. All of the following:
(1) apparently normal prenatal and perinatal development
(2) apparently normal psychomotor development through the first 5 months after birth
(3) normal head circumference at birth
B. Onset of all of the following after the period of normal development:
(1) deceleration of head growth between ages 5 and 48 months
(2) loss of previously acquired purposeful hand skills between ages 5 and 30 months with the subsequent development of stereotyped hand movements (e.g., hand wringing or hand washing)
(3) loss of social engagement early in the course (although often social interaction develops later)
(4) appearance of poorly coordinated gait or trunk movements
(5) severely impaired expressive and receptive language development with severe psychomotor retardation

From American Psychiatric Association. *Diagnostic and Statistical Manual of Mental Disorders.* 4th ed. Text rev. Washington, DC: American Psychiatric Association; copyright 2000, with permission.

hand-wringing; the loss of previously acquired speech; psychomotor retardation; and ataxia. Other stereotypical hand movements may occur, such as licking or biting the fingers and tapping or slapping. The head circumference growth decelerates and produces microcephaly. All language skills are lost, and both receptive and expressive communicative and social skills seem to plateau at developmental levels between 6 months and 1 year. Poor muscle coordination and an apraxic gait with an unsteady and stiff quality develop. All of these clinical features are diagnostic criteria for the disorder (Table 38–5).

Associated features include seizures in up to 75 percent of affected children and disorganized EEGs with some epileptiform discharges in almost all young children with Rett's disorder, even in the absence of clinical seizures. An additional associated feature is irregular respiration, with episodes of hyperventilation, apnea, and breath holding. The disorganized breathing occurs in most patients while they are awake; during sleep, the breathing usually normalizes. Many patients with Rett's disorder also have scoliosis. As the disorder progresses, muscle tone seems to change from an initial hypotonic condition to spasticity to rigidity.

Although children with Rett's disorder may live for well more than a decade after the onset of the disorder, after 10 years, many patients are wheelchair bound, with muscle wasting, rigidity, and virtually no language ability. Long-term receptive and expressive communication and socialization abilities remain at a developmental level of less than 1 year.

Darla was born at term after an uncomplicated pregnancy. An amniocentesis had been obtained because of maternal age and was normal. At birth, Darla was in good condition; weight, height, and head circumference were all near the 50th percentile. Her development during the first months of life was within normal limits. At approximately 8 months of age, her development seemed to stagnate and her interest in the environment, including the social environment, waned. Her developmental milestones then became markedly delayed; she was just starting to walk at her second birthday and had no spoken language. Evaluation at that time revealed that head growth had decelerated. Some self-stimulatory behaviors were present. Marked cognitive and communicative delays were noted on formal testing. Darla began to lose purposeful hand movements and developed unusual hand-washing stereotyped behaviors. By age 6, her EEG was abnormal and purposeful hand movements were markedly impaired. Subsequently, she developed truncal ataxia and breath-holding spells, and motor skills deteriorated further. (Courtesy of Fred Volkmar, M.D.)

Differential Diagnosis

Some children with Rett's disorder receive initial diagnoses of autistic disorder because of the marked disability in social interactions in both disorders, but the two disorders have some predictable differences. In Rett's disorder, a child shows deterioration of developmental milestones, head circumference, and overall growth; in autistic disorder, aberrant development is usually present from early on. In Rett's disorder, specific and characteristic hand motions are always present; in autistic disorder, hand mannerisms may or may not appear. Poor coordination, ataxia, and apraxia are predictably part of Rett's disorder; many persons with autistic disorder have unremarkable gross motor function. In Rett's disorder, verbal abilities are usually lost completely; in autistic disorder, patients use characteristically aberrant language. Respiratory irregularity is characteristic of Rett's disorder, and seizures often appear early; in autistic disorder, no respiratory disorganization is seen, and seizures do not develop in most patients; when seizures do develop, they are more likely in adolescence than in childhood.

Course and Prognosis

Rett's disorder is progressive. The prognosis is not fully known, but patients who live into adulthood remain at a cognitive and social level equivalent to that in the first year of life.

Treatment

Treatment is symptomatic. Physiotherapy has been beneficial for the muscular dysfunction, and anticonvulsant treatment is usually necessary to control the seizures. Behavior therapy, along with medication, may help control self-injurious behaviors, as it does in the treatment of autistic disorder, and it may help regulate the breathing disorganization.

CHILDHOOD DISINTEGRATIVE DISORDER

Childhood disintegrative disorder is characterized by marked regression in several areas of functioning after at least 2 years of apparently normal development. Childhood disintegrative disorder, also called *Heller's syndrome* and *disintegrative psychosis*, was described in 1908 as a deterioration over several months of intellectual, social, and language function occurring in 3- to 4-year-olds with previously normal functions. After the deterioration, the children closely resembled children with autistic disorder.

Epidemiology

Epidemiological data have been complicated by the variable diagnostic criteria used, but childhood disintegrative disorder is estimated to be at least one tenth as common as autistic disorder, and the prevalence has been estimated to be about 1 case in 100,000 boys. The sex ratio is estimated to be between 4 and 8 boys to 1 girl.

Etiology

The cause of childhood disintegrative disorder is unknown, but it has been associated with other neurological conditions, including seizure disorders, tuberous sclerosis, and various metabolic disorders.

Diagnosis and Clinical Features

The diagnosis is made on the basis of features that fit a characteristic age of onset, clinical picture, and course. Cases reported have ranged in onset from ages 1 to 9 years, but in most, the onset is between 3 and 4 years; according to DSM-IV-TR, the minimum age of onset is 2 years (Table 38–6). The onset may be insidious over several months or relatively abrupt, with abilities

Table 38–6
DSM-IV-TR Diagnostic Criteria for Childhood Disintegrative Disorder

A. Apparently normal development for at least the first 2 years after birth as manifested by the presence of age-appropriate verbal and nonverbal communication, social relationships, play, and adaptive behavior.
B. Clinically significant loss of previously acquired skills (before age 10 years) in at least two of the following areas:
   (1) expressive or receptive language
   (2) social skills or adaptive behavior
   (3) bowel or bladder control
   (4) play
   (5) motor skills
C. Abnormalities of functioning in at least two of the following areas:
   (1) qualitative impairment in social interaction (e.g., impairment in nonverbal behaviors, failure to develop peer relationships, lack of social or emotional reciprocity)
   (2) qualitative impairments in communication (e.g., delay or lack of spoken language, inability to initiate or sustain a conversation, stereotyped and repetitive use of language, lack of varied make-believe play)
   (3) restricted, repetitive, and stereotyped patterns of behavior, interests, and activities, including motor stereotypies and mannerisms
D. The disturbance is not better accounted for by another specific pervasive developmental disorder or by schizophrenia.

From American Psychiatric Association. *Diagnostic and Statistical Manual of Mental Disorders.* 4th ed. Text rev. Washington, DC: American Psychiatric Association; copyright 2000, with permission.

diminishing in days or weeks. In some cases, a child displays restlessness, increased activity level, and anxiety before the loss of function. The core features of the disorder include loss of communication skills, marked regression of reciprocal interactions, and the onset of stereotyped movements and compulsive behavior. Affective symptoms are common, particularly anxiety, as is the regression of self-help skills, such as bowel and bladder control.

To receive the diagnosis, a child must exhibit loss of skills in two of the following areas: language, social, or adaptive behavior; bowel or bladder control; play; and motor skills. Abnormalities must be present in at least two of the following categories: reciprocal social interaction, communication skills, and stereotyped or restricted behavior. The main neurological associated feature is seizure disorder.

Bob's early history was within normal limits. By age 2, he was speaking in sentences, and his development appeared to be proceeding appropriately. At age 40 months he abruptly exhibited a period of marked behavioral regression shortly after the birth of a sibling. He lost previously acquired skills in communication and was no longer toilet trained. He became uninterested in social interaction, and various unusual self-stimulatory behaviors became evident. Comprehensive medical examination failed to reveal any conditions that might account for this developmental regression. Behaviorally, he exhibited features of autistic disorder. At follow-up at age 12 he spoke only an occasional single word and was severely retarded. (Courtesy of Fred Volkmar, M.D.)

Differential Diagnosis

The differential diagnosis of childhood disintegrative disorder includes autistic disorder and Rett's disorder. In many cases, the clinical features overlap with autistic disorder, but childhood disintegrative disorder is distinguished from autistic disorder by the loss of previously acquired development. Before the onset of childhood disintegrative disorder (occurring at 2 years or older), language has usually progressed to sentence formation. This skill is strikingly different from the premorbid history of even high-functioning patients with autistic disorder, in whom language generally does not exceed single words or phrases before diagnosis of the disorder. Once the disorder occurs, however, those with childhood disintegrative disorder are more likely to have no language abilities than are high-functioning patients with autistic disorder. In Rett's disorder, the deterioration occurs much earlier than in childhood disintegrative disorder, and the characteristic hand stereotypies of Rett's disorder do not occur in childhood disintegrative disorder.

Course and Prognosis

The course of childhood disintegrative disorder is variable, with a plateau reached in most cases, a progressive deteriorating course in rare cases, and some improvement in occasional cases to the point of regaining the ability to speak in sentences. Most patients are left with at least moderate mental retardation.

39 ▲

Attention-Deficit Disorders

ATTENTION-DEFICIT/HYPERACTIVITY DISORDER

Attention-deficit/hyperactivity disorder (ADHD) is character-ized by a pattern of diminished sustained attention and higher levels of impulsivity in a child or adolescent than expected for someone of that age and developmental level. Whereas in the past, hyperactivity was believed to be the underlying impairing symptom in this disorder, the current consensus is that hyperac-tivity is often secondary to poor impulse control. Impulsivity and hyperactivity share one dimension in today's diagnostic criteria for ADHD. The diagnosis of ADHD is based on the consensus of experts that three observable subtypes—*inattentive*, *hyperactive/ impulsive*, and *combined*—are all manifestations of the same disorder. To meet the criteria for the diagnosis of ADHD, some symptoms must be present before the age of 7 years, although ADHD is not diagnosed in many children until they are older than 7 years when their behaviors cause problems in school and other places. To confirm a diagnosis of ADHD, impairment from inattention and/or hyperactivity-impulsivity must be observable in at least two settings and interfere with developmentally ap-propriate functioning socially, academically, or in extracurric-ular activities. ADHD is not diagnosed when symptoms occur in a child, adolescent, or adult with a pervasive developmental disorder, schizophrenia, or other psychotic disorder.

Epidemiology

Reports on the incidence of ADHD in the United States have varied from 2 to 20 percent of grade-school children. A conser-vative figure is about 3 to 7 percent of prepubertal elementary school children. In Great Britain a lower incidence is reported than in the United States, less than 1 percent. ADHD is more prevalent in boys than in girls, with the ratio ranging from 2:1 to as much as 9:1. First-degree biological relatives (e.g., siblings of probands with ADHD) are at high risk to develop it as well as to develop other disorders, including disruptive behavior disorders, anxiety disorders, and depressive disorders. Siblings of children with ADHD are also at higher risk than the general population to have learning disorders and academic difficulties. The parents of children with ADHD show an increased incidence of hyperkine-sis, sociopathy, alcohol use disorders, and conversion disorder. Symptoms of ADHD are often present by age 3 years, but the diagnosis is generally not made until the child is in a structured school setting, such as preschool or kindergarten, when teacher information is available comparing the attention and impulsivity of the child in question with peers of the same age.

Etiology

Genetic Factors. Evidence for a genetic contribution to the emer-gence of ADHD includes greater concordance in monozygotic than in dizygotic twins. In addition, siblings of hyperactive children have about twice the risk of having the disorder as those in the general population. One sibling may have predominantly hyperactivity symptoms, and oth-ers may have predominantly inattention symptoms. Biological parents of children with the disorder have a higher risk for ADHD than adoptive parents. Children with ADHD are at higher risk of developing conduct disorders, and alcohol use disorders and antisocial personality disorder are more common in their parents than in the general population.

Developmental Factors. Reports in the literature state that September is the peak month for births of children with ADHD with and without comorbid learning disorders. The implication is that prenatal exposure to winter infections during the first trimester may contribute to the emergence of ADHD symptoms in some susceptible children.

BRAIN DAMAGE. It has been speculated that some children affected by ADHD had subtle damage to the central nervous system (CNS) and brain development during their fetal and perinatal periods. The hypothe-sized brain damage may potentially be associated with circulatory, toxic, metabolic, mechanical, or physical insult to the brain during early infancy caused by infection, inflammation, and trauma. Children with ADHD ex-hibit nonfocal (soft) neurological signs at higher rates than those in the general population.

Neurochemical Factors. Many neurotransmitters have been associated with ADHD symptoms. Animal studies have shown that the locus ceruleus, consisting of mainly noradrenergic neurons, plays a major role in attention. The noradrenergic system consists of the central system (originating in the locus ceruleus) and the peripheral sympathetic sys-tem. The peripheral noradrenergic system may be of more importance in ADHD. Thus, a dysfunction in peripheral epinephrine, which causes the hormone to accumulate peripherally, could potentially feed back to the central system and "reset" the locus ceruleus to a lower level. In part, hypotheses about the neurochemistry of the disorder have arisen from the impact of many medications that exert a positive effect on it. The most widely studied drugs in the treatment of ADHD—the stimulants— affect both dopamine and norepinephrine, leading to neurotransmitter hypotheses that include possible dysfunction in both the adrenergic and the dopaminergic systems. Stimulants increase catecholamine concen-trations by promoting their release and blocking their uptake. Stimulants and some tricyclic drugs—for example, desipramine (Norpramin)— reduce levels of urinary 3-methoxy-4-hydroxyphenylglycol, a metabo-lite of norepinephrine. Clonidine (Catapres), a norepinephrine agonist, has been helpful in treating hyperactivity. Other drugs that have reduced hyperactivity include tricyclic drugs and monoamine oxidase inhibitors. Overall, no clear-cut evidence implicates a single neurotransmitter in the development of ADHD, but many neurotransmitters may be involved in the process.

Neurophysiological Factors.   The human brain normally undergoes major growth spurts at several ages: 3 to 10 months, 2 to 4 years, 6 to 8 years, 10 to 12 years, and 14 to 16 years. Some children have a maturational delay in the sequence and manifest symptoms of ADHD that appear to normalize by about age 5 years. A physiological correlate is the presence of a variety of nonspecific abnormal electroencephalogram (EEG) patterns that are disorganized and characteristic of young children. In some cases, the EEG findings normalize over time. A recent study of quantitative EEGs in children with ADHD, in children with undifferentiated attentional problems, and in normal controls indicates that both groups with attentional problems evince increased beta-band relative percentages and decreased rare tone P3000 amplitudes. Increased beta-band percentage or decreased delta-band percentage is associated with increased arousal.

Computed tomographic head scans of children with ADHD show no consistent findings. Studies using positron emission tomography (PET) have found lower cerebral blood flow and metabolic rates in the frontal lobe areas of children with ADHD than in controls. PET scans have also shown that female adolescents with the disorder have globally lower glucose metabolism than both normal control females and males with the disorder. One theory explains these findings by supposing that the frontal lobes in children with ADHD are not adequately performing their inhibitory mechanism on lower structures, an effect leading to disinhibition.

Psychosocial Factors.   Children in institutions are frequently overactive and have poor attention spans. These signs result from prolonged emotional deprivation, and they disappear when deprivational factors are removed, such as through adoption or placement in a foster home. Stressful psychic events, disruption of family equilibrium, and other anxiety-inducing factors contribute to the initiation or perpetuation of ADHD. Predisposing factors may include the child's temperament, genetic-familial factors, and the demands of society to adhere to a routinized way of behaving and performing. Socioeconomic status does not seem to be a predisposing factor.

Diagnosis

The principal signs of inattention, impulsivity, and hyperactivity are based on a detailed history of a child's early developmental patterns along with direct observation of the child, especially in situations that require sustained attention. Hyperactivity may be more severe in some situations (e.g., school) and less marked in others (e.g., one-on-one interviews), and it may be less obvious in pleasant structured activities (sports). The diagnosis of ADHD requires persistent, impairing symptoms of either hyperactivity/impulsivity or inattention that cause impairment in at least two different settings. For example, many children with ADHD have difficulties in school and at home. The diagnostic criteria for ADHD are outlined in Table 39–1.

Other distinguishing features of ADHD are short attention span and easy distractibility. In school, children with ADHD cannot follow instructions and often demand extra attention from their teachers. At home, they often do not comply with their parents' requests. They act impulsively, show emotional lability, and are explosive and irritable.

Children who have hyperactivity as a predominant feature are more likely to be referred for treatment than are children with primarily symptoms of attention deficit. Children with the predominantly hyperactive-impulsive type are more likely to have a stable diagnosis over time and to have concurrent conduct disorder than are children with the predominantly inattentive type

without hyperactivity. Disorders involving reading, arithmetic, language, and coordination can occur in association with ADHD. A child's history may give clues to prenatal (including genetic), natal, and postnatal factors that may have affected the CNS structure or function. Rates of development, deviations in development, and parental reactions to significant or stressful behavioral transitions should be ascertained because they may help clinicians determine the degree to which parents have contributed or reacted to a child's inefficiencies and dysfunctions.

School history and teachers' reports are important in evaluating whether a child's difficulties in learning and school behavior are primarily caused by the child's inability to sustain attention or compromised understanding of the academic material. Additional school difficulties can result from attitudinal or maturational problems, social rejection, and poor self-image because of felt inadequacies. These reports may also reveal how the child has handled these problems. How the child has related to siblings, to peers, to adults, and to free and structured activities gives valuable diagnostic clues to the presence of ADHD and helps identify the complications of the disorder.

The mental status examination may show a secondarily depressed mood but no thought disturbance, impaired reality testing, or inappropriate affect. A child may show great distractibility, perseveration, and a concrete and literal mode of thinking. Indications of visual-perceptual, auditory-perceptual, language, or cognition problems may be present. Occasionally, evidence appears of a basic, pervasive, organically based anxiety, often referred to as *body anxiety*. A neurological examination may reveal visual, motor, perceptual, or auditory discriminatory immaturity or impairments without overt signs of visual or auditory acuity disorders. Children may have problems with motor coordination and difficulty copying age-appropriate figures, rapid alternating movements, right-left discrimination, ambidexterity, reflex asymmetries, and a variety of subtle nonfocal neurological signs (soft signs).

Clinicians should obtain an EEG to recognize the child with frequent bilaterally synchronous discharges resulting in short absence spells. Such a child may react in school with hyperactivity out of sheer frustration. The child with an unrecognized temporal lobe seizure focus can have a secondary behavior disorder. In these instances, several features of ADHD are often present. Identification of the focus requires an EEG obtained during drowsiness and during sleep.

Clinical Features

Attention-deficit/hyperactivity disorder can have its onset in infancy, although it is rarely recognized until a child is at least toddler age. Infants with the disorder are unduly sensitive to stimuli and are easily upset by noise, light, temperature, and other environmental changes. At times, the reverse occurs, and the children are placid and limp, sleep much of the time, and appear to develop slowly in the first months of life. More commonly, however, infants with ADHD are active in the crib, sleep little, and cry a great deal. They are far less likely than normal children to reduce their locomotor activity when their environment is structured by social limits.

In school, children with ADHD may attack a test rapidly but answer only the first two questions. They may be unable to wait to be called on in school and may respond before everyone else.

Table 39–2
Stimulant Medications in the Treatment of Attention-Deficit/Hyperactivity Disorder (ADHD)

Medication	Preparation (mg)	Approximate Duration (hrs)	Recommended Dose
Methylphenidate preparations			
Ritalin	5, 10, 15, 20	3–4	0.3–1 mg/kg t.i.d; up to 60 mg/day
Ritalin-SR	20	8	Up to 60 mg/day
Concerta	18, 36, 54	12	Up to 54 mg q AM
Metadate ER	10, 20	8	Up to 60 mg/day
Metadate CD	20	12	Up to 60 mg q AM
Ritalin LA	5, 10, 15, 20	8	
Dexmethylphenidate preparation			
Focalin	2.5, 5, 10	3–4	Up to 10 mg
Focalin XR	5, 10, 20	6–8	Up to 20 mg
Dextroamphetamine preparations			
Dexedrine	5, 10	3–4	0.15–0.5 mg/kg b.i.d.; up to 40 mg/day
Dexedrine Spansule	5, 10, 15	8	Up to 40 mg/day
Dextroamphetamine and amphetamine salt preparations			
Adderall	5, 10, 20, 30	4–6	0.15–0.5 mg/kg b.i.d.; up to 40 mg/day
Adderall XR	10, 20, 30	12	Up to 40 mg q AM
Proamphetamine preparation			
Lisdexamfetamine	30, 50, 70	8	30–70 mg/day

b.i.d., twice daily; q, every; t.i.d., three times daily.

lisdexamfetamine (Vyvanse) was also released. Advantages of the sustained-release preparations for children are that one dose in the morning will sustain the effects all day, and the child is no longer required to interrupt his or her school day, as well as the physiological advantage that the medication is sustained at an approximately even level in the body throughout the day so that periods of rebound and irritability are avoided. Table 39–2 contains comparative information on these medications. Second-line agents with evidence of efficacy for some children and adolescents with ADHD include atomoxetine (Stratera), a norepinephrine uptake inhibitor, shown to be effective in the treatment of children with ADHD; antidepressants, such as bupropion (Wellbutrin, Wellbutrin SR), venlafaxine (Effexor, Effexor XR); and the α-adrenergic receptor agonists clonidine (Catapres), and guanfacine (Tenex). The U.S. Food and Drug Administration approved the use of dextroamphetamine in children 3 years of age and older and methylphenidate in children 6 years of age and older. These are the two most commonly used pharmacological agents for the treatment of children with ADHD.

A prodrug of amphetamine called lisdexamfetamine was recently approved for ADHD. It has a similar side-effect profile to amphetamine and is prescribed once a day. In children 6 to 12 years of age, the recommended dose is 30 mg/day given in the morning. If required, the dose may be increased incrementally by 20 mg/day at weekly intervals to a maximum of 70 mg/day. It is available in 30-, 50-, or 70-mg extended-release capsules.

TREATMENT OF CNS STIMULANT SIDE EFFECTS. CNS stimulants are generally well tolerated, and the consensus is that once-a-day dosing is preferable with regard to convenience and rebound side effects. A recent study of the long-term tolerability of once-daily mixed amphetamine salts has shown mild side effects, most commonly decreased appetite, insomnia, and headache.

Given the predictable side effects of central stimulant medications, strategies have been developed to ameliorate these problems. For example, a variety of strategies have been suggested by experts for a given child or adolescent with ADHD who re-

sponds favorably to methylphenidate (Concerta) but for whom insomnia has become a significant problem. Suggestions for the management of insomnia in such a case include the use of diphenhydramine (25 to 75 mg), a low dose of trazodone (25 to 50 mg), or the addition of an α-adrenergic agent, such as guanfacine. In some cases, insomnia may attenuate on its own after several months of treatment.

Monitoring Pharmacological Treatment

Stimulants.   At baseline, the most recent American Academy of Child and Adolescent Psychiatry practice parameters recommend the following workup before starting use of stimulant medications: physical examination, blood pressure, pulse, weight, and height. It is recommended that children and adolescents being treated with stimulants have their height, weight, blood pressure, and pulse checked on a quarterly basis and have a physical examination annually.

EVALUATION OF THERAPEUTIC PROGRESS.   Monitoring starts with the initiation of medication. Because school performance is most markedly affected, special attention and effort should be given to establishing and maintaining a close collaborative working relationship with a child's school personnel. In most patients, stimulants reduce overactivity, distractibility, impulsiveness, explosiveness, and irritability. No evidence indicates that medications directly improve any existing impairments in learning, although, when the attention deficits diminish, children can learn more effectively. In addition, medication can improve self-esteem when children are no longer constantly reprimanded for their behavior.

Psychosocial Interventions.   Medication alone is often not sufficient to satisfy the comprehensive therapeutic needs of children with the disorder and is usually but one facet of a multimodality regimen. Social skills groups, training for parents of children with ADHD, and behavioral interventions at school and at home are often efficacious in the overall management of children with ADHD. Evaluation and treatment of coexisting learning disorders or additional psychiatric disorders is important.

Children who are prescribed medications should be taught the purpose of the medication and given the opportunity to reveal their feelings about it. Doing so helps dispel misconceptions about medication use (such as "I'm crazy") and makes it clear that the medication helps the child handle situations better than before. When children are helped to structure their environment, their anxiety diminishes. It is often beneficial for parents and teachers to work together to develop a concrete set of expectations for the child and a system of rewards for the child when the expectations are met.

A common goal of therapy is to help parents of children with ADHD recognize and promote the notion that, although the child may not "voluntarily" exhibit symptoms of ADHD, he or she is still capable of being responsible for meeting reasonable expectations. Parents should also be helped to recognize that, despite their child's difficulties, every child faces the normal tasks of maturation, including significant building of self-esteem when he or she develops a sense of mastery. Therefore, children with ADHD do not benefit from being exempted from the requirements, expectations, and planning applicable to other children. Parental training is an integral part of the psychotherapeutic interventions for ADHD. Most parental training is based on helping parents develop usable behavioral interventions with positive reinforcement that target both social and academic behaviors.

Group therapy aimed at both refining social skills and increasing self-esteem and a sense of success may be very useful for children with ADHD, who have great difficulty functioning in group settings, especially in school. A recent year-long group therapy intervention in a clinical setting for boys with the disorder described the goals as helping the boys improve skills in game playing and feeling a sense of mastery with peers. The boys were first asked to do a task that was fun, in pairs, and then were gradually asked to do projects in a group. They were directed in following instructions, waiting, and paying attention and were praised for successful cooperation. This level of highly structured group therapeutic "play" is developmentally appropriate for these children, who benefit from an increased ability to participate in any group activities.

ATTENTION-DEFICIT/HYPERACTIVITY DISORDER NOT OTHERWISE SPECIFIED

The DSM-IV-TR includes ADHD not otherwise specified as a residual category for disturbances with prominent symptoms of inattention or hyperactivity that do not meet the criteria for ADHD.

ADULT MANIFESTATIONS OF ADHD

Attention-deficit/hyperactivity disorder was historically believed to be a childhood condition resulting in delayed development of impulse control that would be outgrown by adolescence. Only in the last few decades have adults with ADHD been identified, diagnosed, and successfully treated. Longitudi-

nal follow-up has shown that up to 40 to 60 percent of children with ADHD have persistent impairment from symptoms into adulthood. Genetic studies, brain imaging, and neurocognitive and pharmacological studies in adults with ADHD have virtually replicated findings demonstrated in children with ADHD. Increased public awareness and treatment studies within the last decade have led to widespread acceptance of the need for diagnosis and treatment of adults with ADHD.

Epidemiology

Among adults, evidence suggests an approximate 4 percent prevalence of ADHD in the population. ADHD in adulthood is generally diagnosed by self-report, given the lack of school information and observer information available; therefore, it is more difficult to make an accurate diagnosis.

Etiology

ADHD is believed to be largely transmitted genetically, and increasing evidence supports this hypothesis, including the genetic studies, twin studies, and family studies outlined in the child and adolescent ADHD section. Brain imaging studies have obtained data suggesting that adults with ADHD exhibit decreased prefrontal glucose metabolism on PET compared with adults without ADHD. It is unclear whether these data reflect the presence of the disorder or a secondary effect of having ADHD over a period of time. Further studies using single photon emission tomography have revealed increased dopamine transporter (DAT) binding densities in the striatum of the brain in samples of adults with ADHD. This finding may be understood within the context of treatment for ADHD, in that standard stimulant treatment for ADHD, such as methylphenidate, acts to block DAT activity, possibly leading to a normalization of the striatal brain region in individuals with ADHD.

Factors associated with early childhood emergence of ADHD include premature birth, maternal use of nicotine during the pregnancy, and increased serum lead levels. Factors that protect against emergence of ADHD until later in childhood are not known.

Diagnosis and Clinical Features

The clinical phenomenology of ADHD in children that has evolved over the last few decades has resulted in features of inattention and manifestations of impulsivity prevailing as the core of this disorder. A leading figure in the development of criteria for adult manifestations of ADHD is Paul Wender, from the University of Utah, who began his work on adult ADHD in the 1970s. Wender developed criteria that could be applied to adults. They included a retrospective diagnosis of ADHD in childhood and evidence of current impairment from ADHD symptoms in adulthood. Furthermore, evidence exists of several additional symptoms that are typical of adult behavior as opposed to childhood behaviors.

In adults, residual signs of the disorder include impulsivity and attention deficit (e.g., difficulty in organizing and completing work, inability to concentrate, increased distractibility, and sudden decision making without thought of the consequences). Many people with the disorder have a secondary depressive

Table 40–1
DSM-IV-TR Diagnostic Criteria for Oppositional Defiant Disorder

A. A pattern of negativistic, hostile, and defiant behavior lasting at least 6 months, during which four (or more) of the following are present:
   (1) often loses temper
   (2) often argues with adults
   (3) often actively defies or refuses to comply with adults' requests or rules
   (4) often deliberately annoys people
   (5) often blames others for his or her mistakes or misbehavior
   (6) is often touchy or easily annoyed by others
   (7) is often angry and resentful
   (8) is often spiteful or vindictive
Note: Consider a criterion met only if the behavior occurs more frequently than is typically observed in individuals of comparable age and developmental level.
B. The disturbance in behavior causes clinically significant impairment in social, academic, or occupational functioning.
C. The behaviors do not occur exclusively during the course of a psychotic or mood disorder.
D. Criteria are not met for conduct disorder, and, if the individual is age 18 years or older, criteria are not met for antisocial personality disorder.

From American Psychiatric Association. *Diagnostic and Statistical Manual of Mental Disorders.* 4th ed. Text rev. Washington, DC: American Psychiatric Association; copyright 2000, with permission.

These children are often friendless and perceive human relationships as unsatisfactory. Despite adequate intelligence, they do poorly or fail in school, as they withhold participation, resist external demands, and insist on solving problems without others' help. Secondary to these difficulties are low self-esteem, poor frustration tolerance, depressed mood, and temper outbursts. Adolescents may abuse alcohol and illegal substances. Often, the disturbance evolves into a conduct disorder or a mood disorder.

Pathology and Laboratory Examination.   No specific laboratory tests or pathological findings help diagnose oppositional defiant disorder. Because some children with the disorder become physically aggressive and violate the rights of others as they get older, they may share some of the same characteristics under investigation in violent people, such as low serotonin levels in the central nervous system (CNS).

Differential Diagnosis

Because oppositional behavior is both normal and adaptive at specific developmental stages, these periods of negativism must be distinguished from oppositional defiant disorder. Developmental-stage oppositional behavior, which is of shorter duration than oppositional defiant disorder, is neither considerably more frequent nor more intense than that seen in other children of the same mental age.

Oppositional defiant behavior occurring temporarily in reaction to a stress should be diagnosed as an adjustment disorder. When features of oppositional defiant disorder appear during the course of conduct disorder, schizophrenia, or a mood disorder, the diagnosis of oppositional defiant disorder should not be made. Oppositional and negativistic behaviors can also be present in

attention-deficit/hyperactivity disorder (ADHD), cognitive disorders, and mental retardation. Whether a concomitant diagnosis of oppositional defiant disorder should be made depends on the severity, pervasiveness, and duration of such behavior. Some young children who receive a diagnosis of oppositional defiant disorder go on in several years to meet the criteria for conduct disorder. Some investigators believe that the two disorders may be developmental variants of each other, with conduct disorder being the natural progression of oppositional defiant behavior when a child matures. Most children with oppositional defiant disorder, however, do not later meet the criteria for conduct disorder, and up to one fourth of children with oppositional defiant disorder may not meet the diagnosis several years later.

The subtype of oppositional defiant disorder that tends to progress to conduct disorder is one in which aggression is prominent. Most children who have ADHD and conduct disorder develop conduct disorder before the age of 12 years. Most children who develop conduct disorder have a history of oppositional defiant disorder. Overall, the current consensus is that two subtypes of oppositional defiant disorder may exist. One type, which is likely to progress to conduct disorder, includes certain symptoms of conduct disorder (e.g., fighting, bullying). The other type, which is characterized by less aggression and fewer antisocial traits, does not progress to conduct disorder.

Jared, age 8 years, was brought to the clinic for evaluation of misbehavior by his mother. She complained that he has frequent tantrums, usually in response to limits on his behavior or not getting his way. She describes the tantrums as consisting of shouting, cursing, crying, slamming doors, and sometimes throwing books or objects on the floor. She states that these outbursts occur almost daily. She feels that sometimes it seems as though he is trying to provoke her. Recently, he was kicking his foot against his mother's chair and she asked him to stop. He looked at her and continued to kick her chair. She says that she has given up on asking him to pick up his room or help with chores, because it inevitably results in an argument. Jared appears sullen and irritable on interview. He says that it was his mother's fault and she is always after him about one thing or another. He interrupts her several times during the joint interview, saying that she was lying or giving his version of events. His grades at school are excellent, and there are no reports of any behavior problems or disobedience at school. His mother says that he does not have many friends because he has difficulty sharing his things and tends to be bossy. He had a series of ear infections as an infant and occasionally experiences seasonal allergies, but is otherwise in good health, with normal physical development. His mother describes him as being fussy as an infant and difficult to comfort when upset. He is an only child, and his parents separated and divorced when he was 3. He has had no contact with his father since then. His mother was depressed for a year after the divorce until she sought treatment. She has always felt guilty that his father is not in his life and worries that he blames her for not having his father around. She believes his behaviors have become worse since she recently started dating again. (Courtesy of Christopher R. Thomas, M.D.)

Course and Prognosis

The course of oppositional defiant disorder depends largely on the severity of the symptoms and the ability of the child to develop more-adaptive responses to authority. The stability of oppositional defiant disorder varies over time. Persistence of oppositional defiant symptoms poses an increased risk of additional disorders, such as conduct disorder and substance use disorders. Positive outcomes are more likely for intact families who can modify their own expression of demands and give less attention to the child's argumentative behaviors.

About one fourth of all children who receive the diagnosis of oppositional defiant disorder do not continue to meet diagnostic criteria over the next several years. It is not clear in these cases whether the criteria captured children whose behavior was not developmentally abnormal or the disorder spontaneously remitted. Patients in whom the diagnosis persists may remain stable or go on to violate the rights of others and, thus, develop conduct disorder. Such patients should receive guarded prognoses.

An association exists between conduct disorder and later substance use disorders, as well as elevated rates of mood disorders, in children with oppositional defiant disorder, conduct disorder, and ADHD. Parental psychopathology, such as antisocial personality disorder and substance abuse, appears to be more common in families with children who have oppositional defiant disorder than in the general population, which creates additional risks for chaotic and troubled home environments. The prognosis for oppositional defiant disorder in a child depends somewhat on family functioning and the development of comorbid psychopathology.

Treatment

The primary treatment of oppositional defiant disorder is family intervention using both direct training of the parents in child management skills and careful assessment of family interactions. Behavior therapists emphasize teaching parents how to alter their behavior to discourage the child's oppositional behavior and encourage appropriate behavior. Behavior therapy focuses on selectively reinforcing and praising appropriate behavior and ignoring or not reinforcing undesired behavior.

Children with oppositional defiant behavior may also benefit from individual psychotherapy insofar as the child is exposed to a situation with an adult in which to "practice" more-adaptive responses. In the therapeutic relationship, the child can learn new strategies to develop a sense of mastery and success in social situations with peers and families. In the safety of a more "neutral" relationship, children may discover that they are capable of less provocative behavior. Often, self-esteem must be restored before a child with oppositional defiant disorder can make more positive responses to external control. Parent–child conflict strongly predicts conduct problems; patterns of harsh physical and verbal punishment particularly evoke the emergence of aggression and deviance in children. Thus, it is likely that eliminating harsh, punitive parenting and increasing positive parent–child interactions may positively influence the course of oppositional and defiant behaviors.

CONDUCT DISORDER

Children with conduct disorder are likely to demonstrate behaviors in the following four categories: physical aggression or threats of harm to people, destruction of their own property or that of others, theft or acts of deceit, and frequent violation of age-appropriate rules. Conduct disorder is an enduring set of behaviors that evolves over time, usually characterized by aggression and violation of the rights of others. Conduct disorder is associated with many other psychiatric disorders, including ADHD, depression, and learning disorders, and it is also associated with certain psychosocial factors, such as harsh, punitive parenting, family discord, lack of appropriate parental supervision, lack of social competence, and low socioeconomic level. The DSM-IV-TR criteria require three specific behaviors of the 15 listed, which include bullying, threatening, or intimidating others and staying out at night despite parental prohibitions, beginning before 13 years of age. DSM-IV-TR also specifies that truancy from school must begin before 13 years of age to be considered a symptom of conduct disorder. The disorder can be diagnosed in a person older than 18 years only if the criteria for antisocial personality disorder are not met. DSM-IV-TR describes a mild level of the disorder as showing few, if any, conduct problems in excess of those needed to make the diagnosis and conduct problems that cause only minor harm to others. According to DSM-IV-TR, the severe level shows many conduct problems in excess of the minimal diagnostic criteria or conduct problems that cause considerable harm to others.

Epidemiology

Occasional rule breaking and rebellious behavior is common during childhood and adolescence, but in youth with conduct disorder, behaviors that violate the rights of others are repetitive and pervasive. Estimated rates of conduct disorder among the general population range from 1 to 10 percent, with a general population rate of approximately 5 percent. The disorder is more common among boys than girls, and the ratio ranges from 4:1 to as much as 12:1. Conduct disorder occurs with greater frequency in the children of parents with antisocial personality disorder and alcohol dependence than in the general population. The prevalence of conduct disorder and antisocial behavior is associated with socioeconomic factors.

Etiology

No single factor can fully account for a child's antisocial behavior and conduct disorder. Rather, many biopsychosocial factors contribute to development of the disorder.

Parental Factors.   Harsh, punitive parenting characterized by severe physical and verbal aggression is associated with the development of children's maladaptive aggressive behaviors. Chaotic home conditions are associated with conduct disorder and delinquency. Divorce itself is considered a risk factor, but the persistence of hostility, resentment, and bitterness between divorced parents may be the more important contributor to maladaptive behavior. Parental psychopathology, child abuse, and negligence often contribute to conduct disorder. Sociopathy, alcohol dependence, and substance abuse in the parents are associated with conduct disorder in their children. Parents may be so negligent that a child's care is shared by relatives or assumed by foster parents. Many such parents were scarred by their own upbringing and tend to be abusive, negligent, or engrossed in getting their own personal needs met.

Sociocultural Factors.   Socioeconomically deprived children are at higher risk for the development of conduct disorder, as are children and adolescents who grow up in urban environments. Unemployed

Course and Prognosis

In general, the prognosis for children with conduct disorder is most guarded in those who have symptoms at a young age, exhibit the greatest number of symptoms, and express them most frequently. This finding is true partly because those with severe conduct disorder seem to be most vulnerable to comorbid disorders later in life, such as mood disorders and substance use disorders. It stands to reason that the more concurrent mental disorders a person has, the more troublesome his or her life will be. A recent report found that, although assaultive behavior in childhood and parental criminality predict a high risk for incarceration later in life, the diagnosis of conduct disorder per se was not correlated with imprisonment. A good prognosis is predicted for mild conduct disorder in the absence of coexisting psychopathology and the presence of normal intellectual functioning.

Treatment

Multimodality treatment programs that use all the available family and community resources are likely to bring about the best results in efforts to control conduct-disordered behavior. Multimodal treatments can involve the use of behavioral interventions in which rewards may be earned for prosocial and nonaggressive behaviors, social skills training, family education and therapy, and pharmacological interventions. Overall, treatment programs have been more successful in decreasing overt symptoms of conduct, such as aggression, than the covert symptoms, such as lying or stealing. Treatment strategies for young children that focus on increasing social behavior and social competence are believed to reduce aggressive behavior.

An environmental structure that provides support, along with consistent rules and expected consequences, can help control a variety of problem behaviors. The need for reduction of violence and aggression in schools is an important setting for interventions. A thoughtful approach to the management of threats of violence includes provision of a functioning security hierarchy, peer-participant programs, threat assessment, and crisis response initiatives. All of these strategies increase the structure necessary to maintain a safe school environment. The structure can be applied to family life in some cases so that parents become aware of behavioral techniques and grow proficient at using them to foster appropriate behaviors. Families in which psychopathology or environmental stressors prevent parental understanding of the techniques may require parental psychiatric evaluation and treatment before making such an endeavor. When a family is abusive or chaotic, the child may have to be removed from the home to benefit from a consistent and structured environment. School settings can also use behavioral techniques to promote socially acceptable behavior toward peers and to discourage covert antisocial incidents.

Behaviorally based individual psychotherapy targeting problem-solving skills with appropriate rewards can be useful because children with conduct disorder may have a long-standing pattern of maladaptive responses to daily situations. The age at which treatment begins is important because the longer the maladaptive behaviors continue, the more entrenched they become.

Pharmacological treatments for aggression have become more accepted adjunctive treatment in the context of conduct disorder. Overt explosive aggression responds to several medications. Early studies of antipsychotics, most notably haloperidol (Haldol), reported decreased aggressive and assaultive behaviors in children with a variety of psychiatric disorders. Currently, the atypical antipsychotics risperidone (Risperdal), olanzapine (Zyprexa), quetiapine (Seroquel), ziprasidone (Geodon), and aripiprazole (Abilify) have replaced the older antipsychotics because of their comparable efficacy and improved side-effect profiles. Risperidone has been shown to reduce aggression in children with disruptive behavior disorders in placebo-controlled, randomized trials, particularly in populations with pervasive developmental disorders and aggression. Growing evidence suggests that atypical antipsychotics are efficacious in contributing to the management of aggression among children and adolescents.

Long-term effects of the use of these agents are largely unknown and require further investigation. Side effects include sedation, increased prolactin levels (with risperidone use), and extrapyramidal symptoms, including akathisia. In general, however, the atypical antipsychotics appear to be well tolerated. A preliminary study of clozapine (Clozaril), used mainly in the treatment of refractory schizophrenia, has reported decreased aggressive behavior in a sample of treatment-refractory children and adolescents with schizophrenia and aggressive behavior. Lithium (Eskalith) has been reported to have efficacy for some aggressive children with or without comorbid bipolar disorders. Although previous trials suggested that carbamazepine (Tegretol) may help control aggression, a double-blind, placebo-controlled study did not show superiority of carbamazepine over placebo in decreasing aggression. A recent pilot study found that clonidine (Catapres) may decrease aggression. The selective serotonin reuptake inhibitors, such as fluoxetine (Prozac), sertraline (Zoloft), paroxetine (Paxil), and citalopram (Celexa), have been used in an attempt to diminish impulsivity, irritability, and lability of mood, which often occur with conduct disorder. Conduct disorder frequently coexists with ADHD, learning disorders, and, over time, mood disorders and substance-related disorders; thus, the treatment of any concurrent disorders must also be addressed.

DISRUPTIVE BEHAVIOR DISORDER NOT OTHERWISE SPECIFIED

According to DSM-IV-TR, the category of disruptive behavior disorder not otherwise specified can be used for disorders of conduct or oppositional defiant behaviors that do not meet the diagnostic criteria for either conduct disorder or oppositional defiant disorder but in which there is notable impairment (Table 40–3).

Table 40–3
DSM-IV-TR Diagnostic Criteria for Disruptive Behavior Disorder Not Otherwise Specified

This category is for disorders characterized by conduct or oppositional defiant behaviors that do not meet the criteria for conduct disorder or oppositional defiant disorder. For example, include clinical presentations that do not meet full criteria either for oppositional defiant disorder or conduct disorder, but in which there is clinically significant impairment.

From American Psychiatric Association. *Diagnostic and Statistical Manual of Mental Disorders.* 4th ed. Text rev. Washington, DC: American Psychiatric Association; copyright 2000, with permission.

41 ◢

Feeding and Eating Disorders of Infancy or Early Childhood

PICA

In the text revision of the fourth edition of the *Diagnostic and Statistical Manual of Mental Disorders* (DSM-IV-TR), pica is described as persistent eating of nonnutritive substances for at least 1 month. The behavior must be developmentally inappropriate, not culturally sanctioned, and sufficiently severe to merit clinical attention. Pica is diagnosed even when these symptoms occur in the context of another disorder, such as autistic disorder, schizophrenia, or Kleine-Levin syndrome. Pica appears much more frequently in young children than in adults; it also occurs in persons with mental retardation. Among adults, certain forms of pica, including geophagia (clay eating) and amylophagia (starch eating), have been reported in pregnant women.

Epidemiology

A survey of a large clinic population reported that 75 percent of 12-month-old infants and 15 percent of 2- to 3-year-old toddlers placed nonnutritive substances in their mouth. Pica is more common among children and adolescents with mental retardation. It has been reported in up to 15 percent of persons with severe mental retardation. Pica appears to affect both sexes equally.

Etiology

Pica is most often a transient disorder that typically lasts for several months and then remits. In younger children, it is more frequently seen among children with developmental speech and social developmental delays. A substantial number of adolescents with pica exhibited depressive symptoms and use of substances. Several theories have been proposed to explain the phenomenon of pica, but none has been universally accepted. A higher-than-expected incidence of pica seems to occur in the relatives of persons with the symptoms. Nutritional deficiencies have been postulated as causes of pica; in particular circumstances, cravings for nonedible substances have been produced by dietary insufficiencies. For example, cravings for dirt and ice are sometimes associated with iron and zinc deficiencies, which are corrected by their administration. A high incidence of parental neglect and deprivation has been associated with cases of pica. Theories relating children's psychological deprivation and subsequent ingestion of inedible substances have suggested that pica is a compensatory mechanism to satisfy oral needs.

Diagnosis and Clinical Features

Eating nonedible substances repeatedly after 18 months of age is usually considered abnormal. The onset of pica is usually between ages 12 and 24 months, and the incidence declines with age. The specific substances ingested vary with their accessibility, and they increase with a child's mastery of locomotion and the resultant increased independence and decreased parental supervision. Typically, young children ingest paint, plaster, string, hair, and cloth; older children with pica may ingest dirt, animal feces, stones, and paper. The clinical implications can be benign or life threatening, depending on the objects ingested. Among the most serious complications are lead poisoning (usually from lead-based paint), intestinal parasites after ingestion of soil or feces, anemia and zinc deficiency after ingestion of clay, severe iron deficiency after ingestion of large quantities of starch, and intestinal obstruction from the ingestion of hair balls, stones, or gravel. Except in persons with mental retardation, pica usually remits by adolescence. Pica associated with pregnancy is usually limited to the pregnancy itself. The DSM-IV-TR diagnostic criteria for pica are given in Table 41–1.

Pathology and Laboratory Examination

No single laboratory test confirms or rules out a diagnosis of pica, but several laboratory tests are useful because pica has frequently been associated with abnormal indexes. Levels of iron and zinc in serum should always be determined; in many cases of pica, these levels are low and may contribute to the development of pica. Pica may disappear when oral iron and zinc are administered. A patient's hemoglobin level should be determined; if the level is low, anemia can result. In children with pica, the lead level in serum should be determined; lead poisoning can result from ingesting lead. When a child's lead level is high, this condition must be treated.

Differential Diagnosis

The differential diagnosis of pica includes iron and zinc deficiencies. Pica also can occur in conjunction with failure to thrive and several other mental and medical disorders, including schizophrenia, autistic disorder, anorexia nervosa, and Kleine-Levin syndrome. In psychosocial dwarfism, a dramatic but reversible endocrinological and behavioral form of failure to thrive, children often show bizarre behaviors, including ingesting toilet

Table 41–1
DSM-IV-TR Diagnostic Criteria for Pica

A. Persistent eating of nonnutritive substances for a period of at least 1 month.
B. The eating of nonnutritive substances is inappropriate to the developmental level.
C. The eating behavior is not part of a culturally sanctioned practice.
D. If the eating behavior occurs exclusively during the course of another mental disorder (e.g., mental retardation, pervasive developmental disorder, schizophrenia), it is sufficiently severe to warrant independent clinical attention.

From American Psychiatric Association. *Diagnostic and Statistical Manual of Mental Disorders.* 4th ed. Text rev. Washington, DC: American Psychiatric Association; copyright 2000, with permission.

water, garbage, and other nonnutritive substances. A recent case report presented an association of pica with hypersomnolence, lead intoxication, and precocious puberty. Precocious puberty implicates the hypothalamus as a site for at least part of the dysfunction. Lead intoxication is known to be associated with pica as well as several other neuropsychiatric abnormalities in memory and cognitive performance. A few children with autistic disorder and schizophrenia may have pica. For children who exhibit pica along with another medical disorder, both disorders should be coded according to DSM-IV-TR.

In certain regions of the world and among certain cultures, such as the Australian aborigines, rates of pica in pregnant women are reportedly high. According to DSM-IV-TR, however, if such practices are culturally accepted, the diagnostic criteria for pica are not met.

Course and Prognosis

The prognosis for pica is usually good because in children of normal intelligence it generally remits spontaneously within several months. In childhood, pica usually resolves with increasing age; in pregnant women, pica is usually limited to the term of the pregnancy. In some adults, however, especially those with mental retardation, pica can continue for years. Follow-up data on these populations are too limited to permit conclusions.

Treatment

The first step in the treatment of pica is determining the cause whenever possible. When pica is associated with situations of neglect or maltreatment, these circumstances naturally need to be altered. Exposure to toxic substances, such as lead, must also be eliminated. No definitive treatment exists for pica; most treatment is aimed at education and behavior modification. Treatments emphasize psychosocial, environmental, behavioral, and family guidance approaches. An effort should be made to ameliorate any significant psychosocial stressors. When lead is present in the surroundings, it must be eliminated or rendered inaccessible or the child must be moved to new surroundings.

Several behavioral techniques have been used with some effect. The most rapidly successful technique seems to be mild aversion therapy or negative reinforcement (e.g., a mild electric shock, an unpleasant noise, or an emetic drug). Positive reinforcement, modeling, behavioral shaping, and overcorrec-

tion treatment have also been used. Increasing parental attention, stimulation, and emotional nurturance may yield positive results. One study found that pica was negatively correlated with involvement with play materials and occurred most frequently in impoverished environments. In some patients, correcting an iron or zinc deficiency has eliminated pica. Medical complications (e.g., lead poisoning) that develop secondarily to the pica must also be treated.

RUMINATION DISORDER

Rumination can be observed in developmentally normal infants who put their thumb or hand in the mouth, suck their tongue rhythmically, and arch their back to initiate regurgitation. This behavior pattern is not infrequently observed in infants who receive inadequate emotional interaction and have learned to soothe and stimulate themselves through rumination. The onset of the disorder generally occurs after 3 months of age; once the regurgitation occurs, the food may be swallowed or spit out. Infants who ruminate are observed to strain to bring the food back into their mouths and appear to find the experience pleasurable. Infants who are "experienced" ruminators are able to bring up the food through tongue movements and may not spit out the food at all, but hold it in their mouths and reswallow it. The disorder is rare in older children, adolescents, and adults. It varies in severity and is sometimes associated with medical conditions, such as hiatal hernia, that result in esophageal reflux. In its most severe form, the disorder can be fatal.

The diagnosis of rumination disorder can be made whether or not an infant has attained a normal weight for his or her age. Failure to thrive, therefore, is not a necessary criterion of this disorder, but it is sometimes a sequela. According to DSM-IV-TR, the disorder must be present for at least 1 month after a period of normal functioning, and it is not associated with gastrointestinal illness or other general medical conditions.

Epidemiology

Rumination is a rare disorder. It seems to be more common among male infants, and it emerges between 3 months and 1 year of age. It persists more frequently among children and adults with mental retardation. Adults with rumination usually maintain a normal weight. No reliable figures on predisposing factors or familial patterns are available.

Etiology

Rumination and gastroesophageal reflux often coexist, leading to a spectrum of variable contributions from organic and psychological factors for the emergence of the disorder. In some cases, vomiting secondary to gastroesophageal reflux or an acute illness precedes a pattern of rumination that lasts for several months. It appears, for some infants, that the rumination behavior is self-soothing or produces a sense of relief, leading to a continuation of behaviors to bring it about. In those with mental retardation, the disorder may be attributed to self-stimulatory behavior. Psychodynamic theories hypothesize various disturbances in the mother–child relationship as a contributing factor in the development of rumination disorder. The mothers of infants with the disorder have been characterized as immature, exposing the infant to increased levels of marital conflict, leading to understimulation and inadequate emotional attention to the baby. These factors are hypothesized to result in insufficient emotional gratification and stimulation for the infant who seeks to self-stimulate. The rumination is interpreted as the infant's attempt to recreate the feeding process and to provide gratification that the mother does not.

Overstimulation and tension have also been suggested as causes of rumination. A dysfunctional autonomic nervous system may be implicated. As sophisticated and accurate investigative techniques are refined, a substantial number of children classified as ruminators are shown to have gastroesophageal reflux or hiatal hernia.

Behaviorists attribute rumination to the positive reinforcement of pleasurable self-stimulation and to the attention the baby receives from others as a consequence of the disorder.

Diagnosis and Clinical Features

The DSM-IV-TR diagnostic criteria for rumination disorder are given in Table 41–2. DSM-IV-TR notes that the essential feature of the disorder is repeated regurgitation and rechewing of food in which the condition persists for a period of at least 1 month after a period of normal functioning. Partially digested food is brought up into the mouth without nausea, retching, disgust, or associated gastrointestinal disorder. This activity can be distinguished from vomiting by the clear, purposeful movements the infant makes to induce it. The food is then ejected from the mouth or reswallowed. A characteristic position of straining and arching of the back, with the head held back, is observed. The infant makes sucking movements with the tongue and gives the impression of gaining considerable satisfaction from the activity. Usually, the infant is irritable and hungry between episodes of rumination.

Initially, rumination may be difficult to distinguish from the regurgitation that frequently occurs in normal infants. In fully developed cases, however, the diagnosis is obvious. Food or milk is regurgitated without nausea, retching, or disgust and is subjected to what appears to be innumerable pleasurable sucking and chewing movements. The food is then reswallowed or ejected from the mouth.

Although spontaneous remissions are common, severe secondary complications can develop, such as progressive malnutrition, dehydration, and lowered resistance to disease. Failure to thrive, with absence of growth and developmental delays in all areas, can occur. A mortality rate as high as 25 percent has been reported in severe cases. An additional complication is that the mother or caretaker is often discouraged by failure to feed the infant successfully and can become alienated if this is not already the case. Further alienation often occurs as the noxious odor of the regurgitated material leads to avoidance of the infant.

Table 41–2
DSM-IV-TR Diagnostic Criteria for Rumination Disorder

A. Repeated regurgitation and rechewing of food for a period of at least 1 month following a period of normal functioning.
B. The behavior is not due to an associated gastrointestinal or other general medical condition (e.g., esophageal reflux).
C. The behavior does not occur exclusively during the course of anorexia nervosa or bulimia nervosa. If the symptoms occur exclusively during the course of mental retardation or a pervasive developmental disorder, they are sufficiently severe to warrant independent clinical attention.

From American Psychiatric Association. *Diagnostic and Statistical Manual of Mental Disorders.* 4th ed. Text rev. Washington, DC: American Psychiatric Association; copyright 2000, with permission.

Justin was 9 months old when he was referred by a gastroenterologist for a psychiatric evaluation because of concerns that he continued to vomit because of rumination. Justin was born full-term and had developed nicely until he was approximately 6 weeks old, when he began to vomit increasing amounts of milk during and after feedings. He was diagnosed with gastroesophageal reflux, which was treated with thickened feedings and medication. Justin responded well to the treatment; he stopped vomiting almost completely and gained weight adequately. Because Justin was doing so well, his mother decided to go back to work when Justin was 8 months old. She transitioned his care to a young woman who would come to the house during the mother's working hours. Justin started to vomit soon after his mother left the house. The vomiting seemed to increase from day to day in frequency and in intensity, and, after 2 weeks of the mother's return to work, Justin vomited several times daily and was losing weight. He was seen by a gastroenterologist, and during the barium swallow, it was noticed that Justin put his hand in his mouth, which seemed to trigger vomiting. Justin was put back on medication for gastroesophageal reflux, but he continued to vomit with increasing frequency, which led to the psychiatric consultation.

Observation of mother and infant during feeding revealed that, as soon as Justin finished feeding, he put his hand in his mouth and vomited. When his mother restricted his hand, Justin moved his tongue back and forth in a rhythmic manner until he vomited again. This happened repeatedly, and Justin continued the rhythmic tongue movements even when he could not bring up any more milk.

Because of his poor nutritional state and moderate dehydration, Justin was admitted to the hospital, and a nasojejunal tube was inserted for feedings. When Justin was awake, a special nurse or the parents played with him and tried to distract him whenever he attempted to put his hand in his mouth or thrust his tongue rhythmically. Justin became increasingly engaged, and his ruminatory activity decreased accordingly. After 1 week in the hospital, small feedings were started; however, Justin tried to ruminate again, and the oral feedings had to be stopped. At this point, the mother decided to stop working and take Justin home to continue the treatment at home. The mother started small feedings, played with Justin after feedings, and was able to keep him from ruminating. After 4 weeks of slow increments in his feedings, Justin was able to take all his feedings by mouth without ruminating, and the nasojejunal tube could be removed. (Courtesy of Irene Chatoor, M.D.)

Pathology and Laboratory Examination

No specific laboratory examination is pathognomonic of rumination disorder. Clinicians must rule out physical causes of vomiting, such as pyloric stenosis and hiatal hernia, before making the diagnosis of rumination disorder. Rumination disorder can be associated with failure to thrive and varying degrees of starvation. Thus, laboratory measures of endocrinological function (thyroid function tests, dexamethasone-suppression test), serum electrolytes, and a hematological workup help determine the severity of the effects of rumination disorder.

Differential Diagnosis

To make the diagnosis of rumination disorder, clinicians must rule out gastrointestinal congenital anomalies, infections, and other medical illnesses. Pyloric stenosis is usually associated with projectile vomiting and is generally evident before 3 months of age, when rumination has its onset. Rumination has been associated with various mental retardation syndromes in which other stereotypic behaviors and eating disturbances, such as pica, are present. Rumination disorder can occur in patients with other eating disorders, such as bulimia nervosa.

Course and Prognosis

Rumination disorder is believed to have a high rate of spontaneous remission. Indeed, many cases of rumination disorder may develop and remit without ever being diagnosed. Only limited data are available about the prognosis of rumination disorder in adults.

Treatment

The treatment of rumination disorder is often a combination of education and behavioral techniques. Sometimes, an evaluation of the mother–child relationship reveals deficits that can be influenced by offering guidance to the mother. Behavioral interventions, such as squirting lemon juice into the infant's mouth whenever rumination occurs, can be effective in diminishing the behavior. This practice appears to be the most rapidly effective treatment, with rumination reportedly eliminated in 3 to 5 days. In the aversive-conditioning reports on rumination disorder, infants were doing well at 9- or 12-month follow-up, with no recurrence of the rumination and with weight gains, increased activity levels, and increased responsiveness to persons. Rumination may be decreased by the technique of withdrawing attention from the child whenever this behavior occurs. The effectiveness of treatments is difficult to evaluate. Most reported are single-case studies; patients are not randomly assigned to controlled studies.

Treatments include improvement of the child's psychosocial environment, increased tender loving care from the mother or caretakers, and psychotherapy for the mother or both parents. When anatomical abnormalities, such as hiatal hernia, are present, surgical repair may be necessary. If an infant is malnourished and continues to lose most nutrition through rumination, a jejunal tube may need to be inserted before other treatments can be utilized.

Medications are not a standard part of the treatment of rumination. Case reports, however, cite a variety of medications that have been tried, including metoclopramide (Reglan), cimetidine (Tagamet), and antipsychotics such as haloperidol (Haldol) and thioridazine (Mellaril) have been cited to be helpful according to anecdotal reports. One study showed that when infants were allowed to eat as much as they wanted, the rate of rumination decreased.

The treatment of adolescents with rumination disorder is often complex and includes a multidisciplinary approach consisting of individual psychotherapy, nutritional intervention, and pharmacological treatment for the frequent comorbid anxiety and depressive symptoms.

FEEDING DISORDER OF INFANCY OR EARLY CHILDHOOD

Feeding disorder of infancy, a broadly defined maladaptive pattern of eating behaviors in infants, features the interactive process

Table 41–3
DSM-IV-TR Diagnostic Criteria for Feeding Disorder of Infancy or Early Childhood

A. Feeding disturbance as manifested by persistent failure to eat adequately with significant failure to gain weight or significant loss of weight over at least 1 month.
B. The disturbance is not due to an associated gastrointestinal or other general medical condition (e.g., esophageal reflux).
C. The disturbance is not better accounted for by another mental disorder (e.g., rumination disorder) or by lack of available food.
D. The onset is before age 6 years.

From American Psychiatric Association. *Diagnostic and Statistical Manual of Mental Disorders.* 4th ed. Text rev. Washington, DC: American Psychiatric Association; copyright 2000, with permission.

between caregiver and infant. This disorder has variable components that range from food refusal, food selectivity, eating too little, food avoidance, and delayed self-feeding. According to DSM-IV-TR, feeding disorder of infancy or early childhood is a persistent failure to eat adequately, reflected in significant failure to gain weight or in significant weight loss over 1 month. The symptoms are not better accounted for by a medical condition or by another mental disorder and are not caused by lack of food (Table 41–3). The disorder has its onset before the age of 6 years.

Children with feeding disorders have been found to display less affectionate touch, more negative touch, and more rejection of mother's touch than children without feeding problems. In addition, more rejecting maternal responses to the child's touch have also been observed, and children with feeding disorders are more often positioned out of reach of their mothers' arms. Children with feeding disorders are often withdrawn, and touch is diminished during the entire feeding process compared with other children. It is likely that patterns of proximity and touch between mothers and infants during feeding may serve as an index of risk for future feeding difficulties and potential growth failure.

Epidemiology

It is estimated that between 15 and 35 percent of infants and young children have transient feeding difficulties. A recent survey of feeding problems in nursery school children revealed a prevalence of 4.8 percent with equal gender distribution. Children with feeding problems exhibited more somatic complaints, and mothers of affected infants exhibited increased risk of anxiety symptoms. Data from community samples estimate a prevalence of failure-to-thrive syndromes in approximately 3 percent of infants, with approximately half of those infants exhibiting feeding disorders.

Differential Diagnosis

Feeding disorder of infancy must be differentiated from structural problems with the infants' gastrointestinal tract that may be contributing to discomfort during the feeding process. Because feeding disorders and organic causes of swallowing difficulties often coexist, it is important to rule out medical reasons for feeding difficulties. A recent study of videofluoroscopic evaluation of children with feeding and swallowing problems revealed that clinical evaluation was 92 percent accurate in identifying those children at increased risk of aspiration. This type of evaluation is necessary before psychotherapeutic interventions in cases in which a medical contribution to feeding problems is suspected.

Course and Prognosis

Most infants with feeding disorders exhibit symptoms within the first year of life and, with appropriate recognition and intervention, do not go on to develop failure to thrive. When feeding disorders have their onset later, in children 2 to 3 years of age, growth and development can be affected when the disorder lasts for several months. It is estimated that about 70 percent of infants who persistently refuse food in the first year of life continue to have some feeding problems during childhood.

Treatment

Treatments for feeding disorders need to be individualized and include interventions aimed at the infant and mother—most often targeting the interactions between the infant and mother—or caregiver.

If an infant tires before ingesting an adequate amount of nutrition, it may be necessary to begin treatment with the placement of a nasogastric tube for supplemental oral feedings. On the other hand, if the mother or caregiver is unable to participate in the intervention, it may be necessary to include additional caregivers to contribute to feeding the infant. In rare cases, an infant may require hospitalization until adequate nutrition on a daily basis is accomplished.

Most interventions for feeding disorders are aimed at optimizing the interaction between the mother and infant during feedings and identifying any factors that can be changed to promote greater ingestion. The mother is helped to become more aware of the infant's stamina for length of individual feedings,

the infant's biological regulation patterns, and when the infant is fatigued, with a goal of increasing the level of engagement between mother and infant during feeding.

A transactional model of intervention has been proposed by Irene Chatoor, M.D., a leading expert in the field, for infants who exhibit the "difficult" temperamental traits of emotional intensity, stubbornness, lack of hunger cues, irregular eating and sleeping patterns, and strong will in refusing to eat a sufficient amount and who are intensely interested in noneating exploration of their environment. The treatment includes education for the parents regarding the temperamental traits of the infant, exploration of the parents' anxieties about the infant's nutrition, and training for the parents regarding changing their behaviors to promote internal regulation of eating in the infant. Parents are encouraged to feed the infant on a regular basis at 3- to 4-hour intervals and offer only water between meals. The parents are trained to deliver praise to the infant for any self-feeding efforts, regardless of the amount of food ingested. Furthermore, parents are guided to limit any distracting stimulation during meals and give attention and praise to positive eating behaviors rather than intense negative attention to inappropriate behavior during meals. This training process for parents is recommended to be done in an intense manner within a short period of time. Many parents are able to facilitate improved eating patterns in the infant in a short period of time.

For older children with severe feeding disorders resulting in failure-to-thrive syndromes, hospitalization and nutritional supplementation is necessary before optimal psychotherapeutic interventions. Medication is not a standard component of treatment for feeding disorders, although several anecdotal reports have suggested benefit with adjunctive pharmacological agents. One recent case report indicated that in several preadolescents with failure-to-thrive and feeding disorders who received enteral nutritional interventions and were comorbid for anxiety and mood symptoms, the addition of risperidone (Risperdal) was associated with an increase in oral intake and accelerated weight gain.

42

Tic Disorders

Tic disorders are distinguished by the type of tic symptoms, their frequency, and the pattern in which they emerge over time. Tics are abnormal movements or vocalizations that most commonly affect the muscles of the face and neck, such as eye-blinking, head-jerking, mouth-grimacing, or head-shaking. Typical vocal tics include throat-clearing, grunting, snorting, and coughing. Tics are defined as rapid and repetitive muscle contractions resulting in movements or vocalizations that are experienced as involuntary. Children and adolescents may exhibit tic behaviors that occur after a stimulus or in response to an internal urge. Tic disorders comprise a group of neuropsychiatric disorders that generally begin in childhood or adolescence; they have a stable or fluctuating course in childhood and generally wane by adolescence. Although tics are not volitional, in some individuals they may be suppressed for periods.

TOURETTE'S DISORDER

According to the text revision of the fourth edition of the *Diagnostic and Statistical Manual of Mental Disorders* (DSM-IV-TR), tics in Tourette's disorder are multiple motor tics and one or more vocal tics. The tics occur many times a day for more than 1 year. Tourette's disorder causes distress or significant impairment in important areas of functioning. The disorder has an onset before the age of 18 years, and it is not caused by a substance or by a general medical condition.

Georges Gilles de la Tourette (1857–1904) first described a patient with what was later known as Tourette's disorder in 1885, while he was studying with Jean-Martin Charcot in France. De la Tourette noted a syndrome in several patients that included multiple motor tics, coprolalia, and echolalia.

Epidemiology

The lifetime prevalence of Tourette's disorder is estimated to be 4 to 5 per 10,000. More children exhibit this disorder than adults, such that 5 to 30 of 10,000 children are affected, but by adulthood, only 1 to 2 of 10,000 meet diagnostic criteria. The onset of the motor component of the disorder generally occurs by the age of 7 years; vocal tics emerge on average by the age of 11 years. Tourette's disorder occurs about three times more often in boys than in girls.

Etiology

Genetic Factors. Twin studies, adoption studies, and segregation analysis studies all support a genetic cause for Tourette's disorder.

Twin studies indicate that concordance for the disorder in monozygotic twins is significantly greater than that in dizygotic twins. That Tourette's disorder and chronic motor or vocal tic disorder are likely to occur in the same families lends support to the view that the disorders are part of a genetically determined spectrum. The sons of mothers with Tourette's disorder seem to be at the highest risk for the disorder. Evidence in some families indicates that Tourette's disorder is transmitted in an autosomal dominant fashion. Recent studies of a long family pedigree suggest that Tourette's disorder may be transmitted in a bilinear mode; that is, Tourette's disorder appears to be inherited through an autosomal pattern in some families, intermediate between dominant and recessive. A recent study of 174 unrelated probands with Tourette's disorder identified a greater-than-chance occurrence of a rare sequence variant in SLITRK1 believed to be a candidate gene on chromosome 13q31.

A relation is found between Tourette's disorder and attention-deficit/hyperactivity disorder (ADHD); up to half of all patients with Tourette's disorder also have ADHD. A relation also appears between Tourette's disorder and obsessive-compulsive disorder (OCD); up to 40 percent of all individuals with Tourette's disorder also have OCD. In addition, first-degree relatives of persons with Tourette's disorder are at high risk for the development of the disorder, of chronic motor or vocal tic disorder, and of OCD. The presence of symptoms of ADHD in more than half of persons with Tourette's disorder raises questions about a genetic relation between these two disorders.

Neurochemical and Neuroanatomical Factors. Compelling, but indirect, evidence of dopamine system involvement in tic disorders includes the observations that pharmacological agents that antagonize dopamine (haloperidol [Haldol], pimozide [Orap], and fluphenazine [Prolixin]) suppress tics and that agents that increase central dopaminergic activity (methylphenidate [Ritalin], amphetamines, pemoline [Cylert], and cocaine) tend to exacerbate tics. The relation of tics to neurotransmitter systems is complex and not well understood; for example, in some cases, antipsychotic medications, such as haloperidol, are not effective in reducing tics, and the effect of stimulants on tic disorders reportedly varies. In some cases, Tourette's disorder has emerged during treatment with antipsychotic medications.

More direct analyses of the neurochemistry of Tourette's disorder have been possible using brain proton magnetic resonance spectroscopy, a method only recently used to investigate this disorder. A recent investigation examining the cellular neurochemistry of patients with Tourette's disorder using magnetic resonance spectroscopy of the frontal cortex, caudate nucleus, putamen, and thalamus demonstrated that these patients had a reduced amount of choline and *N*-acetylaspartate in the left putamen along with reduced levels of bilaterally in the putamen. In the frontal cortex, patients with Tourette's disorder were found to have lower concentrations of *N*-acetylaspartate bilaterally, lower levels of creatine on the right side, and reduced myoinositol on the left side. These results imply that deficits in the density of neuronal and nonneuronal cells are present in patients with Tourette's disorder.

Endogenous opioids may be involved in tic disorders and OCD. Some evidence indicates that pharmacological agents that antagonize endogenous opiates—for example, naltrexone (ReVia)—reduce tics and attention deficits in patients with Tourette's disorder. Abnormalities in the noradrenergic system have been implicated in some cases by the reduction of tics with clonidine (Catapres). This adrenergic agonist reduces the release of norepinephrine in the central nervous system and, thus, may reduce activity in the dopaminergic system. Abnormalities in the basal ganglia result in various movement disorders, such as Huntington's disease, and are implicated as possible sites of disturbance in Tourette's disorder, OCD, and ADHD.

Immunological Factors and Postinfection.

An autoimmune process that is secondary to streptococcal infections is a potential mechanism for Tourette's disorder. Such a process could act synergistically with a genetic vulnerability for this disorder. Poststreptococcal syndromes have also been associated with one potential causative factor in the development of OCD in children.

Diagnosis and Clinical Features

To make a diagnosis of Tourette's disorder, clinicians must obtain a history of multiple motor tics and the emergence of at least one vocal tic at some point in the disorder. According to DSM-IV-TR, the tics must occur many times a day nearly every day or intermittently for more than 1 year. The average age of onset of tics is 7 years, but tics can occur as early as age 2 years. The onset must occur before the age of 18 years (Table 42–1).

In Tourette's disorder, the initial tics are in the face and neck. Over time, the tics tend to occur in a downward progression. The most commonly described tics are those affecting the face and head, the arms and hands, the body and lower extremities, and the respiratory and alimentary systems. In these areas, the tics take the form of grimacing; forehead puckering; eyebrow-raising; eyelid-blinking; winking; nose-wrinkling; nostril-trembling; mouth-twitching; displaying the teeth; biting the lips and other parts; tongue-extruding; protracting the lower jaw; nodding, jerking, or shaking the head; twisting the neck; looking sideways; head-rolling; hand-jerking; arm-jerking; plucking fingers; writhing fingers; fist-clenching; shoulder-shrugging; foot, knee, or toe shaking; walking peculiarly; body writhing; jumping; hiccupping; sighing; yawning; snuffing; blowing through the nostrils; whistling; belching; sucking or smacking sounds; and clear-

Table 42–1
DSM-IV-TR Diagnostic Criteria for Tourette's Disorder

A. Both multiple motor and one or more vocal tics have been present at some time during the illness, although not necessarily concurrently. (A tic is a sudden, rapid, recurrent, nonrhythmic, stereotyped motor movement or vocalization.)
B. The tics occur many times a day (usually in bouts) nearly every day or intermittently throughout a period of more than 1 year, and during this period there was never a tic-free period of more than 3 consecutive months.
C. The onset is before age 18 years.
D. The disturbance is not due to the direct physiological effects of a substance (e.g., stimulants) or a general medical condition (e.g., Huntington's disease or postviral encephalitis).

From American Psychiatric Association. *Diagnostic and Statistical Manual of Mental Disorders.* 4th ed. Text rev. Washington, DC: American Psychiatric Association; copyright 2000, with permission.

ing the throat. Several assessment instruments are available that are useful in making diagnoses of tic disorders, including comprehensive self-report assessment tools, such as the *Tic Symptom Self Report* and the *Yale Global Tic Severity Scale,* administered by a clinician.

Typically, prodromal behavioral symptoms (e.g., irritability, attention difficulties, and poor frustration tolerance) are evident before, or coincide with, the onset of tics. More than 25 percent of persons in some studies received stimulants for a diagnosis of ADHD before receiving a diagnosis of Tourette's disorder. The most frequent initial symptom is an eye-blink tic, followed by a head tic or a facial grimace. Most complex motor and vocal symptoms emerge several years after the initial symptoms. Coprolalia usually begins in early adolescence and occurs in about one third of all patients. Mental coprolalia—in which a patient thinks a sudden, intrusive, socially unacceptable thought or obscene word—can also occur. In some severe cases, physical injuries, including retinal detachment and orthopedic problems, have resulted from severe tics.

Obsessions, compulsions, attention difficulties, impulsivity, and personality problems have been associated with Tourette's disorder. Attention difficulties often precede the onset of tics, whereas obsessive-compulsive symptoms often occur after their onset. Whether these problems usually develop secondarily to a patient's tics or are caused primarily by the same underlying pathological condition is still being debated. Many tics have an aggressive or sexual component that may result in serious social consequences for the patient. Phenomenologically, tics resemble a failure of censorship, both conscious and unconscious, with increased impulsivity and inability to inhibit a thought from being put into action.

Pathology and Laboratory Examination

No specific laboratory diagnostic test exists for Tourette's disorder, but many patients with Tourette's disorder have nonspecific abnormal electroencephalographic findings. Computed tomography (CT) and magnetic resonance imaging scans have revealed no specific structural lesions, although about 10 percent of all patients with Tourette's disorder show some nonspecific abnormality on CT scans.

Differential Diagnosis

Tics must be differentiated from other disordered movements (e.g., dystonic, choreiform, athetoid, myoclonic, and hemiballismic movements) and the neurological diseases that they characterize (e.g., Huntington's disease, Parkinsonism, Sydenham's chorea, and Wilson's disease). Tremors, mannerisms, and stereotypic movement disorder (e.g., head-banging or body-rocking) must also be distinguished from tic disorders. Stereotypic movement disorders, including movements such as rocking, hand-gazing, and other self-stimulatory behaviors, seem to be voluntary and often produce a sense of comfort, in contrast to tic disorders. Although tics in children and adolescents may or may not feel controllable, they rarely produce a sense of well-being. Compulsions are sometimes difficult to distinguish from complex tics and may be on the same continuum biologically. Tic disorders also occur comorbidly with multiple behavioral and mood disturbances. In a recent survey, the greater the severity of tics, the higher was the probability of both aggressive and depressive symptoms in children. Even in a given child with Tourette's disorder, it has been reported that when there is exacerbation of tic symptoms, behavior and mood also seem to deteriorate. This phenomenon occurs with children who have Tourette's disorder and ADHD and also with those who have depression or oppositional defiant disorders. In children with Tourette's disorder and ADHD, even when the tic disorder had always been mild, a high frequency of disruptive behavior problems and mood disorder still exists. Both autistic children and children with mental retardation may exhibit symptoms similar to those seen in tic disorders, including Tourette's disorder. A greater-than-expected occurrence of Tourette's disorder, autistic disorder, and bipolar disorder also is present.

Before instituting treatment with an antipsychotic medication, clinicians must make a baseline evaluation of preexisting abnormal movements; such medication can mask abnormal movements and, if the movements occur later, they can be mistaken for tardive dyskinesia. Stimulant medications (e.g., methylphenidate, amphetamines, and pemoline) have reportedly exacerbated preexisting tics in some cases. These effects have been reported primarily in some children and adolescents being treated for ADHD. In most but not all cases, after the drug was discontinued, the tics remitted or returned to premedication levels. Most experts suggest that children and adolescents who experience tics while receiving stimulants are probably genetically predisposed and would have experienced tics regardless of their treatment with stimulants. Until the situation is clarified, clinicians should use great caution and should frequently monitor children at risk for tics who are given stimulants.

Course and Prognosis

Tourette's disorder is a childhood-onset neuropsychiatric disorder that includes both motor and vocal tics with a natural history leading to reduction or complete resolution of tic symptoms in most cases by adolescence. During childhood, individual tic symptoms may decrease, persist, or increase, and old symptoms may be replaced by new ones. Severely afflicted persons may have serious emotional problems, including major depressive disorder. Impairment may also be associated with the motor and vocal tic symptoms of Tourette's disorder; however, in many cases, interference in function is exacerbated by comorbid ADHD and OCD, both of which frequently coexist with the disorder. When the these three disorders are comorbid, severe social, academic, and occupational problems may ensue. Although most children with Tourette's disorder will experience a decline in the frequency and severity of tic symptoms during adolescence, no clinical measures exist to predict which children may have persistent symptoms into adulthood. Imaging studies have provided cross-sectional data showing that Tourette's disorder is associated with reduced caudate nucleus volume.

Treatment

Consideration of a child's or adolescent's overall functioning is the first step in determining the most appropriate treatments for tic disorders. Families, teachers, and peers sometimes misinterpret tics as purposeful behaviors, and a child may be treated as if he or she has a "behavior" problem when the tics are actually experienced as involuntary. Treatment should begin with comprehensive education for families so that children are not unwittingly punished for their tic behaviors. Families must also understand the waxing and waning nature of many tic disorders. In mild cases, children with tic disorders who are functioning well socially and academically may not require treatment. In more severe cases, children with tic disorders may be ostracized by peers and have academic work compromised by the disruptive nature of tics, and a variety of treatments must be considered.

Pharmacological interventions have some efficacy in tic suppression, and behavioral interventions such as "habit reversal" techniques are being used to help children and adolescents become more aware of their tics and initiate voluntary movements that can "counter" them. Older children, adolescents, and adults often report tics to be preceded by an unpleasant sensation denoted as a "premonitory urge." Premonitory urge phenomena may play an important role in behavioral interventions, in that a patient's ability to recognize and respond to a premonitory urge can become the basis of replacing the tic behavior with a desired behavior before it emerges. A scale for premonitory urge called the *Premonitory Urge for Tics Scale*, recently devised and examined psychometrically, was found to be internally consistent and correlated with overall tic severity in youth older than 10 years of age.

Other behavioral techniques—including massed (negative) practice, self-monitoring, incompatible response training, and presentation and removal of positive reinforcement, as well as habit reversal treatment—were reviewed by Stanley A. Hobbs. He reported that tic frequency was reduced in many cases, particularly with habit reversal treatment; additional studies are under way to replicate the efficacy of these techniques. Behavioral techniques, including relaxation, may reduce the stress that often exacerbates Tourette's disorder. It is hypothesized that behavioral techniques and pharmacotherapy together have a synergistic effect.

Pharmacotherapy.   Haloperidol and pimozide are the two best-investigated antipsychotic agents in the treatment of Tourette's disorder, although atypical antipsychotics such as risperidone and olanzapine are often chosen as first-line agents due to their safer side-effect profiles. High-potency dopamine receptor antagonists, such as haloperidol, trifluoperazine, and pimozide, have been shown to reduce tics significantly. Up to 80 percent of patients have some favorable response; their symptoms decrease by as much as 70 to 90 percent of baseline frequency. Follow-up studies, however, indicate that only 20 to 30 percent of these patients continue to take long-term maintenance therapy. Discontinuation is often based on the drug's adverse effects, including extrapyramidal effects and dysphoria. The initial daily haloperidol dose for adolescents is usually between 0.25 and 0.5 mg. Haloperidol is not approved for use in children younger than 3 years of age. For children between 3 and 12 years of age, the recommended total daily dose is between 0.05 and 0.075 mg/kg, administered in divided doses either two or three times a day.

The initial dose of pimozide is usually 1 to 2 mg daily in divided doses; the dose may be increased every other day. Most patients are maintained on less than 0.2 mg/kg a day or 10 mg a day, whichever is less. A dose of 0.3 mg/kg a day or 20 mg a day should never be exceeded because of cardiotoxic adverse effects. Pimozide appears to be relatively safe at recommended dosages, with cardiotoxicity limited to prolonged QT-wave intervals. Electrocardiography is needed at baseline and periodically during treatment. Little experience is reported in administering pimozide to children less than 12 years of age.

Clinicians must forewarn patients and families of the possibility of acute dystonic reactions and Parkinsonian symptoms when use of a conventional or atypical antipsychotic medication is to be initiated. Atypical antipsychotics (serotonin-dopamine antagonists), including risperidone and olanzapine, can be initiated as a treatment option instead of the conventional antipsychotics in the hope that adverse effects will be less pervasive. Risperidone has been used in the treatment of Tourette's disorder in doses ranging from 1 to 6 mg per day with some success. Adverse effects include weight gain, sedation, and extrapyramidal adverse effects. Risperidone and pimozide were found to be of equal efficacy in one study of 50 children, adolescents, and adults with Tourette's disorder. Olanzapine is generally well tolerated, although weight gain and reports of cognitive dulling have limited its use. Even with the serotonin-dopamine antagonists, diphenhydramine (Benadryl) or benztropine (Cogentin) may be required to control extrapyramidal adverse effects.

Although not approved by the U.S. Food and Drug Administration for use in Tourette's disorder, several studies reported that clonidine, an α_2-adrenergic agonist, was efficacious; 40 to 70 percent of patients benefited from the medication. In addition to the reduction in tic symptoms, patients may experience less tension and improved attention span. Another α_2-adrenergic agonist, guanfacine (Tenex), has also been used in the treatment of tic disorders. Clonidine has generally been used in doses ranging from 0.05 mg orally thrice daily to 0.1 mg four times daily; guanfacine is usually used in doses ranging from 1 to 4 mg per day. When used in these dose ranges, adverse effects of the α-adrenergic agents include drowsiness, headache, irritability, and occasional hypotension.

In view of the frequent comorbidity of tic behaviors and obsessive-compulsive symptoms or disorders, the selective serotonin reuptake inhibitors (SSRIs) have been used alone or in combination with antipsychotics in the treatment of Tourette's disorder. Some data suggest that SSRIs, such as fluoxetine (Prozac), may be helpful.

Although clinicians must weigh the risks and benefits of using stimulants in cases of severe hyperactivity and comorbid tics, a recent study reported that methylphenidate does not increase the rate or intensity of motor or vocal tics in most children with hyperactivity and tic disorders. A recent study of atomoxetine (Strattera), at doses ranging from 0.5 to 1.5 mg/kg, in the treatment of children and adolescents with ADHD and tic disorders revealed that the atomoxetine did not exacerbate tics and may be associated with some tic reduction. One case report on the use of bupropion (Wellbutrin), an antidepressant of the aminoketone class, indicated increased tic behavior in several children being treated for Tourette's disorder and ADHD. Other antidepressants, such as imipramine (Tofranil) and desipramine (Norpramin, Pertofrane), may decrease disruptive behavior in children with Tourette's disorder but are no longer widely used because of their potentially serious cardiac adverse effects.

CHRONIC MOTOR OR VOCAL TIC DISORDER

In DSM-IV-TR, chronic motor or vocal tic disorder is defined as the presence of either motor tics or vocal tics, but not both. The other features are the same as those of Tourette's disorder, but chronic motor or vocal tic disorder cannot be diagnosed if the criteria for Tourette's disorder have ever been met. According to DSM-IV-TR criteria, the disorder must have its onset before the age of 18 years.

Epidemiology

The rate of chronic motor or vocal tic disorder has been estimated to be from 100 to 1,000 times greater than that of Tourette's disorder. School-age boys are at highest risk, but the incidence is unknown. Although the disorder was once believed to be rare, current estimates of the prevalence of chronic motor or vocal tic disorder range from 1 to 2 percent.

Etiology

Tourette's disorder and chronic motor or vocal tic disorder aggregate in the same families. Twin studies have found a high concordance for either Tourette's disorder or chronic motor tics in monozygotic twins. This finding supports the importance of hereditary factors in the transmission of at least some tic disorders.

Diagnosis and Clinical Features

The onset of chronic motor or vocal tic disorder appears to be in early childhood. The types of tics and their locations are similar to those in transient tic disorder. Chronic vocal tics are considerably rarer than chronic motor tics. The chronic vocal tics are usually much less conspicuous than those in Tourette's disorder. The vocal tics are usually not loud or intense and are not primarily produced by the vocal cords; they consist of grunts or other noises caused by thoracic, abdominal, or diaphragmatic contractions. The DSM-IV-TR diagnostic criteria are given in Table 42–2.

Differential Diagnosis

Chronic motor tics must be differentiated from a variety of other motor movements, including choreiform movements, myoclonus, restless legs syndrome, akathisia, and dystonias. Involuntary vocal utterances can occur in certain neurological disorders, such as Huntington's disease and Parkinson's disease.

Course and Prognosis

Children whose tics start between the ages of 6 and 8 years seem to have the best outcomes. Symptoms usually last for 4 to 6 years

Table 42–2
DSM-IV-TR Diagnostic Criteria for Chronic Motor or Vocal Tic Disorder

A. Single or multiple motor or vocal tics (i.e., sudden, rapid, recurrent, nonrhythmic, stereotyped motor movements or vocalizations), but not both, have been present at some time during the illness.
B. The tics occur many times a day nearly every day or intermittently throughout a period of more than 1 year, and during this period there was never a tic-free period of more than 3 consecutive months.
C. The onset is before age 18 years.
D. The disturbance is not due to the direct physiological effects of a substance (e.g., stimulants) or a general medical condition (e.g., Huntington's disease or postviral encephalitis).
E. Criteria have never been met for Tourette's disorder.

From American Psychiatric Association. *Diagnostic and Statistical Manual of Mental Disorders.* 4th ed. Text rev. Washington, DC: American Psychiatric Association; copyright 2000, with permission.

and stop in early adolescence. Children whose tics involve the limbs or trunk tend to do less well than those with only facial tics.

Treatment

The treatment of chronic motor or vocal tic disorder depends on the severity and frequency of the tics; the patient's subjective distress; the effects of the tics on school or work, job performance, and socialization; and the presence of any other concomitant mental disorder. Psychotherapy may be indicated to minimize the secondary social difficulties caused by severe tics. Several studies found that behavioral techniques, particularly habit reversal treatments, were effective in treating chronic motor or vocal tic disorder. Antianxiety agents have been unsuccessful. Haloperidol has been helpful in some cases, but the risks must be weighed against the possible clinical benefits because of the drug's adverse effects, including the development of tardive dyskinesia.

TRANSIENT TIC DISORDER

In the DSM-IV-TR, transient tic disorder is defined as the presence of a single tic or multiple motor or vocal tics or both. The tics occur many times a day for at least 4 weeks but no longer than 12 months. The other features are the same as those for Tourette's disorder, but transient tic disorder cannot be diagnosed if the criteria for Tourette's disorder or chronic motor or vocal tic disorder have ever been met. According to DSM-IV-TR, the disorder must have its onset before the age of 18 years.

Epidemiology

Transient tic-like movements and nervous muscular twitches are common in children. From 5 to 24 percent of all school-age children have a history of tics. The prevalence of tics as defined here is unknown.

Etiology

Transient tic disorder probably has organic origins, with some tics-combining psychogenic contributions as well. Early-onset tics, which are probably most likely to progress to Tourette's disorder, occur with greater frequency in children with an increased family history of tics. Tics that progress to chronic motor or vocal tic disorder are most likely to have components of both organic and psychogenic origin. Tics of all sorts are *exacerbated* by stress and anxiety, but no evidence indicates that tics are *caused* by stress or anxiety.

Diagnosis and Clinical Features

The DSM-IV-TR criteria for establishing the diagnosis of transient tic disorder are as follows: The tics are single or multiple, motor or vocal. They occur many times a day nearly every day for at least 4 weeks but no longer than 12 consecutive months. The patient has no history of Tourette's disorder or chronic motor or vocal tic disorder. The onset is before age 18 years. The tics do not occur exclusively during substance intoxication, and they are not caused by a general medical condition. The diagnosis should specify whether a single episode or recurrent episodes are present (Table 42–3). Transient tic disorder can be distinguished

Table 42–3
DSM-IV-TR Diagnostic Criteria for Transient Tic Disorder

A. Single or multiple motor and/or vocal tics (i.e., sudden, rapid, recurrent, nonrhythmic, stereotyped motor movements or vocalizations)
B. The tics occur many times a day, nearly every day for at least 4 weeks, but for no longer than 12 consecutive months.
C. The onset is before age 18 years.
D. The disturbance is not due to the direct physiological effects of a substance (e.g., stimulants) or a general medical condition (e.g., Huntington's disease or postviral encephalitis).
E. Criteria have never been met for Tourette's Disorder or Chronic Motor or Vocal Tic Disorder.

Specify if:
Single episode or **Recurrent**

from chronic motor or vocal tic disorder and Tourette's disorder only by observing the symptoms' progression over time.

Course and Prognosis

Motor tics are frequent among young children and, in general, are not associated with severe impairment. Over time, tics either disappear permanently or recur during periods of special stress. Only a small percentage of those with tics develop chronic motor or vocal tic disorder or Tourette's disorder.

Treatment

Whether the tics will disappear spontaneously, progress, or become chronic is unclear at the beginning of treatment. Focusing much attention on mild or infrequent tics may serve to cause undue stress for a child, but if tics are sufficiently severe to cause impairment in social, academic, or emotional function, psychiatric and pediatric neurological examinations are recommended. Psychopharmacology is recommended when symptoms are severe and disabling. Several studies have found that behavioral techniques, particularly habit reversal treatment, are effective in treating transient tics.

TIC DISORDER NOT OTHERWISE SPECIFIED

According to DSM-IV-TR, tic disorder not otherwise specified refers to disorders characterized by tics but not otherwise meeting the criteria for a specific tic disorder (Table 42–4).2

Table 42–4
DSM-IV-TR Diagnostic Criteria for Tic Disorder Not Otherwise Specified

This category is for disorders characterized by tics that do not meet criteria for a specific tic disorder. Examples include tics lasting less than 4 weeks or tics with an onset after age 18 years.

43

Elimination Disorders

Enuresis and encopresis are the two elimination disorders described in the text revision of the fourth edition of *Diagnostic and Statistical Manual of Mental Disorders* (DSM-IV-TR). These disorders are considered after age 4 years for encopresis and after age 5 years for enuresis, when a child is chronologically, developmentally, and physiologically expected to be able to master these skills. Normal development encompasses a range of time in which a given child is able to devote the attention, motivation, and physiological skills to exhibit competency in elimination processes. Encopresis is defined as a pattern of passing feces in inappropriate places, such as in clothing or other places, at least once per month for 3 consecutive months, whether the passage is involuntary or intentional. The child with encopresis typically exhibits dysregulated bowel function, for example, with infrequent bowel movements, constipation, or recurrent abdominal pain and sometimes pain on defecations. Encopresis is a nonorganic condition in a child who is chronologically at least 4 years old. Enuresis is the repeated voiding of urine into clothes or bed, whether the voiding is involuntary or intentional. The behavior must occur twice weekly for at least 3 months or must cause clinically significant distress or impairment socially or academically. The child's chronological or developmental age must be at least 5 years.

ENCOPRESIS

Epidemiology

Incidence rates for encopretic behavior decrease drastically with increasing age. Although the diagnosis is not made until after age 4 years, encopretic behavior is present in 8.1 percent of 3-year-olds, 2.2 percent of 5-year-olds, and 0.75 percent of 10- to 12-year-olds. In Western cultures, bowel control is established in more than 95 percent of children by their fourth birthday and in 99 percent by the fifth birthday. Encopresis is virtually absent in youth with normal intellectual function by the age of 16 years. Males are found to be about six times more likely to have encopresis than females. A significant relation exists between encopresis and enuresis.

Etiology

Encopresis involves an often-complicated interplay between physiological and psychological factors. Although encopresis is considered a nonorganic disorder, a typical child with encopresis may show evidence of chronic constipation, leading to infrequent defecation, withholding of bowel movements, and avoidance of defecation. Children may avoid the pain of having a bowel movement by holding it in, which then leads to impaction and eventual overflow soiling. This pattern is observed in more than 75 percent of children with encopretic behavior. This common set of circumstances in most children with encopresis supports a behavioral intervention with a focus on ameliorating constipation while increasing appropriate toileting behavior. Inadequate training or the lack of appropriate toilet training may delay a child's attainment of continence.

Evidence indicates that some encopretic children have lifelong inefficient and ineffective sphincter control. Other children may soil involuntarily, either because of an inability to control the sphincter adequately or because of excessive fluid caused by a retentive overflow.

Encopresis has been demonstrated to occur with significantly greater frequency among children with known sexual abuse compared with a normal sample of children, and it occurs with greater frequency among children with a variety of psychiatric disturbances compared with controls. Encopresis, however, is not a specific indicator of sexual abuse because it also occurs with increased frequency in nonabused children with other behavioral problems. Some evidence indicates that encopresis in children is associated with measures of maternal hostility and harsh and punitive parenting. A recent study evaluating the frequency of encopresis and enuresis in children with prepubertal and early adolescent bipolar I disorder found a greater prevalence of encopresis among children with bipolar disorder compared with healthy controls; in most cases, however, the encopresis predated the onset of the affective illness.

It is evident that once a given child has developed a pattern of withholding bowel movements with resulting pain with attempts to defecate, a child's fear and resistance to changing the pattern can lead to a power struggle between child and parent over effective toileting behavior. Perpetual battles often aggravate the disorder and frequently cause secondary behavioral difficulties. Many children with encopresis who are not reported to have early behavioral problems end up being socially ostracized and rejected because of the encopresis. The social consequences of soiling can further lead to the development of psychiatric problems. On the other hand, children with encopresis who clearly can control their bowel function adequately but chronically deposit feces of relatively normal consistency in abnormal places are more likely to have a preexisting neurodevelopmental problem, easy distractibility, short attention span, low frustration tolerance, hyperactivity, or poor coordination. Occasionally, a child has a specific fear of using the toilet, leading to a phobia.

In some children, encopresis can be considered secondary, that is, emerging after a period of normal bowel habits in conjunction with a disruptive life event, such as the birth of a sibling or a move to a new home. When encopresis manifests after a long period of fecal continence, it may reflect a response indicative of a developmental regressive behavior, for example, based on a severe stressor, such as a parental separation, loss of a best friend, or an unexpected academic failure.

Psychogenic Megacolon.   Most children with encopresis retain feces and become constipated, either voluntarily or secondarily to painful defecation. In some cases a subclinical preexisting anorectal dysfunction exists that contributes to the constipation. In either case, resulting chronic rectal distention from large, hard fecal masses can cause loss of tone in the rectal wall and desensitization to pressure. Thus, children in this situation become even less aware of the need to defecate, and overflow encopresis occurs, usually with relatively small amounts of liquid or soft stool leaking out.

Anecdotal reports indicate that children whose parenting has been harsh and punitive and who have been severely punished for "accidents" during toilet training are at greater risk of developing encopresis.

Diagnosis and Clinical Features.   According to DSM-IV-TR, encopresis is diagnosed when feces are passed into inappropriate places on a regular basis (at least once a month) for 3 months (Table 43–1). Encopresis may be present in children who have bowel control and intentionally deposit feces in their clothes or other places for a variety of emotional reasons. Anecdotal reports have suggested that occasionally encopresis is attributable to an expression of anger or rage in a child whose parents have been punitive or of hostility at a parent. In a case such as this, once a child develops this inappropriate repetitive behavior eliciting negative attention, it is difficult to break the cycle of continuous negative attention. In other children, sporadic episodes of encopresis can occur during times of stress—for example, proximal to the birth of a new sibling—but in such cases, the behavior is usually transient and does not fulfill the diagnostic criteria for the disorder.

Encopresis can also be present on an involuntary basis in the absence of physiological abnormalities. In these cases, a child may not exhibit adequate control over the sphincter muscles either because the child is absorbed in another activity or because he or she is unaware of the process. The feces may be of normal, near-normal, or liquid consistency. Some involuntary soiling occurs from chronic retaining of stool, which results in liquid overflow. In rare cases, the involuntary overflow of stool results from psychological causes of diarrhea or anxiety disorder symptoms.

The DSM-IV-TR breaks down the types of encopresis into *with* constipation and overflow incontinence and *without* constipation and overflow incontinence. To receive a diagnosis of encopresis, a child must have a developmental or chronological level of at least 4 years of age. If the fecal incontinence is directly related to a medical condition, encopresis is not diagnosed.

Studies have indicated that children with encopresis who do not have gastrointestinal illnesses have high rates of abnormal anal sphincter contractions. This finding is particularly prevalent among children with encopresis with constipation and overflow incontinence who have difficulty relaxing their anal sphincter muscles when trying to defecate. Children with constipation who have difficulties with sphincter relaxation are not likely to respond well to laxatives in the treatment of their encopresis. Children with encopresis without abnormal sphincter tone are likely to improve over a short period.

Table 43–1
DSM-IV-TR Diagnostic Criteria for Encopresis

A. Repeated passage of feces into inappropriate places (e.g., clothing or floor) whether involuntary or intentional.
B. At least one such event a month for at least 3 months.
C. Chronological age is at least 4 years (or equivalent developmental level).
D. The behavior is not due exclusively to the direct physiological effects of a substance (e.g., laxatives) or a general medical condition except through a mechanism involving constipation.

Code as follows:
With constipation and overflow incontinence
Without constipation and overflow incontinence

From American Psychiatric Association. *Diagnostic and Statistical Manual of Mental Disorders.* 4th ed. Text rev. Washington, DC: American Psychiatric Association; copyright 2000, with permission.

Jack was a 9-year-old boy with daily encopresis, enuresis, and a history of hoarding behaviors, along with hiding the feces around the house. He resided with his adoptive parents, having been removed from his biological parents at age 3 years because of neglect, and physical and sexual abuse. He was reported to be cocaine addicted at birth, but was otherwise healthy. His mother was a known drug and alcohol user, and his father had spent time in jail for drug sales. Jack has always been enuretic at night, and when he was younger he had a history of daytime enuresis as well. Jack had a short attention span, was highly impulsive and had great difficulty staying in his seat at school and remaining on task. He had reading difficulties and was placed in a contained special education classroom because of his disruptive behavior as well as his academic difficulties. Jack also qualified for a diagnosis of oppositional defiant disorder. Despite experiencing physical and sexual abuse, he has not experienced flashbacks or other symptoms indicating the presence of posttraumatic stress disorder. Jack is being treated for attention-deficit/hyperactivity disorder (ADHD) and is responding to methylphenidate (Concerta 36 mg per day).

Jack's adoptive family resided in an urban area that had access to a university hospital with an outpatient program that had expertise in the behavioral treatment of encopresis. This program coupled the bowel training method with a psychoeducational component and psychotherapy. It was determined that Jack's encopresis was not of the retentive-overflow type, and the feces were always well formed. Much to the surprise of the psychiatric consultant, several-week outpatient bowel training course coupled with the psychoeducational component and psychotherapy resulted in significant improvement in the frequency of the encopresis. Jack was proud and gave his therapist a diagram of the functioning of the digestive system that was part of the psychoeducational program. In retrospect, it appeared that although there were symbolic aspects to Jack's encopretic behavior, the soiling was ego-dystonic, and he was motivated to change the behavior. (Courtesy of Edwin J. Mikkelsen, M.D. and Caroly Pataki, M.D.)

Pathology and Laboratory Examination

Although no specific test indicates a diagnosis of encopresis, clinicians must rule out medical illnesses, such as Hirschsprung's disease, before making a diagnosis. If it is unclear whether fecal retention is responsible for encopresis with constipation and overflow incontinence, a physical examination of the abdomen is indicated, and an abdominal X-ray can help determine the degree of constipation present. Sophisticated tests to determine whether sphincter tone is abnormal are generally not conducted in simple cases of encopresis.

Differential Diagnosis

In encopresis with constipation and overflow incontinence, constipation can begin as early as the child's first year and can peak between the second and fourth years. Soiling usually begins at age 4 years. Frequent liquid stools and hard fecal masses are found in the colon and the rectum on abdominal palpation and rectal examination. Complications include impaction, megacolon, and anal fissures.

Encopresis with constipation and overflow incontinence can be caused by faulty nutrition; structural disease of the anus, rectum, and colon; medicinal adverse effects; or nongastrointestinal medical (endocrine or neurological) disorders. The chief differential problem is aganglionic megacolon or Hirschsprung's disease, in which a patient may have an empty rectum and no desire to defecate but may still have an overflow of feces. The disorder occurs in 1 in 5,000 children; signs appear shortly after birth.

Given the frequency of comorbid psychiatric disorders and increased incidence of encopresis among children who have been sexually abused, it is imperative to investigate the possibility of sexual and physical abuse during the evaluation of encopresis.

Course and Prognosis

The outcome of encopresis depends on the cause, the chronicity of the symptoms, and coexisting behavioral problems. In many cases, encopresis is self-limiting, and it rarely continues beyond middle adolescence. Encopresis in children who have contributing physiological factors, such as poor gastric motility and an inability to relax the anal sphincter muscles, is more difficult to treat than that in those with constipation but normal sphincter tone.

Encopresis is a particularly repugnant disorder to most persons, including family members; thus, family tension is often high. The child's peers are also sensitive to the developmentally inappropriate behavior and often ostracize the child. A child with encopresis is often scapegoated by peers and shunned by adults. Many of these children have abysmally low self-esteem and are aware of their constant rejection. Psychologically, the child may appear blunted toward the symptoms or may be entrenched in a pattern of encopresis as a mode of expressing anger. The outcome of cases of encopresis is affected by the family's willingness and ability to participate in treatment without being overly punitive and by the child's awareness of when the passage of feces is about to occur.

Treatment

The treatment plan for encopresis cannot be established until a medical assessment of bowel function is completed as well as a full psychiatric assessment. A typical treatment plan for a child with encopresis includes an initial medical plan to address constipation, in most cases, as well as an ongoing behavioral intervention to enhance appropriate bowel behavior and diminish anxiety related to bowel movement. By the time a child is brought for treatment, considerable family discord and distress are common. Family tensions about the symptom must be reduced and a nonpunitive atmosphere established. Similar efforts should be made to reduce the child's embarrassment at school. Many changes of underwear with a minimum of fuss should be arranged. Education of the family and correction of misperceptions that a family may have about soiling must occur before treatment. A useful physiological approach involves a combination of daily laxatives or mineral oil along with a behavioral intervention in which the child sits on the toilet for timed intervals daily and is rewarded for successful defecation. Laxatives are not necessary for children who are not constipated and do have good bowel control, but regular, timed intervals on the toilet may be useful with these children as well.

A recent report confirms the success of an interactive parent–child family guidance intervention for young children with encopresis based on psychological and behavioral interventions for children younger than the age of 9 years.

Supportive psychotherapy and relaxation techniques may be useful in treating the anxieties and other sequelae of children with encopresis, such as low self-esteem and social isolation. Family interventions can be helpful for children who have bowel control but continue to deposit their feces in inappropriate locations. A good outcome occurs when a child feels in control of life events. Coexisting behavior problems predict a poorer outcome. In all cases, proper bowel habits may need to be taught. In some cases, biofeedback techniques have been of benefit.

ENURESIS

Epidemiology

The prevalence of enuresis decreases with increasing age. The diagnosis of enuresis is not made until the chronological and developmental age of 5 years, but enuretic behavior nocturnally and during the daytime is common, with reported prevalence from 2 to 5 percent among school-aged children. Enuretic behavior is considered developmentally appropriate among young toddlers, precluding diagnoses of enuresis; however, enuretic behavior occurs in 82 percent of 2-year-olds, 49 percent of 3-year-olds, 26 percent of 4-year-olds, and 7 percent of 5-year-olds on a regular basis. Prevalence rates vary, however, on the basis of the population studied and the tolerance for the symptoms in various cultures and socioeconomic groups.

Although most children with enuresis do not have a comorbid psychiatric disorder, children with enuresis are at higher risk for the development of a variety of developmental and behavioral disturbances compared with children without enuresis.

Nocturnal enuresis is about 50 percent more common in boys and accounts for about 80 percent of children with enuresis. Diurnal enuresis is also more often seen in boys who often delay voiding until it is too late. The rate of spontaneous resolution of nocturnal enuresis is about 15 percent per year. Nocturnal enuresis consists of a normal volume of voided urine, whereas, when small volumes of urine are voided at night, other medical causes may be present.

Etiology

Most children with nocturnal enuresis do not exhibit neurological conditions that account for the symptoms. Voiding dysfunction in the absence of a specific neurogenic cause is believed to originate from behavioral factors that affect normal voiding habits and inhibit the maturation of normal voluntary control.

The most severe form of dysfunctional voiding is called Hinman's syndrome, and is thought of as a nonneurogenic neurogenic bladder resulting from habitual, voluntary tightening of the external sphincter during urges to urinate. The pattern may be set in a young child who may start out with a normal or overactive detrusor muscle in the bladder but, in any case, repeatedly attempts to prevent leaking or urination when there is an urge to void. Over time, the sensation of the urge to urinate is diminished and the bladder does not empty regularly, leading to enuresis at night when the bladder is relaxed and can empty without resistance. This immature pattern of urinating can account for some cases of enuresis, especially when the pattern has been in place since early childhood. Most children are not enuretic by intention or even with awareness until after they are wet. Physiological factors often play a role in the development of enuresis, and behavioral patterns are likely to maintain the maladaptive urination. Normal bladder control, which is acquired gradually, is influenced by neuromuscular and cognitive development, socioemotional factors, toilet training, and genetic factors. Difficulties in one or more of these areas can delay urinary continence.

Genetic factors are believed to play a role in the expression of enuresis, given that the emergence of enuresis has been found to be significantly greater in first-degree relatives. A longitudinal study of child development found that children with enuresis were about twice as likely to have concomitant developmental delays as those who did not have enuresis. About 75 percent of children with enuresis have a first-degree relative who has or has had enuresis. A child's risk for enuresis has been found to be more than seven times greater if the father was enuretic. The concordance rate is higher in monozygotic twins than in dizygotic twins. A strong genetic component is suggested, and much can be accounted for by tolerance for enuresis in some families and by other psychosocial factors.

Studies indicate that children with enuresis with a normal anatomic bladder capacity report urge to void with less urine in the bladder than children without enuresis. Other studies report that nocturnal enuresis occurs when the bladder is full because of lower-than-expected levels of nighttime antidiuretic hormone. This could lead to a higher-than-usual urine output. Enuresis does not appear to be related to a specific stage of sleep or time of night; rather, bed-wetting appears randomly. In most cases, the quality of sleep is normal. Little evidence indicates that children with enuresis sleep more soundly than other children.

Psychosocial stressors appear to precipitate enuresis in a subgroup of children with the disorder. In young children, the disorder has been particularly associated with the birth of a sibling, hospitalization between the ages of 2 and 4 years, the start of school, the breakup of a family because of divorce or death, and a move to a new home.

Diagnosis and Clinical Features

Enuresis is the repeated voiding of urine into a child's clothes or bed; the voiding may be involuntary or intentional. For the diagnosis to be made, a child must exhibit a developmental or chronological age of at least 5 years. According to DSM-IV-TR, the behavior must occur twice weekly for a period of at least 3 months or must cause distress and impairment in functioning to meet the diagnostic criteria. Enuresis is diagnosed only if the behavior is not caused by a medical condition. Children with enuresis are at higher risk for ADHD compared with the general population. They are also more likely to have comorbid encopresis. DSM-IV-TR and the tenth revision of *International Statistical Classification of Diseases and Related Health Problems* break down the disorder into three types: nocturnal only, diurnal only, and nocturnal and diurnal (Table 43–2).

Pathology and Laboratory Examination

No single laboratory finding is pathognomonic of enuresis, but clinicians must rule out organic factors, such as the presence of urinary tract infections, that may predispose a child to enuresis. Structural obstructive abnormalities may be present in up to 3 percent of children with apparent enuresis. Sophisticated radiographic studies are usually deferred in simple cases of enuresis with no signs of repeated infections or other medical problems.

Differential Diagnosis

To make the diagnosis of enuresis, organic causes of bladder dysfunction must be investigated and ruled out. Organic syndromes, such as urinary tract infections, obstructions, or anatomical conditions, are found most often in children who experience both nocturnal and diurnal enuresis combined with urinary frequency and urgency. The organic features include genitourinary pathology—structural, neurological, and infectious—such as obstructive uropathy, spina bifida occulta, and cystitis; other organic disorders that can cause polyuria and enuresis, such as

Table 43–2
DSM-IV-TR Diagnostic Criteria for Enuresis

A. Repeated voiding of urine into bed or clothes (whether involuntary or intentional).
B. The behavior is clinically significant as manifested by either a frequency of twice a week for at least 3 consecutive months or the presence of clinically significant distress or impairment in social, academic (occupational), or other important areas of functioning.
C. Chronological age is at least 5 years (or equivalent developmental level).
D. The behavior is not due exclusively to the direct physiological effect of a substance (e.g., a diuretic) or a general medical condition (e.g., diabetes, spina bifida, a seizure disorder).

Specify type:
Nocturnal only
Diurnal only
Nocturnal and diurnal

From American Psychiatric Association. *Diagnostic and Statistical Manual of Mental Disorders.* 4th ed. Text rev. Washington, DC: American Psychiatric Association; copyright 2002, with permission.

diabetes mellitus and diabetes insipidus; disturbances of consciousness and sleep, such as seizures, intoxication, and sleep-walking disorder, during which a child urinates; and adverse effects from treatment with antipsychotics (e.g., thioridazine [Mellaril]).

Course and Prognosis

Enuresis is often self-limited, and a child with enuresis may have a spontaneous remission without psychological sequelae. Most such children find their symptoms ego-dystonic and enjoy enhanced self-esteem and improved social confidence when they become continent. About 80 percent of affected children have never achieved a year-long period of dryness. Enuresis after at least one dry year usually begins between the ages of 5 and 8 years; if it occurs much later, especially during adulthood, organic causes must be investigated. Some evidence indicates that late onset of enuresis in children is more frequently associated with a concomitant psychiatric difficulty than is enuresis without at least one dry year. Relapses occur in children with enuresis who are becoming dry spontaneously and in those who are being treated. The significant emotional and social difficulties of these children usually include poor self-image, decreased self-esteem, social embarrassment and restriction, and intrafamilial conflict. The course of children with enuresis may be influenced by whether they receive appropriate evaluation and treatment for common comorbid disorders such as ADHD.

Treatment

A treatment plan for typical enuresis can be developed after organic causes of urinary dysfunction have been ruled out. Modalities that have been used successfully for enuresis include both behavioral and pharmacological interventions. A relatively high rate of spontaneous remission over long periods also occurs. The first step in any treatment plan is to review appropriate toilet training. If toilet training was not attempted, the parents and the patient should be guided in this undertaking. Record-keeping is helpful in determining a baseline and following the child's progress and may itself be a reinforcer. A star chart may be particularly helpful. Other useful techniques include restricting fluids before bed and night-lifting to toilet train the child. Another basic intervention for those children with enuresis and bowel dysfunction is to assess whether chronic constipation is contributing to urinary dysfunction and to consider increasing dietary fiber to diminish constipation.

Behavioral Therapy.   Classic conditioning with the bell (or buzzer) and pad apparatus is generally the most effective treatment for enuresis, with dryness resulting in more than 50 percent of cases. The treatment is equally effective in children with and without concomitant mental disorders, and no evidence suggests symptom substitution. Difficulties may include child and fam-

ily noncompliance, improper use of the apparatus, and relapse. Bladder training—encouragement or reward for delaying micturition for increasing times during waking hours—has also been used. Although sometimes effective, this method is decidedly inferior to the bell and pad.

Pharmacotherapy.   Medication is considered when enuresis is causing impairment in social, family, and school function and behavioral, dietary, and fluid restriction have not been efficacious. When the problem interferes significantly with a child's functioning, several medications can be considered, although the problem often recurs as soon as medications are withdrawn.

Imipramine (Tofranil) is efficacious and has been approved for use in treating childhood enuresis, primarily on a short-term basis. Initially, up to 30 percent of patients with enuresis stay dry, and up to 85 percent wet less frequently than before treatment. The success often does not last, however, and tolerance can develop after 6 weeks of therapy. Once the drug is discontinued, relapse and enuresis at former frequencies usually occur within a few months. The drug's adverse effects, which include cardiotoxicity, are also a serious problem.

The tricyclic drugs are not currently used frequently for enuresis because of their risks and reports of sudden death in several children with ADHD who were taking desipramine (Norpramin, Pertofrane). Desmopressin, an antidiuretic compound that is available as an intranasal spray, has shown some initial success in reducing enuresis. Reduction of enuresis has varied from 10 to 90 percent with the use of desmopressin. In most studies, enuresis recurred shortly after discontinuation of this medication. Adverse effects that can occur with desmopressin include headache, nasal congestion, epistaxis, and stomachache. The most serious adverse effect reported with the use of desmopressin to treat enuresis was a hyponatremic seizure experienced by a child.

Reboxetine (Edronax, Vestra), a norepinephrine reuptake inhibitor with a noncardiotoxic side-effect profile, has recently been investigated as a safer alternative to imipramine in the treatment of childhood enuresis. In one trial, 22 children with socially handicapping enuresis who had not responded to an enuresis alarm, desmopressin, or anticholinergics were administered 4 to 8 mg of reboxetine at bedtime. Of the 22 children, 13 (59 percent) in this open trial achieved complete dryness with reboxetine alone or in combination with desmopressin. Side effects were minimal and did not lead to discontinuation of the medication in this trial. Future placebo-controlled trials are indicated to determine the efficacy of this promising medication in the treatment of enuresis.

Psychotherapy.   Psychotherapy may be useful in dealing with the coexisting psychiatric problems and the emotional and family difficulties that arise secondary to chronic enuresis. Although many psychological and psychoanalytic theories regarding enuresis have been advanced, controlled studies have found that psychotherapy alone is not effective in the short-term treatment of enuresis.

44 ▲

Other Disorders of Infancy, Childhood, and Adolescence

▲ 44.1 Reactive Attachment Disorder of Infancy or Early Childhood

Reactive attachment disorder (RAD) is a clinical disorder characterized by aberrant social behaviors in a young child reflecting an environment of maltreatment that interfered with the development of normal attachment behavior. Unlike most disorders in the text revision of the fourth edition of the *Diagnostic and Statistical Manual of Mental Disorders* (DSM-IV-TR), a diagnosis of RAD is based on the presumption that the etiology is directly linked to environmental deprivation experienced by the child. The diagnosis of RAD is a relatively recent entity, added to the third edition of the DSM (DSM-III) in 1980. The formation of this diagnosis is largely based on the building blocks of attachment theory, which describes the quality of a child's generalized affective relationship with primary caregivers, usually parents. This basic relationship is the product of a young child's need for protection, nurturance, and comfort and the interaction of the parents and child in fulfilling these needs.

The disorder may result in a picture of failure to thrive, in which an infant shows physical signs of malnourishment and does not exhibit the expected developmental motor and verbal milestones. When this is the case, the failure to thrive is coded on Axis III.

EPIDEMIOLOGY

Few data exist on the prevalence, sex ratio, or familial pattern of RAD. It has been estimated to occur in less than 1 percent of the population. Studies have used selected high-risk populations. In a retrospective report of children in one county of the United States who were removed from their homes because of neglect or abuse before the age of 4 years, 38 percent exhibited signs of emotionally withdrawn or indiscriminate RAD. A study in 2004 established the reliability of the diagnosis by reviewing videotaped assessments of children at risk interacting with caregivers along with a structured interview with caregivers. Given that pathogenic care, including maltreatment, occurs more frequently in the presence of general psychosocial risk factors, such as poverty, disrupted families, and mental illness among caregivers, these circumstances are likely to increase the risk

of RAD. In unusual circumstances, however, a caregiver may be fully satisfactory for one child, whereas another child in the same household is maltreated and develops RAD.

ETIOLOGY

The essence of RAD is the malformation of normal attachment behaviors. The inability of a young child to develop normative social interactions that culminate in aberrant attachment behaviors in RAD is inherent in the disorder's definition. RAD is linked to maltreatment, including emotional neglect, physical abuse, or both as well. Grossly pathogenic care of an infant or young child by the caregiver presumably causes the markedly disturbed social relatedness that is usually evident. The emphasis is on the unidirectional cause; that is, the caregiver does something inimical or neglects to do something essential for the infant or child. In evaluating a patient for whom such a diagnosis is appropriate, however, clinicians should consider the contributions of each member of the caregiver-dyad and their interactions. Clinicians should weigh such things as infant or child temperament, deficient or defective bonding, a developmentally disabled or sensorially impaired child, and a particular caregiver–child mismatch. The likelihood of neglect increases with parental mental retardation; lack of parenting skills because of personal upbringing, social isolation, or deprivation and lack of opportunities to learn about caregiving behavior; and premature parenthood (during early and middle adolescence), in which parents are unable to respond to, and care for, an infant's needs and in which the parents' own needs take precedence over their infant's or child's needs. Frequent changes of the primary caregiver—as may occur in institutionalization, repeated lengthy hospitalizations, and multiple foster care placements—may also cause a reactive attachment disorder of infancy or early childhood.

DIAGNOSIS AND CLINICAL FEATURES

Children with RAD may initially be identified by a preschool teacher or by a pediatrician based on direct observation of the child's inappropriate social responses. The diagnosis of RAD is based on documenting evidence of pervasive disturbance of attachment leading to inappropriate social behaviors present before the age of 5 years. The clinical picture varies greatly, depending on a child's chronological and mental ages, but expected social interaction and liveliness are not present. Often, the child is not progressing developmentally or is frankly malnourished.

644

Perhaps the most typical clinical picture of an infant with one form of RAD is the nonorganic failure to thrive. Such infants usually exhibit hypokinesis, dullness, listlessness, and apathy with a poverty of spontaneous activity. Infants look sad, joyless, and miserable. Some infants also appear frightened and watchful, with a radar-like gaze. Nevertheless, they may exhibit delayed responsiveness to a stimulus that would elicit fright or withdrawal from a normal infant (Table 44.1–1). Infants with failure to thrive and RAD appear significantly malnourished, and many have protruding abdomens. Occasionally, foul-smelling, celiac-like stools are reported. In unusually severe cases, a clinical picture of marasmus appears.

The infant's weight is often below the third percentile and markedly below the appropriate weight for his or her height. If serial weights are available, the weight percentiles may have decreased progressively because of an actual weight loss or a failure to gain weight as height increases. Head circumference is usually normal for the infant's age. Muscle tone may be poor. The skin may be colder and paler or more mottled than skin of a normal child. Laboratory findings are usually within normal limits, except for abnormal findings coincident with any malnutrition,

dehydration, or concurrent illness. Bone age is usually retarded. Growth hormone levels are usually normal or elevated, a finding suggesting that growth failure in these children is secondary to caloric deprivation and malnutrition. The children improve physically and gain weight rapidly after they are hospitalized.

Socially, the infants usually show little spontaneous activity and a marked diminution of both initiative toward others and reciprocity in response to the caregiving adult or examiner. Both mother and infant may be indifferent to separation on hospitalization or to termination of subsequent hospital visits. The infants frequently show none of the normal upset, fretting, or protest about hospitalization. Older infants usually show little interest in their environment. They may not play with toys, even if encouraged; however, they rapidly or gradually take an interest in, and relate to, their caregivers in the hospital.

Classic psychosocial dwarfism or psychosocially determined short stature is a syndrome that usually is first manifest in children 2 to 3 years of age. The children are typically unusually short and have frequent growth hormone abnormalities and severe behavioral disturbances. All of these symptoms result from an inimical caregiver–child relationship. The affectionless character may appear when there is a failure, or lack of opportunity, to form attachments before the age of 2 to 3 years. Children cannot form lasting relationships, and their inability is sometimes accompanied by a lack of guilt, an inability to obey rules, and a need for attention and affection. Some children are indiscriminately friendly.

Table 44.1–1
DSM-IV-TR Diagnostic Criteria for Reactive Attachment Disorder of Infancy or Early Childhood

A. Markedly disturbed and developmentally inappropriate social relatedness in most contexts, beginning before age 5 years, as evidenced by either (1) or (2):
   (1) persistent failure to initiate or respond in a developmentally appropriate fashion to most social interactions, as manifest by excessively inhibited, hypervigilant, or highly ambivalent and contradictory responses (e.g., the child may respond to caregivers with a mixture of approach, avoidance, and resistance to comforting, or may exhibit frozen watchfulness)
   (2) diffuse attachments as manifest by indiscriminate sociability with marked inability to exhibit appropriate selective attachments (e.g., excessive familiarity with relative strangers or lack of selectivity in choice of attachment figures)
B. The disturbance in Criterion A is not accounted for solely by developmental delay (as in mental retardation) and does not meet criteria for a pervasive developmental disorder.
C. Pathogenic care as evidenced by at least one of the following:
   (1) persistent disregard of the child's basic emotional needs for comfort, stimulation, and affection
   (2) persistent disregard of the child's basic physical needs
   (3) repeated changes of primary caregiver that prevent formation of stable attachments (e.g., frequent changes in foster care)
D. There is a presumption that the care in Criterion C is responsible for the disturbed behavior in Criterion A (e.g., the disturbances in Criterion A began following the pathogenic care in Criterion C).

Specify type:
   Inhibited type: if Criterion A1 predominates in the clinical presentation
   Disinhibited type: if Criterion A2 predominates in the clinical presentation

From American Psychiatric Association. *Diagnostic and Statistical Manual of Mental Disorders.* 4th ed. Text rev. Washington, DC: American Psychiatric Association; copyright 2000, with permission.

A 6-year-old boy was referred by his adoptive parents because of hyperactivity and disruptive behavior at school. He had been adopted at 5 years of age, after living most of his life in a Romanian orphanage in which he received care from a rotating shift of caregivers. Although he had been below the 5th percentile for height and weight on arrival, he quickly approached the 10th percentile in his new home. However, both of his adoptive parents were frustrated by their inability to "reach him." They had initially worried about a hearing disturbance, although testing and his capacity to engage many adults and children verbally suggested otherwise. He showed interest in anyone and would often follow strangers willingly. He showed little empathy when others were hurt and blandly resisted redirection in school. He was frequently injured because of seemingly reckless behavior, although he had an extremely high tolerance for pain. Intensive intervention focused on problem behaviors at home decreased his self-endangering behavior, although he remained oddly overfriendly and nonempathic at home and in school. The boy was diagnosed with reactive attachment disorder, disinhibited type. (Courtesy of Neil W. Boris, M.D. and Charles H. Zeanah, Jr., M.D.)

PATHOLOGY AND LABORATORY EXAMINATION

Although no single specific laboratory test is used to make a diagnosis, many children with RAD have disturbances of growth and development. Thus, establishing a growth curve and examining the progression of developmental milestones may be helpful in determining whether associated phenomena, such as failure to thrive, are present.

DIFFERENTIAL DIAGNOSIS

The differential diagnosis of RAD must consider other psychiatric disorders that are more likely to arise in conjunction with conditions of maltreatment, including posttraumatic stress disorders, developmental language disorders, and mental retardation syndromes. Metabolic disorders, pervasive developmental disorders, mental retardation, various neurological abnormalities, and psychosocial dwarfism are also considerations in the differential diagnosis. Children with autistic disorder are typically well nourished and of age-appropriate size and weight; they are generally alert and active, despite their impairments in reciprocal social interactions. Moderate, severe, or profound mental retardation is present in about 50 percent of children with autistic disorder, whereas when mental retardation is comorbid with RAD, it is generally in milder forms. Unlike most children with RAD, children with autistic disorder do not improve rapidly if they are removed from their homes and placed in a hospital or other favorable environment. Mentally retarded children may show delays in all social skills. Such children, unlike children with RAD, are usually adequately nourished, their social relatedness is appropriate to their mental age, and they show a sequence of development similar to that seen in normal children.

COURSE AND PROGNOSIS

Most of the data available on the natural course of children with RAD come from follow-up studies of institutionalized children with histories of serious neglect. Findings from these studies suggest that in children with the inhibited patterns of RAD who are adopted into more normative caring environments, the quality of attachment behaviors tends to become more normalized over time. Children with the indiscriminate sociability and disinhibited forms of RAD appear to persist in behavioral patterns of children for years even when they appear to be attached to new caregivers. Children with indiscriminate social behavior tend to exhibit poor peer relationships over time. The prognosis for children with reactive attachment disorders is influenced by the duration and severity of the neglectful and pathogenic parenting and on associated complications, such as failure to thrive. Constitutional and nutritional factors interact in children, who may either respond resiliently to treatment or continue to fail to thrive. Outcomes range from the extremes of death to the developmentally healthy child. In general, the longer a child remains in the adverse environment without adequate intervention, the more the physical and emotional damage and the worse the prognosis. After the pathological environmental situation has been recognized, the amount of treatment and rehabilitation that the family receives affects the child who returns to this family. Children who have multiple problems stemming from pathogenic caregiving may recover physically faster and more completely than they do emotionally.

TREATMENT

Recommendations in the management of RAD must begin with a comprehensive assessment of the current level of safety and adequate caregiving. Thus, the first consideration in treating the disorder is a child's safety. With suspicion of maltreatment currently persisting in the home, the first decision is often whether to hospitalize the child or to attempt treatment while the child remains in the home. If neglect, or emotional, physical, or sexual abuse is suspected, legally, such must be reported to the appropriate law enforcement and child protective services in the area. The child's physical and emotional state and the level of pathological caregiving determine the therapeutic strategy. A determination must be made regarding the nutritional status of the child and the presence of ongoing physical abuse or threat. Hospitalization is necessary for children with malnourishment. Along with an assessment of the child's physical well-being, an evaluation of the child's emotional condition is important. Immediate intervention must address the parents' awareness and capacity to participate in altering the injurious patterns that have ensued. The treatment team must begin to alter the unsatisfactory relationship between the caregiver and child, which usually requires extensive and intensive intervention and education with the mother or with both parents when possible.

Psychosocial interventions for families in which a child has RAD include (1) psychosocial support services, including hiring a homemaker, improving the physical condition of the apartment, or obtaining more adequate housing; improving the family's financial status; and decreasing the family's isolation; (2) psychotherapeutic interventions, including individual psychotherapy, psychotropic medications, and family or marital therapy; (3) educational counseling services, including mother–infant or mother–toddler groups, and counseling to increase awareness and understanding of the child's needs and to increase parenting skills; and (4) provisions for close monitoring of the progression of the patient's emotional and physical well-being. Sometimes, separating a child from the stressful home environment temporarily, as in hospitalization, allows the child to break out of the accustomed pattern. A neutral setting, such as the hospital, is the best place to start with families who are genuinely available emotionally and physically for intervention. If interventions are unfeasible or inadequate or if they fail, placement with relatives or in foster care, adoption, or a group home or residential treatment facility must be considered.

▲ 44.2 Stereotypic Movement Disorder and Disorder of Infancy, Childhood, or Adolescence Not Otherwise Specified

STEREOTYPIC MOVEMENT DISORDER

Stereotypic movements are repetitive voluntary, often rhythmic movements, that occur in normal children, and with increased frequency in children who have received a diagnosis of pervasive developmental disorder and mental retardation syndromes. These movements appear to be purposeless, but in some cases, such as body rocking, head rocking, or hand flapping, they may be either self-soothing or self-stimulating. In other cases, stereotypic movements, such as head banging, face slapping, eye poking, or hand biting, can cause significant self-harm. Nail-biting, thumb-sucking, and nose-picking are generally not included as symptoms of stereotypic movement disorder because they rarely cause impairment.

According to the text revision of the fourth edition of *Diagnostic and Statistical Manual of Mental Disorders* (DSM-IV-TR), stereotypic movement disorder is repetitive, nonfunctional motor behavior that seems to be compulsive. The behavior significantly interferes with normal activities or produces self-inflicted bodily injuries sufficiently severe to require medical care unless the child is protected. For children with mental retardation, the injurious behavior is sufficiently dangerous to become the focus of treatment.

Epidemiology

The incidence of transient stereotypic habits is reported to be about 7 percent in the normal pediatric populations, with a prevalence of about 15 to 20 percent in children under the age of 6 years. After age 6 years, the rates of stereotypic movements in the normal population are unknown, but believed to be negligible. The prevalence of self-injurious behaviors, however, has been estimated to be in the range of 2 to 3 percent among children and adolescents with mental retardation.

Behaviors such as nail-biting are common and affect as many as one half of all school-age children; behaviors such as thumb-sucking and rocking are normal in young children, but are often maladaptive in older children and adolescents. These behaviors usually do not constitute a stereotypic movement disorder; most children who bite their nails function in daily activities without impairment or self-injury. In one pediatric clinic, as many as 20 percent of children had a history of rocking, head-banging, or swaying in one form or another.

Deciding which cases are sufficiently severe to confirm a diagnosis of stereotypic movement disorder may be difficult. The diagnosis is a compilation of many symptoms, and various behaviors must be studied separately to obtain data about prevalence, sex ratio, and familial patterns. It is clear, however, that stereotypic movement disorder is more prevalent in boys than in girls. Stereotypic behaviors are common among children who are mentally retarded; 10 to 20 percent are affected. Self-injurious behaviors occur in some genetic syndromes, such as Lesch-Nyhan syndrome, and also in some patients with Tourette's disorder. Self-injurious stereotypic behaviors are increasingly common in persons with severe mental retardation. Stereotypic behaviors are also common in children with sensory impairments, such as blindness and deafness.

Etiology

The causes of stereotypic movement disorder can be considered from the standpoint of behavioral factors, developmental factors, and functional and neurobiological perspectives. Some stereotypic behaviors in young children can be associated with normal development; for example, up to 80 percent of all normal children show rhythmic activities that phase out by 4 years of age. These rhythmic patterns seem to be purposeful, to provide sensorimotor stimulation and tension release, and to be satisfying and pleasurable to the children. The movements may increase at times of frustration, boredom, and tension.

The progression from early expressions of stereotyped behavior in toddlers to stereotypic movement disorder in older children often reflects disordered development, as in mental retardation or a pervasive developmental disorder. Genetic factors likely play a role in some stereotypic movements, such as the X-linked recessive deficiency of enzymes leading to Lesch-Nyhan syndrome, which has predictable features including mental retardation, hyperuricemia, spasticity, and self-injurious behaviors. Other stereotypic movements (e.g., nail-biting), although often causing minimal or no impairment, seem to run in families. Some stereotypic behaviors seem to emerge or become exaggerated in situations of neglect or deprivation; such behaviors as head-banging have been associated with psychosocial deprivation.

Stereotypic movements seem to be associated with dopamine activity. Neurobiological factors may contribute to the development of stereotypic movement disorders. Dopamine agonists induce or increase stereotypic behaviors, whereas dopamine antagonists decrease them. In one report, four children with attention-deficit/hyperactivity disorder (ADHD) who were treated with a stimulant medication began to bite their nails and fingertips. The nail-biting ceased when the medication was eliminated. Endogenous opioids also have been implicated in producing self-injurious behaviors.

Diagnosis and Clinical Features

The presence of multiple repetitive stereotyped symptoms tends to occur among those most severely afflicted with mental retardation or a pervasive developmental disorder. Patients with multiple stereotyped movements frequently have other significant mental disorders, including disruptive behavior disorders. In extreme cases, severe mutilation and life-threatening injuries can result, and secondary infection and septicemia may follow self-inflicted trauma. The DSM-IV-TR diagnostic criteria for stereotypic movement disorder are listed in Table 44.2–1.

Table 44.2–1
DSM-IV-TR Diagnostic Criteria for Stereotypic Movement Disorder

A. Repetitive, seemingly driven, and nonfunctional motor behavior (e.g., hand shaking or waving, body rocking, head banging, mouthing of objects, self-biting, picking at skin or bodily orifices, hitting own body).
B. The behavior markedly interferes with normal activities or results in self-inflicted bodily injury that requires medical treatment (or would result in an injury if preventive measures were not used).
C. If mental retardation is present, the stereotypic or self-injurious behavior is of sufficient severity to become a focus of treatment.
D. The behavior is not better accounted for by a compulsion (as in obsessive-compulsive disorder), a tic (as in tic disorder), a stereotypy that is part of a pervasive developmental disorder, or hair pulling (as in trichotillomania).
E. The behavior is not due to the direct physiological effects of a substance or a general medical condition.
F. The behavior persists for 4 weeks or longer.

Specify if:
With self-injurious behavior: if the behavior results in bodily damage that requires specific treatment (or that would result in bodily damage if protective measures were not used)

From American Psychiatric Association. *Diagnostic and Statistical Manual of Mental Disorders.* 4th ed. Text rev. Washington, DC: American Psychiatric Association; copyright 2000, with permission.

Head Banging.   Head banging exemplifies a stereotypic movement disorder that can result in functional impairment. According to the DSM-IV-TR, the male-to-female ratio is 3 to 1. Typically, head-banging begins during infancy, between 6 and 12 months of age. Infants strike their heads with a definite rhythmic and monotonous continuity against the crib or another hard surface. They seem to be absorbed in the activity, which can persist until they become exhausted and fall asleep. The head-banging is often transitory, but sometimes persists into middle childhood. Head-banging that is a component of temper tantrums differs from stereotypic head-banging and ceases after the tantrums and their secondary gains have been controlled.

Nail Biting.   Nail biting begins as early as 1 year of age and increases in incidence until age 12. All nails are usually bitten. Most cases are not sufficiently severe to meet the DSM-IV-TR diagnostic criteria. In other cases, children cause physical damage to the fingers themselves, usually by associated biting of the cuticles, which leads to secondary infections of the fingers and nail beds. Nail-biting seems to occur or increase in intensity when a person is either anxious or bored. Some of the most severe nail-biting occurs in those who are severely and profoundly mentally retarded and some patients with paranoid schizophrenia; however, some nail-biters have no obvious emotional disturbance.

Pathology and Laboratory Examination

No specific laboratory measures are helpful in the diagnosis of stereotypic movement disorder.

Victor, a legally blind 14-year-old boy with severe mental retardation, was evaluated when he transferred to a new residential school for children with multiple disabilities. Observed in his classroom, he was noted to be a small boy who appeared younger than his age. He held his hands in his pockets and spun around in place. Periodically, he approached his teacher, kissed her, positioned himself to receive a return kiss, and clearly enjoyed the contact with her. When offered a toy (which had to be held close to his eyes), he took it and manipulated it for awhile. When he was prompted to engage in various tasks that required that he take his hands out of his pockets, he began hitting his head with his hands. If his hands were held by the teacher, he hit his head with his knees. He was adept in contorting himself, so that he could hit or kick himself in almost any position, even while walking. Soon, his face and forehead were covered with black-and-blue marks.

Only sketchy personal history was available. He was a premature baby, with birthweight of 2 pounds. Retinopathy of prematurity and severe mental retardation were diagnosed early in life. His development was delayed in all spheres, and he never developed language. Comprehensive studies did not disclose the etiology of Victor's developmental disabilities other than prematurity. He lived at home and attended a special educational program. His self-injurious behaviors developed early in life, and, when his parents tried to stop him, he became aggressive. Gradually, he became too difficult for them to manage, and, at 3 years of age, he was placed in a special school. The self-abusive and self-restraining (i.e., holding his hands in his pockets) behavior was present throughout his stay there, and, virtually all of the

time, he was on one antipsychotic medication or another. He carried a diagnosis of *cerebral dysfunction*. Although the psychiatrist's notes mentioned improvement in his self-injurious behavior, other notes described it as continuing and fluctuating. He was transferred to the new school because of lack of progress and difficulties in managing him as he became bigger and stronger. His intellectual functioning was within the 34 to 40 intelligence quotient (IQ) range. His adaptive skills were poor. He required full assistance in self-care, could not provide even for his own simple needs, and required constant supervision for his safety.

In a few months, Victor settled into the routine in his new school. His self-injurious behavior fluctuated. It was reduced or even absent when he restrained himself by holding his hands in his pockets or inside his shirt or even by manipulating some object with his hands. If left to himself, he could contort himself, while holding his hands inside his shirt, to such degree that he was nicknamed Pretzel. Because the stereotypic self-injurious and self-restraining behavior interfered with his daily activities and education, it became a primary focus of a behavior modification program. For a few months, he did well, especially when he developed a good relationship with a new teacher, who was firm, consistent, and nurturing. With him, Victor could engage in some school tasks. When the teacher left, Victor regressed. To prevent injuries, the staff started blocking his self-hitting with a pillow. He was offered activities that he liked and in which he could engage without resorting to self-injury. After several months, his antipsychotic medication was slowly discontinued, over a period of 11 months, without any behavioral deterioration. (Courtesy of Bhavik Shah, M.D.)

Differential Diagnosis

The differential diagnosis of stereotypic movement disorder includes obsessive-compulsive disorder (OCD) and tic disorders, both of which are exclusionary criteria in DSM-IV-TR. Although stereotypic movements are voluntary and not spasmodic, it is difficult to differentiate these features from tics in all cases. A recent study of stereotyped movements compared with tics found that stereotyped movements tended to be longer in duration, and displayed more rhythmic qualities than tics. Tics seemed to occur more when a child was in an "alone" condition, rather than when the child was in a play condition, whereas stereotypic movements occurred with the same frequency in these two different conditions. Stereotypic movements are likely to be self-soothing, whereas tics are often associated with distress. In OCD, the compulsions must be ego-dystonic, although this, too, is difficult to discern in young children.

Differentiating dyskinetic movements from stereotypic movements can be difficult. Because antipsychotic medications can suppress stereotypic movements, clinicians must note any stereotypic movements before initiating treatment with an antipsychotic agent. Stereotypic movement disorder may be diagnosed concurrently with substance-related disorders (e.g., amphetamine use disorders), severe sensory impairments, central nervous system and degenerative disorders (e.g., Lesch-Nyhan syndrome), and severe schizophrenia.

Course and Prognosis

The duration and course of stereotypic movement disorder vary, and the symptoms may wax and wane. As many as 80 percent of normal children show rhythmic activities that seem purposeful and comforting and tend to disappear by 4 years of age. When stereotypic movements are present or emerge more severely later in childhood or in a noncomforting manner, they range from brief episodes occurring under stress to an ongoing pattern in the context of a chronic condition, such as mental retardation or a pervasive developmental disorder. Even in chronic conditions, stereotypic behaviors may come and go. In some cases, stereotypic movements are prominent in early childhood and diminish as a child gets older.

The severity of the dysfunction caused by stereotypic movements also varies with the associated frequency, amount, and degree of self-injury. Children who exhibit frequent, severe, self-injurious stereotypic behaviors have the poorest prognosis. Repetitive episodes of head-banging, self-biting, and eye-poking can be difficult to control without physical restraints. Most nail-biting is benign and often does not meet the diagnostic criteria for stereotypic movement disorder. In severe cases in which the nail beds are repetitively damaged, bacterial and fungal infections can occur. Although chronic stereotypic movement disorders can severely impair daily functioning, several treatments help control the symptoms.

Treatment

Treatment modalities yielding the most promising effects include behavioral techniques, such as habit reversal and differential reinforcement of other behavior, as well as pharmacological interventions. A recent report on utilizing both habit reversal (in which the child is trained to replace the undesired repetitive behavior with a more acceptable behavior) and reinforcement for reducing the unwanted behavior indicated that these treatments had efficacy among 12 nonautistic children between 6 and 14 years.

Pharmacologic interventions have been used in clinical practice to minimize self-injury in children whose stereotyped movements caused significant harm to their bodies. In the past, typical antipsychotics were utilized; more recently, however, atypical antipsychotics are favored. Small open-label studies have re- ported benefit of atypical antipsychotics, and case reports have indicated use of serotonin reuptake inhibitor agents in the management of self-injurious stereotypies. Valproic acid has been used clinically, although no current controlled trial supports its use.

The dopamine antagonists have been the commonly used medications for treating stereotypic movements and self-injurious behavior. Phenothiazines have been the most frequently used drugs. Opiate antagonists have reduced self-injurious behaviors in some patients without exposing them to tardive dyskinesia or impaired cognition. Additional pharmacological agents that have been tried in the treatment of stereotypic movement disorder include fenfluramine (Pondimin), clomipramine (Anafranil), and fluoxetine (Prozac). In some reports, fenfluramine diminished stereotypic behaviors in children with autistic disorder; in other studies, the results were less encouraging. Open trials indicate that both clomipramine and fluoxetine may decrease self-injurious behaviors and other stereotypic movements in some patients. Trazodone (Desyrel) and buspirone (BuSpar) have also been tried, with unclear results.

DISORDER OF INFANCY, CHILDHOOD, OR ADOLESCENCE NOT OTHERWISE SPECIFIED

The DSM-IV-TR describes disorder of infancy, childhood, or adolescence not otherwise specified as a category that includes disorders with onset in infancy, childhood, or adolescence that do not meet the criteria for any specific disorder. The DSM-IV-TR diagnostic criteria are shown in Table 44.2–2.

Table 44.2–2
DSM-IV-TR Diagnostic Criteria for Disorder of Infancy, Childhood, or Adolescence Not Otherwise Specified

This category is a residual category for disorders with onset in infancy, childhood, or adolescence that do not meet criteria for any specific disorder in the classification.

From American Psychiatric Association. *Diagnostic and Statistical Manual of Mental Disorders.* 4th ed. Text rev. Washington, DC: American Psychiatric Association; copyright 2000, with permission.

45

Mood Disorders and Suicide in Children and Adolescents

▲ 45.1 Depressive Disorders and Suicide in Children and Adolescents

Depressive disorders occur in children of all ages but are much more prevalent with increasing age. Children and adolescents with depressive disorders often display irritability, withdrawal from family and peers, and deterioration in academic investment, leading to devastating social isolation. The core features of major depressive disorder have striking similarities in children, adolescents, and adults, although developmental factors influence its clinical presentation.

Although suicidal thoughts and behaviors can occur in the context of a depressive disorder, most youth who contemplate, attempt, or complete suicide are not in the midst of a major depression. Most children and adolescents with depressive disorders do not exhibit suicidal behaviors. Thus, it is not clear that optimal treatments for depression mitigate the risks of suicidality among youth in general.

Mood disorders among children and adolescents have been increasingly recognized over the last three decades, and evidence suggests that combined treatment modalities, including medication and cognitive-behavioral strategies, may have the greatest efficacy. Although clinicians and parents have readily acknowledged transient sadness and despair among youth, it has become clear that the full criteria of persistent disorders of mood can occur even in prepubertal children. Two criteria for mood disorders in childhood and adolescence are a disturbance of mood, such as depression or elation, and irritability.

Although diagnostic criteria for mood disorders in the text revision of the fourth edition of the *Diagnostic and Statistical Manual of Mental Disorders* (DSM-IV-TR) are almost identical across all age groups, the expression of disturbed mood varies in children according to their age. Young, depressed children commonly show symptoms that appear less often as they grow older, including mood-congruent auditory hallucinations, somatic complaints, withdrawn and sad appearance, and poor self-esteem. Symptoms that are more common among depressed youngsters in late adolescence than in young childhood are pervasive anhedonia, severe psychomotor retardation, delusions, and a sense of hopelessness. Symptoms that appear with the same frequency regardless of age and developmental status include suicidal ideation, depressed or irritable mood, insomnia, and diminished ability to concentrate.

EPIDEMIOLOGY

Depressive disorders increase in frequency with increasing age in the general population. Mood disorders among preschool-age children are extremely rare; the rate of major depressive disorder in preschoolers is estimated to be about 0.3 percent in the community and 0.9 percent in a clinic setting. Among prepubertal school-age children in the community, the point prevalence is approximately 1 percent. Depression in referred samples of school-age children is about the same in boys as in girls, with some surveys indicating a slightly increased rate among boys. Among adolescents, reported rates of major depression range from 1 to about 6 percent in community samples, and the rate of depression among adolescent females is double the rate in adolescent males. Estimates of cumulative prevalence of depression among older adolescents range between 14 and 25 percent. Reported rates of dysthymic disorder are generally lower than those of major depressive disorder, with rates of 5 of 100,000 in prepubertal children compared with 1 percent for major depressive disorder. School-age children with dysthymic disorder have a high likelihood of developing major depressive disorder at some point after 1 year of the dysthymic disorder. In adolescents, as in adults, dysthymic disorder is reported to occur in about 5 of 1,000 adolescents compared with about 5 percent for major depressive disorder.

Among hospitalized children and adolescents, the rates of major depressive disorder are much higher than in the general community; of these, as many as 20 percent of children and 40 percent of adolescents are depressed.

ETIOLOGY

Considerable evidence indicates that the mood disorders in childhood are the same fundamental diseases experienced by adults.

Molecular Genetic Studies

Two genes have been identified as incurring vulnerability for depressive disorder. The first one, the MAOA gene, is responsible for the functioning of monoamine oxidase, and the second is the serotonin transporter gene (5-HTT). The serotonin transporter gene, which is involved in the process of making serotonin available, is present in homozygous long alleles, a heterozygous one long and one short allele pair, and homozygous short alleles. A large longitudinal study in New Zealand found a relationship of early environmental stress and subsequent depression in children with one or two short alleles, but not in those children in the sample with two long alleles. Because the short alleles are less efficient in transcription, this finding suggests that the availability of the transporter gene may provide a marker for vulnerability to depression. Thus, a stress-diathesis model for the emergence of depression may best fit with these data.

Familiality.
Mood disorders in children, adolescents, and adult patients tend to cluster in the same families. An increased incidence of mood disorders is generally found among children of parents with mood disorders and relatives of children with mood disorders; having one depressed parent probably doubles the risk for offspring. Having two depressed parents probably quadruples the risk of a child having a mood disorder before age 18 years compared with the risk for children with two unaffected parents. Some evidence indicates that the number of recurrences of parental depression increases the likelihood that the children will be affected, but this increase may be only partly related to the affective loading of the parent's own family tree. Similarly, children with the largest number of severe episodes have shown much evidence of dense and deep familial aggregation for major depressive disorder.

Biological Factors.
Studies of prepubertal major depressive disorder and adolescent mood disorder have revealed a variety of biological abnormalities. For example, prepubertal children in an episode of depressive disorder secrete significantly more growth hormone during sleep than do normal children and those with nondepressed mental disorders. These children also secrete significantly less growth hormone in response to insulin-induced hypoglycemia than do nondepressed patients. Both abnormalities persist for at least 4 months of full, sustained clinical response, with the last month in a drug-free state. In contrast, the data conflict regarding cortisol hypersecretion during major depressive disorder; some workers report hypersecretion, and others report normal secretion.

Sleep studies are inconclusive in depressed children and adolescents. Polysomnography shows either no change or changes characteristic of adults with major depressive disorder: reduced rapid eye movement (REM) latency and an increased number of REM periods.

Magnetic Resonance Imaging.
Magnetic resonance imaging (MRI) scans in more than 100 psychiatrically hospitalized children with mood disturbances show a low frontal lobe volume and a high ventricular volume. These results are consistent with MRI findings in adults with major depression insofar as postmortem studies of depressed adults have demonstrated selective loss of frontal lobe cells and frontal lobe serotonin. Damage to the frontal lobes has also been associated with depressive symptoms in patients after stroke. The frontal lobes seem to have multiple connections with the basal ganglia and the limbic system and are also believed to be involved in the neuropathology of depressive symptomatology.

Endocrine Studies.
Thyroid hormone studies have found lower free total thyroxine (FT4) levels in depressed adolescents than in a matched control group. These values were associated with normal thyroid-stimulating hormone. This finding suggests that, although values of thyroid function remain in the normative range, FT4 levels have been shifted downward. These downward shifts in thyroid hormone possibly contribute to the clinical manifestations of depression. Some data suggest that the addition of exogenous thyroid hormone can potentiate the effects of antidepressant medication in adults with depression. Impairment in mood and cognitive function in adults with subclinical hypothyroidism has been found to be corrected with exogenous thyroid hormone.

Social Factors

The finding that identical twins do not have 100 percent concordance suggests a role for nongenetic factors in the emergence of major depressive disorder. Despite a lack of definitive evidence,

given the stress-diathesis hypotheses of depression, genetic vulnerability in combination with a variety of social factors, including level of family conflict, abuse or neglect, conflict, family socioeconomic status, and parental separation or divorce, may play a significant role in the emergence of depressive disorders in children. Evidence indicates that boys whose fathers died before they were 13 years of age are at greater risk than controls to develop depression.

The psychosocial impairment that characterizes depressed children lingers far after recovery from the index episode of depression. These deficits can be compounded by the relatively long duration of at least 1 year for a dysthymic episode and an average of 9 months to 1 year for a depressive episode in a child or adolescent. For an adolescent, a major depressive episode significantly interferes with social and academic skills, which are poorly accomplished or unaccomplished during the episode. Among preschoolers with depressive clinical presentations, the role of environmental influences is likely to have a significant impact on the course and recovery of the young child.

DIAGNOSIS AND CLINICAL FEATURES

Major Depressive Disorder

Major depressive disorder in children is diagnosed most easily when it is acute and occurs in a child without previous psychiatric symptoms. Often, however, the onset is insidious, and the disorder occurs in a child who has had several years of difficulties with hyperactivity, separation anxiety disorder, or intermittent depressive symptoms.

According to the DSM-IV-TR diagnostic criteria for major depressive episode, at least five symptoms must be present for a period of 2 weeks, and there must be a change from previous functioning. Among the necessary symptoms is either a depressed or irritable mood or a loss of interest or pleasure. Other symptoms from which the other four diagnostic criteria are drawn include a child's failure to make expected weight gains, daily insomnia or hypersomnia, psychomotor agitation or retardation, daily fatigue or loss of energy, feelings of worthlessness or inappropriate guilt, diminished ability to think or concentrate, and recurrent thoughts of death. These symptoms must produce social or academic impairment. To meet the diagnostic criteria for major depressive disorder, the symptoms cannot be the direct effects of a substance (e.g., alcohol) or a general medical condition. A diagnosis of major depressive disorder is not made within 2 months of the loss of a loved one, except when marked functional impairment, morbid preoccupation with worthlessness, suicidal ideation, psychotic symptoms, or psychomotor retardation is present.

A major depressive episode in a prepubertal child is likely to be manifest by somatic complaints, psychomotor agitation, and mood-congruent hallucinations. Anhedonia is also frequent, but anhedonia, as well as hopelessness, psychomotor retardation, and delusions, are more common in adolescent and adult major depressive episodes than in those of young children. Adults have more problems with sleep and appetite than depressed children and adolescents. In adolescence, negativistic or frankly antisocial behavior and the use of alcohol or illicit substances can occur and may justify the additional diagnoses of oppositional defiant disorder, conduct disorder, and substance abuse or dependence. Feelings of restlessness, grouchiness, aggression, sulkiness,

reluctance to cooperate in family ventures, withdrawal from social activities, and a desire to leave home are all common in
adolescent depression. School difficulties are likely. Adolescents
may be inattentive to personal appearance and show increased
emotionality, with particular sensitivity to rejection in love relationships.

Children can be reliable reporters about their own behavior,
emotions, relationships, and difficulties in psychosocial functions. They may, however, refer to their feelings by many names.
Clinicians, therefore, must ask children about feeling sad, empty,
low, down, blue, or very unhappy and about feeling like crying
or about having a bad feeling that is present most of the time.
Depressed children usually identify one or more of these terms as
their persistent feeling. Clinicians should assess the duration and
periodicity of the depressive mood to differentiate relatively universal, short-lived, and sometimes frequent periods of sadness,
usually after a frustrating event, from a true, persistent depressive mood. The younger the child, the more imprecise his or her
time estimates are likely to be.

Mood disorders tend to be chronic if they begin early. Childhood onset may be the most severe form of mood disorder and
tends to appear in families with a high incidence of mood disorders and alcohol abuse. The children are likely to have such
secondary complications as conduct disorder, alcohol and other
substance abuse, and antisocial behavior. Functional impairment
associated with a depressive disorder in childhood extends to
practically all areas of a child's psychosocial world; school performance and behavior, peer relationships, and family relationships all suffer. Only highly intelligent and academically oriented children with no more than a moderate depression can
compensate for their difficulties in learning by substantially increasing their time and effort. Otherwise, school performance is
invariably affected by a combination of difficulty concentrating,
slowed thinking, lack of interest and motivation, fatigue, sleepiness, depressive ruminations, and preoccupations. Depression
in a child may be misdiagnosed as a learning disorder. Learning problems secondary to depression, even when long-standing,
are corrected rapidly after a child's recovery from the depressive
episode.

Children and adolescents with major depressive disorder
may have hallucinations and delusions. Usually, these psychotic
symptoms are thematically consistent with the depressed mood,
occur with the depressive episode (usually at its worst), and
do not include certain types of hallucinations (such as conversing voices and a commenting voice, which are specific to
schizophrenia). Depressive hallucinations usually consist of a
single voice speaking to the person from outside of his or her
head, with derogatory or suicidal content. Depressive delusions
center on themes of guilt, physical disease, death, nihilism, deserved punishment, personal inadequacy, and (sometimes) persecution. These delusions are rare in prepuberty, probably because of cognitive immaturity, but are present in about one half
of psychotically depressed adolescents.

Adolescent onset of a mood disorder can be difficult to diagnose when first seen if the adolescent has attempted self-
medication with alcohol or other illicit substances. In a recent
study, 17 percent of young persons with a mood disorder first
received medical attention because of substance abuse. Only after detoxification could the psychiatric symptoms be assessed
properly and the mood disorder diagnosed correctly.

Dysthymic Disorder

Dysthymic disorder in children and adolescents consists in a depressed or irritable mood for most of the day, for more days than
not, over a period of at least 1 year. DSM-IV-TR notes that in children and adolescents, irritable mood can replace the depressed
mood criterion for adults and that the duration criterion is not
2 years but 1 year. According to the DSM-IV-TR diagnostic criteria, at least three of the following symptoms must accompany
the depressed or irritable mood: poor self-esteem, pessimism
or hopelessness, loss of interest, social withdrawal, chronic fatigue, feelings of guilt or brooding about the past, irritability or
excessive anger, decreased activity or productivity, and poor concentration or memory. During the year of the disturbance, these
symptoms do not resolve for more than 2 months at a time. In
addition, the diagnostic criteria for dysthymic disorder specify
that during the first year, no major depressive episode emerges.
To meet the DSM-IV-TR diagnostic criteria for dysthymic disorder, a child must not have a history of a manic or hypomanic
episode. Dysthymic disorder is also not diagnosed if the symptoms occur exclusively during a chronic psychotic disorder or
if they are the direct effects of a substance or a general medical
condition. DSM-IV-TR provides for specification of early onset
(before 21 years of age) or late onset (after 21 years of age).

A child or adolescent with dysthymic disorder may have had a major
depressive episode before developing a dysthymic disorder, but it is much
more common for a child with dysthymic disorder for more than 1 year
to have major depressive episode. In this case, both depressive diagnoses
are given (double depression). Dysthymic disorder in children is known
to have an average age of onset that is several years earlier than the age of
onset of major depressive disorder. Controversy exists among clinicians
and researchers about whether dysthymic disorder is best categorized as
a chronic, insidious version of major depressive disorder or represents
a separate disorder. Occasionally, young persons fulfill the criteria for
dysthymic disorder, except that their episodes last only 2 weeks to several
months, with symptom-free intervals lasting for 2 to 3 months. These
minor mood presentations in children are likely to indicate severe mood
disorder episodes in the future. Knowledge suggests that the longer,
the more recurrent, the more frequent, and perhaps the less related to
social stress these episodes are, the greater is the likelihood of a severe
mood disorder in the future. When minor depressive episodes follow a
significant stressful life event by less than 3 months, it is often part of an
adjustment disorder.

Cyclothymic Disorder

The only difference in the DSM-IV-TR diagnostic criteria for
child or adolescent cyclothymic disorder is that a period of 1
year of numerous mood swings is necessary instead of the adult
criterion of 2 years. Some adolescents with cyclothymic disorder
probably experience bipolar I disorder.

Schizoaffective Disorder

The criteria for schizoaffective disorder in children and adolescents are identical to those in adults. Although some adolescents
and probably some children do fit the criteria for schizoaffective
disorder, little is known about the natural course of their illness,
family history, psychobiology, and treatment. In DSM-IV-TR,
schizoaffective disorder in children is classified as a psychotic
disorder.

Bereavement

Bereavement is a state of grief related to the death of a loved one, which can occur with symptoms characteristic of a major depressive episode. Typical depressive symptoms associated with bereavement include feelings of sadness, insomnia, diminished appetite, and, in some cases, weight loss. Grieving children may become withdrawn and appear sad, and they are not easily drawn into even favorite activities.

In DSM-IV-TR, bereavement is not a mental disorder but is in the category of additional conditions that may be a focus of clinical attention. Children in the midst of a typical bereavement period may also meet the criteria for major depressive disorder when the symptoms persist longer than 2 months after the loss. In some instances, severe depressive symptoms within 2 months of the loss are considered to be beyond the scope of normal grieving, and a diagnosis of major depressive disorder is warranted. Symptoms indicating major depressive disorder exceeding usual bereavement include guilt related to issues beyond those surrounding the death of the loved one, preoccupation with death other than thoughts about being dead to be with the deceased person, morbid preoccupation with worthlessness, marked psychomotor retardation, prolonged serious functional impairment, and hallucinations other than transient perceptions of the voice of the deceased person.

The duration of a normal period of bereavement varies; in children, the duration may depend partly on the support system in place. For example, a child who must be removed from home because of the death of the only parent in the home may feel devastated and abandoned for a long time. Children who lose loved ones may feel that the death occurred because they were bad or did not perform as expected. The reaction to the loss of a loved one can be partly influenced by the child's being prepared for the death because of the chronic illness preceding it.

PATHOLOGY AND LABORATORY EXAMINATION

No single laboratory test is useful in making a diagnosis of a mood disorder. A screening test for thyroid function can rule out the possibility of an endocrinological contribution. Dexamethasone-suppression tests may be performed serially in cases of major depressive disorder to document whether an initial nonsuppressor becomes a suppressor with treatment or with resolution of the symptoms.

DIFFERENTIAL DIAGNOSIS

Substance-induced mood disorder can sometimes be differentiated from other mood disorders only after detoxification. Anxiety symptoms and conduct-disordered behavior can coexist with depressive disorders and frequently can pose problems in differentiating those disorders from nondepressed emotional and conduct disorders.

Of particular importance is the distinction between agitated depressive or manic episodes and attention-deficit/hyperactivity disorder (ADHD), in which the persistent excessive activity and restlessness can cause confusion. Prepubertal children do not show classic forms of agitated depression, such as hand-wringing and pacing. Instead, an inability to sit still and frequent temper tantrums are the most common symptoms. Sometimes, the correct diagnosis becomes evident only after remission of the depressive episode. If a child has no difficulty concentrating, is not hyperactive when recovered from a depressive episode, and is in a drug-free state, ADHD probably is not present.

COURSE AND PROGNOSIS

The course and prognosis of mood disorders in children and adolescents depend on the age of onset, episode severity, and the presence of comorbid disorders. In most cases, younger age of onset, recurrent episodes, and comorbid disorders predict a poorer prognosis. The mean length of an episode of major depression in children and adolescents is about 9 months; the cumulative probability of recurrence is 40 percent by 2 years and 70 percent by 5 years. Reportedly, depressed children who live in families with high levels of chronic conflict are more likely to have relapses. Follow-up studies have found that in 20 to 40 percent of adolescents who have a major depression, bipolar I disorder will develop in a period of 5 years after the index depression. Clinical characteristics of the depressive episode that suggest the highest risk of developing bipolar I disorder include delusionality and psychomotor retardation in addition to a family history of bipolar illness. Depressive disorders are associated with short- and long-term peer relationship difficulties and complications, poor academic achievement, and persistently poor self-esteem. Dysthymic disorder has an even more protracted recovery than major depression; the mean episode length is about 4 years. Early-onset dysthymic disorder is associated with significant risks of comorbidity with major depression (70 percent), bipolar disorder (13 percent), and eventual substance abuse (15 percent). The risk of suicide, which represents 12 percent of mortalities in the adolescent age range, is significant among adolescents with depressive disorders.

TREATMENT

Hospitalization

Safety is the most immediate consideration in evaluating a child or adolescent with major depression, and determining whether hospitalization is indicated to keep the child or adolescent safe becomes the first decision point. Children and adolescents who are depressed and express suicidal thoughts or behaviors are in need of an extended evaluation in the hospital to provide maximal protection against the patient's self-destructive impulses and behavior. Hospitalization also may be needed when a child or adolescent has coexisting substance abuse or dependence.

Psychotherapy

Cognitive-behavioral therapy (CBT) is widely recognized as an efficacious intervention for the treatment of moderately severe depression in children and adolescents. Cognitive-behavioral therapy aims to challenge maladaptive beliefs and enhance problem-solving abilities and social competence. A recent review of controlled cognitive-behavioral studies in children and adolescents revealed that, as with adults, both children and adolescents showed consistent improvement with these methods. Other "active" treatments, including relaxation techniques, were also shown to be helpful as adjunctive treatment for mild to moderate depression. Findings from one large controlled study comparing cognitive-behavioral interventions with nondirective supportive psychotherapy and systemic behavioral family therapy showed that 70 percent of adolescents had some improvement with each of the interventions; cognitive-behavioral intervention had the most rapid effect. Another controlled study comparing a brief course of CBT with relaxation therapy favored the cognitive-behavioral intervention. At a 3- to 6-month follow-up, however, no significant differences existed between the two treatment groups. This effect resulted from relapse in the cognitive-behavioral group, along with continued recovery in some patients in the relaxation group. Factors that seem to interfere with treatment responsiveness include the presence of comorbid anxiety disorder that probably was present before the depressive episode.

Family education and participation are necessary treatment components for children with depression, especially to promote more effective conflict resolution. Because depressed children's psychosocial function can remain impaired for long periods, even after the depressive episode has remitted, long-term social support from families and (in some cases) social skills interventions are helpful. Modeling and role-playing techniques can be useful in fostering good problem-solving skills.

Pharmacotherapy

Pharmacologic agents from among the selective serotonin reuptake inhibitors (SSRIs) are widely accepted as first-line pharmacological intervention for moderate to severe depressive disorders in children and adolescents. Acute randomized clinical trials have demonstrated efficacy of fluoxetine (Prozac), citalopram (Celexa), and sertraline (Zoloft) compared with placebo in the treatment of major depression in children and adolescents. In September 2004, the U.S. Food and Drug Administration received information from their Psychopharmacologic Drug and Pediatric advisory committee indicating, based on their review of reported suicidal thoughts and behavior among depressed children and adolescents who participated in randomized clinical trials with nine different antidepressants, an increased risk of suicidality in those children on active antidepressant medications.

Several reviews since then, however, have concluded that the data do not indicate a significant increase in the risk of suicide or serious suicide attempt after starting treatment with antidepressant drugs. Rather than a worsening effect, antidepressant use was associated with the protective effect against new-onset and ongoing suicidal ideation. One study showed that the rates of suicide attempts in patients treated with an antidepressant were one third of those observed for patients not treated with an antidepressant. In a strongly worded editorial in the *Journal of the American Psychiatric Association* (July 2007) it was concluded that, "It is much more likely that suicidal behavior leads to treatment than that treatment leads to suicidal behavior."

When first-line SSRI medications have not led to improvement, other antidepressant agents are used clinically, although without proven efficacy. For example, bupropion (Wellbutrin) has stimulant properties as well as antidepressant efficacy and has been used for youth with both ADHD and depression. It has few anticholinergic properties or other adverse effects such as sedation. Venlafaxine (Effexor), which blocks both serotonin and norepinephrine uptake, has been used clinically in the treatment of depression in adolescents. Adverse effects are usually mild, and include agitation, nervousness, and nausea. Mirtazapine (Remeron) is also a serotonin and norepinephrine uptake inhibitor with a relatively safe adverse-effect profile, but it has not been used as frequently because of its adverse effect of sedation.

Tricyclic antidepressants are not generally recommended for the treatment of depression in children and adolescents because of the lack of proven efficacy along with the potential risk of cardiac arrhythmia associated with their use.

One possible outcome of treating a depressed child or adolescent with an antidepressant agent is the emergence of behavioral activation or induction of hypomanic symptoms. In these cases, the medication should be discontinued to determine whether the activation resolves with discontinuation of the medication or evolves into a hypomanic or manic episode. Hypomanic symptom responses to antidepressants, however, do not necessarily predict that bipolar disorder has emerged.

Duration of Treatment

Based on longitudinal data and the natural history of major depression in children and adolescents, current recommendations include maintaining antidepressant treatment for 1 year in a depressed child who has achieved a good response and then discontinuing the medication at a time of relatively low stress for a medication-free period.

Pharmacological Treatment Strategies for Resistant Depression

Given the data, the current pharmacological recommendations, taking into account a consensus panel for the Texas Children's Medication Algorithm Project, are to treat first with one of the SSRIs alone and, if no response occurs within a reasonable amount of time—perhaps, up to 3 months—change to another SSRI medication. If a child is not responsive to the second SSRI medication, then either a combination of antidepressants or augmentation strategies may be reasonable choices, as well as an antidepressant from another class of medications.

Electroconvulsive Therapy. Electroconvulsive therapy (ECT) has been used for a variety of psychiatric illnesses in adults, primarily severe depressive and manic mood disorders and catatonia. ECT rarely is used for adolescents, although published case reports indicate its efficacy in adolescents with depression and mania. Case reports suggest that ECT may be a relatively safe and useful treatment for adolescents who have persistent severe affective disorders, particularly with psychotic features, catatonic symptoms, or persistent suicidality.

SUICIDE

In the United States, suicide is the second leading cause of death among adolescents, topped by accidental death and homicide. In all countries, suicide rarely occurs in children who have not reached puberty. In the last 15 years, the rates of both completed suicide and suicidal ideation have decreased among adolescents. This decrease appears to coincide with the increase in SSRI medications prescribed to adolescents with mood and behavioral disturbance. Suicidal ideation, gestures, and attempts are frequently, but not always, associated with depressive disorders. Reports indicate that as many as half of suicidal individuals express suicidal intentions to a friend or a relative within 24 hours before enacting suicidal behavior.

Suicidal ideation occurs in all age groups and with greatest frequency in children and adolescents with severe mood disorders. More than 12,000 children and adolescents are hospitalized in the United States each year because of suicidal threats or behavior, but completed suicide is rare in children younger than 12 years of age. A young child is hardly capable of designing and carrying out a realistic suicide plan. Cognitive immaturity seems to play a protective role in preventing even children who wish they were dead from committing suicide. Completed suicide occurs about five times more often in adolescent boys than in girls, although the rate of suicide attempts is at least three times higher among adolescent girls than among boys. Suicidal ideation is not a static phenomenon; it can wax and wane. The decision to engage in suicidal behavior may be made impulsively without much forethought, or the decision may be the culmination of prolonged rumination.

The method of the suicide attempt influences the morbidity and completion rates, independent of the severity of the intent to die at the time of the suicidal behavior. The most common method of completed suicide in children and adolescents is the use of firearms, which accounts for about two thirds of all suicides in boys and almost one half of suicides in girls. The second-most-common method of suicide in boys, occurring in about one fourth of all cases, is hanging; in girls, about one fourth commit suicide through ingestion of toxic substances. Carbon monoxide poisoning is the next-most-common method of suicide in boys, but it occurs in less than 10 percent; suicide by hanging and carbon monoxide poisoning are equally frequent among girls and account for about 10 percent each. Additional risk factors in suicide include a family history of suicidal behavior, exposure to family violence, impulsivity, substance abuse, and availability of lethal methods.

Epidemiology

Suicide rates in 2000 among boys and girls 10 to 14 years of age were 2.3 and 0.6 per 100,000, respectively, whereas among late adolescent boys and girls the rates increased to 13.2 and 2.8 per 100,000, respectively. Large surveys indicate that, although up to 20 percent of high school students in the United States have experienced suicidal ideation and 10 percent have exhibited suicidal behaviors, only about 2 percent of adolescents who attempt suicide come to medical attention. In the last 15 years, the rates of both completed suicide and suicidal ideation have decreased.

Etiology

Genetic Factors. Completed suicide and suicidal behavior are two to four times more likely to occur in individuals with a first-degree family member with similar behavior.

Biological Factors. Recent studies have documented a reduction in the density of serotonin transporter receptors in the prefrontal cortex and in serotonin receptors among individuals with suicidal behaviors. Neurochemical findings show some overlap between persons with aggressive, impulsive behaviors and those who complete suicide. Low levels of serotonin and its major metabolite, 5-hydroxyindoleacetic acid (5-HIAA), have been found postmortem in the brains of persons who completed suicide. Low levels of 5-HIAA have been found in the cerebrospinal fluid of depressed persons who attempted suicide by violent methods. Alcohol and other psychoactive substances may lower 5-HIAA levels, perhaps increasing the vulnerability for suicidal behavior in an already predisposed person. Low serotonin may turn out to be a marker, rather than a cause, of aggression and suicidal propensity, influencing behavioral responses to stress.

Psychosocial Factors. Although major depressive illness is the most significant risk factor for suicide, increasing its risk by 20 percent, many severely depressed individuals are not suicidal. Various features, including a sense of hopelessness, impulsivity, recurrent substance use, and a history of aggressive behavior, have been associated with an increased risk of suicide. A wide range of psychopathological symptoms can result from exposure to violent and abusive homes. Aggressive, self-destructive, and suicidal behaviors seem to occur with greatest frequency among youth who have endured chronically stressful family lives. Large community studies have provided data suggesting that sexual orientation is a risk factor, with increased rates of suicidal behavior of two to six times among youth who identify themselves as gay, lesbian, or bisexual.

Diagnosis and Clinical Features

The characteristics of adolescents who attempt suicide and those who complete suicides are similar, and as many as 40 percent of suicidal persons have made a previous attempt. Direct questioning of children and adolescents about suicidal thoughts is necessary because studies have consistently shown that parents are frequently unaware of such ideas in their children. Suicidal thoughts (i.e., children talking about wanting to harm themselves) and suicidal threats (e.g., children stating that they want to jump in front of a car) are more common than suicide completion.

Most suicidal youth meet diagnostic criteria for one or more psychiatric disorders, which often include major depressive disorder, manic episodes, and psychotic disorders. Those with mood disorders in combination with substance abuse and a history of aggressive behavior are particularly at high risk. Those without mood disorders who are violent, aggressive, and impulsive may be susceptible to suicide during family or peer conflicts. High levels of hopelessness, poor problem-solving skills, and a history of aggressive behavior are risk factors for suicide. Depression alone is a more serious risk factor for suicide in girls than in boys, but boys often have more severe psychopathology than girls who commit suicide. The profile of an adolescent who commits suicide is occasionally one of high achievement and perfectionistic character traits; such an adolescent may have been humiliated recently by a perceived failure, such as diminished academic performance.

In psychiatrically disturbed and vulnerable adolescents, suicide attempts typically are related to recent stressors. The precipitants of suicidal behavior include conflicts and arguments with family members and boyfriends or girlfriends. Alcohol and other substance use can further predispose an already vulnerable adolescent to suicidal behavior. In other cases, an adolescent attempts suicide in anticipation of punishment after being caught by the police or other authority figures for a forbidden behavior.

About 40 percent of youthful persons who complete suicide had previous psychiatric treatment and about 40 percent had made a previous suicide attempt. A child who has lost a parent by any means before age 13 years is at high risk for mood disorders and suicide. The precipitating factors include loss of face with peers, a broken romance, school difficulties, unemployment, bereavement, separation, and rejection. Clusters of suicides among adolescents who know one another and go to the same school have been reported. Suicidal behavior can precipitate other such attempts within a peer group through identification—so-called copycat suicides. Some studies have found an increase in adolescent suicide after television programs in which the main theme was the suicide of a teenager. In general, however, many other factors are involved, including a necessary substrate of psychopathology.

Treatment

Hospitalization.
Adolescents who come to medical attention because of suicidal attempts must be evaluated before determining whether hospitalization is necessary. Those who fall into high-risk groups should be hospitalized until the acute suicidality is no longer present. Persons at high risk include those who have made previous suicide attempts; boys older than 12 years of age with histories of aggressive behavior or substance abuse; those who have made an attempt with a lethal method, such as a gun or a toxic ingested substance; those with major depressive disorder characterized by social withdrawal, hopelessness, and a lack of energy; girls who have run away from home, are pregnant, or have made an attempt with a method other than ingesting a toxic substance; and any person who exhibits persistent suicidal ideation. A child or an adolescent with suicidal ideation must be hospitalized if a clinician has any doubt about the family's ability to supervise the child or to cooperate with treatment in an outpatient setting. In such a situation, child protective services must be involved before the child can be discharged. When adolescents with suicidal ideation report that they are no longer suicidal, discharge can be considered only after a complete discharge plan is in place.

Psychotherapy.
Scant data exist to evaluate the efficacy of psychotherapy in reducing suicidal behavior among adolescents. Cognitive-behavioral therapy has been shown to be effective in the treatment of depression among adolescents; however, no evidence is available to assess its efficacy in preventing suicidal behavior per se. Dialectical behavior therapy (DBT), a long-term behavioral intervention that can be applied to individuals or groups of patients, has been shown to reduce suicidal behavior in adults but has yet to be investigated in adolescents. Components of DBT include mindfulness training to improve self-acceptance, assertiveness training, instruction on avoiding situations that may trigger self-destructive behavior, and increasing the ability to tolerate psychological distress. This approach warrants investigation among adolescents.

Pharmacotherapy.
Pharmacologic efficacy in the treatment of suicidal behavior has been shown in adults with depression and cluster B personality with SSRI antidepressants and in suicidal adults with bipolar disorder using lithium.

In children and adolescents with major depression, fluoxetine, citalopram, and sertraline have all been shown to have efficacy through randomized clinical trials; however, pharmacologic interventions targeting suicidal behavior has not been investigated in this population. Given the reduction in completed suicide among adolescents over the last decade during the same period in which SSRI antidepressant treatment in this population has markedly risen, it is possible that SSRI antidepressants have been instrumental in this effect. As mentioned earlier, close monitoring for suicidality is mandatory for any child or adolescent being treated with antidepressants.

▲ 45.2 Early-Onset Bipolar Disorders

Bipolar I disorder is being diagnosed with increasing frequency in prepubertal children, with the caveat that "classic" manic episodes are uncommon in this age group, even when depressive symptoms have already appeared. Because few prepubertal children with features of depression and mania or hypomania exhibit discrete mood "cycles," that these children satisfy diagnostic criteria for bipolar disorder remains controversial. These "atypical" manic episodes among prepubertal children are sometimes associated with family histories of classic bipolar I disorder. Features of the mood and behavior disturbances among prepubertal children who are currently diagnosed with bipolar disorder by some clinicians include extreme mood variability, intermittent aggressive behavior, high levels of distractibility, and poor attention span. This constellation of mood and behavior disturbance is often not clearly episodic but fluctuating and appears to be less responsive to mood-stabilizing agents than classic episodes of depression or mania in older adolescents and adults.

Children with atypical hypomanic episodes often have past histories of severe attention-deficit/hyperactivity disorder (ADHD), making the diagnosis of bipolar disorder even more complicated. In general, families with many relatives with ADHD do not have family histories with an increased rate of bipolar I disorder. Children with atypical bipolar disorder function poorly, often require hospitalization, exhibit symptoms of depression, and often have a history of ADHD. How many of these children will develop discrete mood cycling as they mature or whether their clinical pictures will remain consistent over time is under investigation.

According to the text revision of the fourth edition of *Diagnostic and Statistical Manual of Mental Disorders* (DSM-IV-TR), the diagnostic criteria for a manic episode are the same for children and adolescents as for adults (*see* Table 12.1–2). The diagnostic criteria for a manic episode include a distinct period of an abnormally elevated, expansive, or irritable mood that lasts at least 1 week or for any duration if hospitalization is necessary. In addition, during periods of mood disturbance, at least three of the following significant and persistent symptoms must be present: inflated self-esteem or grandiosity, decreased need for sleep, pressure to talk, flight of ideas or racing thoughts, distractibility, an increase in goal-directed activity, and excessive involvement in pleasurable activities that may result in painful consequences. The mood disturbance suffices to cause marked impairment and it is not caused by the direct effect of a substance or a general medical condition. Thus, manic states precipitated by somatic medications (e.g., antidepressants) cannot be interpreted as indicating a diagnosis of bipolar I disorder.

EPIDEMIOLOGY

The prevalence of early-onset bipolar disorder is rare based on the diagnostic criteria in the DSM-IV-TR. Epidemiologic studies in older adolescents have reported lifetime prevalence of bipolar I and II disorders to be approximately 1 percent. A recent epidemiologic survey of current illness in children younger than 13 years of age found no cases of classic bipolar illness.

The most valid diagnosis for prepubertal children with mood lability, extreme irritability, or rapid mood cycling remains controversial. Among adults with bipolar disorder, the 20 to 30 percent who exhibit "mixed mania" are most likely to have a chronic course, absence of discrete episodes, higher risk of suicidal behavior, onset of the disorder in childhood and adolescence, and neuropsychological features similar to those of children with ADHD and show a poorer response to treatment. These phenomenological features appear to be similar to the clinical presentation of the prepubertal children who are more frequently being described as having atypical bipolar disorders. Longitudinal studies are warranted to determine whether children with early-onset atypical bipolar disorders become adults with bipolar disorders with mixed mania.

ETIOLOGY

Genetic Factors

Family studies consistently demonstrate that offspring of a parent with bipolar I disorder have a 25 percent chance of having a mood disorder, and offspring of two parents with bipolar disorder have a 50 to 75 percent risk of developing a mood disorder. The high rates of comorbid ADHD among children with early-onset bipolar disorder has led to questions regarding the cotransmission of these disorders in family members. Offspring of parents with bipolar disorder have been found to have higher rates of ADHD compared with controls. In first-degree relatives of children with bipolar disorder, ADHD occurs with the same rate as in first-degree relatives of children with ADHD only. The combination of ADHD and bipolar disorder was not found as frequently in relatives of children with ADHD only, however, compared with first-degree relatives of children with the combination. These results suggest that childhood bipolar disorder may be distinguished as a subtype of bipolar disorder that emerges in children whose family histories are heavily loaded for bipolar disorder and psychiatric comorbidities, such as ADHD.

DIAGNOSIS AND CLINICAL FEATURES

Early-onset bipolar disorder is characterized by extreme irritability that is severe and persistent and may include aggressive outbursts and violent behavior. Between outbursts, children with this syndrome may continue to be angry or dysphoric. Occasionally, a child with early-onset bipolar disorder may exhibit grandiose thoughts or euphoric mood; for the most part, children with this disorder are predominantly intensely emotional with a fluctuating but overriding negative mood. DSM-IV-TR diagnostic criteria for bipolar disorders in children and adolescents are the same as those used in adults. The clinical picture of early-onset bipolar disorder, however, is complicated by the prevalent comorbid psychiatric disorders.

Comorbidity with ADHD

One of the main sources of diagnostic confusion regarding children with early-onset bipolar disorder is the comorbid ADHD, which is present in 60 to 90 percent of them. One of the reasons for the vast concurrence of these two disorders is that they share many diagnostic criteria, including distractibility, hyperactivity, and talkativeness. Even when the overlapping symptoms are removed from the diagnostic count, 89 percent of children with bipolar disorder continue to meet the full criteria for ADHD. This implies that both disorders with their own distinct features are present in many cases.

Comorbidity with Conduct Disorder

Rates of comorbid conduct disorder have been found to range from 48 to 69 percent among children and adolescents with bipolar disorder. Joseph Biederman found that the two manic symptoms more common in the comorbid group than the bipolar only group were physical restlessness and poor judgment.

Comorbidity with Anxiety Disorders

Children and adolescents with bipolar disorder have been reported to have higher-than-expected rates of panic and other anxiety disorders. Lifetime prevalence of panic disorder was found to be 21 percent among subjects with bipolar disorder compared with 0.8 percent in those without mood disorders. Patients with bipolar disorder with high levels of anxiety symptoms were reported to abuse alcohol and exhibit suicidal behavior.

PATHOLOGY AND LABORATORY EXAMINATION

No specific laboratory indices are helpful in making the diagnosis of bipolar disorders among children and adolescents.

DIFFERENTIAL DIAGNOSIS

A consensus of research studies in children diagnosed with early-onset bipolar disorder suggests that between 80 and 90 percent also meet diagnostic criteria for ADHD. Among youth with adolescent-onset of mania, rates of ADHD have been found to be 60 percent, a rate that is still markedly increased compared with controls. Although childhood ADHD tends to have its onset earlier than pediatric mania, evidence from family studies supports the presence of ADHD and bipolar disorders as highly comorbid in children, and the concurrence is not because of the overlapping symptoms that the two disorders share.

COURSE AND PROGNOSIS

It is not known whether early-onset bipolar disorders have the same natural history over time as bipolar disorders with an onset during adolescence or early adulthood. Investigations of the course of early-onset bipolar disorder have focused on rates of recovery, recurrence, changes in symptoms over time, and predictors of outcome. No differences were found in the rates of recovery for children and adolescents whose diagnosis was bipolar I disorder, bipolar II disorder, or bipolar disorder not otherwise specified; however, those youth whose diagnosis was bipolar disorder not otherwise specified had a significant longer duration of illness before recovery, with less frequent recurrences once they recovered.

All of the existing longitudinal literature on bipolar disorders in early childhood has found that when the illness emerges in young children, recovery rates are lower. In addition, a greater likelihood is seen of mixed states and rapid cycling and higher rates of polarity changes compared with those who develop bipolar disorders in late adolescence or early adulthood. Further investigations are needed to understand the mechanisms by which low socioeconomic status, psychosis, and less well-defined mood episodes predict more changes in polarity and a poorer prognosis.

TREATMENT

Few randomized, placebo-controlled treatment trials have been conducted with youth diagnosed with early-onset bipolar disorder. Therefore, the clinical strategies for youth diagnosed with bipolar disorders continue to include downward extensions of the literature from older adolescent and adult treatment studies of bipolar disorders.

Pharmacotherapy

Mood-stabilizing agents, particularly lithium, has been demonstrated to be an effective treatment for adults with bipolar disorder for acute mania and bipolar depressive states and has been shown to offer prophylactive properties in bipolar disorders. In childhood, controlled trials have provided evidence suggesting that lithium is efficacious in the management of aggression behavior disorders.

A recent randomized clinical trial comparing divalproex (Depakote) and quetiapine (Seroquel), an atypical antipsychotic, in the treatment of 50 adolescent patients with mania suggested that quetiapine is at least as effective as divalproex in the treatment of acute manic symptoms and may work more quickly. Placebo-controlled trials will be necessary to determine whether quetiapine is an effective monotherapy for child and adolescent mania. Other drugs used are lamotrigine (Lamictal) and risperidone (Risperdal).

Psychosocial treatment intervention studies for bipolar disorder among youth using family-focused psychoeducational treatment has been shown to reduce relapse rates. Children and adolescents treated with mood-stabilizing agents in addition to psychosocial intervention showed improvement in depressive symptoms, manic symptoms, and behavioral disturbance over 1 year.

More investigation is needed to determine the most efficacious treatments for early-onset bipolar disorder and its frequent comorbidities.

46

Anxiety Disorders of Infancy, Childhood, and Adolescence

Obsessive-compulsive disorder (OCD) is characterized by the presence of recurrent intrusive thoughts associated with anxiety or tension and/or repetitive purposeful mental or physical actions aimed at reducing fears and tensions caused by obsessions. It has become increasingly evident that the majority of cases of OCD begin in childhood or adolescence. The clinical presentation of OCD in childhood and adolescence is similar to that in adults, and the only alteration in diagnostic criteria in the text revision of the fourth edition of the *Diagnostic and Statistical Manual of Mental Disorders* (DSM-IV-TR) for children is that they do not necessarily demonstrate awareness that their thoughts or behaviors are unreasonable. Pediatric OCD has been investigated with respect to treatment with placebo-controlled trials of pharmacologic agents and cognitive-behavioral therapy (CBT); it is the only childhood anxiety disorder with data showing optimal treatment to include a combination of serotoninergic agents and CBT treatment.

EPIDEMIOLOGY

Obsessive-compulsive disorder is common among children and adolescents, with a point prevalence of about 0.5 percent and a lifetime rate of 1 to 3 percent. The rate of OCD rises exponentially with increasing age among youth, with a rate of 0.3 percent in children between the ages of 5 years and 7 years and rising to 0.6 percent among teens. Rates of OCD among adolescents are greater than rates for disorders such as schizophrenia and bipolar disorder. Among young children with OCD there appears to be a slight male predominance, which diminishes with age.

ETIOLOGY

Genetic Factors

OCD is a heterogeneous disorder that has been recognized for decades to run in families. Family studies have documented an increased risk of at least fourfold in first-degree relatives of individuals with early-onset OCD. In addition, the presence of subclinical symptom constellations in

family members appears to breed true. Molecular genetic studies have suggested linkage to regions of chromosomes 2 and 9 in certain pedigrees with multiple members exhibiting early-onset OCD. Candidate gene studies have been inconclusive. Family studies have pointed to a relationship between OCD and tic disorders such as Tourette's syndrome. OCD and tic disorders are believed to share susceptibility factors along with the concept of a broader "obsessive-compulsive spectrum" including eating disorders, and somatoform disorders may account for expression of repetitive and stereotyped symptoms.

Neuroimmunology

The association of emergence of OCD syndromes following a documented exposure to or infection with group A β-hemolytic streptococcus in a subgroup of children and adolescents has led to the studies of immune responses in OCD. Cases of infection-triggered OCD have been termed pediatric autoimmune neuropsychiatric disorders associated with streptococcus and are believed to represent an autoimmune process such as that of Sydenham's chorea during rheumatic fever. It is hypothesized that exposure to streptococcal bacteria activates the immune system, leading to inflammation of the basal ganglia and resulting in disruption of the cortical-striatal-thalamo-cortical function. Magnetic resonance imaging (MRI) has documented a proportional relationship between the size of the basal ganglia and the severity of OCD symptoms. The presentation of OCD in children and adolescents due to acute exposure to group A β-hemolytic streptococcus represents a minority of OCD cases in this population.

Neurochemistry

Involvement of several neurotransmitter systems, including the serotonin system and the dopamine system, have been postulated to contribute to the emergence of OCD. The observation that serotonin reuptake inhibitors (SSRIs) diminish symptoms of OCD, along with the findings of altered sensitivity to the acute administration of 5-hydroxytryptamine agonists, supports the likelihood that the serotonin system plays a role in OCD. In addition, the dopamine system is believed to be influential in this disorder, especially in light of the frequent comorbidity of OCD with tic disorders in children. Clinical observations have indicated that obsessions and compulsions may be exacerbated during treatment of ADHD (another frequent comorbidity) with stimulant agents. Dopamine antagonists administered along with SSRIs may augment the effectiveness of SSRIs in the treatment of OCD. It is most likely that multiple neurotransmitter systems play a role in OCD.

Neuroimaging

Both computed tomography and MRI of untreated children and adults with OCD have revealed smaller volumes of basal ganglia segments

659

compared to normal controls. In children, there is a suggestion that thalamic volume is increased. Adult studies have provided evidence of hypermetabolism of frontal cortical-striatal-thalamo-cortical networks in untreated individuals with OCD. Of interest, imaging studies before and after treatment have revealed that both medication and behavioral interventions lead to a reduction of orbit frontal and caudate metabolic rates in children and adults with OCD.

DIAGNOSIS AND CLINICAL FEATURES

The most commonly reported obsessions in children and adolescents include extreme fears of contamination—exposure to dirt, germs, or disease—followed by worries related to harm befalling themselves or family members and fear of harming others due to losing control over aggressive impulses. Also commonly reported are obsessional need for symmetry or exactness, hoarding, and excessive religious or moral concerns. Typical compulsive rituals among children and adolescents involve cleaning, checking, counting, repeating behaviors, and arranging items. Associated features in children and adolescents with OCD include avoidance, indecision, doubt, and a slowness to complete tasks. In most cases of OCD among youth, obsessions and compulsions are present. According to DSM-IV-TR, diagnosis of OCD is identical to that of adults, with the modification that, unlike adults, children are not required to recognize that their obsessions or compulsions are excessive or irrational. Table 46.1–1 gives the DSM-IV-TR diagnostic criteria for OCD.

The majority of children who develop OCD have an insidious presentation and may hide their symptoms when possible, whereas a minority of children, particularly boys with early onset, may have a rapid unfolding of multiple symptoms within a few months. OCD is commonly found to be comorbid with other psychiatric disorders, especially other anxiety disorders. There are also higher than expected rates of ADHD and tic disorders, including Tourette's syndrome, among children and adolescents with OCD. Children with comorbid OCD and tic disorders are more likely to exhibit counting, arranging, or ordering compulsions and less likely to manifest excessive washing and cleaning compulsions. The high comorbidity of OCD, Tourette's syndrome, and ADHD has led investigators to postulate a common genetic vulnerability to all three of these disorders. It is important to search for comorbidity in children and adolescents with OCD so that optimal treatments can be administered.

Pathology and Laboratory Examination

No specific laboratory measures are useful in the diagnosis of obsessive-compulsive disorder.

When the onset of obsessions or compulsions is believed to be associated with an exposure to or recent infection with group A β-hemolytic streptococcus, antigens and antibodies to the bacteria can be obtained, although a diagnosis of OCD can not be confirmed on the basis of positive results.

Table 46.1–1
DSM-IV-TR Diagnostic Criteria for Obsessive-Compulsive Disorder

A. Either obsessions or compulsions:
   Obsessions as defined by (1), (2), (3), and (4):
   (1) Recurrent and persistent thoughts, impulses, or images that are experienced, at some time during the disturbance, as intrusive and inappropriate and that cause marked anxiety or distress
   (2) The thoughts, impulses, or images are not simply excessive worries about real-life problems
   (3) The person attempts to ignore or suppress such thoughts, impulses, or images, or to neutralize them with some other thought or action
   (4) The person recognizes that the obsessional thoughts, impulses, or images are a product of his or her own mind (not imposed from without as in thought insertion)
   Compulsions as defined by (1) and (2):
   (1) Repetitive behaviors (e.g., hand washing, ordering, checking) or mental acts (e.g., praying, counting, repeating words silently) that the person feels driven to perform in response to an obsession, or according to rules that must be applied rigidly
   (2) The behaviors or mental acts are aimed at preventing or reducing distress or preventing some dreaded event or situation; however, these behaviors or mental acts either are not connected in a realistic way with what they are designed to neutralize or prevent or are clearly excessive
B. At some point during the course of the disorder, the person has recognized that the obsessions or compulsions are excessive or unreasonable. **Note:** This does not apply to children.
C. The obsessions or compulsions cause marked distress, are time consuming (take more than 1 hour a day), or significantly interfere with the person's normal routine, occupational (or academic) functioning, or usual social activities or relationships.
D. If another Axis I disorder is present, the content of the obsessions or compulsions is not restricted to it (e.g., preoccupation with food in the presence of an eating disorder; hair pulling in the presence of trichotillomania; concern with appearance in the presence of body dysmorphic disorder; preoccupation with drugs in the presence of a substance use disorder; preoccupation with having a serious illness in the presence of hypochondriasis; preoccupation with sexual urges or fantasies in the presence of a paraphilia; or guilty ruminations in the presence of major depressive disorder).
E. The disturbance is not due to the direct physiological effects of a substance (e.g., a drug of abuse, a medication) or a general medical condition.

Specify if:
With poor insight: if, for most of the time during the current episode, the person does not recognize that the obsessions and compulsions are excessive or unreasonable

From American Psychiatric Association. *Diagnostic and Statistical Manual of Mental Disorders.* 4th ed. Text rev. Washington, DC: American Psychiatric Association; copyright 2000, with permission.

DIFFERENTIAL DIAGNOSIS

Developmentally appropriate rituals in the play and behavior of young children must be differentiated from obsessive-compulsive disorder in that age group. Preschoolers often engage in ritualistic play and request a predictable routine, such as bathing, reading stories, or selecting the same stuffed animal at bedtime, to promote a sense of security and comfort. These routines allay developmentally normal fears and lead to reasonable completion of daily activities, in contrast to obsessions or compulsions, which are driven by extreme fears and interfere with normative daily function due to the excessive time that they consume and the extreme distress they cause when not fully completed. The rituals of preschoolers generally become less rigid by the time they enter grade school, and school-aged children usually do not have a surge of anxiety when they encounter small changes in their routine.

Children and adolescents with anxiety disorders such as generalized anxiety disorder, separation anxiety disorder, or social phobia experience more intense worries than children without any anxiety disorders and may express their concerns repeatedly, but these are differentiated from typical obsessions by their more mundane content, whereas obsessions are so excessive that they approach seeming bizarre. A child with generalized anxiety disorder might worry repeatedly about performance on academic examinations, whereas a child with OCD is likely to have intrusive concerns that he or she may lose control and harm a loved one. The compulsions of OCD are not exhibited in other anxiety disorders, but children and adolescents with pervasive developmental disorders often display repetitive behaviors that resemble those of OCD. In contrast to the rituals of OCD, however, children with pervasive developmental disorder are not responding to anxiety, but are more often manifesting stereotyped behaviors that are self-stimulating or self-comforting.

Children and adolescents with tic disorders such as Tourette's syndrome may exhibit complex repetitive compulsive behaviors that are similar to the compulsions seen in OCD. In fact, children and adolescents with tic disorders are at higher risk for the development of concurrent OCD.

In severe cases of OCD, it may be difficult to differentiate whether psychosis is present, given the extreme and bizarre nature that obsessions and compulsions can possess. In adults and often in children and adolescents with OCD, despite the inability to control the obsessions or the irresistible drive to complete the compulsions, insight about their lack of reasonableness is preserved. When insight is present and underlying anxiety can be described even in the face of significant dysfunction due to bizarre obsessions and compulsion, the diagnosis of OCD is suspect.

COURSE AND PROGNOSIS

OCD with an onset in childhood and adolescence is characterized as a chronic, though waxing and waning, disorder with a great variation in severity and outcome. Follow-up studies suggest that up to 50 percent of affected children and adolescents experience recovery from OCD with minimal remaining symptoms. In a recent study of childhood OCD, treatment with sertraline resulted in close to 50 percent of subjects experiencing complete remission and another 25 percent experiencing partial remission with a follow-up time of 1 year. The predictor of the best outcome was

the absence of comorbid disorders, including tic disorders and ADHD. Overall, the prognosis is hopeful for most children and adolescents with mild to moderate OCD. In a minority of cases, however, the OCD diagnosis may be considered a prodrome of a psychotic disorder, which has been found to emerge in up to 10 percent in some samples of children and adolescents with OCD. In children with subthreshold symptoms of OCD, there is a high risk of the development of the full OCD disorder within 2 years. In the majority of studies of childhood OCD, treatment results in improvement if not complete remission in the majority of cases.

TREATMENT

Results from multiple randomized, placebo-controlled trials of both medication and cognitive-behavioral interventions in children and adolescents with OCD show the most successful treatment of this disorder compared to any of the other anxiety disorders of childhood. In a recent multisite National Institute of Health–funded investigation of sertraline and cognitive-behavioral therapy each alone and in combination for the treatment of childhood onset OCD, the Pediatric OCD Treatment Study revealed that the combination was superior to either treatment alone.

Three SSRIs—sertraline (at least 6 years of age), fluoxetine (at least 7 years of age), and fluvoxamine (at least 8 years of age)—have received U.S. Federal Drug Administration approval for the treatment of OCD. The black-box warning for antidepressants used in children for any disorder, including OCD, is applicable, so that close monitoring for suicidal ideation or behavior is mandated when these agents are used in the treatment of childhood OCD.

Cognitive-behavioral therapy geared toward children of varying ages is based on the principle of developmentally appropriate exposure to the feared stimuli coupled with response prevention, leading to diminishing anxiety over time for exposure to feared situations. CBT manuals have been developed to ensure that developmentally appropriate interventions are made and that comprehensive education is provided to the child and parents.

Most treatment guidelines for children and adolescents with mild to moderate OCD recommend a trial of CBT prior to initiating medication. There is evidence that optimal treatment includes the combination of SSRI medication and CBT. In terms of pharmacological interventions, acute treatment of childhood OCD has been shown to occur within 8 to 12 weeks of treatment. The vast majority of children and adolescents who experienced a remission with acute treatment using SSRIs were still responsive over a period of 1 year. Given the lack of data on discontinuation, recommendations for maintaining medication include stabilization and education about relapse risk, and tapering medication during the summer is likely to be advised to minimize academic compromise in case of relapse. For children and adolescents with more-severe or multiple episodes of significant exacerbation of symptoms, treatment for a longer period of time—greater than 1 year—is recommended.

Augmentation strategies enhancing serotonergic effects, for example, atypical antipsychotics such as risperidone, have demonstrated increased response when partial response has been achieved with SSRI agents.

Overall, efficacy of treatment for children and adolescents with OCD is high with appropriate choice of SSRI agent and CBT therapy.

▲ 46.2 Separation Anxiety Disorder, Generalized Anxiety Disorder, and Social Phobia

Anxiety disorders are among the most common disorders in youth, affecting more than 10 percent of children and adolescents at some point in their development. Separation anxiety is a universal human developmental phenomenon emerging in infants less than 1 year of age and marking a child's awareness of a separation from his or her mother or primary caregiver. Normative separation anxiety peaks between 9 months and 18 months and diminishes by about 2.5 years of age, enabling young children to develop a sense of comfort away from their parents in preschool. Separation anxiety, or stranger anxiety as it has been termed, most likely evolved as a human response that has survival value. The expression of transient separation anxiety is also normal in young children entering school for the first time. Approximately 15 percent of young children display intense and persistent fear, shyness, and social withdrawal when faced with unfamiliar settings and people. Young children with this pattern of behavioral inhibition are at higher risk for the development of separation anxiety disorder, generalized anxiety disorder, and social phobia. Behaviorally inhibited children, as a group, exhibit characteristic physiological traits, including higher-than-average resting heart rates, higher morning cortisol levels than average, and low heart rate variability. Separation anxiety disorder is diagnosed when developmentally inappropriate and excessive anxiety emerges related to separation from the major attachment figure. According to the text revision of the fourth edition of the *Diagnostic and Statistical Manual of Mental Disorders* (DSM-IV-TR), separation anxiety disorder requires the presence of at least three symptoms related to excessive worry about separation from the major attachment figures. The worries may take the form of refusal to go to school, fears and distress on separation, repeated complaints of such physical symptoms as headaches and stomachaches when separation is anticipated, and nightmares related to separation issues.

Separation anxiety disorder and selective mutism are the two anxiety disorders found in the child and adolescent section of DSM-IV-TR, although childhood onset of all of the anxiety disorders is frequent. Children who exhibit recurrent excessive worries pertaining to their performance in school and social settings and experience at least one physiological symptom, such as restlessness, poor concentration, or irritability related to their fears, may be diagnosed with generalized anxiety disorder. Children with generalized anxiety disorder tend to feel fearful in multiple settings and expect more-negative outcomes when faced with academic or social challenges compared with peers. Children who experience recurrent extreme anxiety and avoid social situations in which they fear scrutiny or humiliation may meet the DSM-IV-TR diagnostic criteria for social phobia, a disorder that also occurs in adolescents and adults. Children with social phobia experience distress and discomfort in the presence of peers as well as adults. Separation anxiety disorder, generalized anxiety, and social phobia in children are often considered together in a differential diagnosis and in developing treatment strategies because they are highly comorbid and have overlapping symptoms. A child with separation anxiety disorder, generalized anxiety disorder, or social phobia has a 60 percent chance of having at least one of the other two disorders as well. Of children with one of the aforementioned anxiety disorders, 30 percent have all three of them. Children and adolescents may also have other anxiety disorders described among the adult disorders of DSM-IV-TR, including specific phobia, panic disorder, obsessive-compulsive disorder, and posttraumatic stress disorder.

EPIDEMIOLOGY

The prevalence of anxiety disorders has varied with the age group of the children surveyed and the diagnostic instruments used. Lifetime prevalence of any anxiety disorder in children and adolescents ranges from 8.3 to 27 percent. A recent epidemiologic survey using the *Preschool Age Psychiatric Assessment* found that 9.5 percent of preschoolers met DSM-IV-TR criteria for any anxiety disorder, with 6.5 percent exhibiting generalized anxiety disorder, 2.4 percent meeting criteria for separation anxiety disorder, and 2.2 percent meeting criteria for social phobia. The rate of separation anxiety disorder is estimated to be about 4 percent in children and young adolescents. Separation anxiety disorder is more common in young children than in adolescents and has been reported to occur equally in boys and girls. The onset may occur during preschool years but is most common in children 7 to 8 years of age. The rate of generalized anxiety disorder in school-age children is estimated to be approximately 3 percent, the rate of social phobia is 1 percent, and the rate of simple phobias is 2.4 percent. In adolescents, lifetime prevalence for panic disorder was found to be 0.6 percent; the prevalence for generalized anxiety disorder was 3.7 percent.

ETIOLOGY

Biopsychosocial Factors

In very young children, psychosocial factors in conjunction with temperament may influence the degree of separation anxiety that emerges in situations of brief separation and exposure to unfamiliar environments. The relation between temperamental traits and the predisposition to develop anxiety symptoms has been investigated. The temperamental tendency to be unusually shy or to withdraw in unfamiliar situations seems to be an enduring response pattern, and young children with this propensity are at higher risk of developing separation anxiety disorder, generalized anxiety disorder, social anxiety disorders, or all three during their next few years of life.

Neurophysiological correlation is found with behavioral inhibition (extreme shyness); children with this constellation are shown to have a higher resting heart rate and an acceleration of heart rate with tasks requiring cognitive concentration. Additional physiological correlates of behavioral inhibition include elevated salivary cortisol levels, elevated urinary catecholamine levels, and greater papillary dilation during cognitive tasks. The quality of maternal attachment also appears to play a role in the development of anxiety disorder in children. Mothers with anxiety disorders who are observed to show insecure attachment to their children tend to have children with higher rates of anxiety disorders. It is difficult to separate the contribution of the relationship between mother and child from the mother's potential genetic contribution to anxiety. Families in which a child manifests separation anxiety disorder may be close-knit and caring, and the children often seem to be the objects of parental overconcern. External life stresses often coincide with development of the disorder. The death of a relative, a child's illness, a change in a child's environment, or a move to a new neighborhood or school is frequently noted in the histories of children with separation anxiety disorder. In a vulnerable child, these changes probably intensify anxiety.

Social Learning Factors

Fear in response to a variety of unfamiliar or unexpected situations may be unwittingly communicated from parents to children by direct modeling. If a parent is fearful, the child will probably have a phobic adaptation to new situations, especially to a school environment. Some parents appear to teach their children to be anxious by overprotecting them from expected dangers or by exaggerating the dangers. For example, a parent who cringes in a room during a lightning storm teaches a child to do the same. A parent who is afraid of mice or insects conveys the affect of fright to a child. Conversely, a parent who becomes angry with a child when the child expresses fear of a given situation— for example, when exposed to animals—may promote a phobic concern in the child by exposing the child to the intensity of the anger expressed by the parent. Social learning factors in the development of anxiety reactions are magnified when parents have anxiety disorders. These factors may be pertinent in the development of separation anxiety disorder, as well as in generalized anxiety disorder and social phobia. In a recent study of adverse psychosocial events, such as ongoing family conflict, there was no association found between psychosocial hardships and behavioral inhibition among young children. It appears that temperamental predisposition to anxiety disorders emerges as a highly heritable constellation of traits and is not created by psychosocial stressor.

Genetic Factors

Genetic studies of families suggest that genes account for at least one third of the variance in the development of anxiety disorders in children. Thus, temperamental constellation of behavioral inhibition, excessive shyness, the tendency to withdraw from unfamiliar situations, and the eventual emergence of anxiety disorders have a genetic contribution; however, approximately two thirds of young children with behavioral inhibition do not appear to go on to develop anxiety disorders. Family studies have shown that the biological offspring of adults with anxiety disorders are susceptible to parents with panic disorder with agoraphobia, who appear to have an increased risk of having a child with separation anxiety disorder. Separation anxiety disorder and depression in children overlap, and the presence of an anxiety disorder increases the risk of a future episode of a depressive disorder. Current consensus on the genetics of anxiety disorders suggests that what is inherited is a general predisposition toward anxiety, with resulting heightened levels of arousability, emotional reactivity, and increased negative affect, all of which increase the risk for the development of separation anxiety disorder, generalized anxiety disorder, and social phobia.

DIAGNOSIS AND CLINICAL FEATURES

Separation anxiety disorder, generalized anxiety disorder, and social phobia are highly related in children and adolescence because, in most children, if one occurs, another is present as well. Generalized anxiety disorder is the most common anxiety disorder in childhood, but in 30 percent of cases, a child with generalized anxiety disorder also exhibits the other two disorders. Separation anxiety disorder and selective mutism are the two anxiety disorders contained in the childhood section of the DSM-IV-TR; however, most anxiety disorders originate in childhood or adolescence. Diagnostic criteria for separation anxiety disorder, according to DSM-IV-TR, include three of the following symptoms for at least 4 weeks: persistent and excessive worry about losing, or possible harm befalling, major attachment figures; persistent and excessive worry that an untoward event can lead to separation from a major attachment figure; persistent reluctance or refusal to go to school or elsewhere because of fear of separation; persistent and excessive fear or reluctance to be alone or without major attachment figures at home or without significant adults in other settings; persistent reluctance or refusal to go to sleep without being near a major attachment figure or to sleep away from home; repeated nightmares involving the theme of separation; repeated complaints of physical symptoms, including headaches and stomachaches, when separation from major attachment figures is anticipated; and recurrent excessive distress when separation from home or major attachment figures is anticipated or involved (Tables 46.2–1 through 46.2–3).

Alan W was an 8-year-old boy referred for outpatient evaluation by his family physician. He was having trouble sleeping in his room alone at night and was refusing to go to school. Alan expressed recurrent fears that something bad would happen to his mother. He worried that she would get into a car accident or that there would be a fire at home and his mother would be killed. Developmental history showed Alan was anxious and irritable as an infant and toddler. He had trouble adjusting to baby-sitters in the preschool years. There was a history of panic disorder, with agoraphobia in the mother and major depression in the father.

Nighttime was a particularly difficult time at home. While Mrs. W would read to her son and talk with him before bedtime, Alan would often whine and cry, asking to have mother lie in bed with him until he fell asleep. He also expected his mother to be in the master bedroom across the hall from his room throughout the evening. Mrs. W reported that some evenings her son would get up and peek through the crack in the master bedroom door, as frequently as every 10 minutes, to be certain that she was still there. Alan reported frequent bad dreams that his parents were killed or that monsters caught him and took him away from his family forever.

During the daytime, he would shadow his mother around the house. Alan would agree to play a game with his sister in the lower level of the house only if his mother was close by. When Mrs. W went upstairs, he would interrupt the game and follow her upstairs. He was reluctant to sleep at a friend's house; a couple of times he attempted to do this. However, as the evening progressed, he described a queasy sensation

Table 46.2–1
DSM-IV-TR Diagnostic Criteria for Separation Anxiety Disorder

A. Developmentally inappropriate and excessive anxiety concerning separation from home or from those to whom the individual is attached, as evidenced by three (or more) of the following:
   (1) recurrent excessive distress when separation from home or major attachment figures occurs or is anticipated
   (2) persistent and excessive worry about losing, or about possible harm befalling, major attachment figures
   (3) persistent and excessive worry that an untoward event will lead to separation from a major attachment figure (e.g., getting lost or being kidnapped)
   (4) persistent reluctance or refusal to go to school or elsewhere because of fear of separation
   (5) persistently and excessively fearful or reluctant to be alone or without major attachment figures at home or without significant adults in other settings
   (6) persistent reluctance or refusal to go to sleep without being near a major attachment figure or to sleep away from home
   (7) repeated nightmares involving the theme of separation
   (8) repeated complaints of physical symptoms (such as headaches, stomachaches, nausea, or vomiting) when separation from major attachment figures occurs or is anticipated
B. The duration of the disturbance is at least 4 weeks.
C. The onset is before age 18 years.
D. The disturbance causes clinically significant distress or impairment in social, academic (occupational), or other important areas of functioning.
E. The disturbance does not occur exclusively during the course of a pervasive developmental disorder, schizophrenia, or other psychotic disorder and, in adolescents and adults, is not better accounted for by panic disorder with agoraphobia.

Specify if:
Early onset: if onset occurs before age 6 years

From American Psychiatric Association. *Diagnostic and Statistical Manual of Mental Disorders.* 4th ed. Text rev. Washington, DC: American Psychiatric Association; copyright 2000, with permission.

in his stomach, a feeling of sadness, and missing his mother. Subsequently Alan would call home and his parents would pick him up.

On school days, Alan had stomachaches and tried to stay home. He appeared quite distressed and panicky when it was time to separate from his mother. Once at school, he seemed calmer and less anxious, but occasionally was seen in the nurse's office, complaining of nausea and seeking to be sent home. (Courtesy of Gail A. Bernstein, M.D., and Anne E. Layne, Ph.D.)

The essential feature of separation anxiety disorder is extreme anxiety precipitated by separation from parents, home, or other familiar surroundings, whereas in generalized anxiety disorder, fears are extended to negative outcomes for all kinds of events, including academic, peer relationship, and family activities. In generalized anxiety disorder, a child or adolescent experiences at least one recurrent physiological symptom, such as restlessness, poor concentration, irritability, or muscle tension. In social phobia, the child's fears peak during performance situations involving exposure to unfamiliar people or situations. Children and adolescents with social phobia have extreme concerns about being embarrassed, humiliated, or negatively judged. In each of the foregoing anxiety disorders, the child's experience can

Table 46.2–2
DSM-IV-TR Diagnostic Criteria for Generalized Anxiety Disorder

A. Excessive anxiety and worry (apprehensive expectation), occurring more days than not for at least 6 months, about a number of events or activities (such as work or school performance).
B. The person finds it difficult to control the worry.
C. The anxiety and worry are associated with three (or more) of the following six symptoms (with at least some symptoms present for more days than not for the past 6 months). **Note:** Only one item is required in children.
   (1) Restlessness or feeling keyed up or on edge
   (2) Being easily fatigued
   (3) Difficulty concentrating or mind going blank
   (4) Irritability
   (5) Muscle tension
   (6) Sleep disturbance (difficulty falling or staying asleep, or restless unsatisfying sleep)
D. The focus of the anxiety and worry is not confined to features of an Axis I disorder, e.g., the anxiety or worry is not about having a panic attack (as in panic disorder), being embarrassed in public (as in social phobia), being contaminated (as in obsessive-compulsive disorder), being away from home or close relatives (as in separation anxiety disorder), gaining weight (as in anorexia nervosa), having multiple physical complaints (as in somatization disorder), or having a serious illness (as in hypochondriasis), and the anxiety and worry do not occur exclusively during posttraumatic stress disorder.
E. The anxiety, worry, or physical symptoms cause clinically significant distress or impairment in social, occupational, or other important areas of functioning.
F. The disturbance is not due to the direct physiological effects of a substance (e.g., a drug of abuse, a medication) or a general medical condition (e.g., hyperthyroidism) and does not occur exclusively during a mood disorder, psychotic disorder, or a pervasive developmental disorder.

From American Psychiatric Association. *Diagnostic and Statistical Manual of Mental Disorders.* 4th ed. Text rev. Washington, DC: American Psychiatric Association; 2000, with permission.

Table 46.2–3
DSM-IV-TR Diagnostic Criteria for Social Phobia

A. A marked and persistent fear of one or more social or performance situations in which the person is exposed to unfamiliar people or to possible scrutiny by others. The individual fears that he or she will act in a way (or show anxiety symptoms) that will be humiliating or embarrassing. **Note:** In children, there must be evidence of capacity for age-appropriate social relationships with familiar people and the anxiety must occur in peer settings, not just in interactions with adults.

B. Exposure to the feared social situation almost invariably provokes anxiety, which may take the form of a situationally bound or situationally predisposed panic attack. **Note:** In children, the anxiety may be expressed by crying, tantrums, freezing, or shrinking from social situations with unfamiliar people.

C. The person recognizes that the fear is excessive or unreasonable. **Note:** In children, this feature may be absent.

D. The feared social or performance situations are avoided, or else endured with intense anxiety or distress.

E. The avoidance, anxious anticipation, or distress in the feared social or performance situation(s) interferes significantly with the person's normal routine, occupational (academic) functioning, or social activities or relationships with others, or there is marked distress about having the phobia.

F. In individuals under age 18 years, the duration is at least 6 months.

G. The fear or avoidance is not due to the direct physiological effects of a substance (e.g., a drug of abuse, a medication) or a general medical condition, and is not better accounted for by another mental disorder (e.g., panic disorder with or without agoraphobia, separation anxiety disorder, body dysmorphic disorder, a pervasive developmental disorder, or schizoid personality disorder).

H. If a general medical condition or other mental disorder is present, the fear in Criterion A is unrelated to it, (e.g., the fear is not of stuttering, trembling in Parkinson's disease, or exhibiting abnormal eating behavior in anorexia nervosa or bulimia nervosa).

Specify if:
Generalized: If the fears include most social situations (also consider the additional diagnosis of avoidant personality disorder).

From American Psychiatric Association. *Diagnostic and Statistical Manual of Mental Disorders.* 4th ed. Text rev. Washington, DC: American Psychiatric Association; 2000, with permission.

approach terror or panic. The distress is greater than that normally expected for the child's developmental level and cannot be explained by any other disorder. Morbid fears, preoccupations, and ruminations characterize separation anxiety disorder. Children with anxiety disorders overestimate the probability of danger and the likelihood of negative outcome. Children with separation anxiety disorder and generalized anxiety disorder become overly fearful that someone close to them will be hurt or that something terrible will happen to them or their families, especially when they are away from important caring figures. Many children with anxiety disorders are preoccupied with health and worry that their families or friends will become ill. Fears of getting lost, being kidnapped, and losing the ability to be in contact with their families are predominant among children with separation anxiety disorder.

Associated features of anxiety disorders include fear of the dark and imaginary, bizarre worries. Children may have the feeling that eyes are staring at them and monsters are reaching out for them in their bedrooms. Children with anxiety disorders often complain of somatic symptoms and are very sensitive to changes in their bodies. They are often more sensitive than peers and more easily brought to tears. Frequent somatic complaints include gastrointestinal symptoms, nausea, vomiting, and stomachaches; unexplained pain in various parts of the body; sore throats; and flu-like symptoms. Older children typically complain of somatic experiences classically reported by adults with anxiety, such as cardiovascular and respiratory symptoms—palpitations, dizziness, faintness, and feelings of strangulation. Physiological signs of anxiety are a part of the diagnostic criteria for generalized anxiety disorder, but they are more often also experienced by children with separation anxiety and social phobia than the general population. The most common anxiety disorder that coexists with separation anxiety disorder is specific phobia, which occurs in about one third of referred cases of separation anxiety disorder.

Pathology and Laboratory Examination

No specific laboratory measures help in the diagnosis of separation anxiety disorder.

DIFFERENTIAL DIAGNOSIS

Because some degree of separation anxiety is a normal phenomenon in a very young child, clinical judgment must be used in distinguishing normal anxiety from separation anxiety disorder in this age group. In older school-age children, it is apparent when a child is experiencing more than normal distress when school is refused on a regular basis. For children who resist school, it is important to distinguish whether fear of separation, general worry about performance, or more specific fears of humiliation in front of peers or the teacher are driving the resistance. In many cases in which anxiety is the primary obstacle, all three of these feared scenarios come into play. In generalized anxiety disorder, anxiety is not focused on separation. In pervasive developmental disorders and schizophrenia, anxiety about separation may occur but is viewed as caused by these conditions rather than being a separate disorder. When depressive disorders occur in children, the comorbid diagnosis of separation anxiety disorder should also be made when the criteria for both disorders are met; the two diagnoses often coexist. Panic disorder with agoraphobia is uncommon before 18 years of age; the fear is of being incapacitated by a panic attack rather than of separation from parental figures. In some adult cases, however, many symptoms of separation anxiety disorder may be present. In conduct disorder, truancy is common but children stay away from home and do not have anxiety about separation. School refusal is a frequent symptom in separation anxiety disorder but is not pathognomonic of it. Children with other diagnoses, such as simple phobias, social phobias, or fear of failure in school because of learning disorder, also evince school refusal. When school refusal occurs in an adolescent, the severity of the dysfunction is generally greater than when separation anxiety emerges in a young child. Similar and distinguishing characteristics of childhood separation anxiety disorder, generalized anxiety disorder, and social phobia are presented in Table 46.2–4.

Table 46.2–4
Common Characteristics of Selected Anxiety Disorders That Occur in Children

Criteria	Separation Anxiety Disorder	Social Phobia	Generalized Anxiety Disorder
Minimal duration to establish diagnosis	At least 4 wks	No minimum	At least 6 mos
Age of onset	Preschool to 18 yrs	Not specified	Not specified
Precipitating stresses	Separation from significant parental figures, other losses, travel	Pressure for social participation with peers	Unusual pressure for performance, damage to self-esteem, feelings of lack of competence
Peer relationships	Good when no separation is involved	Tentative, overly inhibited	Overly eager to please, peers sought out and dependent relationships established
Sleep	Reluctance or refusal to go to sleep, fear of dark, nightmares	Difficulty in falling asleep at times	Difficulty in falling asleep
Psychophysiological symptoms	Complaints of stomachaches, nausea, vomiting, flu-like symptoms, headaches, palpitations, dizziness, faintness	Blushing, body tension	Stomachaches, nausea, vomiting, lump in the throat, shortness of breath, dizziness, palpitations
Differential diagnosis	Generalized anxiety disorder, schizophrenia, depressive disorders, conduct disorder, pervasive developmental disorders, major depressive disorder, panic disorder with agoraphobia	Adjustment disorder with depressed mood, generalized anxiety disorder, separation anxiety disorder, major depressive disorder, dysthymic disorder, avoidant personality disorder, borderline personality disorder	Separation anxiety disorder, attention-deficit/hyperactivity disorder, social phobia, adjustment disorder with anxiety, obsessive-compulsive disorder, psychotic disorders, mood disorders

Adapted from Sidney Werkman, M.D.

COURSE AND PROGNOSIS

The course and the prognosis of separation anxiety disorder, generalized anxiety, and social phobia are varied and are related to the age of onset, the duration of the symptoms, and the development of comorbid anxiety and depressive disorders. Young children who can maintain attendance in school, after-school activities, and peer relationships generally have a better prognosis than children or adolescents who refuse to attend school or drop out of social activities. A follow-up study of children and adolescents with anxiety disorders over a 3-year period reported that up to 82 percent no longer met criteria for the anxiety disorder at follow-up. Of the group followed, 96 percent of those with separation anxiety disorder had a remission at follow-up. Most children who recovered did so within the first year. Early age of onset and later age at diagnosis were factors that predicted slower recovery. Close to one third of the group studied, however, had developed another psychiatric disorder within the follow-up period, and 50 percent of these children developed another anxiety disorder. Reports have indicated a significant overlap of separation anxiety disorder and depressive disorders. In these complicated cases, the prognosis is guarded. Most follow-up studies have methodological problems and are limited to hospitalized, school-phobic children, not children with separation anxiety disorder per se. Little is reported about the outcome of mild cases, and whether children are seen in outpatient treatment or receive no treatment. Notwithstanding the limitations of the studies, reports indicate that some children with severe school phobia continue to resist attending school for many years.

TREATMENT

The treatment of separation anxiety disorder, generalized anxiety disorder, and social phobia are often considered together, given the frequent comorbidity and overlapping symptomatology of these disorders. A multimodal comprehensive treatment approach may include cognitive-behavioral therapy (CBT), family education, family psychosocial intervention, and pharmacological interventions. A trial of CBT may be applied first, if available, when a child is able to function sufficiently well to engage in daily activities while obtaining this treatment. Evidence from a recent large multisite National Institute of Mental Health investigation (Research Units in Pediatric Psychopharmacology) confirmed the safety and efficacy of fluvoxamine (Luvox) in the treatment of childhood separation anxiety disorder, generalized anxiety disorder, and social phobia. Several other randomized clinical trials have also supported the efficacy of selective serotonin reuptake inhibitor (SSRI) medications in the treatment of child and adolescent anxiety disorders. The U.S. Food and Drug Administration has placed a "black-box" warning on antidepressants, including all of the SSRI agents, used in the treatment of any childhood disorder because of concerns about increased suicidality; however, no individual childhood anxiety study has found a statistically significant increase in suicidal thoughts or behaviors. Clearly, SSRI medications have been shown to be both safe and efficacious in the treatment of childhood anxiety disorders, yet the evidence is not in on whether the optimal treatment approach is to administer CBT first, medication first, or both simultaneously. Cognitive-behavioral therapy is widely accepted as a first-line treatment for a variety of anxiety disorders for children, including separation anxiety disorder, social phobia, and selective mutism. Specific cognitive strategies and relaxation exercises may also be added components of treatment for some children as self-contained strategies to control their anxiety. Family interventions are also frequently critical in the management of separation anxiety disorder, especially in children who refuse to attend school, so that firm encouragement of school attendance is maintained while appropriate support is also provided.

School refusal associated with separation anxiety disorder can be viewed as a psychiatric emergency. A comprehensive treatment plan involves the child, the parents, and the child's peers and school. The child should be encouraged to attend school, but when a return to a full school day is overwhelming, a program should be arranged so the child can progressively increase the time spent at school. Graded contact with an object of anxiety is a form of behavior modification that can be applied to any type of separation anxiety. Some severe cases of school refusal require hospitalization. Cognitive-behavioral modalities include exposure to feared separations and cognitive strategies, such as coping self-statements aimed at increasing a sense of autonomy and mastery.

▲ 46.3 Selective Mutism

Selective mutism is characterized in a child by persistent failure to speak in one or more specific social situations, most typically including the school setting. A child with selective mutism may remain completely silent or near silent, in some cases whispering instead of speaking out loud. The most recent conceptualization of selective mutism highlights the relationship between underlying social anxiety and the resulting failure to speak. Most children with the disorder are completely silent during the stressful situations, whereas some may verbalize almost inaudibly single-syllable words. Children with selective mutism are fully capable of speaking competently when not in a socially anxiety-producing situation. Some children with the disorder communicate with eye contact or nonverbal gestures. These children speak fluently in other situations, such as at home and in certain familiar settings. Selective mutism is believed to be an expression of social phobia because of its expression in selective social situations.

EPIDEMIOLOGY

The prevalence of selective mutism varies with age, with younger children at increased risk for the disorder. One epidemiological study using the criteria of the text revision of the fourth edition of the *Diagnostic and Statistical Manual of Mental Disorders* (DSM-IV-TR) reported a rate of selective mutism in preschoolers to be 0.6 percent. Another large epidemiological survey in the United Kingdom reported a prevalence rate of selective mutism to be 0.69 percent in children 4 to 5 years of age, which dropped to 0.8 percent near the end of the same academic year. Another survey in the United Kingdom identified 0.06 percent of 7-year-olds as having selective mutism. Selective mutism has been estimated to range between 3 and 8 per 10,000 children. Some surveys indicate that it may occur in up to 0.5 percent of schoolchildren. Young children are more vulnerable to the disorder than older ones. Selective mutism appears to be more common in girls than in boys.

ETIOLOGY

Genetic Contribution

Over the last two decades the conceptualization of selective mutism has evolved from one that focused on oppositionality or childhood trauma as possible contributing factors to the current consensus that it has the same etiological factors as lead to the emergence of social phobia. Those, which include genetic factors leading to social phobia and other comorbid anxiety disorders, have histories of delayed onset of speech or speech abnormalities that may be contributory. In a recent survey, 90 percent of children with selective mutism met diagnostic criteria for social phobia. These children showed high levels of social anxiety without notable psychopathology in other areas, according to parent and teacher ratings. Thus, selective mutism may not represent a distinct disorder, but may be better conceptualized as a subtype of social phobia. Similar to families with children who exhibit other anxiety disorders, maternal anxiety, depression, and heightened dependence needs are often noted in families of children with selective mutism.

Parental Interactions

Given the likely higher levels of anxiety disorders in parents of children with selective mutism, anxiety-tinged interpersonal interactions between parents and child may unwittingly serve to promote social anxiety in children with selective mutism. Maternal overprotection and an overly close but ambivalent relationship between parents and a selectively mute child may promote symptoms. Children with selective mutism usually speak freely at home and only exhibit symptoms when under social pressure either in school or other social situations. Some children seem predisposed to selective mutism after early emotional or physical trauma; thus, some clinicians refer to the phenomenon as *traumatic mutism* rather than selective mutism.

Speech and Language Factors

Selective mutism is a psychologically determined inhibition or refusal to speak, yet a higher-than-expected proportion of children with the disorder have a history of speech delay. An interesting finding suggests that children with selective mutism are at higher risk for a disturbance in auditory processing, which may interfere with efficient processing of incoming sounds. For the most part, however, speech and language problems in children with selective mutism are subtle and are exclusionary criteria for the diagnosis of selective mutism.

DIAGNOSIS AND CLINICAL FEATURES

The DSM-IV-TR diagnostic criteria are given in Table 46.3–1. The diagnosis of selective mutism is not difficult to make after it is clear that a child has adequate language skills in some

Table 46.3–1
DSM-IV-TR Diagnostic Criteria for Selective Mutism

A. Consistent failure to speak in specific social situations (in which there is an expectation for speaking, e.g., at school) despite speaking in other situations.
B. The disturbance interferes with educational or occupational achievement or with social communication.
C. The duration of the disturbance is at least 1 month (not limited to the first month of school).
D. The failure to speak is not due to a lack of knowledge of, or comfort with, the spoken language required in the social situation.
E. The disturbance is not better accounted for by a communication disorder (e.g., stuttering) and does not occur exclusively during the course of a pervasive developmental disorder, schizophrenia, or other psychotic disorder.

From American Psychiatric Association. *Diagnostic and Statistical Manual of Mental Disorders.* 4th ed. Text rev. Washington, DC: American Psychiatric Association; copyright 2000, with permission.

environments but not in others. The mutism may have developed gradually or suddenly after a disturbing experience. The age of onset can range from 4 to 8 years. Mute periods are most commonly manifested in school or outside of the home; in rare cases, a child is mute at home but not in school. Children who exhibit selective mutism may also have symptoms of separation anxiety disorder, school refusal, and delayed language acquisition. Because social anxiety is almost always present in children with selective mutism, behavioral disturbances, such as temper tantrums and oppositional behaviors, may also occur in the home.

Pathology and Laboratory Examination

No specific laboratory measures are useful in the diagnosis or treatment of selective mutism.

DIFFERENTIAL DIAGNOSIS

Differential diagnosis of children who are silent in social situations emphasizes ruling out pervasive developmental disorders, such as autism. Once it is confirmed that the child is fully capable of speaking in certain situations that are comfortable but not in school and other social situations, an anxiety-related disorder comes to mind. Shy children may exhibit a transient muteness in new, anxiety-provoking situations. These children often have histories of not speaking in the presence of strangers and of clinging to their mothers. Most children who are mute on entering school improve spontaneously and may be described as having transient adaptational shyness. Selective mutism must also be distinguished from mental retardation, pervasive developmental disorders, and expressive language disorder. In these disorders, the symptoms are widespread, and no one situation exists in which the child communicates normally; the child may have an inability, rather than a refusal, to speak. In mutism secondary to conversion disorder, the mutism is pervasive. Children introduced into an environment in which a different language is spoken may

be reticent to begin using the new language. Selective mutism should be diagnosed only when children also refuse to converse in their native language and when they have gained communicative competence in the new language but refuse to speak it.

COURSE AND PROGNOSIS

Many very young children with early symptoms of selective mutism in the transitional period when entering preschool may have a spontaneous improvement over a number of months and never fulfill criteria for the full disorder. Children with selective mutism are often abnormally shy during preschool years, but the onset of the full disorder is usually not until age 5 or 6 years. The most common pattern is that children speak almost exclusively at home with the nuclear family but not elsewhere, especially not at school. Consequently, they may have academic difficulties and even failure. Children with selective mutism are generally shy, anxious, and vulnerable to the development of depression. Most children with mild forms of anxiety disorder, including selective mutism, remit with or without treatment. With recent data suggesting that fluoxetine (Prozac) may influence the course of selective mutism, recovery may be enhanced. Children in whom the disorder persists often have difficulty forming social relationships. Teasing and scapegoating by peers may cause them to refuse to go to school. Some children with this severe social phobia are characterized by rigidity, compulsive traits, negativism, temper tantrums, and oppositional and aggressive behavior at home. Other children with the disorder tolerate the feared situation better by communicating with gestures, such as nodding, shaking the head, and saying "Uh-huh" or "No." Most cases last for only a few weeks or months, but some cases persist for years. In one follow-up study, about one half of the children improved within 5 to 10 years. Children who do not improve by age 10 years appear to have a long-term course and a worse prognosis than those who do improve by that age. As many as one third of children with selective mutism, with or without treatment, may develop other psychiatric disorders, particularly other anxiety disorders and depression.

TREATMENT

Published data on the successful treatment of children with selective mutism are very scant, yet solid evidence indicates that children with social phobia respond to various selective serotonin reuptake inhibitor agents (SSRIs), and cognitive-behavioral treatments are under investigation in a multisite, randomized, placebo-controlled trial of children with anxiety disorders.

In the absence of data to support an approach utilizing therapy or medication alone or in combination, a multimodal approach using psychoeducation for the family, cognitive-behavioral therapy, and SSRI medication as needed is recommended. Preschool children may also benefit from a therapeutic nursery. For school-age children, individual cognitive-behavioral therapy is recommended as a first-line treatment. Family education and cooperation are beneficial. SSRI medication is now an accepted component of treatment when psychosocial interventions do not suffice to manage symptoms.

47

Early-Onset Schizophrenia

Childhood-onset schizophrenia (COS) is a rare and severe form of schizophrenia characterized by an onset of psychotic symptoms by age 12 years, believed to represent a subgroup of affected individuals with an increased heritable etiology. Children diagnosed with COS have high rates of premorbid developmental abnormalities that appear to be nonspecific markers of severe early impaired neurodevelopment. Recent imaging studies have provided data to suggest that children with COS have decreased anterior cingulated gyrus (ACG) volumes with age, unlike controls, and an absence of the normal decreased left- to right-ACG volume asymmetry. These structural differences are hypothesized to be related to abnormal neurodevelopment influencing attention and emotion regulation, which are characteristic of some cognitive impairments in psychosis. The frequency of COS is reported to be less than 1 case in 10,000 children, whereas among adolescents between the ages of 13 and 18 years, the frequency of schizophrenia is markedly increased. Schizophrenia with childhood onset has the same core phenomenological features as schizophrenia in adolescence and adulthood; however, extremely high rates of comorbid psychiatric disorders, including attention-deficit/hyperactivity disorder (ADHD), depressive disorders, and separation anxiety disorder, are seen in children and adolescents with COS.

EPIDEMIOLOGY

Schizophrenia in prepubertal children is exceedingly rare; it is estimated to occur in less than 1 of 10,000 children. In adolescents, the prevalence of schizophrenia is estimated to be 50 times that in younger children, with probable rates of 1 to 2 per 1,000. Boys seem to have a slight preponderance among children diagnosed with schizophrenia, with an estimated ratio of about 1.67 boys to 1 girl. Boys often become identified at a younger age than girls. It has been estimated that 0.1 to 1 percent present before age 10 years, with 4 percent presenting before 15 years of age. The rate of onset increases sharply during adolescence. Schizophrenia rarely is diagnosed in children younger than 5 years of age. Psychotic symptoms usually emerge insidiously, and the diagnostic criteria are met gradually over time. Occasionally, the onset of schizophrenia is sudden and occurs in a previously well-functioning child. Schizophrenia also may be diagnosed in a child who has had chronic difficulties and then experiences a significant exacerbation. The prevalence of schizophrenia among the parents of children with schizophrenia is about 8 percent, which is close to twice the prevalence in the parents of patients with adult-onset schizophrenia.

Schizotypal personality disorder is similar to schizophrenia in its inappropriate affects, excessive magical thinking, odd be-

liefs, social isolation, ideas of reference, and unusual perceptual experiences, such as illusions. Schizotypal personality disorder, however, does not have psychotic features; still, the disorder seems to aggregate in families with adult-onset schizophrenia. Therefore, the relation between the two disorders is unclear.

ETIOLOGY

The etiology of COS has multiple contributing factors, and estimates of its heritability are as high as 80 percent. COS is a severe form of schizophrenia, which may increase its likelihood of heritability to among the highest of estimates. Genetic studies provide substantial evidence for a significant genetic basis in the development of schizophrenia. The precise mechanisms of transmission of schizophrenia are not well understood. It is known to be up to eight times more prevalent among first-degree relatives of those with schizophrenia than in the general population. Adoption studies of patients with adult-onset schizophrenia have shown that schizophrenia occurs in the biological relatives, not the adoptive relatives. Additional genetic evidence is supported by higher concordance rates for schizophrenia in monozygotic twins than in dizygotic twins. Higher rates of schizophrenia are found among relatives of those with childhood-onset schizophrenia than among relatives of those with adult-onset schizophrenia. A recent case report identified a rare genetic occurrence in which an offspring received two chromosome homologues from the same parent (uniparental isodisomy) of chromosome 5, already implicated in several linkage studies to be associated with schizophrenia in a child with COS.

Currently, no reliable method can identify persons at the highest risk for schizophrenia in a given family. Neurodevelopmental abnormalities and higher-than-expected rates of neurological soft signs and impairments in sustaining attention and in strategies for information processing appear among children at high risk. Increased rates of disturbed communication styles are found in families with a member with schizophrenia. Recent reports have documented marked neuropsychological deficits in attention, working memory, and premorbid intelligence quotient (IQ) among children who develop schizophrenia and its spectrum disorders. High expressed emotion, characterized by overly critical responses in families, has been shown to be correlated with increased relapse rates among patients with schizophrenia.

Recent studies have documented gray matter loss in the brains of children with COS that started in the parietal region and proceeded frontally to dorsolateral prefrontal and temporal cortices, including superior temporal gyri. Magnetic resonance imaging (MRI) studies of 12 children with COS at baseline, and at follow-up 5 years later, were compared with normal controls. Children with COS showed severe bilateral frontal gray matter loss over the 5-year period that occurred in a dorsal-to-ventral pattern across the medial hemispheres. Frontal regions were most affected, whereas cingulated-limbic regions were less vulnerable, which correlates with the brain areas responsible for the cognitive and metabolic dysfunction typically observed in schizophrenia. Children and adolescents with schizophrenia are more likely to have a premorbid history of social rejection, poor peer relationships, clingy, withdrawn behavior, and academic trouble than individuals with adult-onset schizophrenia. Some children with schizophrenia first seen in middle childhood have early histories of motor milestones and delayed language acquisition that are similar to some symptoms of autistic disorder. The mechanisms of biological vulnerability and environmental influences producing manifestations of schizophrenia are under investigation.

DIAGNOSIS AND CLINICAL FEATURES

All of the symptoms included in adult-onset schizophrenia may be manifest in children with the disorder. The onset is frequently insidious; after first exhibiting inappropriate affects of unusual behavior, a child may take months or years to meet all of the diagnostic criteria for schizophrenia. Children who eventually meet the criteria often are socially rejected and clingy and have limited social skills. They may have histories of delayed motor and verbal milestones and do poorly in school, despite normal intelligence. Although children with schizophrenia and autistic disorder may be similar in their early histories, children with schizophrenia have normal intelligence and do not meet the criteria for a pervasive developmental disorder.

According to DSM-IV-TR, a child with schizophrenia may experience deterioration of function, along with the emergence of psychotic symptoms, or the child may never achieve the expected level of functioning (see Table 10–1). Auditory hallucinations commonly occur in children with schizophrenia. They may hear several voices making an ongoing critical commentary, or command hallucinations may tell children to kill themselves or others. The voices may be bizarre, identified as "a computer in my head," "Martians," or the voice of someone familiar, such as a relative. Visual hallucinations are experienced by a significant number of children with schizophrenia and often are frightening; the children may see the devil, skeletons, scary faces, or space creatures. Transient phobic visual hallucinations also occur in traumatized children who do not eventually have a major psychotic disorder.

Delusions are present in more than one half of children with schizophrenia; the delusions take various forms, including persecutory, grandiose, and religious. Delusions increase in frequency with increased age. Blunted or inappropriate affects appear almost universally in children with schizophrenia. Children with schizophrenia may giggle inappropriately or cry without being able to explain why. Formal thought disorders, including loosening of associations and thought blocking, are common features among children with schizophrenia. Illogical thinking and poverty of thought are also often present. Unlike adults with schizophrenia, children with schizophrenia do not have poverty of speech content, but they speak less than other children of the same intelligence and are ambiguous in the way in which they refer to persons, objects, and events. The communication deficits observable in children with schizophrenia include unpredictably changing the topic of conversation without introducing the new topic to the listener (loose associations). Children with schizophrenia also exhibit illogical thinking and speaking and tend to underuse self-initiated repair strategies to aid in their communication. When an utterance is unclear or vague, normal children attempt to clarify their communication with repetitions, revision, and more detail. Children with schizophrenia, on the other hand, fail to aid communication with revision, fillers, or starting over. These deficits may be conceptualized as negative symptoms in childhood schizophrenia.

The core phenomena for schizophrenia seem to be the same among various age groups, but a child's developmental level influences the presentation of the symptoms. Delusions of young children are less complex, therefore, than those of older children. Age-appropriate content, such as animal imagery and monsters, is likely to be a source of delusional fear in children. Other features that seem to occur frequently in children with schizophrenia are poor motor functioning, visuospatial impairments, and attention deficits.

The DSM-IV-TR delineates five types of schizophrenia: paranoid, disorganized, catatonic, undifferentiated, and residual.

A 12-year-old boy developed concerns that his parents might be poisoning his food. Over the next year, his symptoms progressed with increased fearfulness, preoccupation with food, and beliefs that Satan and voices from the radio and television were sending him bad thoughts. During this time, his parents also observed bizarre behaviors, including talking and yelling to himself, perseverating about devils and demons, assaulting family members because he thought they were evil, and attempting to hurt himself because he believed it would please God. No predominant mood symptoms or any history of substance abuse were found.

Developmentally, he was the product of a full-term pregnancy complicated by a difficult labor and forceps delivery. His early motor and speech milestones were normal. As a younger child, he tended to be quiet and socially awkward. His intelligence was felt to be in the normal range, but academic testing was consistently below grade level.

He has had no significant medical problems. An organic work-up included normal serum chemistries, thyroid functions, toxicology screen, ceruloplasmin, and brain MRI. His family psychiatric history was significant for depression in a maternal aunt and a completed suicide in a maternal great-grandparent. His symptoms have not significantly improved in the 5 years subsequent to the onset of his illness. He has been hospitalized nine times, including placement in a long-term residential program. He has been on numerous antipsychotic medications, both traditional neuroleptics and atypical agents, and numerous other agents, including selective serotonin reuptake inhibitors (SSRIs) and mood stabilizers. His mental status examination continued to display tangential and disorganized thinking, paranoid delusions, loose associations, perseverative speech patterns, and a flat, at times inappropriate, affect. His time has generally been spent pacing and muttering to himself, with no social interaction with others unless initiated by adults. Some improvement was finally noted with clozapine (Clozaril) therapy, although he remained symptomatic. (Courtesy of Jon M. McClellan, M.D.)

PATHOLOGY AND LABORATORY EXAMINATIONS

No specific laboratory tests are diagnostically specific for COS. Although neuroimaging studies are converging to suggest that children with COS have decreased ACG volumes with age and an absence of the normal decreased left- to right-ACG volume asymmetry, this research cannot be used as an index for diagnosis. High incidences of pregnancy and birth complications have been reported in the histories of children with schizophrenia, but no specificity has been found in these risks for childhood schizophrenia. Electroencephalogram studies have not been helpful in distinguishing children with schizophrenia from other children. Although data exist to suggest that hypoprolinemia is associated with the risk of schizoaffective disorder because of an alteration on chromosome 22q11, no association has been found of hyperprolinemia with COS.

DIFFERENTIAL DIAGNOSIS

The differential diagnosis of COS includes autistic disorder, bipolar disorders, depressive psychotic disorders, multicomplex developmental syndromes, Asperger's syndrome, drug-induced psychosis, and psychotic states caused by organic disorders. Children with COS have been shown to have multiple, frequently occurring concurrent disorders, including ADHD, oppositional defiant disorder, and depression. Children with schizotypal personality disorder have some traits in common with children who meet diagnostic criteria for schizophrenia. Blunted affect, social isolation, eccentric thoughts, ideas of reference, and bizarre behavior can be seen in both disorders; however, in schizophrenia, overt psychotic symptoms, such as hallucinations, delusions, and incoherence, must be present at some point. When they are present, they exclude a diagnosis of schizotypal personality disorder. Hallucinations alone, however, are not evidence of schizophrenia; patients must show either a deterioration of function or an inability to meet an expected developmental level to warrant the diagnosis of schizophrenia. Auditory and visual hallucinations can appear as self-limited events in nonpsychotic young children who are faced with extreme psychosocial stressors, such as the breakup of their parents, and in children experiencing a major loss or significant change in lifestyle.

Psychotic phenomena are common among children with major depressive disorder, in which both hallucinations and, less commonly, delusions may occur. The congruence of mood with psychotic features is most pronounced in depressed children, although children with schizophrenia may also seem sad. The hallucinations and delusions of schizophrenia are more likely to have a bizarre quality than those of children with depressive disorders. In children and adolescents with bipolar I disorder, it often is difficult to distinguish a first episode of mania with psychotic features from schizophrenia if the child has no history of previous depressions. Grandiose delusions and hallucinations are typical of manic episodes, but clinicians often must follow the natural history of the disorder to confirm the presence of a mood disorder. Pervasive developmental disorders, including autistic disorder with normal intelligence, often share some features with schizophrenia. Most notably, difficulty with social relationships, an early history of delayed language acquisition, and ongoing communication deviance occur in both disorders;

however, hallucinations, delusions, and formal thought disorder are core features of schizophrenia and are not expected features of pervasive developmental disorders. Pervasive developmental disorders usually are diagnosed by 3 years of age, but schizophrenia with childhood onset can rarely be diagnosed before 5 years of age.

Alcohol and other substance abuse sometimes can result in a deterioration of function, psychotic symptoms, and paranoid delusions. Use of amphetamines, lysergic acid diethylamide, and phencyclidine may lead to a psychotic state. A sudden, flagrant onset of paranoid psychosis is more suggestive of substance-induced psychotic disorder than an insidious onset. Medical conditions that can induce psychotic features include thyroid disease, systemic lupus erythematosus, and temporal lobe disease.

COURSE AND PROGNOSIS

Important predictors of the course and outcome of early-onset schizophrenia include the child's level of functioning before the onset of schizophrenia, the age of onset, IQ, response to pharmacologic interventions, how much functioning the child regained after the first episode, and the amount of support available from the family. Children with developmental delays, learning disorders, lower IQ, and premorbid behavioral disorders, such as ADHD and conduct disorder, seem to respond less well to medication treatment of schizophrenia and are likely to have the most guarded prognoses. In a long-term outcome study of patients with schizophrenia with onset before 14 years of age, the worst prognoses occurred in children with schizophrenia that was diagnosed before they were 10 years of age and who had preexisting personality disorders.

TREATMENT

The treatment of COS requires a multimodal approach, including pharmacological interventions, family education, social skills interventions, and appropriate educational placement. Current research suggests that, in adolescents and young adults, early interventions during the prodrome of schizophrenia with atypical antipsychotics and psychosocial support may improve symptoms and delay or prevent progression to full-blown schizophrenia. Investigation is needed on the recognition of prodromal states of COS to assess the benefits of very early interventions. Current treatments for COS are based on very limited data. Antipsychotic medications are indicated, given the degree of impairment in both social relationships and academic function exhibited by children with schizophrenia. Children with COS may have less robust responses to antipsychotic medications than adolescents and adults with the same disorder. Family education and ongoing family interventions are critical to maximize the level of support that the family can give the patient. The proper educational setting for the child is also important because social skills deficits, attention deficits, and academic difficulties often accompany childhood schizophrenia.

Pharmacotherapy

Second-generation antipsychotics are first-line treatment for children and adolescents with schizophrenia, having replaced the dopamine receptor antagonists because of their more favorable side-effect profiles. The serotonin-dopamine agonists, including risperidone (Risperdal), olanzapine (Zyprexa), and clozapine (Clozaril), differ from the conventional antipsychotics in that they act as serotonin receptor antagonists with some dopamine (D_2) activity but without a predominance of D_2-receptor antagonism. They are hypothesized to be more effective in reducing positive and negative symptoms of schizophrenia and incur less risk of causing extrapyramidal adverse effects. Additional atypical antipsychotics, such as quetiapine (Seroquel), ziprasidone (Geodon), and aripiprazole (Abilify), are also serotonin-dopamine antagonists that are used in clinical practice for children and adolescents with psychotic disorders who do not respond to other atypical antipsychotics. A limited evidence base exists to inform the treatment of COS with the atypical antipsychotics, and a need is seen for randomized clinical trials in this patient population.

Children and adolescents who are treated with antipsychotic medications are at risk for withdrawal dyskinesia. The long-term adverse effects, including tardive dyskinesia, are perpetual risks for any patients treated with an antipsychotic medication.

Psychotherapy

Psychosocial interventions aimed at family education and patient and family support are recognized as critical components of the treatment plan for COS. Psychotherapists who work with children with schizophrenia must take into account a child's developmental level. They must continually support the child's good reality testing and be sensitive to the child's sense of self. Long-term intensive and supportive psychotherapy combined with pharmacotherapy is the most effective approach to this disorder.

48

Child Psychiatry: Additional Conditions That May Be a Focus of Clinical Attention

BORDERLINE INTELLECTUAL FUNCTIONING

Intellectual functioning of a child or adolescent is influenced by multiple factors, including birth history of full-term gestation, neonatal head circumference, learning, nutritional status, and brain development after birth. Brain parameters, parental head circumference, and prenatal nutrition are most correlated with the head circumference of the newborn. In a sample of Chilean school-age children, those born with small head circumference of at least two standard deviations below the mean (microcephalic) were most likely to present with lower overall brain volume, compromised intellectual and scholastic functions, and poor nutrition. Although intellectual quotients (IQs) are generally believed to be stable over time, in some cases, a single measurement of intellectual functioning does not accurately predict intellectual function in all areas over the long term. For example, a follow-up study conducted to investigate the stability of IQ measurement in a group of dyslexic adolescents and young adults who were tested at age 12 years and retested after a mean interval of 6.5 years found the following differences over time: Compared with first IQ tests, for the teens and young adults, the retests showed a significant relative decrease in verbal IQ (VIQ), which was interpreted as either poor reliability of the test or a loss of ability based on diminished experience with reading and writing compared with same-age peers over time. Performance IQ (PIQ), however, was found to be significantly increased, leading to the hypothesis that a compensatory process had been developed by these children with dyslexia, such as a more visual or creative way to process information, leading to greater success on performance test items. The conclusion was that a single IQ test in childhood may not be a fully accurate predictor of later abilities and that potential interventions to help children with disabilities such as dyslexia keep up academically with peers may have implications for final IQ and intellectual functioning.

Borderline intellectual functioning, according to the text revision of the fourth edition of the *Diagnostic and Statistical Manual of Mental Disorders* (DSM-IV-TR), is a category that can be used when the focus of clinical attention is on a child or adolescent with IQ in the 71 to 84 range. The intellectual functioning of children plays a major role in their adjustment to school, social relationships, and family function. Children who cannot quite understand class work and may also be slow in understanding rules of games and the social rules of their peer group are often bitterly rejected. Some children with borderline intellectual functioning can mingle socially better than they can keep up academically in class. In these cases, the strengths of these children may be peer relationships, especially if they excel at sports, but eventually, their academic struggles will take a toll on self-esteem if they are not appropriately remediated.

Etiology

Genetic factors are increasingly being found to play a role in intellectual deficits. Environmental deprivation and infectious and toxic exposures can also contribute to cognitive impairment. Twin and adoption studies support the hypothesis that many genes contribute to the development of a given IQ. Specific infectious processes (e.g., congenital rubella), prenatal exposures (e.g., fetal alcohol syndrome), and specific chromosomal abnormalities (e.g., fragile X syndrome) result in mental retardation.

Diagnosis

The DSM-IV-TR contains the following statement about borderline intellectual functioning:

This category can be used when the focus of clinical attention is associated with borderline intellectual functioning, that is, an IQ in the 71 to 84 range. Differential diagnosis between Borderline Intellectual Functioning and Mental Retardation (an IQ of 70 or below) is especially difficult when the coexistence of certain mental disorders (e.g., Schizophrenia) is involved. Coding note: This is categorized on a V Code.

Treatment

The goals of treatment are to maximize educational and vocational placements so that individuals can develop the most optimal practical adaptive skills, social skills, and self-esteem. The goal is to improve the match between the person's capabilities and lifestyle. After the underlying problem becomes known to the therapist, psychiatric treatment can be useful. Many persons with borderline intellectual functioning can function at a superior level in some areas while being markedly deficient in others.

By directing such persons to appropriate areas of endeavor, by pointing out socially acceptable behavior, and by teaching them living skills, the therapist can help improve their self-esteem.

ACADEMIC PROBLEM

The DSM-IV-TR refers to an academic problem as a problem that is not caused by a mental disorder or, if caused by a mental disorder, is sufficiently severe to warrant clinical attention. This diagnostic category is used when a child or adolescent is having significant academic difficulties that are not deemed to be caused by a specific learning disorder or communication disorder or directly related to a psychiatric disorder. Nevertheless, intervention is necessary because the child's achievement in school is significantly impaired. A child or adolescent of normal intelligence and who is free of a learning disorder or a communication disorder but is failing in school or doing poorly falls into this category.

Etiology

Many psychological factors contribute to a child's confidence, competence, and academic success. In the absence of a specific learning disorder to account for the academic difficulty or primary psychiatric disorder responsible for the academic compromise, subclinical states of anxiety or depression or peer and family stressors such as divorce, marital discord, abuse, or mental illness in a family member may interrupt academic production. Children who are troubled by social isolation, identity issues, preoccupation with sexuality, or extreme shyness may withdraw from full participation in academic activities. Academic problems may be the result of a confluence of multiple contributing factors and may occur in adolescents who were previously high academic achievers. School is the main social and educational venue for children and adolescents. Success and acceptance in the school setting depend on children's physical, cognitive, social, and emotional adjustment. Children's general coping mechanisms in many developmental tasks usually are reflected in their academic and social success in school. Boys and girls must cope with the process of separation from parents, adjustment to new environments, adaptation to social contacts, competition, assertion, intimacy, and exposure to unfamiliar attitudes. A corresponding relation often exists between school performance and how well these tasks are mastered.

Anxiety can play a major role in interfering with children's academic performances. Anxiety can hamper their abilities to perform well on tests, to speak in public, and to ask questions when they do not understand something. Some children are so concerned about the way in which others view them that they cannot attend to their academic tasks. For some children, conflicts about success and fears of the consequences imagined to accompany the attainment of success can hamper academic success. Sigmund Freud described persons with such conflicts as "those wrecked by success." For example, an adolescent girl may be unable to succeed in school because she fears social rejection, the loss of perceived femininity, or both, and she may perceive success as being involved with aggression and competition with boys.

Depressed children also may withdraw from academic pursuits; they require specific interventions to improve their academic performances and to treat their depression. Children who do not have major depressive disorder but who are consumed by family problems, such as financial troubles, marital discord between their parents, and mental illness in family members, may be distracted and unable to attend to academic tasks. Children who receive mixed messages from their parents about accepting criticism and redirection from their teachers can become confused and unable to perform well in school. The loss of the parents as the primary and predominant teachers in a child's life can result in identity conflicts for some children. Some students lack a stable sense of self and cannot identify goals for themselves, a situation that leads to a sense of boredom or futility.

Cultural and economic background can play a role in how well accepted a child feels in school and can affect the child's academic achievement. Familial socioeconomic level, parental education, race, religion, and family functioning can influence a child's sense of fitting in and can affect preparation to meet school demands.

Schools, teachers, and clinicians can share insights about how to foster productive and cooperative environments for all students in a classroom. Teachers' expectations about their students' performance influence these performances. Teachers serve as agents whose varying expectations can shape the differential development of students' skills and abilities. Such conditioning early in school, especially when negative, can disturb academic performance. A teacher's affective response to a child, therefore, can prompt the appearance of an academic problem. Most important is a teacher's humane approach to students at all levels of education, including medical school.

Diagnosis

The DSM-IV-TR contains the following statement about the category of academic problem:

> This category can be used when the focus of clinical attention is an academic problem that is not due to a mental disorder or, if due to a mental disorder, is sufficiently severe to warrant independent clinical attention. An example is a pattern of failing grades or of significant underachievement in a person with adequate intellectual capacity in the absence of a learning or a communication disorder or any other mental disorder that would account for the problem.

A 15-year-old boy was admitted to an intensive outpatient program for evaluation of insidiously declining grades at school, isolative behavior, and anhedonia occurring for the first time over the course of the last semester at high school. The patient had no previous psychiatric history and was in good health. School reports showed his full-scale IQ to be 100 and revealed no previous behavior or academic problems. Interviews with family and patient revealed that the boy had an intact family with no apparent or unusual conflicts noted and that his mother found evidence of drug paraphernalia—cigarette papers, small pipe, matches, and a suspicious-looking dried substance in his bedroom. When confronted, the patient revealed a 6-month use of marijuana. A primary diagnosis of cannabis abuse, in addition to academic problem, was made. Referral to a therapeutic drug and alcohol program was immediately implemented. (Courtesy of Frank John Ninivaggi, M.D.)

Treatment

The initial step in determining a useful intervention for an academic problem is a comprehensive diagnostic evaluation. Identifying and addressing family-, school-, and peer-related stressors are critical. Substance use disorders must be carefully ruled out, as well as concurrent psychiatric disorders that may require treatment before improvement in academic function. An individualized educational plan evaluation and meeting may be requested in writing to the school so that specific educational testing can be integrated into the assessment of the overall academic problem and educational accommodations can be considered.

Psychosocial intervention may be applied successfully for scholastic difficulties related to poor motivation, poor self-concept, and underachievement. Early efforts to relieve the problem are critical: Sustained problems in learning and school performance frequently are compounded and precipitate severe difficulties. Feelings of anger, frustration, shame, loss of self-respect, and helplessness—emotions that most often accompany school failures—damage self-esteem emotionally and cognitively, disabling future performance and clouding expectations for success. Generally, children with academic problems require either school-based intervention or individual attention.

Tutoring is an effective technique for dealing with academic problems and should be considered in most cases. Tutoring has proved of value in preparing for objective multiple-choice examinations, such as the *Scholastic Aptitude Test* and the *Medical College Aptitude Test*. Taking such examinations repetitively and using relaxation skills are two behavioral techniques of great value in diminishing anxiety.

CHILDHOOD OR ADOLESCENT ANTISOCIAL BEHAVIOR

According to DSM-IV-TR, child or adolescent antisocial behavior refers to behavior that is not caused by a mental disorder and includes isolated antisocial acts, not a pattern of behavior. This category covers many acts by children and adolescents that violate the rights of others, such as overt acts of aggression and violence and covert acts of lying, stealing, truancy, and running away from home. Certain antisocial acts, such as fire setting, possession of a weapon, or a severe act of aggression toward another child, require intervention for even a single occurrence. Sometimes, children without a pattern of recurrent aggression or antisocial behavior become involved in occasional less severe behaviors that nevertheless require some intervention. The DSM-IV-TR definition of conduct disorder requires a repetitive pattern of at least three antisocial behaviors for at least 6 months, but childhood or adolescent antisocial behavior may consist of isolated events that do not constitute a mental disorder but do become the focus of clinical attention. The emergence of occasional antisocial symptoms is common among children who have a variety of mental disorders, including psychotic disorders, depressive disorders, impulse-control disorders, disruptive behavior, and attention-deficit disorders, such as attention-deficit/hyperactivity disorder and oppositional defiant disorder.

A child's age and developmental level affect the manifestations of disturbed conduct and influence the likelihood that a child meets the diagnostic criteria for a conduct disorder as opposed to childhood antisocial behavior. Therefore, a child of 5 or 6 years of age is not likely to meet the criteria for three antisocial symptoms—for example, physical confrontations, the use of weapons, and forcing someone into sexual activity—but a single symptom, such as initiating fights, is common in children 5 to 6 years of age. The term *juvenile delinquent* is defined by the legal system as a youth who has violated the law in some way, but the term does not imply that the youth meets the criteria for a mental disorder.

Epidemiology

Estimates of antisocial behavior range from 5 to 15 percent of the general population and somewhat less among children and adolescents. Reports have documented a higher frequency of antisocial behaviors in urban settings than in rural areas. In one report, the risk of coming into contact with the police for antisocial behavior was estimated to be 20 percent for teenage boys and 4 percent for teenage girls.

Etiology

Antisocial behaviors can occur in the context of a mental disorder or in its absence. Antisocial behavior is multidetermined and occurs most frequently in children or adolescents with many risk factors. Among the most common risk factors are harsh and physically abusive parenting, parental criminality, and a child's tendency toward impulsive and hyperactive behavior. Protective factors can attenuate the risk of antisocial behaviors by exerting an independent influence on strengthening core aspects of functioning and thereby decreasing risk. Protective factors can include high intelligence, an easy or self-directed temperament, high levels of social skill, competence in school or in other domains of artistic or athletic skill, and, finally, a strong bond with at least one parent. Additional associated features of children and adolescents with antisocial behavior are low IQ, academic failure, and low levels of adult supervision. (See Chapter 29 for a discussion of genetic and social factors as causes of adult antisocial behavior.)

Psychological Factors.   If their parenting is poor, children experience emotional deprivation, which leads to low self-esteem and unconscious anger. When children are not given any limits, their consciences are deficient because they have not internalized parental prohibitions that account for superego formation. Therefore, they have so-called *superego lacunae*, which allow them to commit antisocial acts without guilt. At times, such children's antisocial behavior is a vicarious source of pleasure and gratification for parents who act out their own forbidden wishes and impulses through their children. A consistent finding in persons who perform repeated acts of violent behavior is a history of physical abuse.

Diagnosis and Clinical Features

The DSM-IV-TR contains the following statement about childhood or adolescent antisocial behavior:

> This category can be used when the focus of clinical attention is antisocial behavior in a child or adolescent that is not due to a mental disorder (e.g., Conduct Disorder or an Impulse-Control Disorder). Examples include isolated antisocial acts of children or adolescents (not a pattern of antisocial behavior).

The childhood behaviors most associated with antisocial behavior are theft, incorrigibility, arrests, school problems, impulsiveness, promiscuity, oppositional behavior, lying, suicide attempts, substance abuse, truancy, running away, associating with undesirable persons, and staying out late at night. The more symptoms present in childhood, the greater is the probability of adult antisocial behavior; however, the presence of many symptoms also indicates the development of other mental disorders in adult life.

Differential Diagnosis

Substance-related disorders (including alcohol, cannabis, and cocaine use disorders), bipolar I disorder, and schizophrenia in childhood often manifest themselves as antisocial behavior.

A 9-year-old child was arrested by police for breaking into a local hardware store. He was accompanied by two friends. The three had ridden their bikes in a suburban neighborhood until after dark and engaged in a play of "cops and robbers," taking turns in pursuing and being pursued. To make the game more lifelike, one of the three suggested that they actually break into this store, whose owner was a somewhat gruff and intimidating man. The three decided that such an adventure would be quite exciting and proceeded to smash in the glass door with a brick. Shortly after the glass broke, the police arrived and arrested them. Parents were called to come and to collect their children. None of the three had any previous contact with the police or any social service agency. Although they previously engaged in some mischief in the neighborhood, such as throwing toilet paper on people's houses and egging cars, none of the three had any serious infractions of societal rules, and none of the three boys had any more of these events cluster in the past few months. One of them had a history of ADHD and some learning difficulties at school, whereas the other two boys had no particular risk factors for the persistence of antisocial behavior. The antisocial activities of the child with ADHD progressed to the point of fulfilling conduct disorder criteria in early adolescence. Much of his future acting out consisted of drug-related offenses, that is, the use and sales of drugs, stealing, and other covert delinquent activities. The two boys without risks proceeded to develop through a normative, turbulent, and lively adolescence without any further legal involvement. (Courtesy of Hans Steiner, M.D., and Niranjan Karnik, M.D., Ph.D.)

Treatment

Antisocial behavior does not specifically represent a corresponding psychiatric disorder; therefore, a comprehensive psychiatric assessment and the context in which the antisocial behavior emerged must be conducted to delineate the place of the antisocial behavior with respect to any comorbid psychopathology.

Disturbances of conduct frequently accompany the onset of various other psychiatric disorders. The first step in determining the appropriate treatment for a child or an adolescent who is manifesting antisocial behavior is to evaluate the need to treat any coexisting mental disorder, such as bipolar I disorder, a psychotic disorder, or a depressive disorder, that may be contributing to the antisocial behavior. The treatment of antisocial behavior usually involves behavioral management, which is most effective when the patient is in a controlled environment in a structured day or residential setting. In less severe situations, the child's family

members are able to manage the symptoms in collaboration with the clinician by utilizing a cooperative behavioral program.

In some cases, special educational settings are necessary to provide the essential monitoring and feedback necessary to diminish the undesired behaviors. In some cases, even regular school classroom teachers can help modify antisocial behavior in the classroom. Rewards for prosocial behaviors and positive reinforcement for the control of unwanted behaviors have merit.

Medications generally are not used in patients with rare or occasional antisocial behaviors, especially when no comorbid psychiatric disorders exist. Medications have been used with some success when repetitive episodes of explosive behavior, aggression, or violent outbursts ensue. Lithium (Eskalith), divalproex (Depakote) and atypical antipsychotics such as risperidone (Risperdal), olanzapine (Zyprexa), quetiapine (Seroquel), ziprasidone (Geodon), or aripiprazole (Abilify) may reduce explosive behavior and rage outbursts. For young children who are sensitive to the extrapyramidal side effects of antipsychotics, chlorpromazine (Thorazine), despite its sedating properties, may be better tolerated and more efficacious in managing acute aggression. The use of diphenhydramine (Benadryl) or lorazepam (Ativan) may be helpful as adjunctive medications in the short-term control of aggressive behavior. When symptoms of ADHD, such as hyperactivity and impulsivity, are contributing factors, short- or long-acting methylphenidate agents (Ritalin, Concerta), or short- or long-acting amphetamine and amphetamine salts (Adderall, Adderall XR) may help to reduce impulsivity and decrease aggression.

It is more difficult to treat children and adolescents who exhibit long-term patterns of antisocial behavior, particularly covert behaviors, such as stealing and lying. Group therapy in the context of residential treatment centers has been used for these behaviors, and cognitive problem-solving approaches are potentially helpful.

IDENTITY PROBLEM

The conceptualization of identity encompasses cognitive, psychodynamic, psychosexual, neurobiological, and cultural development. The developmentalist Erik Erikson proposed, in writings collected in his book *Identity and the Life Cycle*, that the central task of adolescence is to achieve a sense of self-sameness and continuity in time. The normative developmental process for an adolescent was conceptualized by Erikson as an adolescent crisis of identity. The transition between a childhood identity and the process of accepting a more mature sense of self is the resolution of the crisis. The notion of an identity crisis in adolescence gained widespread attention by clinicians and the popular media during the late 1960s and early 1970s when many adolescents were displaying rejection of mainstream cultural values and ideas and demonstrating alternate lifestyles.

The concept of *identity disorder* as a psychiatric diagnosis was embraced in the 1980s when the DSM-III was devised, as a disorder usually first evident in childhood. It was meant to include adolescents who presented with "severe subjective distress regarding uncertainty about a variety of issues relating to identity" to the point at which they became impaired. So, according to DSM-IV-TR, *identity problem* refers to uncertainty about issues, such as goals, career choice, friendships, sexual behavior, moral values, and group loyalties. An identity problem can cause severe distress for a young person and can lead a person to seek psychotherapy or guidance. Identity problem, however, is not recognized as a mental disorder in DSM-IV-TR. It sometimes manifests in the context of such mental disorders as mood disorders, psychotic disorders, and borderline personality disorder.

Epidemiology

No reliable information is available regarding predisposing factors, familial pattern, sex ratio, or prevalence, but problems with identity formation seem to be a result of life in modern society. Today, children and adolescents often experience great instability in family life, problems with identity formation, conflicts between adolescent peer values and the values of parents and society, and exposure through the media and education to various moral, behavioral, and lifestyle possibilities.

Etiology

The causes of identity problems often are multifactorial and include the pressures of a highly dysfunctional family and the influences of coexisting mental disorders. In general, adolescents with major depressive disorder, psychotic disorders, and other mental disorders report feeling alienated from family members and experience some turmoil. Children who have had difficulty mastering expected developmental tasks all along are likely to have difficulty with the pressure to establish a well-defined identity during adolescence. Erikson used the term *identity versus role diffusion* to describe the developmental and psychosocial tasks challenging adolescents to incorporate past experiences and present goals into a coherent sense of self.

Diagnosis and Clinical Features

The DSM-IV-TR contains the following statement about identity problem:

> This category can be used when the focus of clinical attention is uncertainty about multiple issues relating to identity such as long-term goals, career choice, friendship patterns, sexual orientation and behavior, moral values, and group loyalties.

The essential features of identity problem seem to revolve around the question, "Who am I?" Conflicts are experienced as irreconcilable aspects of the self that the adolescent cannot integrate into a coherent identity. As Erikson described the identity problem, a young person manifests severe doubting and an inability to make decisions, a sense of isolation, inner emptiness, a growing inability to relate to others, disturbed sexual functioning, a distorted time perspective, a sense of urgency, and the assumption of a negative identity. The associated features frequently include marked discrepancy between the adolescent's self-perception and the views that others have of the adolescent; moderate anxiety and depression that are usually related to inner preoccupation, rather than external realities; and self-doubt and uncertainty about the future, with either difficulty making choices or impulsive experiments in an attempt to establish an independent identity. Some persons with identity problem join cult-like groups.

Differential Diagnosis

Identity problem must be differentiated from a mental disorder (e.g., borderline personality disorder, schizophreniform disor-

der, schizophrenia, or a mood disorder). At times, what initially seems to be an identity problem may be the prodromal manifestations of one of these disorders. Intense but normal conflicts associated with maturing, such as adolescent turmoil and midlife crisis, may be confusing, but they usually are not associated with marked deterioration in school, in vocational or social functioning, or with severe subjective distress. Considerable evidence indicates that adolescent turmoil often is not a phase that is outgrown but an indication of true psychopathology.

Course and Prognosis

The onset of identity problem most frequently occurs in late adolescence as teenagers separate from the nuclear family and attempt to establish an independent identity and value system. The onset usually is characterized by a gradual increase in anxiety, depression, regressive phenomena (e.g., loss of interest in friends, school, and activities), irritability, sleep difficulties, and changes in eating habits. The course usually is relatively brief as developmental lags respond to support, acceptance, and the provision of a psychosocial moratorium.

Extensive prolongation of adolescence with continued identity problem can lead to the chronic state of role diffusion, which may indicate a disturbance of early developmental stages and the presence of borderline personality disorder, a mood disorder, or schizophrenia. An identity problem usually resolves by the mid-20s. If it persists, the person with the identity problem may be unable to make career commitments or lasting attachments.

Cory, an 8-year-old girl, was adopted in Taiwan at 10 months of age by a white midwestern couple. As she grew, her vulnerability to separations became increasingly more pronounced. Even the possibility that her adoptive mother would leave her for the day triggered what appeared to be dramatic disruptions in Cory's reality contact, as well as outbursts of rage and misbehavior in school. She pleaded with her mother to care for the many aches and pains that plagued her. If her mother stayed with her, they could both enjoy the girl's favorite game—the mother playing the part of an Asian queen, with Cory as her beloved princess. Yet, the girl's demands, including the requirements of "royalty," were so exhausting that, at times, the mother would seek relief at her own mother's home in a nearby town.

Such "abandonment" would more than perturb the idyllic fantasy of the queen and her princess. Without the love, protection, and presence of the queen, Cory herself changed, turning into a "Chinese bitch." Later, in therapy, she discussed how a vivid fantasy would come to her at times of separation. In this fantasy, a witch, a vicious vixen of mixed Caucasian and Asian features, taunted Cory and threatened to drag her down into a bottomless pit.

Cory hated this witch nearly as much as she hated the "Chinese bitch" she herself became. She hated, in particular, the rage and anguish that overwhelmed her. To punish the "bitch," she would hit herself and poke at her skin until it bled.

By the time she reached adolescence, Cory's self-mutilating behavior was firmly established. She responded to frustration, separations, or perceived threats of abandonment

The sessions consisted of psychoeducational approaches concerning John's developmental level of functioning and the way he perceived and experienced his environment. His parents were helped to recognize and handle John's problems, as well their own conflicts, and strategies were proposed for facilitating John's development. At termination, it was agreed that John would return to see the therapist for one follow-up session every 3 months in the first year and every 6 months in the following 2 years. At the 2-year follow-up, it was apparent that John had improved academically and had resumed his outside activities, such as sports. He remained sensitive to rejection, but he was able to use the skills he had learned to manage those feelings. (Courtesy of Euthymia D. Hibbs, Ph.D.)

Cognitive-behavioral therapy (CBT) is an amalgam of behavioral therapy and cognitive psychology. It emphasizes how children may use thinking processes and cognitive modalities to reframe, restructure, and solve problems. A child's distortions are addressed by generating alternative ways of dealing with problematic situations. Cognitive-behavioral strategies have been shown in multiple studies to be effective in the treatment of child and adolescent mood disorders, OCD, and anxiety disorders. A recent study compared a family-focused CBT—the "Building Confidence Program"—with traditional child-focused CBT with minimal family involvement for children with anxiety disorders. Both interventions included coping skills training and in vivo exposure, but the family CBT intervention also included parent communication training. Compared with the child-focused CBT, family CBT was associated with greater improvement on independent evaluators' ratings and parent reports of child anxiety but not on children's self-reports of improvement. Family-focused CBT has also been used in the treatment of pediatric bipolar disorder with promising success.

One of the limiting factors in providing CBT to children with OCD, anxiety disorders, and depressive disorders is the lack of sufficient numbers of trained child and adolescent cognitive-behavioral therapists, and a recent study addressed the issue of the feasibility of combining a CBT via clinic-plus-Internet condition. Children who received the clinic-plus Internet condition showed significantly greater reductions in anxiety from pre- to posttreatment condition and maintained gains for a period of 12 months compared with children who received no active treatment but were on a wait-list condition. The Internet treatment was acceptable to families, and dropout rate was minimal.

A recent study of a CBT in conjunction with an attachment-based family therapy used in adolescents with anxiety disorders and their families showed that significant improvements could be achieved by using individual CBT along with a family therapy condition. Participants followed at 6 to 9 months after the treatment showed significant decreases in anxiety and depressive symptoms. Cognitive-behavior therapy has now been shown in multiple randomized clinical trials to have efficacy in the treatment of anxiety disorders in children and adolescents. Using a variety of components, including behavioral exposure, cognitive restructuring, and psychoeducation, CBT has been shown to be adaptable to a variety of formats, including individual, family, and group treatment.

Remedial, educational, and patterning psychotherapy is focused on teaching new attitudes and patterns of behavior to children who persist in using immature and inefficient patterns that are often presumed to be caused by a maturational lag. Supportive psychotherapy is particularly helpful in enabling a well-adjusted youngster to cope with emotional turmoil engendered by a crisis. It also is used with disturbed youngsters whose less-than-adequate ego functioning may be seriously disrupted by an expressive-exploratory mode or by other forms of therapeutic intervention.

At the beginning of most psychotherapy, regardless of a patient's age and the nature of the therapeutic interventions, the principal therapeutic elements perceived by patients tend to be supportive as a consequence of therapists' universal efforts to be reliably and sensitively responsive. In fact, some therapy may never proceed beyond the supportive level, whereas other therapy develops an expressive-exploratory or behavioral modification flavor on top of the supportive foundation.

Preschool-age children are sometimes treated through the parents, a process called *filial therapy*. Therapists using the strategy should be alert to the possibility that apparently successful filial treatment can obscure a significant diagnosis because patients are not treated directly. The first case of filial therapy was that of Little Hans, reported by Freud in 1905. Hans was a 5-year-old phobic child who was treated by his father under Freud's supervision.

Although historically psychotherapy had its roots in psychodynamic theories, current evidence has shown that cognitive-behavioral therapeutic techniques are efficacious in the treatment of anxiety disorders and mood disorders in youth. Children generally are unaware of these unreal dangers, their fear of them, and the psychological defenses they use to avoid both the danger and the fear. With the awareness that is facilitated, patients can evaluate the usefulness of their defensive maneuvers and can relinquish unnecessary maneuvers that constitute the symptoms of their emotional disturbance.

Child psychoanalysis, an intensive, uncommon form of psychoanalytic psychotherapy, works on unconscious resistance and defenses during three to four sessions a week. Under these circumstances, therapists anticipate unconscious resistance and allow transference manifestations to mature to a full transference neurosis through which neurotic conflicts are resolved. Interpretations of dynamically relevant conflicts are emphasized in psychoanalytic descriptions, and elements that are predominant in other types of psychotherapies are not overlooked. Indeed, in all psychotherapy, children should derive support from the consistently understanding and accepting relationship with their therapists. Remedial educational guidance is provided when necessary.

Probably the most vivid examples of the integration of psychodynamic and behavioral approaches, although they are not always explicitly conceptualized as such, appear in the milieu of child and adolescent psychiatric therapy in inpatient, residential, and day treatment facilities. Behavioral change is initiated in these settings, and its repercussions are explored concurrently in individual psychotherapeutic sessions, so that the action in one arena and the information stemming from it augment and illuminate what occurs in the other arena.

DIFFERENCES BETWEEN CHILDREN AND ADULTS

Logic suggests that psychotherapy with children, who generally are more flexible than adults and who have simpler defenses and other mental mechanisms, should consume less time than comparable treatment of adults. Experience usually does not confirm this expectation, because children usually lack some elements that contribute to successful treatment. A child, for example, typically does not seek help. As a consequence, one of a therapist's first tasks is to stimulate a child's motivation for treatment. Children commonly begin therapy involuntarily, often without the benefit of true parental support. Although parents may want their children to be helped or changed, the desire often is generated by frustrated anger toward the children. Typically, the anger is accompanied by relative insensitivity to what therapists perceive as the children's need and the basis for a therapeutic alliance. Therefore, whereas adult patients frequently perceive advantages in getting well, children may envision therapeutic change as nothing more than conforming to a disagreeable reality, an attitude that heightens the likelihood of their perceiving a therapist as the parent's punitive agent. This is hardly the most fertile soil in which to nurture a therapeutic alliance.

Children have a limited capacity for self-observation, with the notable exception of some obsessive children who resemble adults in this ability. Such obsessive children, however, usually isolate the vital emotional components. In exploratory-interpretative psychotherapies, the development of a capacity for ego splitting—that is, simultaneous emotional involvement and self-observation—is most helpful. Only by identifying with a trusted adult and in alliance with this adult can children approach such an ideal. A therapist's gender and the relatively superficial aspects of the therapist's demeanor may be important elements in the development of a trusting relationship with a child.

Recognition of the importance of play constituted a major forward stride in these efforts.

PLAYROOM

The structure, design, and furnishing of the playroom are important. Some therapists maintain that the toys should be few, simple, and carefully selected to facilitate the communication of fantasy. Other therapists suggest that a wide variety of playthings should be available to increase the range of feelings that children can express. These contrasting recommendations have been attributed to differences in therapeutic methods. Some therapists tend to avoid interpretation, even of conscious ideas, whereas others recommend the interpretation of unconscious content directly and quickly.

Therapists tend to change their preferences in equipment as they accumulate experience and develop confidence in their abilities. Although special equipment—such as genital dolls, amputation dolls, and see-through anatomically complete (except for genitalia) models—has been used in therapy, many therapists have observed that the unusual nature of such items risks making children wary and suspicious of a therapist's motives. Until dolls available to children in their homes include genitalia, the psychological content that special dolls are designed to elicit may be more available at the appropriate time with conventional dolls.

Although the choices of play materials vary among therapists, the following equipment can constitute a well-balanced playroom or play area: multigenerational families of flexible but sturdy dolls of various races; additional dolls representing special roles and feelings, such as police officer, doctor, and soldier; dollhouse furnishings with or without a dollhouse; toy animals; puppets; paper, crayons, paint, and blunt-ended scissors; a sponge-like ball; clay or something comparable; tools such as rubber hammers, rubber knives, and guns; building blocks, cars, trucks, and airplanes; and eating utensils. The toys should enable children to communicate through play. Therapists should avoid toys and materials that are fragile or break easily, that can result in physical injury to a child, or that can increase a child's guilt.

INITIAL APPROACH

Various approaches are associated with each therapist's individual style and perception of children's needs, from approaches in which a therapist endeavors to direct children's thought content and activity (release therapy, some behavior therapy, and certain educational patterning techniques) to exploratory methods in which a therapist endeavors to follow children's leads. Although children determine the focus, therapists structure the situation. Encouraging children to say whatever they wish and to play freely, as in exploratory psychotherapy, establishes a definite structure. Therapists create an atmosphere in which they get to know all about a child—the good side as well as the bad side, as children would put it. A therapist may communicate to a child that the child's response elicits neither anger nor pleasure but only understanding from the therapist. Such an assertion does not imply that therapists have no emotions, but it assures the young patient that the therapist's personal feelings and standards are subordinate to understanding the youngster.

THERAPEUTIC INTERVENTIONS

Psychotherapy with children and adolescents generally is more directed and active than it often is with adults. Children usually cannot synthesize histories of their lives, but they are excellent reporters of their current internal states. Even with adolescents, a therapist often takes an active role, is somewhat less open-ended than with adults, and offers more direction and advocacy than with adults. A child or adolescent therapist often makes exclamations and expresses confrontations in which attention is directed to data of which patients are cognizant. A therapist may use interpretations, designed to expand patients' conscious awareness of themselves, by making explicit the elements that have previously been expressed implicitly in the patients' thoughts, feelings, and behavior. Beyond interpretation, therapists may educatively offer new information to which patients have not been exposed previously. At the most active end of the continuum are advising, counseling, and directing, which are designed to help patients adopt a course of action or a conscious attitude.

Nurturing and maintaining a therapeutic alliance may require educating children about the process of therapy. Another educational intervention may entail assigning labels to affects that have not been part of a youngster's experience. Rarely does therapy have to compensate for a real absence of education about acceptable decorum and playing games. Children usually are not in therapy because they have never been exposed to educational efforts, but are there because repeated educational efforts have hyperactivity disorder and cognitive-behavioral group interventions for depressed children and for children with bereavement problems or eating disorders. In these more specialized groups, the issues are more specific, and actual tasks (as in social skills groups) can be practiced within the group. Some residential and day treatment units use group psychotherapy techniques. Group psychotherapy in schools for underachievers and children from low socioeconomic levels has relied on reinforcement and on modeling theory in addition to traditional techniques and has been supplemented by parent groups.

In controlled conditions, residential treatment units have been used for specific studies in group psychotherapy, such as behavioral contracting. Behavioral contracting with reward-punishment reinforcement provides positive reinforcements among preadolescent boys with severe concerns in basic trust, low self-esteem, and dependence conflicts. Somewhat akin to formal residential treatment units are social group work homes. For children who undergo many psychological assaults before placement, supportive group psychotherapy offers ventilation and catharsis, but more often it succeeds in letting children become aware of the enjoyment of sharing activities and developing skills.

Public schools—also a structured environment, although not usually considered the best site for group psychotherapy—have been used by several workers. Group psychotherapy as group counseling readily lends itself to school settings. One such group used gender- and problem-homogeneous selection for groups of six to eight students, who met once a week during school hours over 2 to 3 years.

INDICATIONS

Many indications exist for the use of group psychotherapy as a treatment modality. Some indications are situational; a therapist may work in a reformatory setting, in which group psychotherapy seems to reach adolescents better than individual treatment does. Another indication is time economics; more patients can be reached in a given time by the use of groups than by individual therapy. Group therapy best helps a child at a given age and developmental stage and with a given type of problem. In young age groups, children's social hunger and their potential need for peer acceptance help determine their suitability for group therapy. Criteria for unsuitability are controversial and have been loosened progressively.

PARENT GROUPS

In group psychotherapy, as in most treatment procedures for children, parental difficulties can present obstacles. Sometimes, uncooperative parents refuse to bring a child or to participate in their own therapy. The extreme of this situation reveals itself when severely disturbed parents use a child as their channel of communication to work out their own needs. In such circumstances, a child is in the unfortunate position of receiving positive group experiences that seem to create havoc at home.

Parent groups, therefore, can be a valuable aid to group psychotherapy for their children. A recent study showed that a cognitive-behavioral group intervention for parents can teach them how to utilize therapeutic interventions successfully with their anxiety-disordered children. Parents of children in therapy often have difficulty understanding their children's ailments, discerning the line of demarcation between normal and pathological behavior, relating to the medical establishment, and coping with

feelings of guilt. Parent groups assist in these areas and help members formulate guidelines for action.

▲ 49.3 Residential, Day, and Hospital Treatment

Current national trends in available treatment and delivery systems for children and adolescents with psychiatric disorders indicate a significant decline in the availability of child and adolescent inpatient beds. Given that there are just less than 10 million children and adolescents with psychiatric disorders, questions arise about the most effective ways of providing them with psychiatric care. Given the paucity of psychiatric inpatient units for children and adolescents, those children with severe psychiatric conditions may turn to residential treatment centers and various types of intensive outpatient programs or partial hospital treatment programs. Residential treatment centers and facilities are appropriate settings for children and adolescents with mental disorders who require a highly structured and supervised setting for a substantial time. Such settings have the advantage of providing a stable, consistent environment with a high level of psychiatric monitoring that is less intensive than that in a hospital. Children and adolescents with serious psychiatric disturbances often end up in residential facilities because of difficulties managing their own psychiatric problems and because of family situations in which appropriate supervision and parenting are impossible. Residential settings offer many treatments, including behavioral management, psychotherapy, medication, special education, and the therapeutic milieu itself. Children and adolescents who benefit from residential settings have a wide variety of psychiatric problems and commonly have difficulty with impulse control and structuring their time. Many residents of such programs also have families with serious psychiatric, financial, and parenting difficulties. Given the multitude of treatment modalities available for children and adolescents with psychiatric disorders, including cognitive-behavioral and interpersonal individual therapies, social skills and cognitive-behavioral group therapies, family education and therapy, psychopharmacology, special educational services, and therapeutic recreational therapies, residential facilities are even more critical in providing the setting in which to conduct the evidence-based research for the these interventions.

Partial hospitalization has been used more frequently with the advent of managed care as an alternative to hospitalization to provide short-term crisis stabilization or as a step-down from inpatient treatment for children and adolescents with psychiatric disorders. Day treatment programs, sometimes used interchangeably with the term *partial hospitalization*, are designed to serve the needs of children and adolescents with severe disorders who require interventions focused on improved level of function but who do not meet criteria of medical necessity to be in the hospital. A variety of intensive outpatient programming constitutes a day treatment program. One of the key ingredients of a day treatment program is the provision of a therapeutic day that optimally includes an educational component. Day treatment programs are excellent alternatives for children and adolescents who require more intensive support, monitoring, and supervision than is available in the community but who can live successfully at home if they receive the proper level of intervention. In most cases, children and adolescents who attend day hospital programs have serious mental disorders and might warrant psychiatric hospitalization without the program's support. Family therapy, group and individual psychotherapy, psychopharmacology, behavioral management programs, and special education are integral parts of these programs.

Tammy, age 13, was first seen in a pediatric emergency department on a Saturday morning by a psychiatry resident who determined that, although she had continued suicidal ideation, she did not have a specific plan and could be treated without hospitalization. Over the weekend, the resident contacted Tammy and her family twice by phone and arranged for her to be admitted to a partial hospital program on Monday morning. During her first few days in the program, she was monitored closely by the staff, and her suicide potential was evaluated at the end of each day by the medical director. During the first week, her suicidal ideation resolved in response to the support and structure of the program. At the end of her second week in the partial hospital program, she was stabilized, started on antidepressant medication, and transitioned to outpatient family and group therapy after stated commitments to follow up by the patient and her parents. The use of partial hospitalization prevented a psychiatric inpatient admission for this acutely symptomatic adolescent. (Courtesy of Laurel J. Kiser, Ph.D., M.B.A., Jerry Heston M.D., and David Pruitt, M.D.)

HOSPITALIZATION

Psychiatric hospitalization is needed when a child or adolescent exhibits dangerous behavior, is contemplating suicide, or is experiencing an exacerbation of a psychotic disorder or another serious mental disorder. Safety, stabilization, and effective treatment are the goals of hospitalization. Recently, the length of stay for child and adolescent psychiatric patients has decreased because of financial pressures and increased availability of day treatment programs. Psychiatric hospitalization may be some children's first opportunity to experience a stable, safe environment. Hospitals often are the most appropriate places to start use of new medications, and they provide an around-the-clock setting in which to observe a child's behavior. Children may show remission of some symptoms by virtue of their removal from a stressful or abusive environment. After a child has been observed for several weeks, the best treatment and disposition may become clear.

RESIDENTIAL TREATMENT

More than 20,000 emotionally disturbed children are in residential treatment centers in the United States, and this number is increasing. Deteriorating social conditions, particularly in cities, often make it impossible for a child with a serious mental disorder to live at home. In these cases, residential treatment centers serve a real need. They provide a structured living environment in which children may form strong attachments to, and receive

commitments from, staff members. The purpose of the center is to provide treatment and special education for children and their families.

Indications

Most children who are referred for residential treatment have had multiple evaluations by professionals, such as school psychologists, outpatient psychotherapists, juvenile court officials, or state welfare agency staff. Attempts at outpatient treatment and foster home placement usually precede residential treatment. Sometimes, the severity of a child's problems or the inability of a family to provide for the child's needs prohibits sending a child home. Many children sent to residential treatment centers have disruptive behavior problems in addition to other problems, including mood disorders and psychotic disorders. In some cases, serious psychosocial problems, such as physical or sexual abuse, neglect, indigence, or homelessness, necessitate out-of-home placement. The age range of the children varies among institutions, but most children are between 5 and 15 years of age. Boys are referred more frequently than girls.

An initial review of data enables the intake staff to determine whether a particular child is likely to benefit from the treatment program; often, for every child accepted for admission, three are rejected. The next step usually involves interviews with the child and the parents by various staff members, such as a therapist, a group-living worker, and a teacher. Psychological testing and neurological examinations are given, when indicated, if they have not already been performed. The child and parents should be prepared for these interviews.

Group Living

Most of a child's time in a residential treatment setting is spent in group living. The group-living staff consists of child-care workers who offer a structured environment that forms a therapeutic milieu; the environment places boundaries and limitations on the children. Tasks are defined within the limits of children's abilities; incentives, such as additional privileges, encourage them to progress rather than regress. In milieu therapy, the environment is structured, limits are set, and a therapeutic atmosphere is maintained.

The children often select one or more staff members with whom to form a relationship; through this relationship, they express, consciously and unconsciously, many of their feelings about their parents. The child-care staff should be trained to recognize such transference reactions and to respond to them in a way that differs from the children's expectations, which are based on their previous or even current relationships with their parents.

Education

Children in residential treatment frequently have severe learning disorders, disruptive behavior, and attention-deficit disorder (ADHD). Usually, the children cannot function in a regular community school and consequently need a special on-grounds school. A major goal of the on-grounds school is to motivate children to learn. The educational process in residential treatment is complex.

Table 49.4–1
Common Psychoactive Drugs in Childhood and Adolescence

Drug	Indications	Dosage	Adverse Reactions and Monitoring
Antipsychotics: also known as *major tranquilizers, neuroleptics* Divided into (1) high-potency, low-dose, e.g., haloperidol (Haldol), pimozide (Orap), trifluoperazine (Stelazine), thiothixene (Navane); (2) low-potency, high-dose (more sedating), e.g., chlorpromazine (Thorazine); and (3) atypicals, e.g., risperidone (Risperdal), olanzapine (Zyprexa), quetiapine (Seroquel), and clozapine (Clozaril)	Psychoses; agitated self-injurious behaviors in MR, PDDs, CD, and Tourette's disorder—haloperidol and pimozide Clozapine—refractory schizophrenia in adolescence	All can be given in two to four divided doses or combined into one dose after gradual buildup Haloperidol: child 0.5–6 mg/day, adolescent 0.5–16 mg/day Clozapine: dose not determined in children; <600 mg/day in adolescents Risperidone: 1–3 mg/day Olanzapine: 2.5–10 mg/day Quetiapine: 25–500 mg/day	Sedation, weight gain, hypotension, lowered seizure threshold, constipation, extrapyramidal symptoms, jaundice, agranulocytosis, dystonic reaction, tardive dyskinesia Hyperprolactinemia with atypicals except quetiapine Monitor blood pressure, CBC count, LFTs, and prolactin if indicated; with thioridazine, pigmentary retinopathy is rare but dictates a ceiling of 800 mg in adults and proportionally lower in children; with clozapine, weekly WBC counts for development of agranulocytosis and EEG monitoring because of lowering of seizure threshold
Stimulants Dextroamphetamine (Dexedrine) and amphetamine-dextroamphetamine (Adderall), FDA approved for children ≥3 yrs Methylphenidate (Ritalin, Concerta) and pemoline (Cylert), FDA approved for children ≥6 yrs	In ADHD for hyperactivity, impulsivity, and inattentiveness Narcolepsy	Dextroamphetamine and methylphenidate are generally given at 8 AM and noon Dextroamphetamine: about half the dose of methylphenidate Methylphenidate: 10–60 mg/day or up to about 0.5 mg/kg per dose Adderall: about half the dose of methylphenidate	Insomnia, anorexia, weight loss (possibly growth delay), rebound hyperactivity, headache, tachycardia, precipitation or exacerbation of tic disorders With pemoline, monitor LFTs because hepatotoxicity and liver failure are possible
Daytrana patch	ADHD	15, 20, 30 mg Wear for 9 hrs/day	Skin irritation
Nonstimulants Atomoxetine (Straterra)	ADHD	Begin with 0.5 mg/kg up to 1.8 mg/kg	Abdominal pain, loss of appetite
Mood stabilizers Lithium: considered an antimanic drug; also has antiaggression properties	Studies support use in MR and CD for aggressive and self-injurious behaviors; can be used for same in PDD; also indicated for early-onset bipolar disorder	600–2,100 mg in two or three divided doses; keep blood levels to 0.4–1.2 mEq/L	Nausea, vomiting, polyuria, headache, tremor, weight gain, hypothyroidism Experience with adults suggests renal function monitoring
Divalproex (Depakote)	Bipolar disorder, aggression	Up to about 20 mg/kg per day; therapeutic blood level range appears to be 50–100 µg/mL	Monitor CBC count and LFTs for possible blood dyscrasias and hepatotoxicity Nausea, vomiting, sedation, hair loss, weight gain, possibly polycystic ovaries
Carbamazepine (Tegretol): an anticonvulsant	Aggression or dyscontrol in MR or CD Bipolar disorder	Start with 10 mg/kg per day, can build to 20–30 mg/kg per day; therapeutic blood-level range appears to be 4–12 mg/day	Drowsiness, nausea, rash, vertigo, irritability; monitor CBC count and LFTs for possible blood dyscrasias and hepatotoxicity; must obtain blood concentrations

(continued)

Table 49.4–1
(Continued)

Drug	Indications	Dosage	Adverse Reactions and Monitoring
Antidepressants			
Tricyclic antidepressants: imipramine (Tofranil), nortriptyline (Pamelor), clomipramine (Anafranil)	Major depressive disorder, separation anxiety disorder, bulimia nervosa, enuresis; sometimes used in ADHD, sleepwalking disorder, and sleep terror disorder Clomipramine is effective in childhood OCD and sometimes in PDD	Imipramine: start with divided doses totaling about 1.5 mg/kg per day; can build up to not more than 5 mg/kg per day and eventually combine in one dose, which is usually 50–100 mg before sleep Clomipramine: start at 50 mg/day; can raise to not more than 3 mg/kg per day or 200 mg/day	Dry mouth, constipation, tachycardia, arrhythmia
Selective serotonin reuptake inhibitors: fluoxetine (Prozac), sertraline (Zoloft), fluvoxamine (Luvox), paroxetine (Paxil), citalopram (Celexa)	OCD; may be useful in major depressive disorder, anorexia nervosa, bulimia nervosa, repetitive behaviors in MR or PDD	Less than adult doses	Nausea, headache, nervousness, insomnia, dry mouth, diarrhea, drowsiness, disinhibition
Bupropion (Wellbutrin)	ADHD	Start low and titrate up to between 100 and 250 mg/day	Disinhibition, insomnia, dry mouth, gastrointestinal problems, tremor, seizures
Anxiolytics			
Benzodiazepines			
Clonazepam (Klonopin)	Panic disorder, generalized anxiety disorder	0.5–2.0 mg/day	Drowsiness, disinhibition
Alprazolam (Xanax)	Separation anxiety disorder	Up to 1.5 mg/day	Drowsiness, disinhibition
Buspirone (BuSpar)	Various anxiety disorders	15–90 mg/day	Dizziness, upset stomach
α_2-Adrenergic receptor agonists			
Clonidine (Catapres)	ADHD, Tourette's disorder, aggression	Up to 0.4 mg/day	Bradycardia, arrhythmia, hypertension, withdrawal hypotension
Guanfacine (Tenex)	ADHD	0.5–3.0 mg/day	Same as with clonidine plus headache, stomachache
β-Adrenergic receptor antagonist (β-blocker)			
Propranolol (Inderal)	Explosive aggression	Start at 20–30 mg/day and titrate	Monitor for bradycardia, hypotension, bronchoconstriction Contraindicated in asthma and diabetes
Other agents			
Naltrexone (ReVia)	Hyperactivity or self-injurious behavior in autism or MR	0.5–1.0 mg/kg per day	Drowsiness, vomiting, anorexia, headache, nasal congestion, hyponatremic seizures
Desmopressin (DDAVP)	Nocturnal enuresis	20–40 μg intranasally	Headache, nasal congestion, hyponatremic seizures (rare)

ADHD, attention-deficit/hyperactivity disorder; CBC, complete blood count; CD, conduct disorder; EEG, electroencephalogram; FDA, U.S. Food and Drug Administration; LFT, liver function test; MR, mental retardation; OCD, obsessive-compulsive disorder; PDD, pervasive development disorder; WBC, white blood cell.

Psychosurgery for severe and intransigent OCD is virtually absent from the literature in children and adolescents.

No controlled studies provide evidence that food allergies or sensitivities play a role in childhood mental disorders. Diets that eliminate food additives, colorings, and sugar are difficult to maintain and usually have no effect. Megavitamin therapy has not been shown to influence behavioral disorders (unless the child has a frank vitamin deficiency) and can cause serious adverse effects.

Significant advances have been made in scientific studies assessing the efficacy and safety of pharmacological agents in the treatment of childhood psychiatric disorders, and, given the trend of increased use of psychotropic medications in the treatment of childhood disorders, future large multisite studies are needed to confirm optimal pharmacological treatments and combinations of psychosocial and pharmacological treatments.

▲ 49.5 Psychiatric Treatment of Adolescents

Psychiatric treatment is indicated for an adolescent in whom is found a disturbance of thought, affect, or behavior to the point that it disrupts normal functioning. For adolescents, this includes influences on eating, sleeping, and school function, as well as relationships with family and peers. A variety of serious psychiatric disorders, including schizophrenia, bipolar disorder, eating disorders, and substance abuse, typically have their onset during adolescence. In addition, the risk for completed suicide drastically increases in adolescence. Although some stress is virtually universal in adolescence, most teenagers without mental disorders can cope well with the environmental demands. Teenagers with preexisting mental disorders may experience exacerbations during adolescence and may become frustrated, alienated, and demoralized.

DIAGNOSIS

Questions to be asked regarding adolescents' stage-specific tasks are the following: What degree of separation from their parents have they achieved? What sort of identities are evolving? How do they perceive their past? Do they perceive themselves as responsible for their own development or as only the passive recipients of their parents' influences? How do they perceive themselves with regard to the future, and how do they anticipate their future responsibilities for themselves and others? Can they think about the varying consequences of different ways of living? How do they express their sexual and affectionate interests? These tasks occupy all adolescents and normally are performed at varying times.

Adolescents' family and peer relationships must be evaluated. Do they perceive and accept both good and bad qualities in their parents? Do they see their peers and boyfriends or girlfriends as separate persons with needs and identities of their own, or do others exist only for the adolescents' own needs?

A respect for, and (if possible) some actual understanding of, an adolescent's subcultural and ethnic background are essential. For example, in some groups, depression is acceptable; in other groups, overt depression is a sign of weakness and is masked by antisocial acts, substance misuse, and self-destructive risks. A psychiatrist need not be of the same race or group identity as a given adolescent to treat him or her effectively. Respect and knowledgeable concern are human qualities and are not group restricted.

INTERVIEWS

Whenever circumstances permit, both an adolescent patient and his or her parents should be interviewed. Other family members also may be included, depending on their involvement in the teenager's life and difficulties. Clinicians should see the adolescent first, however; preferential treatment helps avoid the appearance of being the parents' agent. In psychotherapy with an older adolescent, the therapist and the parents usually have little contact after the initial part of the therapy because ongoing contact inhibits the adolescent's desire to open up.

Interview Techniques

All patients' test and mistrust therapists, but adolescents often manifest these reactions crudely, intensely, provocatively, and for prolonged periods. Clinicians must establish themselves as trustworthy and helpful adults to promote a therapeutic alliance. They should encourage adolescents to tell their own stories, without interrupting to check discrepancies; such a tactic seems as though the clinician is correcting and expressing disbelief. Clinicians should ask patients for explanations and theories about what happened. Why did these behaviors or feelings occur? When did things change? What caused the identified problems to begin when they did?

Sessions with adolescents generally follow the adult model; the therapist sits across from the patient. In early adolescence, however, board games (e.g., checkers) may help to stimulate conversation in an otherwise quiet, anxious patient.

Language is crucial. Even when a teenager and a clinician come from the same socioeconomic group, their languages are seldom the same. Psychiatrists should use their own language, explain any specialized terms or concepts, and ask for an explanation of unfamiliar in-group jargon or slang. Many adolescents do not talk spontaneously about illicit substances and suicidal tendencies but do respond honestly to a therapist's questions. A therapist may need to ask specifically about each substance and the amount and frequency of its use.

The sexual histories and current sexual activities of adolescents are increasingly important pieces of information for adequate evaluation. The nature of adolescents' sexual behaviors often is a vignette of their whole personality structures and ego development, but a long time may elapse in therapy before adolescents begin to talk about their sexual behavior.

The parents of a 13-year-old boy noted that it was difficult for him to get up in the morning. He seemed as though he was not sleeping. When asked about his sleep, he was reluctant to answer and simply indicated that he was having "a little trouble" falling asleep at night. His parents began watching him and found that he was up until 2 or 3 AM. He was getting up out of bed numerous times. They also found that he took longer and longer time in the bathroom. In school, he often missed classes and was found in the bathroom. When confronted, he disclosed that he had developed a number of bedtime rituals that took longer and longer to complete because if he did them incorrectly, he had to repeat them. They included checking the locks on the windows and doors, placing objects in the "right" places on his dresser, and repeating a prayer 16 times. He also revealed that when in the bathroom, he had to wash his hands a certain way and dry them "just so," or he feared something terrible would happen. His psychiatric evaluation revealed significant obsessive-compulsive disorder (OCD) and social phobia. Treatment was initiated, including use of a selective serotonin reuptake inhibitor (SSRI), cognitive-behavioral therapy (CBT), and problem-solving family therapy. Over the course of 6 months, his OCD responded well to the combination of medications and CBT, and the family learned ways of helping him both at home and in school. (Courtesy of Eugene V. Beresin, M.D. and Steven C. Schlozman, M.D.)

TREATMENT

Individual Psychotherapy

Individual psychosocial modalities with an evidence base for efficacy with adolescents include cognitive-behavioral treatments for psychiatric disorders, such as anxiety disorders, mood disorders, and OCD. Interpersonal therapy is a technique that has been applied to mood disorders in adolescents. Few adolescent patients are trusting or open without considerable time and testing, and it is helpful to anticipate the testing period by letting patients know that it is to be expected and is natural and healthy. Pointing out the likelihood of therapeutic problems—for instance, impatience and disappointment with the psychiatrist, with the therapy, with the time required, and with the often intangible results—may help keep problems under control. Therapeutic goals should be stated in terms that adolescents understand and value. Although they may not see the point in exercising self-control, enduring dysphoric emotions, or forgoing impulsive gratification, they may value feeling more confidently than in the past and gain more control over their lives and the events that affect them.

Typical adolescent patients need a real relationship with a therapist they can perceive as a real person. The therapist becomes another parent because adolescents still need appropriate parenting or reparenting. Thus, a professional who is impersonal and anonymous is a less useful model than one who can accept and respond rationally to an angry challenge or confrontation without fear or false conciliation—one that can impose limits and controls when adolescents cannot, can admit mistakes and ignorance, and can openly express the gamut of human emotions. Adolescents perceive as indifference or collusion a failure to take a stand about self-damaging and self-destructive behavior or to respond actively to manipulative and dishonest behavior.

Countertransference reactions can be intense in psychotherapeutic work with adolescents, and therapists must be aware of them. An adolescent often expresses hostile feelings toward adults, such as parents and teachers. A therapist may react with overidentification with the adolescent or with the parents. Such reactions are determined, at least in part, by a therapist's experiences during adolescence or, when applicable, his or her experiences as a parent.

Individual outpatient therapy is appropriate for adolescents whose problems are manifest in conflicted emotions and non-dangerous behavior, who are not too disorganized to be maintained outside a structured setting, and whose families or other living environments are not sufficiently disturbed to negate the influence of therapy. Such therapy characteristically focuses on intrapsychic conflicts and inhibitions; on the meanings of emotions, attitudes, and behavior; and on the influence of the past and the present. Antianxiety agents can be considered in adolescents whose anxiety may be high at certain times during psychotherapy, but adolescents' potential for abusing these drugs must be weighed carefully.

Psychopharmacotherapy and Combined Therapy

Randomized clinical trials have provided evidence of the superiority of CBT in combination with SSRI medication in the treatment of mood disorders, OCD, and, most likely, anxiety disorders in adolescents.

Attention-deficit/hyperactivity disorder (ADHD) in adolescents has not been studied systematically with regard to effectiveness of combination treatment with CBT. In the Mutimodal Treatment Study of Children with ADHD, psychosocial interventions did not add to the efficacy of the stimulant treatments for the core symptoms of ADHD. Other outcome measures of psychosocial improvements are needed, however, in future studies of combination treatment. Psychostimulants, such as methylphenidate (Ritalin, Concerta), dextroamphetamine (Dexedrine) and amphetamine salts (Adderall, Adderall XR), however, have been found to be efficacious in adolescents in the treatment of ADHD.

Advances in drug development have widened the choice of medications with which to treat mood disorders (e.g., SSRIs) and schizophrenia (e.g., serotonin-dopamine antagonists, including risperidone [Risperdal], olanzapine [Zyprexa], and clozapine [Clozaril]). Although these medications have been used to treat adolescent disorders, systematic research is required to determine the efficacy and safety profiles of these medications for treatment of adolescent psychopathology.

A comprehensive workup is needed before starting psychopharmacotherapy with adolescents, including a physical examination; blood tests to evaluate hematological, kidney, liver, thyroid, and other physiological functions; and an electrocardiogram to measure cardiac function. Neurological assessment with an electroencephalogram is necessary if seizure disorder is suspected or if the medication is likely to lower the seizure threshold.

A 17-year-old girl complained of episodes of rapid heartbeat, sweating, trembling, and fears of going out alone to the shopping mall. She had entered her senior year in high school, was considering her choice of colleges, and was planning to take her college entrance examination. Her parents wanted her to maintain the family tradition and go to the college from which her mother graduated. Psychoanalytically oriented outpatient treatment and treatment with an SSRI were instituted to alleviate the panic disorder symptoms. The psychotherapy focused on the patient's conflicts with her parents, highlighting her chronic concern that she could not meet parental expectations and fears of her independence. Medication appeared to reduce symptoms of tachycardia, tremulousness, and preoccupation with lack of competence. Psychotherapy was maintained for 8 months during her last year in high school. (Courtesy of Cynthia R. Pfeffer, M.D.)

Group Psychotherapy

In many ways, group psychotherapy is a natural setting for adolescents. Most teenagers are more comfortable with peers than with adults. A group diminishes the sense of unequal power between the adult therapist and the adolescent patient. Participation varies, depending on an adolescent's readiness. Not all interpretations and confrontations should come from the parent-figure therapist; group members often are adept at noticing symptomatic behavior in each other, and adolescents may find it easier to hear and consider critical or challenging comments from their peers.

Group psychotherapy usually addresses interpersonal and current life issues. Some adolescents, however, are too fragile for group psychotherapy or have symptoms or social traits that are too likely to elicit peer group ridicule; they need individual therapy to attain sufficient ego strength to struggle with peer relationships. Conversely, other adolescents must resolve interpersonal issues in a group before they can tackle intrapsychic issues in the intensity of one-on-one therapy.

Family Therapy

Family therapy is the primary modality when adolescents' difficulties mainly reflect a dysfunctional family (e.g., teenagers with school refusal, runaways). The same may be true when developmental issues, such as adolescent sexuality and striving for autonomy, trigger family conflicts or when family pathology is severe, as in cases of incest and child abuse. In these instances, adolescents usually need individual therapy as well, but family therapy is mandatory if an adolescent is to remain in the home or return to it. Serious character pathology, such as that underlying antisocial and borderline personality disorders, often develops from highly pathogenic early parenting. Family therapy is strongly indicated whenever possible for such disorders, but most authorities consider it adjunctive to intensive individual psychotherapy when individual psychopathology has become so internalized that it persists regardless of the current family status.

Inpatient Treatment

Residential treatment schools often are preferable for long-term therapy, but hospitals are more suitable for emergencies, although some adolescent inpatient hospital units also provide educational, recreational, and occupational facilities for long-term patients. Adolescents whose families are too disturbed or incompetent, who are dangerous to themselves or others, who are out of control in ways that preclude further healthy development, or who are seriously disorganized require, at least temporarily, the external controls of a structured environment.

Long-term inpatient therapy is the treatment of choice for severe disorders that are considered wholly or largely psychogenic in origin, such as major ego deficits that are caused by early massive deprivation and that respond poorly or not at all to medication. Severe borderline personality disorder, for example, regardless of the behavioral symptoms, requires a full-time corrective environment in which regression is possible and safe and in which ego development can take place. Psychotic disorders in adolescence often require hospitalization, but psychotic adolescents often respond to appropriate medication, so that therapy usually is feasible in an outpatient setting, except during exacerbation. Adolescent patients with schizophrenia who exhibit a long-term deteriorating course may require hospitalization periodically.

Day Hospitals

In day hospitals, which have become increasingly popular, adolescents spend the day in class, individual and group psychotherapy, and other programs, but they go home in the evenings. Day hospitals are less expensive than full hospitalization and usually are preferred by patients.

CLINICAL PROBLEMS
Atypical Puberty

Pubertal changes that occur 2.5 years earlier or later than the average age are within the normal range. Body image is so important to adolescents, however, that extremes of the norm may be distressing to some, either because markedly early maturation subjects them to social and sexual pressures for which they are unready or because late maturation makes them feel inferior and excludes them from some peer activities. Medical reassurance, even if based on examination and testing to rule out pathophysiology, may not suffice. An adolescent's distress may show as sexual or delinquent acting out, withdrawal, or problems at school that are sufficiently serious to warrant therapeutic intervention. Therapy also may be prompted by similar disturbances in some adolescents who fail to achieve peer-valued stereotypes of physical development despite normal pubertal physiology.

Substance-Related Disorders

Some experimentation with psychoactive substances is almost ubiquitous among adolescents, especially if this category of behavior includes alcohol use. Most adolescents, however, do not become abusers, particularly of prescription drugs and illegal substances. Any regular substance abuse represents disturbance. Substance abuse sometimes is self-medication against depression or schizophrenic deterioration, and sometimes it signals a character disorder in teenagers whose ego deficits render them unequal to the stresses of puberty and the tasks of adolescence. Some substances, including cocaine, have a physiologically reinforcing action that acts independently of preexisting psychopathology. When substance abuse covers an underlying illness or is a maladaptive response to current stresses or disturbed family dynamics, treatment of the underlying cause may diminish the substance use; in most cases of significant abuse, however, the drug-taking behavior typically requires intervention. Substance abuse treatments typically include a 12-step program with behavioral monitoring to accomplish sobriety as well as the ability to verbalize regarding the motivations for substance use. These philosophies are adapted to inpatient, intensive outpatient, and once-a-week outpatient treatment.

Suicide

Suicide is currently the second leading cause of death among adolescents. Many hospital admissions of adolescents result from suicidal ideation or behavior. Among adolescents who are not psychotic, the highest suicidal risks occur in those who have a history of parental suicide, who are unable to form stable attachments, who display impulsive behavior, and who abuse alcohol or other substances. Many adolescents who complete suicide have backgrounds that include long-standing family conflict and social problems since early childhood and the escalation of subjective distress under the pressure of a sudden perceived conflict or loss. Early childhood loss of parents also can increase the risk of depression in adolescence. Adolescents who are susceptible to rapid and extreme mood swings and a history of impulsive behavior are at greater risk to respond to despair with impulsive suicide attempts. In addition, alcohol and other substances are known added risks for suicidal behavior in adolescents with suicidal ideations. The developmentally predictable "omnipotent" attitudes of adolescents may cloud the immediate sense of permanence of death that result in impulsive self-destructive behavior in adolescents.

During a psychiatric evaluation of an adolescent with suicidal thoughts, plans and past attempts must be discussed directly when the concern arises and information is not volunteered. Recurring suicidal thoughts should be taken seriously, and a clin-ician must evaluate the imminent clinical danger requiring in-patient hospitalization versus an adolescent's ability to engage in an agreement or contract mandating that the adolescent will seek help before engaging in self-destructive behavior. Adolescents typically are honest in their refusal of such agreements, and, in such cases, hospitalization is indicated. Hospitalization of a suicidal adolescent by a clinician is an act of serious, protective concern. See Section 45.1 for a more complete discussion of suicide in adolescents.

Geriatric Psychiatry

Old age is not a disease. It is a phase of the life cycle characterized by its own developmental issues, many of which are concerned with loss of physical agility and mental acuity, friends and loved ones, and status and power. At the same time, old age is associated with the accumulation of wisdom and the opportunity to pass that on to future generations, one of the tasks that informs Erik Erikson's view of healthy old age as a time of integrity and not a time of despair. In contrast to this group of the well-old, there are the sick-old, persons with mental or physical disorders, or both, that impair their ability to function or even survive. This group is the concern of geriatric psychiatry, which deals with preventing, diagnosing, and treating psychological disorders in older adults. The American Board of Psychiatry and Neurology established geropsychiatry (from the Greek *geros* ["old age"] and *iatros* ["physical"]) as a subspecialty in 1991, and today geriatric psychiatry is one of the fastest growing fields in psychiatry.

Prevalence data for mental disorders in elderly persons vary widely, but a conservatively estimated 25 percent have significant psychiatric symptoms. The number of mentally ill elderly persons was estimated to be about 9 million in the year 2005. That figure is expected to rise to 20 million by the middle of the century.

STRESSORS

High-ranking stresses of aging include acute and chronic medical illnesses, the concomitant use of therapeutic drugs, and the complicating drug–drug and drug–disease interactions. Thus, geriatric psychiatrists must be able to recognize the physical and mental ills of their patients, as well as have skills in the social sciences, knowledge of the health care delivery system, and information about the availability of financial and social supports, especially nursing homes. Moreover, self-assessment of health is associated with income. The loss of one's job, including voluntary and involuntary retirement, carries with it the loss of financial resources, social status, and much of the person's social network; the loss of contemporaries through death, illness, and migration brings both psychological deprivation of an intimate love object and a void that usually remains unfilled; forming new relationships that result in marriage is difficult in old age. In part, because of their greater life expectancy, older women are more likely to live alone than older men. Physical limitations and the loss of friends are frequently associated with restricted mobility, which leads to further social isolation and increased difficulty in pursuing the tasks of daily living, such as procuring food and clothing and maintaining one's shelter. Often, homes are lost because of financial strains and the inability to perform home upkeep. Many middle class widows, for example, have had to move from the five- to ten-room family homes that they occupied for most of their lives to one-half of a room in a residential extended-care facility for the elderly. In addition to losing most of their worldly possessions and social support, they also lose their privacy and their sense of self-worth.

Poverty in the Aged

A strong correlation exists between poverty and increased rates of mental and physical illness in the elderly. For workers 65 years and older, the median earned income in 2005 was $15,000. Although the overall rate of poverty is relatively low, it remains high for women, minorities, the less well educated, and those older than 80 years. Of Americans 65 years or older, 28 percent had incomes of less than $10,000 in 2005, whereas 10 percent had incomes of $50,000 or more. Earnings from work continue to be an important source of income for older Americans, especially those younger than age 70 years. Although a trend was seen toward earlier retirement from about 1960 to 1985, over the last 20 years more Americans have continued to work at older ages. In 2005, median earnings for individuals of age 55 to 61 years who worked were $34,000, whereas median earned income for workers of age 62 to 64 years was $27,000.

PSYCHIATRIC EXAMINATION OF THE OLDER PATIENT

Psychiatric history taking and the mental status examination of older adults follow the same format as those of younger adults; however, because of the high prevalence of cognitive disorders in older persons, psychiatrists must determine whether a patient understands the nature and purpose of the examination. When a patient is cognitively impaired, an independent history should be obtained from a family member or caretaker. The patient still should be seen alone—even in cases of clear evidence of impairment—to preserve the privacy of the doctor–patient relationship and to elicit any suicidal thoughts or paranoid ideation, which may not be voiced in the presence of a relative or nurse.

When approaching the examination of the older patient, it is important to remember that older adults differ markedly from one another. The approach to examining the older patient must take into account whether the person is a healthy 75-year-old who recently retired from a second career or a frail 96-year-old who just lost his or her only surviving relative with the death of a 75-year-old caregiving daughter.

Psychiatric History

A complete psychiatric history includes preliminary identification (name, age, sex, marital status), chief complaint, history of the present illness, history of previous illnesses, personal history, and family history. A review of medications (including over-the-counter medications) that the patient is using or has used in the recent past is also important.

Patients older than age 65 years often have subjective complaints of minor memory impairments, such as forgetting persons' names and misplacing objects. Minor cognitive problems also can occur because of anxiety in the interview situation. These age-associated memory impairments are of no significance; the term *benign senescent forgetfulness* has been used to describe them.

Mental Status Examination

The mental status examination offers a cross-sectional view of how a patient thinks, feels, and behaves during the examination. With older adults, a psychiatrist may not be able to rely on a single examination to answer all of the diagnostic questions. Repeat mental status examinations may be needed because of fluctuating changes in the patient's family.

Functional Assessment.
Patients older than 65 years of age should be evaluated for their capacity to maintain independence and to perform the activities of daily life, which include toileting, preparing meals, dressing, grooming, and eating. The degree of functional competence in their everyday behaviors is an important consideration in formulating a treatment plan for these patients.

MEMORY. Memory usually is evaluated in terms of immediate, recent, and remote memory. Immediate retention and recall are tested by giving the patient six digits to repeat forward and backward. The examiner should record the result of the patient's capacity to remember. Persons with unimpaired memory usually can recall six digits forward and five or six digits backward. The clinician should be aware that the ability to do well on digit-span tests is impaired in extremely anxious patients. Remote memory can be tested by asking for the patient's place and date of birth, the patient's mother's name before she was married, and names and birthdays of the patient's children.

In cognitive disorders, recent memory deteriorates first. Recent memory assessment can be approached in several ways. Some examiners give the patient the names of three items early in the interview and ask for recall later. Others prefer to tell a brief story and ask the patient to repeat it verbatim. Memory of the recent past also can be tested by asking for the patient's place of residence, including the street number; the method of transportation to the hospital; and some current events. If the patient has a memory deficit, such as amnesia, careful testing should be performed to determine whether it is retrograde amnesia (loss of memory before an event) or anterograde amnesia (loss of memory after the event). Retention and recall also can be tested by having the patient retell a simple story. Patients who confabulate make up new material in retelling the story.

Medical History.
Elderly patients have more concomitant, chronic, and multiple medical problems and take more medications than younger adults; many of these medications can influence their mental status. The medical history includes all major illnesses, traumata, hospitalizations, and treatment interventions. The psychiatrist should also be alert to underlying medical illness. Infections, metabolic and electrolyte disturbances, and myocardial infarction and stroke may first be manifested by psychiatric symptoms. Depressed mood, delusions, and hallucinations may precede other symptoms of Parkinson's disease by many months. On the other hand, a psychiatric disorder can also cause such somatic symptoms as weight loss, malnutrition, and inanition of severe depression.

Careful review of medications (including over-the-counter medications, laxatives, vitamins, tonics, and lotions) and even recently discontinued substances is extremely important. Drug effects can be long lasting and may induce depression (e.g., antihypertensives), cognitive impairment (e.g., sedatives), delirium (e.g., anticholinergics), and seizures (e.g., neuroleptics). The review of medications must include sufficient detail to identify misuse (overdose, underuse) and relate medication use to special diets. A dietary history is also important; deficiencies and excesses (e.g., protein, vitamins) can influence physiological function and mental status.

EARLY DETECTION AND PREVENTION STRATEGIES

Many age-related illnesses develop insidiously and gradually progress over the years. The most common cause of late-life cognitive impairment, Alzheimer's disease, is characterized neuropathologically by a gradual accumulation of neuritic plaques and neurofibrillary tangles in the brain. Clinically, a progression of cognitive decline is seen, which begins with mild memory loss and ends with severe cognitive and behavioral deterioration.

Because it will likely be easier to prevent neural damage than to repair it once it occurs, investigators are developing strategies for early detection and prevention of age-related illnesses, such as Alzheimer's disease. Considerable progress has been made in the detection component of this strategy, using brain-imaging technologies, such as positron emission tomography and functional magnetic resonance imaging, in combination with genetic risk measures. With these approaches, subtle brain changes can be detected that progress and can be followed over time. Such surrogate markers allow clinical scientists to track disease progression and to test novel treatments designed to decelerate brain aging. Clinical trials of cholinesterase inhibitor drugs, anticholesterol drugs, antiinflammatory drugs, and others (e.g., vitamin E) are in progress to determine whether such treatments delay the onset of Alzheimer's disease or the progression of brain metabolic or cognitive decline.

MENTAL DISORDERS OF OLD AGE

The National Institute of Mental Health's Epidemiologic Catchment Area (ECA) program has found that the most common mental disorders of old age are depressive disorders, cognitive disorders, phobias, and alcohol use disorders. Older adults also have a high risk for suicide and drug-induced psychiatric symptoms. Many mental disorders of old age can be prevented, ameliorated, or even reversed. Of special importance are the reversible causes of delirium and dementia; if not diagnosed accurately and treated in a timely fashion, however, these conditions can progress to an irreversible state requiring a patient's institutionalization. Use of a comprehensive battery is preferable for confident determination of presence and type of dementia or other cognitive disorder in elderly persons; in some circumstances, however, administering a several-hour battery is not possible.

Several psychosocial risk factors also predispose older persons to mental disorders. These risk factors include loss of social roles, loss of autonomy, the deaths of friends and relatives, declining health, increased isolation, financial constraints, and decreased cognitive functioning.

Many drugs can cause psychiatric symptoms in older adults. These symptoms can result from age-related alterations in drug absorption, a prescribed dose that is too large, not following instructions and taking too large a dose, sensitivity to the medication, and conflicting regimens presented by several physicians. Almost the entire spectrum of mental disorders can be caused by drugs.

Dementing Disorders

Only arthritis is a more common cause of disability among adults of age 65 years and older than dementia, a generally progressive and irreversible impairment of the intellect, the prevalence of which increases with age. About 5 percent of persons in the United States older than age 65 years have severe dementia, and 15 percent have mild dementia. Of persons older than age 80 years, about 20 percent have severe dementia. Known risk factors for dementia are age, family history, and female sex. (See Section 7.3.)

Depressive Disorders

Depressive symptoms are present in about 15 percent of all older adult-community residents and nursing home patients. Age itself is not a risk factor for the development of depression, but being widowed and having a chronic medical illness are associated with vulnerability to depressive disorders. Late-onset depression is characterized by high rates of recurrence.

The common signs and symptoms of depressive disorders include reduced energy and concentration, sleep problems (especially early-morning awakening and multiple awakenings), decreased appetite, weight loss, and somatic complaints. The presenting symptoms may be different in older depressed patients from those seen in younger adults because of an increased emphasis on somatic complaints in older persons. Older persons are particularly vulnerable to major depressive episodes with melancholic features, characterized by depression, hypochondriasis, low self-esteem, feelings of worthlessness, and self-accusatory trends (especially about sex and sinfulness) with paranoid and suicidal ideation.

Schizophrenia

Schizophrenia usually begins in late adolescence or young adulthood and persists throughout life. Although first episodes diagnosed after age 65 years are rare, a late-onset type beginning after age 45 years has been described. Women are more likely to have a late onset of schizophrenia than men. Another difference between early-onset and late-onset schizophrenia is the greater prevalence of paranoid schizophrenia in the late-onset type. About 20 percent of persons with schizophrenia show no active symptoms by age 65 years; 80 percent show varying degrees of impairment. Psychopathology becomes less marked as patients age. (See Chapter 10.)

Delusional Disorder

The age of onset of delusional disorder usually is between ages 40 and 55 years, but it can occur at any time during the geriatric period. Delusions can take many forms; the most common are persecutory—patients believe that they are being spied on, followed, poisoned, or harassed in some way. Persons with delusional disorder may become violent toward their supposed persecutors. Some persons lock themselves in their rooms and live reclusive lives. Somatic delusions, in which persons believe they have a fatal illness, also can occur in older persons. In one study of persons older than 65 years of age, pervasive persecutory ideation was present in 4 percent of persons sampled.

Anxiety Disorders

The anxiety disorders include panic disorder, phobias, obsessive-compulsive disorder, generalized anxiety disorder, acute stress disorder, and posttraumatic stress disorder. Anxiety disorders begin in early or middle adulthood, but some appear for the first time after age 60 years. An initial onset of panic disorder in older persons is rare, but can occur. The ECA study determined that the 1-month prevalence of anxiety disorders in persons of age 65 years and older is 5.5 percent. By far the most common disorders are phobias (4 to 8 percent). The rate for panic disorder is 1 percent.

Somatoform Disorders

Somatoform disorders, characterized by physical symptoms resembling medical diseases, are relevant to geriatric psychiatry because somatic complaints are common among older adults. More than 80 percent of persons older than 65 years of age have at least one chronic disease—usually arthritis or cardiovascular problems. After age 75 years, 20 percent have diabetes and an average of four diagnosable chronic illnesses that require medical attention.

Alcohol and Other Substance Use Disorder

Older adults with alcohol dependence usually give a history of excessive drinking that began in young or middle adulthood. They usually are medically ill, primarily with liver disease, and are either divorced, widowed, or are men who never married. Many have arrest records and are numbered among homeless persons. A large number have chronic dementing illness, such as Wernicke's encephalopathy and Korsakoff's syndrome. Of nursing home patients, 20 percent have alcohol dependence.

Sleep Disorders

Advanced age is the most important factor associated with the increased prevalence of sleep disorders. Sleep-related phenomena reported more frequently by older than by younger adults are sleeping problems, daytime sleepiness, daytime napping, and the use of hypnotic drugs. Clinically, older persons experience higher rates of breathing-related sleep disorder and medication-induced movement disorders than younger adults.

Changes in sleep structure among persons older than 65 years of age involve both rapid eye movement (REM) sleep and non-REM (NREM) sleep. The REM changes include the redistribution of REM sleep throughout the night, more REM episodes, shorter REM episodes, and less total REM sleep. The NREM changes include the decreased amplitude of delta waves, a lower percentage of stages 3 and 4 sleep, and a higher percentage of stages 1 and 2 sleep. In addition, older persons experience increased awakening after sleep onset.

Much of the observed deterioration in the quality of sleep in older persons is caused by the altered timing and consolidation of sleep. For example, with advanced age, persons have a lower amplitude of circadian rhythms, a 12-hour sleep-propensity rhythm, and shorter circadian cycles.

SUICIDE RISK

Elderly persons have a higher risk for suicide than any other population. The suicide rate for white men older than the age of 65 years is five times higher than that of the general population. One third of elderly persons report loneliness as the principal reason for considering suicide. Approximately 10 percent of elderly individuals with suicidal ideation report financial problems, poor medical health, or depression as reasons for suicidal thoughts. Psychological studies suggest that most elderly persons who commit suicide have had a psychiatric disorder, most commonly depression. Psychiatric disorders of suicide victims, however, often do not receive medical or psychiatric attention. More elderly suicide victims are widowed and fewer are single, separated, or divorced than is true of younger adults. Violent methods of suicide are more common in the elderly, and alcohol use and psychiatric histories appear to be less frequent. The most common precipitants of suicide in older individuals are physical illness and loss, whereas problems with employment, finances, and family relationships are more frequent precipitants in younger adults.

Hearing Loss

About 30 percent of persons older than the age of 65 years have significant hearing loss (presbycusis). After age 75 years, that figure rises to 50 percent. Causes vary. Clinicians should be sensitive to hearing loss in patients who complain they can hear but cannot understand what is being said or who ask that questions be repeated. Most elderly persons with hearing loss can be treated with hearing aids.

Elder Abuse

An estimated 10 percent of persons older than 65 years of age are abused. Elder abuse is defined by the American Medical Association as "an act or omission which results in harm or threatened harm to the health or welfare of an elderly person." Mistreatment includes abuse and neglect—physically, psychologically, financially, and materially. Sexual abuse does occur. Acts of omission include withholding food, medicine, clothing, and other necessities.

Family conflicts and other problems often underlie elder abuse. The victims tend to be very old and frail. They often live with their assailants, who may be financially dependent on the victims. Both the victim and the perpetrator tend to deny or minimize the presence of abuse. Interventions include providing legal services, housing, and medical, psychiatric, and social services.

SPOUSAL BEREAVEMENT

Demographic data suggest that 51 percent of women and 14 percent of men older than the age of 65 years will be widowed at least once. Spousal loss is among the most stressful of all life experiences. As a group, older adults appear to have a more favorable outcome than expected following the death of a spouse. Depressive symptoms peak within the first few months after a death but decline significantly within a year. A relationship exists between spousal loss and subsequent mortality. Elderly survivors of spouses who committed suicide are especially vulnerable, as are those with psychiatric illness.

PSYCHOPHARMACOLOGICAL TREATMENT OF GERIATRIC DISORDERS

The major goals of the pharmacological treatment of older persons are to improve the quality of life, maintain persons in the community, and delay or avoid their placement in nursing homes. Individualization of dosing is the basic tenet of geriatric psychopharmacology.

Alterations in drug doses are required because of the physiological changes that occur as persons age. Renal disease is associated with decreased renal clearance of drugs; liver disease

results in a decreased ability to metabolize drugs; cardiovascular disease and reduced cardiac output can affect both renal and hepatic drug clearance; and gastrointestinal disease and decreased gastric acid secretion influence drug absorption. As a person ages, the ratio of lean to fat body mass also changes. With normal aging, lean body mass decreases and body fat increases. Changes in the ratio of lean to fat body mass that accompany aging affect the distribution of drugs. Many lipid-soluble psychotropic drugs are distributed more widely in fat than in lean tissue, so a drug's action can be unexpectedly prolonged in older persons. Similarly, changes in end-organ or receptor-site sensitivity must be taken into account. In older persons, the increased risk of orthostatic hypotension from psychotropic drugs is related to reduced functioning of blood pressure–regulating mechanisms.

As a general rule, the lowest possible dose should be used to achieve the desired therapeutic response. Clinicians must know the pharmacodynamics, pharmacokinetics, and biotransformation of each drug prescribed and the effects of the interaction of the drug with other drugs that a patient is taking.

PSYCHOTHERAPY FOR GERIATRIC PATIENTS

The standard psychotherapeutic interventions—such as insight-oriented psychotherapy, supportive psychotherapy, cognitive therapy, group therapy, and family therapy—should be available to geriatric patients. Common age-related issues in therapy involve the need to adapt to recurrent and diverse losses (e.g., the deaths of friends and loved ones), the need to assume new roles (e.g., the adjustment to retirement and the disengagement from previously defined roles), and the need to accept mortality. Psychotherapy helps older persons to deal with these issues and the emotional problems surrounding them and to understand their behavior and the effects of their behavior on others. In addition to improving interpersonal relationships, psychotherapy increases self-esteem and self-confidence, decreases feelings of helplessness and anger, and improves the quality of life. Geriatric psychotherapy has the general aim of assisting older adults to have minimal complaints, to help them make and keep friends of both sexes, and to have sexual relations when they have interest and capacity.

Life Review or Reminiscence Therapy

Robert Butler and others have noted the universal tendency of the aging person to reflect on, and reminisce about, the past. Reminiscence is characterized by the progressive return of memories of past experiences, especially those that were meaningful and conflictual. To varying degrees, elderly patients in therapy reminisce about the past, search for meaning in their lives, and strive for some resolution of past interpersonal and intrapsychic conflicts. Life review therapy systematically enhances this reminiscing process and makes it more conscious and deliberate. The therapist may guide the process by encouraging the patient to write or tape a biography with review of special events and turning points. Techniques include reunions with family and good friends and looking through memorabilia, such as scrapbooks or picture albums. This technique has been reported to resolve old problems, increase tolerance of conflict, relieve guilt and fears, and enhance self-esteem, creativity, generosity, and acceptance of the present.

51 ▲

End-of-Life Care

▲ 51.1 Palliative Care

Palliative care (from Latin *palliere*, "to cloak") is concerned with treating the dying patient. It is geared to the relief of pain and suffering; it is not designed to cure. Physicians able to deal with death and dying are able to communicate effectively in several areas: diagnosis and prognosis; the nature of terminal illness; advance directives about life-sustaining treatment; hospice care; legal and ethical issues; grief and bereavement; and psychiatric care. Palliative care physicians must also be skilled in pain management, especially in the use of powerful opioids—the gold standard of drugs used for pain relief. In 1991 the American Board of Pain Medicine was established to ensure that physicians treating patients in pain were both qualified to do so and were kept up to date on the latest advances in the field.

COMMUNICATION

After a diagnosis and prognosis have been made, physicians need to talk to the patient and the patient's family. Formerly, doctors subscribed to a conspiracy of silence, believing that their patients' chances for recovery would improve if they knew less because news of impending death might bring despair. The current practice is now one of honesty and openness toward patients; in fact, the question is not whether to tell the patient, but when and how. The American Hospital Association in 1972 drafted the Patient's Bill of Rights, declaring that patients have the "right to obtain complete, current information regarding diagnosis, treatment and prognosis in terms the patient can be reasonably expected to understand."

Breaking Bad News

When breaking news of impending death to the patient, as when relating any bad news, diplomacy and compassion should be guiding principles. Often, bad news is not completely related during one meeting, but rather is presented so that it can be absorbed gradually over a series of separate conversations. Advance preparations, including scheduling sufficient time for the visit, researching pertinent information, such as test results and facts about the case, and even arranging furniture appropriately can make the patient feel more comfortable.

Telling the Truth

Tactful honesty is the doctor's most important aid. Honesty, however, need not preclude hope or guarded optimism. It is important to be aware

that if 85 percent of patients with a particular disease die in 5 years, 15 percent are still alive after that time. The principles of doing good and not doing harm inform the decision of whether to tell the patient the truth. In general, most patients want to know the truth about their condition. Various studies of patients with malignancies show that 80 to 90 percent want to know their diagnosis.

Doctors, however, should ask patients how much they want to know because some persons do not want to know all the facts about their illness. Such patients, if told the truth, deny that they ever were told, and they cannot participate in end-of-life decisions, such as the use of life-sustaining equipment. The patients who openly request that they not be given "bad news" are often those who most fear death. Physicians should deal with these fears directly, but if the patient still cannot bear to hear the truth, someone closely related to the patient must be informed.

Brain Death and Persistent Vegetative State

Brain death is associated with the loss of higher brain functions (e.g., cognition) and all brain stem function (e.g., pupillary and reflex eye movement), respiration, and gag and corneal reflexes. Determination of brain death is a generally accepted criterion for death. Some clinicians advocate an absence of brain waves on electroencephalography to confirm the diagnosis.

Persistent vegetative state is defined by the American Academy of Neurology as a condition in which there is no awareness of self or environment associated with severe neurological damage. Medical treatment provides no benefits to patients in a persistent vegetative state, and once the diagnosis is established, do not resuscitate (DNR) and do not intubate (DNI) orders can be followed and life-sustaining methods (e.g., feeding tubes, ventilators) can be removed.

Advance Directives

Advance directives are wishes and choices about medical intervention when the patient's condition is considered terminal. Advance directives, which are legally binding in all 50 states, include three types: living will, health care proxy, and DNR and DNI orders.

Living Will. In a living will, a patient who is mentally competent gives specific instructions that doctors must follow when the patient cannot communicate them because of illness. These instructions may include rejection of feeding tubes, artificial airways, or any other measures to prolong life.

Health Care Proxy. Also known as *durable power of attorney*, the health care proxy gives another person the power to make medical decisions if the patient cannot do so. That person, also known as the surrogate, is empowered to make all decisions about terminal care on the basis of what he or she thinks the patient would want.

Do Not Resuscitate and Do Not Intubate Orders.

These orders prohibit doctors from attempting to resuscitate (DNR) or intubate (DNI) the patient who is in extremis. DNR and DNI orders are made by the patient who is competent to do so. They can be made part of the living will or expressed by the health care proxy.

Psychiatric Consultation.

Psychiatric consultation is indicated for patients who become severely anxious, suicidal, depressed, or overtly psychotic. In each instance, appropriate psychiatric medication can be prescribed to provide relief. Patients who are suicidal do not always have to be transferred to a psychiatric service. An attendant or nurse can be assigned to the patient on a 24-hour basis (one-on-one coverage). In such instances, the relationship that develops between the observer and the patient may have therapeutic overtones, especially with patients whose depression is related to a sense of abandonment. Patients who are terminal and who are at high risk for suicide are usually in pain. When pain is relieved, suicidal ideation is likely to diminish. A careful evaluation of suicide potential is required for all patients. A premorbid history of past suicide attempts is a high risk factor for suicide in terminally ill patients. In patients who become psychotic, impaired cognitive function secondary to metastatic lesions to the brain must always be considered. Such patients respond to antipsychotic medications, and psychotherapy may also be of use.

PAIN MANAGEMENT

Types of Pain

Dying patients are subject to several different kinds of pain. The distinctions are important because they call for different treatment strategies; somatic and visceral pain are responsive to opiates, whereas neuropathic and sympathetically maintained pain may require adjuvant medications in addition to opiates. Most patients with advanced cancer, for example, have more than one kind of pain and require complex treatment regimens.

Treatment of Pain

It cannot be overemphasized that pain management should be aggressive, and treatment should be multimodal. In fact, a good pain regimen may require several drugs or the same drug used in different ways and administered via different routes. For example, intravenous morphine can be supplemented by self-administered oral "rescue" doses, or a continuous epidural drip can be supplemented by bolus intravenous doses. Transdermal patches may provide baseline concentrations in patients for whom intravenous or oral intake is difficult. Patient-controlled analgesia systems for intravenous opiate administration result in better pain relief with lower amounts dispensed than in staff-administered dosing.

Opioids commonly cause delirium and hallucinations. A frequent mechanism of psychotoxicity is the accumulation of drugs or metabolites whose duration of analgesia is shorter than their plasma half-life (morphine, levorphanol [Levo-Dromoran], and methadone [Dolophine]). Use of drugs such as hydromorphone (Dilaudid), which have half-lives closer to their analgesic duration, can relieve the problem without loss of pain control. Cross-tolerance is incomplete between opiates; hence, several should be tried in any patient, with the dose lowered when switching drugs.

The benefits of maintenance analgesia administration in terminally ill patients compared with as-needed administration cannot be overemphasized. Maintenance dosing improves pain control, increases drug efficiency, and relieves patient anxiety, whereas as-needed orders allow pain to increase while waiting for the drug to be given. Moreover, as-needed analgesia administration perversely sets up the patient for staff complaints about drug-seeking behavior. Even when maintenance treatment is used, extra doses of medication should be available for breakthrough pain, and repeated use of these medications should signal the need to raise the maintenance dose. Depending on their previous experiences with opioid analgesics and their weight, it is not unusual for some patients to require 2 g or more of morphine per day for relief of symptoms.

Knowing doses of different drugs and different routes of administration is important to avoid accidental undermedication. For example, when changing a patient from intramuscular to oral morphine use, the intramuscular dose must be multiplied by 6 to avoid causing the patient pain and provoking drug-seeking behavior. Many adjuvant drugs used for pain are psychotropics with which psychiatrists are familiar, but, in some cases, their analgesic effect is separate from their primary psychotropic effect. Commonly used adjuvants include antidepressants, mood stabilizers (e.g., gabapentin) phenothiazines, butyrophenones, antihistamines, amphetamines, and steroids. They are particularly important in neuropathic and sympathetically maintained pain, for which they can be the mainstay of treatment.

Other developments in pain management include more-intrusive procedures, such as nerve blocks or the use of continuous epidural infusions. In addition, radiation therapy, chemotherapy, and even surgical resection can be considered as pain management modalities in palliative care. Short courses of radiotherapy or chemotherapy can be used to shrink tumors or manage metastatic lesions that cause pain or impairment. In patients with end-stage Hodgkin's disease, for example, systemic chemotherapy can improve the patient's quality of life by decreasing tumor burden. Surgical resection of invasive tumors, most notably breast carcinomas, can be useful for the same reason.

Medical Use of Marijuana.

An effective treatment for nausea and vomiting associated with chemotherapy is the use of Δ-tetrahydrocannabinol (THC), the active ingredient of marijuana. Oral synthetic cannabinoid, dronabinol (Marinol), is used in 1- to 2-mg doses every 8 hours. The use of marijuana cigarettes to deliver THC is believed to be more effective than pills. Proponents say that its absorption is faster and antiemetic properties are more potent via the pulmonary system. Repeated attempts to legalize marijuana cigarettes for medical use have met with only limited success in the United States.

Legal Issues Regarding Opioids.

The American Medical Association supports the position that patients with a terminal condition require substantial doses of opioids on a regular basis and should not be denied drugs for fear of producing physical dependence. A similar view is endorsed in *Goodman and Gilman's The Pharmacological Basis of Therapeutics* as follows:

The physician should not wait until the pain becomes agonizing; no patient should ever wish for death because of a physician's reluctance to use adequate amounts of effective opioids. Accordingly, physicians who treat the terminally ill should not be intimidated by legal oversight.

This is especially important because the Drug Enforcement Administration (DEA) is considering examining the prescribing practices of physicians who care for terminally ill patients. A strongly worded editorial in the *New England Journal of Medicine* (January 5, 2006) criticized the DEA for its involvement with what constitutes acceptable medical practice for dying patients on the grounds that the DEA's federal mandate is limited to combating criminal substance abuse, not monitoring the care of dying patients. Physicians must be vigilant and forceful in protecting their rights to administer opioids to treat patients for intractable pain.

HOSPICE CARE

In 1967 the founding of St. Christopher's Hospice in England by Cicely Saunders launched the modern hospice movement. In 1983, Medicare began reimbursing hospice care. Medicare hospice guidelines emphasize home care, with benefits provided for a broad spectrum of physician, nursing, psychosocial, and spiritual services at home or, if necessary, in a hospital or nursing home. To be eligible, the patient must be physician certified as having 6 months or less to live. By electing hospice care, patients agree to receive palliative rather than curative treatment. Many hospice programs are hospital based, sometimes in separate units and sometimes in the form of hospice beds interspersed throughout the facility. Other program models include free-standing hospices and programs, hospital-affiliated hospices, nursing home hospice care, and home care programs. Nursing homes are the site of death for many elderly patients with incurable chronic illness, yet dying nursing home residents have limited access to palliative and hospice care.

CHILD END-OF-LIFE CARE

After accidents, cancer is the second-most-common cause of death in children. Although many childhood cancers are treatable, palliative care is necessary for children with cancers that are not. Children require more support than adults in coping with death. On average, a child does not view death as permanent until the age of about 10 years; before that, death is viewed as a sleep or separation. Therefore, children should be told only what they can understand; if they are capable, they should be involved in the decision-making process about treatment plans. Ensuring that patients are pain free and physically comfortable is just as important for children as it is for adults.

A unique aspect of end-of-life care in children involves addressing their fear of being separated from their parents. It is helpful to have parents participate in end-of-life care tasks within their capacities. Family sessions with the child in attendance allow feelings to emerge and questions to be answered.

SPIRITUAL ISSUES

The inclusion of a section on religious or spiritual problems in the text revision of the fourth edition of the *Diagnostic and Statistical Manual of Mental Disorders* (DSM-IV-TR) is but one sign of increasing awareness of the importance of this area to patients and families, as well as many staff members. Several studies have shown that religious beliefs are often associated with mature and active coping methods, and the field of psychological and spiritual interfaces in terminally ill patients is spawning a whole new area of psychological research within the traditional medical establishment. The psychiatric consultant should inquire about faith, its meaning, associated religious practices, and impact on the coping response. It can be a source of strength or guilt at all stages of the disease, ranging from the earliest "What did I do to cause this?" through "Will God give me only what I can carry?" to the poignant life review of the late stage. It is often a primary

factor in the reactions to suicidality and in attitudes toward terminal care decisions. Mental health professionals should deal with these areas in an un-self-conscious and noncondescending manner and work to help patients fully integrate this aspect of their personality into their current crisis. The professional should also work in harmony with the patient's spiritual guide, if one is available. Sometimes, an experienced, effective chaplain working with the appropriate patient can achieve positive results more directly than any psychotherapy. The following case exemplifies how creative pastoral care can relieve suffering.

> A young woman was admitted to a hospice in a terminal state. She was experiencing a severe depression, which she attributed to not being able to see her oldest daughter receive her first communion. Arrangements were made for a ceremonial communion for her daughter to take place at the hospice. After the ceremony, the patient's mood improved markedly as one of her fears was alleviated and a religious need was satisfied. As her mood improved, she was able to address other unresolved issues and have quality visits with her children in her remaining days. (From O'Neil MT. Pastoral care. In: Cimino JE, Brescia MJ, eds. *Calvary Hospital Model for Palliative Care in Advanced Cancer*. Bronx, NY: Palliative Care Institute; 1998, with permission.)

▲ 51.2 Euthanasia and Physician-Assisted Suicide

EUTHANASIA

From the Greek term for good death, euthanasia means compassionately allowing, hastening, or causing the death of another. Generally, someone resorts to euthanasia to relieve suffering, maintain dignity, and shorten the course of dying when death is inevitable. Euthanasia can be *voluntary* if the patient has requested it or *involuntary* if the decision is made against the patient's wishes or without the patient's consent. Euthanasia can be *passive*—simply withholding heroic lifesaving measures—or *active*—deliberately taking a person's life. Euthanasia assumes that the intent of the physician is to aid and abet the patient's wish to die.

Arguments for euthanasia revolve around patient autonomy and dignified dying. One of the most dramatic ways patients can exercise their right to self-determination is by asking that life-sustaining treatment to be withdrawn. If the patient is mentally competent, physicians must respect such wishes. Proponents of active, voluntary euthanasia argue that the same rights should be extended to patients who are not on life-sustaining treatment but also choose to have their physicians help them die.

Opponents of euthanasia also provide strong ethical and medical justification for their position. First, active euthanasia, even if the patient voluntarily requests it, is a form of killing and should never be sanctioned. Second, many patients who request aid in dying may be suffering from depression, which, when treated, will change the patient's mind about wanting to die.

Most medical, religious, and legal groups in the United States oppose euthanasia. Both the American Psychiatric Association (APA) and the American Medical Association (AMA) condemn active euthanasia as illegal and contrary to medical ethics; however, few individuals have been convicted of euthanasia. Most physicians and medical groups in other parts of the world also oppose legalizing euthanasia. In the United Kingdom, for example, the British Medical Association believes that euthanasia is "alien to the traditional ethos and moral focus of medicine" and, if legalized, "would irrevocably change the context of health care for everyone, but especially for the most vulnerable."

The World Medical Association issued the following declaration on euthanasia in October 1987:

Euthanasia, that is, the act of deliberately ending the life of a patient, even at his own request or at the request of his close relatives, is unethical. This does not prevent the physician from respecting the will of a patient to allow the natural process of death to follow its course in the terminal phase of sickness.

In 2002, the World Medical Association reissued a resolution condemning euthanasia as "unethical" and urging all doctors and medical associations to refrain from the practice.

Similarly, the New York State Committee on Bioethical Issues issued a statement declaring its opposition to euthanasia. The Committee stated that the physician has an obligation to relieve pain and suffering and to promote the dignity and autonomy of dying patients in their care, including providing effective palliative treatment, even though it may occasionally hasten death. Physicians, however, should not perform active euthanasia or participate in assisted suicide. The Committee felt that support, comfort, respect for patient autonomy, good communication, and adequate pain control would dramatically decrease the demand for euthanasia and assisted suicide. They argued that the societal risks of involving physicians in medical interventions to cause a patient's death were too great to condone active euthanasia or physician-assisted suicide. In response to shifting public opinion and lobbying groups with different views, challenges to the constitutionality of laws that banned physician-assisted death in Washington State and New York State were sent to the U.S. Supreme Court. In June 1997, the Court unanimously held that terminally ill patients do not have the right to physician aid in dying. The ruling, however, left room for continuing debate and future policy initiates at the state level.

PHYSICIAN-ASSISTED SUICIDE

In the United States, most of the debate centers on physician-assisted suicide rather than on euthanasia. Some have argued that physician-assisted suicide is a humane alternative to active euthanasia in that the patient maintains more autonomy, remains the actual agent of death, and may be less likely to be coerced. Others feel that the distinctions are capricious, in that the intent in both cases is to bring about a patient's death. Indeed, it may be difficult to justify providing a lethal dose of medication to a terminally ill patient (physician-assisted suicide) while ignoring the desperate pleas of another patient who may be even more ill and distressed but who cannot complete the act because of problems with swallowing, dexterity, or strength.

Several degrees are seen to which a physician may assist the suicidal patient to end his or her life. Physician-assisted suicide can involve providing information on ways of committing suicide, supplying a prescription for a lethal dose of medication or a means of inhaling a lethal amount of carbon monoxide, or, perhaps, even providing a suicide device that the patient can operate.

The controversy over physician-assisted suicide came to national attention surrounding the activities of retired pathologist Jack Kevorkian, who, in 1989, provided his suicide machine to a 54-year-old woman with probable Alzheimer's disease. After the woman killed herself with his device, Kevorkian was charged with first-degree murder. The charges were dismissed because Michigan had no law against physician-assisted suicide. Following that first case, Kevorkian assisted in several more suicides, often for persons he had met on only a few occasions, and frequently for persons who did not have a terminal illness. Claiming to have helped more than 130 people take their lives, Kevorkian was arrested, tried, and convicted; he was sent to prison in 1999 and was released in 2006. His attorneys and followers applaud his courage in easing pain and suffering; his detractors counter that he is a serial mercy killer. Opponents of Kevorkian's methods charge that, without safeguards, consultations, and thorough psychiatric evaluations, patients may search out suicide not because of terminal illness or intractable pain but because of untreated depressive disorders. They argue that suicide rarely occurs in the absence of psychiatric illness. Finding more-effective treatments for pain and depression rather than inventing more-sophisticated devices to help desperate patients kill themselves defines compassionate and effective physician care.

In 1994, Oregon passed a ballot initiative legalizing physician-assisted suicide (Death with Dignity Act), making Oregon the first state in the United States to permit assisted suicides. An assessment of the first 4 years revealed the following: Patients dying from physician-assisted suicide represent approximately 8 of 10,000 deaths. The most common underlying illnesses were cancer, amyotrophic lateral sclerosis, and chronic lower respiratory disease. The three most common end-of-life concerns were loss of autonomy (85 percent), a decreasing ability to participate in activities that made life enjoyable (77 percent), and losing control of bodily functions (63 percent). Eighty percent of the patients were enrolled in hospice programs, and 91 percent died at home. The prescribing physician was present in 52 percent of the cases.

In 2001, U.S. Attorney General John Ashcroft attempted to prosecute Oregon doctors who helped terminally ill patients die, claiming that doctor-assisted suicide is not a legitimate medical purpose. The case was brought to the Supreme Court, which, in 2006, supported the Oregon law and said the "authority claimed by the attorney general is both beyond his expertise and incongruous with the statutory purposes and design."

Despite the abhorrence that many physicians and medical ethicists express regarding physician-assisted suicide, poll after poll shows that as many as two thirds of Americans favor the legalization of physician-assisted suicide in certain circumstances, and evidence even indicates that the formerly uniform opposition to physician-assisted suicide within the medical community has eroded. Consistent with their positions on active euthanasia, the AMA, APA, and American Bar Association, however, continue to oppose physician-assisted suicide. Recently, the American College of Physicians–American Society of Internal Medicine (ACP-ASIM) expressed its commitment to improving

For example, privilege does not exist at all in military courts, regardless of whether the physician is military or civilian and whether the privilege is recognized in the state in which the court martial takes place.

Confidentiality

A long-held premise of medical ethics binds physicians to hold secret all information given by patients. This professional obligation is called *confidentiality*. Confidentiality applies to certain populations and not to others; a group that is within the circle of confidentiality shares information without receiving specific permission from a patient. Such groups include, in addition to the physician, other staff members treating the patient, clinical supervisors, and consultants.

A subpoena can force a psychiatrist to breach confidentiality, and courts must be able to compel witnesses to testify for the law to function adequately. A subpoena is an order to appear as a witness in court or at a deposition. Physicians usually are served with a *subpoena duces tecum*, which requires that they also produce their relevant records and documents. Although the power to issue subpoenas belongs to a judge, they are routinely issued at the request of an attorney representing a party to an action.

In bona fide emergencies, information may be released in as limited a way as feasible to carry out necessary interventions. Sound clinical practice holds that a psychiatrist should make the effort, time allowing, to obtain the patient's permission anyway and should debrief the patient after the emergency.

As a rule, clinical information may be shared with the patient's permission—preferably written permission, although oral permission suffices with proper documentation. Each release is good for only one piece of information, and permission should be reobtained for each subsequent release, even to the same party. Permission overcomes only the legal barrier, not the clinical one; the release is permission, not obligation. If a clinician believes that the information may be destructive, the matter should be discussed, and the release may be refused, with some exceptions.

Child Abuse.   In many states, all physicians are legally required to take a course on child abuse for medical licensure. All states now legally require that psychiatrists, among others, who have reason to believe that a child has been the victim of physical or sexual abuse make an immediate report to an appropriate agency. In this situation, confidentiality is decisively limited by legal statute on the ground that potential or actual harm to vulnerable children outweighs the value of confidentiality in a psychiatric setting. Although many complex psychodynamic nuances accompany the required reporting of suspected child abuse, such reports generally are considered ethically justified.

HIGH-RISK CLINICAL SITUATIONS

Suicidal Patients

Psychiatrists may be sued when their patients commit suicide, particularly when psychiatric inpatients kill themselves. Psychiatrists are assumed to have more control over inpatients, making the suicide preventable.

The evaluation of suicide risk is one of the most complex, dauntingly difficult clinical tasks in psychiatry. Suicide is a rare event. In our current state of knowledge, clinicians cannot accurately predict when or if a patient will commit suicide. No professional standards exist for predicting who will or will not commit suicide. Professional standards do exist for assessing suicide risk, but at best, only the degree of suicide risk can be judged clinically following a comprehensive psychiatric assessment.

A review of the case law on suicide reveals that certain affirmative precautions should be taken with a suspected or confirmed suicidal patient. For example, failing to perform a reasonable assessment of a suicidal patient's risk for suicide or implement an appropriate precautionary plan will likely render a practitioner liable. The law tends to assume that suicide is preventable if it is foreseeable. Courts closely scrutinize suicide cases to determine if a patient's suicide was foreseeable. Foreseeability is a deliberately vague legal term that has no comparable clinical counterpart, a common-sense rather than a scientific construct. It does not (and should not) imply that clinicians can predict suicide. Foreseeability should not be confused with preventability, however. In hindsight, many suicides seem preventable that were clearly not foreseeable.

Violent Patients

Psychiatrists who treat violent or potentially violent patients may be sued for failure to control aggressive outpatients and for the discharge of violent inpatients. Psychiatrists can be sued for failing to protect society from the violent acts of their patients if it was reasonable for the psychiatrist to have known about the patient's violent tendencies and if the psychiatrist could have done something that could have safeguarded the public. In the landmark case *Tarasoff v. Regents of the University of California*, the California Supreme Court ruled that mental health professionals have a duty to protect identifiable, endangered third parties from imminent threats of serious harm made by their outpatients. Since then, courts and state legislatures have increasingly held psychiatrists to a fictional standard of having to predict the future behavior (dangerousness) of their potentially violent patients. Research has consistently demonstrated that psychiatrists cannot predict future violence with any dependable accuracy.

The duty to protect patients and endangered third parties should be considered primarily a professional and moral obligation and, only secondarily, a legal duty. Most psychiatrists acted to protect both their patients and others threatened by violence long before *Tarasoff*.

If a patient threatens harm to another person, most states require that the psychiatrist perform some intervention that might prevent the harm from occurring. In states with duty-to-warn statutes, the options available to psychiatrists and psychotherapists are defined by law. In states offering no such guidance, health care providers are required to use their clinical judgment and act to protect endangered third persons. Typically, a variety of options to warn and protect are clinically and legally available, including implementing voluntary hospitalization, implementing involuntary hospitalization (if civil commitment requirements are met), warning the intended victim of the threat, notifying the police, adjusting medication, and seeing the patient more frequently. Warning others of danger, by itself, is usually insufficient. Psychiatrists should consider the *Tarasoff* duty to be a national standard of care, even if they practice in states that do not have a duty to warn and protect.

HOSPITALIZATION

All states provide for some form of involuntary hospitalization. Such action usually is taken when psychiatric patients present a danger to themselves or others in their environment to the extent that their urgent need for treatment in a closed institution is evident. Certain states allow involuntary hospitalization when patients are unable to care for themselves adequately.

The statutes governing hospitalization of persons who are mentally ill generally have been designated commitment laws, but psychiatrists have long considered the term to be undesirable. *Commitment* legally means a warrant for imprisonment. The American Bar Association and the American Psychiatric Association have recommended that the term *commitment* be replaced by the less offensive and more accurate term *hospitalization*, which most states have adopted. Although this change in terminology does not correct the punitive attitudes of the past, the emphasis on hospitalization is in keeping with psychiatrists' views of treatment rather than punishment.

Procedures of Admission

Four procedures of admission to psychiatric facilities have been endorsed by the American Bar Association to safeguard civil liberties and to make sure that no person is railroaded into a mental hospital. Although each of the 50 states has the power to enact its own laws on psychiatric hospitalization, the procedures outlined here are gaining much acceptance.

Informal Admission. Informal admission operates on the general hospital model, in which a patient is admitted to a psychiatric unit of a general hospital in the same way that a medical or surgical patient is admitted. Under such circumstances, the ordinary doctor–patient relationship applies, with the patient free to enter and to leave–even against medical advice.

Voluntary Admission. In cases of voluntary admission, patients apply in writing for admission to a psychiatric hospital. They may come to the hospital on the advice of a personal physician, or they may seek help on their own. In either case, patients are admitted if an examination reveals the need for hospital treatment. The patient is free to leave, even against medical advice.

Temporary Admission. Temporary admission is used for patients who are so senile or so confused that they require hospitalization and are not able to make decisions on their own and for patients who are so acutely disturbed that they must be admitted immediately to a psychiatric hospital on an emergency basis. Under the procedure, a person is admitted to the hospital on the written recommendation of one physician. Once the patient has been admitted, the need for hospitalization must be confirmed by a psychiatrist on the hospital staff. The procedure is temporary because patients cannot be hospitalized against their will for more than 15 days.

Involuntary Admission. Involuntary admission involves the question of whether patients are suicidal—and, thus, a danger to themselves—or homicidal—and, thus, a danger to others. Because these persons do not recognize their need for hospital care, the application for admission to a hospital may be made by a relative or a friend. Once the application is made, the patient must be examined by two physicians, and if both physicians confirm the need for hospitalization, the patient can then be admitted.

Involuntary hospitalization involves an established procedure for written notification of the next of kin. Furthermore, the patients have access at any time to legal counsel, who can bring the case before a judge. If the judge does not think that hospitalization is indicated, the patient's release can be ordered.

Involuntary admission allows a patient to be hospitalized for 60 days. After this time, if the patient is to remain hospitalized, the case must be reviewed periodically by a board consisting of psychiatrists, nonpsychiatric physicians, lawyers, and other citizens not connected with the institution. In New York State, the board is called the Mental Health Information Service.

Persons who have been hospitalized involuntarily and who believe that they should be released have the right to file a petition for a writ of habeas corpus. Under law, a writ of habeas corpus can be proclaimed by those who believe that they have been illegally deprived of liberty. The legal procedure asks a court to decide whether a patient has been hospitalized without due process of law. The case must be heard by a court at once, regardless of the manner or the form in which the motion is filed. Hospitals are obligated to submit the petitions to the court immediately.

RIGHT TO TREATMENT

Among the rights of patients, the right to the standard quality of care is fundamental. This right has been litigated in highly publicized cases in recent years under the slogan of "right to treatment."

In 1966, Judge David Bazelon, speaking for the District of Columbia Court of Appeals in *Rouse v. Cameron*, noted that the purpose of involuntary hospitalization is treatment and concluded that the absence of treatment draws into question the constitutionality of the confinement. Treatment in exchange for liberty is the logic of the ruling. In this case, the patient was discharged on a writ of habeas corpus, the basic legal remedy to ensure liberty. Judge Bazelon further held that, if alternative treatments that infringe less on personal liberty are available, involuntary hospitalization cannot take place.

Alabama Federal Court Judge Frank Johnson was more venturesome in the decree he rendered in 1971 in *Wyatt v. Stickney*. The *Wyatt* case was a class-action proceeding brought under newly developed rules that sought not release but treatment. Judge Johnson ruled that persons civilly committed to a mental institution have a constitutional right to receive such individual treatment as will give them a reasonable opportunity to be cured or to have their mental condition improved. Judge Johnson set out minimal requirements for staffing, specified physical facilities and nutritional standards, and required individualized treatment plans.

RIGHT TO REFUSE TREATMENT

The right to refuse treatment is a legal doctrine that holds that, except in emergencies, persons cannot be forced to accept treatment against their will. An emergency is defined as a condition in clinical practice that requires immediate intervention to prevent death or serious harm to the patient or another person or to prevent deterioration of the patient's clinical state.

In the 1976 case of *O'Connor v. Donaldson*, the Supreme Court ruled that harmless mentally ill patients cannot be confined against their will without treatment if they can survive outside. According to the Court, a finding of mental illness alone cannot or perhaps thought the act was correct, a delusion causing the defendant to act in legitimate self-defense.

Jeffery Dahmer killed 17 young men and boys between June 1978 and July 1991. Most of his victims were either homosexual or bisexual. He would meet and select his prey at gay bars or bathhouses and then lure them by offering them money for posing for photographs or simply to enjoy some beer and videos. Then he would drug them, strangle them, masturbate on the body or have sex with the corpse, and dismember the body and dispose of it. Sometimes, he would keep the skull or other body parts as souvenirs.

On July 13, 1992, Dahmer changed his plea to guilty by means of insanity. That Dahmer could plan his murders and systematically dispose of the bodies convinced the jury, however, that he was able to control his behavior. All of the testimony bolstered the notion that, as with most serial killers, Dahmer knew what he was doing and knew right from wrong. Finally, the jury did not accept the defense that Dahmer experienced a mental illness to the degree that it had disabled his thinking or behavioral controls. Dahmer was sentenced to 15 consecutive life terms or a total of 957 years in prison. He was killed by an inmate on November 28, 1994.

Irresistible Impulse. In 1922, a committee of jurists in England reexamined the M'Naghten rule. The committee suggested broadening the concept of insanity in criminal cases to include the irresistible impulse test, which rules that a person charged with a criminal offense is not responsible for an act if the act was committed under an impulse that the person was unable to resist because of mental disease. The courts have chosen to interpret this concept in such a way that it has been called the *policeman-at-the-elbow law*. In other words, the court grants an impulse to be irresistible only when it can be determined that the accused would have committed the act even if a policeman had been at the accuser's elbow. To most psychiatrists, this interpretation is unsatisfactory because it covers only a small, special group of those who are mentally ill.

Model Penal Code. In its model penal code, the American Law Institute recommended the following test of criminal responsibility: Persons are not responsible for criminal conduct if, at the time of such conduct, as a result of mental disease or defect, they lacked substantial capacity either to appreciate the criminality (wrongfulness) of their conduct or to conform their conduct to the requirement of the law. The term *mental disease or defect* does not include an abnormality manifest only by repeated criminal or otherwise antisocial conduct.

Subsection 1 of the American Law Institute rule contains five operative concepts: mental disease or defect, lack of substantial capacity, appreciation, wrongfulness, and conformity of conduct to the requirements of law. The rule's second subsection, stating that repeated criminal or antisocial conduct is not, of itself, to be taken as mental disease or defect, aims to keep the sociopath or psychopath within the scope of criminal responsibility.

Guilty but Mentally Ill. Some states have established an alternative verdict of guilty but mentally ill. Under guilty but mentally ill statutes, this alternative verdict is available to the jury if the defendant pleads not guilty by reason of insanity. Under an insanity plea, four outcomes are possible: not guilty, not guilty by reason of insanity, guilty but mentally ill, and guilty.

The problem with guilty but mentally ill is that it is an alternative verdict without a difference. It is basically the same as finding the defendant just plain guilty. The court must still impose a sentence on the convicted person. Although the convicted person supposedly receives psychiatric treatment, if necessary, this treatment provision is available to all prisoners.

OTHER AREAS OF FORENSIC PSYCHIATRY

Emotional Damage and Distress

A rapidly rising trend in recent years is to sue for psychological and emotional damage, both secondary to physical injury or as a consequence of witnessing a stressful act and from the suffering endured under the stress of such circumstances as concentration camp experiences. The German government heard many of these claims from persons detained in Nazi camps during World War II. In the United States, the courts have moved from a conservative to a liberal position in awarding damages for such claims. Psychiatric examinations and testimony are sought in these cases, often by both the plaintiffs and the defendants.

Recovered Memories

Patients alleging recovered memories of abuse have sued parents and other alleged perpetrators. In a number of instances, the alleged victimizers have sued therapists who, they claim, negligently induced false memories of sexual abuse. In an about-face, some patients have recanted and joined forces with others (usually their parents) to sue therapists.

Courts have handed down multimillion-dollar judgments against mental health practitioners. A fundamental allegation in these cases is that the therapist abandoned a position of neutrality to suggest, to persuade, to coerce, and to implant false memories of childhood sexual abuse. The guiding principle of clinical risk management in recovered memory cases is maintenance of therapist neutrality and establishment of sound treatment boundaries.

Ethics in Psychiatry

Ethical guidelines and a knowledge of ethical principles help psychiatrists avoid *ethical conflicts* (which can be defined as tension between what one wants to do and what is ethically right to do) and think through *ethical dilemmas* (conflicts between ethical perspectives or values).

Ethics deals with the relations between people in different groups and often entails balancing rights. *Professional ethics* refers to the appropriate way to act when in a professional role. Professional ethics derives from a combination of morality, social norms, and the parameters of the relationship people have agreed to have.

Most professional organizations and many business groups have codes of ethics that reflect a consensus about the general standards of appropriate professional conduct. The American Medical Association's *Principles of Medical Ethics* and the American Psychiatric Association's *Principles of Medical Ethics with Annotations Especially Applicable to Psychiatry* articulate ideal standards of practice and professional virtues of practitioners. These codes include exhortations to use skillful and scientific techniques, to self-regulate misconduct within the profession, and to respect the rights and needs of patients, families, colleagues, and society. A summary of these principles is provided in Table 53–1.

Table 53–1
The Principles of Medical Ethics with Annotations Especially Applicable to Psychiatry

Each of the AMA principles of medical ethics printed separately (in italics) along with annotations especially applicable to psychiatry.

Preamble
The medical profession has long subscribed to a body of ethical statements developed primarily for the benefit of the patient. As a member of this profession, a physician must recognize responsibility not only to patients but also to society, to other health professionals, and to self. The following Principles, adopted by the American Medical Association, are not laws but standards of conduct, which define the essentials of honorable behavior for the physician.

Section 1
A physician shall be dedicated to providing competent medical service with compassion and respect for human dignity.[a]

1. A psychiatrist shall not gratify his/her own needs by exploiting a patient. The psychiatrist shall be ever vigilant about the impact that his/her conduct has upon the boundaries of the doctor–patient relationship and thus upon the well-being of the patient. These requirements become particularly important because of the essentially private, highly personal, and sometimes intensely emotional nature of the relationship with the psychiatrist.
2. A psychiatrist should not be a party to any type of policy that excludes, segregates, or demeans the dignity of any patient because of ethnic origin, race, sex, creed, age, socioeconomic status, or sexual orientation.
3. In accord with the requirements of law and accepted medical practice, it is ethical for a physician to submit his/her work to peer review and to the ultimate authority of the medical staff executive body and the hospital administration and its governing body.
4. A psychiatrist should not be a participant in a legally authorized execution.

Section 2
A physician shall deal honestly with patients and colleagues, and strive to expose those physicians deficient in character or competence, or who engage in fraud or deception.

1. The requirement that the physician conduct himself/herself with propriety in his/her profession and in all the actions of his/her life is especially important for the psychiatrist because the patient tends to model his/her behavior on that of his/her psychiatrist by identification. Further, the necessary intensity of the treatment relationship may tend to activate sexual and other needs and fantasies of both patient and psychiatrist, while weakening the objectivity necessary for control. Additionally, the inherent inequality in the doctor–patient relationship may lead to exploitation of the patient. Sexual activity with a current or former patient is unethical.
2. The psychiatrist should diligently guard against exploiting information furnished by the patient and should not use the unique position of power afforded by the psychotherapeutic situation to influence patients in any way not directly relevant to the treatment goals.
3. A psychiatrist who regularly practices outside his/her area of professional competence should be considered unethical. Determination of professional competence should be made by peer review boards or other appropriate bodies.
4. Special consideration should be given to psychiatrists who, due to illness, jeopardize the welfare of their patients and their own reputations and practices. It is ethical, even encouraged, for another psychiatrist to intercede in such situations.
5. Psychiatric services, like all medical services, are dispensed in the context of a contractual arrangement between the patient and the treating physician. The provisions of the contractual arrangement, which are binding on both the physician and the patient, should be explicitly established.

(continued)

Index

Page numbers followed by *t* indicate tables.

AA. *See* Alcoholics Anonymous
AAS. *See* Anabolic-androgenic steroid
Abilify. *See* Aripiprazole
Abnormal swallowing syndrome,
    sleep-related, 358
Abortion, 406
Abuse
  child, 414–418, 437
    clinical features of, 414–417
    confidentiality and, 704
    diagnosis of, 414–417
    differential diagnosis of, 417
    epidemiology of, 414
    factitious disorder by proxy and, 287
    physical, 414–415
    preventing, 418
    reporting, 418
    sexual, 415–416
    treatment of, 417–418
  elder, 697
  physical
    adult, 418–419
    child, 414–415, 437
  problems related to, 414–420
  sexual
    adult, 419
    child, 415–416, 437
    incest as, 416
    rape, 419
    statutory rape, 416
    spousal, 418–419
Academic problems, 674–675
Acamprosate (Campral), 502, 503–504
  alcohol-related disorder, 104*t*, 105
  substance-related disorder, 89
Acculturation problems, 426–427
Acebutolol (Sectral), 477
  dosing, 478
Acetylcholine, schizophrenia and, 159
Acquired immune deficiency syndrome (AIDS)
  dementia related to, 80
  fetal transmission of, 141
  HIV blood tests and, 17
  HIV infection and development of, 80–81
  pediatric, 438
  suicide and, 82
  treatment, 83
    psychotherapy, 84
ACT. *See* Assertive community treatment
Acute stress disorder, 258–263
  adjustment disorder differential diagnosis
    and, 373
  clinical features, 261–262

comorbidity, 258
course, 262
diagnosis, 259–261
differential diagnosis, 262
dissociative amnesia differential diagnosis
  and, 295
DSM-IV-TR diagnostic criteria, 259–260,
  260*t*
epidemiology, 258
etiology, 258–259
prognosis, 262
treatment, 263
Adapin. *See* Doxepin
Adaptive functioning, 575
Adderall. *See*
    Dextroamphetamine-amphetamine salt
ADHD. *See* Attention-deficit/hyperactivity
  disorder
Adjustment disorder(s), 371–374
  with anxiety, 372
  clinical features, 372–373
  course, 373
  with depressed mood, 372
  diagnosis, 372–373, 372*t*
  differential diagnosis, 373
  with disturbance of conduct, 373
  epidemiology, 371
  etiology, 371–372
    family factors in, 372
    genetic factors in, 372
    psychodynamic factors in, 371–372
  HIV-related, 82
  with mixed anxiety-depressive disorder,
    372–373
  with mixed disturbance of motions and
    conduct, 373
  prognosis, 373
  treatment, 373–374
    pharmacotherapy, 374
    psychotherapy, 373–374
  unspecified, 373
Adolescent(s)
  AIDS in, 438
  antisocial behavior in, 675–676
  anxiety disorders, 659–668
    separation, 662–667, 664*t*
  bereavement in, 653
  bipolar disorder in, 656–658
  clinical interviews, 569
  clinical problems, 692–693
  cyclothymic disorder in, 652
  depression in, 214–215
  depressive disorders in, 650–654

disorder of, NOS, 649, 649*t*
dissociative identity disorder in, 300
dysthymic disorder in, 652
GAD, 662–667, 664*t*
gender identity disorders in, 328–329
  treatment of, 329
hospitalization of, 684–686
major depressive disorder in, 651–652
mania in, 215
mood disorders in, 650–658
OCD, 659–662, 660*t*
psychiatric treatment of, 690–693
  psychotherapy, 691–692
psychiatry, 3–4
psychotherapy, 679–684
PTSD in, 261, 438
puberty, atypical, 692
schizoaffective disorder in, 652
selective mutism, 667–668, 668*t*
social phobias, 662–667, 665*t*
substance-related disorder, 692
suicide in, 436, 654–656, 692–693
working in, 424
Adrenal disorder(s), 78
  psychosomatic medicine and, 397–398
Adrenal hyperplasia, congenital virilizing, 330
α-adrenergic receptor antagonists, 475–477
  adverse reactions, 476
  clinical guidelines, 476–477
  Clonidine, 475–477
  dosing, 476–477
  drug interactions, 476
  Guanfacine, 475–477
  laboratory interferences, 476
  overdose, 476
  pharmacological actions, 475
  precautions, 476
  psychiatric emergency, 435
  sexual dysfunction and, 313
  therapeutic indications, 475–476
  withdrawal, 476
β-adrenergic receptor antagonists, 477–478
  adverse reactions, 478
  clinical guidelines, 478
  dosing, 478
  drug interactions, 478
  pharmacological actions, 477,
    477*t*
  precautions, 478
  sexual dysfunction and, 313
  therapeutic indications, 477–478
Adrenoleukodystrophy, 578
Adulthood, 4–5